MRI of the Abdomen and Pelvis

MRI OF THE ABDOMEN AND PELVIS

A TEXT-ATLAS

Richard C. Semelka, M.D.
University of North Carolina

Susan M. Ascher, M.D.
Georgetown University

Caroline Reinhold, M.D.
McGill University

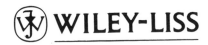

WILEY-LISS

A JOHN WILEY & SONS, INC., PUBLICATION

New York • Chichester • Weinheim • Brisbane • Singapore • Toronto

While the authors, editors, and publisher believe that drug selection and dosage and the specification and usage of equipment and devices set forth in this book are in accord with current recommendations and practice at the time of publication, they accept no legal responsibility for any errors or omissions, and make no warrant, express or implied, with respect to material contained herein. In view of ongoing research, equipment modifications, changes in governmental regulations and the constant flow of information relating to drug therapy, drug reactions, and the use of equipment and devices, the reader is urged to review and evaluate the information provided in the package insert or instructions for each drug, piece of equipment, or device for, among other things, any changes in the instructions or indication of dosage or usage and for added warnings and precautions.

Library of Congress Cataloging in Publication Data:

Semelka, Richard C.
    MRI of the abdomen and pelvis : a text-atlas / by Richard C.
Semelka, Susan M. Ascher, Caroline Reinhold.
      p.   cm.
    ISBN 0-471-16164-0 (cloth : alk. paper)
    1. Abdomen--Magnetic resonance imaging--Atlases.   2. Pelvis-
-Magnetic resonance imaging--Atlases.   I. Ascher, Susan M.
II. Reinhold, Caroline.   III. Title.
    [DNLM: 1. Abdomen--atlases.   2. Pelvis--atlases.   3. Magnetic
Resonance Imaging--methods--atlases.   WI 17 S471m 1997]
RC944.S45   1997
617.5′507548--DC21
DNLM/DLC
for Library of Congress   96-46195
                                                                      CIP

Printed in the United States of America

10 9 8 7 6 5 4 3 2 1

The first accomplishment is to have an untroubled spirit. The second is to look things in the face and know them for what they are.

Marcus Aurelius

CONTENTS

CONTRIBUTORS

RICHARD C. SEMELKA, M.D., Associate Professor, Director of Magnetic Resonance Services, Department of Radiology, University of North Carolina, Chapel Hill, North Carolina.

SUSAN M. ASCHER, M.D., Associate Professor, Associate Director Body MRI, Department of Radiology, Georgetown University, Washington, D.C.

CAROLINE REINHOLD, M.D., Assistant Professor, Director Body MRI, Montreal General Hospital, McGill University, Montreal, Canada.

PATRICE M. BRET, M.D., Professor and Chairman, Department of Radiology, McGill University, Montreal, Canada.

ELIZABETH D. BROWN, M.D., Radiology Resident, University of North Carolina, Chapel Hill, North Carolina.

DEREK A. BURDENY, M.D., Abdominal Imaging Fellow, University of North Carolina, Chapel Hill, North Carolina.

LARA B. EISENBERG, M.D., Radiology Resident, University of North Carolina, Chapel Hill, North Carolina.

BENOIT P. GALLIX, M.D., Abdominal Imaging Fellow, Montreal General Hospital, McGill University, Montreal, Canada.

RAHEL A. HUCH BÖNI, M.D., Assistant Professor, Department of Radiology, University Hospital of Zurich, Zurich, Switzerland.

NIKOLAOS L. KELEKIS, M.D., MRI Research Fellow, University of North Carolina, Chapel Hill, North Carolina.

TARA C. NOONE, M.D., Radiology Resident, University of North Carolina, Chapel Hill, North Carolina.

ERIC K. OUTWATER, M.D., Associate Professor, Department of Radiology, Thomas Jefferson University Hospital, Philadelphia, Pennsylvania.

SUVIPAPUN WORAWATTANAKUL, M.D., MRI Research Fellow, University of North Carolina, Chapel Hill, North Carolina.

PREFACE

The fundamental principles of diagnostic magnetic resonance imaging (MRI) of the abdomen and pelvis are good image quality, reproducibility of image quality, good conspicuity of disease, and comprehensive imaging information. This text-atlas illustrates a complete range of diseases of the abdomen and pelvis applying these principles. As MRI is an evolving modality, the key to optimized examination protocols is to incorporate or substitute new techniques that reflect these principles and achieve them in a time-efficient manner. This work describes imaging approaches obtained on state-of-the-art 1.5 T MRI systems emphasizing the use of phased-array surface multicoils and new, fast imaging sequences. Although this level of image quality may be obtainable only on these types of MRI systems, the principles of imaging strategies and the appearances of disease entities apply to all MRI systems. Emphasis in the text is placed on the imaging protocols currently considered most beneficial for the investigation of various disease processes.

MRI is highly accurate for the investigation of the majority of malignant abdominopelvic diseases and performs well in the evaluation of inflammatory disease. The advances that have rendered MRI so effective include high-quality breath-hold and breathing-independent imaging and the routine use of intravenous gadolinium administration. The reproducibility of high-quality images has advanced MRI from the status of a modality that can also demonstrate abdominopelvic disease to the modality of choice for detecting an expanding list of disease entities. This may ultimately result in earlier diagnosis and earlier appropriate patient management and may translate into health care savings. The future challenges for MRI are to reduce examination time while maintaining the range of diagnostic information, which should herald a greater role for MRI investigation of abdominopelvic disease.

ACKNOWLEDGEMENTS

The authors would like to acknowledge Hedvig Hricak, M.D., Ph.D., Shirley McCarthy, M.D., Ph.D., Leslie Scoutt, M.D., Charles B. Higgins, M.D., Alexander R. Margulis, M.D., Anne McBride Curtis, M.D., Joseph K. T. Lee, M.D., Milton Lautatzis, M.D., Coralie Shaw, M.D., Donald G. Mitchell, M.D., J. Patrick Shoenut, B.Sc., Richard H. Patt, M.D., Ann E. Aldis, M.D., George M. Kintzen, M.D., Mostafa Atri, M.D., Micheline Thibodeau, M.D., Margaret A. Fraser-Hill, M.D., Howard M. Greenberg, M.D., Robert K. Zeman, M.D., and our referring physicians for their support.

RICHARD C. SEMELKA, M.D.
SUSAN M. ASCHER, M.D.
CAROLINE REINHOLD, M.D.

MRI of the Abdomen and Pelvis

GENERAL CONSIDERATIONS FOR PERFORMING MAGNETIC RESONANCE STUDIES OF THE ABDOMEN AND PELVIS

R. C. SEMELKA, M.D., S. M. ASCHER, M.D., AND C. REINHOLD, M.D.

High image quality, reproducibility of image quality, and good conspicuity of disease require the use of sequences that are robust, reliable, and avoid artifacts. Maximizing these principles to achieve high-quality diagnostic MR images usually requires the use of fast scanning techniques. Therefore, the important goal of shorter examination time may also be achieved with the same principles that maximize diagnostic quality. With the decrease of imaging times for individual sequences, a variety of sequences may be employed to take advantage of the major strength of magnetic resonance imaging (MRI), which is comprehensive information on disease processes.

Respiration and bowel peristalsis are the major artifacts that have lessened the reproducibility of MRI. Breathing-independent sequences and breath-hold sequences form the foundation of high-quality MRI studies of the abdomen. Breathing artifact is less problematic in the pelvis, and high-spatial and contrast-resolution imaging have been the mainstay for maximizing image quality for pelvis studies.

Disease conspicuity depends on the principle of maximizing the difference in signal intensities between diseased tissues and the background tissue. For disease processes situated within or adjacent to fat, this is readily performed by manipulating the signal intensity of fat, which can range from low to high in signal intensity on both T1-weighted and T2-weighted images. For example, diseases that are low in signal intensity on T1-weighted images, such as peritoneal fluid or retroperitoneal fibrosis, are most conspicuous on T1-weighted sequences in which fat is high in signal intensity (i.e., sequences without fat suppression). Conversely, diseases, which are high in signal intensity, such as subacute blood or proteinaceous fluid, are more conspicuous if fat is rendered low in signal intensity with the use of fat-suppression techniques. On T2-weighted images, diseases, which are low in signal intensity, such as fibrous tissue, are most conspicuous on sequences in which background fat is high in signal intensity, such as echo-train, spin-echo sequences. Diseases, which are moderate to high in signal intensity, such as lymphadenopathy or ascites, are most conspicuous using sequences in which fat signal intensity is low, such as fat-suppressed sequences.

Gadolinium chelate enhancement may be routinely useful since it provides at least two further imaging parameters that are able to detect and characterize disease, specifically the pattern of blood delivery (i.e., capillary enhancement) and the size and/or rapidity of drainage of the interstitial space (i.e., interstitial enhancement). Capillary-phase image acquisition is achieved by using a short-duration sequence initiated immediately after gadolinium injection. Spoiled gradient-echo (SGE) sequences, performed as multisection acquisition, is an ideal sequence to use for capillary phase imaging. The majority of focal mass lesions are best evaluated in the capillary phase of enhancement, particularly lesions that do not distort the margins of the organs in which they are located (e.g., focal liver, spleen, or pancreatic lesions). Images acquired 2 to 10 minutes following contrast administration are in the interstitial phase of enhancement. Diseases that are superficial, spreading, or inflammatory in nature are generally well-shown on interstitial-phase images. Examples of diseases well-shown on interstitial-phase images include peritoneal metastases, cholangio-carcinoma, ascending cholangitis, inflammatory bowel disease, and abscesses.

More extensive description of physical principles of various sequences is given elsewhere [1]. Description of sequences well-suited for the investigation of abdominal disease is given in the following discussion.

T1-WEIGHTED SEQUENCES

T1-weighted sequences are routinely useful for investigating diseases of the abdomen, and supplement T2-weighted images for investigating disease of the pelvis. The primary information that precontrast T1-weighted images provide includes (1) information on abnormally increased fluid content or fibrous tissue content that appears low in signal intensity on T1-weighted images, and (2) information on the presence of subacute blood or concentrated protein, which are both high in signal intensity. T1-weighted sequences obtained without fat suppression also demonstrate the presence of fat as high signal intensity tissue.

Spoiled Gradient-Echo (SGE) Sequences

SGE sequences are the most important and versatile sequences for studying abdominal disease. They provide true T1-weighted imaging and, with the use of phased-array multicoil imaging, may be used to replace longer duration sequences such as the T1-weighted spin-echo (SE) sequence. Image parameters for SGE are (1) relatively long repetition time (TR) (approximately 150 msec)

to maximize signal-to-noise ratio and the number of sections that can be acquired in one multisection acquisition and (2) the shortest in-phase echo time (TE) (approximately 6.0 msec at 1.0 T and 4.2 to 4.5 msec at 1.5 T) to maximize signal-to-noise ratio and the number of sections per acquisition [2]. For routine T1-weighted images, in-phase TE may be preferable to the shorter out-of-phase echo times (4.0 msec at 1.0 T and 2.2 to 2.4 msec at 1.5 T), to avoid both phase-cancellation artifact around the borders of organs and fat-water phase cancellation in tissues containing both fat and water protons. Flip angle should be approximately 70 to 90 degrees to maximize T1-weighted information. Using the body coil, the signal-to-noise ratio of SGE sequences is usually suboptimal with section thickness less than 8 mm, whereas with the phased-array multicoil, section thickness of 5 mm results in diagnostically adequate images. On new MRI machines up to 22 sections may be acquired in a 20-second breath-hold.

In addition to its use as precontrast T1-weighted images, SGE should be routinely used for capillary-phase image acquisition following gadolinium administration for investigation of the liver, spleen, pancreas, and kidneys. SGE may also be modified as a single-shot technique using the minimum TR to achieve breathing-independent images for noncooperative patients (Fig. 1.1).

SGE sequences can be performed as three-dimensional (3D) acquisition, which can be used both for volumetric imaging of organs such as the liver and for pre- and postgadolinium administration. Gadolinium-enhanced 3D gradient-echo sequences also are the most clinically effective techniques for MR angiography (MRA) of the body (see Chapter 10 on the Retroperitoneum and Body Wall).

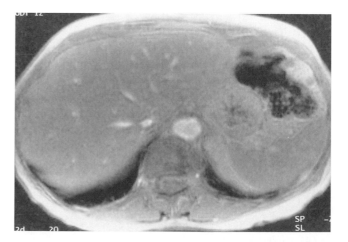

FIG. 1.1 Single-section SGE. Transverse 90-second postgadolinium single-section SGE image obtained during patient respiration. Image quality of the liver appears acceptable using this breathing-independent sequence. Gadolinium opacification of hepatic veins, inferior vena cava (IVC), and aorta are appreciated

Fat-Suppressed SGE Sequences

Fat-suppressed (FS) SGE sequences are routinely used as precontrast images for evaluating the pancreas and for the detection of subacute blood. Image parameters are similar to those for standard SGE; however, it is advantageous to employ a lower out-of-phase echo time (2.2 to 2.5 msec at 1.5 T), primarily to benefit from additional fat-attenuating effects, but also to increase signal-to-noise ratio and the number of sections per acquisition. On state-of-the-art MRI machines fat-suppressed-SGE may acquire 22 sections in a 20-second breath-hold with reproducible uniform fat suppression.

Fat-suppressed-SGE images are used to acquire interstitial-phase gadolinium-enhanced images. The complementary roles of gadolinium enhancement, which generally increases the signal intensity of disease tissue, and fat suppression, which diminishes the competing high signal intensity of background fat are particularly effective at maximizing conspicuity of diseased tissue. The principle of maximizing signal difference between diseased tissue and background tissue is achieved in the majority of MRI examinations with this approach.

If fat-suppressed-SGE sequencing cannot be performed on an MRI system, then fat-suppressed spin-echo sequencing can be substituted, with little loss of diagnostic information.

Out-of-Phase SGE Sequences

Out-of-phase (opposed-phase) SGE images are useful for demonstrating diseased tissue in which fat and water protons are present within the same voxel. The most common indications are for detecting the presence of fatty liver and lipid within adrenal masses to characterize them as adenomas. Another useful feature is that the generation of a phase-cancellation artifact around high-signal-intensity masses, located in water-based tissues, confirms that these lesions are fatty. Examples of this include angiomyolipomas of the kidney and ovarian dermoids.

Magnetization-Prepared Rapid-Acquisition Gradient-Echo (MP-RAGE) Sequences

MP-RAGE sequences include turbo fast low-angle shot (turboFLASH). These techniques are generally performed as a single shot with image acquisition duration of 1 to 2 seconds, which renders them relatively breathing independent. Magnetization preparation is currently performed with a 180 inversion pulse to achieve T1-weighted information. The inversion pulse may be either slice or nonslice selective. The advantage of a slice-selective inversion pulse is that no time delay is required between acquisition of single sections in multiple single-section acquisition. A stack of single-section images can be ac-

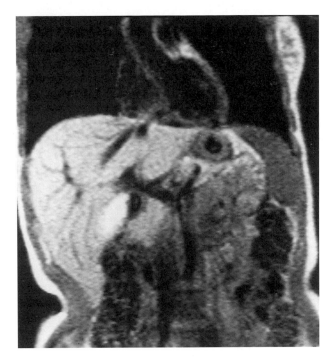

F IG . 1.2 Nonslice-selective MP-RAGE. A coronal image through the liver demonstrates good T1-weighting, evidenced by a moderately high-signal-intensity liver and moderately low-signal-intensity spleen (*arrow*). The infracardiac portion of the left lobe is artifact-free. Blood vessels in the liver and the cardiac chambers are seen signal-void.

quired in a rapid fashion. This is important for dynamic gadolinium-enhanced studies. A nonslice-selective inversion pulse results in slightly better image quality, particularly because flowing blood is signal-void (Fig. 1.2). Approximately 3 seconds of tissue relaxation are required between acquisition of individual sections, which limits the usefulness of this sequence for dynamic gadolinium-enhanced acquisitions. Current versions of MP-RAGE are limited because of low signal-to-noise varying signal intensity and contrast between sections, unpredictable bounce-point boundary artifacts due to signal-nulling effects caused by the inverting 180 pulse, and unpredictable nulling of tissue enhanced with gadolinium. Research is ongoing to alleviate these problems with MP-RAGE so that it may assume a more important clinical role. Routine use of a high quality MP-RAGE sequence would further increase the reproducibility of MR image quality by obviating the need for breath-holding, particularly in patients unable to suspend respiration.

T2-WEIGHTED SEQUENCES

The predominant information provided by T2-weighted sequences are (1) the presence of increased fluid in diseased tissue, which results in high signal intensity, (2) the presence of chronic fibrotic tissue, which results in low signal intensity and (3) the presence of iron deposition, which results in low signal intensity.

Echo-Train Spin-Echo Sequences

Echo-train spin-echo sequences are termed fast spin-echo, turbo spin-echo, or Rapid Acquisition with Relaxation Enhancement (RARE) sequences. The principle of echo-train spin-echo sequences is to summate multiple echoes within the same repetition time interval to decrease examination time, increase spatial resolution, or both. Echo-train spin-echo has achieved widespread use because of these advantages. The eagerness to adopt these sequences stems from the fact that conventional T2 spin-echo sequences are lengthy and thus suffer from patient motion and increased examination time, factors that are lessened with echo-train spin-echo. With the advantages of echo-train spin-echo, disadvantages also occur. The major disadvantage is that T2 differences between tissues are minimized. This generally is not problematic in the pelvis due to substantial differences in the T2 values between diseased and normal tissue. In the liver, however, the T2 difference between diseased and background liver may be small, and the T2-averaging effects of summated multiple echoes blur this T2 difference. These effects are most commonly observed with hepatocellular carcinoma. Fortunately, diseases with T2 values similar to those of liver generally have lower T1 values than liver, so that lesions poorly visualized on echo-train spin-echo are apparent on SGE or immediate postgadolinium SGE images.

Echo-train spin-echo, and T2-weighted sequences in general, are important for evaluating the liver and pelvis. T2-weighted sequences are often useful for the pancreas, but the role for other organs/tissues, particularly the bowel and peritoneum, has been limited due to motion artifacts from respiration and bowel peristalsis. The introduction of breathing-independent single shot T2-weighted sequences has increased the role of T2-weighted images for investigation of these other organs/tissues.

Fat is high in signal intensity on echo-train spin-echo sequences in comparison to conventional spin-echo sequences in which fat is intermediate in signal intensity. It is important to recognize this difference, particularly in the setting of recurrent malignant disease versus fibrosis for pelvic malignancies. The literature, in general, uses the internal standard of comparing diseased tissue with background tissue. As such recurrent malignant disease in the pelvis (e.g., cervical, endometrial, bladder, or rectal cancer) generally appears high in signal intensity because of the high-signal-intensity relationship to the moderately low-signal-intensity fat on conventional spin-echo sequences. In contrast, fat is high in signal intensity on echo-train spin-echo images, and recurrent disease will invariably be lower in signal intensity. Caution must

therefore be exercised not to interpret recurrent disease as fibrotic tissue because of an a priori knowledge that recurrence is higher in signal intensity than background fat. Fat may also be problematic in the liver because fatty liver will be high in signal intensity on echo-train spin-echo sequences, thereby diminishing contrast with the majority of liver lesions, which are generally high in signal intensity on T2-weighted images. It may be essential to use fat suppression on T2-weighted echo-train spin-echo sequences for liver imaging.

Echo-train spin-echo sequences, acquired as contiguous thin 2D sections or as a thick 3D volume slab, form the basis for MR cholangiography (see Chapter 3 on the Gallbladder and Biliary System) and MR urography (see Chapter 9 on Kidneys).

Single Shot Echo-Train Spin-Echo Sequence

Single shot echo-train spin-echo sequence (e.g.: Half-fourier Snapshot Turbo Spin-Echo (HASTE)) sequence is a breathing independent T2-weighted sequence that has had a substantial impact on abdominal imaging [3]. HASTE is a single-shot technique with a 400 msec image acquisition time in which K space is filled in one data acquisition using half-fourier reconstruction (Fig. 1.3). Use of an effective echo time of 60 msec is recommended for bowel-peritoneal disease, and an effective echo time of 103 msec is recommended for liver-biliary disease. Other parameters are a repetition time that is infinite and echo time length of 104. A stack of sections should be acquired in single-section mode in one breath-hold to avoid slice misregistration. Motion artifacts from respiration and bowel peristalsis are obviated; chemical-shift artifact is negligible; and susceptibility artifact from air in bowel, lungs, and other locations is minimized, such that bowel wall is clearly demonstrated. Similarly, suscep-

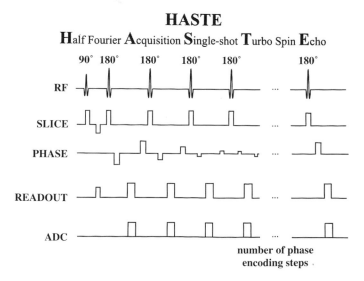

HASTE
Half Fourier Acquisition Single-shot Turbo Spin Echo

FIG. 1.3 HASTE sequence timing diagram.

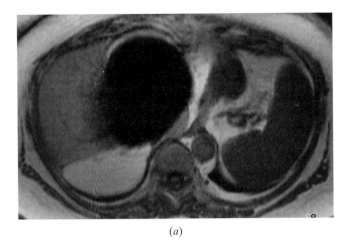

(a)

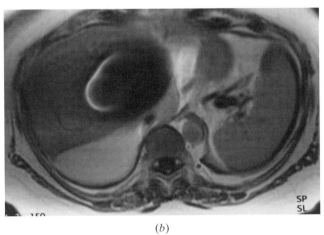

(b)

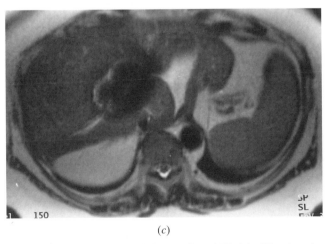

(c)

FIG. 1.4 Metallic susceptibility artifact. SGE (*a*), T1 spin-echo (T1-SE) (*b*), and HASTE (*c*) images. Severe susceptibility artifact is present on the gradient-echo image (*a*) with the result that the images of the liver are not interpretable. T1-SE (*b*) is relatively resistant to image degradation by susceptibility artifact; however substantial artifact still renders much of the liver uninterpretable. The HASTE image (*c*) is the least sensitive MR sequence, and less sensitive than CT, imaging for artifacts generated by metallic devices. Only a small portion of the liver is not interpretable with HASTE (*c*).

tibility artifact from metallic devices such as surgical clips or hip prostheses is minimal (Fig. 1.4). All of these effects render HASTE an attractive sequence for evaluating abdominal disease.

Fat-Suppression (FS) Single Shot Echo-Train Spin-Echo Sequence

FS-HASTE may be useful for investigating focal liver disease to attenuate the high signal intensity of fatty infiltration, if present. Fatty liver is high in signal intensity on echo-train spin-echo sequences, in particular on HASTE, which lessens the detectability of high-signal-intensity metastases. Diminishing fat signal intensity with fat suppression accentuates the high signal intensity of focal liver lesions (Fig. 1.5). FS-HASTE is also useful for evaluat-

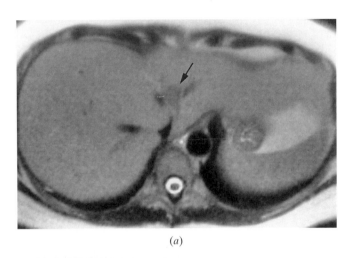

(a)

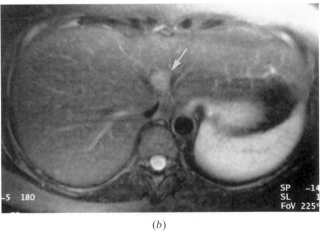

(b)

FIG. 1.5 Focal liver lesion in a fatty liver. HASTE (*a*) and FS-HASTE (*b*). The liver appears high in signal intensity on the HASTE image (*a*) due to the presence of fatty liver. A focal liver lesion (focal nodular hyperplasia) is identified which is mildly lower in signal intensity than liver parenchyma. On the FS-HASTE image (*b*), the liver has decreased in signal intensity, and the liver lesion (*arrow, b*) now appears moderately high in signal intensity relative to liver. Good liver-spleen contrast is also apparent on the fat-suppressed image (*b*), with no liver-spleen contrast on the nonsuppressed sequence (*a*).

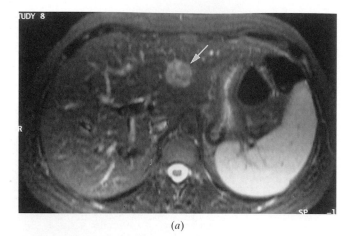

(a)

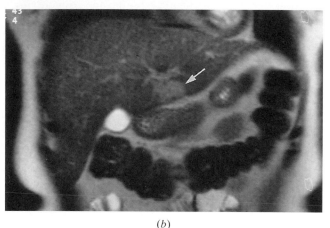

(b)

FIG. 1.6 TurboSTIR and HASTE. Transverse turboSTIR (*a*) and coronal HASTE (*b*) images in a patient with colon cancer liver metastases. A moderately high-signal-intensity metastasis is present in the left lobe of the liver on the turboSTIR (*arrow, a*). Background fat is nulled. The liver metastasis is also shown on the coronal HASTE image (*arrow, b*). Background fat is high in signal intensity. Variations in the signal intensity of the background fat provide differing contrast relationships.

ing the biliary tree. Fat suppression appears to diminish the image quality of bowel due to susceptibility artifact and is not recommended for bowel studies.

Turbo Short Tau Inversion Recovery (TurboSTIR) Sequence

TurboSTIR is a short-duration T2-type sequence that can be performed in a breath-hold [4]. Five sections may be acquired in a 20-second breath-hold. Lesion conspicuity is high for focal liver lesions, but image quality generally is fair. As the sequence is fundamentally different from HASTE, it may be useful to combine both short-duration sequences for the liver in place of longer, nonbreath-hold echo-train spin-echo (Fig. 1.6).

IMAGING STRATEGIES

A major strength of MRI is the variety of information types that the modality is able to generate. As a result, MRI is able to provide comprehensive information on organ systems and disease entities. The use of a diverse group of sequences minimizes the risk of not detecting disease or misclassifying disease. This is a reflection of the fact that the more different information that is acquired, the less likely it is that disease will escape detection. Attention to length of examination is critical because longer examinations result in fewer patients who can be examined and a decrease in patient cooperation. Ideally, many of the different sequences employed should be of short duration and breath-hold or breathing independent. An attempt should be made to achieve this goal in protocol design. Another consideration is reproducibility of examination protocols. Efficient operation of an MRI system requires set protocols that can be run relatively independently of physician intervention, which serves to speed up examinations, render exams reproducible, and increase utilization by familiarity with a standard approach.

The protocol of MRI studies that investigate the abdomen and pelvis in the same setting may be rendered most efficient by acquiring a complete study of the upper abdomen initially, using precontrast SGE and T2-weighted FS-echo-train spin-echo and serial postgadolinium SGE and FS-SGE images, then acquiring the pelvis study including postgadolinium FS-SGE and T2-weighted high-resolution sequences. Comprehensive examination of all organs and tissues in the abdomen and pelvis can be achieved with this technique (Fig. 1.7). This approach minimizes table motion and repositioning of the phased-array coil, which are time-consuming procedures. Although it is not generally desired to acquire T2-weighted images after gadolinium, the presence of concentrated low-signal-intensity gadolinium in the bladder on T2-weighted images may in fact be beneficial by increasing conspicuity of bladder involvement from malignant pelvic diseases. The liver is the organ that benefits the most from immediate postgadolinium imaging, and imaging protocols should be designed in a fashion to image the liver immediately following gadolinium administration. If, however, liver metastases are unlikely and the pelvis is the major focus of investigation, studies can be structured to acquire immediate postgadolinium images of the pelvis (e.g., for the evaluation of bladder tumors).

The phased-array coil is initially placed over the upper abdomen, and image acquisition is centered over the liver. With the patient positioned in the bore of the magnet, gadolinium is injected as a forceful hand bolus injection over 5 seconds, followed by injection of a normal saline flush over 3 seconds. Image acquisition is initiated immediately after the normal saline flush with the SGE sequence. Following the postgadolinium se-

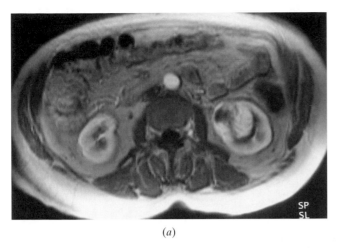

(a)

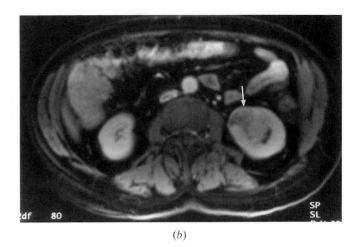

(b)

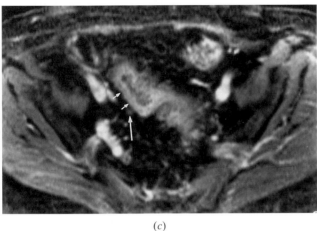

(c)

FIG. 1.7 Combined abdominopelvic MRI examination. Immediate postgadolinium SGE (*a*) and 90-second postgadolinium FS-SGE (*b*) images of the kidneys and 3-minute postgadolinium FS-SGE (*c*) image of the pelvis. These images were obtained in an abdominopelvic MRI examination for staging of colon cancer of the sigmoid colon. Images acquired of the upper abdomen in the first part of the examination demonstrated no liver metastases; however, a 3-cm renal cancer arising in the left kidney (*arrow, b*) was identified, which possessed the typical imaging features of renal-cell cancer. In the second part of the study, examination of the pelvis, the sigmoid colon cancer is well-defined (*small arrows, c*). The serosal surface is slightly irregular, and small regional lymph nodes (*arrow, c*) are present. Comprehensive evaluation of the entire abdomen and pelvis permitted accurate staging of the sigmoid colon cancer with concurrent serendipitous detection of a renal cancer.

quences of the upper abdomen, the phased-array coil is then shifted over the pelvis and the table is repositioned for image acquisition centered over the pelvis. Initial pelvic images should be the T1-weighted images in order to utilize the presence of gadolinium before too much washout has occurred (e.g., within 10 minutes). T2-weighted images then follow. This approach sacrifices precontrast SGE images of the pelvis. The major disadvantage is that hemorrhagic pelvic lesions may not be demonstrated, but in practice this mainly decreases the ability to detect endometriosis. When investigation of endometriosis is required, then precontrast FS-SGE images would be obtained and a dedicated pelvis protocol would be performed.

Tables 1.1 to 1.18 show the current protocols that are useful for the investigation of abdominopelvic disease when imaging at 1.5 T using a phased-array multicoil.

The sequence protocols are designed for a Siemens system. Venxor specific variations in imaging parameters should be employed as needed. Variations in TR/TE/flip angle for SGE sequences should generally be avoided. Imaging parameters of echo-train spin-echo sequences

are more flexible, with minor changes resulting in no substantial loss of diagnostic information. With the use of phased-array multicoils both slice thickness and FOV can be substantially refered for many protocols (e.g.: slice thickness of 5 mm for the pancreas, adrenals and pelvis, and FOV of 200 mm for the pelvis).

Serial MRI Examination

MRI is currently considered the most expensive imaging modality, which has hampered its appropriate utilization. The expense of MRI studies can be dramatically reduced by decreasing study time and the number of sequences employed. This may be done most reasonably in the setting of follow-up examinations. Depending on the amount of information needed, a follow-up study that employs coronal HASTE, transverse precontrast SGE, and immediate and 45-second postgadolinium SGE provides relatively comprehensive information in a 5-minute study time. Even more curtailed examination can be performed if only change in size is examined for. An adrenal mass or lymphadenopathy may be adequately followed by

Table 1.1 Liver (Short Version)

Sequence	Plane	TR	TE	FOV	Thickness/ Gap	Flip	Matrix
Localizer							
HASTE	Coronal	∞	103	320–400	8–10 mm/25%	90° Refocusing angle: 130°–180°	192 × 256
SGE	Coronal	140	4	320–400	8–10 mm/25%	80°	128 × 256
Fat-suppressed HASTE	Transverse	∞	103	320–400	8–10 mm/25%	90° Refocusing angle: 130°–180°	144 × 256
SGE	Transverse	140	4	320–400	8–10 mm/25%	80°	128 × 256
SGE out-of-phase	Transverse	140	2	320–400	8–10 mm/25%	80°	128 × 256
SGE 1, 45 sec postGd	Transverse	140	4	320–400	8–10 mm/25%	80°	128 × 256
Fat-suppressed SGE 90-sec postGd	Transverse	140	2–4	320–400	8–10 mm/25%	80°	128 × 256
SGE 5-min postGd	Transverse	140	4	320–400	8–10 mm/25%	80°	128 × 256

Note: Breath-hold TurboSTIR. may be used in place of T2 fat-suppressed HASTE.

Table 1.2 Liver

Sequence	Plane	TR	TE	FOV	Thickness/ Gap	Flip	Matrix
Localizer							
T2 fat-suppressed ETSE	Transverse	3000–4500	20, 90	320–400	8–10 mm/25%	180°	144 × 256
HASTE	Coronal	∞	103	320	8–10 mm/30%	90° Refocusing angle: 130°–180°	192 × 256
SGE	Coronal	140	4	320–400	8–10 mm/25%	80°	128 × 256
SGE out-of-phase	Transverse	140	2	320–400	8–10 mm/25%	80°	128 × 256
SGE	Transverse	140	4	320–400	8–10 mm/25%	80°	128 × 256
SGE 1, 45 sec postGd	Transverse	140	4	320–400	8–10 mm/25%	80°	128 × 256
Fat-suppressed SGE 90-sec postGd	Transverse	140	2–4	320–400	8–10 mm/25%	80°	128 × 256
SGE 5-min postGd	Transverse	140	4	320–400	8–10 mm/25%	80°	128 × 256

Note: use 3/4 rectangular FOV. For patients who cannot breath-hold, substitute:
(a) T1 Fat suppressed SE for precontrast SGE
(b) Slice selective MP-RAGE pre and postGd for SGE pre and 1, 45-sec postGd
(c) T1 Fat suppressed SE for 90, sec and 5-min postGd SGE and fat-suppressed SGE
For rectal cancer: if sacral invasion is suspected add fat-suppressed to T2 high-resolution ETSE.

Table 1.3 Liver and Pancreas

Sequence	Plane	TR	TE	FOV	Thickness/ Gap	Flip	Matrix
Localizer							
T2 Fat-suppressed ETSE (Liver)	Transverse	3000–4500	20, 90	320–400	8–10 mm/25%	180°	144 × 256
HASTE (liver-pancreas)	Coronal	∞	103	400	8 mm/30%	90° Refocusing angle: 130°–180°	192 × 256
HASTE (liver-pancreas)	Transverse	140	4	320–400	8 mm/30%	90° Refocusing angle: 130°–180°	192 × 256
SGE fat-suppressed (pancreas)	Transverse	140	2–4	320–400	8–10 mm/25%	80°	128 × 256
SGE out-of-phase (Liver)	Transverse	140	4	320–400	8–10 mm/25%	80°	128 × 256
SGE (liver-pancreas)	Transverse	140	4	320–400	8–10 mm/25%	80°	128 × 256
SGE 1, 45 sec postGd (liver-pancreas)	Transverse	140	4	320–400	8–10 mm/25%	80°	128 × 256
Fat-suppressed SGE 90-sec postGd (pancreas)	Transverse	140	2–4	320–400	8–10 mm/25%	80°	144 × 256
SGE 5-min (liver)	Transverse	140	4	320–400	8–10 mm/25%	80°	128 × 256

Note: For patients who cannot breath-hold substitute:
(a) T1 fat-suppressed SE for SGE and fat-suppressed SGE
(b) Slice-selective MP-RAGE transverse for SGE, 1, 45 sec postGd SGE
(c) Ti fat-suppressed SE for 90 sec, fat-suppressed SGE and SGE 5 min

Table 1.4 Liver and Kidney

Sequence	Plane	TR	TE	FOV	Thickness/ Gap	Flip	Matrix
Localizer							
T2 fat-suppressed ESTE (liver)	Transverse	3000–4500	20, 90	320–400	8–10 mm/25%	180°	144 × 256
HASTE (liver-kidney)	Coronal	∞	103	450	8–10 mm/25%	80°	128 × 256
Fat-suppressed SGE (kidney)	Transverse	140	2–4	320	8–10 mm/25%	80°	144 × 256
SGE (liver-kidney)	Transverse	140	4	320–400	8–10 mm/25%	80°	128 × 256
SGE 1, 45 sec postGd (liver-kidney)	Transverse	140	4	320–400	8–10 mm/25%	80°	128 × 256
Fat-suppressed SGE 90 sec (kidney)	Transverse	140	2–4	320–400	8–10 mm/25%	80°	144 × 256
Fat-suppressed SGE (kidney)	Sagittal	140	2–4	320	8–10 mm/25%	80°	128 × 256
SGE 5-min (liver)	Transverse	140	4	320–400	8–10 mm/25%	80°	128 × 256

Note: For patients who cannot breath-hold substitute:
(a) T1 fat-suppressed SE for SGE and fat-suppressed SGE
(b) Slice-selective MP-RAGE transverse for SGE, 1, 45 sec Gd SGE
(c) Ti fat-suppressed SE for 90 sec fat-suppressed SGE and SGE 5 min

Table 1.5 Liver and Pelvis

Sequence	Plane	TR	TE	FOV	Thickness/ Gap	Flip	Matrix
Localizer							
T2 fat-suppressed ETSE (liver)	Transverse	3000– 4500	20, 90	320–400	8–10 mm/25%	180°	144 × 256
SGE (liver)	Coronal	140	4	320–400	8–10 mm/25%	800	128 × 256
SGE out-of-phase (liver)	Transverse	140	2	320–400	8–10 mm/25%	800	128 × 256
HASTE (liver)	Coronal	∞	103	320	8 mm/30%	90° Refocusing angle: 130°–180°	198 × 256
SGE (liver)	Transverse	140	4	320–400	8–10 mm/25%	800	128 × 256
SGE (liver) 1, 45 sec postGd	Transverse	140	4	320–400	8–10 mm/25%	800	128 × 256
Fat-suppressed SGE 90 sec postGd (liver-midabdomen)	Transverse	140	2–4	320–400	8–10 mm/25%	800	128 × 256
SGE (liver) 5-min postGd	Transverse	140	4	320–400	8–10 mm/25%	800	128 × 256
Fat-suppressed SGE (pelvis)	Transverse	140	2–4	400	8 mm/25%	80°	128 × 256
Fat-suppressed SGE (pelvis)	Sagittal	140	2–4	400	8 mm/25%	80°	128 × 256
T2 high-resolution ETSE (pelvis)	Transverse	4300	130	320	6–8 mm/25%	180°	270 × 512
T2 high-resolution ETSE (pelvis)	Sagittal	4300	130	320	8 mm/25%	180°	270 × 512

Note: Use 6/8 rectangular FOV. For patients who cannot breath-hold, substitute:
(a) T1 fat-suppressed SE for precontrast SGE
(b) slice-selective MP-RAGE pre and postGd for SGE pre and 1, 45 sec postGd
(c) T1 fat-suppressed SE for 90, sec and 5 min postGd SGE and fat-suppressed SGE
For rectal cancer; if sacral invasion is suspected, add fat-suppression to T2 echo-train spin-echo high resolution.

Table 1.6 Abdomen (Agitated Noncooperative)

Sequence	Plane	TR	TE	FOV	Thickness/ Gap	Flip	Matrix
Localizer							
HASTE	Coronal	∞	60	320–450	8–10 mm/25%	90° Refocusing angle: 130°–180°	192 × 256
Slice selective MP-RAGE	Coronal	11	450–500	450	8–10 mm/25%	15°	128 × 256
Post Gd slice selective MP-RAGE (wait 9 sec)	Coronal	11	450–500	450	8–10 mm/25%	15°	128 × 256
PostGd slice-selective turbo SGE	Coronal	11	450–500	450	8–10 mm/25%	15°	128 × 256

Note: The pelvis also requires sagittal HASTE.

Table 1.7 Pancreas

Sequence	Plane	TR	TE	FOV	Thickness/Gap	Flip	Matrix
Localizer							
HASTE (liver)	Coronal	∞	103	400	8 mm/25%	90° Refocusing angle: 130°–180°	192 × 256
HASTE (liver-pancreas)	Transverse	∞	103	320–400	8 mm/30%	90° Refocusing angle: 130°–180°	192 × 256
Fat-suppressed SGE (pancreas)	Transverse	140	2–4	320–400	8 mm/25%	80°	128 × 256
SGE (liver-pancreas)	Transverse	140	4	320–400	8–10 mm/25%	80°	128 × 256
SGE (pancreas) 1, 45 sec postGd	Transverse	140	4	320–400	8–10 mm/25%	80°	128 × 256
Fat-suppressed SGE 90-sec (pancreas)	Transverse	140	2–4	320–400	8–10 mm/25%	80°	144 × 256
SGE (liver) 5 min	Transverse	140	4	320–400	8–10 mm/25%	80°	128 × 256

Note: For patients who cannot breath-hold substitute:
(a) T1 fat-suppressed SE for SGE and fat-suppressed SGE
(b) Slice-selective MP-RAGE transverse (no rectangular FOV, slice thickness > 8 mm) for SGE, 1, 45 sec postGd SGE
(c) T1 fat-suppressed SE for 90 sec, fat-suppressed SGE and SGE 5 min

Table 1.8 Bowel

Sequence	Plane	TR	TE	FOV	Thickness/Gap	Flip	Matrix
Localizer							
SGE (abdomen)	Coronal	140	4	320–400	8–10 mm/25%	80°	128 × 256
HASTE (abdomen)	Coronal	∞	60	320–400	8 mm/30%	90° Refocusing angle: 130°–180°	192 × 256
HASTE (abdomen)	Transverse	∞	60	320–400	8 mm/30%	90° Refocusing angle: 130°–180°	192 × 256
SGE (abdomen)	Transverse	140	4	320–400	8–10 mm/25%	80°	128 × 256
Fat-suppressed SGE	Transverse	140	2–4	320–400	8 mm/25%	80°	128 × 256
Fat-suppressed SGE (5 sec postGd)	Transverse	140	2–4	320–400	8–10 mm/25%	80°	128 × 256
Fat-suppressed SGE	Coronal/Sagittal	140	2–4	320–400	8 mm/25%	80°	128 × 256

Note: For rectal cancer, use T2 high-resolution echo-train spin-echo sagittal + transverse, do not use HASTE.

Table 1.9 Adrenal

Sequence	Plane	TR	TE	FOV	Thickness/Gap	Flip	Matrix
SGE diaphragm to aortic bifurcation)	Transverse	140	4		8 mm/25%	800	128 × 256
T2 fat-suppressed ETSE	Transverse	3000–4500	20, 90	320–400	5 mm/25%	180°	128 × 256
Fat-suppressed SGE	Transverse	140	2–4	320–400	7 mm/25%	80°	128 × 256
SGE out-of-phase	Transverse	140	2	320–400	8 mm/25%	80°	128 × 256
SGE-1, 45 sec postGd	Transverse	140	4	320–400	8 mm/25%	800	128 × 256
Fat-suppressed SGE 90 sec	Transverse	140	2–4	320–400	7 mm/25%	80°	128 × 256

Table 1.10 Kidney

Sequence	Plane	TR	TE	FOV	Thickness/Gap	Flip	Matrix
Localizer							
Fat-suppressed SGE	Transverse	140	2–4	320–400	8–10 mm/25%	80°	144 × 256
SGE	Transverse	140	4	320–400	8–10 mm/25%	800	128 × 256
SGE 1 sec postGd	Transverse	140	4	320–400	8–10 mm/25%	800	128 × 256
Fat-suppressed SGE 45 sec	Transverse	140	2–4	320–400	8–10 mm/25%	80°	144 × 256
Fat-suppressed SGE 90 sec postGd	Transverse	140	4	320–400	8–10 mm/25%	800	128 × 256
Fat-suppressed SGE 3 min postGd	Sagittal or Coronal	140	4	320–400	8–10 mm/25%	80°	128 × 256

Note: If possible, cover liver as well as kidneys on 1 sec postGd SGE.
Renal artery studies require fat-suppressed SGE 1 sec postGd transverse 5 mm/0% and fat-suppressed SGE coronal 5 mm/0% gap.

Table 1.11 Abdominal Aorta

Sequence	Plane	TR	TE	FOV	Thickness/Gap	Flip	Matrix
Localizer							
SGE (diaphragm to bifurcation of femoral arteries)	Transverse	140	4	320–400	8–10 mm/25%	80°	128 × 256
3D FISP (diaphragm to bifurcation of femoral arteries (with 3–6 sec post injection)	Coronal	5	2	300–450	2 mm/32–52 partitions	30°	128 × 256
Fat-suppressed SGE (diaphragm to bifurcation of femoral arteries)	Transverse	140	2–4	320–400	6–8 mm/0%	80°	144 × 256
Fat-suppressed SGE (diaphragm to bifurcation of femoral arteries)	Transverse	140	2–4	320–400	6–8 mm/0%	80°	144 × 256

Table 1.12 Male: Screening Abdomen and Pelvis

Sequence	Plane	TR	TE	FOV	Thickness/Gap	Flip	Matrix
Localizer	Coronal	15	5	450	10 mm/0%	10°	160 × 256
SGE (liver)	Coronal	140	4	450	10 mm/20%	80°	128 × 256
HASTE (liver)	Coronal	∞	103	320	8 mm/30%	90° Refocusing angle: 130°–180°	192 × 256
SGE (liver)	Transverse	140	4	320–400	8–10 mm/25%	80°	128 × 256
SGE-Gd 1, 45 sec (liver)	Transverse	140	4	320–400	10 mm/25%	80°	128 × 256
Fat-suppressed SGE (Liver-mid abdomen)	Transverse	140	2–4	320–400	10 mm/25%	80°	128 × 256
Fat-suppressed SGE-Gd (pelvis)	Transverse	140	2–4	320–400	10 mm/25%	80°	128 × 256
Fat-suppressed SGE-Gd (pelvis)	Sagittal	140	2–4	320–400	8 mm/20%	80°	128 × 256
T2 high-resolution ETSE (pelvis)	Transverse	3000–4500	130	320–400	6 mm/25%	180°	144 × 256

Note: Phased-array imaging of upper abdomen is followed by phase-array imaging of pelvis.
For a short version, substitute HASTE for T2 turbo in pelvis.

Table 1.13 Prostate

Sequence	Plane	TR	TE	FOV	Thickness/Gap	Flip	Matrix
Localizer							
T2 high-resolution ETSE	Transverse	4000	103	320–400	5 mm/25%	900	144 × 256
SGE (pelvis)	Transverse	140	4	320–400	7 mm/25%	900	144 × 256
T2 high-resolution ETSE (pelvis)	Sagittal	3000–4500	130	320–400	5 mm/25%	900	144 × 256
SGE (mid abdomen)	Transverse	140	4	320–400	10 mm/25%	800	128 × 256
Fat-suppressed SGE 10 sec postGD (pelvis)	Transverse	140	2–4	300	8–10 mm/25%	80°	128 × 256
Fat-suppressed SGE (mid abdomen)	Transverse	140	2–4	300	8–10 mm/25%	80°	128 × 256

Note: All sequences should be RECFOV.

Table 1.14 Female: Screening Abdomen and Pelvis

Sequence	Plane	TR	TE	FOV	Thickness/Gap	Flip	Matrix
Localizer							
SGE (abdomen)	Coronal	140	4	500	10 mm/20%	80°	128 × 256
HASTE (abdomen)	Coronal	∞	103	320	8 mm/30%	90° Refocusing angle: 130°–180°	192 × 256
SGE (liver)	Transverse	140	4	320	8–10 mm/25%	80°	128 × 256
SGE 1, 45 sec (liver)	Transverse	140	4	320	10 mm/25%	80°	128 × 256
Fat suppressed SGE-Gd (mid abdomen)	Transverse	140	2–4	320	10 mm/25%	80°	128 × 256
Fat-suppressed SGE-Gd (pelvis)	Transverse	140	2–4	320	10 mm/25%	80°	128 × 256
T2 high-resolution ETSE (pelvis)	Sagittal	3000–4500	130	320	6 mm/25%	180°	144 × 256
T2 high-resolution ETSE (pelvis)	Transverse	3500	19–93	320	8–10 mm/25%	180°	144 × 256

Note: For the short version, substitute HASTE for T2 echo-train spin-echo in pelvis.

Table 1.15 Uterus, (Benign Disease)

Sequence	Plane	TR	TE	FOV	Thickness/Gap	Flip	Matrix
Localizer							
T2 high-resolution ETSE (pelvis)	Transverse	3000–4500	130	320–400	5 mm/25%	180°	270 × 512
T2 high-resolution ETSE (pelvis)	Sagittal	3000–4500	130	320–400	5 mm/25%	180°	270 × 512
SGE (pelvis)	Transverse	140	4	320–400	8 mm/25%	800	128 × 256
SGE (pelvis)	Sagittal	140	4	320–400	7 mm/25%	800	128 × 256

Table 1.16 Endometrial/Cervical Cancer

Sequence	Plane	TR	TE	FOV	Thickness/ Gap	Flip	Matrix
Localizer	Coronal	15	5	450	10 mm/0%	10°	160 × 256
HASTE (liver)	Coronal	∞	60	320	8 mm/30%	90° Refocusing angle: 130°–180°	192 × 256
SGE (liver)	Transverse	140	4	320–400	8–10 mm/20%	80°	128 × 256
SGE-Gd 1, 45 sec (liver)	Transverse	140	4	320–400	8–10 mm/25%	80°	128 × 256
Fat-suppressed SGE (liver-mid-abdomen)	Transverse	140	2–4	320	10 mm/25%	80°	128 × 256
Fat-suppressed SGE (pelvis)	Transverse	140	2–4	320	8 mm/25%	80°	128 × 256
Fat-suppressed SGE (pelvis)	Sagittal	140	2–4	320	8 mm/25%	80°	128 × 256
T2 high-resolution ETSE (pelvis)	Transverse	3000–4500	130	320	5 mm/25%	180°	270 × 512
T2 high-resolution ETSE (pelvis)	Sagittal	3000–4500	130	320	5 mm	180°	270 × 512

precontrast SGE alone, or, in the case of an adrenal adenoma, in combination with out-of-phase SGE.

Noncooperative Patients

Special attention to the noncooperative patient is required. In general, noncooperative patients fall into the categories of those who cannot suspend respiration, but breathe in a regular fashion, and those who cannot suspend respiration and cannot breathe regularly. The most common patient population that fits into the first group are sedated pediatric patients. Agitated patients are the most commonly encountered who fit into the second group. Imaging strategies differ for each.

In patients who breathe regularly, substitution of breath-hold images (e.g., SGE) can be made readily with breathing-averaged spin-echo images, the image quality of which is improved by using fat suppression. Additionally, breathing-independent T2-weighted HASTE is useful, as is T1-weighted MP-RAGE or single-section SGE if dynamic gadolinium-enhanced images are required (Fig. 1.8).

In patients who are agitated, breathing-independent T2-weighted HASTE and T1-weighted MP-RAGE or sin-

Table 1.17 Endometriosis

Sequence	Plane	TR	TE	FOV	Thickness/ Gap	Flip	Matrix
Localizer							
T2 high-resolution fat-suppressed (Pelvis)	Transverse	3000–4500	130	320–400	5 mm/25%	90°–130°	144 × 256
T2 high-resolution turbo SE (pelvis)	Sagittal	3000–4500	130	320–400	5 mm/25%	90°	144 × 256
T1 SGE (pelvis)	Transverse	140	4	320–400	8 mm/25%	80°	128 × 256
T1 fat-suppressed SGE (pelvis)	Transverse	140	2–4	320–400	8 mm/25%	90°–130°	128 × 256
T1 fat-suppressed SGE (pelvis)	Sagittal	140	2–4	320–400	8 mm/25%	80°	128 × 256

Table 1.18 Ovarian Cancer

Sequence	Plane	TR	TE	FOV	Thickness/Gap	Flip	Matrix
Localizer							
T2 ETSE fat-suppressed (liver)	Transverse	3000	20, 90	320–400	8–10 mm/25%	180°	144 × 256
HASTE (liver)	Coronal	∞	103	320	8 mm/30%	90° Refocusing angle: 130°–180°	192 × 256
SGE (liver)	Transverse	140	4	320	8–10 mm/25%	80°	128 × 256
SGE (liver) 1 sec postGd	Transverse	140	4	320	8–10 mm/25%	80°	128 × 256
Fat-suppressed SGE (upper abdomen)	Transverse	140	2–4	320–400	8–10 mm/25%	80°	128 × 256
Fat-suppressed SGE (upper abdomen)	Coronal	140	2–4	320	8–10 mm/25%	80°	128 × 256
Fat-suppressed SGE (lower abdomen/pelvis)	Transverse	140	2–4	320	8 mm/25%	80°	128 × 256
Fat-suppressed SGE (lower abdomen/pelvis)	Sagittal	140	2–4	320	8 mm/25%	80°	128 × 256
T2 ETSE high-resolution (pelvis)	Transverse	3000–4500	130	320	7–8 mm/25%	180°	270 × 512

Note: If this is initial presentation T2 echo-train spin-echo sagittal should be added to the pelvis.

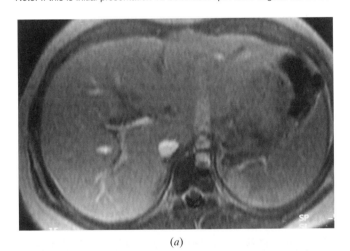

(a)

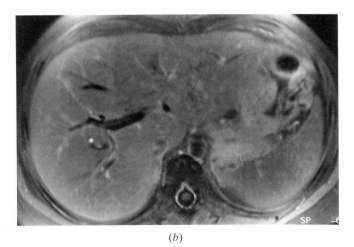

(b)

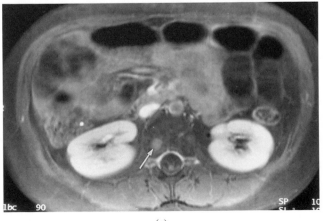

(c)

FIG. 1.8 Noncooperative patient who can breathe regularly. Dynamic gadolinium-enhanced breathing-independent MP-RAGE (*a*), and interstitial-phase gadolinium-enhanced FS-SE (*b,c*) images. Patients who cannot suspend respiration but can breathe regularly, such as this sedated pediatric patient, can be well-examined by a combination of breathing-averaged sequences (*b,c*) and breathing-independent sequences for dynamic image acquisition following gadolinium administration (*a*). A high-signal-intensity focus in a lumbar vertebral body is apparent, which represents a focal deposit of leukemia (*arrow, c*).

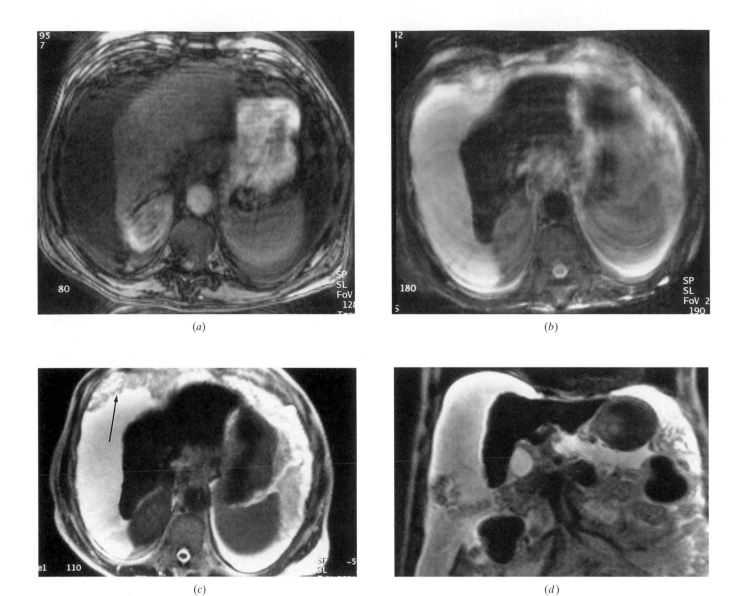

(a)

(b)

(c)

(d)

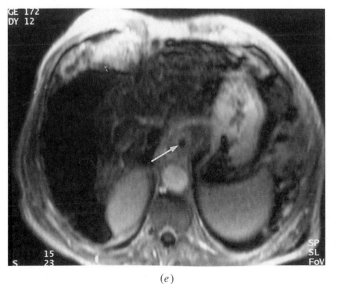

(e)

FIG. 1.9 Noncooperative agitated patient. SGE (*a*), FS-ETSE (*b*), HASTE (*c*), coronal HASTE (*d*), and 90-second postgadolinium slice-selective MP-RAGE (*e*) images. Severe ghosting artifact from respiration is present on both breath-hold (*a*) and breathing-averaged (*b*) MR sequences, reflecting the fact that the patient could neither suspend respiration nor breathe in a regular fashion. Transverse HASTE image (*c*) at the same level as the breathing-averaged T2-weighted ETSE image (*b*) shows clear definition of liver, spleen, stomach, and top of right kidney. The liver is shrunken, irregular in contour, and low in signal intensity. The spleen is relatively normal in size and signal intensity. The combination of these findings is compatible with idiopathic he-mochromatosis. A large volume of ascites is present, which is high in signal intensity on the breathing-independent T2-weighted images (*c,d*) and low in signal intensity on the breathing-independent T1-weighted image (*e*). Hypertrophy of the omentum is well-shown on the breathing independent HASTE sequence (*long arrow, c*) but not apparent on the breathing-averaged T2-weighted image at the same level (*b*). In addition, inflammatory tissue surrounding the esophagus is clearly defined on the breathing-independent sequences (*c,e*) but poorly defined on longer duration sequences (*a,b*). The lumen of the esophagus is defined as a signal void structure within the inflammatory tissue (*arrow, e*).

gle-section SGE pre- and postgadolinium administration should be performed (Fig. 1.9).

REFERENCES

1. Brown MA, Semelka RC: MRI: basic principles and applications. New York: Wiley-Liss, 1995.

2. Semelka RC, Willms AB, Brown MA, Brown ED, Finn JP: Comparison of breath-hold T1-weighted MR sequences for imaging of the liver. J Magn Reson Imaging 4:759–765, 1994.

3. Semelka RC, Kelekis NL, Thomasson D, Brown MA, Laub GA: HASTE MR imaging: Description of technique and preliminary results in the abdomen. J Magn Reson Imaging 6:698–699, 1996.

4. Gaa J, Hutabu H, Jenkins RL, Finn JP, Edelman RR: Liver masses: replacement of conventional T2-weighted spin echo MR imaging with breath-hold MR imaging. Radiology 200:459–464, 1996.

LIVER

R. C. SEMELKA, M.D. AND N. L. KELEKIS, M.D.

NORMAL ANATOMY

The liver is divided into right and left hepatic lobes, each composed of two segments. The right lobe is divided into anterior and posterior segments, and the left lobe is divided into medial and lateral segments. The caudate lobe is a separate smaller lobe that derives its arterial supply from both the right and left hepatic arteries and has venous drainage directly into the inferior vena cava.

The separation into right and left lobes is defined by the middle hepatic vein superiorly and by the gallbladder fossa inferiorly. The division of the right lobe into anterior and posterior segments is defined by the right hepatic vein. The division of the left lobe into medial and lateral segments is defined superiorly by the left hepatic vein and inferiorly by the fissure for the ligamentum teres.

A more recent nomenclature [1] divides the liver into segments based on portal venous supply and hepatic venous drainage. This classification system described by Couinaud introduces a plane to create superior and inferior subsegments of the anterior and posterior segments of the right lobe defined by the right portal vein, and another plane to create superior and inferior subsegments of the lateral segment of the left lobe defined by the left portal vein. This classification is widely used because it defines the liver into segments that are surgically resectable.

The liver contains three fissures: (1) the interlobular fissure, (2) the fissure for the ligamentum teres (left inter-segmental fissure), and (3) the fissure for the ligamentum venosum. The interlobar fissure is an incomplete fissure, occasionally identified on lower topographic sections of the liver situated in the plane of cleavage defined by the gallbladder fossa. The fissure for the ligamentum teres is a continuation at the falciform ligament. The fissure for the ligamentum venosum has a transverse orientation and is present at the level of contact between the lateral segment of the left lobe and the caudate lobe.

The vascular anatomy of the liver includes the hepatic arterial system, portal venous system, and hepatic venous system. Intrahepatic portal triads include branches of the portal vein, hepatic arteries, and bile ducts. Those structures are situated in the central portion of lobes and segments. Hepatic veins are located between segments and are not accompanied by other structures. Figure 2.1 illustrates normal anatomy.

MRI TECHNIQUE

The current standard MRI examination of the liver includes a T1-weighted sequence, a T2-weighted sequence, and a contrast-enhanced sequence. The most comprehensive contrast administration approach is the use a nonspecific extracellular contrast agent, gadolinium chelate, as a rapid bolus injection with serial imaging using a spoiled gradient-echo (SGE) sequence.

A variety of sequences exist that generate T1- and

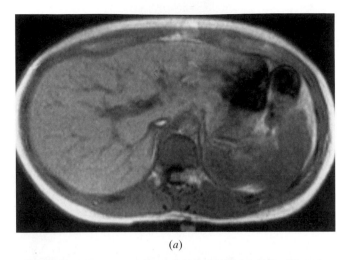

(a)

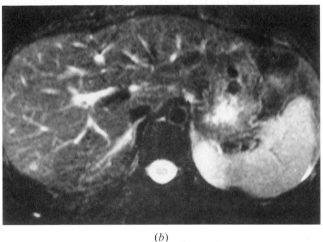

(b)

FIG. 2.1 Normal liver. SGE (a) and T2-weighted fat-suppressed SE (b) images. The liver is higher in signal intensity than spleen on the T1-weighted image (a) and lower in signal than normal, noniron-deposited spleen on the T2-weighted image (b).

T2-weighted images. Field strength and gradient factors of the MRI machine generally dictate the type of sequences employed. At lower field strength (<1 T) spin-echo sequences are generally used because of gradient strength and signal-to-noise ratio limitations. At high field strength (≥1 T) gradient-echo sequences are generally used for T1-weighted sequences, and echo-train sequences are used for T2-weighted sequences. The following is a brief discussion of sequences, emphasizing techniques employed on state-of-the-art high field systems.

T1-Weighted Sequences

The most common techniques used for T1-weighted images are spin-echo, inversion recovery, SGE (e.g., fast low-angle shot [FLASH] or fast multiplanar spoiled gradient echo [FMSPGR]), and inversion-recovery magnetization-prepared snapshot (e.g., turboFLASH) techniques.

Adequate T1-weighting is achieved by ensuring that repetition time is short (≤500 msec for spin-echo and ≤170 msec for SGE sequences) and echo time is short (15 msec with spin-echo and ≤7 msec for SGE sequences). Breathing artifact is the most problematic artifact in abdominal MRI. A variety of compensation techniques are employed to control this artifact in sequences such as spin-echo sequences that are nonbreath-hold. These include respiratory compensation, multiple averaging, fat suppression, anterior saturation, and, most recently, navigator echoes.

On high field MRI systems, the breath-hold SGE sequence performs well for T1-weighted imaging. The advantages of this sequence include fast data acquisition, robust sequence performance, avoidance of breathing artifact, complete coverage of the liver in one breath-hold, and good T1-weighting (see Fig. 2.1). Effective parameters for this sequence include relatively long repetition time (e.g., 100 to 150 msec), which allows acquisition of sufficient sections in one breath-hold for complete liver coverage and a high signal-to-noise ratio; lowest in-phase echo time (6 msec at 1.0 T, 4 msec at 1.5 T), which allows acquisition of multiple sections, a high signal-to-noise ratio, and true T1-weighting; and a flip angle of approximately 90° (range of 60° to 90°), the advantages of which are a good signal-to-noise ratio and adequate T1-weighting. One signal average and a matrix of 128 to 170 by 256 (phase encoding by frequency encoding) are also recommended. This sequence generates 14 to 22 sections in a 20-second breath-hold period. The other important use of SGE sequencing is for dynamic gadolinium chelate imaging. It is usually advisable to use an in-phase echo time on SGE images for contrast-enhanced studies in order to avoid (1) confusing variations in signal intensity based on fatty infiltration of the liver and (2) black-ring phase-cancellation artifact that will mask capsular-based disease.

The drawback of SGE sequencing is that it requires patient cooperation to suspend respiration for 20 seconds. In patients who cannot suspend respiration, the spin-echo sequence is effective if the patient breathes at a regular rate. In patients who cannot suspend respiration and who are unable to breathe regularly or are agitated, breathing-independent techniques such as turboFLASH or SGE sequences acquired in a single-section fashion using the minimum repetition time are necessary. Work is currently going on to increase the image quality of turboFLASH because this sequence suffers from low signal-to-noise ratio and spatial resolution, and image quality is not uniformly reliable.

T2-Weighted Imaging

T2-weighted imaging is most frequently performed as conventional spin-echo or echo-train spin-echo sequences (e.g., fast spin-echo or turbo spin-echo sequences). Echo-train techniques are currently employed more frequently on state-of-the-art MRI systems because of the shorter sequence duration, which can be utilized to decrease data acquisition time, increase spatial resolution, or both. Short tau inversion recovery (STIR) also may be used to acquire T2-weighted type information. As with spin-echo sequences this can be modified as an echo-train sequence (e.g., turboSTIR). Both turbo spin-echo and turboSTIR imaging may be performed in a breath-hold period to avoid breathing artifact. A variation of the turbo spin-echo sequence termed half-fourier acquisition single-shot turbo spin-echo (HASTE) has been developed recently, which acquires individual image sections in less than 1 second. Current implementations of this sequence result in robust, reproducible image quality that are breathing independent.

Chemically selective fat suppression is a useful addition to T2-weighted imaging because it reduces phase artifact, removes chemical shift artifact, and improves the dynamic range of tissue signal intensities (see Fig. 2.1). The use of chemically selective fat suppression may be particularly important with echo-train spin-echo sequences. Fat is high in signal intensity on these sequences, and fatty liver will therefore be high in signal intensity, reducing the conspicuity of high-signal-intensity focal lesions. Because fatty liver is common in the presence of a number of focal liver lesions such as metastatic disease, fat suppression should be routinely employed with echo train sequences for imaging the liver.

Out-Of-Phase (Opposed-Phase) Imaging

Out-of-phase imaging is an effective approach for the detection of fatty infiltration in the liver and is useful for characterizing focal lesions as focal fatty infiltration. It is reasonable to routinely include an out-of-phase sequence for liver examinations because the sequence is rapidly acquired in one breath-hold, and fatty liver is a common entity that often has clinical implications. Out-of-phase imaging is best performed as an SGE technique with the lowest possible out-of-phase echo time (4 msec at 1.0 T and 2 msec at 1.5 T). This approach results in a good signal-to-noise ratio and the maximum number of sections per acquisition, and prevents confusion between fatty liver and iron-deposited liver. In the presence of fatty infiltration, the liver is higher in signal intensity on the longer in-phase echo-time images than on the lower out-of-phase echo-time images, whereas in an iron-deposited liver, the liver is lower in signal intensity on the longer in-phase echo-time images than on the shorter out-of-phase echo-time images. In fatty liver, the signal intensity of the liver varies in a cyclical fashion with the liver low in signal on out-of-phase echo time and higher in signal intensity on in-phase echo time due to phase cycling of fat and water, whereas in an iron-deposited liver, magnetic susceptibility effects increase progressively with increasing echo time.

The addition of chemically selective fat suppression to a low-echo-time out-of-phase sequence is an effective approach to maximize fat attenuation. Fat-suppressed T1-weighted SGE sequence is useful in combination with gadolinium administration to look for either capsular-based or bile-duct disease. In general, image acquisition between 90 seconds and 5 minutes maximizes conspicuity of these disease processes.

MR Angiography (MRA)

MRA is occasionally useful in the examination of liver disease, especially in the setting of hepatic cirrhosis, to examine for portal vein patency or presence of varices. Time-of-flight, phase-contrast, or gadolinium enhanced gradient-echo techniques can be used for this purpose. The recent implementation of gadolinium-enhanced three-dimensional (3D) Fast Imaging with Steady State Precession (FISP) and gadolinium-enhanced 3D water excitation SGE sequences has facilitated the delineation of the portal venous system (Fig. 2.2) and of the origin and anatomical relationships of the hepatic artery, which may be useful for surgical planning of hepatic resection.

Contrast Enhancement

In current clinical practice, gadolinium chelates are frequently employed as liver contrast agents. These agents are nonspecific extracellular space agents.

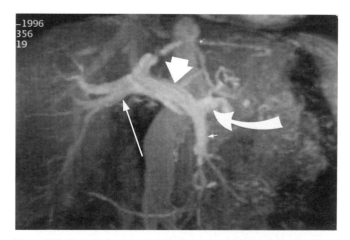

F IG. 2.2 Portal venous system. Anteroposterior projection from 3D maximum-intensity projection (MIP) reconstruction of a set of coronal bolus gadolinium enhanced breath-hold 3D FISP 2 mm-thin sections. Superior mesenteric vein (*small arrow*), splenic vein (*curved arrow*), main portal vein (*large arrow*), and intrahepatic portal veins (*long arrow*) are well-defined on this gadolinium-enhanced 3D FISP image.

Gadolinium chelates are distributed initially within the intravascular compartment and diffuse rapidly throughout the extracellular (vascular plus interstitial) space in a distribution similar to that of water-soluble iodinated contrast agents. These agents cause T1-shortening of adjacent water molecules, which results in tissue brightening on T1-weighted images. Gadolinium enhancement is visually similar to iodine contrast enhancement on computed tomography (CT) images. This analogous appearance facilitates MR image interpretation for diagnosticians familiar with CT image interpretation.

Gadolinium chelates should be used with dynamic scanning techniques to maximize detection and characterization of liver lesions. The best results are achieved using the SGE technique as a single breath-hold with complete liver coverage [2–5].

The following phases of enhancement are important for lesion detection and characterization:

1. *Capillary* (arterial, presinusoidal)-*phase images* are especially important for detecting hypervascular malignancies (e.g., hepatocellular carcinoma and metastases from hypervascular primary tumors such as, islet-cell tumors, renal cancer, pheochromocytoma, carcinoid, and leiomyosarcoma). These images are acquired immediately after a rapid bolus injection of gadolinium chelate, with the patient positioned in the magnet bore. Optimal timing of this sequence is demonstrated by the presence of contrast in hepatic arteries and in portal veins, but not within hepatic veins (Fig. 2.3). At this phase of enhancement the normal pancreas and renal cortex are enhanced intensely, renal medulla is minimally enhanced, and normal spleen has an arciform or serpiginous enhancement. Although gadolinium is present in portal veins, the majority of the gadolinium within the liver has been delivered by hepatic arteries at this early enhancement phase. Specific enhancement features of various hepatic lesions are best shown on these images because over time many focal lesions tend to enhance throughout their substance and approach the signal intensity of liver. Image acquisition timed at approximately 6 seconds earlier demonstrates gadolinium present only in hepatic arteries (Fig. 2.4). This phase is less ideal because the liver is essentially unenhanced and the blood supply of hepatic lesions is not visualized.

2. *Portal-phase images* show maximal hepatic enhancement and maximal contrast between liver and hypovascular lesions. These images are acquired approximately 1 minute following contrast agent administration. All hepatic vessels are enhanced at this phase of enhancement, and demonstration of vascular patency is usually well-shown on these images.

3. *Equilibrium* (delayed, interstitial) *images* are acquired 2 or more minutes after injection of contrast material, by which time contrast material has diffused into the interstitium of non-CNS (central nervous system) tissues. Delayed contrast enhancement is particularly prominent in edematous tissues such as neoplasms, areas of inflammation, and fibrosis. The concurrent use of frequency-selective fat suppression is useful to increase conspicuity of these types of disease processes on interstitial-phase images. Images acquired between 5 and 10 minutes after injection permit sufficient time for many hemangiomas to fill in, which serves to increase observer confidence of lesion characterization.

New contrast agents that have tissue-specific properties are currently under investigation. These include agents which accumulate within hepatocytes (e.g., manganese (Mn)-DPDP gadolinium (Gd)-EOB-DTPA, Gd-DTPA-BOPTA) [6–8], within reticuloendothelial cells (e.g., superparamagnetic iron oxide particles) [9–11] or within the blood pool (e.g., ultrasmall paramagnetic iron oxide particles) [12]. Other agents are targeted to cell membrane antigens [13].

Regarding hepatocyte specific agents, Mn-DPDP, Gd-EOB-DTPA, and Gd-DTPA-BOPTA are all T1-relaxation-enhancing agents that cause an increase in the signal intensity of normal liver tissue (Fig. 2.5) and hepatocyte-containing tumors and are not taken up by nonhepatocyte-continuing masses (hemangioma, metastases) on T1-weighted images. To achieve hepatocellular enhancement, image acquisition is usually performed less than 15 minutes after contrast injection. The advantages of T1-relaxation agents include these: (1) They can be used with SGE, which results in robust, reproducible image quality with complete liver coverage in one breath-hold, and (2) they do not result in artifacts, such as susceptibility artifact, which can mask small lesions. All these agents have both renal and hepatobiliary excretion. Both Gd-EOB-DTPA and Gd-DTPA-BOPTA can be used to acquire early perfusional information, similar in appearance to standard gadolinium chelates, and late (>15-minute) hepatocyte enhancement [15]. The early perfusional information may be used for lesion characterization with the additional benefit of improved lesion detection. The late images may be used for lesion detection with some additional information on characterization to distinguish hepatocyte-containing from nonhepatocyte-containing tumors. Although hepatocyte-specific agents permit distinction between hepatocyte containing tumors (e.g., adenoma, focal nodular hyperplasia [FNH], hepatocellular carcinoma) and nonhepatocyte-containing tumors (e.g., hemangioma, metastases), it is generally more important to distinguish between benign and malignant tumors within these categories. Early perfusional information generally achieves this goal.

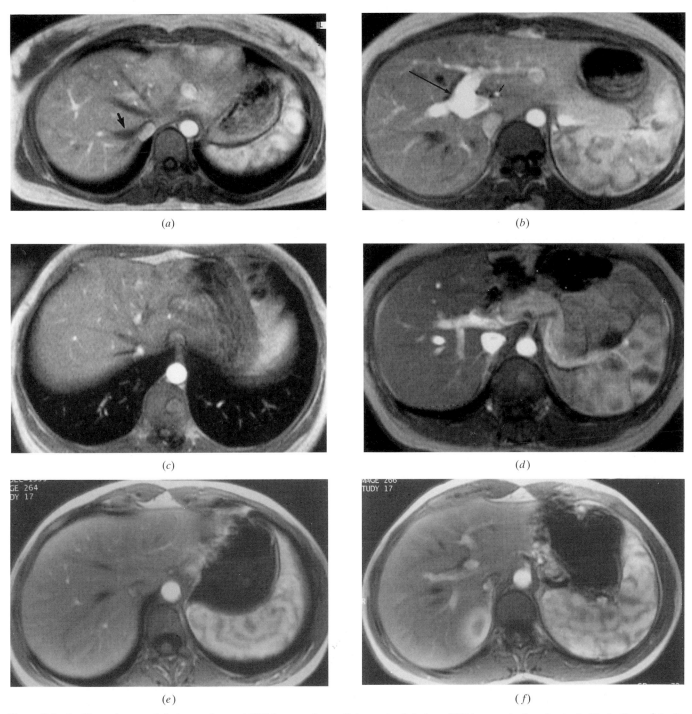

F I G . 2.3 Capillary-phase gadolinium enhanced SGE images. Immediate postgadolinium SGE images in 3 patients (*a,b*), (*c,d*), and (*e,f*), respectively. Images acquired from the higher tomographic sections (*a,c,e*) demonstrate absence of gadolinium in hepatic veins (*arrow, a*), and images acquired from the more inferior tomographic sections (*b,d,f*) demonstrate presence of gadolinium in hepatic arteries (*small arrow, b*) and portal veins (*long arrow, b*).

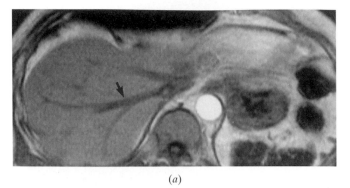

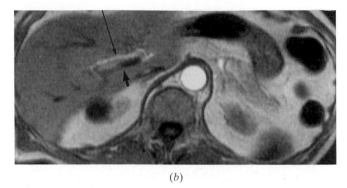

(a)   (b)

F I G . 2.4 Hepatic arterial-phase gadolinium-enhanced SGE images. SGE images acquired from superior (*a*) and more inferior (*b*) tomographic sections demonstrate absence of contrast in hepatic veins (*arrow, a*) and portal veins (*arrow, b*) and the presence of contrast in hepatic arteries (*long arrow, b*). The liver is essentially unenhanced at this early phase of enhancement.

Regarding reticuloendothelial cell-specific contrast agents, superparamagnetic iron oxide particles are T2-relaxation-enhancing agents that lower the signal intensity of normal reticuloendothelial cells containing liver tissue on T2-weighted images, and do not alter the signal intensity of mass lesions that do not contain reticuloendothelial cells (e.g., hemangiomas, metastases). This results in an increase in the conspicuity of liver tumors that are moderately high in signal intensity on T2-weighted images (Fig. 2.5). Overall image quality is improved by imaging with a proton density-weighted sequence with a shorter echo time (e.g., 30 to 60 msec) and standard repetition time for a T2-weighted sequence (>2,000 msec). The high signal-to-noise ratio of proton density sequences complements the T2-shortening effect of the contrast agent, which maximizes lesion conspicuity. Susceptibility artifact may potentially interfere with detection of subcentimeter lesions such as metastases.

Regarding ultrasmall paramagnetic iron oxide particles, these agents have blood pool effects that may be helpful in detecting or characterizing vascular lesions such as hemangiomas. Ring enhancement has been described using this agent, and the specificity of this finding has yet to be determined [12].

The applications and roles for new contrast agents will ultimately depend on how they compare with non-

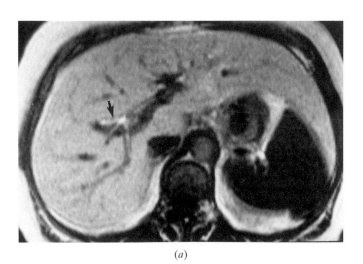

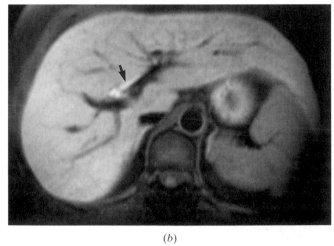

(a)   (b)

F I G . 2.5 Mn-DPDP-enhancement and iron oxide enhancement. Mn-DPDP-enhanced SGE (*a*) and Mn-DPDP-enhanced T1-weighted fat-suppressed spin-echo (*b*) images in a normal patient. Normal liver homogeneously enhances with Mn-DPDP due to its T1-shortening effect. Excretion of Mn-DPDP in the biliary system is shown as high signal intensity fluid in biliary ducts (*arrow, a,b*). Nonenhanced (*a*) and iron oxide particulate-enhancer (*b*) T2-weighted fat suppressed echo-train spin-echo images in a second patient who has liver metastases. Following contrast administration, a greater number of less than 1 cm metastases are identified in the liver (*small arrows, b*).

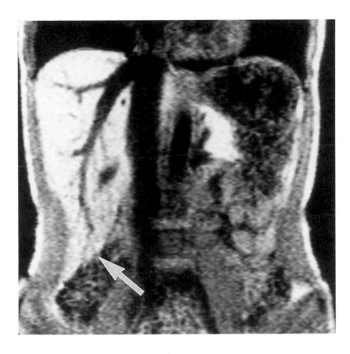

FIG. 2.7 Riedel's lobe. Coronal MP-RAGE (turboFLASH) image shows elongation of the inferior aspect of the right lobe of the liver (*arrow*).

specific extracellular gadolinium chelates. Recent studies have compared contrast agents in an attempt to define clinical uses [7,14–15].

NORMAL VARIATIONS

A number of normal variations in liver size and shape occur. Common variations include horizontal elongation of the lateral segment of the left lobe, hypoplasia of the left lobe, and vertical elongation of the right lobe, termed *Riedel's lobe.* An elongated lateral segment may wrap around the anterior aspect of the upper abdomen and extend laterally to the spleen. A clear distinction between liver and spleen may be made with T2-weighted images in which normal spleen is high in signal intensity and distinct from the lower signal intensity liver (Fig. 2.6). Hypoplasia of the left lobe does not generally result in diagnostic difficulties, although it may simulate a left

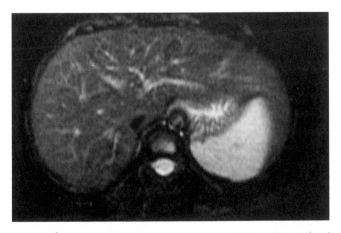

FIG. 2.6 Elongated lateral segment of the left lobe. T2-weighted fat-suppressed spin-echo image demonstrates an elongated lateral segment that extends lateral to the spleen. Clear distinction is made between lower-signal-intensity liver and moderately high-signal-intensity spleen.

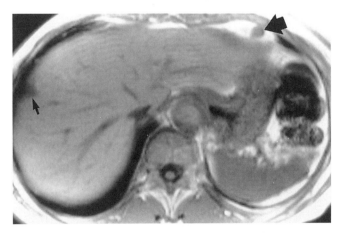

FIG. 2.8 Diaphragmatic insertion. SGE image demonstrates a wedge-shape defect along the lateral superior margin of the liver (*arrow*). Diaphragmatic insertions are usually multiple but may be single as in this case. Incidental note is made of a subdiaphragmatic lymph node (*large arrow*).

hepatectomy, which clinical history readily establishes. Riedel's lobe is a common finding and is more frequently observed in women. The importance of correct identification of a Riedel's lobe is to avoid confusion with hepatomegaly. Transverse and coronal images are effective at demonstrating this variant, and coronal images are useful for excluding an exophytic mass lesion such as hepatic adenoma or metastasis (Fig. 2.7).

Diaphragmatic insertions are not an uncommon finding along the lateral aspect of the liver. They tend to be multiple and closely related to overlying ribs, having wedge-shaped margins with the capsular surface of the liver (Fig. 2.8). Insertions are low in signal on T1- and T2-weighted images. These features help to distinguish diaphragmatic insertions from peripheral mass lesions.

PARTIAL HEPATECTOMY

Imaging findings in the setting of partial hepatectomy vary depending on the remoteness of the resection. Magnetic susceptibility artifact is often present along the resection margin of the liver. Hyperplasia of the remaining liver may be appreciated as early as 3 months after surgery. Partial hepatectomy of the right lobe is a common procedure. Within 1 year, general enlargement of the left lobe occurs, and hypertrophy of the medial segments creates the appearance of a small pseudo right lobe (Fig. 2.9).

◼ DISEASE OF THE HEPATIC PARENCHYMA

MASS LESIONS

Benign Masses

Cysts
Hepatic cysts are common lesions and frequently multiple. Simple cysts are congenital in origin, believed to arise from aberrant bile ducts or to be acquired, such as from obstructed bile ducts caused by inflammatory hyperplasia. Cysts are more frequently found in females. Cysts are homogeneous, well-defined lesions that possess a sharp margin with liver and are usually oval-shaped, although slight variations are common [16]. Occasionally, cysts are so closely grouped that they resemble a multicystic mass.

Cysts are low in signal intensity on T1-weighted images and high in signal intensity on T2-weighted images and retain signal intensity on longer echo time (e.g. >120 msec) T2-weighted images. Cysts do not enhance with gadolinium on MR images (Fig. 2.10). Delayed postgado-

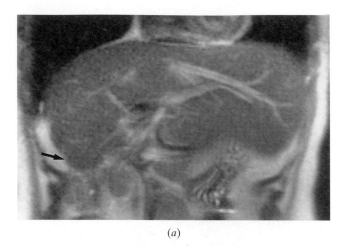

(a)

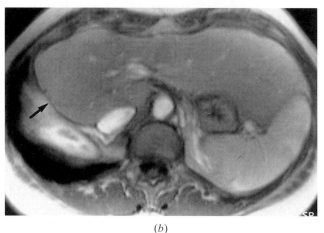

(b)

FIG. 2.9 Liver regeneration following right hepatectomy. Coronal HASTE (*a*) and immediate postgadolinium SGE (*b*) images. The lateral segment of the left lobe is enlarged and rounded in contour (*a,b*). Hypertrophy of the medial segment results in an appearance of a pseudo right lobe (*arrow, a*). A relatively sharp resection margin is noted (*arrow, b*) with no abnormal tissue apparent.

linium images (up to 5 minutes) may be useful to ensure that lesions are cysts and not poorly vascularized metastases that show gradual enhancement [17]. An advantage of MRI over computed tomography (CT) imaging in the characterization of cysts is that on gadolinium-enhanced MR images cysts are nearly signal-void, whereas cysts on contrast-enhanced CT images are a light gray in attenuation. Single shot breathing independent T2-weighted sequences (e.g., HASTE) are particularly effective at showing small (25 mm) cysts. MRI is particularly valuable when lesions are small and the patient has a known primary malignancy.

The vast majority of liver cysts are simple in type. Therefore, the majority are low in signal intensity on T1-weighted images and nearly signal-void on postgadolinium images.

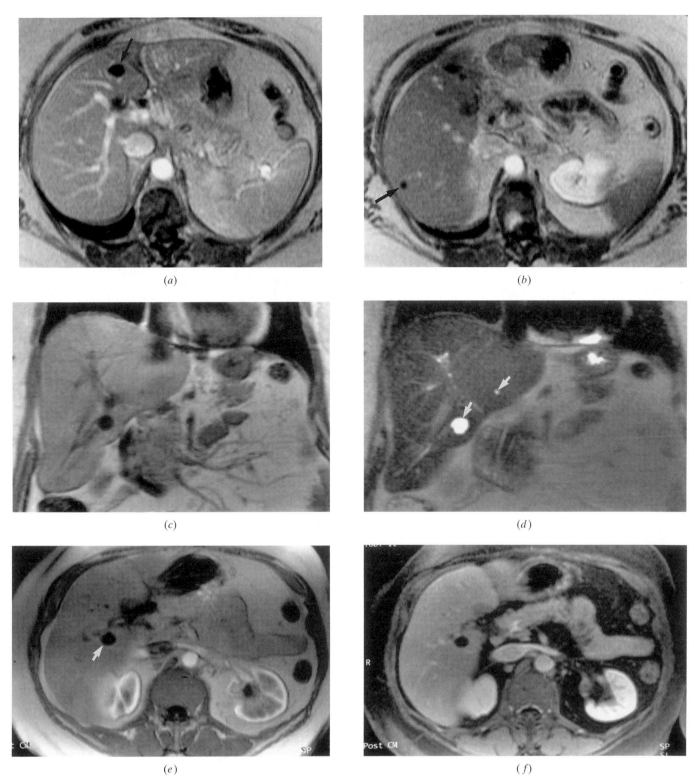

F I G . 2.10 Liver cysts. Five-minute postgadolinium SGE images (*a,b*) demonstrate a 1-cm sharply demarcated signal-void cyst in the medial segment and a 5-mm sharply demarcated signal void cyst in the posterior segment of the right lobe (*arrow, b*). Coronal SGE (*c*), coronal HASTE (*d*), immediate postgadolinium SGE (*e*), and 90 second postgadolinium fat-suppressed SGE (*f*) images in a second patient. A 2-mm and a 10-mm cysts are present on coronal images (*arrows, d*). Cysts measuring < 5 mm are most clearly shown on HASTE images. Cysts are low-signal intensity on T1-weighted images (*c*) and high signal on T2-weighted images (*d*). The 10mm cyst (*arrow, e*) is signal void on early (*e*) and later (*f*) postgadolinium images.

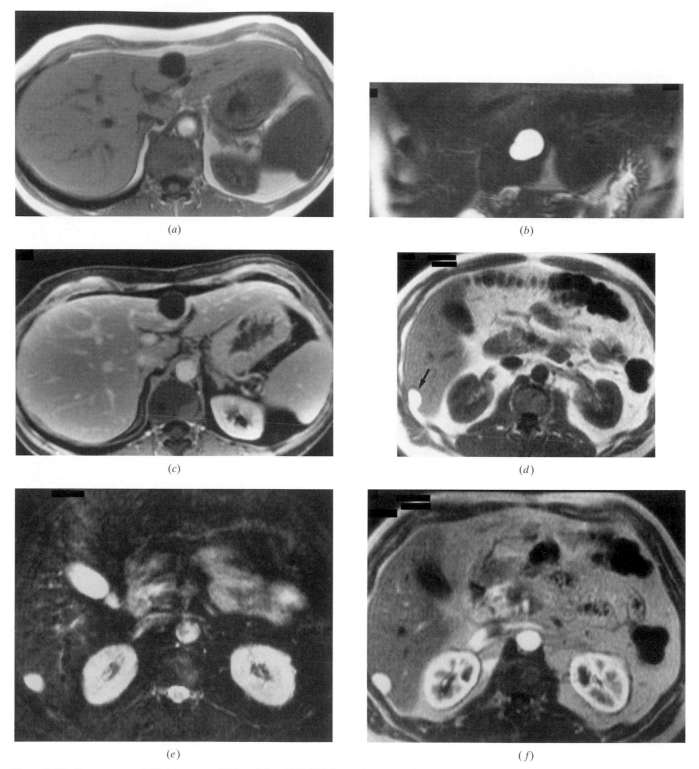

(a)

(b)

(c)

(d)

(e)

(f)

FIG. 2.11 Foregut cyst. SGE (*a*), coronal T2-weighted HASTE (*b*) and 90-second postgadolinium fat-suppressed SGE (*c*) images. A 3-cm cystic lesion is noted in the medial segment superiorly, adjacent to the lateral segment. The lesion extends beyond the contour of the liver and has a thin perceptible wall, features that are characteristic of foregut cysts. SGE (*d*), T2-weighted fat-suppressed spin-echo (*e*), and immediate postgadolinium SGE (*f*) images in a second patient demonstrate a 1.5-cm lesion along the lateral inferior aspect of the right lobe of the liver (*arrow, d*). The lesion is sharply demarcated and is high in signal intensity on the T1- (*d*) and T2-weighted (*e*) images and does not change in shape or appearance following gadolinium administration (*f*). The lesion extends beyond the contour of the liver. The high concentration of mucin in the cyst accounts for the high signal intensity on the T1-weighted images.

Foregut Cysts

Foregut cysts are congenital in origin and not uncommon. These cysts are most frequently located at the anterosuperior margin of the liver, but may be situated elsewhere, superficially along the external surface of the liver, typically at intersegmental locations. Foregut cysts range from hypo- to hyperintense on T1-weighted images, are hyperintense on T2-weighted images, and do not enhance with gadolinium [18,19]. The presence of mucin in these cysts results in high signal intensity on T1-weighted images, with the increase in signal intensity dependent on the concentration of mucin. The characteristic features of these cysts are that they bulge the liver contour and possess a perceptible enhancing cyst wall on postgadolinium images (Fig. 2.11). The presence of a cystic lesion with an enhancing wall and extension beyond the contour of the liver may also be observed in malignant diseases such as ovarian cancer. Absent history of peritoneal spreading malignancy and lack of malignant disease elsewhere are necessary information to establish the diagnosis of foregut cyst on imaging studies.

Autosomal Dominant Polycystic Kidney Disease

The liver is the most common extrarenal organ in which cysts occur in patients with autosomal dominant polycystic kidney disease. These cysts vary in number and size, but tend to be multiple and smaller than the renal cysts, measuring less than 2 cm (Fig. 2.12). They generally do not distort hepatic architecture and do not undergo hemorrhage. Extensive hepatic replacement with large cysts has been described [20].

Extramedullary Hematopoiesis

Extramedullary hematopoiesis may appear as focal hepatic masses in the setting of hereditary disorders of hematopoiesis or in long-standing hematologic malignancies. Masses tend to be homogeneous and moderately high in signal intensity on T2-weighted images and enhance in a diffuse homogeneous fashion on immediate postgadolinium images.

Angiomyolipomas

Angiomyolipomas are uncommon primary benign tumors in the liver. Tumors do not have as high an associa-

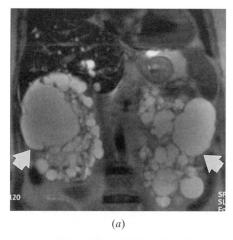

(a)

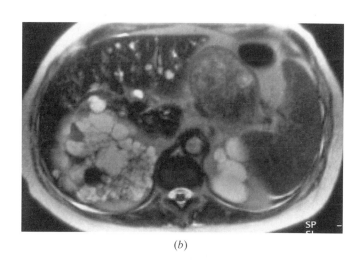

(b)

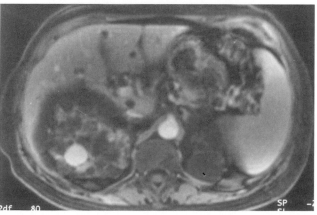

(c)

FIG. 2.12 Liver cysts in polycystic kidney disease. Coronal HASTE (a), transverse HASTE (b), and 90-second postgadolinium fat-suppressed SGE (c) images. The kidneys are massively enlarged and contain multiple cysts of varying size with no definable renal parenchyma (arrows, a). Multiple <1-cm cysts are present and scattered throughout the liver that are high in signal intensity on T2-weighted images (a,b) and do not enhance following gadolinium administration (c).

tion with tuberous sclerosis as that observed with renal angiomyolipomas. Hepatic angiomyolipomas frequently have a high fat content and are high in signal intensity on T1-weighted images and decrease in signal intensity on fat-suppressed images. Angiomyolipomas also may have a low fat content and may appear as moderately low in signal intensity on T1-weighted images and moderately high in signal intensity on T2-weighted images, enhancing in a diffuse heterogeneous fashion on immediate postgadolinium SGE images (Fig. 2.13) [21]. This enhancement pattern is most commonly observed in hepatocellular carcinoma and represents the appearance of well-defined tumors of hepatic origin. Angiomyolipomas are well-defined, sharply marginated masses.

Lipomas

Hepatic lipomas are rarer than angiomyolipomas. Tumors are commonly multiple and appear as fatty tumors that are high in signal intensity on T1-weighted sequences and low in signal intensity on fat-suppressed techniques (Fig. 2.14) [22]. These lesions show negligible enhancement on postgadolinium images.

Hemangiomas

Hemangiomas are the most common benign hepatic neoplasm, with an autopsy incidence between 0.4 and 20 percent [23,24]. Hemangiomas are more frequent in females. They rarely manifest clinically and are usually detected in the investigation of other disease. The great

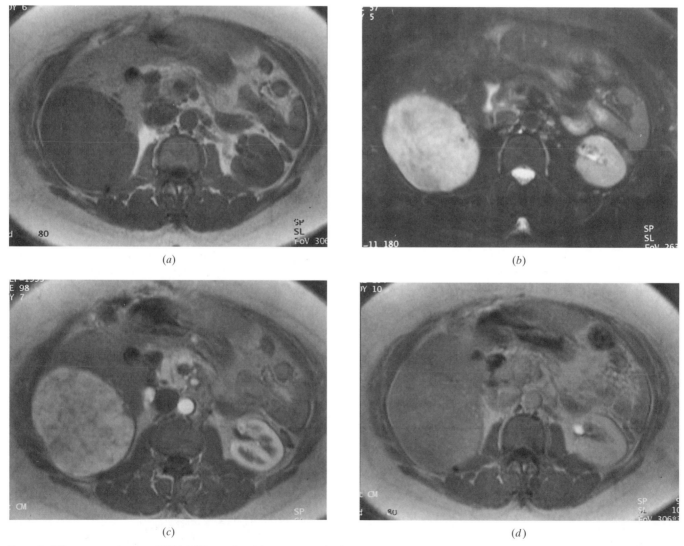

(a) (b)

(c) (d)

F I G. 2.13 Angiomyolipoma. SGE (a), T2-weighted fat-suppressed echo-train spin-echo (b), immediate (c), and 90-second (d) postgadolinium SGE images. The angiomyolipoma is moderately hypointense on the T1-weighted image (a), moderately hyperintense with slight heterogeneity on the T2-weighted image (b), and enhances in an intense diffuse heterogeneous fashion on the immediate postgadolinium SGE image (c). By 90 seconds after gadolinium (d), the lesion has faded in signal intensity to slightly higher than background liver. This angiomyolipoma is unusual in that it contains minimal fat. The diffuse heterogeneous enhancement is typical of tumors of hepatic origin.

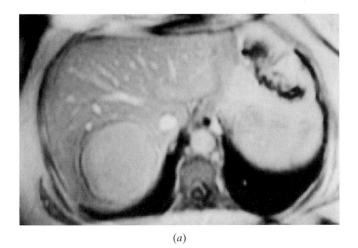

(a)

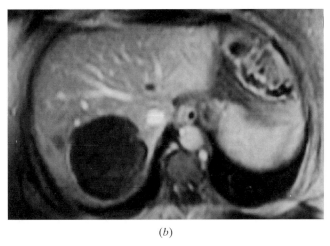

(b)

F IG . 2.14 Lipoma. Gadolinium enhanced SGE (a) and gadolinium-enhanced fat suppressed SGE (b) images. A 6-cm lipoma is present that is uniformly high in signal intensity on the nonsuppressed image (a) and is uniformly low in signal intensity on the fat-suppressed image (b).

ripheral nodular fashion on dynamic serial gadolinium-enhanced MR images with slow progressive complete or nearly complete fill-in of the entire lesion by 10 minutes [29–31]. Serial gadolinium-enhanced SGE images have been shown to be effective in distinguishing benign from malignant hepatic masses [32,33].

The MRI appearances of small (<1.5 cm), medium (1.5 to 5.0 cm), and large (>5.0 cm) hemangiomas have been reported in a multi-institutional study [34]. Among the 154 hemangiomas in 66 patients, 81 lesions were small, 56 medium, and 17 large. Hemangiomas were multiple in 68 percent of patients. All lesions were high in signal intensity on T2-weighted images. Three types of enhancement patterns were observed: (1) uniform high signal intensity immediately following contrast (Type 1), (2) peripheral nodular enhancement with centripetal progression to uniform high signal intensity (Type 2), and (3) peripheral nodular enhancement with centripetal progression and a persistent central scar (Type 3). Type 1 enhancement was observed only in small tumors. Type 2 and Type 3 enhancements were observed in all size categories. Type 3 enhancement was observed in 16 of 17 large tumors. A variation in the Type 2 enhancement pattern is that contrast enhancement may spread at a fairly rapid rate with complete enhancement at 1 to 2 minutes [34]. Similar findings also have been described in an Asian patient population [35].

Small hemangiomas most commonly demonstrate Type 2 enhancement. The peripheral nodules of enhancement are typically very small (Fig. 2.15). Type 1 enhancement is the next most common pattern. Type 3 enhancement is uncommonly observed in small hemangiomas (Fig. 2.16). These lesions are difficult to distinguish from other types of liver lesions, specifically liver metastases, and MRI follow-up is generally required.

majority of these lesions are cavernous hemangiomas, but in rare instances they may be capillary. Cavernous hemangiomas are composed primarily of large vascular lakes and channels (see Fig. 2.25). Some of these channels undergo thrombosis and fibrous organization [25]. Hemangiomas are multiple in at least 50 percent of patients. They may coexist with focal nodular hyperplasia lesions in the setting of the multiple focal nodular hyperplasia syndrome [26].

Hemangiomas have long T1 and T2 values, so they are low in signal intensity on T1-weighted images and high in signal intensity on T2-weighted images, maintaining signal intensity on longer echo times (e.g., >120 msec) [27,28]. Hemangiomas have well-defined round or lobular borders [27,28]. Small lesions typically appear round, whereas larger lesions have a lobular margin. However, T2 measurements are substantially shorter than those of cysts. Hemangiomas typically enhance in a pe-

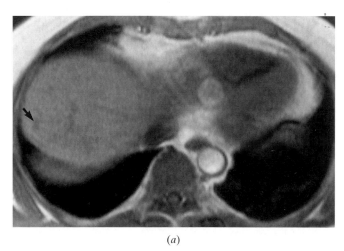

(a)

F IG . 2.15 Small hemangiomas, Type 2 enhancement. SGE (a), T2-weighted fat-suppressed echo-train spin-echo (b), immediate (c), and five minute (d) postgadolinium SGE images.

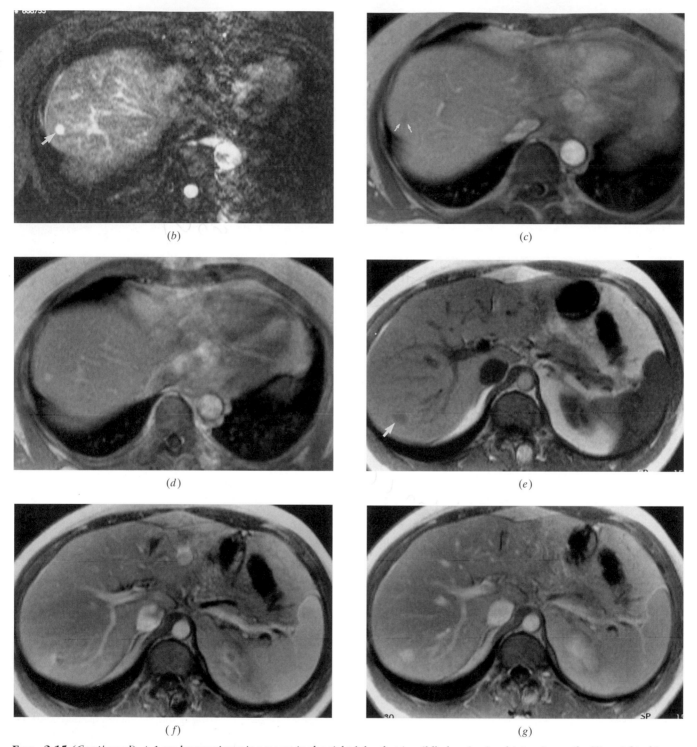

(b)

(c)

(d)

(e)

(f)

(g)

FIG. 2.15 (*Continued*) A 1-cm hemangioma is present in the right lobe that is mildly low in signal intensity on the T1-weighted image (*arrow, a*), high in signal intensity on the T2-weighted image (*arrow, b*), demonstrates peripheral nodular enhancement (*arrows, c*) on the early post contrast image (*c*), and is uniformly homogeneous and moderately high in signal intensity on the delayed image (*d*). SGE (*e*), immediate (*f*), and 90-second (*g*) postgadolinium images in a second patient demonstrate a 1-cm lesion that is moderately hypointense on the T1-weighted image (*arrow, e*), develops peripheral nodular enhancement on the immediate postgadolinium image (*f*), and is uniform and moderately high in signal intensity on the 90-second postgadolinium image (*g*).

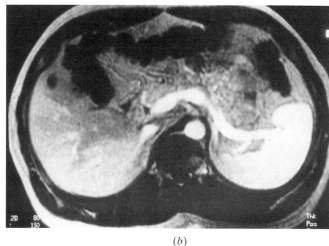

(a)

(b)

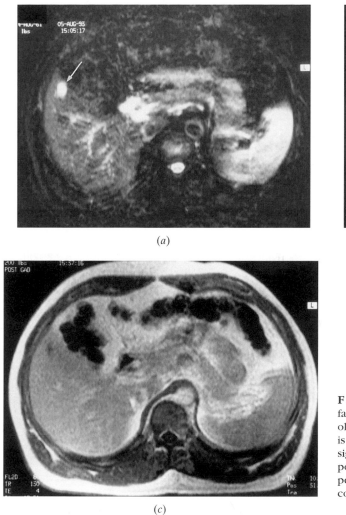

(c)

FIG. 2.16 Small hemangioma, Type 3 enhancement. T2-weighted fat-suppressed spin-echo (a), immediate (b), and 10 minute (c) postgadolinium SGE images. A 1.5-cm lesion is present in the right lobe that is high in signal intensity on the T2-weighted image (*arrow, a*), nearly signal-void with subtle small peripheral nodules on the immediate postgadolinium image (b), and shows peripheral enhancement with persistence of central low signal intensity on the delayed image (c) consistent with a central scar.

The great majority of medium-sized hemangiomas exhibit Type 2 enhancement (Fig. 2.17), and these represent the classic hemangiomas. Type 3 enhancement is the next most common enhancement pattern (Fig. 2.18). Type 1 enhancement is exceedingly rare to nonexistent.

Lesions larger than 1.5 cm with Type 1 enhancement either represent well-differentiated tumors of hepatocellular origin or hypervascular liver metastases.

Giant hemangiomas most frequently have a central scar [34,38]; virtually all giant hemangiomas have Type

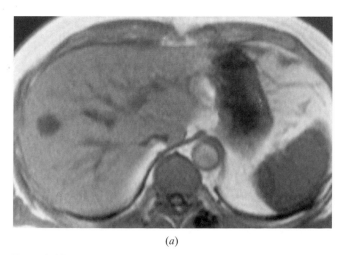

(a)

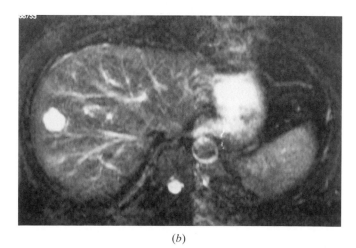

(b)

FIG. 2.17 Medium-sized hemangiomas, Type 2 enhancement. SGE (a), T2-weighted fat-suppressed echo-train spin-echo (b), immediate (c), and 10-minute (d) postgadolinium SGE images.

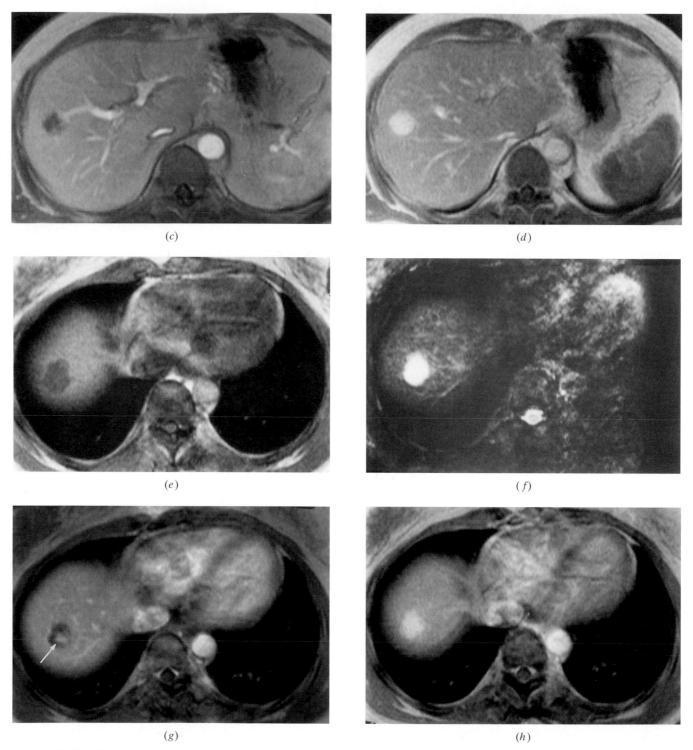

(c)

(d)

(e)

(f)

(g)

(h)

FIG. 2.17 (*Continued*) A 2.1-cm hemangioma is moderately low in signal intensity on the T1-weighted image (*a*), high in signal intensity on the T2-weighted image (*b*), enhances in a peripheral nodular fashion on the immediate postgadolinium image (*c*), and is uniform and high in signal intensity on the delayed postgadolinium image (*d*). SGE (*e*), T2-weighted fat-suppressed echo-train spin-echo (*f*), 45-second (*g*), and 10-minute (*h*) postgadolinium SGE images in a second patient. A 2.5-cm hemangioma is present that demonstrates the same signal-intensity features as the hemangioma in the prior patient. In this patient, the early postcontrast image demonstrates one predominant enhancing nodule that is almost central in location (*arrow, g*).

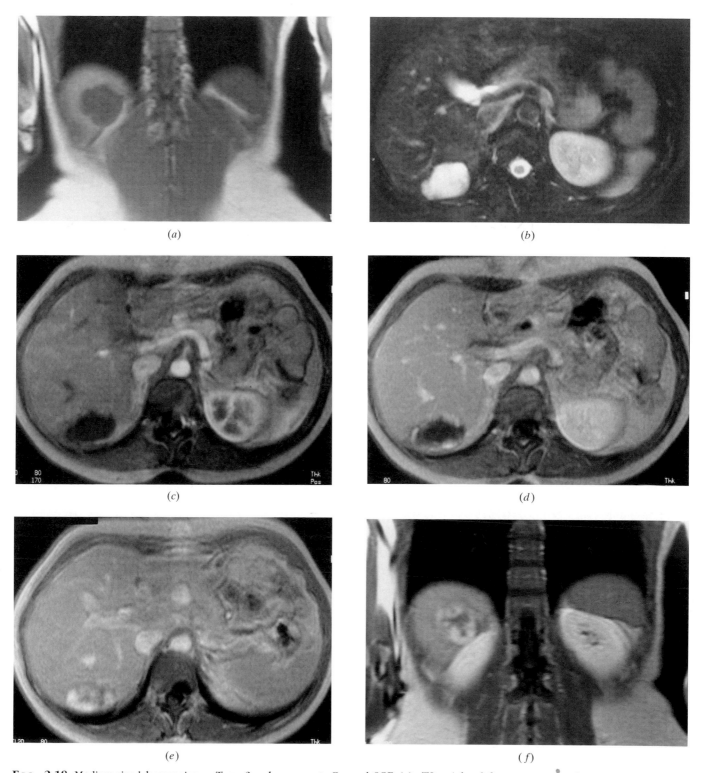

FIG. 2.18 Medium-sized hemangioma, Type 3 enhancement. Coronal SGE (*a*), T2-weighted fat-suppressed echo-train spin-echo (*b*), immediate (*c*), 90-second (*d*), 10-minute transverse (*e*), and coronal (*f*) SGE images. The hemangioma is moderately low in signal intensity on the T1-weighted image (*a*), high in signal intensity on the T2-weighted image (*b*), and demonstrates peripheral nodular enhancement (*c*) that progresses centripetally (*d*). Persistent central low signal intensity is present on the delayed images (*e,f*) consistent with a central scar.

3 enhancement (Fig. 2.19). Absence of a central scar should raise the concern that the mass may represent another lesion. Large hemangiomas frequently have mildly complex signal intensity on T2-weighted images with the frequent presence of low signal strands. Large hemangiomas in rare instances may compress adjacent portal veins resulting in transient segmental increased enhancement on immediate postgadolinium images secondary to autoregulatory increased hepatic arterial supply (Fig. 2.20). On rare occasions, large hemangiomas may also hemorrhage.

The most distinctive imaging feature of hemangiomas is the demonstration of a discontinuous ring of nodules immediately after gadolinium administration [32,34,36]. Nodular enhancement is most frequently eccentric in location. However, central enhancement may

occur. The appearance of central enhancement is rare for all histological types of tumors, and it occurs by early filling of a large central lake by a narrow feeding vessel. Hemangiomas may fade in signal intensity over time, but they will fade in a homogeneous fashion with no evidence of peripheral or heterogeneous washout [32,34]. Hemangiomas may fade in signal to isointensity with liver, but will not fade to hypointensity. Small hemangiomas with Type 1 enhancement may be indistinguishable from hypervascular malignant liver lesions such as hepatocellular carcinomas or leiomyosarcoma. Small hemangiomas are high in signal intensity on T2-weighted images, whereas small hepatocellular carcinomas are often near isointensity. Small hypervascular metastases may appear identical in appearance to small hemangioma on all sequences. Usually, however, a large lesion is also

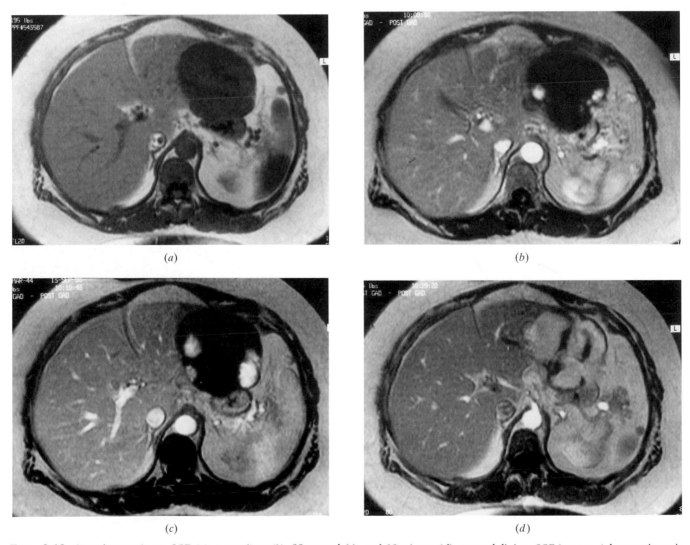

(a)   (b)   (c)   (d)

FIG. 2.19 Giant hemangioma. SGE (*a*), immediate (*b*), 90-second (*c*), and 10-minute (*d*) postgadolinium SGE images. A hemangioma is present in the left lobe that is moderately low in signal intensity on the T1-weighted image, demonstrates peripheral nodular enhancement in a discontinuous ring on the immediate postcontrast image (*b*), and gradually enhances in a centripetal fashion (*c*) with persistent low signal intensity centrally at 10 minutes (*d*), findings consistent with a central scar.

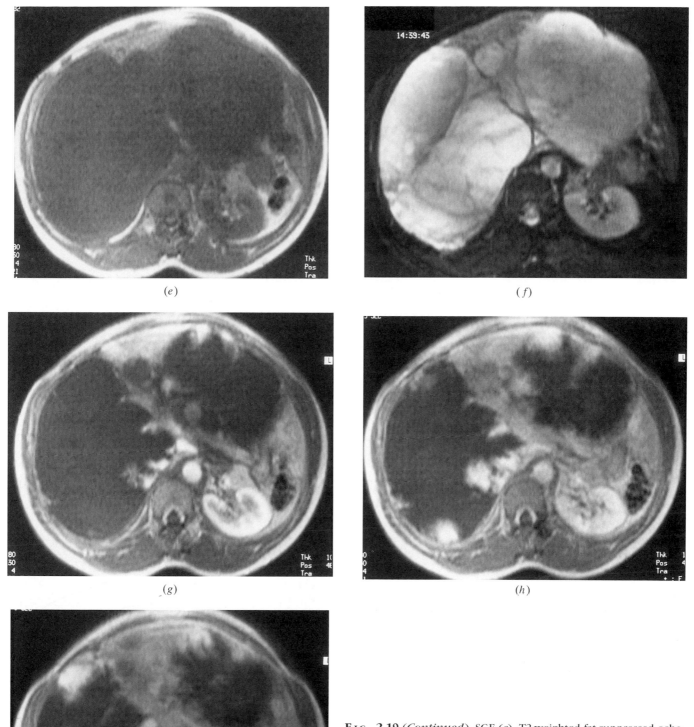

(e)

(f)

(g)

(h)

(i)

FIG. 2.19 (*Continued*) SGE (*e*), T2-weighted fat-suppressed echo-train spin-echo (*f*), immediate (*g*), 90-second (*h*), and 5-minute (*i*) postgadolinium SGE images in a second patient. The liver is largely replaced with massive hemangiomas. They are moderately low in signal intensity on the T1-weighted image (*e*), high in signal intensity with multiple low-signal-intensity linear strands on the T2-weighted image (*f*), and demonstrate peripheral nodular enhancement (*g*) that progresses centrally (*h*). Large central unenhanced regions persist on the 5 minute image (*i*). Low-signal-intensity linear strands are common on T2-weighted images in giant hemangiomas and represent bands of collagenous tissue. This patient underwent liver transplantation because of the extensive hepatic replacement by hemangiomas.

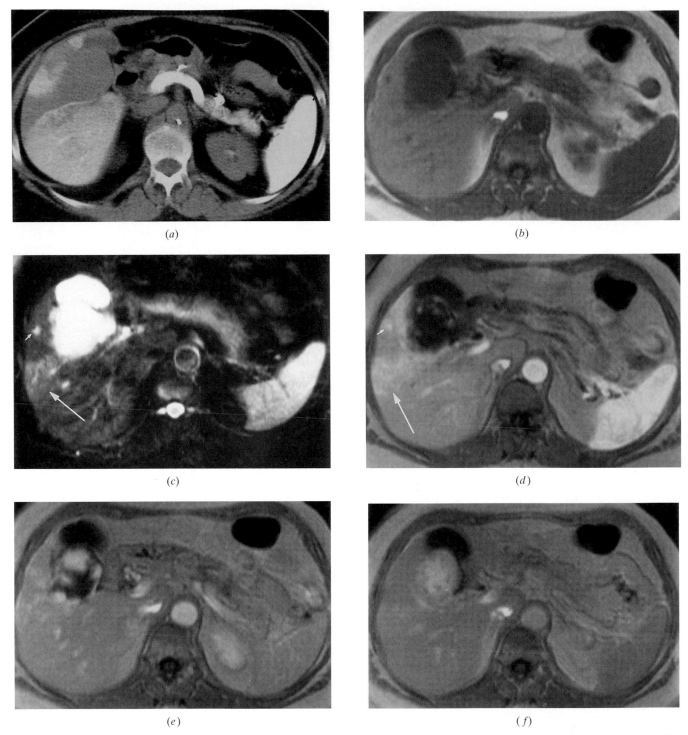

FIG. 2.20 Hemangioma compressing portal vein. Spiral CTAP (*a*), SGE (*b*), T2-weighted fat-suppressed echo-train spin-echo (*c*), immediate (*d*), 90-second (*e*), and 10-minute (*f*) postgadolinium SGE images. A 6-cm lesion is present in the anterior segment of the right lobe that causes distal wedge-shaped diminished portal venous perfusion on the CTAP image (*a*), findings that were considered consistent with a malignant tumor. The tumor is moderately low in signal intensity on the T1-weighted image (*b*), high in signal intensity on the T2-weighted image (*c*), and has peripheral nodular enhancement on the immediate postgadolinium image (*d*) that progresses in a centripetal fashion (*e*) to hyperintensity at 10 minutes (*f*) with small central low-signal-intensity foci consistent with a central scar. The perfusion defect observed on the CTAP image is noted to be wedge-shaped and minimally hyperintense on the T2-weighted image (*long arrow, c*), enhancing in a transient fashion greater than adjacent liver on the immediate postgadolinium image (*d*), findings consistent with portal vein compression.

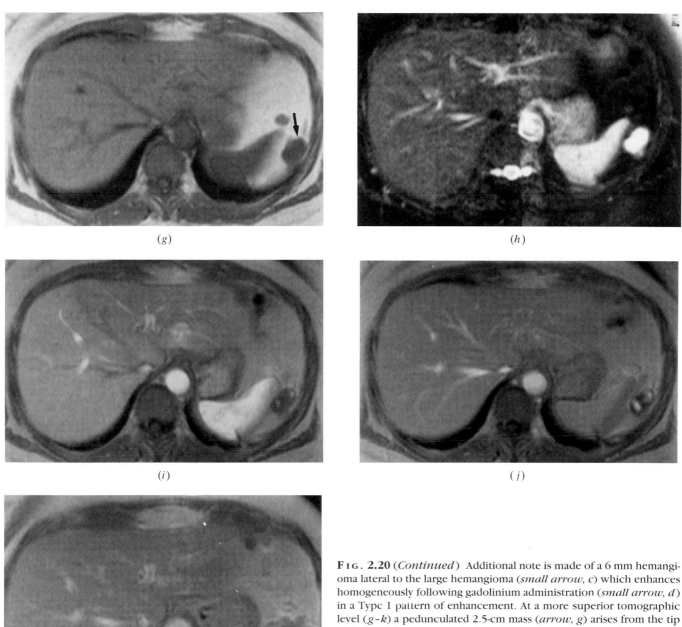

(g)

(h)

(i)

(j)

(k)

Fig. 2.20 (*Continued*) Additional note is made of a 6 mm hemangioma lateral to the large hemangioma (*small arrow, c*) which enhances homogeneously following gadolinium administration (*small arrow, d*) in a Type 1 pattern of enhancement. At a more superior tomographic level (*g–k*) a pedunculated 2.5-cm mass (*arrow, g*) arises from the tip of the lateral segment of the liver. The mass is moderately low in signal intensity on the SGE image (*g*), high in signal intensity on the T2-weighted fat-suppressed echo-train spin-echo image (*h*), enhances in a peripheral nodular fashion on the immediate postgadolinium SGE image (*i*) with centripetal progression on the 90-second postgadolinium SGE image (*j*) and is hyperintense with small low-signal-intensity foci on the 10-minute postgadolinium SGE image (*k*). Hemangiomas are multiple in approximately 68 percent of patients.

present that will exhibit the enhancement features of either a hemangioma or a metastasis, so that the histology of the small lesions may be inferred.

Chemotherapy-treated liver metastases, when treatment has been initiated within 2 to 9 months, may resemble the appearance of hemangiomas. This presumably reflects a histological response to chemotherapy due to less aggressive growth and angiogenesis. Angiosarcomas may resemble hemangiomas; central hemorrhage and less orderly nodular progressive enhancement are features consistent with angiosarcoma. Clinical history is important because patients with hypervascular malignant liver lesions usually have a known primary tumor [37] and the use of chemotherapy can be established.

Advantages of MRI over CT imaging in the evaluation of hemangiomas include (1) the ability to image the entire liver in the same phase of contrast enhancement, which is useful when multiple lesions are present, (2) greater lesion enhancement on contrast enhanced images such that lesions are comparatively brighter than background liver, and (3) superior detection of small hemangiomas.

Reports have shown that hemangiomas may be reliably distinguished from metastases on T2-weighted images based on the smooth lobular margins of hemangiomas and the higher calculated T2 values (mean of 140 msec) [39]. Although this may be true in the majority of patients, cumulative experience from many centers has shown that T2-weighted images alone may not allow characterization of small tumors nor allow reliable distinction between hemangiomas and hypervascular malignant tumors (such as leiomyosarcoma and islet-cell tumors). Therefore, the routine combination of T2-weighted information with serial gadolinium-enhanced SGE may be useful in order to increase observer confidence for establishing the correct diagnosis, and also to maximize evaluation of other hepatic and extrahepatic diseases.

Hepatic Adenomas

Approximately 90 percent of hepatic adenomas occur in young adult women [40,41]. These lesions are associated with the use of birth control pills or the presence of other hepatocellular stimulating agents, including the use of anabolic steroids and abnormal carbohydrate metabolism as in familial diabetes mellitus, galactosemia, and glycogen storage disease Type 1 [26]. Tumors may be multiple in 10 to 20 percent of the cases [26]. Adenomas are derived primarily from hepatocytes. Histologically, the typical features of adenomas are a thin pseudocapsule, intracellular glycogen and bile deposition, lack of architecture, paucity of mature bile ducts, and degenerative necrosis [26,40]. Necrosis and hemorrhage are frequent causes of pain. Hemorrhage, on occasion, may be massive and life-threatening. Adenomas not uncommonly contain substantial fat and may, on occasion, contain central fibrosis and resemble FNH [26].

The typical MRI appearance of an adenoma is a lesion that varies in signal intensity from mildly hypointense to moderately hyperintense on T1-weighted images, and is mildly hyperintense on T2-weighted images (Fig. 2.21). The degree of high signal intensity on T1-weighted images reflects the quantity of fat they contain. Tumors may decrease in signal intensity on out-of-phase or fat-suppressed images due to their fat content (Fig. 2.22) [42]. Homogeneous drop in signal intensity on out-of-phase images is a feature of fat-containing adenomas. At present experience is lacking whether fat-containing well differentiated hepatocellular carcinomas may diminish homogeneously in signal intensity. Adenomas may be nearly isointense with liver on all imaging sequences reflecting similarity to liver parenchyma. Tumors also may have mixed high signal intensity on T1- and T2-weighted images due to the presence of hemorrhage [42,43] (Fig. 2.23). Characteristically, tumors have a transient blush immediately after gadolinium chelate admin-

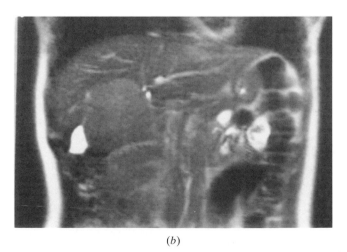

(a)   (b)

FIG. 2.21 Hepatic adenoma. SGE (*a*), coronal HASTE (*b*), T2-weighted fat-suppressed echo-train spin-echo (*c*), immediate (*d*), and 90-second (*e*) postgadolinium SGE images.

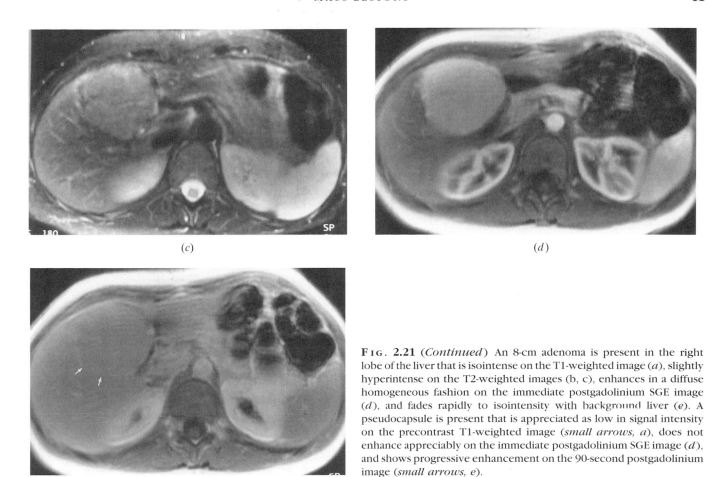

(c)

(d)

(e)

FIG. 2.21 (*Continued*) An 8-cm adenoma is present in the right lobe of the liver that is isointense on the T1-weighted image (*a*), slightly hyperintense on the T2-weighted images (b, c), enhances in a diffuse homogeneous fashion on the immediate postgadolinium SGE image (*d*), and fades rapidly to isointensity with background liver (*e*). A pseudocapsule is present that is appreciated as low in signal intensity on the precontrast T1-weighted image (*small arrows, a*), does not enhance appreciably on the immediate postgadolinium SGE image (*d*), and shows progressive enhancement on the 90-second postgadolinium image (*small arrows, e*).

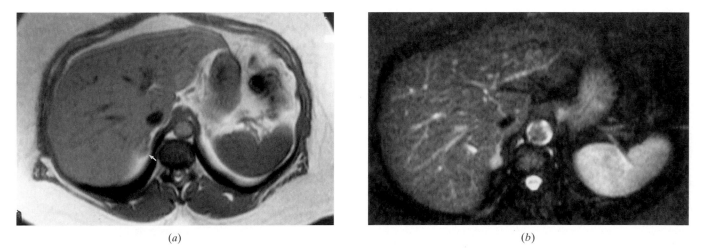

(a)

(b)

FIG. 2.22 Hepatic adenoma. SGE (*a*), T2-weighted fat-suppressed echo-train spin-echo (*b*), out-of-phase SGE (*c*), immediate (*d*), and 90-second (*e*) postgadolinium SGE images. No focal liver lesions are apparent on the T1- (*a*) or T2-weighted (*b*) images.

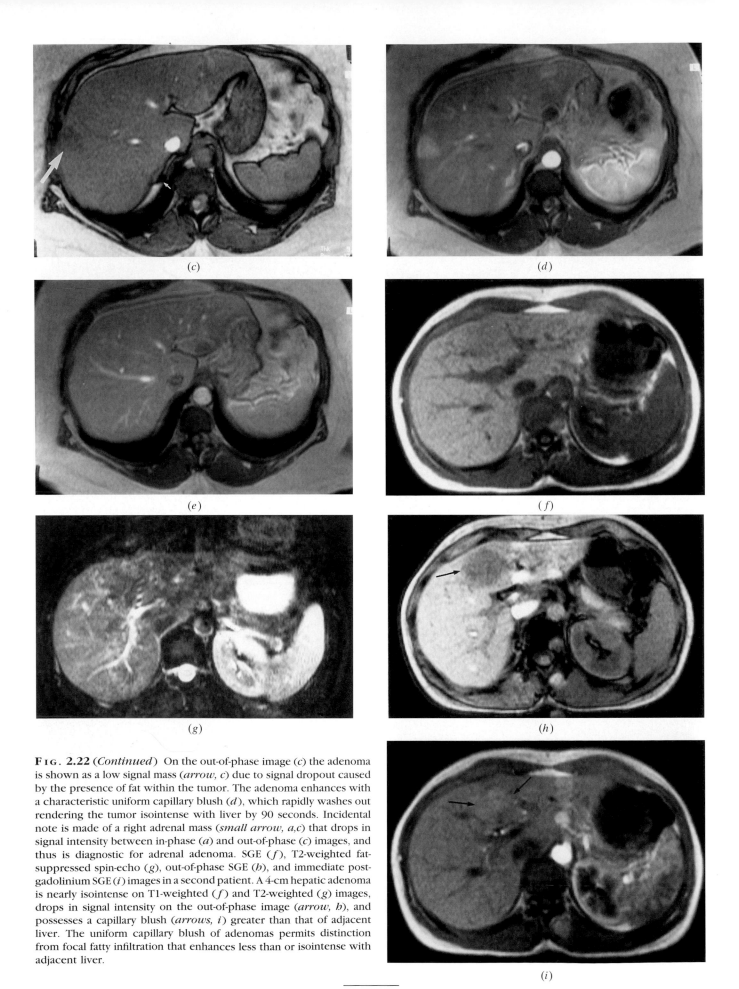

(c)

(d)

(e)

(f)

(g)

(h)

Fig. 2.22 (*Continued*) On the out-of-phase image (*c*) the adenoma is shown as a low signal mass (*arrow, c*) due to signal dropout caused by the presence of fat within the tumor. The adenoma enhances with a characteristic uniform capillary blush (*d*), which rapidly washes out rendering the tumor isointense with liver by 90 seconds. Incidental note is made of a right adrenal mass (*small arrow, a,c*) that drops in signal intensity between in-phase (*a*) and out-of-phase (*c*) images, and thus is diagnostic for adrenal adenoma. SGE (*f*), T2-weighted fat-suppressed spin-echo (*g*), out-of-phase SGE (*h*), and immediate post-gadolinium SGE (*i*) images in a second patient. A 4-cm hepatic adenoma is nearly isointense on T1-weighted (*f*) and T2-weighted (*g*) images, drops in signal intensity on the out-of-phase image (*arrow, h*), and possesses a capillary blush (*arrows, i*) greater than that of adjacent liver. The uniform capillary blush of adenomas permits distinction from focal fatty infiltration that enhances less than or isointense with adjacent liver.

(i)

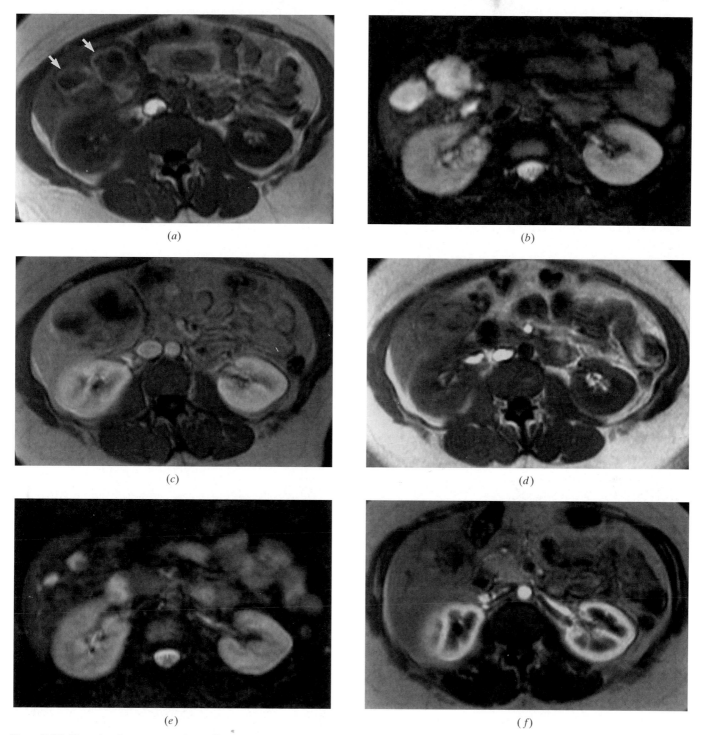

Fig. 2.23 Hepatic adenoma complicated by hemorrhage. SGE (*a*), T2-weighted fat-suppressed spin-echo (*b*), and immediate postgadolinium SGE (*c*) images. An 8-cm mass arises from the inferior aspect of the right lobe of the liver. Regions within the mass possess high signal intensity peripheral rims on the T1-weighted image (*arrows, a*) and high signal intensity on the T2-weighted image (*b*) consistent with blood. Heterogeneous enhancement of the nonhemorrhagic portions of the mass is identified on the immediate postgadolinium image (*c*). The patient discontinued birth control pills and on the 3-month follow-up study the mass has decreased in size to 3.5 cm and is heterogeneously high in signal intensity on the T1-weighted SGE (*d*) and T2-weighted fat-suppressed spin-echo (*e*) images consistent with subacute blood. The peripheral, viable portion of the tumor enhances greater than background liver on the immediate postgadolinium SGE image (*f*).

istration that fades by 1 minute (see Fig. 2.21). Coexistent fatty infiltration of the liver is not uncommon. Because adenomas contain hepatocytes, hepatocyte-specific contrast agents (e.g., Mn-DPDP) will be taken up by these tumors [44].

Focal Nodular Hyperplasia (FNH)

FNH most commonly occurs in adult females, although 10 to 20 percent of cases occur in men [41]. These tumors are not related to the use of birth control pills, and they are solitary in two-thirds of cases. Multiple lesions may be encountered as part of the multiple FNH syndrome, which consists of more than two FNH lesions and one or more of the following lesions: hepatic hemangiomas, dysplastic systemic arteries, CNS vascular malformations, meningiomas and astrocytomas [45]. It is believed that FNH arises from a vascular malformation. FNH contains

hepatocytes, bile-duct elements, Kupffer cells, and fibrous tissue [40]; and commonly possesses a central scar. Two subtypes exist: (1) the solid type, which is the most common type, characterized by the presence of a central fibrous stalk with an enlarged artery that may be inconspicuous or absent in lesions smaller than 1 cm, and (2) the telangiectatic type, characterized by the presence of multiple blood spaces centrally with more abundant and smaller arteries than in the solid type, and usually part of the multiple FNH syndrome [26]. FNH generally does not contain fatty tissue. However, background liver tissue may be fatty, and a collar of higher concentration perilesional fatty infiltration has been described [46]. FNH has not been shown to have malignant potential, and hemorrhage is exceedingly rare, encountered only in large lesions [26,41].

The most common appearance on noncontrast MR images is slight hypointensity on T1-weighted images and

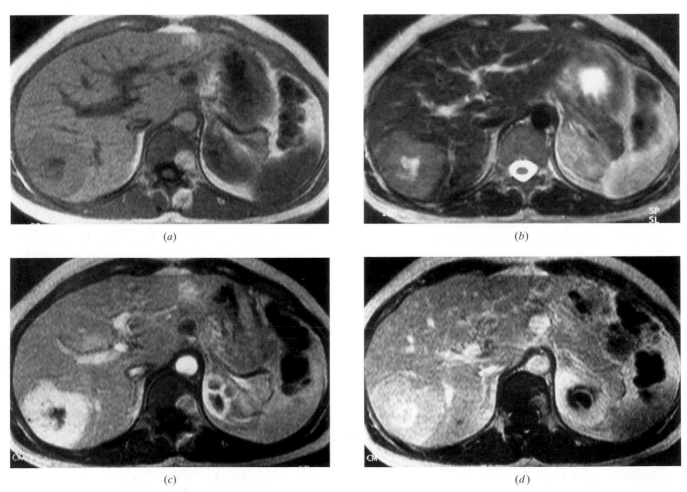

(a)

(b)

(c)

(d)

FIG. 2.24 Focal nodular hyperplasia. SGE (*a*), T2-weighted echo-train spin-echo (*b*), immediate (*c*), and 5-minute (*d*) postgadolinium SGE images. A 5.5-cm mass is present in the right lobe of the liver. The tumor is mildly hypointense on the T1-weighted image (*a*) and mildly hyperintense on the T2-weighted image (*b*). A central scar is present that is low in signal intensity on the T1-weighted image (*a*) and high in signal intensity on the T2-weighted image (*b*). On the immediate postgadolinium image (*c*) the tumor enhances with a uniform capillary blush, whereas the central scar remains low in signal intensity. On the delayed postgadolinium image (*d*) the tumor fades to near isointensity with background liver while the central scar shows delayed enhancement.

slight hyperintensity on T2-weighted images, although tumors may be nearly isointense on both of these sequences. Unlike adenomas, FNH rarely has higher signal intensity than liver on T1-weighted images. High signal intensity of the central scar on T2-weighted images is a characteristic feature of FNH, but is observed in only 10 to 49 percent of patients [47–50]. Although the central scar is usually high in signal intensity on T2-weighted images, it is not infrequently low in signal intensity [47,51]. The signal intensity of the scar presumably reflects age and volume of fibrous tissue and blood vessels. FNH enhances with an intense uniform blush on immediate postgadolinium images and fades rapidly to near isointensity (typically at 1 minute after contrast) (Fig. 2.24) [52,53]. When observed, the central scar is low in signal intensity on immediate postgadolinium images and gradually enhances to hyperintensity over time (see Fig. 2.24) [53]. This enhancement pattern is that of scar tissue independent of location. Fatty liver is not uncommon in the presence of FNH, and the tumor may be mildly hypointense on in-phase T1-weighted images and hyperintense on out-of-phase images (Fig. 2.25). Lesions that are isointense on all precontrast images may be appreciated only on the immediate postgadolinium SGE image as a mass that transiently enhances in a uniform homogeneous fashion (Fig. 2.26).

Adenomas and FNH may be distinguished by the following features: the presence of a pseudocapsule, internal hemorrhage, or fat, which are more typical for adenomas, and a central scar that shows delayed enhancement, which is more typical for FNH [42]. Both lesions have an early transient tumor blush on gadolinium enhanced images [29,52,53], and both may take up Mn-DPDP [44,54]. A uniform capillary blush and uptake of Mn-DPDP must be cautiously interpreted because they are features of well-differentiated tumors of hepatocellular origin, including well-differentiated or early hepatocellular carcinoma.

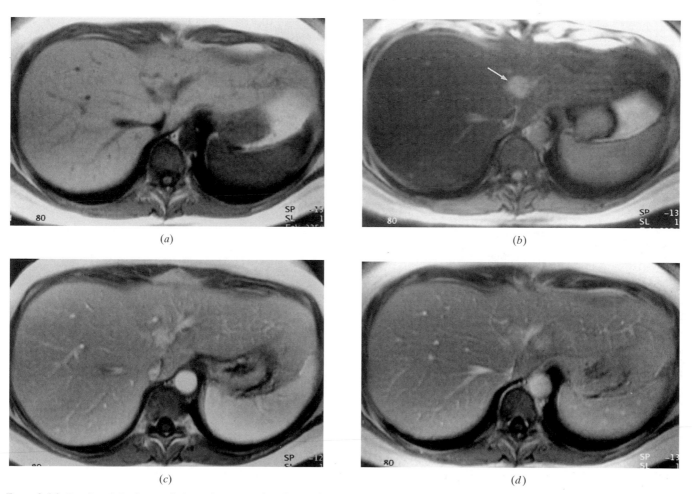

(a)

(b)

(c)

(d)

FIG. 2.25 Focal nodular hyperplasia with surrounding fatty infiltration. SGE (*a*), out-of-phase SGE (*b*), immediate (*c*), and 90-second (*d*) postgadolinium SGE images. A 2-cm focal nodular hyperplasia is present in the medial segment that is hypointense on the in-phase T1-weighted image (*a*) and hyperintense on the out-of-phase T1-weighted image (*arrow, b*) due to signal dropout of the fatty liver. The tumor enhances with a uniform capillary blush on the immediate postgadolinium image (*c*) and fades in signal intensity by 90 seconds (*d*).

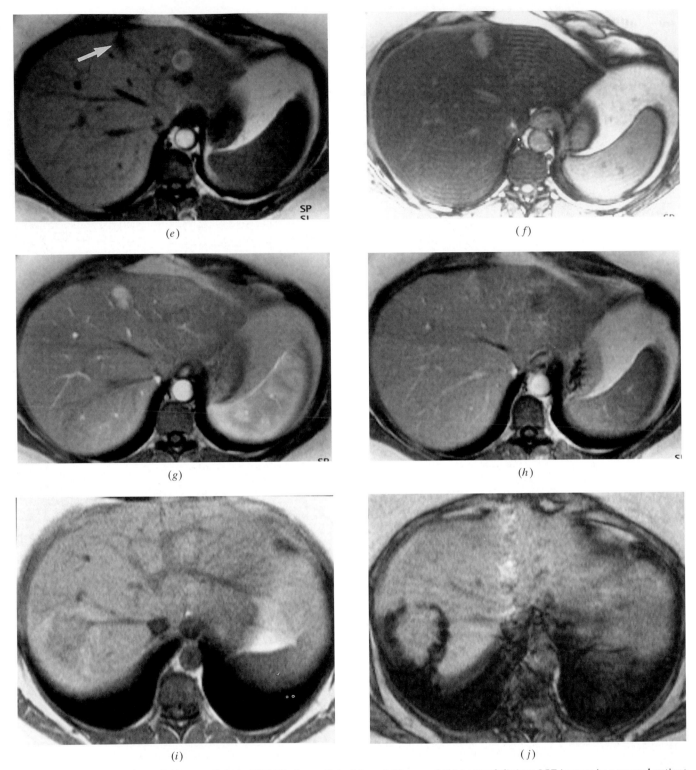

(e)   *(f)*

(g)   *(h)*

(i)   *(j)*

F IG. 2.25 (*Continued*) SGE (*e*), out-of-phase SGE (*f*), immediate (*g*), and 90-second (*h*) postgadolinium SGE images in a second patient with diffuse fatty infiltration and a 2-cm focal nodular hyperplasia in the medial segment (*arrow, e*). The identical imaging findings are present as those shown on the prior patient. A 4-cm focal nodular hyperplasia in a third patient demonstrates a collar of condensed fatty infiltration. The perilesional fat is moderately high in signal intensity on the in-phase SGE image (*i*) and drops to nearly signal-void on the out-of-phase SGE image (*j*).

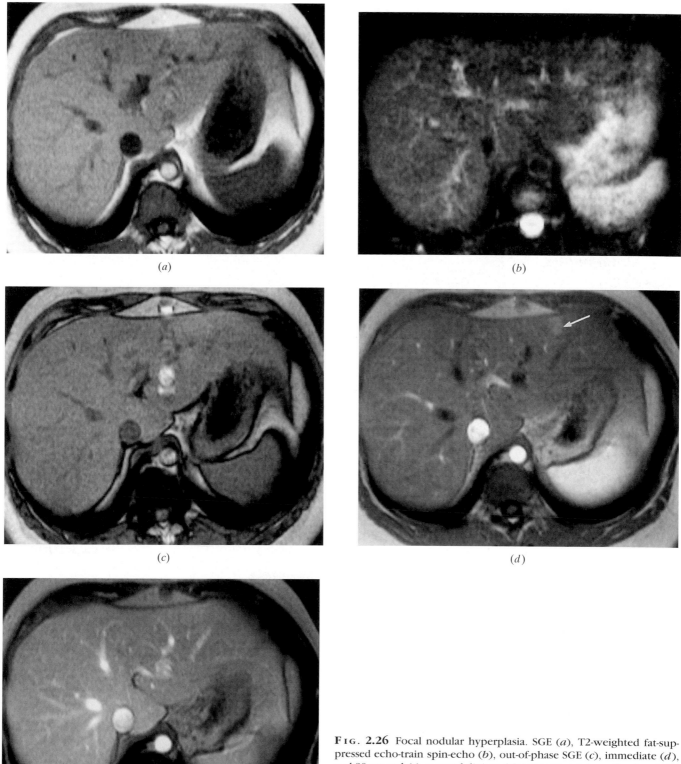

(a)

(b)

(c)

(d)

(e)

FIG. 2.26 Focal nodular hyperplasia. SGE (*a*), T2-weighted fat-suppressed echo-train spin-echo (*b*), out-of-phase SGE (*c*), immediate (*d*), and 90-second (*e*) postgadolinium SGE images. A 1.5-cm focal nodular hyperplasia is present in the lateral segment that is isointense on T1-weighted (*a*), T2-weighted (*b*), and out-of-phase (*c*) images. The tumor is only visualized on the immediate postgadolinium SGE image by the presence of a capillary blush (*arrow, d*). The tumor fades by 90 seconds to isointensity with background liver (*e*).

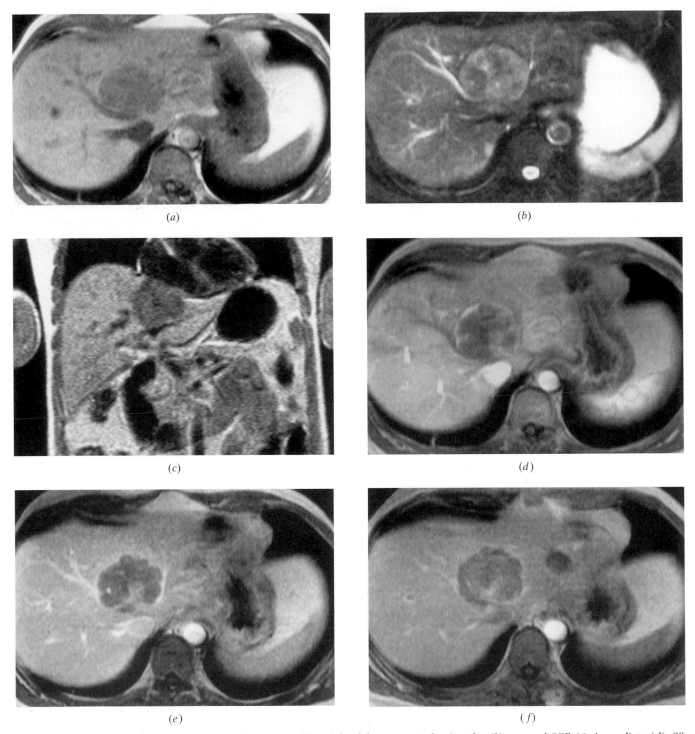

(a)

(b)

(c)

(d)

(e)

(f)

FIG. 2.27 Liver metastases, imaging protocol. SGE (*a*), T2-weighted fat-suppressed spin-echo (*b*), coronal SGE (*c*), immediate (*d*), 90-second (*e*), and 10 minute (*f*) postgadolinium SGE images. A comprehensive imaging protocol to evaluate for liver metastases should include a T1-weighted sequence (*a*), a T2-weighted sequence (*b*), a coronal sequence (*c*), and immediate (*d*), portal venous-phase (*e*), and delayed (*f*) postgadolinium SGE sequences. This lesion possesses the typical imaging features of a colon cancer metastasis. It is mildly hypointense on the T1-weighted image (*a*), heterogeneous and moderately hyperintense on the T2-weighted image (*b*), develops ring enhancement on the immediate postgadolinium image (*d*) and progresses in enhancement over time (*e*,*f*).

Malignant Masses

Liver Metastases

Liver metastases are the most common malignant tumors of the liver. Optimal hepatic imaging evaluation involves both detection and characterization of focal lesions [29,54–56]. Detection involves identification of the presence of lesions and the segmental extent of liver involvement [55]. Demonstration that malignant disease has limited hepatic involvement may have a substantial impact on patient management. Survival of patients with colorectal metastases may be improved by partial hepatectomy if metastases are localized to three or fewer segments [58,59]. MRI is superior to CT imaging in the evaluation of the liver [5,29,37,60–62]. The current challenge is whether the superior performance of MRI translates into an effect on patient management, outcome, and health care costs. New MR sequences, phased-array surface coils, and tissue-specific MR contrast agents suggest that MRI may further exceed the diagnostic ability of CT imaging.

An imaging protocol including T1-weighted SGE, T2-weighted, and serial gadolinium-enhanced SGE images acquired with whole liver coverage per acquisition achieves good lesion detection (T2-weighted and immediate postgadolinium SGE images) and characterization (T2-weighted and serial postgadolinium SGE images) (Fig. 2.27). The use of fat suppression on T2-weighted sequences is advisable because it facilitates detection of subcapsular lesions [63]. Fat suppression is especially important to apply on echo-train spin-echo sequences. Fat is high in signal on echo-train spin-echo sequences, with the result that fatty liver is high in signal intensity, and conspicuity of coexistent metastases is diminished. Fatty liver is not uncommon in the setting of liver metasta-

ses, because fatty metamorphosis occurs as a response to the presence of metastases. On out-of-phase SGE images, liver metastases may appear high in signal intensity due to signal drop of background liver parenchyma (Fig. 2.28). On occasion, this may facilitate lesion detection, particularly if lesions are intrinsically high in signal intensity (Fig. 2.29). The acquisition of at least one sequence in the coronal plane may be of value to evaluate the superior and inferior margins of the liver, particularly the infracardiac portion of the left lobe [64]. Breath-hold techniques such as SGE, HASTE, or both are useful for this purpose (Fig. 2.30).

A previous study, which compared nonspiral dynamic contrast-enhanced CT imaging and MRI employing T2-weighted fat-suppressed spin-echo, SGE, and dynamic serial post gadolinium SGE images in 73 patients with clinically suspected liver disease, demonstrated greater lesion detection and characterization by MRI (Fig. 2.31). Lesion detection was greatest with T2 fat suppression (T2-FS) (272 lesions) and contrast-enhanced SGE (244 lesions) images, which was statistically greater than with CT (220 lesions) and SGE (219 lesions) images ($p < .03$) [29]. Lesion characterization was greatest with contrast-enhanced SGE images (236 lesions) ($p < .01$), followed by CT (199 lesions), SGE (164 lesions), and T2-FS (144 lesions) images. A more recent comparison, between these MRI sequences and dynamic nonspiral contrast-enhanced CT images, in 20 patients with solitary hepatic metastases detected by CT imaging, demonstrated that MRI detected more than 1 lesion in 6 out of 20 (30%) of patients [5].

Characterization of liver lesions is important because patients with known primary malignancies commonly have small hepatic lesions that are benign cysts or hemangiomas. A previous report described the detection of

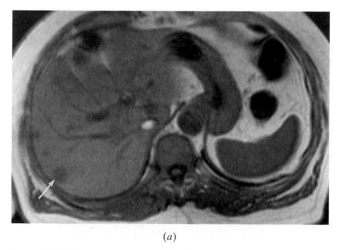

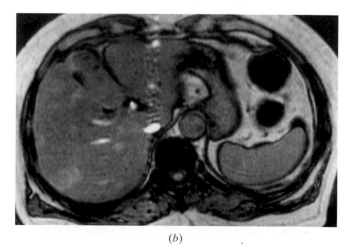

(a)

(b)

FIG. 2.28 Liver metastases in fatty liver. SGE (a) out-of-phase SGE (b) and immediate postgadolinium SGE (c) images. Multiple low-signal-intensity metastases are present in the liver on the in-phase T1-weighted image (arrow, a). On the out-of-phase T1-weighted image (b), the liver diminishes in signal intensity rendering the metastases mildly high in signal intensity relative to liver.

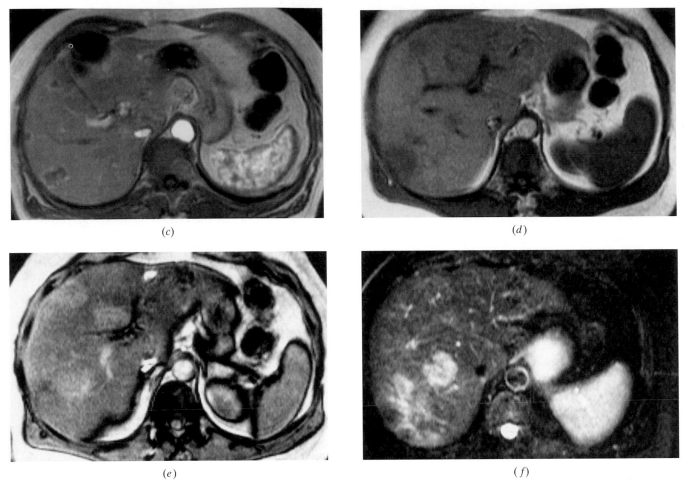

(c)   (d)

(e)   (f)

F I G . 2.28 (*Continued*) Immediate postgadolinium SGE image (c) shows that the lesions enhance with a uniform peripheral ring consistent with metastases. SGE (d), out-of-phase SGE (e) and T2-weighted fat-suppressed spin-echo (f) in a second patient with colon cancer liver metastases. Liver metastases are low in signal intensity on the T1-weighted image (d). The liver drops in signal intensity of the out-of-phase image (e) due to fatty infiltration, rendering the metastases moderately high in signal intensity. The fat-suppressed T2-weighted image demonstrates good conspicuity of liver metastases as fat suppression decreases the signal intensity of the liver rendering the higher signal metastases more conspicuous.

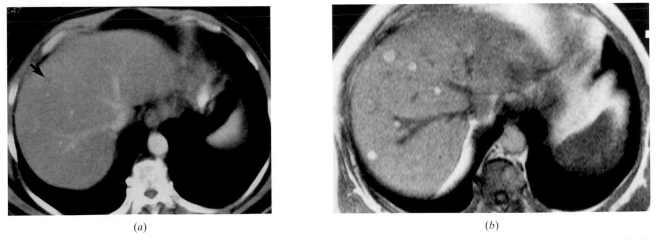

(a)   (b)

F I G . 2.29 Melanoma metastases in a fatty liver, comparison of spiral CT imaging and MRI. Spiral CT (a), SGE (b), out-of-phase SGE (c), and T2-weighted fat-suppressed spin-echo (d) images. A solitary melanoma metastasis is apparent on the spiral CT image (*arrow, a*).

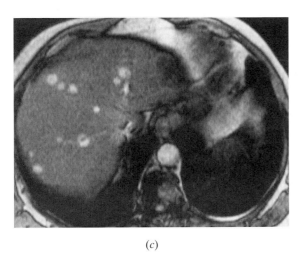

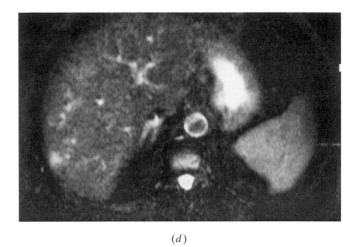

(c)

(d)

FIG. 2.29 (*Continued*) Multiple mildly hyperintense metastases smaller than 1 cm are identified on the SGE image (*b*), and these high-signal-intensity lesions become more conspicuous on the out-of-phase image (*c*). Lesions are apparent on the T2-weighted image, but not as clearly shown (*d*). Fatty infiltration has resulted in a signal drop of liver on the out-of-phase image (*c*), which has increased the conspicuity of the high T1-weighted signal intensity liver metastases.

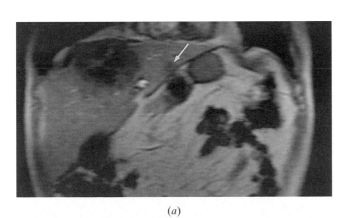

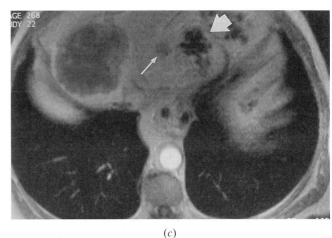

(a)

(c)

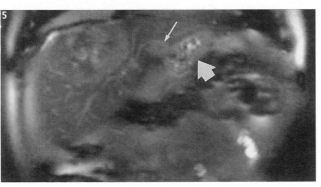

(b)

FIG. 2.30 Liver metastases, coronal images. Coronal slice-selective MP-RAGE (*a*), coronal fat-suppressed HASTE (*b*), and 45-second postgadolinium SGE (*c*) images. A 6-cm colon cancer metastasis is present in the medial segment that is heterogeneous and low in signal intensity on the T1-weighted image (*a*), and heterogeneous and mildly hyperintense on the T2-weighted image (*b*). A 1-cm capsular based metastasis is identified in the lateral segment (*arrows a,b*) that has signal-intensity features similar to those of the larger metastasis. Close proximity to the stomach (*large arrow, b*) is appreciated. The transverse postgadolinium image (*c*) demonstrates ring enhancement around the large heterogeneously low-signal-intensity metastasis. Ring enhancement is also appreciated around the small lesion (*arrow, c*). This lesion could easily be mistaken for a partial volume artifact with the nearby stomach (*large arrow, c*) on transverse sections.

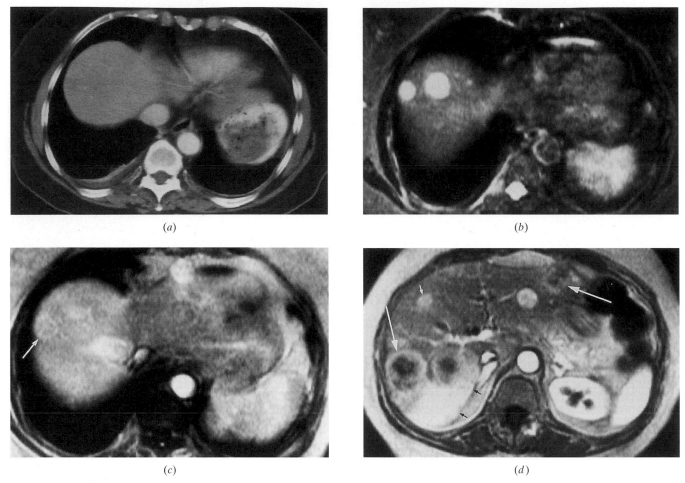

(a)   *(b)*

(c)   *(d)*

F I G . 2.31 Liver metastases, dynamic contrast-enhanced CT imaging versus MRI. Dynamic contrast-enhanced CT (*a*), T2-weighted fat-suppressed spin-echo (*b*), and immediate postgadolinium SGE (*c,d*) images. Few lesions are apparent on the dynamic contrast-enhanced CT image, including no lesions at the dome of the liver (*a*). At this tomographic level two well-defined high-signal-intensity masses are identified on the T2-weighted image (*b*). These lesions are distinguished from hemangiomas by the demonstration of uniform ring enhancement on the immediate postgadolinium image (*arrow, c*). On the immediate postgadolinium image from a more inferior tomographic section (*d*), multiple ring enhancing (*long arrows, d*) and uniform enhancing (*short arrow, d*) metastases are identified. Intense ill-defined perilesional enhancement is present (*black arrows, d*), which is commonly observed with colon cancer liver metastases.

small (<15 mm) lesions in 254 of 1,454 patients who underwent CT examination [65]. The majority of patients (82%) with liver lesions in this study had a known primary tumor, yet lesions in 51 percent of these patients were benign. Another report described a large series of cancer patients in whom 41.8 percent of detected focal liver lesions were benign [66]. Patients may have a variety of lesions that can be multiple and scattered throughout the liver. Therefore, the whole organ coverage per acquisition of SGE permits optimal evaluation of the entire liver in distinct phases of enhancement using serial image acquisition following gadolinium administration. In the presence of multiple liver lesions, the distinction of benign and malignant lesions is of critical importance and is well-performed by MRI (Fig. 2.32).

Comparison between spiral CT arterial portography (CTAP) and MRI employing the aforementioned se-

quences for diagnostic accuracy, cost, and effect on patient management recently has been reported involving a population of 26 patients referred for hepatic surgery with suspected limited malignant disease [67]. Regarding lesion detection, CTAP and MRI, respectively, showed 185 and 176 true-positive malignant lesions, 15 and 0 false-positive malignant lesions, 0 and 18 true-negative malignant lesions, and 13 and 22 false-negative malignant lesions. Regarding segmental involvement, CTAP and MRI, respectively, showed 107 and 105 true-positive segments, 11 and 0 false-positive segments, 80 and 91 true-negative segments, and 4 and 6 false-negative segments. A significant difference in specificity of segmental involvement was observed between MRI (1.0 ± 0) and CTAP (0.88 ± 0.05) ($p < 0.03$). Total procedural cost was $3,499 for CTAP and $1,224 for MRI. CTAP findings did not alter patient management over MRI in any patient,

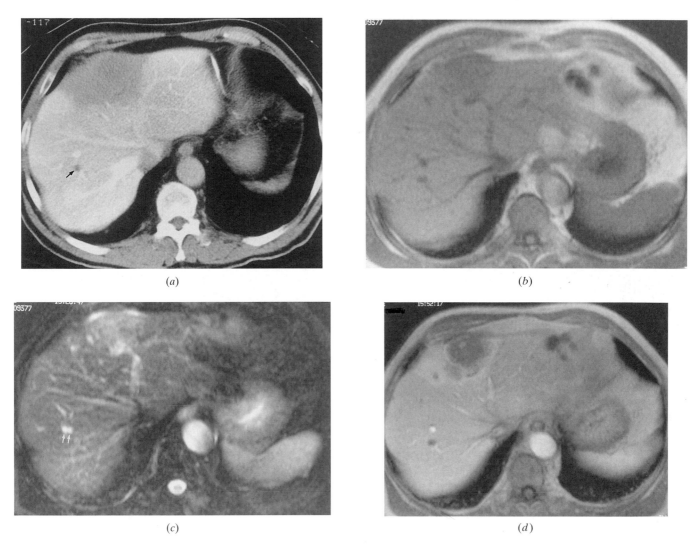

(a)

(b)

(c)

(d)

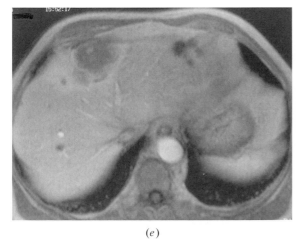

(e)

FIG. 2.32 Liver metastasis with coexistent cysts, spiral CTAP, and MRI comparison. Spiral CTAP (*a*), SGE (*b*), T2-weighted fat-suppressed spin-echo (*c*), immediate (*d*), and 5-minute (*e*) postgadolinium SGE images. The CTAP image (*a*) demonstrates a large perfusional defect in the medial segment related to a colon cancer metastasis. A 6-mm lesion in the anterior segment (*arrow, a*) was interpreted as one of several similar-appearing small lesions consistent with metastases scattered throughout the remainder of the liver. The MR images demonstrate a 4-cm mass in the medial segment with the imaging features of a colon cancer metastasis, including transient ill-defined perilesional enhancement on the immediate postgadolinium image (*d*). The lesion in the anterior segment represents two 3-mm juxtaposed cysts (*arrows, c*) that are small, sharply marginated, low in signal intensity on the T1-weighted image (*b*), and high in signal intensity on the T2-weighted image (*c*). Lack of enhancement on early (*d*) and later (*e*) postgadolinium-enhanced images are diagnostic for cysts. The remaining small liver lesions scattered throughout the liver were all shown to be cysts on MR images. The patient was operated on based on the MRI findings of a solitary liver metastases and multiple coexistent cysts. Intraoperative sonography-guided aspiration demonstrated that these small lesions were cysts. MRI was more diagnostically accurate than CTAP and had a greater effect on patient management.

whereas MRI findings resulted in a change in patient management over CTAP findings in 7 patients, which was significant ($p = 0.015$). The results of this study showed that state-of-the-art MRI has higher diagnostic accuracy and greater effect on patient management than spiral CTAP and is 64 percent less expensive. A major problem with CTAP is the frequent occurrence of perfusion defects that can resemble a focal mass. Perfusion defects are generally not problematic on MR images (Fig. 2.33). Perfusion defects also can mask the presence of metastases on CTAP images (Fig. 2.34).

We have recently reported a comparison between MRI using T2-weighted fat-suppressed echo-train spin-echo and immediate postgadolinium SGE with single-phase spiral CT for the detection and characterization of hepatic lesions in 89 patients [68]. Regarding true-positive lesion detection, 295 and 519 lesions were detected on spiral CT and MR images, respectively, which was significantly different on a patient by patient basis ($p <$ 0.001). More lesions were detected on MR than on spiral CT in 44 of 89 patients (49.4 percent), and 11 of these 44 patients had lesions shown on MRI in whom no lesions were apparent on CT images. No patients had true positive lesions shown on spiral CT that were not shown on MRI. Regarding lesion characterization, 129 and 486 lesions were characterized on spiral CT and MRI images, respectively, which was significantly different on a patient by patient basis ($p < 0.001$). More lesions were characterized on MR than CT images in 68 (76.4 percent) patients. Regarding effect on patient management, chart review with physician interview demonstrated that findings on MRI provided information that altered patient management as compared to findings on spiral CT in 57 patients. Retrospective clinical evaluation by the surgical and medical oncologist showed that MRI was considered to have a greater effect on patient management than spiral CT in 58 and 55 patients, respectively.

Metastases vary substantially in appearance on T1-

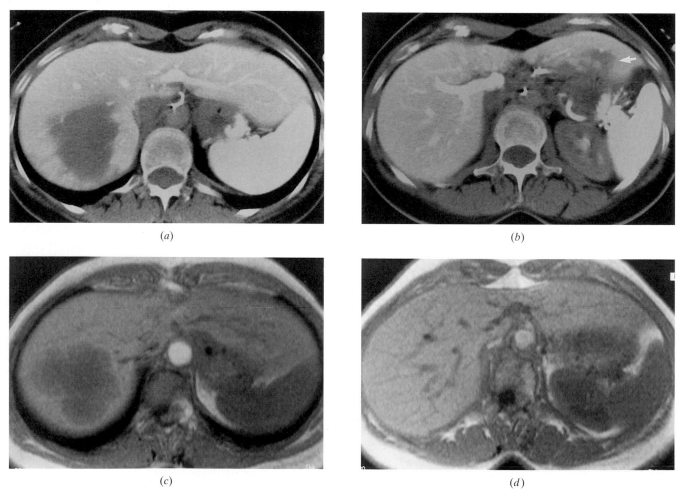

(a)

(b)

(c)

(d)

FIG. 2.33 Liver metastases, spiral CT arterial portography versus MRI. Spiral CTAP (a,b), SGE (c,d), T2-weighted fat-suppressed spin-echo (e,f) and immediate postgadolinium SGE (g,h) images from superior (a,c,e,g) and more inferior (b,d,f,h) tomographic sections. A large metastasis is present in the right lobe of the liver shown on all imaging techniques (a,c,e,g). A second metastasis was suspected on the CTAP image (arrow, b) in the lateral segment. No lesion was identified in this location on any MRI sequence.

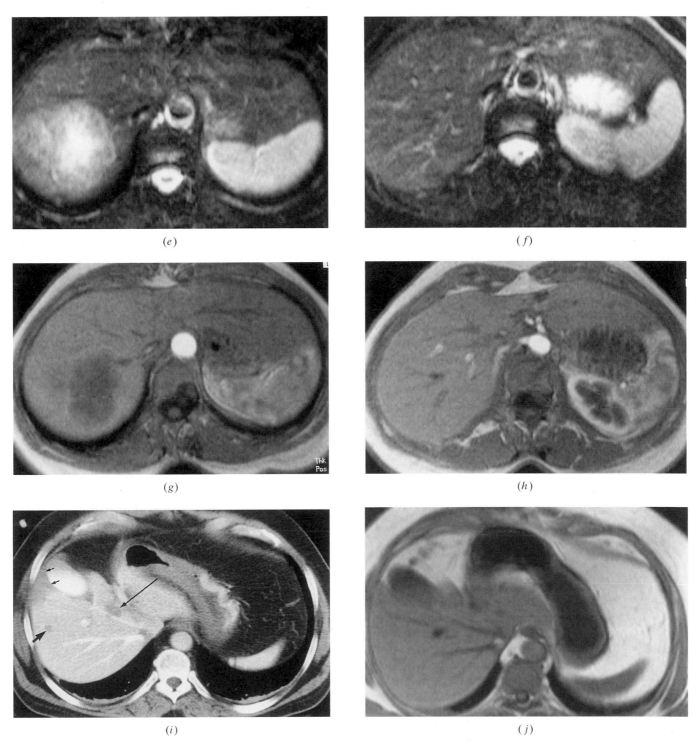

(e)

(f)

(g)

(h)

(i)

(j)

FIG. 2.33 (*Continued*) CTAP findings would have precluded surgery. However, the decision to operate was based on MRI findings. No liver metastasis was identified in the lateral segment by surgical palpation or intraoperative sonography. The patient is disease-free for more than 2 years since right hepatectomy. MRI was more accurate and had a greater impact on patient management and outcome than CTAP. Spiral CTAP (*i*), SGE (*j*), T2-weighted fat-suppressed spin-echo (*k*), and immediate postgadolinium SGE (*l*) images in a second patient with liver metastases from colon cancer. Spiral CTAP and MR images demonstrate an 8-mm metastasis in the anterior segment of the right lobe (*arrow, i,k*) and a perfusional abnormality related to a metastasis in the anterior segment of the right lobe (*short arrows, i,l*).

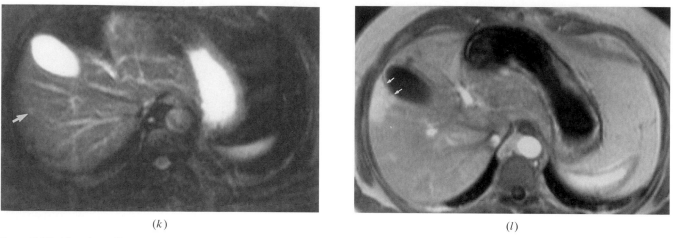

(k)   (l)

FIG. 2.33 (*Continued*) A focal defect interpreted as metastasis on the CTAP image (*long arrow, l*) is apparent in the medial segment, but is not identified on any of the MR images (*j–l*). No metastasis in this location was identified at surgery and intraoperative sonography.

and T2-weighted images. Borders are usually irregular but may be sharp. Lesion shape is frequently irregular but may be round or oval. Metastases generally are moderately low in signal intensity on T1-weighted images and modestly high in signal intensity on T2-weighted images. Some metastases, particularly vascular metastases from islet-cell tumors, leiomyosarcoma pheochromocytoma, and renal-cell cancer or necrotic metastases may be high in signal intensity on T2-weighted images, rendering distinction from hemangiomas difficult [27,37,69].

Metastases do not have the classical enhancement patterns of benign lesions (i.e., no enhancement as seen with cysts, peripheral nodular enhancement as seen with hemangiomas, or, in metastases greater than 2 cm, transient immediate postgadolinium homogeneous blush as seen with FNH or adenomas) [29,32,33,37,52,53]. Transient tumor blush, however, is commonly observed in small (<2 cm) hypervascular metastases. The most common enhancement feature of metastases is a peripheral ring of enhancement on immediate postgadolinium chelate SGE images [37,69]. This enhancement pattern reflects the underlying pathophysiology in which metastases parasitize surrounding hepatic arterial blood supply [70]. Central progression of contrast enhancement is com-

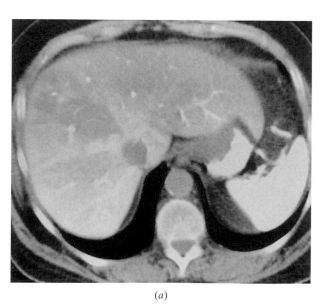

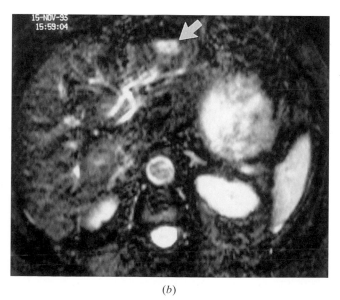

(a)   (b)

FIG. 2.34 Liver metastases perfusional defect. Spiral CTAP (*a*) and T2-weighted fat-suppressed spin-echo (*b*) images. Multiple large perfusional defects are present on the CTAP image (*a*) with the entire left lobe exhibiting diminished perfusion. A 1.5-cm liver metastasis is present on the T2-weighted image (*arrow, b*), which was masked by the perfusion defect on the CTAP image.

mon. Irregular or peripheral contrast washout is also observed [32,37,71], and is common in hypervascular metastases.

Certain histological types of metastases have distinctive enhancement or morphological features. Metastases from colorectal cancer typically develop a cauliflower-type appearance when tumors exceed 3 cm in diameter (Fig. 2.35). Ill-defined increased perilesional and subsegmental enhancement is common with colorectal cancer and pancreatic ductal adenocarcinoma metastases, but less common with other metastases, including hypervascular tumors such as islet-cell tumors or renal-cell carcinomas. This likely is due to a vasculitis induced by a substance elaborated by the tumors, which may be mucin. Metastases from squamous-cell lung cancer not uncommonly are well-defined rounded masses that have a high-signal-intensity rim and low-signal-intensity center on T2-weighted images and show intense enhancement of the outer rim on early postgadolinium images (Fig. 2.36). Squamous-cell carcinomas from other sites of origin also have a tendency to be rounded and have uniform ring enhancement on the immediate postgadolinium SGE images (see Fig. 2.36). Poorly differentiated adenocarcinomas frequently demonstrate numerous metastases smaller than 2 cm scattered throughout the entire liver. These metastases are typically high in signal intensity on T2-weighted images and show peripheral ring enhancement on immediate postgadolinium images (Fig. 2.37).

Metastases may undergo hemorrhage which may result in differing high- and low-signal-intensity lesions on T1- and T2-weighted images. Coagulative necrosis may produce central low signal intensity on T2-weighted images surrounded by higher signal intensity viable tumor [72]. This appearance may be observed with colorectal metastases. Melanoma metastases usually are a mixture of high- and low-signal-intensity lesions on T1- and T2-

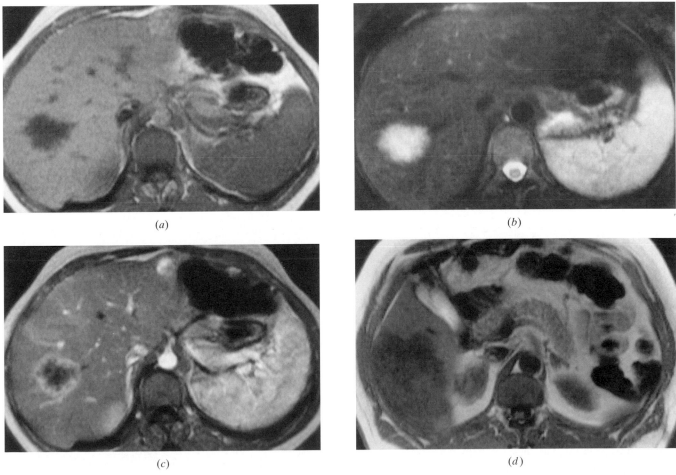

(a)

(b)

(c)

(d)

FIG. 2.35 Liver metastases from colon cancer. SGE (a), T2-weighted fat-suppressed echo-train spin-echo (b) and immediate postgadolinium SGE (c) images. An irregularly marginated mass is present in the right lobe that is moderately low in signal intensity on the T1-weighted image (a), moderately high in signal intensity on the T2-weighted image (b), and demonstrates intact ring enhancement on the immediate postgadolinium image (c) with an irregular inner margin to the ring. A faint region of ill-defined transient increased enhancement is present on the immediate postgadolinium image (c). SGE (d) and immediate postgadolinium SGE (e) images in a second patient with a large colon cancer metastasis in the right lobe of the liver.

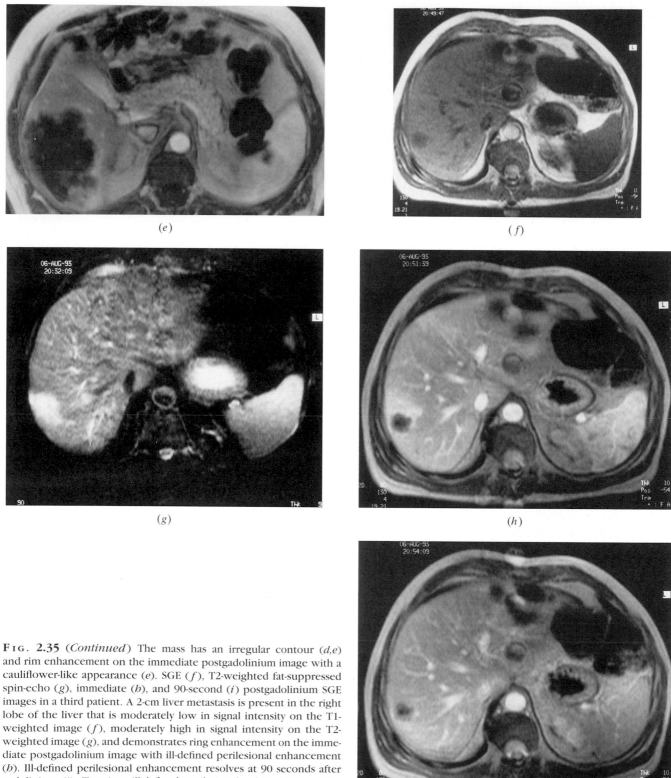

(e)

(f)

(g)

(h)

(i)

FIG. 2.35 (*Continued*) The mass has an irregular contour (*d,e*) and rim enhancement on the immediate postgadolinium image with a cauliflower-like appearance (*e*). SGE (*f*), T2-weighted fat-suppressed spin-echo (*g*), immediate (*h*), and 90-second (*i*) postgadolinium SGE images in a third patient. A 2-cm liver metastasis is present in the right lobe of the liver that is moderately low in signal intensity on the T1-weighted image (*f*), moderately high in signal intensity on the T2-weighted image (*g*), and demonstrates ring enhancement on the immediate postgadolinium image with ill-defined perilesional enhancement (*h*). Ill-defined perilesional enhancement resolves at 90 seconds after gadolinium (*i*). Transient ill-defined perilesional enhancement and a cauliflower-like shape are typical for colon cancer metastases.

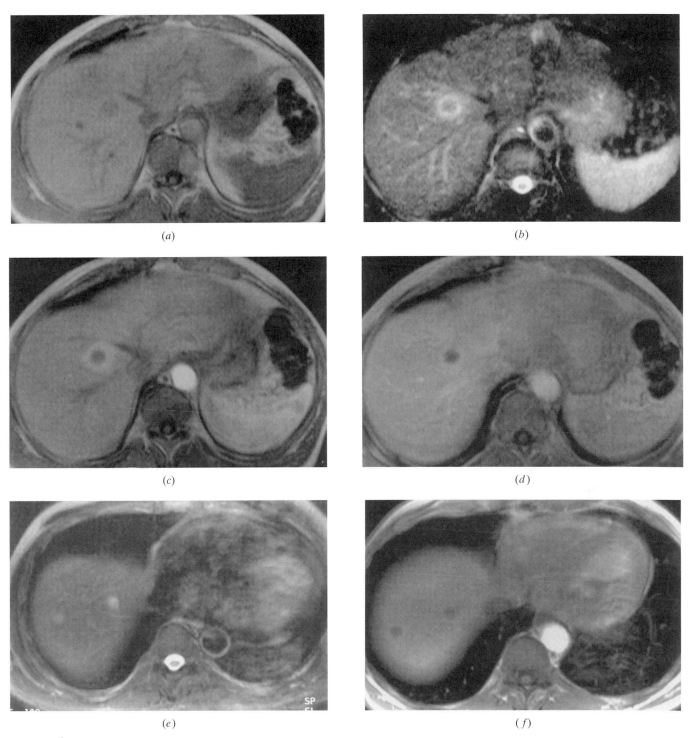

FIG. 2.36 Liver metastasis, squamous cell lung cancer. SGE (*a*), T2-weighted fat-suppressed echo-train spin-echo (*b*), immediate (*c*), and 90-second (*d*) postgadolinium SGE images. A well-defined 2-cm metastasis is present in the anterior segment of the right lobe that is mildly low in signal intensity on the T1-weighted image (*a*), has a moderately high signal-intensity ring with central isointensity on the T2-weighted image (*b*), shows uniform ring enhancement on the image postgadolinium SGE image (*c*), and fades over time with negligible central enhancement (*d*). The enhancing ring on the immediate postgadolinium image (*c*) corresponds to the high-signal-intensity rim on the T2-weighted image (*b*). This is a typical appearance for liver metastases from squamous-cell lung cancer. Liver metastases from esophageal squamous-cell cancer in a second patient shown on T2-weighted echo-train spin-echo (*e*), immediate (*f*), and 90-second (*g*) postgadolinium SGE images.

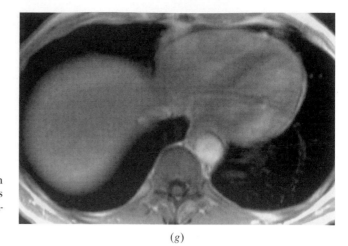

(g)

F I G . 2.36 (*Continued*) The metastases are round, well-defined, high in signal on the T2-weighted image (*e*), enhance with uniform rings on the immediate postgadolinium SGE image (*f*), and become isointense with liver at 90 seconds (*g*).

weighted images due to the paramagnetic property of melanin (Fig. 2.38) [72]. Metastases from mucin-producing tumors such as ovarian cancer or macrocystic cystadenocarcinoma of the pancreas may result in liver metastases that are high in signal intensity on T1-weighted images due to the protein content (Fig. 2.39). Metastases that are active in protein synthesis, such as in the produc-

tion of enzymes or hormones (e.g., carcinoid tumors) may be high in signal intensity on T1-weighted images due to the presence of a high concentration of protein (Fig. 2.40).

Capsular-based metastases occur in the setting of tumors that metastasize by intraperitoneal spread. Ovarian cancer most commonly results in capsular-based

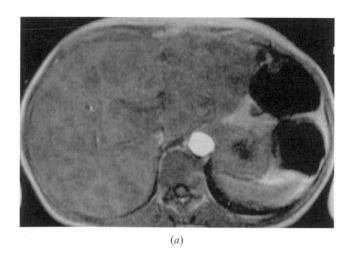

(a)

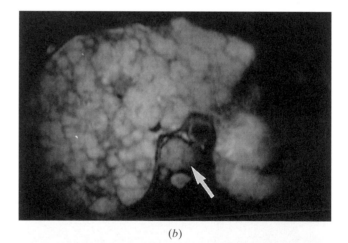

(b)

F I G . 2.37 Liver metastases, poorly differentiated cell type. SGE (*a*), T2-weighted fat-suppressed echo-train spin-echo (*b*) and immediate postgadolinium SGE (*c*) images. The liver is extensively replaced by numerous metastatic lesions smaller than 2 cm. Lesions are mildly low in signal intensity on the T1-weighted image (*a*), high in signal intensity on the T2-weighted image (*b*), and demonstrate intact ring enhancement on the immediate postgadolinium image (*c*). High signal intensity is also apparent in the bone marrow on the T2-weighted image (*arrow, b*), which represents bone metastases. Poorly differentiated or anaplastic malignancies not uncommonly result in this pattern of liver metastases. This patient has small-cell lung cancer.

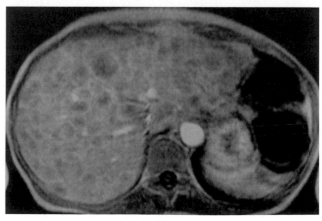

(c)

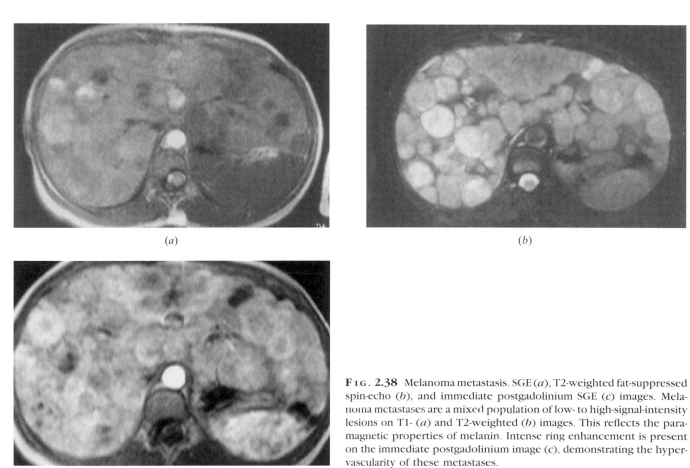

(a)

(b)

(c)

F IG . 2.38 Melanoma metastasis. SGE (*a*), T2-weighted fat-suppressed spin-echo (*b*), and immediate postgadolinium SGE (*c*) images. Melanoma metastases are a mixed population of low- to high-signal-intensity lesions on T1- (*a*) and T2-weighted (*b*) images. This reflects the paramagnetic properties of melanin. Intense ring enhancement is present on the immediate postgadolinium image (*c*), demonstrating the hypervascularity of these metastases.

(a)

(b)

F IG . 2.39 High T1-weighted signal mucin-producing liver metastases, ovarian cancer. SGE (*a*) and 90-second postgadolinium SGE (*b*) images. A large capsular-based metastasis is present along the lateral margin of the liver (*black arrows, a*), and a smaller subcapsular metastasis is present in the spleen (*white arrow, a*).

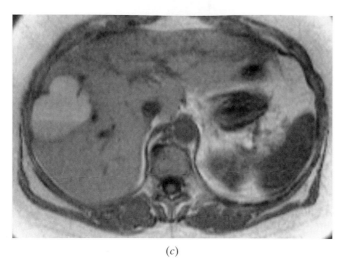

(c)

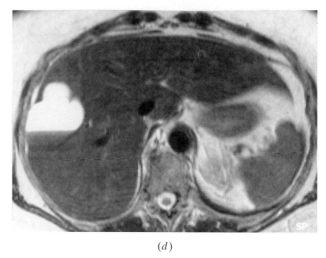

(d)

FIG. 2.39 (*Continued*) The metastases are high in signal intensity due to high mucin content, and enhancement of cyst walls is present on postgadolinium images (*b*). The spleen is nearly signal-void on these T1-weighted images due to transfusional hemosiderosis. SGE (*a*) and T2-weighted echo-train spin-echo (*b*) in a second patient demonstrate a cystic ovarian metastasis located superficially in the right lobe of the liver. The high mucin content of the cystic metastasis renders it high in signal intensity on the T1-weighted image (*c*). On the T2-weighted image (*d*), low-signal-intensity material layers in the dependent portion of the metastasis.

metastases (see Fig. 2.39), followed by colon cancer. A variety of malignancies, however, can produce capsular-based metastases (Fig. 2.41).

Hypovascular Metastases. Primary tumors that not uncommonly result in hypovascular metastases include colorectal cancer, transitional-cell cancer, and carcinoid tumors. Lymphoma and hepatocellular carcinomas are other malignant lesions that are occassionally hypovascular. Malignant hypovascular metastases possess a diminished blood supply usually as a result of a

fibrous-collagenous tumor matrix, necrosis, or monotonous dense cellularity.

Lesions usually are low in signal on T1- and T2-weighted images, signal features that are comparable to those of muscle or fibrous tissue. They are hypointense relative to liver on T1-weighted images, and are often nearly isointense on T2-weighted images [73]. These tumors are usually most conspicuous on portal-phase gadolinium-enhanced SGE images (Fig. 2.42) [73]. Hypovascular metastases may contain a large volume of extracellular fluid and mimic the appearance of cysts (i.e., high signal

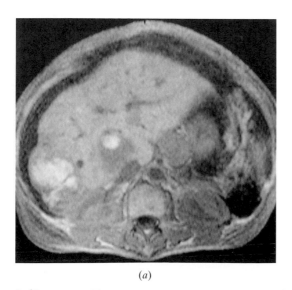

(a)

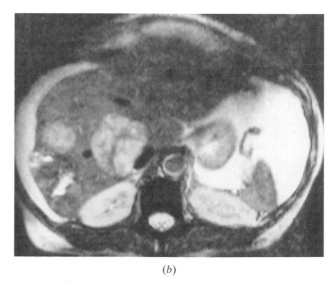

(b)

FIG. 2.40 Carcinoid liver metastases. SGE (*a*) and T2-weighted fat-suppressed spin-echo (*b*) images. Metastases are heterogeneous with mixed high signal intensity on T1- (*a*) and T2-weighted (*b*) images. The high signal intensity on the T1-weighted image reflects a high protein concentration due to protein synthesis from hormone production.

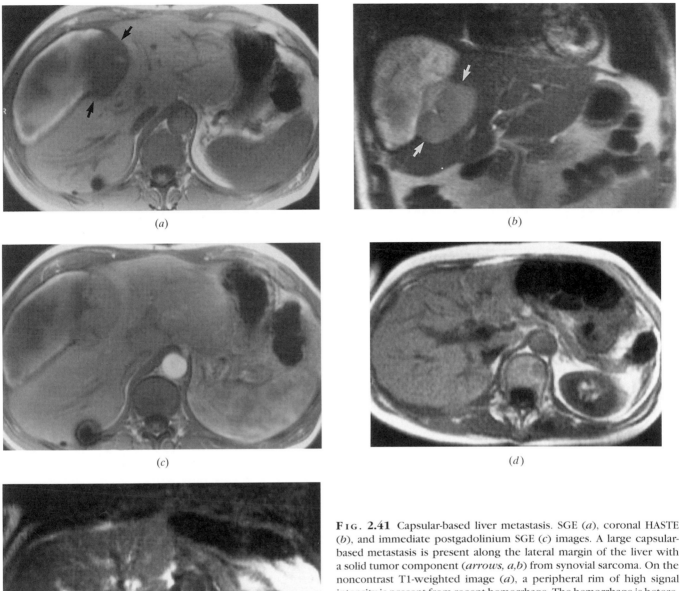

(a)

(b)

(c)

(d)

(e)

Fig. 2.41 Capsular-based liver metastasis. SGE (*a*), coronal HASTE (*b*), and immediate postgadolinium SGE (*c*) images. A large capsular-based metastasis is present along the lateral margin of the liver with a solid tumor component (*arrows, a,b*) from synovial sarcoma. On the noncontrast T1-weighted image (*a*), a peripheral rim of high signal intensity is present from recent hemorrhage. The hemorrhage is heterogeneous on the T2-weighted image (*b*). On the immediate postgadolinium image (*c*), the solid tumor component enhances uniformly. SGE (*d*) and T2-weighted fat-suppressed spin-echo (*e*) images in a second patient with capsular-based metastases from colon cancer. Capsular-based metastases are subtle on the SGE image (*d*) but are very conspicuous on the fat-suppressed T2-weighted image (*arrows, e*) due to the intrinsic high signal intensity of the masses and removal of the competing signal of fat.

intensity on T2-weighted images and nearly signal-void immediately following gadolinium administration). Delayed postgadolinium images demonstrate that lesion borders become indistinct and lesions decrease in size due to peripheral enhancement (Fig. 2.43).

Hypervascular Metastases. The malignancies that most commonly result in hypervascular liver metastases include renal, carcinoid, islet-cell, leiomyosarcoma, and melanoma [37]. Malignancies that occasionally result in hypervascular liver metastases include bowel, breast,

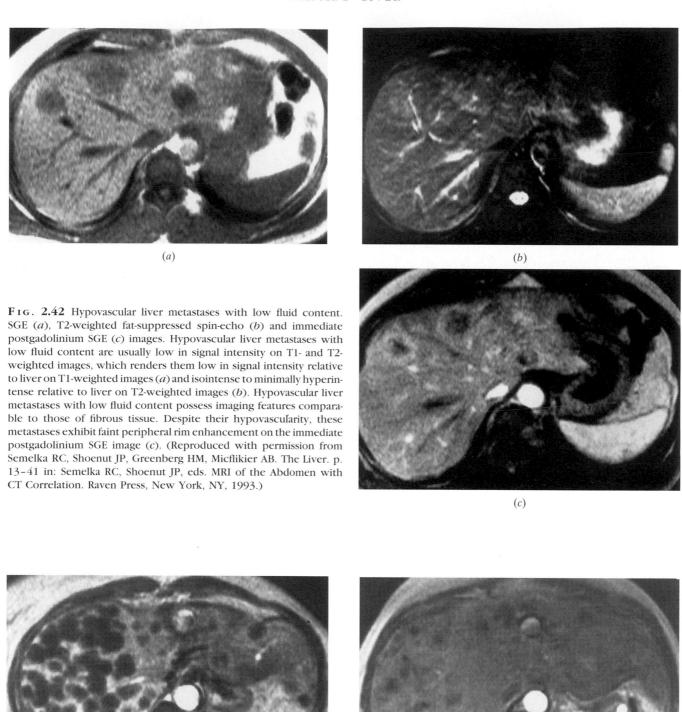

(a)

(b)

FIG. 2.42 Hypovascular liver metastases with low fluid content. SGE (a), T2-weighted fat-suppressed spin-echo (b) and immediate postgadolinium SGE (c) images. Hypovascular liver metastases with low fluid content are usually low in signal intensity on T1- and T2-weighted images, which renders them low in signal intensity relative to liver on T1-weighted images (a) and isointense to minimally hyperintense relative to liver on T2-weighted images (b). Hypovascular liver metastases with low fluid content possess imaging features comparable to those of fibrous tissue. Despite their hypovascularity, these metastases exhibit faint peripheral rim enhancement on the immediate postgadolinium SGE image (c). (Reproduced with permission from Semelka RC, Shoenut JP, Greenberg HM, Micflikier AB. The Liver. p. 13–41 in: Semelka RC, Shoenut JP, eds. MRI of the Abdomen with CT Correlation. Raven Press, New York, NY, 1993.)

(c)

(a)

(b)

FIG. 2.43 Hypovascular liver metastases with high fluid content. Immediate (a) and 10-minute (b) postgadolinium SGE images. Hypovascular liver metastases with a high fluid content are low in signal intensity on T1-weighted images and high in signal intensity on T2-weighted images (not shown). On immediate postgadolinium images (a) they may appear well-defined and nearly signal-void, mimicking the appearance of cysts. On delayed postgadolinium images (b) these lesions will partially enhance and decrease in size, permitting correct characterization. (Reproduced with permission from Semelka RC, Shoenut JP, Greenberg HM, Micflikier AB. The Liver. p. 13–41 in: Semelka RC, Shoenut JP, eds. MRI of the Abdomen with CT Correlation. Raven Press, New York, NY, 1993.)

and lung cancer. Hypervascular metastases are generally high in signal intensity on T2-weighted images and possess an intense peripheral ring of enhancement immediately following gadolinium administration (Fig. 2.44) [32,37,69]. In many of these lesions, contrast will progress in a centripetal fashion [37]. Dynamic serial gadolinium-enhanced MR images are particularly important for lesion detection and characterization in patients with known vascular primary tumors (Fig. 2.45). Vascular metastases from gastrinomas enhance with a uniform peripheral ring pattern on immediate postgadolinium images (Fig. 2.46). These metastases have a particular propensity to fade peripherally on more delayed images [67]. Vascular metastases from renal-cell cancer, bowel cancer, carcinoid, or nongastrinoma islet-cell tumors tend to be irregular in size and shape and to enhance with a thick irregular rim that may gradually fill in. Enhancement of hypervascular metastases is better shown on MR than on CT images due to the higher sensitivity of MRI for gadolinium chelates, the more compact bolus of contrast delivered to

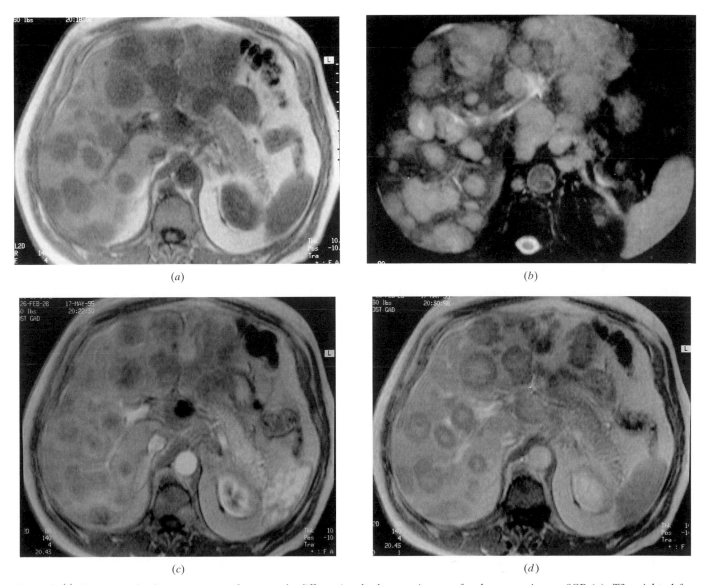

(a)

(b)

(c)

(d)

FIG. 2.44 Hypervascular liver metastases from poorly differentiated adenocarcinoma of unknown primary. SGE (*a*), T2-weighted fat-suppressed echo-train spin-echo (*b*), immediate (*c*) and 2-minute (*d*) postgadolinium SGE images. The liver contains numerous metastases scattered throughout all segments that are well-defined and moderately low in signal intensity on T1-weighted images (*a*), are moderately high in signal intensity on T2-weighted images (*b*), and have prominent thick uniform rings of enhancement on immediate postgadolinium images (*c*). Peripheral washout with centripetal progression of enhancement is noted on the delayed postcontrast image (*d*). Peripheral washout is common in hypervascular tumors that possess uniform intense rings of enhancement on immediate postgadolinium images.

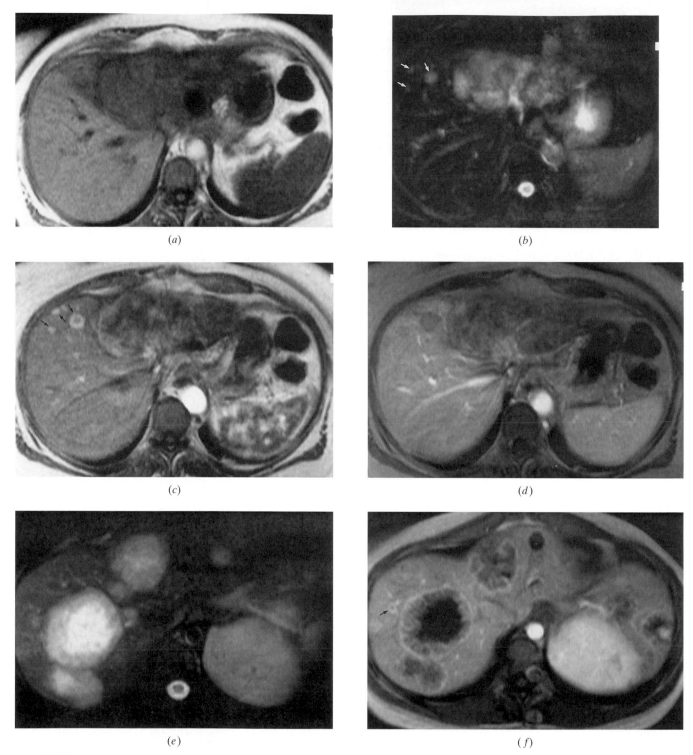

(a)

(b)

(c)

(d)

(e)

(f)

FIG. 2.45 Hypervascular liver metastases. SGE (a), T2-weighted fat-suppressed spin-echo (b), immediate (c), and 90-second (d) postgadolinium SGE images. A 7-cm metastasis is identified in the left lobe of the liver (a–d). Several metastases smaller than 1 cm are present in the medial and anterior segments. These small metastases are not visible on the T1-weighted image (a), are moderately high in signal intensity on the T2-weighted image (arrows, b), enhance intensely on the immediate postgadolinium image (arrow, c) and washout and are lower in signal intensity than liver, on the 90-second postgadolinium image (d). On the immediate postgadolinium image the smallest lesions enhance homogeneously, whereas the 1-cm metastasis has ring enhancement. T2-weighted fat suppressed spin-echo (e), immediate (f), and 10-minute (g) postgadolinium SGE images in a second patient with ovarian cancer. Multiple varying-sized metastases are scattered throughout the liver. The largest metastasis is high in signal intensity centrally on the T2-weighted image (e) due to central necrosis.

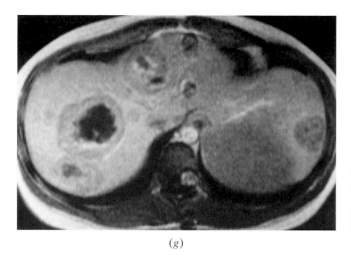

(g)

FIG. 2.45 (*Continued*) Metastases are better shown on the immediate postgadolinium image and appear as multiple hypervascular lesions with ring enhancement. Ring enhancement is appreciated in metastases as small as 6 mm (*arrow, f*). Peripheral washout of metastases is apparent on the 10-minute postgadolinium image (*g*).

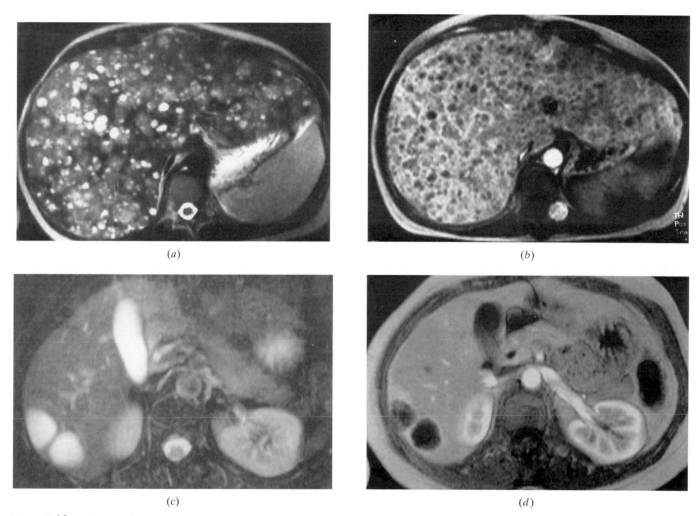

(a)

(b)

(c)

(d)

FIG. 2.46 Hypervascular liver metastases from islet cell tumors. Transverse 512 resolution T2-weighted echo-train spin-echo (*a*) and immediate postgadolinium SGE (*b*) images in a patient with gastrinoma. Numerous metastases smaller than 1 cm are scattered throughout all segments, many of which are well-defined and high in signal intensity on the T2-weighted image (*a*). The immediate postgadolinium image (*b*) demonstrates that the metastases have intact ring enhancement. T2-weighted fat-suppressed spin-echo (*c*) and immediate postgadolinium SGE (*d*) images in a second patient who has an untyped islet cell tumor. The metastases are well-defined round masses that are high in signal intensity on the T2-weighted image (*a*) and have calculated T2 values of 160 msec. On the immediate postgadolinium image (*d*), the lesions possess intact rings of enhancement that are a feature of metastases and not of hemangiomas. Prior outside MRI performed with conventional spin-echo techniques, and original outside interpretation of percutaneous biopsy specimen suggested the diagnosis of hemangiomas. On the gadolinium-enhanced images, hypervascular cystic liver metastases and a 2-cm islet-cell tumor in the head of the pancreas were shown. The histology specimen was reexamined, and the diagnosis of islet-cell tumor was confirmed.

the hepatic parenchyma, and the better temporal resolution for dynamic image acquisition (Fig. 2.47).

Features that are more consistent with malignant lesions than hemangiomas are (1) early intense peripheral ring, (2) uniformity of the thickness of the ring, (3) jagged or serrated internal margin of the ring rather than a lobular margin, and (4) peripheral washout of the ring with presence of more central enhancement [32,33,37,69,71]. Fea-

tures that are more consistent with hemangiomas are (1) discontinuous nodular ring of enhancement on immediate postgadolinium images and (2) progressively increased intensity of enhancement between immediately and 90 seconds after gadolinium administration.

Small hypervascular metastases frequently enhance in a uniform fashion and fade to near isointensity by 1 minute (see Fig. 2.47) [37]. Some small hemangiomas

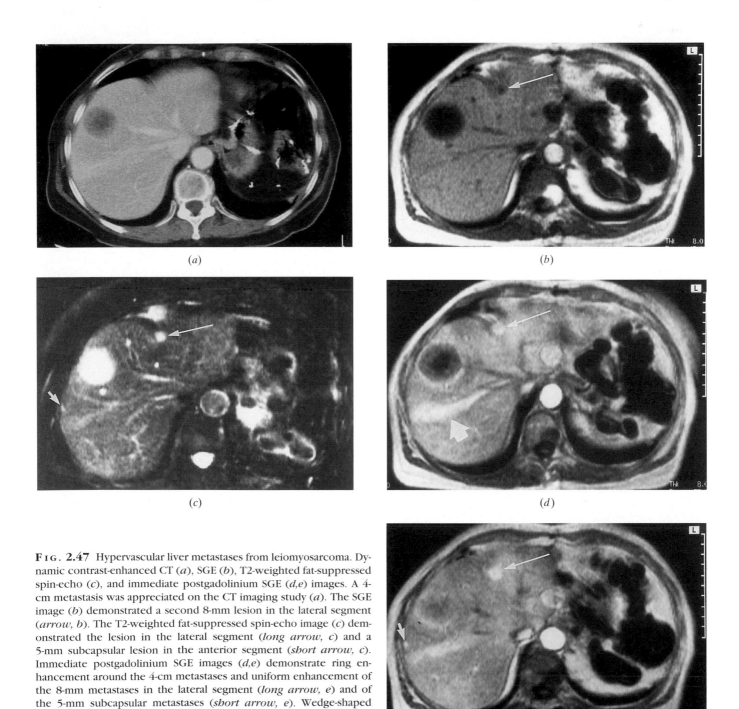

(a)

(b)

(c)

(d)

(e)

FIG. 2.47 Hypervascular liver metastases from leiomyosarcoma. Dynamic contrast-enhanced CT (a), SGE (b), T2-weighted fat-suppressed spin-echo (c), and immediate postgadolinium SGE (d,e) images. A 4-cm metastasis was appreciated on the CT imaging study (a). The SGE image (b) demonstrated a second 8-mm lesion in the lateral segment (arrow, b). The T2-weighted fat-suppressed spin-echo image (c) demonstrated the lesion in the lateral segment (long arrow, c) and a 5-mm subcapsular lesion in the anterior segment (short arrow, c). Immediate postgadolinium SGE images (d,e) demonstrate ring enhancement around the 4-cm metastases and uniform enhancement of the 8-mm metastases in the lateral segment (long arrow, e) and of the 5-mm subcapsular metastases (short arrow, e). Wedge-shaped transient increased enhancement is present in the posterior segment (large arrow, d), which is also faintly apparent on the CT image (a).

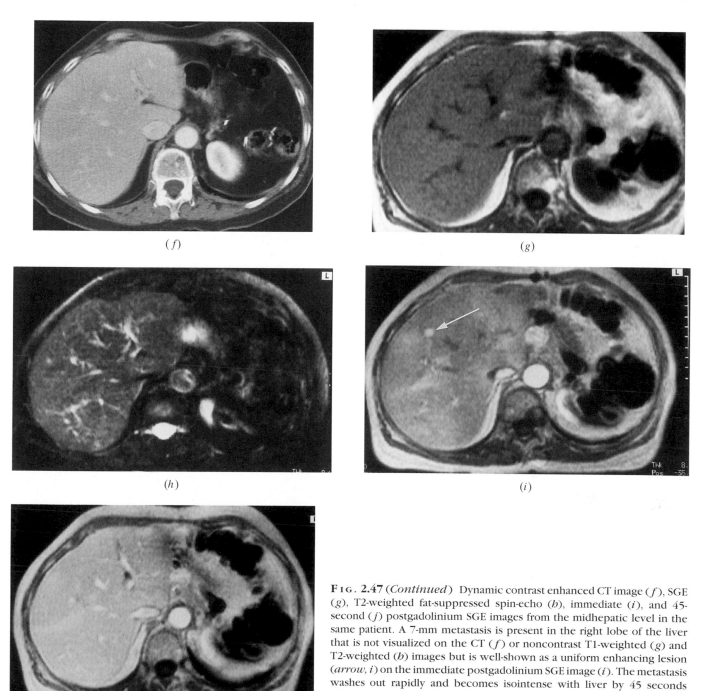

(f)

(g)

(h)

(i)

(j)

FIG. 2.47 (*Continued*) Dynamic contrast enhanced CT image (*f*), SGE (*g*), T2-weighted fat-suppressed spin-echo (*h*), immediate (*i*), and 45-second (*j*) postgadolinium SGE images from the midhepatic level in the same patient. A 7-mm metastasis is present in the right lobe of the liver that is not visualized on the CT (*f*) or noncontrast T1-weighted (*g*) and T2-weighted (*h*) images but is well-shown as a uniform enhancing lesion (*arrow, i*) on the immediate postgadolinium SGE image (*i*). The metastasis washes out rapidly and becomes isointense with liver by 45 seconds (*j*). Small hypervascular malignant lesions commonly are shown only on capillary phase images.

may enhance as rapidly; however, hemangiomas tend to retain contrast and remain high in signal intensity for a more prolonged period. Most often at least one lesion greater than 2 cm in diameter is present that possesses more typical enhancement of metastases or hemangiomas, which permits inference of the nature of the smaller lesions. The capillary phase of enhancement is the most important phase of image acquisition both for detection

and characterization, and later phases assist with lesion characterization.

Infected Liver Metastases. Infected metastases may occur in the liver and most commonly arise from colon cancer metastases. The high content of intraluminal bacteria within the colon accounts for this association. The underlying mechanism presumably is embolization of coliform bacteria with tumor cells. Infected metastases may simulate the clinical picture and imaging features of liver abscesses. Infected metastases tend to have thickened irregular walls, have heterogeneous intermediate signal intensity on T2-weighted images, and enhance more centrally on delayed images (Fig. 2.48). Abscesses tend to have thinner walls, have higher signal intensity on T2-weighted images, and do not enhance centrally. Both types of lesions will show transient ill-defined perilesional enhancement reflecting a hyperemic response in the liver.

Lymphoma

Lymphomatous involvement of the liver occurs as a primary or secondary tumor in patients with non-Hodgkin's and Hodgkin's lymphoma. Non-Hodgkin's lymphoma more frequently results in focal hepatic lesions, but involvement with Hodgkin's disease is not uncommon. Lesions are typically low in signal intensity on T1-weighted images, but vary in signal intensity from low to moderately high on T2-weighted images. Enhancement on immediate postgadolinium images tends to parallel the signal intensity on T2-weighted images; lesions that are low in signal intensity on T2-weighted images tend to enhance in a diminished fashion (Fig. 2.49), whereas lesions that are high in signal intensity tend to enhance in a substantial fashion (Fig. 2.50) [74]. As with liver metastases, enhancement on immediate postgadolinium images usually is predominantly peripheral, which reflects parasitization of surrounding hepatic parenchymal arterial blood supply. Lymphomatous lesions may possess transient ill-defined perilesional enhancement on

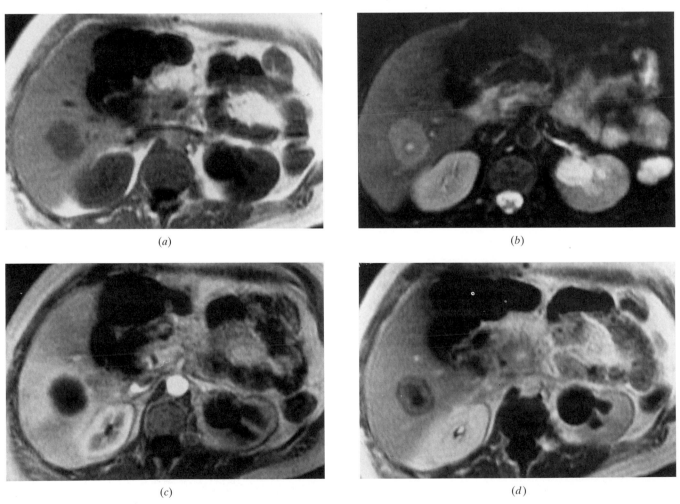

(a)

(b)

(c)

(d)

FIG. 2.48 Infected liver metastases. SGE (a), T2-weighted fat-suppressed SE (b), immediate (c), and 10-minute (d) postgadolinium SGE images. This patient with colon cancer and clinical findings of sepsis has a 4-cm infected metastasis in the right lobe of the liver. The tumor has ill-defined margins and is moderately low in signal intensity on the T1-weighted image (a) and minimally hyperintense on the T2-weighted image with a small central focus of high signal intensity (b). On the immediate postgadolinium image (c), the infected metastasis shows ring enhancement with prominent ill-defined perilesional enhancement. The 10-minute postcontrast image (d) shows some centripetal enhancement with peripheral washout resulting in a low-signal-intensity outer border. Chronic obstruction of the left renal collecting system is caused by entrapment of the ureter by the carcinoma arising in the sigmoid colon.

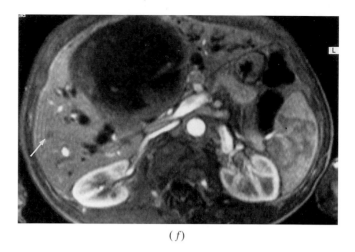

(e)

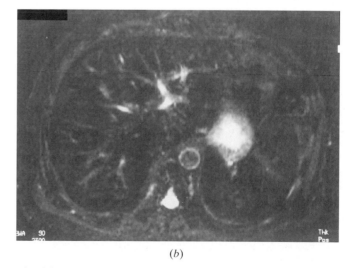

(f)

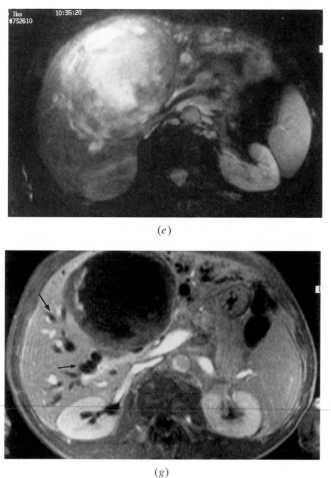

(g)

FIG. 2.48 (*Continued*) T2-weighted fat-suppressed echo-train spin-echo (*e*), immediate (*f*), and 2-minute (*g*) delayed postgadolinium SGE images in a second patient. A 14-cm metastases superinfected by Listeria is present in the left lobe of the liver. The infected metastasis is heterogeneous, high in signal on the T2-weighted image (*e*), and demonstrates enhancement of the thick irregular wall on the immediate postgadolinium image (*f*), with progressive enhancement on the interstitial-phase image (*g*). Additional metastases smaller than 1 cm are evident only on the immediate postgadolinium images (*arrow, f*). The mass caused obstruction of the biliary tree at the level of the porta hepatis resulting in substantial intrahepatic dilatation (*arrows, g*).

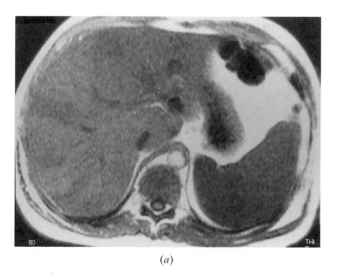

(a)

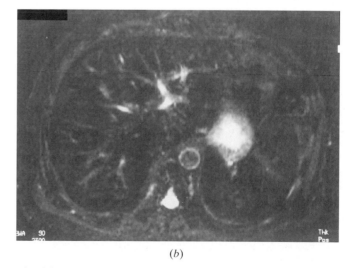

(b)

FIG. 2.49 Hepatic lymphoma, low T2-weighted signal. SGE (*a*), T2-weighted fat-suppressed spin-echo (*b*), immediate (*c*), and 90-second (*d*) postgadolinium SGE images. The SGE image (*a*) demonstrates wedge-shaped regions of low signal intensity representing increased iron deposition.

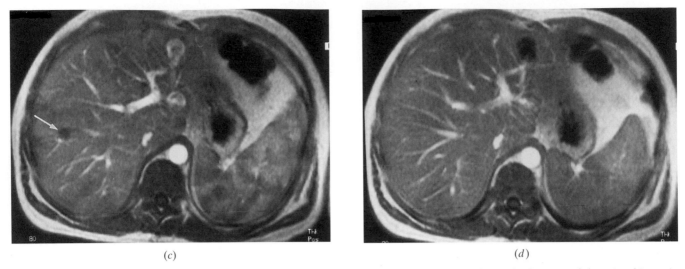

(c)

(d)

FIG. 2.49 (*Continued*) On the T2-weighted image (*b*), the liver and spleen demonstrate transfusional siderosis with low signal intensity of the liver and spleen. On the immediate postgadolinium image (*c*), focal low-signal-intensity masses (*arrow, c*) of diffuse histiocytic lymphoma are shown. On the 90-second postgadolinium image (*d*), these masses enhance to isointensity with hepatic parenchyma.

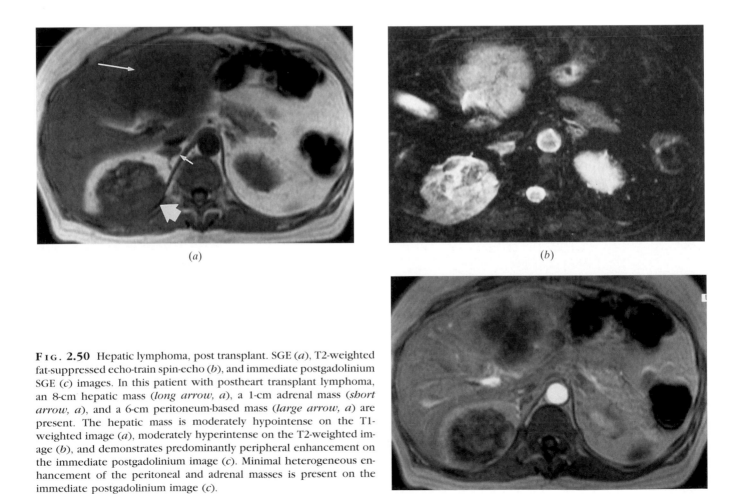

(a)

(b)

(c)

FIG. 2.50 Hepatic lymphoma, post transplant. SGE (*a*), T2-weighted fat-suppressed echo-train spin-echo (*b*), and immediate postgadolinium SGE (*c*) images. In this patient with postheart transplant lymphoma, an 8-cm hepatic mass (*long arrow, a*), a 1-cm adrenal mass (*short arrow, a*), and a 6-cm peritoneum-based mass (*large arrow, a*) are present. The hepatic mass is moderately hypointense on the T1-weighted image (*a*), moderately hyperintense on the T2-weighted image (*b*), and demonstrates predominantly peripheral enhancement on the immediate postgadolinium image (*c*). Minimal heterogeneous enhancement of the peritoneal and adrenal masses is present on the immediate postgadolinium image (*c*).

immediate postgadolinium images independent of the degree of enhancement of the lesions themselves. Presumably, this occurs secondary to a vasculitis induced in adjacent liver parenchyma (Fig. 2.51).

Primary hepatic lymphoma is considerably rarer than secondary involvement. Primary lymphoma usually occurs as a solitary relatively large mass. Tumors are moderately low in signal intensity on T1-weighted images, are mild to moderately high in signal on T2-weighted images, and show relatively diffuse enhancement on immediate postgadolinium SGE images (Fig. 2.52), analogous to primary hepatic tumors of other histologic types.

Multiple Myeloma

Focal deposits of multiple myeloma may occur rarely in the liver, most often in the setting of disseminated disease. Lesions are often small, measuring approximately 1 cm in diameter. They are slightly hyperintense on T1-weighted images and minimally hyperintense on T2-weighted images (Fig. 2.53) [75]. The hyperintensity on T1-weighted images likely reflects the increased protein production for the synthesis of Bence-Jones protein. Focal hepatic lesions are observed most commonly in light-chain multiple myeloma.

Hepatocellular Carcinoma (HCC)

HCC is the most common primary malignancy of the liver and occurs most frequently in males. In North America HCC tends to arise in a previously damaged liver and is most commonly seen in patients with alcoholic cirrhosis, chronic active hepatitis, viral hepatitis, and hemochromatosis. HCC is common in Asia because of the prevalence of viral hepatitis. Hepatic architecture tends to be less distorted in patients with viral hepatitis than in patients with alcoholic cirrhosis. As livers may not appear cirrhotic, a high index of suspicion for HCC is recommended in patients with focal liver masses and underlying viral hepatitis. HCC is solitary in approximately 50 percent, multifocal in approximately 40 percent, and diffuse in less than 10 percent of cases. Reports from Japan have shown that HCCs may arise both de novo and through progressive steps of cellular atypia [76]. Tumors are considered to arise from dysplastic nodules and to progress in a stepwise fashion to early HCC, early-advanced HCC, and finally, advanced HCC. A recent multi-institutional report has proposed a new nomenclature for nodular hepatocellular lesions in which premalignant hepatocellular lesions are defined as dysplastic nodule low grade and dysplastic nodule high grade [26]. In North

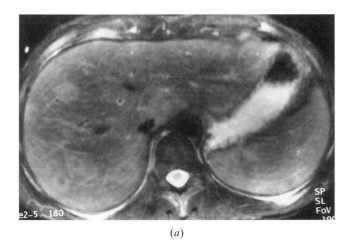

(a)

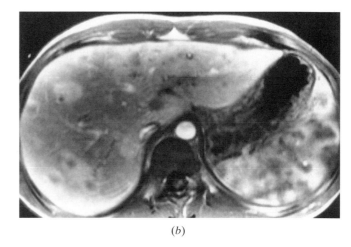

(b)

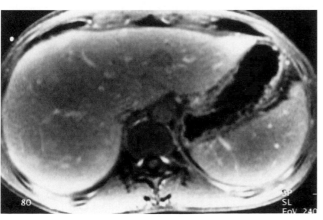

(c)

FIG. 2.51 Hodgkin's lymphoma. T2-weighted fat-suppressed echo-train spin-echo (a), immediate postgadolinium SGE (b), and 90-second postgadolinium fat-suppressed SGE (c) images. Multiple focal mass lesions smaller than 2 cm are present throughout the liver that possess mildly hyperintense rims on the T2-weighted image (a) and demonstrate ring enhancement with regions of ill-defined perilesional enhancement on the immediate postgadolinium image (b). Arciform enhancement of the spleen is present on the immediate postgadolinium image with no evidence of focal low-signal-intensity masses (b). By 90 seconds after gadolinium (c) many of the hepatic masses have become isointense with liver.

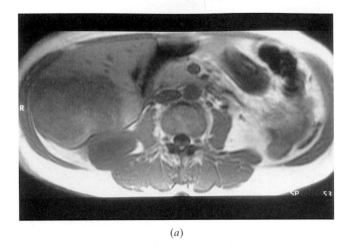

(a)

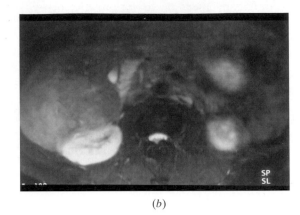

(b)

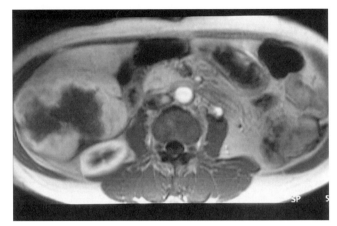

(c)

FIG. 2.52 Primary hepatic lymphoma. SGE (a), T2-weighted fat-suppressed echo-train spin echo (b), and immediate postgadolinium SGE (c) images. An 8-cm primary hepatic lymphoma is present in the right lobe of the liver. The tumor is moderately hypointense on the T1-weighted image (a), mildly hyperintense on the T2-weighted image (b), and demonstrates thick irregular multilayered peripheral enhancement on the immediate postgadolinium image (c).

America, most HCCs are advanced at the time of diagnosis.

Histologically, HCCs commonly have prominent vascularity. Imaging early after contrast injection facilitates the detecting of these tumors based on their vascularity. Because of the greater sensitivity of MRI to gadolinium than CT imaging to iodine contrast, MRI frequently demonstrates HCCs, particularly tumors smaller than 1.5 cm, better than CT imaging (Figs. 2.54 and 2.55). CT imaging is recognized as limited for the detection of unsuspected HCC in cirrhotic patient [77].

Oi et al [78] compared multiphase helical CT with MRI using dynamic gadolinium administration. They reported that early-phase gadolinium enhanced images detected 140 nodules compared to 106 nodules detected by early phase helical CT. In another report, Yamashita et al [79] reported that immediate postgadolinium SGE was superior to arterial phase helical CT for the detection of HCC using ROC analysis.

On MR images, HCCs may have a variety of signal patterns on T1- and T2-weighted images. The most fre-quent appearance is minimally low in signal intensity on T1-weighted images and moderately high in signal intensity on T2-weighted images (see Fig. 2.54) [80–88]. HCCs may, however, range from hypo- to hyperintense on T1- and T2-weighted images. Early HCC is frequently high in signal intensity on T1-weighted images and isointense on T2-weighted images [83,86]. High signal intensity on T1-weighted images on occasion is due to the presence of fat. However, many of these tumors do not contain fat. Copper-binding protein or high protein content may be responsible for the high signal intensity (Fig. 2.56) [84,86,89]. In early advanced hepatocellular carcinoma, the appearance of a low-signal-intensity nodule within a high-signal-intensity nodule (nodule within nodule) has been described on T1-weighted images [90]. This reflects the development of a low-signal high-grade tumor within a high-signal low-grade tumor. HCCs are commonly hypervascular and enhance in a diffuse heterogeneous fashion [4,37,91]. The appearance on capillary-phase gadolinium-enhanced images often permits distinction of HCC from metastatic disease because HCCs

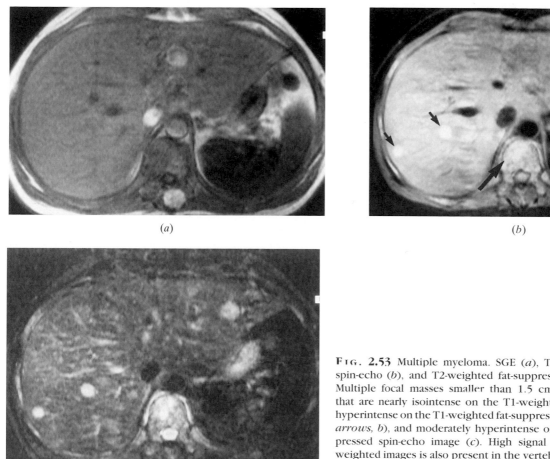

(a)

(b)

(c)

FIG. 2.53 Multiple myeloma. SGE (a), T1-weighted fat-suppressed spin-echo (b), and T2-weighted fat-suppressed spin-echo (c) images. Multiple focal masses smaller than 1.5 cm are present in the liver that are nearly isointense on the T1-weighted image (a), moderately hyperintense on the T1-weighted fat-suppressed spin-echo image (*black arrows, b*), and moderately hyperintense on the T2-weighted fat-suppressed spin-echo image (c). High signal intensity on T1- and T2-weighted images is also present in the vertebral body this tomographic section (*large arrow, b*) due to myelomatous involvement.

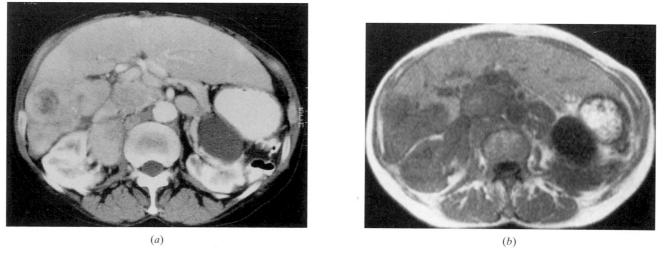

(a)

(b)

FIG. 2.54 Multifocal HCC with adenopathy, spiral CT imaging and MRI comparison. Spiral CT (a), SGE (b), T2-weighted fat-suppressed spin-echo (c), immediate postgadolinium SGE (d), and 45-second postgadolinium SGE (e) images. On the CT image (a), an HCC is identified in the right lobe with multiple nodes in the porta hepatis and retroperitoneum. Precontrast SGE image (a) demonstrates the HCC as a moderately low-signal-intensity mass in the right lobe and the lymph nodes as moderately low in signal intensity.

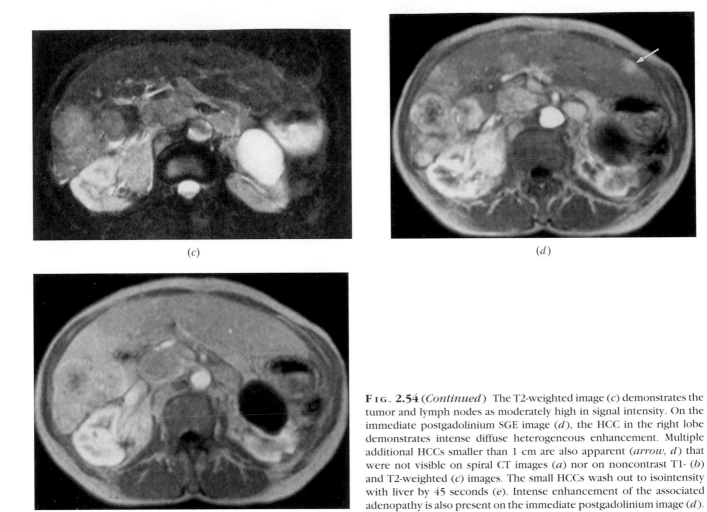

(c)

(d)

(e)

FIG. 2.54 (*Continued*) The T2-weighted image (c) demonstrates the tumor and lymph nodes as moderately high in signal intensity. On the immediate postgadolinium SGE image (d), the HCC in the right lobe demonstrates intense diffuse heterogeneous enhancement. Multiple additional HCCs smaller than 1 cm are also apparent (*arrow, d*) that were not visible on spiral CT images (a) nor on noncontrast T1- (b) and T2-weighted (c) images. The small HCCs wash out to isointensity with liver by 45 seconds (e). Intense enhancement of the associated adenopathy is also present on the immediate postgadolinium image (d).

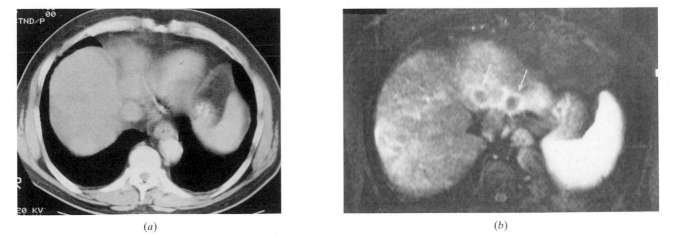

(a)

(b)

FIG. 2.55 Multifocal HCC, CT-MR imaging comparison. Contrast-enhanced spiral CT (a), T2-weighted fat-suppressed spin-echo (b) and immediate postgadolinium SGE (c) images. The contrast enhanced spiral CT image demonstrates a solitary HCC in a patient with 8 HCC tumors. No tumors are evident on this tomographic section (a). T2-weighted fat-suppressed spin-echo demonstrates two 1.8-cm HCCs at this level that have high-signal-intensity peripheral rims and are isointense centrally (*arrows, b*).

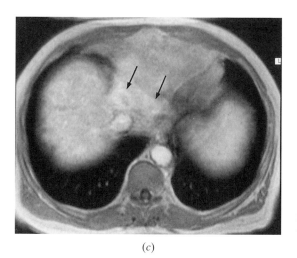

(c)

F IG. 2.55 (*Continued*) On the immediate postgadolinium image (*c*), these tumors enhance in a predominantly ring fashion (*arrows, c*).

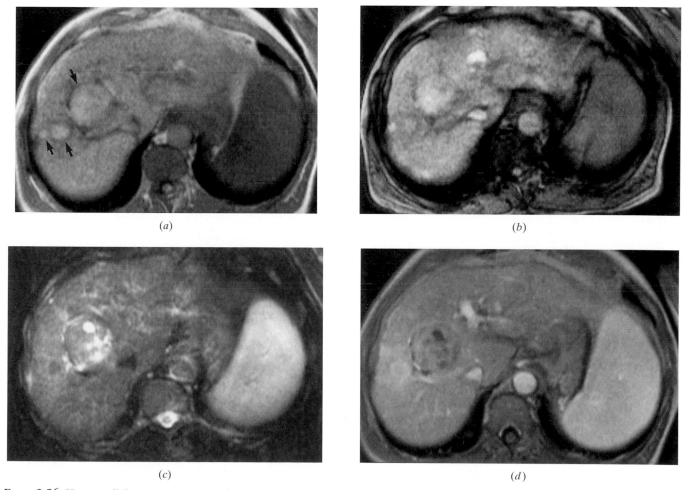

(a)   (b)

(c)   (d)

F IG. 2.56 Hepatocellular carcinoma, multifocal with high signal intensity on T1-weighted images. SGE (*a*), out-of-phase SGE (*b*), T2-weighted fat-suppressed spin-echo (*c*), and immediate postgadolinium SGE (*d*) images. Multiple HCCs are present that are high in signal intensity on the T1-weighted image (*arrows, a*) and do not drop in signal nor develop a phase-cancellation artifact on the out-of-phase image (*b*), which excludes the presence of fat. The small HCCs are isointense with liver on the T2-weighted image, whereas the large tumor is heterogeneous and mildly hyperintense (*c*). On the immediate postgadolinium image the small HCCs exhibit predominantly peripheral enhancement, whereas the larger HCC has diffuse heterogeneous enhancement. A low-signal-intensity pseudocapsule is appreciated around the larger HCC on all imaging sequences.

typically demonstrate enhancing stroma throughout the entire tumor (Fig. 2.57), whereas metastases have peripheral enhancement [37]. The primary hepatic origin of HCC presumably results in a blood supply similar to and in continuity with background liver, explaining the early diffuse heterogeneous enhancement. The degree of vascularity of HCCs may vary substantially: Many are hypervascular, but some neoplasms are very hypovascular [88]. Hypovascular tumors are variable in signal intensity on T1-weighted images but are nearly isointense on T2-weighted images, and these tumors are frequently well-differentiated (Fig. 2.58) [73,88]. Lesion size and number are best evaluated on combined T1- and T2-weighted images and immediate postgadolinium enhanced SGE images, because tumors vary in signal intensity on non-contrast images [37,86,88], and this combination of sequences increases observer confidence. Small tumors (<1.5 cm) are often only apparent on immediate postgadolinium SGE images (Fig. 2.59). Therefore, detecting the

presence of small satellite HCCs requires the acquisition of capillary-phase SGE images. Margins in large tumors are usually best seen on T2-weighted images and are less distinct on gadolinium-enhanced MR images.

Occasionally, no abnormal morphological features are apparent in a cirrhotic liver on imaging studies. Therefore, any mass lesion that enhances in a diffuse heterogeneous fashion immediately after gadolinium should be regarded as a possible malignant hepatocellular tumor.

Diffuse infiltration with HCC may be difficult to recognize on imaging studies because the findings may be subtle or may simulate the appearance of scarring. The most common appearance of diffuse infiltrative hepatocellular carcinoma is mottled with punctate high intensity on T2-weighted images and mottled punctate intense enhancement on capillary-phase gadolinium-enhanced images (Fig. 2.60). The mottled liver texture is more readily appreciated on capillary-phase images. Diffuse infiltration may also appear as irregular linear strands that

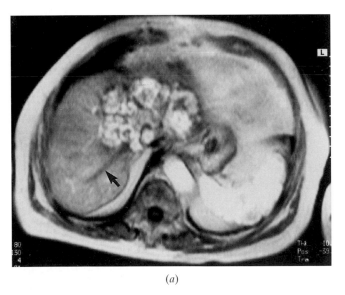

(a)

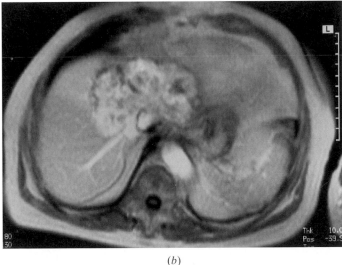

(b)

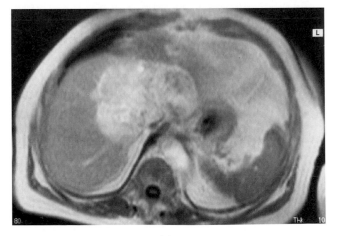

(c)

FIG. 2.57 Hepatocellular carcinoma, solitary hypervascular tumor. Immediate (*a*), 90-second (*b*), and 10-minute (*c*) postgadolinium SGE images. An 8-cm tumor is present superiorly in the liver that demonstrates hypervascular diffuse heterogeneous enhancement on the immediate postgadolinium image (*a*). Hepatic veins are unopacified (*arrow, a*) confirming that image acquisition is in the capillary phase of enhancement. On the 90-second postgadolinium image (*b*), the tumor becomes more homogeneous in enhancement. By 10 minutes (*c*), the tumor is homogeneously enhanced and remains high in signal intensity relative to liver. The heterogeneity of the diffuse enhancement on the immediate post contrast image is an important feature of malignant primary hepatocellular tumors that measure more than 3 cm in diameter and distinguishes them from benign tumors that enhance homogeneously.

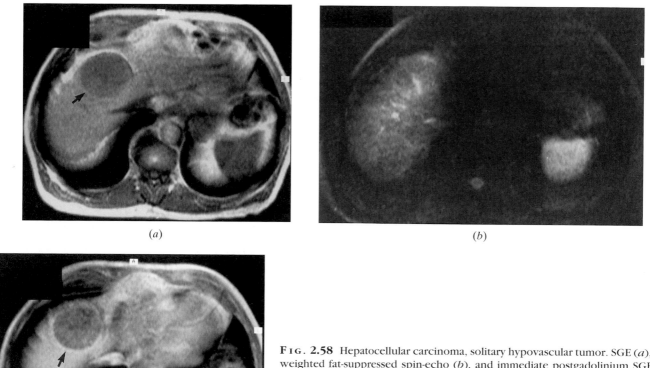

(a)

(b)

(c)

FIG. 2.58 Hepatocellular carcinoma, solitary hypovascular tumor. SGE (*a*), T2-weighted fat-suppressed spin-echo (*b*), and immediate postgadolinium SGE (*c*) images. A 6-cm solitary HCC is present in the liver (*arrow, a*) that is low in signal intensity on the T2-weighted image (*b*) and enhances minimally in a diffuse fashion with enhancement of tumor capsule on the immediate postgadolinium image (*arrow, c*). The hypovascular nature of the tumor results in low signal intensity on T1-weighted, T2-weighted, and immediate postgadolinium images and renders the tumor well-visualized on precontrast and immediate postcontrast T1-weighted images and poorly visualized on T2-weighted images. The low signal intensity on the T2-weighted image renders the HCC nearly isointense with liver.

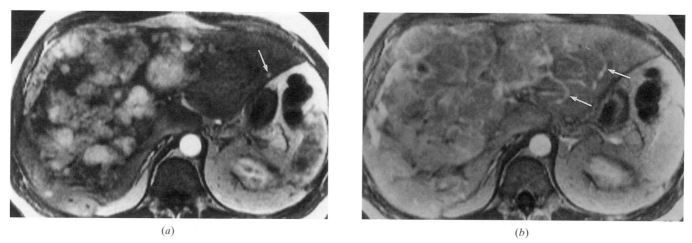

(a)

(b)

FIG. 2.59 Hypervascular HCC with small satellite tumors. Immediate (*a*) and 90-second (*b*) postgadolinium SGE images. Intense diffuse heterogeneous enhancement of a 15-cm HCC is present on the immediate postgadolinium image (*a*). Multiple additional small HCCs are apparent including tumors as small as 3 mm (*arrow, a*). By 90 seconds after gadolinium (*b*), the large tumor has washed out in a heterogeneous fashion with prominent abnormal curvilinear hepatic veins apparent (*arrow, b*). The small HCC has become isointense with liver at this time.

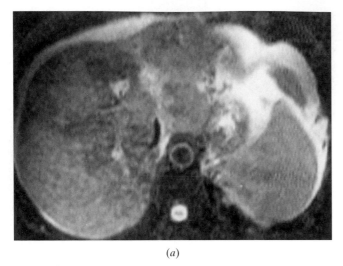

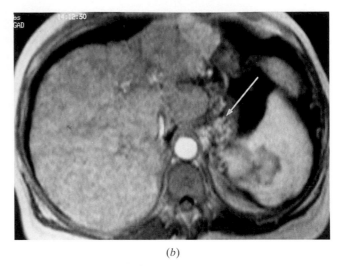

(a)   (b)

FIG. 2.60 Hepatocellular carcinoma, diffuse infiltrative type. T2-weighted fat-suppressed echo-train spin-echo (*a*) and immediate postgadolinium SGE (*b*) images. Mottled diffuse high signal intensity is present throughout the liver on the T2-weighted image (*a*). Diffuse mottled heterogeneous enhancement is appreciated on the immediate postgadolinium image (*b*) that represents the diffuse infiltrative HCC. This mottled signal intensity is the most common MRI appearance for diffuse infiltrative HCC. Occasionally, diffuse infiltrative HCC will appear as low in signal intensity on T2-weighted images and very low in signal intensity on the postgadolinium images. Prominent varices are present along the lesser curvature of the stomach (*arrow, b*).

are hypo- to isointense on T1-weighted images, and iso- to moderately hyperintense on T2-weighted images. On immediate postgadolinium images these tumor strands tend to enhance less than adjacent liver, although more intense enhancement also occurs. Late increased enhancement of the tumor strands may reflect fibrous composition.

A characteristic feature of HCC is tumor extension into the venous system. Tumor extension into portal veins occurs most frequently (Fig. 2.61), but hepatic venous extension also occurs (Fig. 2.62). This feature is observed

in fewer than 50 percent of cases, but is common with large and advanced tumors. Diffusely infiltrative HCC very commonly has associated venous thrombosis. Pseudocapsules are not uncommonly observed in HCC, especially in early or well-differentiated tumors. The typical signal intensity of a pseudocapsule is hypointensity on T1-weighted images, minimal hyperintensity on T2-weighted images, low signal intensity on immediate postgadolinium images and increased enhancement on delayed images [4].

Many HCCs will take up Mn-DPDP, and well-differ-

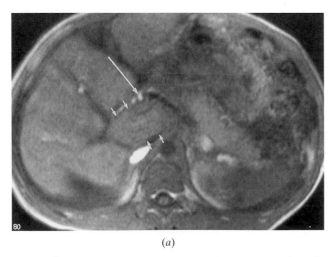

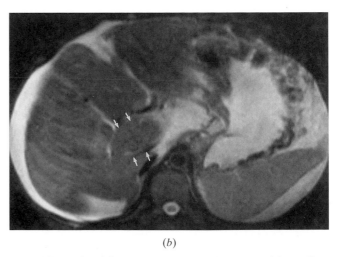

(a)   (b)

FIG. 2.61 Hepatocellular carcinoma with portal-vein thrombosis. SGE (*a*), T2-weighted fat-suppressed spin-echo (*b*), and immediate postgadolinium SGE (*c*) images. The portal vein is expanded with tumor thrombus (*small arrows, a,b*), which is nearly isointense with liver on T1- (*a*) and T2-weighted (*b*) images. Tumor thrombus enhances in a diffuse heterogeneous fashion (*arrows, c*) on the immediate postgadolinium image (*c*).

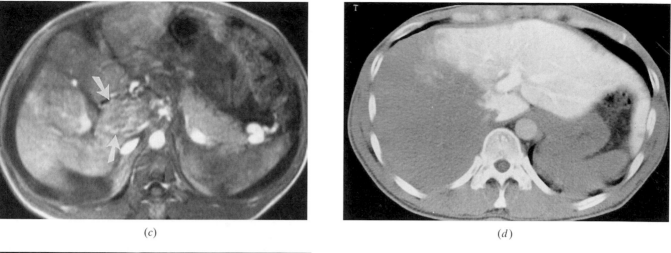

(c)

(d)

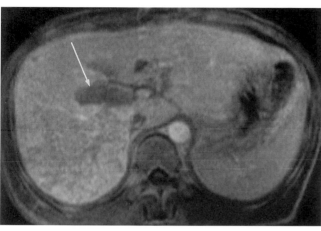

(e)

FIG. 2.61 (*Continued*) The hepatic artery is identified as a small high-signal tubular structure on the precontrast and immediate post-gadolinium SGE images (*long arrow, a*). Heterogeneous enhancement of the liver on the immediate postgadolinium image (*c*) reflects a combination of vascular abnormality from portal-vein thrombosis and heterogeneous enhancement of diffusely infiltrative HCC. A substantial volume of ascites is present that is high in signal intensity on the T2-weighted image (*b*) and low in signal intensity on pre- and postcontrast T1-weighted images (*a,c*). Portal-vein thrombosis in a second patient with HCC shown on spiral CTAP (*d*) and immediate postgadolinium SGE (*e*) images. On the CTAP image (*d*), nonopacification of the right hemiliver is present due to thrombosis of the right portal vein. The immediate postgadolinium SGE image demonstrates a tumor thrombus that expands the right portal vein (*arrow, e*). Diffuse heterogeneous mottled enhancement of the right lobe of the liver is present on the MR image (*e*), which is a typical appearance for diffusely infiltrative HCC.

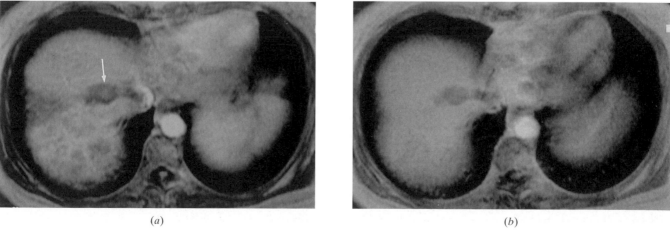

(a)

(b)

FIG. 2.62 Hepatocellular carcinoma with hepatic-vein thrombosis. Pictured are 45- (*a*) and 90-second (*b*) postgadolinium SGE images. On the 45-second postgadolinium image (*a*) tumor thrombus is apparent in the middle hepatic vein as low-signal-intensity material that expands the vein (*arrow, a*). Diffuse heterogeneous enhancement is noted in the right lobe that represents diffuse infiltrative HCC. Distal to the thrombosed hepatic vein, a wedge-shaped perfusion defect is identified. On the 90-second image (*b*) the tumor thrombus maintains low signal intensity compared to liver. However, the perfusion defect has resolved, and the diffuse HCC is more isointense with background liver.

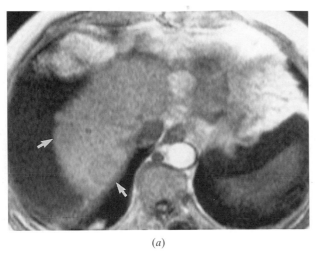

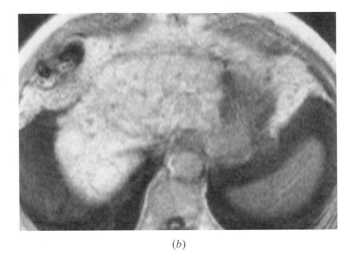

(a)   *(b)*

FIG. 2.63 Hepatocellular carcinoma, Mn-DPDP enhancement. SGE (*a*) and 30-minute post-Mn-DPDP SGE (*b*) images. Subtle low-signal-intensity mass lesions are apparent on the precontrast image (*arrows, a*). Following Mn-DPDP enhancement (*b*) the HCCs enhance slightly more intensely than background liver rendering the tumors minimally hyperintense. A pseudocapsule is appreciated around the more posterior tumor on both the precontrast and postcontrast images.

entiated HCC may take up more Mn-DPDP than surrounding liver, reflecting persistent hepatocellular function with decreased biliary clearance (Fig. 2.63) [44,54,92].

Fibrolamellar HCC. An uncommon variety of HCC is the fibrolamellar HCC. This tumor is unusual in that it occurs in younger patients, frequently females, without underlying cirrhosis [89]. This tumor is biologically distinct from other HCCs and exhibits slow growth. Prognosis is better than for other forms of HCC [93].

Fibrolamellar HCCs are generally large, solitary tumors that are heterogeneous and low in signal intensity on T1-weighted images and heterogeneous and high in signal intensity on T2-weighted images. A central scar, which may have a radiating appearance, has large low-signal components on T2-weighted images that do not enhance with gadolinium on delayed images. Enhancement of the tumor is diffuse heterogeneous and intense on immediate postgadolinium SGE images (Fig. 2.64) [94].

Peripheral Cholangiocarcinoma

Peripheral cholangiocarcinoma is an uncommon entity that presents as a focal hepatic mass lesion. The tumor is frequently large at presentation [95]. The tumor resembles

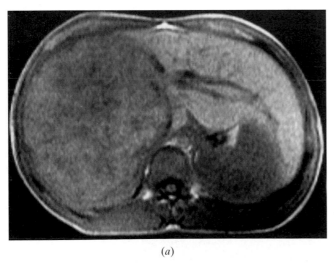

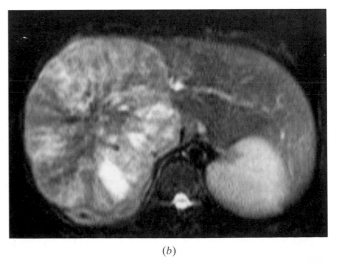

(a)   *(b)*

FIG. 2.64 Fibrolamellar hepatocellular carcinoma. SGE (*a*), T2-weighted fat-suppressed spin-echo (*b*), immediate (*c*) and 10-minute (*d*) postgadolinium SGE images. A 14-cm fibrolamellar hepatocellular carcinoma is present in this adolescent male with no history of liver disease and 1 year duration of gynecomastia. The tumor is hypointense on the T1-weighted image with a low signal intensity central scar (*a*) and heterogeneously hyperintense on the T2-weighted image (*b*) with the central radiating scar largely low in signal intensity.

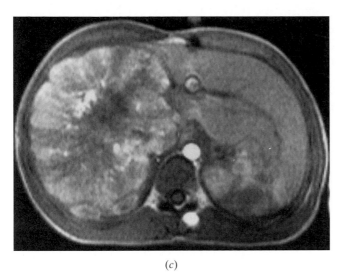

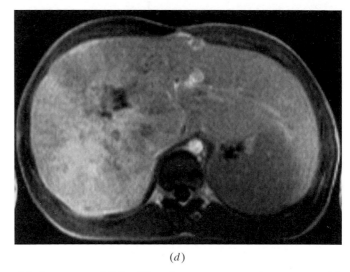

(*c*)   (*d*)

FIG. 2.64 (*Continued*) On the immediate postgadolinium SGE image (*c*), the tumor exhibits diffuse heterogeneous enhancement with negligible enhancement of the radiating scar. On the 10-minute image (*d*), the bulk of the tumor has become isointense with background liver. Portions of the central scar are higher in signal intensity than surrounding tissue while other parts remain low in signal.

HCC in appearance with low signal intensity on T1-weighted and moderate signal intensity on T2-weighted images [94]. High signal on T1-weighted images, pseudocapsule, and invasion into portal and hepatic veins are common with HCC and rarely seen with cholangiocarcinoma. Biliary and extrinsic portal vein obstruction are more common with cholangiocarcinoma. Enhancement with gadolinium varies from minimal to intense diffuse heterogeneous enhancement immediately following contrast administration (Fig. 2.65), with minimal enhancement most commonly observed. Persistent enhancement on delayed images is not uncommon [96]. The hepatic origin of the tumor likely explains the early diffuse heterogeneous enhancement. (For a description of extrahe-

patic cholangiocarcinoma see Chapter 3 on Gallbladder and Biliary System.) Mixed cholangiocarcinoma-HCC tumors occur, and their appearance is generally indistinguishable from that of HCC, with a tendency to be hypervascular (Fig. 2.66).

Biliary Cystadenoma/Cystadenocarcinoma

These rare tumors form a heterogeneous group. The tumors typically are quite large and have a multilocular cystic appearance [43,97–99]. They frequently have solid nodules associated with cystic components (Fig. 2.67) [100]. Mucin content occasionally renders these tumors high in signal intensity on T1-weighted images [43,99]. Solid components of the tumor demonstrate early hetero-

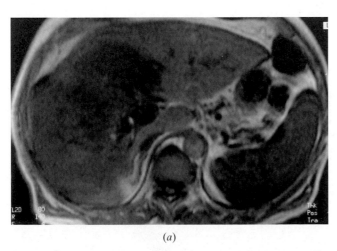

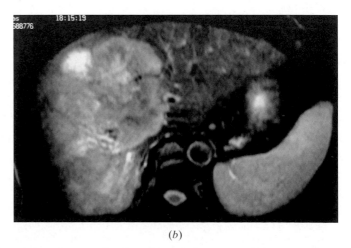

(*a*)   (*b*)

FIG. 2.65 Peripheral cholangiocarcinoma. SGE (*a*), T2-weighted fat-suppressed spin-echo (*b*) and immediate postgadolinium SGE (*c*) images. A 14-cm tumor is present in the right lobe of the liver that is moderately low in signal intensity on the T1-weighted image (*a*), moderately high in signal intensity on the T2-weighted image (*b*),

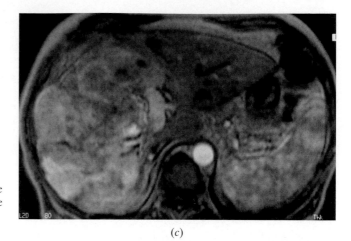

(c)

FIG. 2.65 (*Continued*) and that enhances in an intense diffuse heterogeneous fashion on the immediate postgadolinium SGE image (*c*). The appearance resembles that of an HCC.

geneous enhancement, often in a minimal fashion, which is a pattern consistent with tumors of hepatic origin.

Angiosarcoma

Angiosarcoma is a rare vascular malignancy, the malignant counterpart to hemangioma. Internal hemorrhage is relatively common. Angiosarcoma may be high signal intensity on T2-weighted images [101,102] and demonstrate peripheral nodular enhancement with centripetal progression, and therefore can mimic the appearance of hemangioma (Fig. 2.68). The frequent presence of hemorrhage, which results in heterogeneous low signal

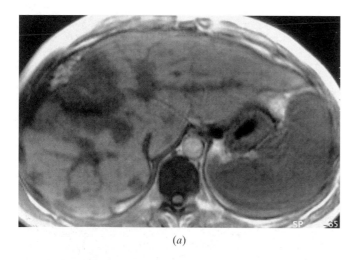

(a)

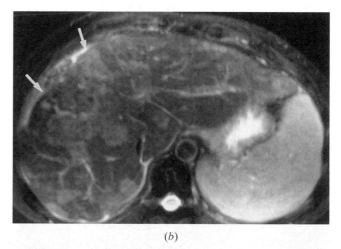

(b)

FIG. 2.66 Mixed HCC-cholangiocarcinoma. SGE (*a*), T2-weighted fat-suppressed spin-echo (*b*), and immediate postgadolinium SGE (*c*) images. A large 14-cm tumor is centered in the medial segment, and multiple small satellite lesions are scattered throughout the remainder of the liver. The tumors are moderately low in signal intensity on the T1-weighted image (*a*), moderately high in signal on the T2-weighted image (*b*), and enhance intensely immediately after gadolinium administration (*c*). Capsular retraction is also noted (*arrows, b*).

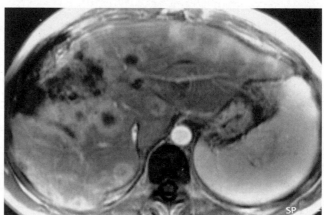

(c)

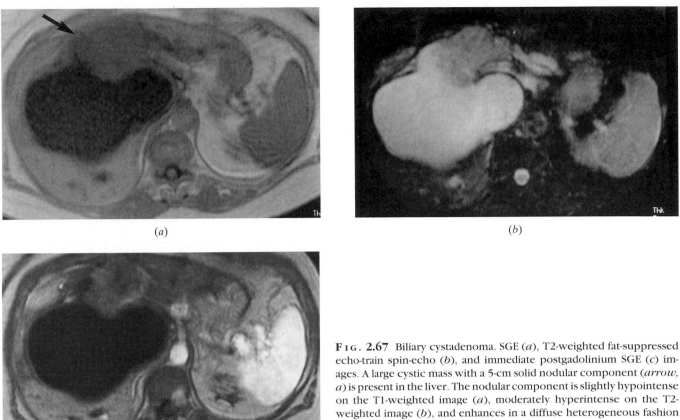

(a)

(b)

(c)

FIG. 2.67 Biliary cystadenoma. SGE (a), T2-weighted fat-suppressed echo-train spin-echo (b), and immediate postgadolinium SGE (c) images. A large cystic mass with a 5-cm solid nodular component (arrow, a) is present in the liver. The nodular component is slightly hypointense on the T1-weighted image (a), moderately hyperintense on the T2-weighted image (b), and enhances in a diffuse heterogeneous fashion on the immediate postgadolinium image (c). Diffuse heterogeneous enhancement on immediate postgadolinium images is a feature of tumors of hepatic origin.

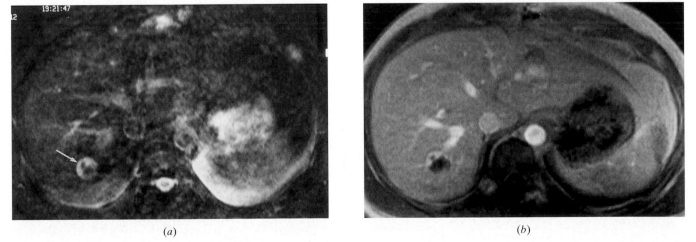

(a)

(b)

FIG. 2.68 Angiosarcoma. T2-weighted fat-suppressed echo-train spin-echo (a), 90-second (b), and 10-minute (c) postgadolinium SGE images. A 2-cm angiosarcoma is present in the right lobe of the liver. The mass is well-defined and largely hyperintense on the T2-weighted image (arrow, a) with a central region of low signal intensity due to hemorrhage. On the 90-second postgadolinium image (b), peripheral nodular enhancement is present. By 10 minutes after contrast (c), nodular enhancement has progressed centripetally, with a central nonenhanced area that corresponds to the region of hemorrhage on the T2-weighted image.

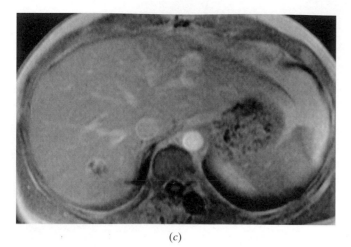

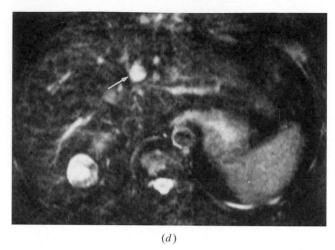

(c)   (d)

FIG. 2.68 (*Continued*) Angiosarcomas mimic the appearance of hemangiomas. The presence of hemorrhage in this case is a common finding in angiosarcomas and rare in hemangiomas. Interval increase in size of this tumor is identified on a follow-up study obtained 1 month later shown on T2-weighted fat-suppressed echo-train spin-echo (d). Increase in size of a second tumor is also present. Rapid growth is compatible with angiosarcomas and not with hemangiomas. A change in the signal intensity of the larger mass on the T2-weighted image (d) is also noted between studies due to aging of the central hemorrhage.

intensity on T2-weighted images, and lack of central enhancement due to hemorrhage are distinguishing features (see Fig. 2.68).

Hemangioendothelioma

Hemangioendothelioma is a rare primary vascular tumor of the liver. Two types of these tumors occur, one predominantly found in the pediatric population (infantile hemangioendothelioma) less than 1 year of age, and another found in adults (epithelioid hemangioendothelioma). The infantile form of this tumor follows a benign course with lesions spontaneously involuting between 1 and 2 years of age. These tumors tend to be numerous similar-size tumors that are uniformly hyperintense on T2-weighted images and enhance homogeneously on interstitial-phase gadolinium-enhanced images (Fig. 2.69). Epithelioid hemangioendotheliomas occur in adult patients and tend to be low grade malignant tumors that

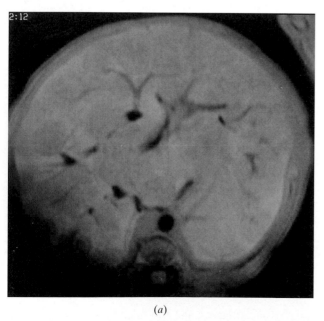

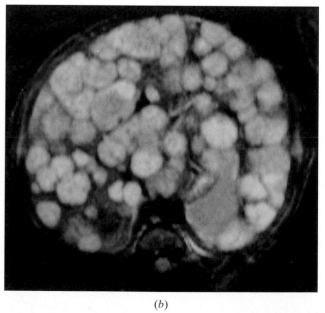

(a)   (b)

FIG. 2.69 Infantile hemangioendothelioma and epithelioid hemangioendothelioma. T1-weighted fat-suppressed spin-echo (a), T2-weighted fat-suppressed spin-echo (b) and gadolinium-enhanced T1-weighted fat-suppressed spin-echo (c) images. The liver in this 9-month-old male is extensively replaced with focal mass lesions smaller than 1 cm that are low in signal intensity on the T1-weighted image (a), high in signal intensity on the T2-weighted image (b), and that enhance homogeneously on the interstitial-phase gadolinium enhanced image (c).

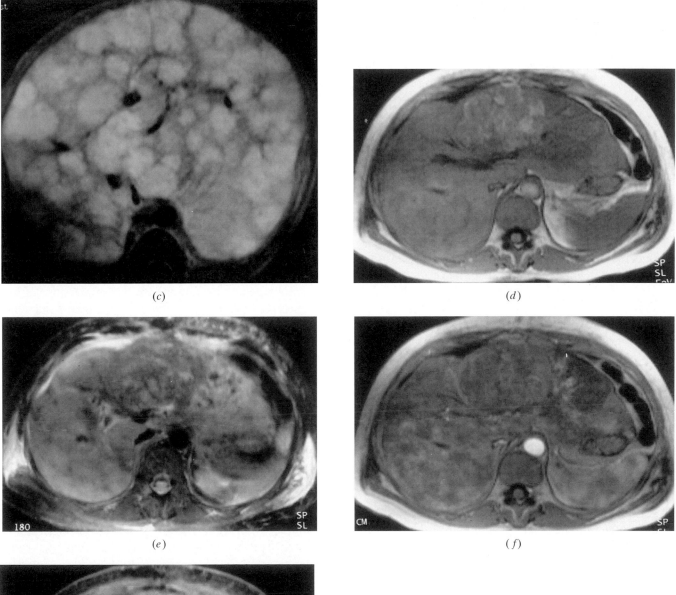

(c)

(d)

(e)

(f)

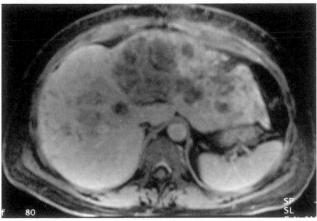

(g)

F IG . 2.69 (*Continued*) This appearance is characteristic for hemangioendothelioma in neonatal patients. SGE (*d*), T2-weighted fat-suppressed echo-train spin-echo (*e*), immediate postgadolinium SGE (*f*), and 90-second postgadolinium fat-suppressed SGE (*g*) images in an adult patient with epithelioid hemangioendotheliosarcoma. Extensive liver involvement with a multifocal malignant epithelioid hemangioendotheliosarcoma is present. Regions of high signal intensity are present in the largest mass on the T1-weighted image (*d*). The tumor is heterogeneous and isointense to minimally hyperintense on the T2-weighted image (*e*). Enhancement is diffuse heterogeneous on the immediate postgadolinium image (*f*) with heterogeneous washout on the 90-second postcontrast image (*g*). The MRI appearance of this epitheloid hemangioendotheliosarcoma resembles HCC.

are usually multifocal with tumors of varying size [101,102]. These tumors are heterogeneous in signal intensity on T2-weighted images and demonstrate irregular rim or diffuse heterogeneous enhancement on immediate postgadolinium images. The appearance is similar to that of hepatocellular carcinoma, particularly in tumors with aggressive growth patterns (Fig. 2.69).

Posttreatment Malignant Liver Lesions

Malignant liver lesions may be treated by a number of interventions, including resection, intravenous chemotherapy, intra-arterial chemotherapy, alcohol injection, cryotherapy, and chemoembolization [103–121]. The appearance of hepatic parenchyma and malignant liver lesions following therapeutic interventions has been described. However, studies involving large series and serial posttreatment imaging are few in number [105–112,114,116–120]. None of these studies has been performed with dynamic gadolinium-enhanced SGE imaging. In the evaluation of the posttreatment liver, the time course of benign posttreatment tissue changes, primarily tissue injury and granulation tissue, and the appearance of persistent or recurrent disease must be ascertained. As with postradiation or postsurgical changes in other tissues and organ systems, the distinction between benign and malignant disease usually can be made with certainty beyond 1 year following treatment. At this time point, benign disease usually exhibits regular or linear margins, low signal intensity on T2-weighted images, and minimal enhancement. In comparison, malignant disease tends to appear more irregular, nodular, or mass-like, with moderately high signal intensity on T2-weighted images and moderate enhancement. The immediate postgadolinium images are most effective at defining pathophysiological changes that reflect successful response or recurrence. Certain features of treatment-related changes depend on the form of therapy. The following discussion describes some of those features.

Resection
Following resection, malignancy may recur along the margin of resection, or separate focal lesions may develop in the remainder of the liver [105,112,114,116–120]. Tumor development along the resection margin is not an uncommon mode of recurrence of hepatocellular carcinoma or metastases following resection. After approximately 3 months, the immediate postsurgical changes of moderately high signal intensity on T2-weighted images and mild ill-defined enhancement on early postgadolinium SGE images, which are present in a linear distribution along the resection margin, begin to resolve. Tumor recurrence, in distinction, has a nodular margin that is moderately high in signal intensity on T2-weighted images and exhibits moderately intense early enhancement on

postgadolinium images. These features progress over time.

Development of separate focal lesions occurs more commonly in the setting of surgical resection for metastatic disease. These lesions appear identical to untreated malignant lesions.

Intravenous Chemotherapy
A number of chemotherapeutic agents are currently utilized in the treatment of focal liver lesions. The number of agents and their cytotoxic effectiveness for the treatment of malignant disease continue to progress dramatically. At present, commonly used chemotherapeutic regimens for the treatment of liver metastases are 5-fluorouracil based. The mechanisms of tumor cell control are complex and probably involve a number of pathways. Recent research has focused on the antiangiogenesis of some of these agents.

The time course and variation in appearance of metastases that have responded to chemotherapy have not been fully elucidated. One report described the appearance of liver metastases treated by intravenous chemotherapy in 34 patients on serial MRI studies [106]. In that report a good prognosis was associated with increased signal intensity of the lesions on T1-weighted images and decreased signal intensity on T2-weighted images, and a poor prognosis was reflected by a decreased signal intensity on T1-weighted images and increased signal intensity on T2-weighted images. Metastases that do not respond grow in size. Features of mild response may be stability of lesion size and signal intensity on T2-weighted, precontrast, and postcontrast T1-weighted images. Regarding subacute changes of successful chemotherapy response, one report described the appearance of liver metastases 2 to 7 months following initiation of chemotherapy [122]. In that report, liver metastases became more well-defined and higher in signal intensity on T2-weighted images, showing peripheral nodular enhancement with progressive enhancement and hyperintensity relative to liver on 10-minute delayed images (Fig. 2.70). The appearance was considered to mimic that of hemangiomas. Underlying pathophysiology was presumed to reflect alteration in tumor physiology and blood supply to a less aggressive pattern, with antitumor angiogenesis a possible underlying mechanism. Continued resolution of metastatic lesions result in progressive decrease in signal intensity on T2-weighted images and progressive decrease in contrast enhancement (Fig. 2.71).

The appearance of chronic healed metastases is comparable to the appearance of treated focal lesions of other causes, such as infection. The chronic healed phase of lesion response usually develops at least 1.5 years after initiation of treatment. Chronic healed lesions possess an irregular polygonal margin frequently associated with retraction of surrounding liver parenchyma. If they are superficial in location, capsular retraction develops, which is readily apparent. Chronic healed lesions contain mature fibrous tissue which has a low fluid content and is hypovascular. The appearance of these lesions on MR images is low signal intensity on T1-weighted images (moderately hypointense with liver) and low signal intensity on T2-weighted images (negligibly hypointense to isointense with liver), exhibiting negligible early enhancement (substantially hypointense to liver) with progressive enhancement on delayed 10-minute images

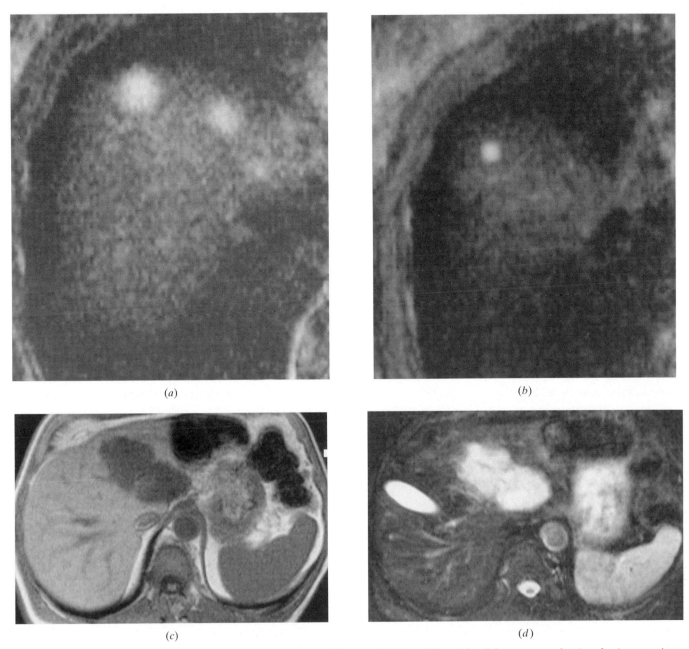

(a)

(b)

(c)

(d)

F I G . 2.70 Chemotherapy-treated metastases within 7 months of therapy initiation. T2-weighted fat-suppressed spin-echo image prior to chemotherapy (a) and T2-weighted fat-suppressed spin-echo image 3 months after initiation of chemotherapy (b). On the pretreatment examination (a), two metastases are evident in the dome of the liver. The metastases have slightly ill-defined margins and are moderate in signal intensity. The large metastases measure 1.5 cm and the smaller are 1 cm in size. Three months after initiation of chemotherapy, the larger metastasis has decreased in size to 4 mm, has well-defined margins, and is hyperintense on the T2-weighted image (b). In a second patient, SGE (c), T2-weighted fat-suppressed spin-echo (d), 90-second (e), and 10-minute (f) postgadolinium SGE images demonstrate two 4-cm metastases. The metastases are well-defined, low in signal intensity on the T1-weighted image (c), high in signal intensity on the T2-weighted image (d), and demonstrate peripheral irregular enhancement (e) that progresses centripetally.

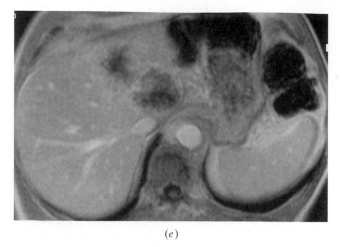

(e)

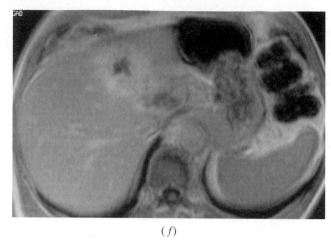

(f)

FIG. 2.70 (*Continued*) The lesions appear hyperintense relative to the liver with a low-signal-intensity central scar at 10 minutes (*f*). In both patients, the appearance of these subacute treated metastases (2 to 7 months after initiation of chemotherapy) mimic the appearance of hemangiomas. History of chemotherapy treatment for liver metastasis is critical to obtain in patients with lesions that resemble hemangiomas.

(isointense to moderately hyperintense). The fibrotic process of chronic healed metastases may be very extensive in the presence of numerous liver metastases, such that a hepatic cirrhosis-type liver appearance may develop [110,112]. This occurs most commonly in the setting of breast cancer metastases (Fig. 2.72).

During the course of chemotherapy, lesions develop acute granulation tissue that may mask the appearance of coexistent viable tumor. Successful resolution of metastases should not be considered to have occurred until lesions are in the chronic healed phase.

Alcohol Injection/Cryotherapy

Both alcohol injection and cryotherapy have been employed to ablate focal lesions by localized nonspecific cytotoxicity [107]. Immediately following treatment, a ne-

crotic cavity is created, which develops an enhancing rim of granulation tissue. With successful treatment, shrinkage of the cavity develops in the subacute phase by tissue retraction and gradual growth of granulation tissue into the space. Response to alcohol injection has been described using MRI [105,107,109]. On MR images, tumors that are successfully ablated exhibit a regular thin margin of inflammatory tissue that enhances substantially on immediate postgadolinium images (Fig. 2.73). This appearance persists for approximately 3 months, after which progressive decrease in rim enhancement and lesion size occurs. Persistent tumor is reflected by irregularity of the wall of the treated lesion with the area of thickening representing persistent or recurrent tumor (see Fig. 2.73) [105,107–109]. The tumor will appear moderate in signal intensity on T2-weighted images and dem-

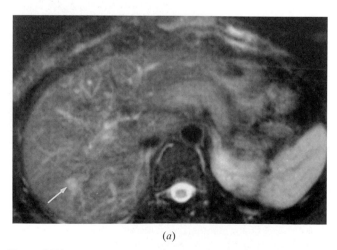

(a)

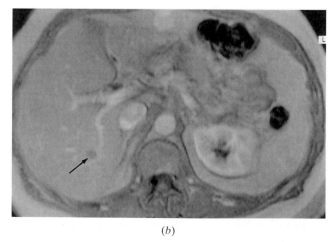

(b)

FIG. 2.71 Liver metastases, chronic, (>1 year) postchemotherapy treatment. T2-weighted fat-suppressed echo-train spin-echo (*a*) and immediate postgadolinium SGE (*b*) images. A 7-mm lesion is present in the right lobe of the liver that is minimally hyperintense on the T2-weighted image (*arrow, a*) and that demonstrates negligible enhancement on the immediate postgadolinium SGE image (*arrow, b*).

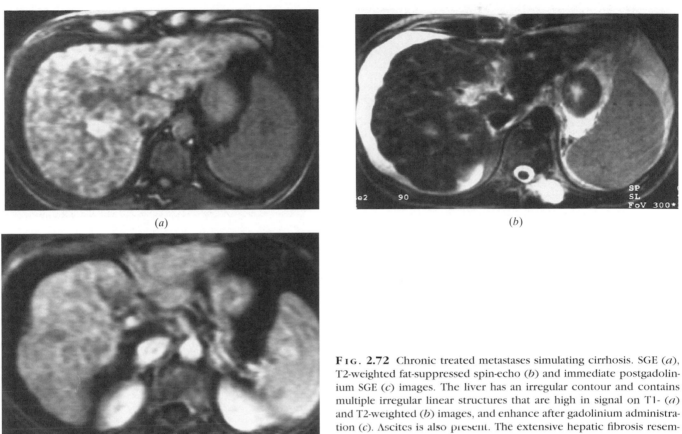

FIG. 2.72 Chronic treated metastases simulating cirrhosis. SGE (*a*), T2-weighted fat-suppressed spin-echo (*b*) and immediate postgadolinium SGE (*c*) images. The liver has an irregular contour and contains multiple irregular linear structures that are high in signal on T1- (*a*) and T2-weighted (*b*) images, and enhance after gadolinium administration (*c*). Ascites is also present. The extensive hepatic fibrosis resembles cirrhosis.

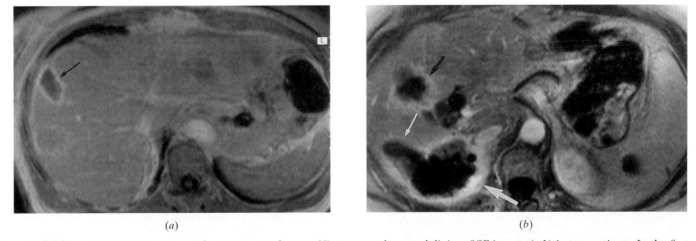

FIG. 2.73 Liver metastases, postcryotherapy, acute changes. Ninety-second postgadolinium SGE images (*a,b*) in two patients. In the first patient (*a*), a cryotherapy defect is present in the right lobe (*arrow, a*) that has a uniform-thickness enhancing wall in continuity with enhancing liver capsule of similar thickness. In the acute stage this appearance is compatible with tumor ablation and formation of acute granulation tissue along the cavity wall. The oblong shape of the defect corresponds to the direction of placement of the cryotherapy device. In the second patient (*b*), a cryotherapy tract (*thin white arrow, b*) is noted in continuity with a necrotic cavity. Portions of the cavity wall are thick and irregular (*large white arrow, b*). A second cryotherapy defect is noted in a more anterior location (*black arrow, b*). The cavity wall is thick and irregular. The presence of thick irregular walls after treatment are consistent with persistent disease.

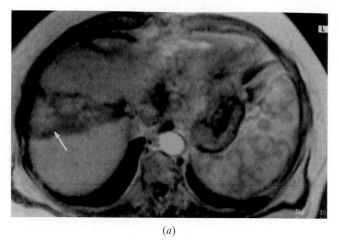

(a)

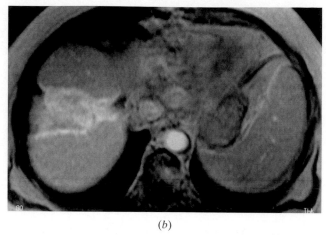

(b)

FIG. 2.74 Liver metastases, postcryotherapy chronic changes with recurrent disease. Immediate (*a*) and 10-minute (*b*) postgadolinium SGE images. A large wedge-shaped defect is present in the superior aspect of the liver that enhances minimally on the immediate postgadolinium image (*a*) and shows delayed enhancement at 10 minutes (*b*). This enhancement pattern is consistent with fibrosis. Focal irregular regions of soft tissue are identified within the wedge-shaped tissue (*arrow, a*) that represent adenocarcinoma.

onstrate moderately intense enhancement on immediate postgadolinium images (Fig. 2.74).

Chemoembolization

The pathophysiological principle underlying hepatic arterial chemoembolization is that a malignant tumor possesses greater hepatic arterial supply than liver parenchyma. Therefore, cytotoxic agents are taken up by the tumor to a greater extent than by the liver [114]. Complete response is evident early (within 1 month) following chemoembolization by the demonstration of a lack of enhancing tumor foci. Changes on T2-weighted images depend on the fluid content of the lesions, which is diminished following successful treatment because the therapy is directed at inflowing blood and results in ischemic necrosis. Successfully treated lesions enhance negligibly on immediate postgadolinium SGE images (Fig.

2.75). In a previous report [104], 27 tumors treated with chemoembolization were low in signal on T2-weighted and postgadolinium T1-weighted images. All of these tumors were necrotic at biopsy. Partial response appears as a decrease in tumor size; with residual tumor showing increased signal intensity on T2-weighted images and enhancement on immediate postgadolinium images. Substantial variation does occur, reflecting variation in the degree of response and the time course of healing.

Future Direction

Blood pool contrast agents have been developed recently. One report demonstrated the relationship between contrast enhancement and capillary permeability following liver irradiation, with the implication that the physiological effects of increased capillary permeability

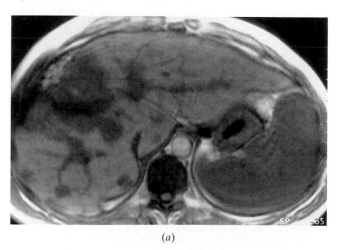

(a)

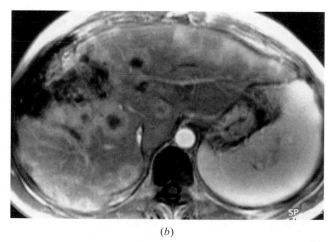

(b)

FIG. 2.75 Liver metastases, before and after chemoembolization. SGE (*a*) and immediate postgadolinium SGE (*b*) images before chemoembolization, and immediate postgadolinium SGE image (*c*) 1 month after chemoembolization. On the pretreatment images (*a,b*), an 8-cm tumor and multiple tumors smaller than 2.5 cm are present throughout the liver. Prominent ring enhancement is present in these tumors (*b*).

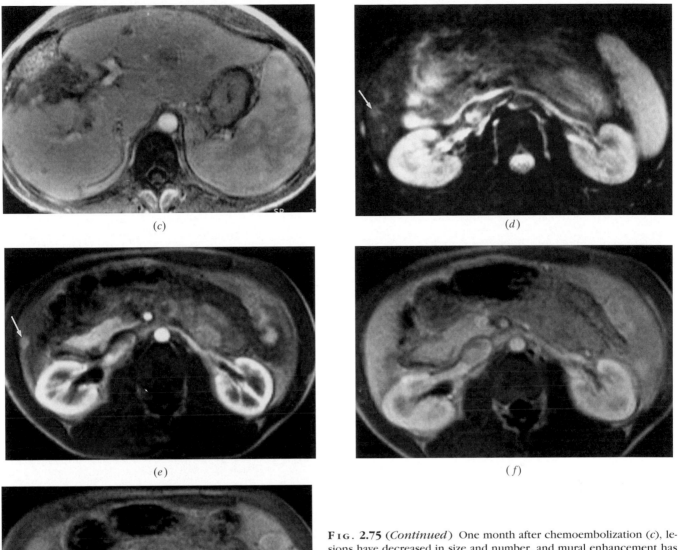

(c)

(d)

(e)

(f)

(g)

FIG. 2.75 (*Continued*) One month after chemoembolization (*c*), lesions have decreased in size and number, and mural enhancement has markedly diminished (*d*). T2-weighted fat-suppressed spin-echo (*d*), immediate (*e*), and 45 second (*f*) postgadolinium SGE images in a second patient before chemoembolization. This patient with recurrent fibrolamellar HCC possesses multiple liver lesions that are modestly high in signal intensity on T2-weighted images (*arrow, c*), show intense uniform enhancement immediately after gadolinium administration (*arrow, d*), and fade rapidly to isointensity with liver by 45 seconds (*e*). Immediate postgadolinium SGE image acquired 1 month after chemoembolization (*g*), shows complete lack of enhancement of the lesion that now has polygonal angular margins (*arrow, g*), consistent with scarring.

may have an impact on the timing of therapeutic regimens [115].

Summary

The evaluation of treatment response of malignant liver lesions using MRI is potentially an important future application. Immediate postgadolinium SGE is particularly effective at demonstrating response, presumably because it reflects changes in tumor angiogenesis and demonstrates patterns of granulation tissue enhancement that vary with age. Further investigation is required to evaluate the time course of response to intervention and patterns of response.

DIFFUSE LIVER PARENCHYMAL DISEASE

Cirrhosis

Cirrhosis results in irreversible hepatic fibrosis that bridges the spaces between portal tracts and destroys underlying hepatic architecture [123]. The most common underlying causes in North America include alcoholism, viral hepatitis, and idiopathic hemochromatosis. Fibrosis and occasionally mild iron deposition occur in cirrhotic livers, which decrease hepatic signal intensity on T1- and T2-weighted images. Many cirrhotic livers contain regions of low signal intensity on T1-weighted images and high signal intensity on T2-weighted images secondary to hepatocellular damage, inflammation, or both [124,125]. Tiny peribiliary cysts also occur in cirrhotic livers [126–128].

Regenerative nodules result from grossly distorted hepatic architecture and heterogeneous regeneration. In the presence of hepatocellular dysplasia they are identified as dysplastic nodules of low or high grade according to the recent classification system for nodular hepatocellular lesions by the International Working Party [26]. At present, there are no reports that describe distinguishing features between regenerative and dysplastic nodules on imaging studies. MRI demonstrates regenerative nodules with greater conspicuity than that shown by other imaging modalities. On T2-weighted images, regenerative nodules are low in signal intensity relative to high signal intensity inflammatory fibrous septa or damaged liver [129]. Approximately 25 percent of regenerative nodules accumulate iron more than the surrounding hepatic parenchyma, facilitating their identification as low in signal on T2-weighted spin-echo images and T2*-weighted gradient-echo images [130]. Regenerative nodules are particularly well-shown on early postgadolinium SGE images as low-signal foci because hepatic parenchyma enhances greater than iron-containing nodules (Fig. 2.76). Irregular linear high-signal abnormalities may be observed on T2-weighted images in cirrhotic livers [131]. These represent bands of fibrous tissue and exhibit a characteristic enhancement pattern on serial postgadolinium SGE images: minimal enhancement on immediate postgadolinium images, and delayed increased enhancement (Fig. 2.77).

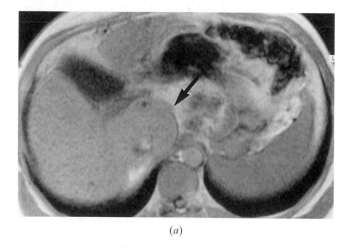

(a)

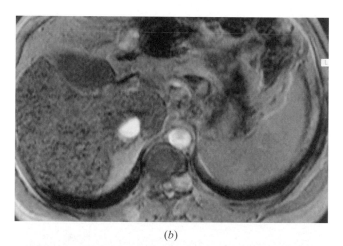

(b)

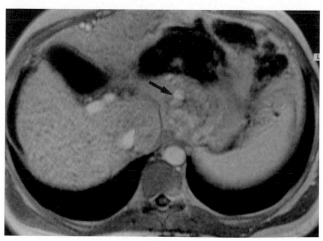

(c)

FIG. 2.76 Cirrhosis with regenerative nodules. SGE (*a*), SGE with longer echo time (*b*), and 45-second postgadolinium SGE (*c*) images. Multiple small low-signal-intensity regenerative nodules are identified on the SGE image (*a*). The presence of iron in these nodules results in susceptibility artifact and increased conspicuity using a longer TE sequence (*b*). Nodules enhance negligibly on early postgadolinium images (*c*) and are rendered conspicuous due to greater enhancement of background liver (*c*). Varies along the lesser curvature are well-shown on portal-phase postcontrast images (*arrow, c*). Enlargement of the caudate lobe (*arrow, a*) is also appreciated.

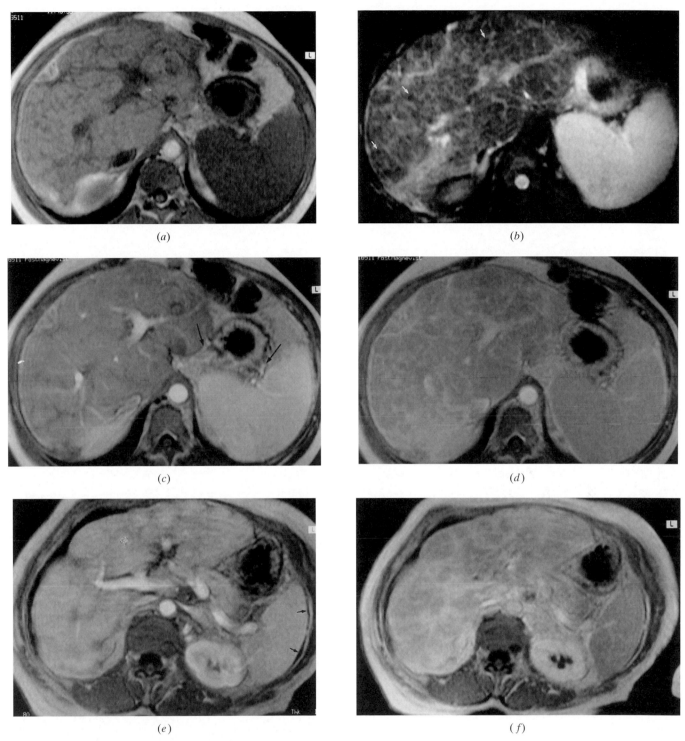

FIG. 2.77 Cirrhosis with regenerative nodules and fibrosis. SGE (*a*), T2-weighted fat-suppressed spin-echo (*b*), immediate (*c*), and 10-minute (*d*) postgadolinium SGE images. The SGE image (*a*) demonstrates irregular hepatic contour and contains prominent low-signal-intensity reticular markings that represent fibrous cirrhosis. On the T2-weighted image (*b*), the liver is mildly low in signal intensity and the linear fibrosis is moderately high in signal intensity. Low-signal-intensity regenerative nodules are also identified (*arrows, b*). On the immediate postgadolinium image (*c*), the liver enhances relatively homogeneously with minimal enhancement of the fibrotic tissue. On the 10-minute post contrast image (*d*), the reticular fibrotic markings have become hyperintense relative to background liver. The spleen is noted to be enlarged, and varices are identified on the immediate postgadolinium image along the lesser and greater curvatures of the stomach (*arrows, c*). Immediate (*e*) and 10 minute (*f*) postgadolinium SGE images in a second patient with cirrhosis and prominent fibrotic tissue. On the immediate postgadolinium image (*e*), fibrotic tissue enhances substantially less than background liver and appears low in signal intensity. Fibrotic tissue demonstrates delayed enhancement greater than background liver on the 10-minute postcontrast image (*f*). Ascites is present that appears nearly signal-void on these post contrast T1-weighted images (*e,f*) with a moderate volume of ascites present along the liver capsule, and a thin layer of ascites identified along the splenic capsule (*arrows, e*).

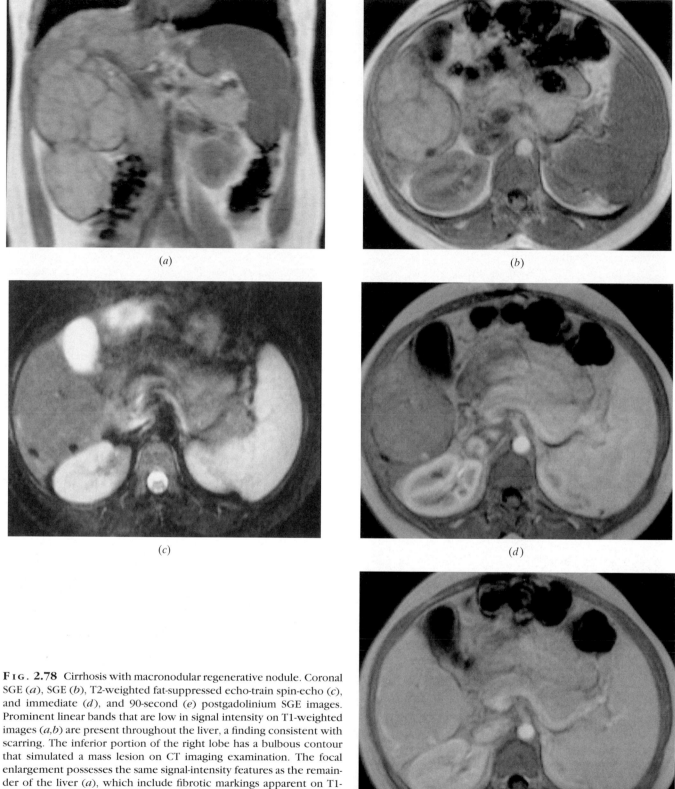

(a)

(b)

(c)

(d)

(e)

FIG. 2.78 Cirrhosis with macronodular regenerative nodule. Coronal SGE (*a*), SGE (*b*), T2-weighted fat-suppressed echo-train spin-echo (*c*), and immediate (*d*), and 90-second (*e*) postgadolinium SGE images. Prominent linear bands that are low in signal intensity on T1-weighted images (*a,b*) are present throughout the liver, a finding consistent with scarring. The inferior portion of the right lobe has a bulbous contour that simulated a mass lesion on CT imaging examination. The focal enlargement possesses the same signal-intensity features as the remainder of the liver (*a*), which include fibrotic markings apparent on T1-weighted images (*a*), homogeneous intermediate signal intensity on the T2-weighted image (*c*), early diminished enhancement of scar tissue (*d*), and more uniform enhancement on the 90-second images (*e*).

Atrophy of the right lobe and the medial segment of the left lobe is most severe in cirrhotic livers. Relative sparing of the caudate lobe and lateral segment of the left lobe are often present, and these segments may undergo hypertrophy. The combination of scarring, atrophy, and regeneration may involve any segment of the liver and result in a bizarre hepatic contour that can simulate tumor mass (Fig. 2.78). Often the hypertrophic region in the liver possesses imaging and enhancement features comparable to those in the remainder of the liver, thus aiding the correct diagnosis.

Portal hypertension results from obstruction at presinusoidal (e.g., portal vein), sinusoidal (e.g., cirrhosis), postsinusoidal (e.g., hepatic vein), or multiple levels [132]. The most common cause of portal hypertension is cirrhosis. Portal hypertension causes or exacerbates complications of cirrhosis such as variceal bleeding, ascites, and splenomegaly. Portosystemic shunts may be identified using 2D time-of-flight techniques or gadolinium-enhanced SGE sequences. Gadolinium-enhanced 3D SGE imaging, alone or with fat suppression, is a particularly effective technique. Direction of flow may be determined by using 2D phase-contrast techniques, or directional information may be derived by observing time-of-flight effects in the main portal vein and correlating it with time-of-flight effects in the aorta and inferior vena cava (IVC). The latter technique is best performed by acquiring superior and inferior multislice slabs, the bottom and top respectively, of the two slabs obtained at the level of the porta hepatis.

In the early stages of portal hypertension, the portal venous system dilates, but flow is maintained. Later, substantial portosystemic shunting develops, reducing the volume of flow to the liver and decreasing the size of the portal vein. With advanced portal hypertension, portal flow may reverse and become hepatofugal. Thrombosis of the portal veins may develop with development of collaterals referred to as cavernous transformation (Fig. 2.79).

Portal varices arise from increased portal pressure, and portal blood is shunted into systemic veins, bypassing hepatic parenchyma. Nutrients absorbed from the gastrointestinal (GI) tract are metabolized less effectively, and hepatic function decreases. Toxic metabolites, such as ammonia, accumulate in the blood and result in clinical manifestations such as hepatic encephalopathy. Diminished portal flow to the liver parenchyma is a major factor in the production of liver atrophy and prevention of regeneration [133], and portosystemic shunting may play a role in the development of hepatic atrophy in advanced cirrhosis. Esophageal varices are a serious complication because they may rupture and produce life-threatening hemorrhage. Flow-sensitive gradient-echo or gadolinium-enhanced SGE images are very effective at demonstrating varices as high-signal tubular structures (Fig. 2.80). Varices are particularly conspicuous using fat-suppression SGE as the competing high signal intensity of fat is removed. These sequences are more sensitive than contrast angiography, endoscopy, or contrast-enhanced CT imaging for detecting varices [134].

Acute disease processes, such as hepatitis, may be superimposed on cirrhosis. Acute inflammation or acute vascular disturbance may be shown as areas of transient patchy enhancement on immediate postgadolinium SGE images (Fig. 2.81).

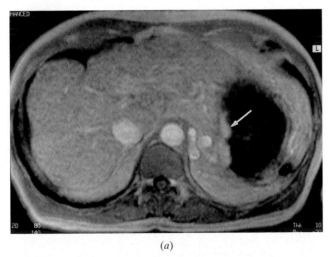
(a)

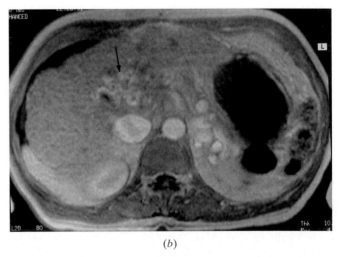
(b)

F IG. 2.79 Cirrhosis, varices. Forty-five-second postgadolinium SGE images (*a,b*) demonstrate a cirrhotic liver with irregular contour and multiple low-signal-intensity regenerative nodules smaller than 5 mm. Prominent varices are present along the lesser curvature, which are well-shown on the portal-phase postgadolinium images. Multiple small serpiginous enhancing structures are present in the porta hepatis (*arrow, b*) that reflect cavernous transformation of the portal vein. A prominent varix is also present within the gastric wall along the lesser curvature (*arrow, a*). Signal-void ascites is also present (*a,b*).

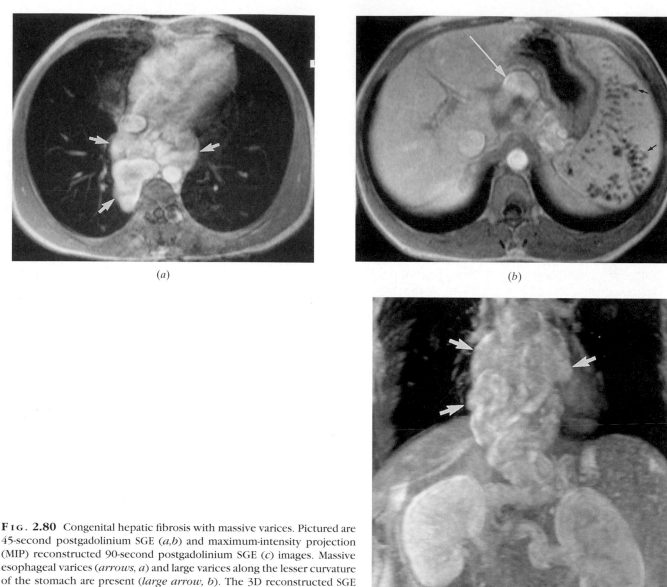

(a)

(b)

(c)

FIG. 2.80 Congenital hepatic fibrosis with massive varices. Pictured are 45-second postgadolinium SGE (*a,b*) and maximum-intensity projection (MIP) reconstructed 90-second postgadolinium SGE (*c*) images. Massive esophageal varices (*arrows, a*) and large varices along the lesser curvature of the stomach are present (*large arrow, b*). The 3D reconstructed SGE images demonstrate the craniocaudal extent of esophageal varices (*arrows, c*). Gamna-Gandy bodies are present in the spleen (*small arrows, b*).

Iron Overload

Iron is deposited in the liver by several mechanisms. Iron overload within tissues reduces T2 and T2* relaxation times substantially. MRI is sensitive and specific for iron overload and for its regional distribution [135]. Because normal liver is more intense than skeletal muscle on virtually all pulse sequences and skeletal muscle is unaffected by iron overload, skeletal muscle is a reliable internal reference tissue for detecting and quantifying decreased hepatic signal intensity [136]. If images with sufficiently short echo times are obtained, estimation of T2 relaxation time may help quantify iron overload, providing a useful parameter for monitoring the response to therapeutic phlebotomy or chelation [137–139]. Condi-

tions associated with increased hepatic iron, and therefore with decreased hepatic signal intensity, include idiopathic (primary) hemochromatosis, transfusional iron overload, hemolytic anemia, and cirrhosis.

Idiopathic Hemochromatosis. Idiopathic hemochromatosis results from increased gastrointestinal absorption and parenchymal deposition of dietary iron [140]. Iron accumulates in the liver, pancreas, heart, and other organs. Causes of death in these patients include cirrhosis, hepatocellular carcinoma, diabetes mellitus and congestive cardiomyopathy. Early in the disease process, iron accumulation is restricted to the liver (Fig. 2.82) [141]. Disease detection at this stage, with institution of

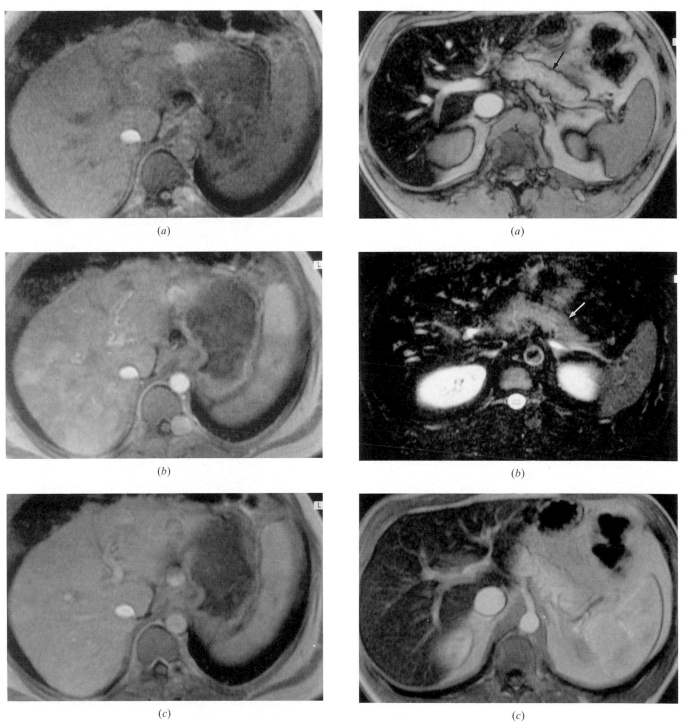

(a)

(b)

(c)

(a)

(b)

(c)

FIG. 2.81 Cirrhosis, transient early enhancement. SGE (*a*), immediate (*b*), and 45-second (*c*) postgadolinium SGE images. Normal signal intensity of the liver is present on the T1-weighted image (*a*). Ill-defined, regions of blotchy enhancement smaller than 2 cm are present on the immediate postgadolinium image (*b*), which resolve by 45 seconds (*c*). The presence of enhancing tissue immediately after contrast raises the concern of HCC in a cirrhotic patient. Diffuse HCC usually results in a mottled enhancement pattern with smaller foci of enhancing tissue. However, this cannot be definitively excluded on the basis of this study. The underlying cause for this appearance is an associated vascular abnormality that may occur in the setting of superimposed acute hepatitis.

FIG. 2.82 Idiopathic hemochromatosis, early disease. Out-of-phase SGE (*a*), T2-weighted echo train spin-echo (*b*), and immediate postgadolinium SGE (*c*) images. The liver is low in signal intensity on noncontrast T1-weighted (*a*) and T2-weighted (*b*) images consistent with substantial iron deposition. The spleen is relatively normal in signal intensity on these sequences reflecting that iron is not in the RES but in hepatocytes. The pancreas (*arrow a,b*) is normal in signal intensity on noncontrast images and enhances normally with gadolinium. Iron deposition limited to the liver is consistent with early precirrhotic disease.

phlebotomy therapy, may result in a normal life expectancy. Over time, iron deposition progresses to involve other organs, primarily the pancreas and heart. In advanced disease, decreased signal intensity of the liver and pancreas occurs, with persistence of normal signal intensity of the spleen on T2-weighted and T2*-weighted images (Fig. 2.83). The presence of iron deposition in the pancreas correlates with irreversible changes of cirrhosis in the liver.

Some patients who present with HCC have previously unsuspected hemochromatosis [135]. Because tumor cells do not contain excess iron [142,143] they are well-shown as high-signal-intensity masses relative to iron-overloaded liver on MR images. In a patient with hemochromatosis, nonsiderotic nodules that are not hemangiomas or cysts should be considered as HCC because regenerative nodules in these patients contain iron. Dysplastic nodules in patients with increased hepatic iron may contain a differing concentration of iron than surrounding hepatic parenchyma.

Transfusional iron overload. Transfusional iron overload is the most common form of excess iron deposition in North America. Iron deposition in the reticuloendothelial system (RES) results in low signal intensity of the spleen, liver, and bone marrow on MR images best shown on T2- or T2*-weighted images.

Iron overload from multiple transfusions is distinguished from idiopathic hemochromatosis by the observation that iron accumulates primarily within reticuloen-

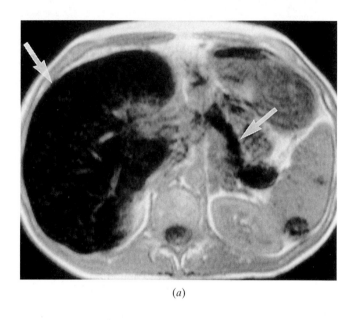

(a)

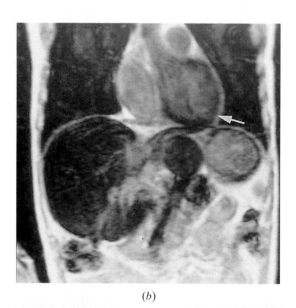

(b)

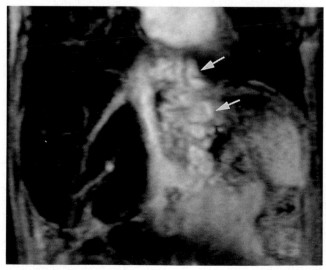

(c)

F IG . 2.83 Idiopathic hemochromatosis, advanced disease. SGE (*a*), coronal SGE (*b*), and coronal 45-second postgadolinium SGE (*c*) images. The precontrast T1-weighted image (*a*) demonstrates signal-void liver and pancreas (*arrows, a*). The coronal SGE image (*b*) also demonstrates low-signal-intensity left ventricular myocardium (*arrow, b*). On the 45-second postgadolinium image (*c*) a clear definition of multiple enhanced varices is shown (*arrows, c*), which is compatible with portal hypertension secondary to cirrhosis.

dothelial cells of the liver and spleen in transfusional iron overload, sparing hepatocytes, pancreas, and other parenchyma. In mild forms of transfusional siderosis signal loss is appreciated only on T2- and T2*-weighted images, and signal intensity on T1-weighted images appears relatively normal (Fig. 2.84). In moderate to severe forms of iron deposition the T2-shortening effect of iron is so great that it results in low signal on T1-weighted images as well (Fig. 2.85). In massive iron overload (e.g., greater than 100 units) direct tissue deposition may occur in other cells and tissues (Fig. 2.86) [135,141]. Transfusional overload is usually distinguishable from idiopathic hemochromatosis by the evaluation of pancreatic and splenic signal intensity. Signal intensity of the spleen is usually normal with idiopathic hemochromatosis, wheras signal intensity of the pancreas is normal with most cases of transfusional overload. This distinction has clinical importance because reticuloendothelial iron is less toxic than hepatocellular iron overload.

Hemolytic Anemia.
Hepatic signal intensity in patients with hemolytic anemia varies, based on the rate of reincorporation of iron into the bone marrow, the rate of absorption of oral iron, and the transfusional history. Patients with thalassemia vera have increased absorption of oral iron and in the absence of blood transfusions will develop erythrogenic hemochromatosis primarily affecting the liver [144]. The appearance is generally indistinguishable from idiopathic hemochromatosis. Patients with heterozygous forms of hemolytic anemias may not have low enough red blood cell counts or hemoglobin levels to necessitate transfusion, and may therefore de-

velop this pattern of iron overload (Fig. 2.87). The majority of patients have received blood transfusions and therefore also develop coexisting transfusional iron overload (Fig. 2.88). Patients with sickle cell anemia have rapid turnover of hepatic iron, and will have normal hepatic signal intensity unless they have undergone recent blood transfusions [144]. Renal cortical signal intensity may be decreased due to filtration and tubular absorption of free hemoglobin, the severity of which is not dependent on transfusional history [141]. Iron overload in the liver and renal cortex is typically seen in patients with paroxysmal nocturnal hemoglobinuria [135].

Cirrhosis.
Hepatocellular iron is not uncommonly increased mildly in patients with cirrhosis, particularly those with cirrhosis secondary to ethanol abuse. The degree of signal loss of the liver is not as great as that seen with idiopathic hemochromatosis or transfusional siderosis.

Coexisting fat and iron deposition.
Fat and iron deposition may occur concurrently within the liver. Coexisting fat and iron deposition may be demonstrated by using gradient-echo MR images with multiple echo times. In the presence of iron, signal intensity of the liver will decrease steadily as echo time increases due to T2* effects. At out-of-phase echo times both higher than and lower than the echo time for in-phase images, a disproportionate drop of liver signal intensity will occur relative to spleen due to fat-water phase cancellation. The combined observations that liver and spleen are nearly signal-void on T2-weighted images, which reflects iron deposi-

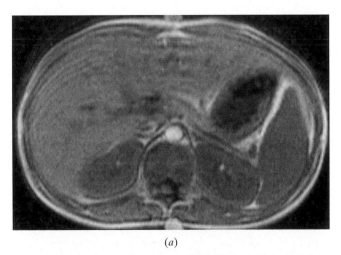

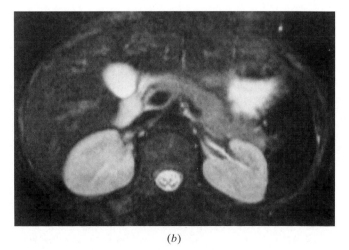

(a)   (b)

FIG. 2.84 Transfusional siderosis, mild. SGE (*a*) and T2-weighted fat-suppressed echo-train spin-echo (*b*) images. Signal intensity of the liver, spleen, and pancreas appears normal on the T1-weighted image (*a*). On the T2-weighted image (*b*), the liver and spleen are low in signal intensity and the pancreas is normal in signal intensity. Iron deposition in the liver and spleen that results in signal loss appreciated only on T2-weighted images and not on T1-weighted images is compatible with mild transfusional siderosis.

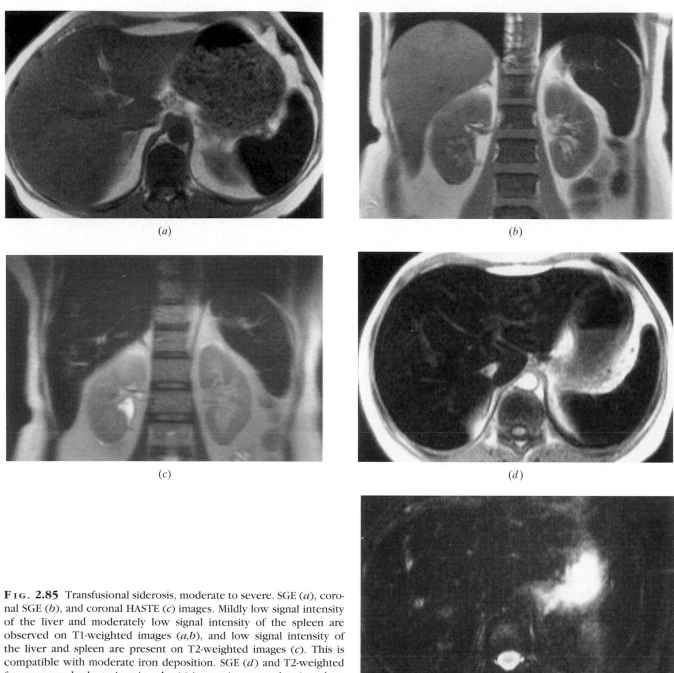

(a) *(b)* *(c)* *(d)* *(e)*

FIG. 2.85 Transfusional siderosis, moderate to severe. SGE (*a*), coronal SGE (*b*), and coronal HASTE (*c*) images. Mildly low signal intensity of the liver and moderately low signal intensity of the spleen are observed on T1-weighted images (*a,b*), and low signal intensity of the liver and spleen are present on T2-weighted images (*c*). This is compatible with moderate iron deposition. SGE (*d*) and T2-weighted fat-suppressed echo-train spin-echo (*e*) images in a second patient demonstrate very low signal intensity of the liver and spleen on T1- and T2-weighted images consistent with severe iron deposition.

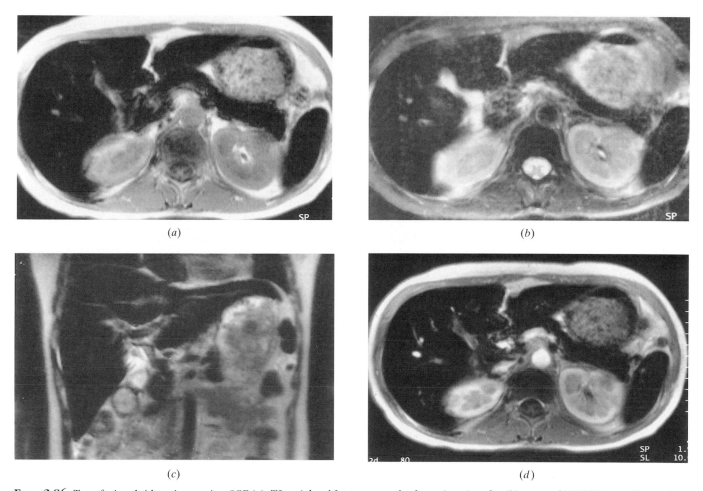

(a)

(b)

(c)

(d)

F I G. 2.86 Transfusional siderosis, massive. SGE (*a*), T2-weighted fat-suppressed echo-train spin-echo (*b*), coronal HASTE (*c*), and immediate postgadolinium SGE (*d*) images. Massive iron deposition is present in the liver, spleen and pancreas (*a–c*), demonstrated by signal-void liver, spleen, and pancreas. Blooming artifact is apparent surrounding the pancreas (*a*). These organs remain signal-void after gadolinium administration (*d*).

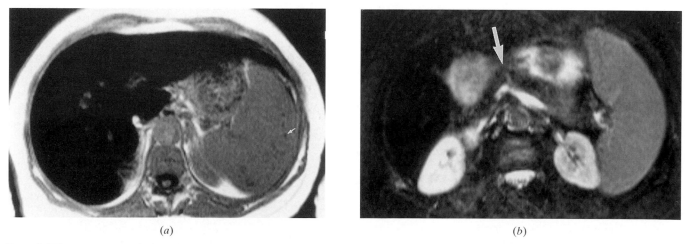

(a)

(b)

F I G. 2.87 Heterozygous thalassemia. SGE (*a*), T2-weighted fat-suppressed spin-echo (*b*), 45-second (*c*), and 90-second (*d*) postgadolinium SGE images. The liver demonstrates severe iron deposition and is signal-void on T1- (*a*) and T2-weighted (*b*) images. The spleen is greatly enlarged and shows negligible iron deposition, but does contain Gamna-Gandy bodies (*arrow, a*). The pancreas is modestly low in signal intensity (*arrow, b*).

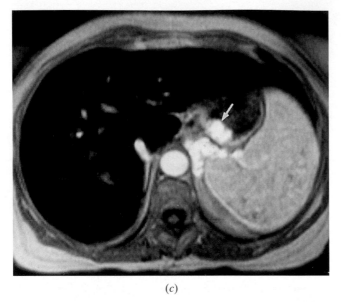

(c)

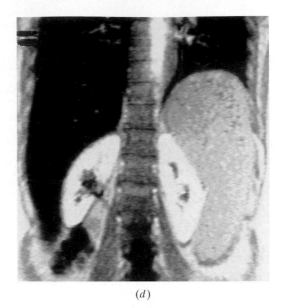

(d)

F IG . 2.87 (*Continued*) Varices along the lesser curvature and within the gastric wall (*arrow, c*) are clearly shown on the 45-second postgadolinium images. Splenomegaly (*d*), Gamma-Gandy bodies and varices are secondary to portal hypertension. The pattern of iron deposition reflects increased intestinal absorption without transfusional siderosis, which is a common appearance for heterozygous hemolytic anemias that do not require blood transfusion.

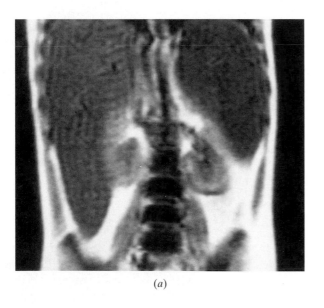

(a)

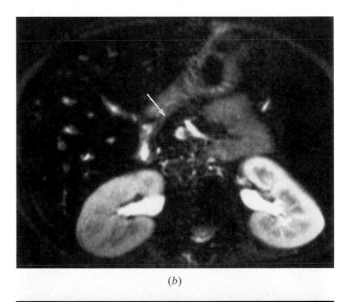

(b)

F IG . 2.88 Alpha thalassemia. Coronal SGE (*a*) and T2-weighted fat-suppressed echo-train spin-echo (*b*) images. Enlargement of the liver and spleen are apparent on the T1-weighted image (*a*). These organs are also lower in signal intensity than psoas muscle on the T1- and T2-weighted images consistent with severe iron deposition in the RES. Vertebral bodies are nearly signal-void, which also reflects RES iron deposition. The pancreas is nearly signal-void (*arrow, b*), reflecting coexistent iron deposition into tissues. SGE image (*c*) through the pelvis shows nearly signal-void pelvic bones secondary to iron deposition.

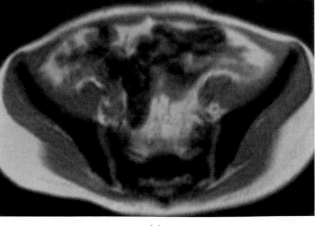

(c)

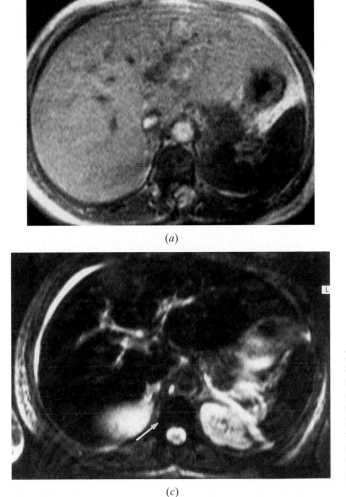

(a)

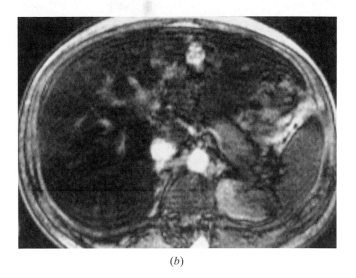

(b)

(c)

FIG. 2.89 Coexistent iron and fatty deposition. SGE (*a*), out-of-phase SGE (*b*), and T2-weighted fat-suppressed spin-echo (*c*) images. On the in-phase T1-weighted image (*a*), the liver and spleen have a normal signal intensity pattern, with the liver higher in signal intensity than the spleen. On the longer-echo-time out-of-phase SGE image (*b*), the liver drops in signal intensity below that of spleen, which is consistent with fatty infiltration. On the T2-weighted image (*c*), the liver, spleen, and bone marrow (*arrow, c*) are nearly signal-void, which is consistent with coexistent iron deposition. Ascites is well-shown as high-signal-intensity fluid along the liver margin on the T2-weighted image (*c*).

tion, and that liver drops in signal intensity relative to spleen comparing out-of-phase to in-phase SGE images, which reflects fat deposition, is also diagnostic for coexistent iron and fat deposition (Fig. 2.89).

Fatty Liver

Fat (primarily triglyceride) may accumulate within hepatocytes in patients with a variety of conditions, including diabetes mellitus, obesity, and malnutrition, or following exposure to ethanol or other chemical toxins. Fatty change may be uniform, patchy, focal, or spare foci of normal liver. At times focal fatty infiltration or focal regions of normal liver within fatty liver may mimic the appearance of mass lesions.

Fatty liver may interfere with the detection of focal liver masses on CT images or sonography [144,146]. MRI is particularly effective in evaluating the liver of patients with fatty liver for the presence of focal lesions such as metastases. In this setting, nonfat-suppressed T1-weighted images and fat-suppressed T2-weighted images are useful to maximize the contrast between the liver

and lesions. On nonfat-suppressed T1-weighted images, the liver may be higher in signal intensity than normal liver, maximizing the contrast with low-signal-intensity masses, whereas on fat-suppressed T2-weighted images fatty liver is lower in signal intensity than normal liver, maximizing the contrast with moderately high-signal-intensity masses.

Out-of-phase SGE imaging is a highly accurate technique to examine for the presence of fatty liver, particularly in the circumstance of distinguishing focal fat from neoplastic masses [147,148]. Demonstration that a lesion, which is isointense or hyperintense to liver on in-phase SGE images, loses signal homogeneously on out-of-phase images, is highly diagnostic for focal fat (Fig. 2.90). Focal normal liver in the setting of diffuse fatty infiltration of the liver is shown by a focus of high signal intensity in a background of diminished liver on out-of-phase images (Fig. 2.91).

The morphology of focal fatty infiltration permits distinction from fat within tumors such as HCC, adenoma, regenerative nodule, angiomyolipoma, or lipoma. Al-

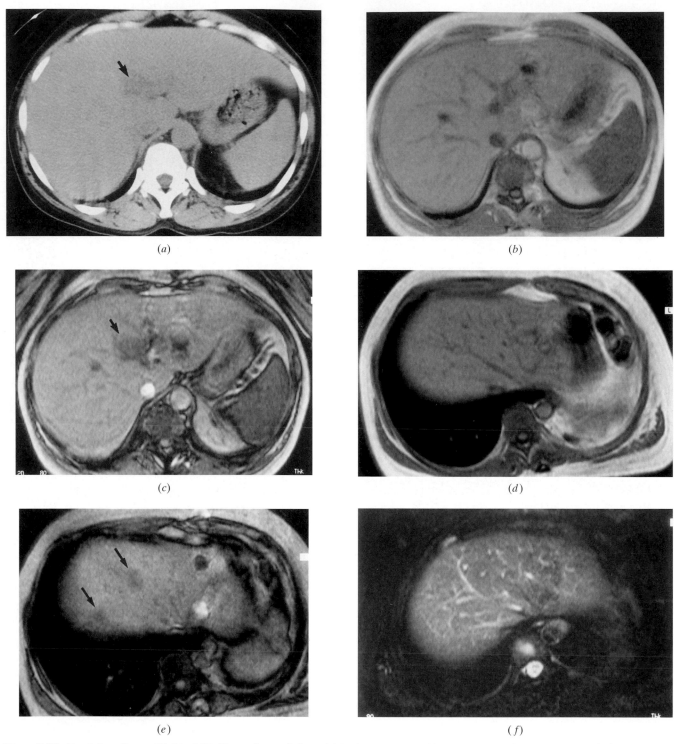

(a)

(b)

(c)

(d)

(e)

(f)

F IG . 2.90 Focal fatty liver. CT (*a*), SGE (*b*), and out-of-phase SGE (*c*) images. A CT image acquired in a patient with breast cancer demonstrates a low-density lesion in the medial segment (*arrow, a*). The in-phase T1-weighted image (*b*) shows no lesion in this location, whereas on the out-of-phase image (*c*), signal drop occurs in the central region of the medial segment (*arrow, c*), which is diagnostic for focal fatty infiltration. SGE (*d*), out-of-phase SGE (*e*) and T2-weighted fat-suppressed echo-train spin-echo (*f*) images in a second patient. Previous ultrasound study in this young boy with acute myelogeneous leukemia demonstrated two liver lesions. No liver lesions are apparent on the in-phase T1-weighted image (*d*). On the out-of-phase image (*e*), two focal low-signal rounded masses are apparent (*arrows, e*). The T2-weighted image (*f*) does not reveal any lesions. No tumor blush was apparent on immediate postgadolinium images (not shown). Identification of lesions only on out-of-phase SGE images is diagnostic for fatty infiltration.

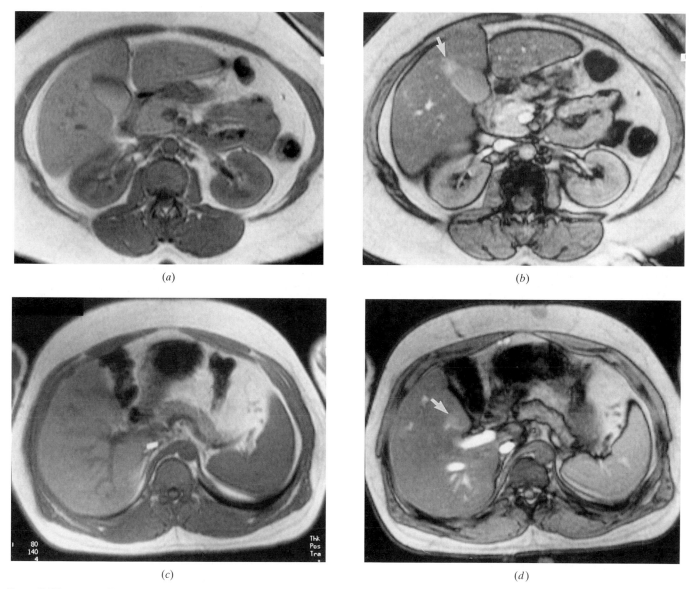

(a)

(b)

(c)

(d)

FIG. 2.91 Fatty infiltration with focal sparing. SGE (*a*) and out-of-phase SGE (*b*) images. Homogeneous signal of the liver is present on the T1-weighted image (*a*). On the out-of-phase SGE image (*b*) the liver drops in signal with a focus of higher signal liver adjacent to the gallbladder (*arrow, b*) representing focal normal liver. SGE (*c*) and out-of-phase SGE (*d*) images in a second patient. The liver is normal in signal intensity on the in-phase image (*c*). On the out-of-phase image (*d*), the liver drops in signal intensity relative to the spleen, with focal sparing present on the tip of the medial segment (*arrow, d*).

though some well-differentiated HCCs contain lipid, most HCCs with high signal intensity on T1-weighted images do not [149]. Hemorrhage, melanin, copper, and protein may be associated with nonfatty masses with high signal intensity on T1-weighted images. Out-of-phase images distinguishes between these tumors and lipid-containing masses or focal fatty infiltration. HCC that contains lipid tends to be better defined than focal fatty infiltration, is often encapsulated, is most commonly not homogeneously fatty, and usually contains some elements with high signal intensity on fat-suppressed T2-weighted im-

ages. Hepatic adenoma may most closely resemble focal fatty infiltration of all focal hepatic lesions since this tumor may have relatively uniform fat content. Demonstration of a capillary blush on immediate postgadolinium SGE images establishes the diagnosis of adenoma. Angiomyolipoma and lipoma may be virtually composed of fat and therefore not drop in signal intensity on out-of-phase images, but will demonstrate a phase-cancellation artifact at the boundary with water-containing liver tissue. These tumors will lose signal when fat-suppression techniques are used.

HEPATIC VASCULAR DISORDERS

Portal Venous Thrombosis

Portal vein thrombosis may be demonstrated by using black-blood techniques (e.g., spin-echo techniques with superior and inferior saturation pulses) and bright-blood techniques (e.g., time-of-flight gradient-echo or gadolinium-enhanced SGE). A combination of both approaches is often useful to increase diagnostic confidence. Portal veins may be occluded by tumor thrombus, bland thrombus, or extrinsic compression. MRI usually is able to distinguish between these entities. Tumor and bland thrombus may be distinguished from each other by the observation that tumor thrombus is higher in signal intensity on T2-weighted images, is soft-tissue signal intensity on time-of-flight gradient-echo images, and enhances with gadolinium (Fig. 2.92). In comparison, bland thrombus is low in signal intensity on T2-weighted and time-of-flight gradient-echo images, and does not enhance with gadolinium (Fig. 2.93). Tumor thrombus is most commonly caused by hepatocellular carcinoma, although it may also occur with metastases. Bland thrombus may be observed in the setting of cirrhosis and various inflammatory/infectious processes involving organs in the portal circulation, with pancreatitis being the most common disease process. Increased enhancement of the vein wall is appreciated in the setting of infected bland thrombus.

Extrinsic compression of portal veins is most commonly caused by malignant tumors, but may occur with benign tumors such as hemangiomas. Cholangiocarcinoma, in particular, has a propensity to cause extrinsic compression and obstruction of portal veins. Lobar or segmental portal vein obstruction caused by tumor may result in discrete wedge-shaped regions of increased signal intensity on T2-weighted images and on immediate postgadolinium SGE images [147,150–154]. Increased signal intensity on T2-weighted images may reflect some degree of hepatocellular injury. Decreased blood supply results in decreased size of hepatocytes, which increases the proportion of liver volume occupied by the vascular and interstitial spaces. Obstruction of the portal vein may also cause atrophy, with compensatory hypertrophy of other segments [147,150]. Collateral periportal veins may maintain portal perfusion when the main portal vein is thrombosed. In time, this network of collateral venous channels dilates and the thrombosed portal vein retracts, producing cavernous transformation [155,156].

After administration of intravenous gadolinium, transient increased enhancement of hepatic parenchyma may be apparent in areas with decreased portal perfusion during the capillary phase of enhancement (see Figs. 2.92, and 2.93) [68,157]. A recent report found exact correlation between perfusion defects on CTAP with regions of transient high signal intensity on immediate postgadolinium SGE images in eight patients (Fig. 2.94) [157]. These findings showed that regions with absent or diminished portal venous supply received increased hepatic arterial supply. This paradoxical increased enhancement of hepatic parenchyma distal to an obstructed portal vein branch largely reflects increased hepatic arterial supply due to an autoregulatory mechanism. Segments with obstructed portal venous supply and increased hepatic arterial supply enhance intensely because gadolinium delivered in the first pass is more concentrated in hepatic

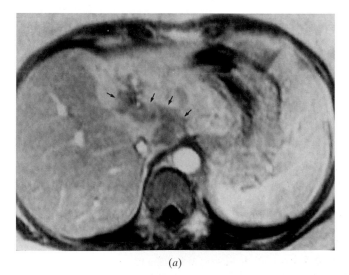

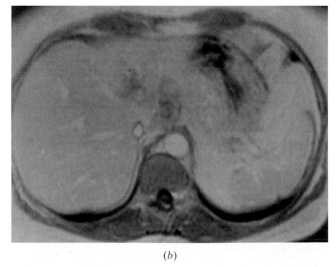

(*a*)   (*b*)

FIG. 2.92 Portal-vein thrombosis, secondary to tumor. Immediate (*a*) and 90-second (*b*) postgadolinium SGE images. A liver metastasis is present in the caudate lobe and the lateral segment with heterogeneously enhancing thrombus extending into the left portal vein (*arrows, a*). On the immediate postgadolinium image (*a*), there is increased enhancement of the left lobe, which equilibrates by 90 seconds (*b*).

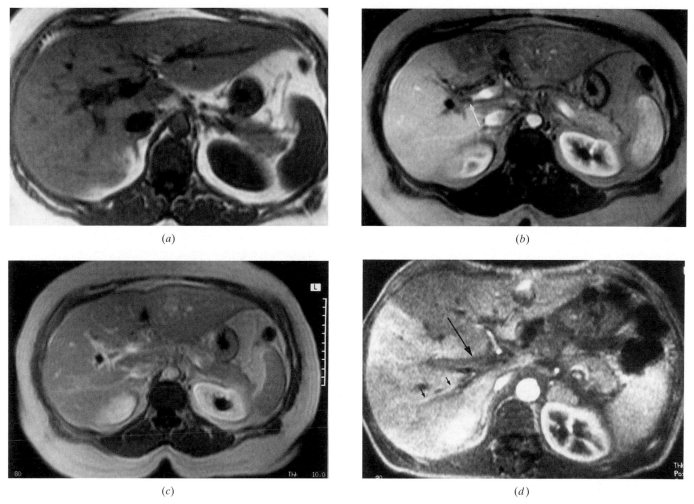

F IG. 2.93 Portal-vein thrombosis, blood thrombus. SGE (*a*), immediate (*b*), and 2-minute (*c*) postgadolinium SGE images in a patient with ascending cholangitis. The SGE image (*a*) demonstrates a normal-signal-intensity liver. On the immediate postgadolinium image (*b*), increased enhancement of the right lobe of the liver is apparent, with signal-void thrombus (*arrow, b*) identified in continuity with the gadolinium-containing high-signal right portal vein. Liver parenchymal enhancement equilibrates by 2 minutes (*c*). Immediate postgadolinium SGE image (*d*) in a second patient with pancreatitis demonstrates transient increased enhancement of the right lobe of the liver. A patent high-signal right hepatic artery is seen (*small arrows, d*); a low-signal-intensity thrombus is present in the right portal vein (*long arrow, d*).

arteries than in portal veins and is delivered earlier by hepatic arteries than by portal veins. In time, concentration of gadolinium in hepatic arteries and portal veins equilibrates, which explains the transient nature of the increased enhancement.

Hepatic Venous Thrombosis

Budd-Chiari Syndrome. The Budd-Chiari syndrome results from obstruction of venous outflow from the liver, resulting in portal hypertension, ascites, and progressive hepatic failure. Hepatic venous outflow often is not completely eliminated since a variety of accessory hepatic veins may drain above or below the site of obstruction. In some cases, obstruction may even be segmental or subsegmental. Although the disease most commonly involves major hepatic veins, demonstration of

patent central hepatic veins may be observed because small or intermediate-sized veins may be occluded in isolation [158]. In the chronic setting, regions with completely obstructed hepatic venous outflow will develop shunting of blood from hepatic veins and arteries to portal veins, producing reversed portal venous flow [153,159–161]. The involved liver parenchyma is thereby deprived of portal vein supply. Hepatic regeneration, hypertrophy, and atrophy depend in part on the degree of portal perfusion [133]. Budd-Chiari syndrome most often results in atrophy of peripheral liver, which experiences severe venous obstruction, and hypertrophy of the caudate lobe and central liver, which are relatively spared.

Absence of hepatic veins may be demonstrated by techniques in which flowing blood is signal-void or by techniques in which flowing blood is high is signal inten-

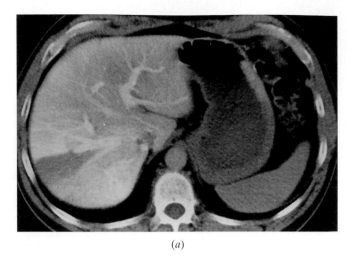

(a)

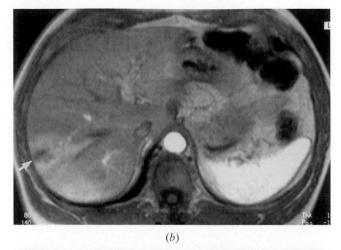

(b)

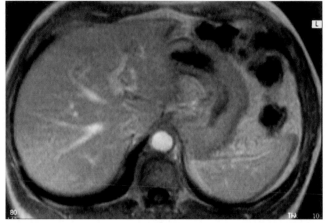

(c)

FIG. 2.94 Perfusional abnormality related to colon cancer liver metastasis. Spiral CTAP (*a*), immediate (*b*), and 90-second (*c*) postgadolinium SGE images. The CTAP image (*a*) demonstrates a wedge-shaped perfusion defect in the right lobe of the liver. On the immediate postgadolinium SGE image (*b*), wedge-shaped increased enhancement is present surrounding a peripheral 2-cm liver metastasis (*arrow, b*). By 90 seconds after gadolinium (*c*), both the perfusion defect and the metastases have equilibrated with liver. (Reproduced with permission from [87].)

sity such as time-of-flight techniques or portal-phase gadolinium-enhanced SGE sequences. Generally, a combination of both approaches results in the highest diagnostic accuracy.

On dynamic gadolinium-enhanced MR images, the peripheral atrophic liver in Budd-Chiari syndrome may enhance to a greater or lesser extent than normal or hypertrophied liver. In acute onset Budd-Chiari syndrome the peripheral liver enhances less than central liver, presumably due to acute increased tissue pressure with resultant diminished blood supply from both hepatic arterial and portal venous systems (Fig. 2.95) [162]. Increased enhancement of peripheral liver may be seen in chronic Budd-Chiari syndrome and may reflect a combination of decreased portal perfusion and dilatation of hepatic sinusoids. The hypertrophied central liver, if less enhanced than the peripheral atrophied liver, may resemble a focal mass. Regional differences in signal intensity due to atrophy, congestion, and/or iron deposition may also be apparent on various MR sequences.

In the chronic setting, hepatic venous obstruction produces hepatic ischemia, which may result in the devel-

opment of nodular regenerative hyperplasia [163,164]. The nodules are usually round and of variable size, having high signal intensity on T1-weighted images and intermediate or low signal intensity on T2-weighted images, similar to that of adenomatous hyperplastic (macroregenerative) nodules (Fig. 2.96) [165]. Nodules tend to possess intense enhancement on immediate postgadolinium SGE images.

Varices are usually prominent in chronic Budd-Chiari syndrome and are well-shown on gadolinium-enhanced SGE images. These vessels tend to be most intensely enhanced on portal-phase images. Extensive portosystemic varices, as observed in other chronic liver diseases, are also present. Curvilinear intrahepatic collaterals and capsular-based collaterals are characteristic of chronic Budd-Chiari syndrome (see Fig. 2.96).

Hepatic Venous Thrombosis Related to Tumor.
Hepatic-vein thrombosis also may occur in the setting of malignant disease. HCC is the cancer most commonly associated with hepatic-vein thrombosis. Tumor thrombosis demonstrates gadolinium enhancement, whereas

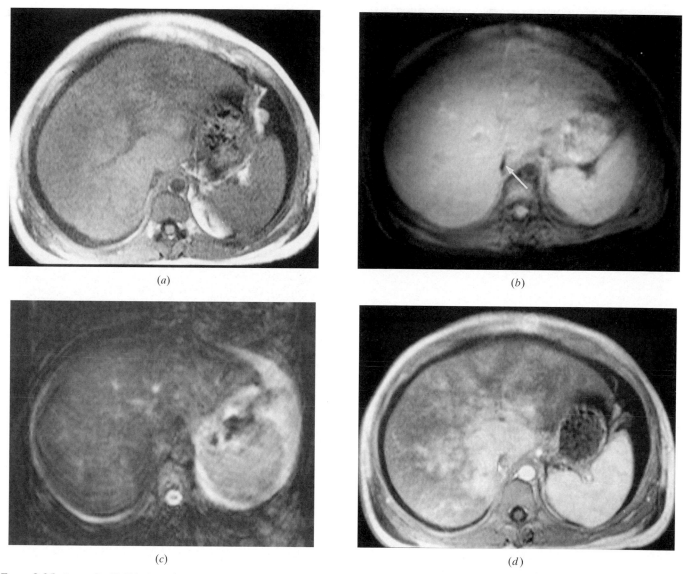

(a) (b)

(c) (d)

F IG. 2.95 Acute Budd-Chiari syndrome. SGE (*a*), proton-density fat-suppressed spin-echo (*b*), T2-weighted fat-suppressed spin-echo (*c*), and immediate postgadolinium SGE (*d*) images. On the precontrast T1-weighted image (*a*), the caudate lobe and central portion of the liver are normal in signal intensity, whereas the peripheral liver is low in signal intensity. The proton-density image (*b*) acquired at the expected level of the hepatic veins demonstrates absence of hepatic veins and a compressed IVC (*arrow, b*). The T2-weighted image (*c*) shows normal signal intensity of the caudate lobe and central liver, and heterogeneous higher signal intensity of the peripheral liver. On the immediate postgadolinium SGE image (*d*), the caudate lobe and central liver enhance intensely, whereas peripheral liver is low in signal intensity. (Reproduced with permission from [162].)

bland thrombus does not enhance. As with the Budd-Chiari syndrome, the degree of enhancement of liver parenchyma that has thrombosed hepatic veins depends on the acuity of the thrombosis. In acute thrombosis involved parenchyma enhances less than surrounding liver. In chronic thrombosis enhancement is more variable and may be increased.

Hepatic Arterial Obstruction

Hepatic arterial obstruction is much less common than either portal venous or hepatic venous obstruction. Hepatic arterial obstruction is most commonly seen in the setting of hepatic transplants. In patients without transplants, embolic occlusion is the most common cause of hepatic arterial compromise. Diminished enhancement of involved hepatic parenchyma is apparent on early postcontrast images.

Preeclampsia-Eclampsia

Preeclampsia may result in the hemolytic anemia, elevated liver function tests, and low platelets (HELLP) syndrome, which may cause peripheral vascular occlusions of the liver or hepatic hematoma [166]. MR images show peripheral wedge-like defects on postgadolinium images

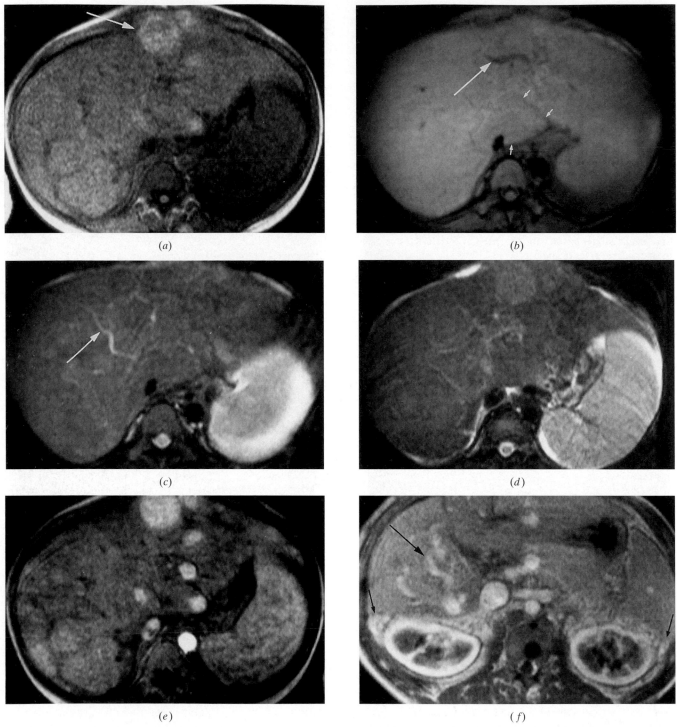

(a)

(b)

(c)

(d)

(e)

(f)

F IG . 2.96 Chronic Budd-Chiari syndrome. SGE (*a*), proton-density fat-suppressed spin-echo (*b*), T2-weighted fat-suppressed spin-echo (*c,d*) and immediate postgadolinium SGE (*e*) images. On T1-weighted images (*a*), multiple well-defined high-signal-intensity mass lesions representing adenomatous hyperplasia are identified, the largest measuring 3.5 cm in diameter (*arrow, a*). The proton-density image at the expected level of the hepatic veins (*b*), demonstrates absence of hepatic veins, with intrahepatic curvilinear venous collaterals in their stead (*arrow, b*). Enlargement of the caudate lobe is shown (*small arrows, b*). The T2-weighted image (*c*) taken from a slightly higher tomographic section demonstrates curvilinear intrahepatic collaterals (*arrow, c*) with absence of hepatic veins. The immediate postgadolinium image (*d*) acquired at the same tomographic level as the precontrast images (*a,d*) shows intense enhancement of the adenomatous hyperplastic nodules, with multiple enhancing nodules apparent that were not visualized on precontrast images. Slight heterogeneity of hepatic enhancement is present. However, the enhancement pattern is distinctly different from that of acute Budd-Chiari syndrome. Immediate postgadolinium SGE image (*f*) in a second patient with chronic Budd-Chiari syndrome. Extensive abdominal collaterals are present (*arrows, f*) including curvilinear intrahepatic collaterals (*long arrow, f*).

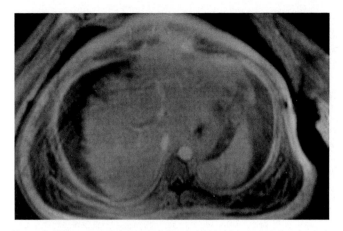

FIG. 2.97 HELLP syndrome. The 45-second postgadolinium SGE image demonstrates an abnormal serrated margin of the liver and massive ascites. Liver changes reflect ischemic injury.

and heterogeneous high signal intensity on T2-weighted images from edema and, in more severe disease, infarction (Fig. 2.97). Hematoma appears as a peripheral fluid collection with signal intensity depending on the age of the blood products, which usually are deoxyhemoglobin or intracellular methemoglobin, reflecting the acuity of the disease process.

Congestive Heart Failure

Patients with congestive heart failure may present with hepatomegaly and hepatic enzyme elevations. On early dynamic contrast-enhanced CT or MR images, the liver may enhance in a mosaic fashion with a reticulated pattern of low-signal-intensity linear markings. By 1 minute past contrast the liver becomes more homogeneous. The suprahepatic IVC is frequently enlarged with enlargement of the hepatic veins. Contrast injected in a brachial vein may appear earlier in the hepatic veins and suprahepatic IVC than in the portal veins and infrahepatic IVC, reflecting reflux of contrast from the heart (Fig. 2.98).

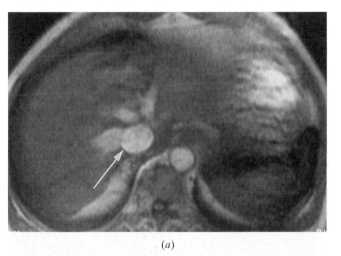

(a)

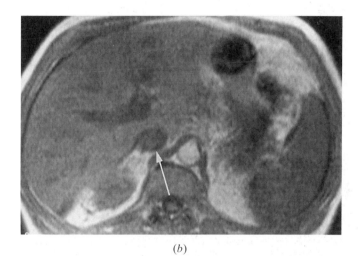

(b)

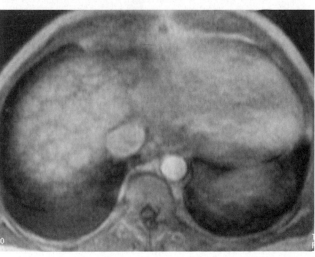

(c)

FIG. 2.98 Mosaic enhancement secondary to congestive heart failure. Immediate (a,b), 45-second (c,d) and 90-second (e) postgadolinium SGE images. The immediate postgadolinium images (a,b) demonstrate the presence of gadolinium early in the arterial phase of enhancement with no enhancement of the abdominal organs due to the low cardiac output state of the patient. Reflux of gadolinium into the dilated suprahepatic IVC and hepatic veins is present (arrow, a) with no contrast present in the infrahepatic IVC (arrow, b).

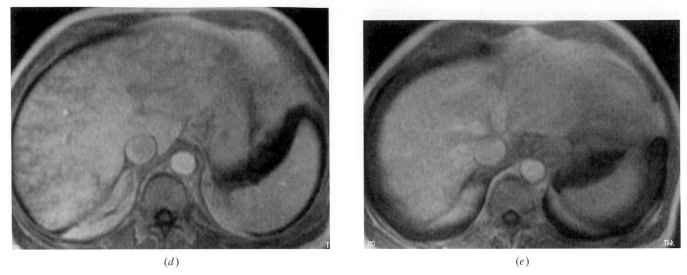

(d)   (e)

FIG. 2.98 (*Continued*) On the 45-second postgadolinium images (*c,d*) a mosaic enhancement pattern is present throughout the liver. This mosaic enhancement resolves on the 90-second postgadolinium image (*e*).

Portal Venous Air

Portal venous air, usually a serious condition associated with bowel ischemia, appears as signal-void foci within distal branches of the portal vein in the nondependent portion of the liver (typically the left lobe) on all imaging sequences. Magnetic susceptibility artifact may also be identified. Air is best appreciated using a combination of high resolution T2-weighted echo train spin-echo and postgadolinium T1-weighted images in which air will be signal-void on both sets of images. The air is most clearly shown on the postcontrast T1-weighted images (Fig.

2.99), and the T2-weighted images confirm the fact that the tubular structures contain signal-void air rather than high-signal fluid.

Air in the Biliary Tree

Air in the biliary tree is usually a relatively benign condition unlike air in portal veins. Air in the biliary tree is less peripheral than air in the portal veins, and is more clearly observed as branching tubular structures conforming to the biliary tree. Air is most commonly observed in the left biliary ducts, reflecting the patient's supine

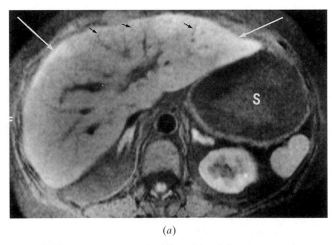
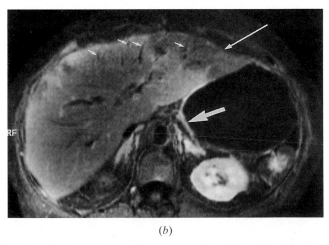

(a)   (b)

FIG. 2.99 Portal venous air. T1-weighted fat-suppressed spin-echo (*a*) and gadolinium-enhanced interstitial-phase T1-weighted fat-suppressed spin-echo (*b*) images. On the precontrast T1-weighted fat-suppressed image (*a*), subtle, linear, signal-void, short, vertically oriented markings are present (*small arrows, a*). Regions of peripheral hepatic high signal intensity are present reflecting hemorrhage (*long arrows, a*). The stomach (*s*) is dilated. On the gadolinium-enhanced T1-weighted fat-suppressed spin-echo image (*b*), the vertically oriented peripheral collections of portal venous air are more clearly defined (*small arrows, b*). Regions that were hyperintense on the precontrast image are shown to have diminished enhancement (*long arrow, b*). The dilated stomach shows increased mural enhancement (*large arrow, b*) consistent with ischemic changes. Portal venous air was signal-void and poorly seen on T2-weighted images (not shown); fluid would be high in signal intensity and well-shown on T2-weighted images.

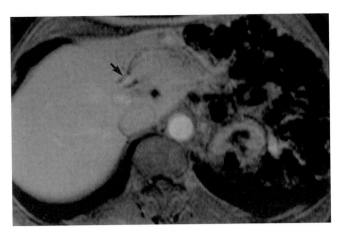

F I G . **2.100** Biliary tree air. Ninety-second postgadolinium SGE image in a patient with a choledochojejunostomy shows signal-void, tubular structures with an arborized pattern (*arrow*). This biliary tree air is more central in location than the portal venous air. The T2-weighted image (not shown) demonstrates signal-void, poorly shown bile ducts consistent with air-containing rather than fluid-containing ducts.

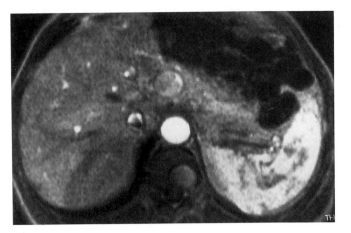

F I G . **2.101** Transient heterogeneous enhancement. Immediate postgadolinium SGE image demonstrates transient heterogeneous hepatic enhancement. Transient heterogeneous enhancement is commonly associated with homogeneous enhancement of the spleen, which is not, however, present in this case. (Reproduced with permission from Semelka RC, Shoenut JP, Greenburg, HM, Micflikier AB. The Liver. p. 13–41 in: Semelka RC, Shoenut JP, eds. MRI of the Abdomen with CT Correlation. Raven Press, New York, 1993.)

position in the bore of the magnet. Air in the biliary tree is signal-void on all MR sequences (Fig. 2.100).

Heterogeneous Hepatic Parenchymal Enhancement

Heterogeneous hepatic parenchymal enhancement is usually observed as a transient phenomenon on immediate postgadolinium enhanced images. This abnormality occurs in a generalized patchy fashion with the presence of wedge-shaped regions of increased enhancement that are conforming to subsegmental distributions (Fig. 2.101). The etiology of this abnormality is presently unknown, but presumably it reflects an imbalance between hepatic arterial and portal venous blood supply with increased hepatic arterial supply to subsegments of increased enhancement. This is frequently not related to focal fatty infiltration, but is commonly associated with homogeneous enhancement of the spleen on immediate postgadolinium images. Liver enzyme elevations of a minor degree may be observed [167]. The concomitant splenic enhancement abnormality may imply an underlying immunological basis for this phenomenon.

Viral Hepatitis

Viral hepatitis may cause severe disease, resulting in acute hepatitis, chronic hepatitis, or cirrhosis. Hepatitis B, C, or delta are parenterally transmitted, and all may result in these conditions. Acute hepatitis is diagnosed by clinical and serologic studies. Imaging studies are generally not performed unless the clinical picture is complicated. Acute hepatitis may result in heterogeneous hepatic signal intensity, which is most apparent on T2-weighted images and immediate postgadolinium images.

Periportal edema is present, and periportal lymph nodes are occasionally identified. In patients with chronic hepatitis, imaging studies are more commonly obtained, usually to detect the presence of cirrhosis or HCC. On T2-weighted images, chronic active hepatitis often has periportal high signal intensity, corresponding to inflammation. This is a nonspecific finding observed in a number of hepatobiliary and pancreatic diseases [168]. Focal inflammatory changes or fibrosis may develop in chronic active hepatitis, resulting in diffuse or regional high signal intensity on T2-weighted images [169,170] and heterogeneous enhancement on SGE images (Fig. 2.102). Enlarged periportal lymph nodes are common in patients with viral hepatitis.

Radiation-Induced Hepatitis

The liver may be included in radiation portals for a variety of malignancies. Edema may develop within 6 months of radiation injury. Edema appears as decreased signal intensity on T1-weighted images and increased signal intensity on T2 weighted images [171,172]. Fat usually is decreased within the radiation portal in patients with fatty liver (Fig. 2.103) [173,174]. This reflects decreased delivery of triglycerides due to diminished portal flow. Increased enhancement is apparent on delayed postgadolinium SGE images in radiation damaged liver. Increased enhancement is more conspicuous when fat-suppression techniques are used (see Fig. 2.103). This increased enhancement is related to leaky capillaries in early radiation injury and represents granulation tissue in late injury.

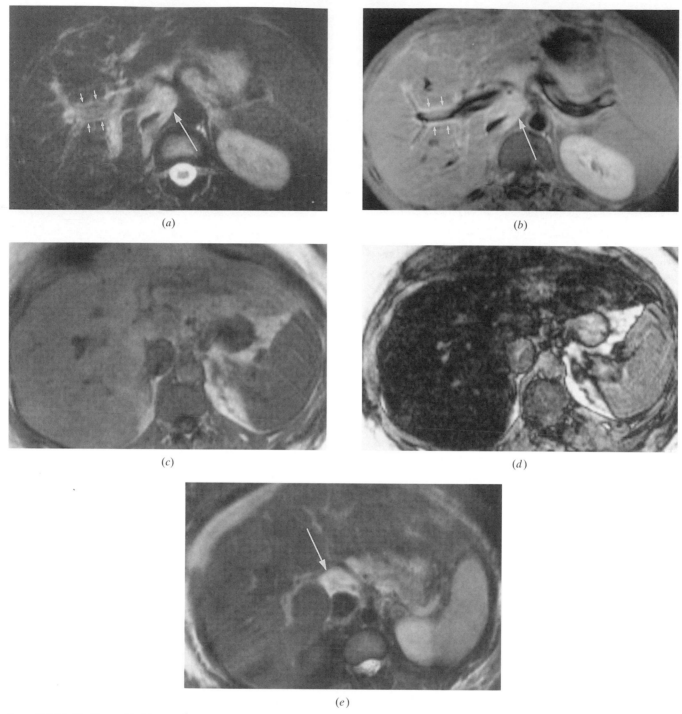

(a)

(b)

(c)

(d)

(e)

FIG. 2.102 Viral hepatitis. T2-weighted fat-suppressed spin-echo (*a*) and interstitial-phase gadolinium-enhanced T1-weighted fat-suppressed spin-echo (*b*) images in a patient with human immunodeficiency virus (HIV) infection and positive serology for hepatitis B and C. On the T2-weighted image (*a*) porta hepatis and para-aortic lymph nodes (*arrow, a*) are clearly shown as high-signal-intensity masses in a lower-signal-intensity background. High signal within the liver in a periportal distribution is also present (*small arrows, a*). This periportal abnormality identified on the T2-weighted image is shown to be enhancing tissue (*small arrows, b*) on the gadolinium-enhanced T1-weighted fat-suppressed image (*b*). Gadolinium enhancement distinguishes periportal inflammatory or neoplastic tissue from edema that would appear signal-void after contrast. Enhancement of adenopathy (*arrow, b*) is also appreciated. Viral hepatitis in a second patient shown on SGE (*c*), out-of-phase SGE (*d*) and T2-weighted fat-suppressed spin-echo (*e*) images. The liver is slightly heterogeneous on the T1-weighted image (*c*). On the out-of-phase image (*d*), the liver drops dramatically in signal intensity due to fatty infiltration. Periportal lymph nodes (*arrow, e*) are well-shown on the T2-weighted fat-suppressed spin-echo image (*e*). The presence of ascites is shown as high-signal-intensity fluid along the liver capsule.

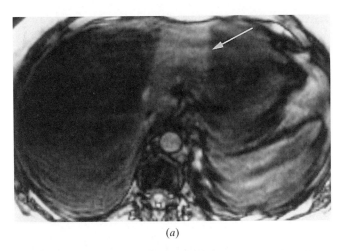

(a)

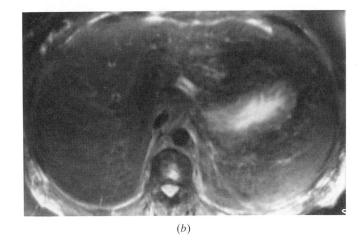

(b)

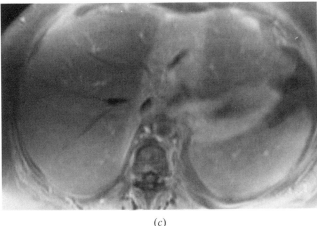

(c)

FIG. 2.103 Radiation damage. Out-of-phase SGE (*a*), T2-weighted fat-suppressed spin-echo (*b*), and gadolinium-enhanced T1-weighted fat-suppressed spin-echo (*c*) images in a patient who had undergone radiation therapy for a vertebral body metastasis. The out-of-phase image shows low-signal-intensity fatty replaced liver with a central, vertically oriented band of higher signal-intensity nonfatty liver (*arrow, a*). Similar findings are apparent on the fat-suppressed T2-weighted image (*b*), with subtle higher signal intensity of the central band of nonfatty liver The gadolinium-enhanced T1-weighted fat-suppressed image demonstrates increased enhancement of the radiation-damaged liver, which may reflect radiation-induced vasculitis.

INFLAMMATORY PARENCHYMAL DISEASE

Sarcoidosis

Focal involvement of the liver and spleen with noncaseating granulomas in sarcoidosis is well-demonstrated on MR images. Sarcoid granulomas are small (approximately 1 cm in diameter) rounded lesions low in signal intensity on T1- and T2-weighted images, and enhance in a diminished, delayed fashion on gadolinium-enhanced SGE images (Fig. 2.104) [175,176]. The diminished enhancement reflects the hypovascular nature of the granuloma. Occasionally, the spleen may be lower in signal intensity than liver on T2-weighted images [175].

Inflammatory Pseudotumor

Inflammatory liver pseudotumor is an inflammatory process that may result in systemic symptomatology, includ-ing fever, weight loss, malaise, and right upper quadrant pain [177]. Inflammatory liver pseudotumor is often mistaken for liver malignancy. The disease responds to steroid administration, and the prognosis is usually good, although fatal outcome also has been reported [178]. The lesions are usually solitary, although in 20 percent of the cases they have been reported to be multiple [177]. Histopathologic findings include proliferation of connective tissue with chronic inflammatory cell infiltration by plasma cells, lymphocytes, and histiocytes [177]. Masses are generally less than 2 cm in diameter and are slightly ill-defined. Tumors are mildly hyperintense on T2-weighted images and are best shown as patchy, rounded regions of transient increased enhancement on immediate post-gadolinium images (Fig. 2.105) [179]. Occasionally tumors may be large and the diffuse heterogeneous enhancement may mimic the appearance of MCC (Fig. 2.105).

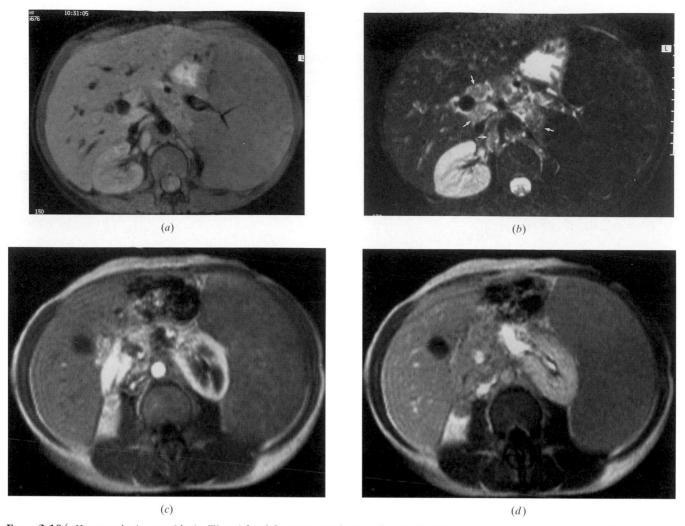

(a)

(b)

(c)

(d)

FIG. 2.104 Hepatosplenic sarcoidosis. T1-weighted fat-suppressed spin-echo (*a*), T2-weighted fat-suppressed spin-echo (*b*), immediate (*c*), and 5-minute (*d*) postgadolinium SGE images. The spleen is massively enlarged, and contains multiple nodules smaller than 1 cm that are low in signal intensity on precontrast T1-weighted images (*a*), low in signal intensity on T2-weighted images (*b*), and that demonstrate negligible enhancement on early postgadolinium images (*c*) with gradual enhancement over time (*d*). Extensive retroperitoneal, celiac, and periportal lymphadenopathy is also present (*a,b*), which has a speckled appearance on the T2-weighted image (*arrows, b*).

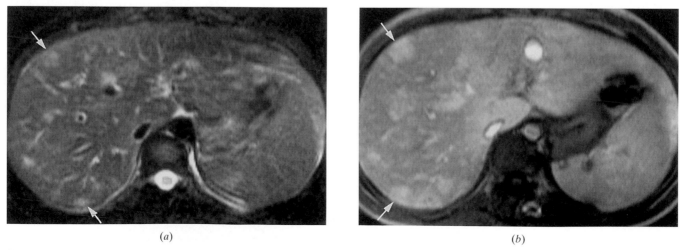

(a)

(b)

FIG. 2.105 Inflammatory pseudotumor. T2-weighted fat-suppressed spin-echo (*a*), immediate (*b*), and 90-second (*c*) postgadolinium SGE images. No definite lesions are apparent on the precontrast T1-weighted image (not shown). Occasional, mildly hyperintense ill-defined lesions are present on the T2-weighted image (*arrows, a*).

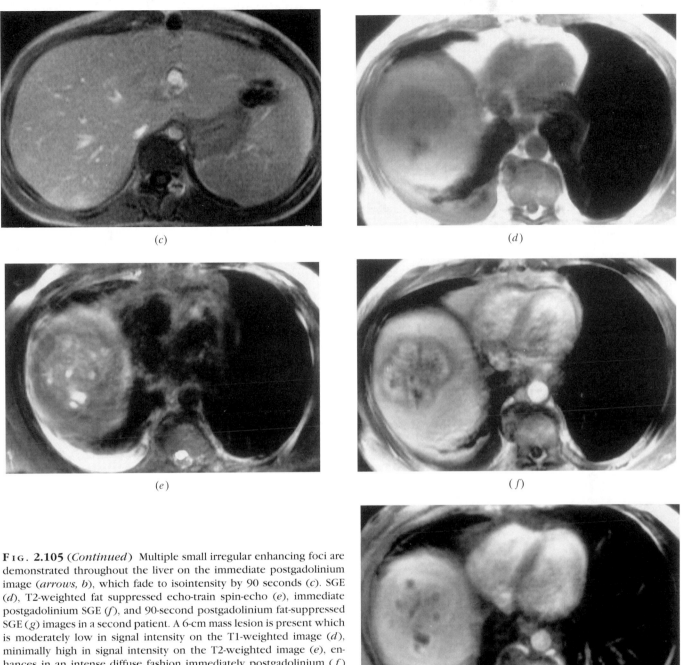

(c)

(d)

(e)

(f)

(g)

Fig. 2.105 (*Continued*) Multiple small irregular enhancing foci are demonstrated throughout the liver on the immediate postgadolinium image (*arrows, b*), which fade to isointensity by 90 seconds (*c*). SGE (*d*), T2-weighted fat suppressed echo-train spin-echo (*e*), immediate postgadolinium SGE (*f*), and 90-second postgadolinium fat-suppressed SGE (*g*) images in a second patient. A 6-cm mass lesion is present which is moderately low in signal intensity on the T1-weighted image (*d*), minimally high in signal intensity on the T2-weighted image (*e*), enhances in an intense diffuse fashion immediately postgadolinium (*f*) and becomes more homogeneous and lower in signal on later images (*g*). The appearance resembles HCC, however the liver is not cirrhotic. The patient also presented with fever and malaise, which are symptoms often observed in patients with inflammatory pseudotumor.

INFECTIOUS PARENCHYMAL DISEASE

Abscesses

Pyogenic abscess

Pyogenic abscesses usually occur in the context of recent surgery, Crohn's disease, appendicitis, and diverticulitis [180]. Characteristic gadolinium-enhanced MRI findings are low signal lesions with enhancing capsules [181]. Abscesses typically have perilesional enhancement with indistinct outer margins on immediate postgadolinium SGE images due to a hyperemic inflammatory response in adjacent liver (Fig. 2.106). The higher sensitivity of MRI to gadolinium chelates than of CT imaging to iodinated agents renders dynamic gadolinium-enhanced MRI a useful technique for patients in whom a distinction between simple cysts and multiple abscesses cannot be made on the basis of CT imaging examination. Metastases may mimic the appearance of hepatic abscesses since both may have prominent rim enhancement. Metastases may also mimic abscesses clinically if they become superinfected. The diagnosis of infected metastases should be entertained when the lesion wall is thicker than 5 mm and has nodular components. Bacterial abscesses commonly are associated with portal-vein thrombosis (see Fig. 2.106).

Nonpyogenic Abscess

Amebic Abscess. Amebic abscess may arise in patients who live in or have traveled to tropical climates. Presenting features include pain, fever, weight loss, nausea and vomiting, diarrhea, and anorexia [182]. Lesions are usually solitary and are prone to invade the diaphragm with development of an empyema [183]. Lesions are encapsulated and demonstrate substantial enhancement of the capsule on gadolinium-enhanced images, which permits differentiation from liver cysts (Fig. 2.107).

Echinococcal Disease

Echinococcus granulosus is the causative organism for hydatid cysts and is the type of echinococcus indigenous in North America. The typical appearance is an intrahepatic encapsulated multicystic lesion with daughter cysts arranged peripherally within the larger cyst. Satellite cysts located exterior to the fibrinous membrane of the main

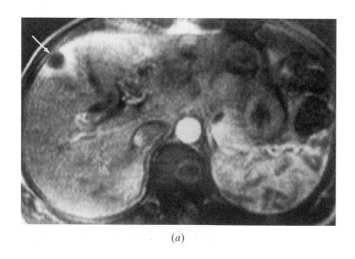

(a)

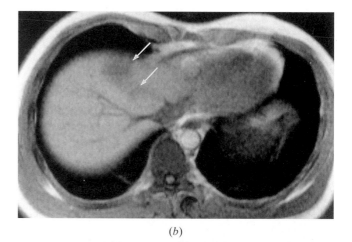

(b)

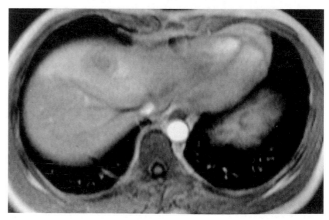

(c)

FIG. 2.106 Hepatic bacterial abscesses. Immediate postgadolinium SGE image (*a*) in a patient with appendiceal abscess demonstrates a thin-walled abscess in the liver (*arrow, a*) with prominent perilesional enhancement. SGE (*b*) and immediate postgadolinium SGE (*c*) images in a patient with fusibacterium liver abscesses.

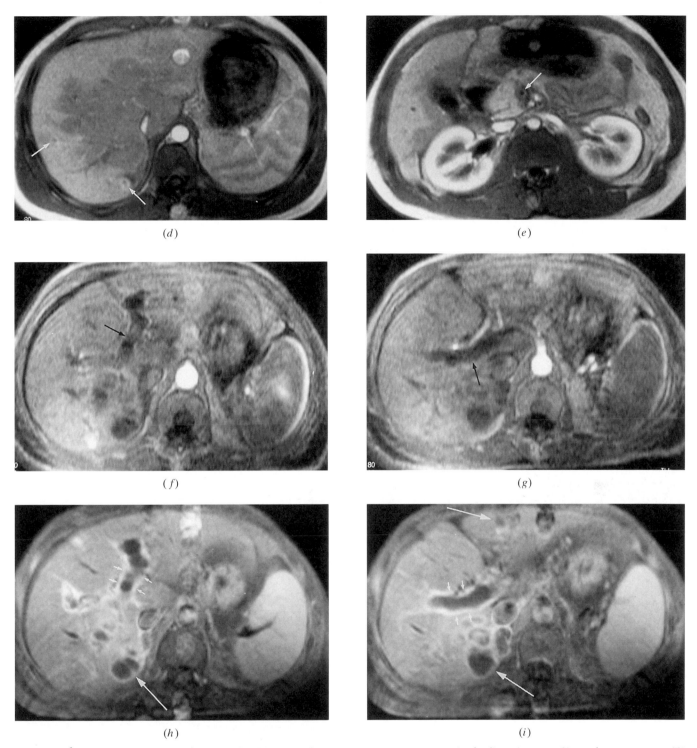

(d)

(e)

(f)

(g)

(h)

(i)

F IG . 2.106 (*Continued*) Two slightly ill-defined low-signal-intensity masses are present in the liver (*arrows, b*) on the precontrast T1-weighted image (*b*). Immediately after gadolinium administration (*c*), the lesions demonstrate substantial perilesional enhancement. The larger lesion demonstrates an outer low-signal rim surrounding an enhancing ring. Immediate postgadolinium SGE images from cranial (*d*) and caudal (*e*) locations through the liver in a third patient. Abnormal diminished central enhancement is present in the liver (*d*) due to portal-vein thrombosis. Small abscesses with enhancing rings (*arrows, d*) are present. On the more inferior tomographic image (*e*), thrombus is identified in the superior mesenteric vein with enhancement of the vein wall (*arrow, e*) reflecting infection of the thrombus. Immediate postgadolinium SGE (*f,g*) and interstitial-phase gadolinium-enhanced T1-weighted fat-suppressed spin-echo (*h,i*) images in a fourth patient obtained at the level of the left (*f,h*) and right (*g,i*) portal veins. The left (*arrow, f*) and right (*arrow, g*) portal veins are expanded with low-signal thrombus on the immediate postgadolinium images. On the gadolinium-enhanced fat-suppressed images, enhancement of the walls of the portal veins is present (*small arrows, h,i*) reflecting the infected nature of the thrombus. The abscesses in the right and left lobes of the liver are well-seen on the interstitial-phase images as low-signal-intensity irregularly shaped cystic masses with enhancing rims (*long arrow, h,i*).

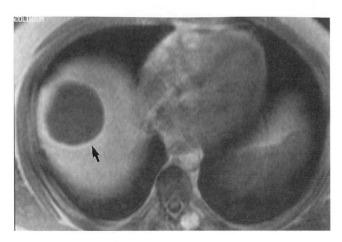

FIG. 2.107 Amebic abscess. Immediate postgadolinium SGE image demonstrates a 7-cm cystic lesion located in the right lobe of the liver superiorly. The amebic abscess has a prominent enhancing wall (*arrow*) confirming that it is not a simple cyst.

hepatic cyst are not uncommon and have been reported in 16 percent of hydatid cysts in a series of 185 patients [182]. The fibrous capsule and internal septations are well-shown on T2-weighted images and gadolinium-enhanced T1-weighted images. Lesions are frequently complex, with mixed low signal intensity on T1-weighted images and mixed high signal intensity on T2-weighted images due to the presence of proteinaceous and cellular debris (Fig. 2.108). Calcification of the cyst wall and internal calcifications are frequently identified on CT images, but calcification may not be distinguishable from the fibrous tissue of the capsule on MR images.

Mycobacterial Infection

Hepatic infection caused by tuberculosis is on the increase, reflecting, in part, an increase in numbers of patients who are immunocompromised, such as patients with HIV infection. Focal hepatic lesions typically are small and multiple with an appearance similar to that of fungal lesions (see next section). Infection frequently predilects the portal triads and spreads in a superficial infiltrating fashion. This can be visualized as periportal

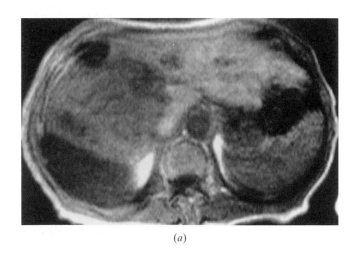

(*a*)

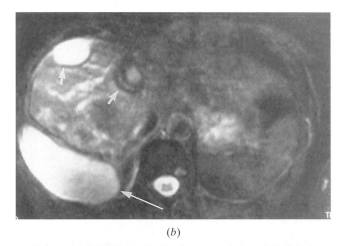

(*b*)

FIG. 2.108 Hydatid cyst. SGE (*a*), T2-weighted fat-suppressed spin-echo (*b*) and immediate postgadolinium SGE (*c*) images. Heterogeneous low-signal-intensity cystic lesions are present on the T1-weighted image (*a*). On the T2-weighted image (*b*) the largest cyst is heterogeneous and moderate in signal intensity and contains peripherally arranged daughter cysts (*arrows, b*). A satellite cyst is also present (*long arrow, b*). The cyst does not enhance after gadolinium administration (*c*).

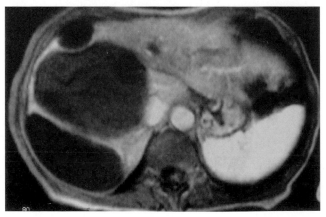

(*c*)

high signal intensity on T2-weighted fat-suppressed images and gadolinium-enhanced T1-weighted fat-suppressed images (Fig. 2.109). Associated porta hepatis nodes are common.

Fungal Infection

Fungal microabscesses are observed as a complication of immunosuppression or an immunocompromised state [184,185]. Patients on medical therapy for acute myelogeneous leukemia (AML) are particularly susceptible to this infection. The most common infecting organism is *Candida albicans,* but other fungi may be found. Acute hepatosplenic candidiasis involves the liver and spleen, with renal involvement occurring in less than 50 percent of patients. Patient survival depends on early diagnosis. Liver lesions are frequently smaller than 1 cm and subcap-

sular in location. The small size and peripheral nature of these lesions make them difficult to detect with CT imaging or standard spin-echo MR sequences. Patients with AML undergo multiple blood transfusions, so the liver and spleen are low in signal intensity on T1-weighted and T2-weighted images [186,188]. T2-weighted fat-suppressed spin-echo sequences are effective at detecting these lesions because of the high conspicuity of this sequence for small lesions and the absence of chemical shift artifact that may mask small peripheral lesions. STIR images also show these lesions well due to the fat-nulling effect of this sequence [186]. MRI employing T2-weighted fat-suppression and dynamic gadolinium-enhanced SGE images has been shown to be more sensitive for the detection of hepatosplenic candidiasis than contrast-enhanced CT imaging [187]. Acute lesions of fungal disease

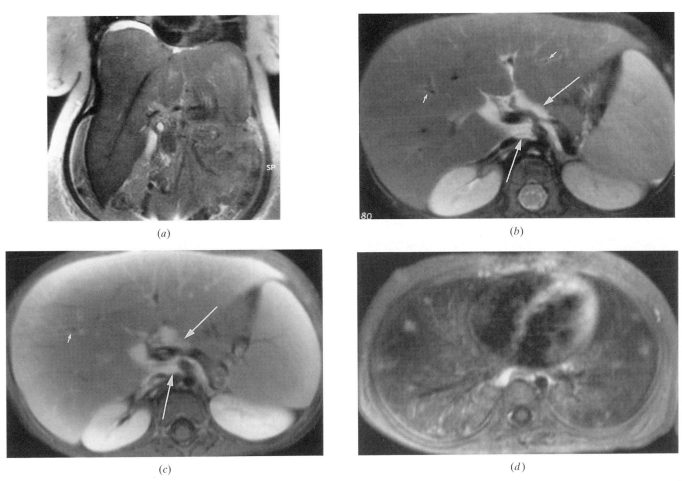

(a)

(b)

(c)

(d)

F IG . 2.109 Mycobacterium avium intracellulare (MAI) hepatic infection. Coronal HASTE (*a*), T2-weighted echo-train spin-echo (*b*) and interstitial-phase gadolinium-enhanced T1-weighted fat-suppressed spin-echo (*c*) images. The coronal image (*a*) demonstrates hepatomegaly (*a*). On the fat-suppressed T2-weighted image (*b*), high-signal-intensity substance is present in the porta hepatis (*long arrows, b*) and extends along periportal tracks (*short arrows, b*). After gadolinium administration, enhancing porta hepatis tissue is clearly shown on the fat-suppressed image (*long arrows, c*), and enhancement is also noted on the periportal tissue. Periportal distribution is a common pattern of involvement with MAI. Gadolinium-enhanced, gated T1-weighted fat-suppressed spin-echo image (*d*) of the lungs demonstrates a ground glass appearance with irregularly marginated 1-cm enhancing nodules consistent with MAI lung infection.

are abscesses and therefore are high in signal intensity on T2-weighted images. They also may be seen on gadolinium-enhanced T1-weighted images as signal-void foci with no appreciable abscess wall enhancement (Fig. 2.110). The abscence of abscess wall reflects the patient's neutropenic state. After institution of antifungal antibiotics, successful response may be demonstrated. Central high signal develops within lesions on T1-weighted and T2-weighted images that enhances with gadolinium, representing granulomatous formation. In addition, a distinctive dark perilesional ring is observed on all sequences, which represents migration of iron-laden macrophages to the periphery of lesions (Fig. 2.111) [189]. This may

represent a good prognostic finding, reflecting the patient's ability to mount an immune response. MRI also demonstrates chronic healed lesions that have responded to antifungal therapy [187]. These lesions are irregularly shaped and low in signal. Chronic healed lesions are hypointense on T1-weighted images, and are generally isointense and poorly shown on T2-weighted images (Fig. 2.112). The lesions are most conspicuous as low-signal-intensity defects with angulated margins on immediate postgadolinium SGE images. Capsular retraction also may be observed adjacent to the lesions. This constellation of imaging features is consistent with chronic scar formation.

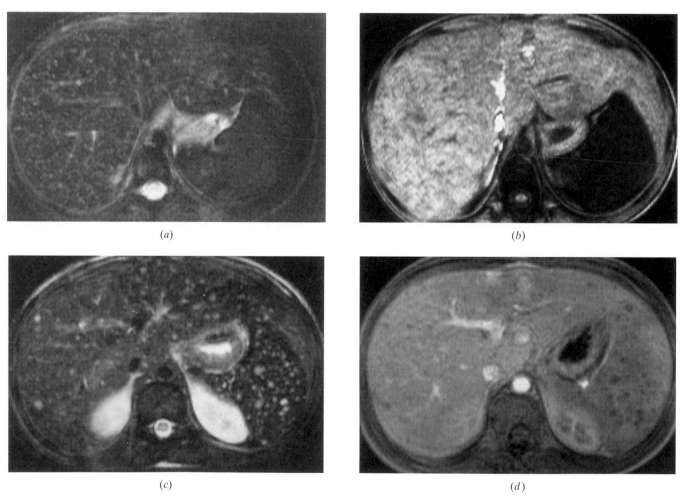

(a)   (b)   (c)   (d)

FIG. 2.110 Acute hepatosplenic candidiasis. T2-weighted fat-suppressed echo-train spin-echo (a) and immediate postgadolinium SGE (b) images. On the T2-weighted images (a), multiple well-defined high-signal-intensity foci smaller than 1 cm are scattered throughout the hepatic parenchyma with a smaller number of similar lesions apparent in the spleen. On the immediate postgadolinium image (b) the liver lesions are nearly signal-void and do not show ring or perilesional enhancement. T2-weighted fat-suppressed echo-train spin-echo (c) and immediate postgadolinium SGE (d) images in a second patient. Multiple well-defined high signal intensity lesions smaller than 1 cm are scattered throughout the liver and spleen on the T2-weighted image (c). Lesions are nearly signal-void and do not show ring or perilesional enhancement on the immediate postgadolinium image (d).

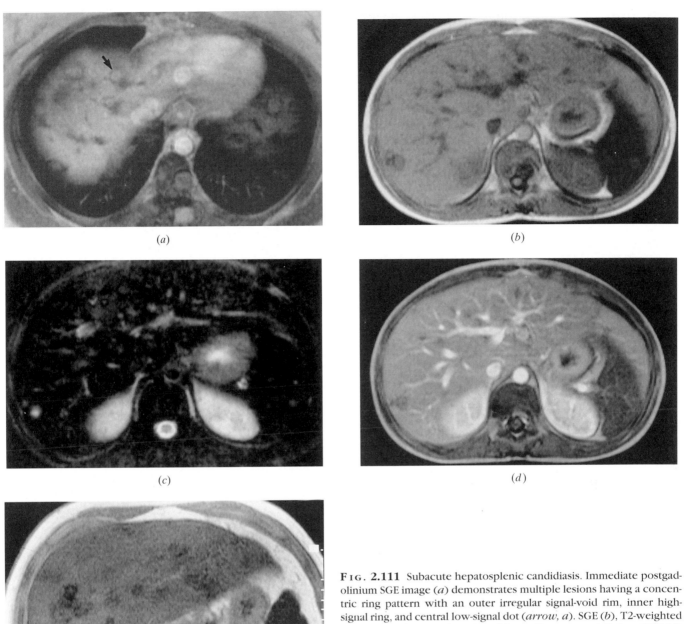

(a)

(b)

(c)

(d)

(e)

F IG. 2.111 Subacute hepatosplenic candidiasis. Immediate postgadolinium SGE image (*a*) demonstrates multiple lesions having a concentric ring pattern with an outer irregular signal-void rim, inner high-signal ring, and central low-signal dot (*arrow, a*). SGE (*b*), T2-weighted fat-suppressed spin-echo (*c*) and immediate postgadolinium SGE (*d*) images in a second patient. Multiple concentric ring lesions are evident, which are best shown on precontrast and immediate postgadolinium SGE images (*b,d*). The outer low-signal-intensity ring is not appreciated on T2-weighted images (*c*) because the perilesional iron deposition blends in with the background RES iron deposition. SGE (*e*), out-of-phase SGE (*f*), and coronal 45-second postgadolinium SGE (*g*) images in a third patient. Multiple concentric ring lesions are scattered throughout the liver on the SGE image (*e*).

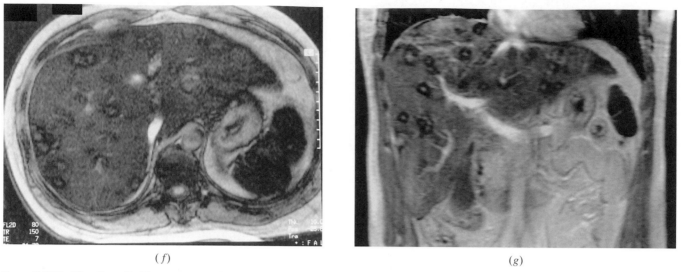

(f)   (g)

FIG. 2.111 (*Continued*) The outer signal-void ring becomes more prominent on the longer echo-time out-of-phase image (*f*) due to magnetic susceptibility artifact from iron. Lesion appearance is largely unchanged on the postgadolinium image (*g*).

TRAUMA

Hepatic trauma may be well-shown on MR images. Hemoperitoneum may be shown as peritoneal fluid with blood products of varying signal intensity on T1-weighted and T2-weighted images reflecting blood products of differing age. Liver lacerations are demonstrated as linear hepatic defects. Intraparenchymal hemorrhage will appear as intraparenchymal fluid with varying signal intensity on T1-weighted and T2-weighted images (Fig. 2.113). The specific appearance of early hemorrhage is low signal intensity on T2-weighted images due to the presence of deoxyhemoglobin or intracellular methemoglobin. The specific appearance of subacute hemorrhage is high signal intensity on T1-weighted and T2-weighted images due to the presence of extracellular methemoglobin.

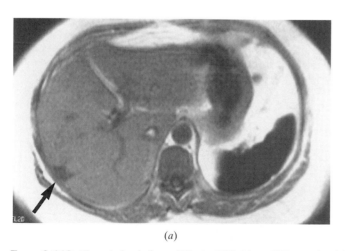

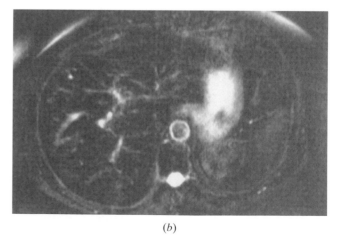

(a)   (b)

FIG. 2.112 Chronic healed candidiasis. SGE (*a*) and T2-weighted fat-suppressed spin-echo (*b*) images. An irregular polygonal low-signal lesion is present in the right lobe of the liver on the T1-weighted image (*arrow, a*). On the T2-weighted image (*b*) the area of fibrosis has similar signal intensity to that of background liver and is not definable.

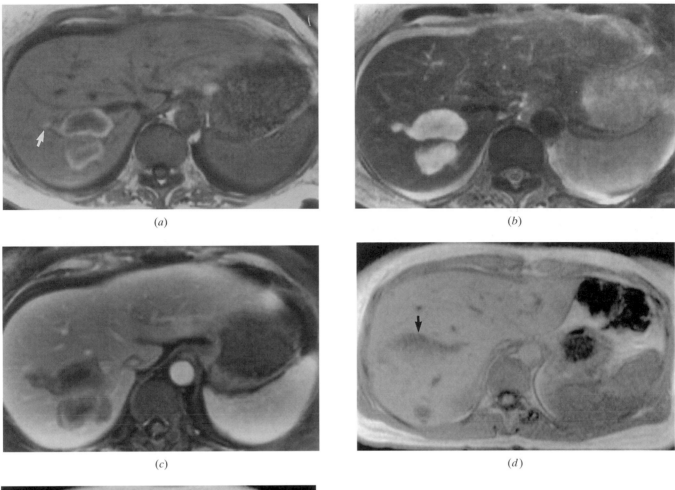

(a)   (b)

(c)   (d)

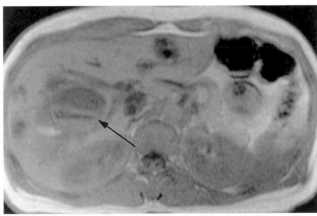

(e)

FIG. 2.113 Hepatic trauma. SGE (*a*), T2-weighted fat-suppressed echo-train spin-echo (*b*) and 45-second postgadolinium SGE (*c*) images. Two hematomas are present in the liver that demonstrate a peripheral ring of high signal intensity on the precontrast T1-weighted image (*a*), which is diagnostic for subacute hematomas. A high-signal-intensity laceration tract is also noted (*arrow, a*). The hematomas are minimally heterogeneous and hyperintense on the T2-weighted image (*b*). The hematomas do not enhance after gadolinium (*c*), but the extracellular methemoglobin ring remains hyperintense. Precontrast SGE (*d,e*) and T2-weighted fat-suppressed echo-train spin-echo (*f,g*) images acquired in a second patient from two tomographic levels, (*d,f*) and (*e,g*). An acute liver laceration is present (*arrow, d*) through the right lobe of the liver, which contains fluid that is dark and bright (oxyhemoglobin) and dark and dark (deoxyhemoglobin) on T1-weighted and T2-weighted images, respectively.

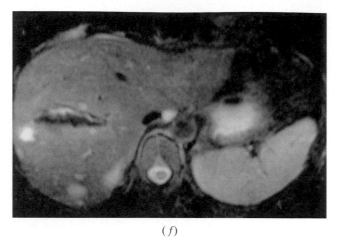

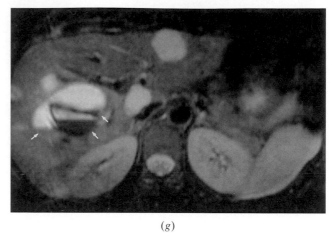

(f)	(g)

FIG. 2.113 (*Continued*) Hemorrhage has extended into two liver cysts that contain a combination of acute blood products including oxyhemoglobin (dark on T1-weighted and bright on T2-weighted images; *thin arrow, e*) and intracellular methemoglobin (bright on T1-weighted and dark on T2-weighted images; *short arrows, g*).

HEPATIC TRANSPLANTATION

MRI provides useful information for preoperative and postoperative evaluation of livers in transplant patients. Preoperatively, patency of the inferior vena cava, portal vein, hepatic artery, and common bile duct may be evaluated, and the presence of malignant disease determined [134,190]. Malignant tumors evaluated for possible transplantation may be evaluated for extent of hepatic involvement and the presence of porta hepatis nodes or distant disease.

The most common cause of early liver graft failure is rejection. Early diagnosis is essential to allow modification of immunosuppressive therapy [191]. The differential diagnosis of rejection includes biliary obstruction, cholangitis, ischemic injury, viral infection, and drug toxicity.

Periportal signal abnormalities are frequently present in transplanted livers. The typical appearance is tissue that is low in signal intensity on T1-weighted images and high in signal intensity on T2-weighted images. Abnormal tissue is most substantial in the porta hepatis and extends along the branching portal tracts into the liver parenchyma [192]. This represents lymphocytic infiltration due to rejection in many cases, but may also be caused by dilated lymphatics due to impaired drainage following surgery [193]. When the periportal tissue appears mass-like, posttransplant lymphoproliferative disease may be present (Fig. 2.114). Inflammatory periportal tissue also may be observed in acute hepatitis following biliary surgery in various benign or malignant diseases, and in portal adenopathy [168].

Vascular complications such as portal vein or IVC

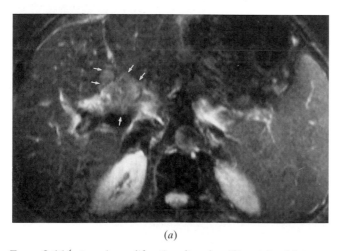

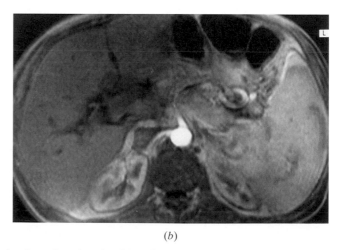

(a)	(b)

FIG. 2.114 Lymphoproliferative disorder. T2-weighted fat-suppressed echo-train spin-echo (*a*) and immediate postgadolinium SGE (*b*) images. A 3-cm mass is present in the porta hepatis that is moderate in signal intensity on the T2-weighted image (*arrows, a*) and that enhances minimally with gadolinium.

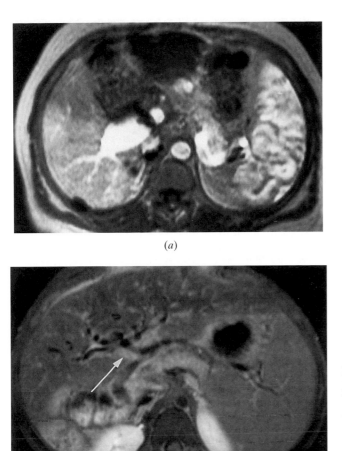

(a)

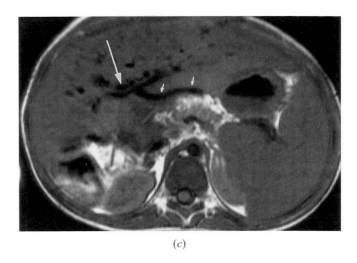

(c)

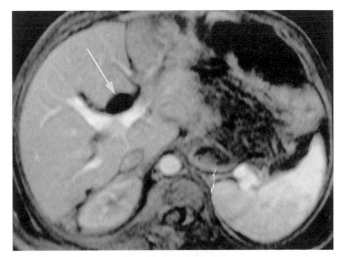

(b)

FIG. 2.115 Hepatic transplant, portal vein complications. Immediate postgadolinium SGE image (a) demonstrates dilation of the right portal vein secondary to anastomotic stenosis. T1-weighted spin-echo (b) and gadolinium-enhanced T1-weighted fat-suppressed spin-echo (c) images in a pediatric patient with a trisegmental transplant. A patent hepatic arterial graft (*small arrows, b*) and biliary ducts (*long arrow, b*) are evident. There is no evidence of a patent portal vein. Enhancing inflammatory tissue is present in the porta hepatis and in the expected location of the portal vein (*long arrow, c*).

thrombosis or hepatic artery stenosis are important causes of graft failure [194]. Portal vein and IVC patency can be diagnosed reproducibly on MR images (Fig. 2.115) [195]. Stenosis of veins is not uncommon and does not necessarily lead to graft failure. Hepatic artery patency can be documented by MRI in most cases. The ability of the gadolinium-enhanced 3D FISP technique to demonstrate stenosis is not presently known. Stenosis or obstruction of the biliary tree (Fig. 2.116) may be shown using techniques that render bile low in signal, high in signal (MR cholangiography), or as a combination of both.

Fluid collections are commonly observed after hepatic transplantation. Bile leaks may develop, sometimes associated with biliary strictures. Mucocele of the cystic duct remnant may occur and appears as a focal fluid collection adjacent to the hepatic duct [196]. MRI is able to distinguish between hematomas and other fluid collections in hepatic transplants because extracellular methemoglobin in subacute hematomas is higher in signal on T1-weighted images than other fluid.

FIG. 2.116 Liver transplant, biliary duct stenosis. Transverse 45-second postgadolinium fat-suppressed SGE image. Dilation of the common hepatic duct (*arrow*) is present secondary to anastomotic stenosis.

MRI demonstrates a variety of morphological abnormalities in transplanted livers, and is able to identify various causes of graft failure. At present, however, no specific MRI findings have been identified to establish or quantify transplant rejection or hepatocellular function. In the future, hepatocyte specific contrast agents may play a role in this determination.

CONCLUSIONS

MRI is an excellent modality to evaluate diffuse liver disease and to detect and characterize focal liver masses. Although MRI may exceed spiral CT imaging for many of these evaluations, due to the high cost of MRI it may be prudent to limit its use to circumstances in which the superiority of MRI may have a substantial impact on patient management. Among all focal liver lesions, MRI has greater impact on patient management than CT imaging in the evaluation of hypervascular malignant lesions such as hepatocellular carcinoma or metastases from hypervascular primary tumors. MRI may be the most accurate nonoperative imaging modality for evaluating patients with suspected limited involvement of the liver with malignant disease who are considered candidates for partial hepatic resection. MRI is also the imaging modality of choice for the detection of hepatosplenic candidiasis. No other modality can exceed the accuracy of MRI for the evaluation of diffuse liver disease, so MRI should be used to investigate patients with suspected iron deposition or fatty infiltration. In many settings, however, MRI may be adequately employed as a problem-solving modality to characterize and determine the extent of focal liver lesions. It is also clear that patients who are not candidates for contrast-enhanced CT examination (e.g., patients with poor renal function or contrast allergy) should be studied with MRI.

REFERENCES

1. Gazelle GS, Haaga JR: Hepatic neoplasms: Surgically relevant segmental anatomy and imaging techniques. Am J Roentgenol 158:1015–1018, 1992.
2. Edelman RR, Siegel JB, Singer A, Dupuis K, Longmaid HE: Dynamic MR imaging of the liver with Gd-DTPA: Initial clinical results. Am J Roentgenol 153:1213–1219, 1989.
3. Low RN, Francis IR, Sigeti JS, Foo TK: Abdominal MR imaging: Comparison of T2-weighted fast and conventional spin-echo, and contrast-enhanced fast multiplanar spoiled gradient-recalled imaging. Radiology 186:803–811, 1993.
4. Mahfouz AE, Hamm B, Wolf KJ: Dynamic gadopentetate dimeglumine-enhanced MR imaging of hepatocellular carcinoma. Eur Radiol 3:453–458, 1993.
5. Semelka RC, Shoenut JP, Ascher SM, Kroeker MA, Greenberg HM, Yaffe CS, Micflikier AB: Solitary hepatic metastasis: Comparison of dynamic contrast-enhanced CT and MR imaging with fat-suppressed T2-weighted, breath-hold T1-weighted FLASH, and dynamic gadolinium-enhanced FLASH sequences. J Magn Reson Imaging 4:319–323, 1994.
6. Caudana R, Morana G, Pirovano GP, Nicoli N, Portuese A, Spinazzi A, Di Rito R, Pistolesi GF: Focal malignant hepatic lesions: MR imaging enhanced with gadolinium benzoxypropionictetra-acetate (BOPTA)—preliminary results of phase II clinical application. Radiology 199:513–520, 1996.
7. Kettritz U, Schlund JF, Wilbur K, Eisenberg LB, Semelka RA: Comparison of gadolinium cheletes with Managanese-DPDP for liver lesion detection and characterization—preliminary results. Magn Reson Imag (in press).
8. Hamm B, Staks T, Muhler A, Bollow M, Taupitz M, Frenzel T, Wolf KJ, Weinmann HJ, Lange L: Phase I clinical evaluation of Gd-EOB-DTPA as a hepatobiliary MR contrast agent: Safety, pharmacokinetics, and MR imaging. Radiology 195:785–792, 1995.
9. Hagspiel KD, Neidl KF, Eichenberger AC, Weder W, Marincek B: Detection of liver metastases: Comparison of superparamagnetic iron oxide-enhanced and unenhanced MR imaging at 1.5 T with dynamic CT, intraoperative US, and percutaneous US. Radiology 196:471–478, 1995.
10. Ros PR, Freeny PC, Marms SE, et al: Hepatic MR imaging with ferumoxides: A multicenter clinical trial of the safety and efficacy in the detection of focal hepatic lesions. Radiology 196:481–488, 1995.
11. Yamamoto H, Yamashita Y, Yoshimatsu S, Baba Y, Hatanaka Y, Murakami R, Nishiharu T, Takahashi M, Higashida Y, Moribe N: Hepatocellular carcinoma in cirrhotic livers: Detection with unenhanced and iron oxide-enhanced MR imaging. Radiology 195:106–112, 1995.
12. Saini S, Edelman RR, Sharma P, Li W, Mayo-Smith W, Slater GJ, Eisenberg PJ, Hahn PF: Blood-pool MR contrast material for detection and characterization of focal hepatic lesions: Initial clinical experience with ultrasmall superparamagnetic iron oxide (AMI-227). Am J Roentgenol 164:1147–1152, 1995.
13. Weissleder R, Lee AS, Fischman AJ, Reimer P, Shen T, Wilkinson R, Callahan RJ, Brady TJ: Polyclonal human immunoglobulin G labeled with polymeric iron oxide: Antibody MR imaging. Radiology 181:245–249, 1991.
14. Vogl TJ, Hammerstingl R, Schwarz W, et al: Superparamagnetic iron oxide-enhanced versus godolinium-enhanced MR imaging for differential diagnosis of focal liver lesions. Radiology 198:881–887, 1996.
15. Vogl TJ, Kummel S, Hammerstingl R, Schellenbeck M, Schumacher G, Balzer T, Schwarz W, Muller PK, Bechstein WO, Mack MG, Sollner O, Felix R: Liver tumors: Comparison of MR imaging with Gd-EOB-DTPA and Gd-DTPA. Radiology 200:59–67, 1996.
16. Barnes PA, Thomas JL, Bernardino ME: Pitfalls in the diagnosis of hepatic cysts by computed tomography. Radiology 141:129–133, 1981.
17. Semelka RC, Shoenut JP, Greenberg HM, Mickflickier AB: The liver. In: Semelka RC, Shoenut JP (eds.). MRI of the Abdomen with CT Correlation. New York: Raven Press, pp. 13–41, 1993.
18. Kadoya M, Matsui O, Nakanuma Y, Yoshikawa J, Arai K, Takashima T, Amano M, Kimura M: Ciliated hepatic foregut cyst: Radiologic features. Radiology 175:475–477, 1990.
19. Shoenut JP, Semelka RC, Levi C, Greenberg H: Ciliated hepatic foregut cysts: US, CT, and contrast-enhanced MR imaging. Abdom Imaging 19:150–152, 1994.
20. Itai Y, Ebihara R, Eguchi N, Saida Y, Kurosaki Y, Minami M, Araki T: Hepatobiliary cysts in patients with autosomal dominant polycystic kidney disease: Prevalence and CT findings. Am J Roentgenol 164:339–342, 1995.
21. Worawattanakul S, Kelekis NL, Semelka RC, Woosley JT: Hepatic angiomyolipoma with minimal fat content: MR demonstration. Magn Reson Imaging 14:687–689, 1996.

22. Garant M, Reinhold C: Answer to the case of the month #36. Hepatic lipoma. Can Assoc Radiol J 47:140–142, 1996.

23. Craig J, Peters R, Edmondson H: Tumors of the liver and intrahepatic bile ducts. In Hartman H, Sobin L (eds.). Atlas of Tumor Pathology. Volume second series, fascicle 26. Washington D.C.: Armed Forces Institute of Pathology, 1989.

24. Karhunen PJ. Benign hepatic tumours and tumour like conditions in men. J Clin Pathol 39:183–188, 1986.

25. Mitsuodo K, Watanabe Y, Saga T, et al: Nonenhanced hepatic cavernous hemangioma with multiple calcifications: CT and pathologic correlation. Abdom Imaging 20:459–461, 1995.

26. International Working Party: Terminology of nodular hepatocellular lesions. International Working Party. Hepatology 22:983–993, 1995.

27. Li KC, Glazer GM, Quint LE, Francis IR, Aisen AM, Ensminger WD, Bookstein FL: Distinction of hepatic cavernous hemangioma from hepatic metastases with MR imaging. Radiology 169:409–415, 1988.

28. Lombardo DM, Baker ME, Spritzer CE, Blinder R, Meyers W, Herfkens RJ: Hepatic hemangiomas vs. metastases: MR differentiation at 1.5 T. Am J Roentgenol 155:55–59, 1990.

29. Semelka RC, Shoenut JP, Kroeker MA, Greenberg HM, Simm FC, Minuk GY, Kroeker RM, Micflikier AB: Focal liver disease: Comparison of dynamic contrast-enhanced CT and T2-weighted fat-suppressed, FLASH, and dynamic gadolinium-enhanced MR imaging at 1.5 T. Radiology 184:687–694, 1992.

30. Schmiedl U, Kolbel G, Hess CF, Klose U, Kurtz B: Dynamic sequential MR imaging of focal liver lesions: Initial experience in 22 patients at 1.5 T. J Comput Assist Tomogr 14:600–607, 1990.

31. Quinn SF, Benjamin GG: Hepatic cavernous hemangiomas: Simple diagnostic sign with dynamic bolus CT. Radiology 182:545–548, 1992.

32. Whitney WS, Herfkens RJ, Jeffrey RB, McDonnell CH, Li KC, Van Dalsem WJ, Low RN, Francis IR, Dabatin JF, Glazer GM: Dynamic breath-hold multiplanar spoiled gradient-recalled MR imaging with gadolinium enhancement for differentiating hepatic hemangiomas from malignancies at 1.5 T. Radiology 189:863–870, 1993.

33. Hamm B, Thoeni RF, Gould RG, Bernardino ME, Luning M, Saini S, Mahfouz AE, Taupitz M, Wolf KJ: Focal liver lesions: Characterization with nonenhanced and dynamic contrast material-enhanced MR imaging. Radiology 190:417–423, 1994.

34. Semelka RC, Brown ED, Ascher SM, Patt RH, Bagley AS, Li W, Edelman RR, Shoenut JP, Brown JJ: Hepatic hemangiomas: A multiinstitutional study of appearance on T2-weighted and serial gadolinium-enhanced gradient-echo MR images. Radiology 192:401–406, 1994.

35. Kim TK, Choi BI, Han JK, Jang H, Han MC: Optimal MR imaging protocol for hepatic hemangiomas: Comparison of T2-weighted fast and conventional SE and serial Gd-DTPA-enhanced GRE techniques. Radiology 197(P):175, 1995.

36. Mitchell DG, Saini S, Weinreb J, De Lange EE, Runge VM, Kuhlman JE, Parisky Y, Johnson CD, Brown JJ, Schnall M, et al: Hepatic metastases and cavernous hemangiomas: Distinction with standard- and triple-dose gadoteridol-enhanced MR imaging. Radiology 193:49–57, 1994.

37. Larson RE, Semelka RC, Bagley AS, Molina PL, Brown ED, Lee JK: Hypervascular malignant liver lesions: Comparison of various MR imaging pulse sequences and dynamic CT. Radiology 192:393–399, 1994.

38. Choi BI, Han MC, Park JH, Kim SH, Han MH, Kim CW: Giant cavernous hemangioma of the liver: CT and MR imaging in 10 cases. Am J Roentgenol 152:1221–1226, 1989.

39. McFarland EG, Mayo-Smith WW, Saini S, Hahn PF, Goldberg MA, Lee MJ: Hepatic hemangiomas and malignant tumors: improved differentiation with heavily T2-weighted conventional spin-echo MR imaging. Radiology 193:43–47, 1994.

40. Kerlin P, Davis GL, McGill DB, Weiland LH, Adson MA, Sheedy PFD: Hepatic adenoma and focal nodular hyperplasia: Clinical, pathologic, and radiologic features. Gastroenterology 84:994–1002, 1983.

41. Shortell CK, Schwartz SI: Hepatic adenoma and focal nodular hyperplasia. Surg Gynecol Obstet 173:426–431, 1991.

42. Paulson EK, McClellan JS, Washington K, Spritzer CE, Meyers WC, Baker ME: Hepatic adenoma: MR characteristics and correlation with pathologic findings. Am J Roentgenol 163:113–116, 1994.

43. Powers C, Ros PR, Stoupis C, Johnson WK, Segel KH: Primary liver neoplasms: MR imaging with pathologic correlation. Radiographics 14:459–482, 1994.

44. Hamm B, Vogl TJ, Branding G, Schnell B, Taupitz M, Wolf KJ, Lissner J: Focal liver lesions: MR imaging with Mn-DPDP—initial clinical results in 40 patients. Radiology 182:167–174, 1992.

45. Wanless IR, Albrecht S, Bilbao J, Frei JV, Heathcote EJ, Roberts EA, Chiasson D: Multiple focal nodular hyperplasia of the liver associated with vascular malformations of various organs and neoplasia of the brain: A new syndrome. Mod Pathol 2:456–462, 1989.

46. Eisenberg LB, Warshauer DM, Woosley JT, Cance WG, Bunzendahl H, Semelka RC. CT and MRI of hepatic focal nodular hyperplasia with peripheral steatosis. J Comput Assist Tomogr 19:498–500, 1995.

47. Lee MJ, Saini S, Hamm B, Taupitz M, Hahn PF, Seneterre E, Ferrucci JT: Focal nodular hyperplasia of the liver: MR findings in 35 proved cases. Am J Roentgenol 156:317–320, 1991.

48. Vilgrain V, Flejou JF, Arrive L, Belghiti J, Najmark D, Menu Y, Zins M, Vuillerme MP, Nahum H: Focal nodular hyperplasia of the liver: MR imaging and pathologic correlation in 37 patients. Radiology 184:699–703, 1992.

49. Schiebler ML, Kressel HY, Saul SH, Yeager BA, Axel L, Gefter WB: MR imaging of focal nodular hyperplasia of the liver. J Comput Assist Tomogr 11:651–654, 1987.

50. Haggar AM, Bree RL: Hepatic focal nodular hyperplasia: MR imaging at 1.0 and 1.5 T. J Magn Reson Imaging 2:85–88, 1992.

51. Shamsi K, De Schepper A, Degryse H, Deckers F: Focal nodular hyperplasia of the liver: Radiologic findings. Abdom Imaging 18:32–38, 1993.

52. Mahfouz AE, Hamm B, Taupitz M, Wolf KJ: Hypervascular liver lesions: Differentiation of focal nodular hyperplasia from malignant tumors with dynamic gadolinium-enhanced MR imaging. Radiology 186:133–138, 1993.

53. Mathieu D, Rahmouni A, Anglade MC, Falise B, Beges C, Gheung P, Mollet JJ, Vasile N: Focal nodular hyperplasia of the liver: Assessment with contrast-enhanced turboFLASH MR imaging. Radiology 180:25–30, 1991.

54. Vogl TJ, Hamm B, Schnell B, McMahon C, Branding G, Lissner J, Wolf KJ: Mn-DPDP enhancement patterns of hepatocellular lesions on MR images. J Magn Reson Imaging 3:51–58, 1993.

55. Rummeny EJ, Wernecke K, Saini S, Vassallo P, Wiesmann W, Oestmann JW, Kivelitz D, Reers B, Reiser MF, Peters PE: Comparison between high-field-strength MR imaging and CT for screening of hepatic metastases: A receiver operating characteristic analysis. Radiology 182:879–886, 1992.

56. Nelson RC, Chezmar JL, Sugarbaker PH, Murray DR, Bernardino ME: Preoperative localization of focal liver lesions to specific liver segments: Utility of CT during arterial portography. Radiology 176:89–94, 1990.

57. Mirowitz SA, Lee JK, Gutierrez E, Brown JJ, Heiken JP, Eilenberg SS: Dynamic gadolinium-enhanced rapid acquisition spin-echo MR imaging of the liver. Radiology 179:371–376, 1991.

58. Sugarbaker PH, Kemeny N: Management of metastatic cancer to the liver. Adv Surg 22:1–56, 1989.

59. Hughes KS, Rosenstein RB, Songhorabodi S, Adson MA, Ilstrup DM, Fortner JG, Maclean BJ, Foster JH, Daly JM, Fitzherbert D,

et al: Resection of the liver for colorectal carcinoma metastases: A multi-institutional study of long-term survivors. Dis Colon Rectum 31:1–4, 1988.

60. Stark DD, Wittenberg J, Butch RJ, Ferrucci JT, Jr: Hepatic metastases: Randomized, controlled comparison of detection with MR imaging and CT. Radiology 165:399–406, 1987.

61. Zeman RK, Dritschilo A, Silverman PM, Clark LR, Garra BS, Thomas DS, Ahlgren JD, Smith FP, Korec SM, Nauta RJ, et al: Dynamic CT vs. 0.5 T MR imaging in the detection of surgically proven hepatic metastases. J Comput Assist Tomogr 13:637–644, 1989.

62. Vassiliades VG, Foley WD, Alarcon J, Lawson T, Erickson S, Kneeland JB, Steinberg HV, Bernardino ME: Hepatic metastases: CT versus MR imaging at 1.5 T. Gastrointest Radiol 16:159–163, 1991.

63. Semelka RC, Hricak H, Bis KG, Werthmuller WC, Higgins CB: Liver lesion detection: Comparison between excitation-spoiling fat suppression and regular spin-echo at 1.5 T. Abdom Imaging 18:56–60, 1993.

64. de Lange EE, Mugler JP III, Bosworth JE, DeAngelis GA, Gay SB, Hurt NS, Berr SS, Rosenblatt JM, Merickel LW, Harris EK: MR imaging of the liver: Breath-hold T1-weighted MP-GRE compared with conventional T2-weighted SE imaging—lesion detection, localization, and characterization. Radiology 190:727–736, 1994.

65. Jones EC, Chezmar JL, Nelson RC, Bernardino ME: The frequency and significance of small (less than or equal to 15 mm) hepatic lesions detected by CT. Am J Roentgenol 158:535–539, 1992.

66. Bruneton JN, Raffaelli C, Maestro C, Padovani B: Benign liver lesions: Implications of detection in cancer patients. Eur Radiol 5:387–390, 1995.

67. Semelka RC, Worawattanakul S, Kelekis NL, et al: Liver lesion detection and characterization. Comparison of single-phase spiral CT and current MR techniques. Radiology 201(P):145, 1996.

68. Semelka RC, Schlund JF, Molina PL, Willms AG, Kahlenberg M, Mauro MA, Weeks SM, Cance WG: Malignant liver lesions: Comparison of spiral CT arterial portography and MR imaging for diagnostic accuracy, cost, and effect on patient management. J Magn Reson Imaging 1:39–43, 1996.

69. Semelka RC, Cumming MJ, Shoenut JP, Magro CM, Yaffe CS, Kroeker MA, Greenberg HM: Islet cell tumors: Comparison of dynamic contrast-enhanced CT and MR imaging with dynamic gadolinium enhancement and fat suppression. Radiology 186:799–802, 1993.

70. Lin G, Lunderquist A, Hagerstrand I, Boijsen E: Postmortem examination of the blood supply and vascular pattern of small liver metastases in man. Surgery 96:517–526, 1984.

71. Mahfouz AE, Hamm B, Wolf KJ: Peripheral washout: A sign of malignancy on dynamic gadolinium-enhanced MR images of focal liver lesions. Radiology 190:49–52, 1994.

72. Outwater E, Tomaszewski JE, Daly JM, Kressel HY: Hepatic colorectal metastases: Correlation of MR imaging and pathologic appearance. Radiology 180:327–332, 1991.

73. Semelka RC, Bagley AS, Brown ED, Kroeker MA: Malignant lesions of the liver identified on T1- but not T2-weighted MR images at 1.5 T. J Magn Reson Imaging 4:315–318, 1994.

74. Kelekis NL, Semelka RC, Siegelman ES, Ascher SM, Outwater EK, Woosley TJ, Reinhold C, Mitchell DG: Focal hepatic lymphoma: MR demonstration using current techniques including gadolinium enhancement. J Magn Reson Imaging (submitted).

75. Kelekis NL, Warshauer DM, Semelka RC, Sallah AS: Nodular liver involvement in light chain multiple myeloma: Appearance on US and MRI. Clin Imaging. In press.

76. Choi BI, Takayasu K, Han MC: Small hepatocellular carcinomas and associated nodular lesions of the liver: Pathology, pathogenesis, and imaging findings. Am J Roentgenol 160:1177–1187, 1993.

77. Miller WJ, Baron RL, Dodd GD III, Federle MP: Malignancies in patients with cirrhosis: CT sensitivity and specificity in 200 consecutive transplant patients. Radiology 193:645–650, 1994.

78. Oi H, Murakami T, Kim T, Matsushita M, Kishimoto H, Nakamura H: Dynamic MR imaging and early-phase helical CT for detecting small intrahepatic metastases of hepatocellular carcinoma. Am J Roentgen 166:369–374, 1996.

79. Yamashita Y, Mitsuzaki K, Yi T, et al: Small heptacellular carcinoma in patients with chronic liver damage: Prospective comparison of detection with dynamic MR imaging and helical CT of the whole liver. Radiology 200:79–84, 1996.

80. Rummeny E, Weissleder R, Stark DD, Saini S, Compton CC, Bennett W, Hahn PF, Wittenberg J, Malt RA, Ferrucci JT: Primary liver tumors: Diagnosis by MR imaging. Am J Roentgenol 152:63–72, 1989.

81. Matsui O, Kadoya M, Kameyama T, Yoshikawa J, Arai K, Gabata T, Takashima T, Nakanuma Y, Terada T, Ida M: Adenomatous hyperplastic nodules in the cirrhotic liver: Differentiation from hepatocellular carcinoma with MR imaging. Radiology 173:123–126, 1989.

82. Rosenthal RE, Davis PL: MR imaging of hepatocellular carcinoma at 1.5 tesla. Gastrointest Radiol 17:49–52, 1992.

83. Hirai K, Aoki Y, Majima Y, Abe H, Nakashima O, Kojiro M, Tanikawa K: Magnetic resonance imaging of small hepatocellular carcinoma. Am J Gastroenterol 86:205–209, 1991.

84. Kadoya M, Matsui O, Takashima T, Nonomura A: Hepatocellular carcinoma: Correlation of MR imaging and histopathologic findings. Radiology 183:819–825, 1992.

85. Muramatsu Y, Nawano S, Takayasu K, Moriyama N, Yamada T, Yamasaki S, Hirohashi S: Early hepatocellular carcinoma: MR imaging. Radiology 181:209–213, 1991.

86. Ebara M, Watanabe S, Kita K, Yoshikawa M, Sugiura N, Ohto M, Kondo F, Kondo Y: MR imaging of small hepatocellular carcinoma: Effect of intratumoral copper content on signal intensity. Radiology 180:617–621, 1991.

87. Itoh K, Nishimura K, Togashi K, Fujisawa I, Noma S, Minami S, Sagoh T, Nakano Y, Itoh H, Mori K, et al: Hepatocellular carcinoma: MR imaging. Radiology 164:21–25, 1987.

88. Yamashita Y, Fan ZM, Yamamoto H, Matsukawa T, Yoshimatsu S, Miyazaki T, Sumi M, Harada M, Takahashi M: Spin-echo and dynamic gadolinium-enhanced FLASH MR imaging of hepatocellular carcinoma: Correlation with histopathologic findings. J Magn Reson Imaging 4:83–90, 1994.

89. Kelekis NL, Semelka RC, Woosley JT: Malignant lesions of the liver with high signal intensity on T1-weighted MR images. J Magn Reson Imaging 6:291–294, 1996.

90. Winter TC III, Takayasu K, Muramatsu Y, Furukawa H, Wakao F, Koga H, Sakamoto M, Hirohashi S, Freeny PC: Early advanced hepatocellular carcinoma: Evaluation of CT and MR appearance with pathologic correlation. Radiology 192:379–387, 1994.

91. Yoshida H, Itai Y, Ohtomo K, Kokubo T, Minami M, Yashiro N: Small hepatocellular carcinoma and cavernous hemangioma: Differentiation with dynamic FLASH MR imaging with Gd-DTPA. Radiology 171:339–342, 1989.

92. Liou J, Lee JK, Borrello JA, Brown JJ: Differentiation of hepatomas from nonhepatomatous masses: Use of MnDPDP-enhanced MR images. Magn Reson Imaging 12:71–79, 1994.

93. Craig JR, Peters RL, Edmondson HA, Omata M: Fibrolamellar carcinoma of the liver: A tumor of adolescents and young adults with distinctive clinico-pathologic features. Cancer 46:372–379, 1980.

94. Corrigan K, Semelka RC: Dynamic contrast-enhanced MR imaging of fibrolamellar hepatocellular carcinoma. Abdom Imaging 20:122–125, 1995.

95. Hamrick-Turner J, Abbitt PL, Ros PR: Intrahepatic cholangiocarcinoma: MR appearance. Am J Roentgenol 158:77–79, 1992.

96. Low RN, Sigeti JS, Francis IR, Weinman D, Bower B, Shimakawa A, Foo TK: Evaluation of malignant biliary obstruction: Efficacy of fast multiplanar spoiled gradient-recalled MR imaging vs. spin-

echo MR imaging, CT, and cholangiography. Am J Roentgenol 162:315–323, 1994.

97. Choi BI, Lim JH, Han MC, Lee DH, Kim SH, Kim YI, Kim CW: Biliary cystadenoma and cystadenocarcinoma: CT and sonographic findings. Radiology 171:57–61, 1989.

98. Kokubo T, Itai Y, Ohtomo K, Itoh K, Kawauchi N, Minami M: Mucin-hypersecreting intrahepatic biliary neoplasms. Radiology 168:609–614, 1988.

99. Palacios E, Shannon M, Solomon C, Guzman M: Biliary cystadenoma: Ultrasound, CT, and MRI. Gastrointest Radiol 15:313–316, 1990.

100. Buetow PC, Buck JL, Pantongrag-Brown L, Ros PR, Devaney K, Goodman ZD, Cruess DF: Biliary cystadenoma and cystadenocarcinoma: Clinical-imaging-pathologic correlations with emphasis on the importance of ovarian stroma. Radiology 196:805–810, 1995.

101. Buetow PC, Buck JL, Ros PR, Goodman ZDLC: Malignant vascular tumors of the liver: Radiologic-pathologic correlation. Radiographics 14:153–166, quiz 167–158, 1994.

102. Ohtomo K, Araki T, Itai Y, Monzawa S, Ohba H, Nogata Y, Hihara T, Koizumi K, Uchiyama G: MR imaging of malignant mesenchymal tumors of the liver. Gastrointest Radiol 17:58–62, 1992.

103. Arrive L, Hricak H, Goldberg HI, Thoeni RF, Margulis ARLC: MR appearance of the liver after partial hepatectomy. Am J Roentgenol 152:1215–1220, 1989.

104. Bartolozzi C, Lencioni R, Caramella D, Falaschi F, Cioni R, DiCoscio G: Hepatocellular carcinoma: CT and MR features after transcatheter arterial embolization and percutaneous ethanol injection. Radiology 191:123–128, 1994.

105. Bartolozzi C, Lencioni R, Caramella D, Mazzeo S, Ciancia EM: Treatment of hepatocellular carcinoma with percutaneous ethanol injection: Evaluation with contrast-enhanced MR imaging. Am J Roentgenol 162:827–831, 1994.

106. Giovagnoni A, Paci E, Terilli F, Cellerino R, Piga A: Quantitative MR imaging data in the evaluation of hepatic metastases during systemic chemotherapy. J Magn Reson Imaging 5:27–32, 1995.

107. Lee MJ, Mueller PR, Dawson SL, Gazelle SG, Hahn PF, Goldberg MA, Boland GWLC: Percutaneous ethanol injection for the treatment of hepatic tumors: Indications, mechanism of action, technique, and efficacy. Am J Roentgenol 164:215–220, 1995.

108. Nagel HS, Bernardino MELC: Contrast-enhanced MR imaging of hepatic lesions treated with percutaneous ethanol ablation therapy. Radiology 189:265–270, 1993.

109. Sironi S, De Cobelli F, Livraghi T, Villa G, Zanello A, Taccagni G, DelMaschio ALC: Small hepatocellular carcinoma treated with percutaneous ethanol injection: Unenhanced and gadolinium-enhanced MR imaging follow-up. Radiology 192:407–412, 1994.

110. Shirkhoda A, Baird S: Morphologic changes of the liver following chemotherapy for metastatic breast carcinoma: CT findings. Abdom Imaging 19:39–42, 1994.

111. Soyer P, Bluemke DA, Zeitoun G, Marmuse JP, Levesque MLC: Detection of recurrent hepatic metastases after partial hepatectomy: Value of CT combined with arterial portography. Am J Roentgenol 162:1327–1330, 1994.

112. Young ST, Paulson EK, Washington K, Gulliver DJ, Vredenburgh JJ, Baker ME: CT of the liver in patients with metastatic breast carcinoma treated by chemotherapy: Findings simulating cirrhosis. Am J Roentgenol 163:1385–1388, 1994.

113. Harned RK, II, Chezmar JL, Nelson RC: Recurrent tumor after resection of hepatic metastases from colorectal carcinoma: Location and time of discovery as determined by CT. Am J Roentgenol 163:93–97, 1994.

114. Lang EK, Brown CL, Jr: Colorectal metastases to the liver: Selective chemoembolization. Radiology 189:417–422, 1993.

115. Scwickert HC, Stiskal M, Roberts TPL, van Dijke CF, Mann J, Muehler A, Shames DM, Demsar F, Disston A, Brasch RC: Contrast-enhanced MR imaging assessment of tumor capillary permeability: Effect of irradiation on delivery of chemotherapy. Radiology 198:893–898, 1996.

116. Matsumoto R, Selig AM, Colucci VM, Jolesz FALC: MR monitoring during cryotherapy in the liver: Predictability of histologic outcome. J Magn Reson Imaging 3:770–776, 1993.

117. Matsumoto R, Oshio K, Jolesz FALC: Monitoring of laser and freezing-induced ablation in the liver with T1-weighted MR imaging. J Magn Reson Imaging 2:555–562, 1992.

118. Vogl TJ, Muller PK, Hammerstingl R, et al: Malignant liver tumors treated with MR imaging-guided laser-induced thermotherapy: Technique and prospective results. Radiology 196:257–265, 1995.

119. Kuszyk BS, Choti MA, Urban BA, Chambers TP, Bluemke DA, Sitzmann JV, Fishman EKLC: Hepatic tumors treated by cryosurgery: Normal CT appearance. Am J Roentgenol 166:363–368, 1996.

120. McLoughlin RF, Saliken JF, McKinnon G, Wiseman D, Temple W: CT of the liver after cryotherapy of hepatic metastases: Imaging findings. Am J Roentgenol 165:329–332, 1995.

121. Marn CS, Andrews JC, Francis IR, Hollett MD, Walker SC, Ensminger WD: Hepatic parenchymal changes after intraarterial Y-90 therapy: CT findings. Radiology 187:125–128, 1993.

122. Burdeny DA, Semelka RC, Kelekis NL, Kettritz U, Woosley JT, Cance WG, Lee JKT: Chemotherapy treated liver metastases which resemble hemangiomas on MR images. J Comput Assist Tomogr (submitted).

123. Popper H: Pathologic aspects of cirrhosis. A review. Am J Pathol 87:228–264, 1977.

124. Lehmann B, Fanucci E, Gigli F, Uhlenbrock D, Bartolozzi C: Signal suppression of normal liver tissue by phase corrected inversion recovery: A screening technique. J Comput Assist Tomogr 13:650–655, 1989.

125. Marti-Bonmati L, Talens A, del Olmo J, de Val A, Serra MA, Rodrigo JM, Ferrandez A, Torres V, Rayon M, Vilar JS: Chronic hepatitis and cirrhosis: Evaluation by means of MR imaging with histologic correlation. Radiology 188:37–43, 1993.

126. Baron RL, Campbell WL, Dodd GDr: Peribiliary cysts associated with severe liver disease: Imaging-pathologic correlation. Am J Roentgenol 162:631–636, 1994.

127. Itai Y, Ebihara R, Tohno E, Tsunoda HS, Kurosaki Y, Saida Y, Doy M: Hepatic peribiliary cysts: Multiple tiny cysts within the larger portal tract, hepatic hilum, or both. Radiology 191:107–110, 1994.

128. Terayama N, Matsui O, Hoshiba K, Kadoya M, Yoshikawa J, Gabata T, Takashima T, Terada T, Nakanuma Y, Shinozaki K, et al: Peribiliary cysts in liver cirrhosis: US, CT, and MR findings. J Comput Assist Tomogr 19:419–423, 1995.

129. Ohtomo K, Itai Y, Ohtomo Y, Shiga J, Iio M: Regenerating nodules of liver cirrhosis: MR imaging with pathologic correlation. Am J Roentgenol 154:505–507, 1990.

130. Terada T, Nakanuma Y: Survey of iron-accumulative macroregenerative nodules in cirrhotic livers. Hepatology 10:851–854, 1989.

131. Mitchell DG, Lovett KE, Hann HW, Ehrlich S, Palazzo J, Rubin R: Cirrhosis: Multiobserver analysis of hepatic MR imaging findings in a heterogeneous population. J Magn Reson Imaging 3:313–321, 1993.

132. Groszmann RJ, Atterbury CE: The pathophysiology of portal hypertension: A basis for classification. Semin Liver Dis 2:177–186, 1982.

133. Starzl TE, Francavilla A, Halgrimson CG, Francavilla FR, Porter KA, Brown TH, Putnam CW: The origin, hormonal nature, and action of hepatotrophic substances in portal venous blood. Surg Gynecol Obstet 137:179–199, 1973.

134. Finn JP, Edelman RR, Jenkins RL, Lewis WD, Longmaid HE, Kane RA, Stokes KR, Mattle HP, Clouse ME: Liver transplantation: MR angiography with surgical validation. Radiology 179:265–269, 1991.

135. Siegelman ES, Mitchell DG, Rubin R, Hann HW, Kaplan KR, Steiner RM, Rao VM, Schuster SJ, Burk DL, Jr., Rifkin MD: Parenchymal versus reticuloendothelial iron overload in the liver: Distinction with MR imaging. Radiology 179:361–366, 1991.

136. Chezmar JL, Nelson RC, Malko JA, Bernardino ME: Hepatic iron overload: Diagnosis and quantification by noninvasive imaging. Gastrointest Radiol 15:27–31, 1990.

137. Gomori JM, Horev G, Tamary H, Zandback J, Kornreich L, Zaizov R, Freud E, Krief O, Ben-Meir J, Rotem H, et al: Hepatic iron overload: Quantitative MR imaging. Radiology 179:367–369, 1991.

138. Kim IY, Mitchell DG, Vinitski S, Consigny PM, Hann HW, Rifkin MD, Rubin R: MR imaging of hepatic iron overload in rat. J Magn Reson Imaging 3:67–70, 1993.

139. Thomsen C, Wiggers P, Ring-Larsen H, Christiansen E, Dalhoj J, Henriksen O, Christoffersen P: Identification of patients with hereditary haemochromatosis by magnetic resonance imaging and spectroscopic relaxation time measurements. Magn Reson Imaging 10:867–879, 1992.

140. McLaren G, Muir W, Kellermeyer R: Iron overload disorders: Natural history, pathogenesis, diagnosis and therapy. Crit Rev Clin Lab Sci 19:205–226, 1984.

141. Siegelman ES, Mitchell DG, Semelka RC: Abdominal iron deposition: Metabolism, MR findings, and clinical importance. Radiology 199:13–22, 1996.

142. Terada T, Kadoya M, Nakanuma Y, Matsui O: Iron-accumulating adenomatous hyperplastic nodule with malignant foci in the cirrhotic liver. Histopathologic, quantitative iron, and magnetic resonance imaging in vitro studies. Cancer 65:1994–2000, 1990.

143. Terada T, Nakanuma Y: Iron-negative foci in siderotic macroregenerative nodules in human cirrhotic liver. A marker of incipient neoplastic lesions. Arch Pathol Lab Med 113:916–920, 1989.

144. Siegelman ES, Outwater E, Hanau CA, Ballas SK, Steiner RM, Rao VM, Mitchell DG: Abdominal iron distribution in sickle cell disease: MR findings in transfusion and nontransfusion dependent patients. J Comput Assist Tomogr 18:63–67, 1994.

145. Kreft BP, Tanimoto A, Baba Y, Zhao L, Chen J, Middleton MS, Compton CC, Finn JP, Stark DD: Diagnosis of fatty liver with MR imaging. J Magn Reson Imaging 2:463–471, 1992.

146. Yates CK, Streight RA: Focal fatty infiltration of the liver simulating metastatic disease. Radiology 159:83–84, 1986.

147. Mitchell DG: Focal manifestations of diffuse liver disease at MR imaging. Radiology 185:1–11, 1992.

148. Mitchell DG, Kim I, Chang TS, Vinitski S, Consigny PM, Saponaro SA, Ehrlich SM, Rifkin MD, Rubin R: Fatty liver. Chemical shift phase-difference and suppression magnetic resonance imaging techniques in animals, phantoms, and humans. Invest Radiol 26:1041–1052, 1991.

149. Mitchell DG, Palazzo J, Hann HW, Rifkin MD, Burk DL, Jr., Rubin R: Hepatocellular tumors with high signal on T1-weighted MR images: Chemical shift MR imaging and histologic correlation. J Comput Assist Tomogr 15:762–769, 1991.

150. Itai Y, Ohtomo K, Kokubo T, Okada Y, Yamauchi T, Yoshida H: Segmental intensity differences in the liver on MR images: A sign of intrahepatic portal flow stoppage. Radiology 167:17–19, 1988.

151. Lorigan JG, Charnsangavej C, Carrasco CH, Richli WR, Wallace S: Atrophy with compensatory hypertrophy of the liver in hepatic neoplasms: Radiographic findings. Am J Roentgenol 150:1291–1295, 1988.

152. Carr DH, Hadjis NS, Banks LM, Hemingway AP, Blumgart LH: Computed tomography of hilar cholangiocarcinoma: A new sign. Am J Roentgenol 145:53–56, 1985.

153. Itai Y, Murata S, Kurosaki Y: Straight border sign of the liver: Spectrum of CT appearances and causes. Radiographics 15:1089–1102, 1995.

154. Schlund JF, Semelka RC, Kettritz U, Eisenberg LB, Lee JKT: Transient increased segmental hepatic enhancement distal to portal vein obstruction on dynamic gadolinium-enhanced gradient echo MR images. J Magn Reson Imaging 5:375–377, 1995.

155. De Gaetano AM, Lafortune M, Patriquin H, De Franco A, Aubin B, Raradis K: Cavernous transformation of the portal vein: Patterns of intrahepatic and splachnic collateral circulation detected with Doppler sonography. Am J Roentgenol 165:1151–1156, 1995.

156. Nakao N, Miura K, Takahashi H, Miura T, Ashida H, Ishikawa Y, Utsunomiya J: Hepatic perfusion in cavernous transformation of the portal vein: Evaluation by using CT angiography. Am J Roentgenol 152:985–986, 1989.

157. Schlund JF, Semelka RC, Kettritz U, Weeks SM, Kahlenberg M, Cance WG: Correlation of perfusion abnormalities on CTAP and immediate postintravenous gadolinium-enhanced gradient echo MRI. Abdom Imaging 21:49–52, 1996.

158. Miller WJ, Federle MP, Straub WH, Davis PL: Budd-Chiari syndrome: Imaging with pathologic correlation. Abdom Imaging 18:329–335, 1993.

159. Mathieu D, Vasile N, Menu Y, Van Beers B, Lorphelin JM, Pringot J: Budd-Chiari syndrome: Dynamic CT. Radiology 165:409–413, 1987.

160. Murata S, Itai Y, Hisashi K, Nakajima K, et al: Effect of temporary occlusion of the hepatic vein on dual blood supply in the liver: Evaluation with spiral CT. Radiology 195:351–356, 1995.

161. Pollard JJ, Nebesar RA: Altered hemodynamics in the Budd-Chiari syndrome demonstrated by selective hepatic and selective splenic angiography. Radiology 89:236–243, 1967.

162. Noone T, Semelka RC, Woosley JT, Pisano ED: Ultrasound and MR findings in acute Budd-Chiari syndrome with histopathologic correlation. J Comput Assist Tomogr 20:819–822, 1996.

163. Castellano G, Canga F, Solis-Herruzo JA, Colina F, Martinez-Montiel MP, Morillas JD: Budd-Chiari syndrome associated with nodular regenerative hyperplasia of the liver. J Clin Gastroenterol 11:698–702, 1989.

164. de Sousa JM, Portmann B, Williams R: Nodular regenerative hyperplasia of the liver and the Budd-Chiari syndrome. Case report, review of the literature and reappraisal of pathogenesis. J Hepatol 12:28–35, 1991.

165. Soyer P, Lacheheb D, Caudron C, Levesque M: MRI of adenomatous hyperplastic nodules of the liver in Budd-Chiari syndrome. J Comput Assist Tomogr 17:86–89, 1993.

166. Rooholamini SA, Au AH, Hansen GC, Kioumehr F, Dadsetan MR, Chow PP, Kurzel RB, Mikhail G: Imaging of pregnancy-related complications. Radiographics 13:753–770, 1993.

167. Brown JJ, Borrello JA, Raza HS, Balfe DM, Baer AB, Pilgram TK, Atilla S: Dynamic contrast-enhanced MR imaging of the liver: Parenchymal enhancement patterns. Magn Reson Imaging 13:1–8, 1995.

168. Matsui O, Kadoya M, Takashima T, Kameyama T, Yoshikawa J, Tamura S: Intrahepatic periportal abnormal intensity on MR images: An indication of various hepatobiliary diseases. Radiology 171:335–338, 1989.

169. Itai Y, Ohtomo K, Kokubo T, Minami M, Yoshida H: CT and MR imaging of postnecrotic liver scars. J Comput Assist Tomogr 12:971–975, 1988.

170. Stark DD, Goldberg HI, Moss AA, Bass NM: Chronic liver disease: Evaluation by magnetic resonance. Radiology 150:149–151, 1984.

171. Unger EC, Lee JK, Weyman PJ: CT and MR imaging of radiation hepatitis. J Comput Assist Tomogr 11:264–268, 1987.

172. Yankelevitz DF, Knapp PH, Henschke CI, Nisce L, Yi Y, Cahill P: MR appearance of radiation hepatitis. Clin Imaging 16:89–92, 1992.

173. Cutillo DP, Swayne LC, Cucco J, Dougan H: CT and MR imaging in cystic abdominal lymphangiomatosis. J Comput Assist Tomogr 13:534–536, 1989.

174. Garra BS, Shawker TH, Chang R, Kaplan K, White RD: The ultrasound appearance of radiation-induced hepatic injury. Correlation

with computed tomography and magnetic resonance imaging. J Ultrasound Med 7:605–609, 1988.

175. Kessler A, Mitchell DG, Israel HL, Goldberg BB: Hepatic and splenic sarcoidosis: Ultrasound and MR imaging. Abdom Imaging 18:159–163, 1993.

176. Warshauer DM, Semelka RC, Ascher SM: Nodular sarcoidosis of the liver and spleen: Appearance on MR images. J Magn Reson Imaging 4:553–557, 1994.

177. Shek TW, Ng IO, Chan KW: Inflammatory pseudotumor of the liver. Report of four cases and review of the literature. Am J Surg Pathol 17:231–238, 1993.

178. Horiuchi R, Uchida T, Kojima T, Shikata T: Inflammatory pseudotumor of the liver. Clinicopathologic study and review of the literature. Cancer 65:1583–1590, 1990.

179. Kelekis NL, Warshauer DM, Semelka RC, Eisenberg LB, Woosley JT: Inflammatory pseudotumor of the liver: Appearance on contrast enhanced helical CT and dynamic MR images. J Magn Reson Imaging 5:551–553, 1995.

180. Bertel CK, van Heerden JA, Sheedy PFd: Treatment of pyogenic hepatic abscesses. Surgical vs. percutaneous drainage. Arch Surg 121:554–558, 1986.

181. Mendez RJ, Schiebler ML, Outwater EK, Kressel HY: Hepatic abscesses: MR imaging findings. Radiology 190:431–436, 1994.

182. Ralls PW, Henley DS, Colletti PM, Benson R, Raval JK, Radin DR, Boswell WD, Jr., Halls JM: Amebic liver abscess: MR imaging. Radiology 165:801–804, 1987.

183. Landay MJ, Setiawan H, Hirsch G, Christensen EE, Conrad MR: Hepatic and thoracic amaebiasis. Am J Roentgenol 135:449–454, 1980.

184. Shirkhoda A, Lopez-Berestein G, Holbert JM, Luna MA: Hepatosplenic fungal infection: CT and pathologic evaluation after treatment with liposomal amphotericin B. Radiology 159:349–353, 1986.

185. Lewis JH, Patel HR, Zimmerman HJ: The spectrum of hepatic candidiasis. Hepatology 2:479–487, 1982.

186. Cho JS, Kim EE, Varma DG, Wallace S: MR imaging of hepatosplenic candidiasis superimposed on hemochromatosis. J Comput Assist Tomogr 14:774–776, 1990.

187. Semelka RC, Shoenut JP, Greenberg HM, Bow EJ: Detection of acute and treated lesions of hepatosplenic candidiasis: Comparison of dynamic contrast-enhanced CT and MR imaging. J Magn Reson Imaging 2:341–345, 1992.

188. Lamminen AE, Anttila VJ, Bondestam S, Ruutu T, Ruutu PJ: Infectious liver foci in leukemia: Comparison of short-inversion-time inversion-recovery, T1-weighted spin-echo, and dynamic gadolinium-enhanced MR imaging. Radiology 191:539–543, 1994.

189. Kelekis NL, Semelka RC, Jeon HJ, Sallah AS, Shea TC, Woosley JT: Dark ring sign: Finding in patients with fungal liver lesions and transfusional hemosiderosis undergoing treatment with antifungal antibiotics. Magn Reson Imaging 14:615–618, 1996.

190. Nghiem HV, Winter TC III, Mountford MC, Mack LA, Yuan C, Coldwell DM, Althaus SJ, Carithers RL, Jr., McVicar JP, Freeny PC: Evaluation of the portal venous system before liver transplantation: Value of phase-contrast MR angiography. Am J Roentgenol 164:871–878, 1995.

191. Demetris AJ, Lasky S, Van Thiel DH, Starzl TE, Dekker A: Pathology of hepatic transplantation: A review of 62 adult allograft recipients immunosuppressed with a cyclosporine/steroid regimen. Am J Pathol 118:151–161, 1985.

192. Lang P, Schnarkowski P, Grampp S, van Dijke C, Gindele A, Steffen R, Neuhaus P, Felix R: Liver transplantation: Significance of the periportal collar on MRI. J Comput Assist Tomogr 19:580–585, 1995.

193. Marincek B, Barbier PA, Becker CD, Mettler D, Ruchti C: CT appearance of impaired lymphatic drainage in liver transplants. Am J Roentgenol 147:519–523, 1986.

194. Wozney P, Zajko AB, Bron KM, Point S, Starzl TE: Vascular complications after liver transplantation: A 5-year experience. Am J Roentgenol 147:657–663, 1986.

195. Dalen K, Day DL, Ascher NL, Hunter DW, Thompson WM, Castaneda-Zuniga WR, Letourneau JG: Imaging of vascular complications after hepatic transplantation. Am J Roentgenol 150:1285–1290, 1988.

196. Zajko AB, Bennett MJ, Campbell WL, Koneru B: Mucocele of the cystic duct remnant in eight liver transplant recipients: Findings at cholangiography, CT, and US. Radiology 177:691–693, 1990.

GALLBLADDER AND BILIARY SYSTEM

C. REINHOLD, M.D.,[1] P. M. BRET, M.D.,[2] AND R. C. SEMELKA, M.D.[3]

C holedocholithiasis and malignant bile-duct obstruction are the most clinically important common diseases involving the biliary tree. Cholelithiasis accounts for over 90 percent of gallbladder pathology, and the majority of cases are diagnosed with a high degree of accuracy using ultrasound. Other imaging techniques play a secondary role in the diagnosis of gallbladder disease and are indicated either in a specific clinical context or as problem-solving modalities. For evaluating the bile ducts, a wide range of imaging techniques have been advocated. Although ultrasound and computed tomography (CT) imaging are used in the initial evaluation of patients with symptoms and signs referable to the pancreaticobiliary system, direct opacification of the biliary tree and pancreatic duct is often needed. Current techniques for direct visualization of the biliary tree include endoscopic retrograde cholangiopancreatography (ERCP) and, to a lesser extent, percutaneous transhepatic cholangiography (THC). Significant advantages of ERCP are that it provides unparalleled resolution and allows the implementation of therapeutic measures at the time of initial diagnosis. Although generally considered a safe procedure, ERCP is associated with morbidity and mortality rates of 7 percent and 1 percent, respectively [1]. In addition, unsuccessful cannulation of the common bile duct (CBD) or pancreatic duct occurs in 3 to 9 percent of cases

[1,2]. To date, the role of MRI in diagnosing diseases of the biliary tract has been limited. However, the recent development of fast imaging sequences and MR cholangiography has generated new interest in applying these techniques to evaluating the biliary system. Fast imaging techniques allow the upper abdomen to be scanned during a single breath-hold and are best suited to the study of tissue enhancement after intravenous (IV) contrast injection. MR cholangiography, on the other hand, provides direct visualization of the biliary tract similar to that of endoscopic retrograde cholangiography. However, as opposed to direct cholangiography, MR cholangiography is noninvasive and does not require the administration of contrast medium.

NORMAL ANATOMY

The gallbladder is an oval-shaped organ located in the gallbladder fossa, which is situated inferiorly between the right and left lobes of the liver. The anatomical components of the gallbladder are the fundus, body, neck, and cystic duct. The cystic duct joins the common hepatic duct to form the common bile duct. The normal gallbladder wall should not exceed 3 mm in thickness. The gallbladder can vary substantially in size and shape. Its position can vary from deep in the interlobar fissure (intrahepatic gallbladder) to substantially inferior extension below the liver. The intrahepatic bile ducts are a component of the intrahepatic portal triad. The biliary tree is an arborized system. Subsegmental branches join to form segmental branches, which join to form right and left bile ducts, which join at the level of the porta hepatis to form the common hepatic duct (CHD). The CHD joins with the cystic duct superior to the head of the pancreas to form the common bile duct (CBD). The CBD enters the head of the pancreas and in close approximation to the pancreatic duct enters the duodenum through the sphincter of Oddi.

MRI TECHNIQUE

General Guidelines

MRI examinations of the gallbladder should be performed after the patient has fasted for at least 8 to 12 hours in order to promote filling of the gallbladder. When imaging the bile ducts, a period of fasting is also advantageous for the following reasons: (1) The gallbladder may serve as a landmark and is easier to identify if physiologically distended; (2) an empty stomach will minimize motion-related artifacts in the upper abdomen; and (3) intestinal peristalsis may be diminished. Oral agents are not routinely administered because in the vast majority of patients there is a sufficient amount of physiologic fluid outlining the duodenum to facilitate its identification.

MR cholangiography has developed into a useful technique for the evaluation of the biliary system. Currently, high quality 2D or 3D long TR/TE echo-train spin-echo sequences (Fig. 3.1) and single-shot echo-train sequences (Fig. 3.2) are particularly effective approaches. Although the presence of surgical clips in the right upper quadrant is not a contraindication to MR imaging, surgical clips may result in signal-void artifacts (Fig. 3.3). Clip artifacts may be differentiated from choledocholithiasis by their extension beyond the borders of the bile ducts and, at times, by the presence of a curvilinear area of high signal at the periphery arising from magnetic susceptibility artifact. The major problem with clip artifacts is the potential masking of disease.

IV or intramuscular injections of an antispasmodic

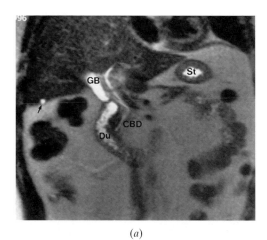

(a)

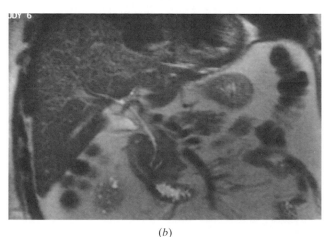

(b)

F I G . 3.2 Normal biliary tree. Half-fourier acquisition single-shot turbo spin-echo (HASTE) image (*a*) demonstrates clear definition of the normal biliary tree. The second part of the duodenum (*Du*) is well-outlined by a small amount of physiologic fluid in this fasting patient. Incidentally, a small liver cyst (*arrow, a*) is present in the right lobe. HASTE image (*b*) in a second adult patient demonstrates comparable visualization of the CBD.

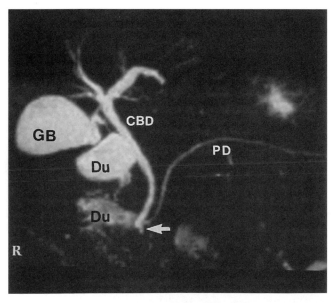

F I G . 3.1 Normal MR cholangiopancreatogram. Heavily T2-weighted, 3D echo-train spin-echo sequence, acquired with respiratory triggering. Coronal maximum intensity projection (MIP) reconstruction shows the normal intra- and extrahepatic bile ducts including the ampullary portion (*arrow*) of the common bile duct (CBD). The entire pancreatic duct (PD) is also well visualized. Du, duodenum; GB, gallbladder. (Courtesy Dr. Olivier Pellet, University of Lyon, France).

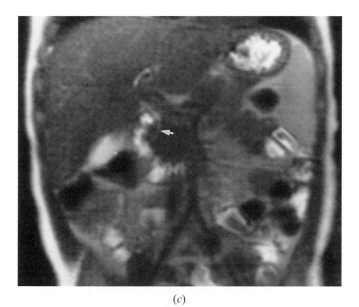

(c)

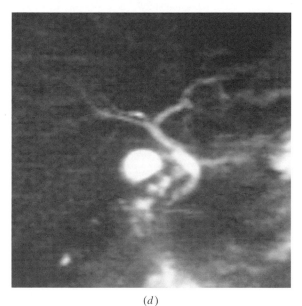

(d)

FIG. 3.2 (*Continued*) HASTE image (*c*) in a 1-year-old child demonstrates good visualization of the CBD (*arrow, c*) despite the lack of patient cooperation. Coronal 3D MIP reconstruction image (*d*) from a set of oblique coronal HASTE sections in a fourth subject reveals good demonstration of the biliary tree. CBD, common bile duct; GB, gallbladder; St, stomach.

agent (if not medically contraindicated) can be administered at the onset of the examination to decrease motion artifacts from bowel peristalsis. The use of a torso phased-array multicoil provides an increased signal-to-noise (S/N) ratio and should be used when available.

Imaging Protocols

MRI techniques for imaging the biliary system may be tailored for improved delineation of either the duct walls

and surrounding soft tissues or the biliary fluid within the ducts. Imaging of the biliary lumen requires optimal contrast between the biliary fluid and surrounding tissues and generally employs bright signal biliary fluid techniques. Pulse sequences that generate bright-signal biliary fluid, using heavily T2-weighted sequences, have received considerable clinical interest and are referred to as *MR cholangiography*. The large variety of proposed MR cholangiographic sequences and the lack of available clinical data are clear indicators that the technique is still in its infancy. In the ensuing discussion on the various MR cholangiographic techniques, a perspective is provided on some of the advantages and limitations of each.

An alternative approach to obtaining bright-signal biliary fluid is the use of T1 relaxation-enhancing intravenous contrast, which is substantially excreted in bile. Manganese(Mn)-DPDP and gadolinium(Gd)-EOB-DTPA are examples of these agents [3–8]. The high signal of contrast-enhanced bile permits good visualization of the biliary tree (Fig. 3.4). These agents, however, are not yet widely available, and their clinical role is yet to be determined.

In addition to generating bright-signal biliary fluid, techniques that result in black-signal biliary fluid can also achieve optimal contrast between the biliary fluid and surrounding tissues. To achieve optimal black-fluid techniques, an intravenous gadolinium chelate is administered, and images are acquired at least 1 minute after contrast administration. This ensures that all hepatic blood vessels contain gadolinium, such that only the biliary fluid will appear as signal-void [9,10]. T1-weighted

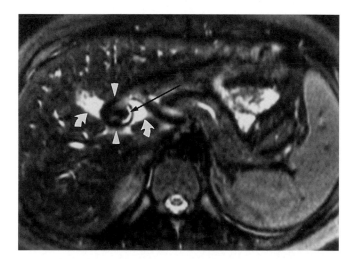

FIG. 3.3 Surgical clip artifact. MR cholangiogram. Heavily T2-weighted, 2D echo-train spin-echo sequence. Axial source image demonstrates a round signal-void artifact (*arrowheads*) at the level of the common hepatic duct (*curved arrows*) resulting in a pseudostone appearance. Note that the signal-void artifact due to the clip extends beyond the borders of the common hepatic duct and has a curvilinear area of high signal intensity at its periphery (*long thin arrow*).

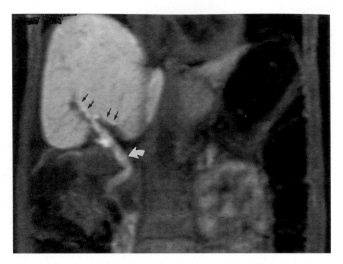

FIG. 3.4 Manganese(Mn)-DPDP-enhanced normal biliary tree. Coronal Mn-DPDP-enhanced SGE image. The normal intrahepatic (*small arrows*) and extrahepatic (*curved arrow*) bile ducts demonstrate increased signal intensity due to the T1-relaxation of the Mn-DPDP, which is substantially excreted in the bile. Note also the higher signal intensity of the normal liver.

spoiled gradient-echo (SGE) sequences with fat saturation are particularly suited to achieve this effect, because spin-echo sequences frequently show mixed signal in blood vessels. The addition of gradient-moment nulling to spin-echo sequences results in increased signal intensity of blood vessels and can be performed in addition to the SGE sequence in patients unable to cooperate with breath-holding [11]. The advantage of using a black-signal biliary fluid technique is that it allows optimal depiction of the bile-duct walls. Black-signal biliary fluid techniques are not suited for delineating the luminal contents of bile ducts, such as choledocholithiasis, and are therefore best used in conjunction with MR cholangiographic techniques (Fig. 3.5).

Conventional MRI

MRI examinations of the gallbladder and bile ducts should be tailored to the clinical situation. Conventional MRI techniques frequently combine the use of T1- and T2-weighted sequences. T2-weighted sequences can be obtained using spin-echo (SE) or echo-train spin-echo (e.g., fast spin-echo or turbo spin-echo) sequences. Advantages of the echo-train spin-echo sequences include (1) an increase in the bile-to-liver signal-intensity ratio and (2) improved conspicuity of the gallbladder contours due to shorter acquisition times, and consequently, decreased motion artifacts. T2-weighted sequences are primarily used to evaluate the soft tissues surrounding the biliary tree and the wall of the gallbladder, and may provide supplementary information on the status of the bile-duct walls. The addition of gradient-moment nulling to conventional T2-weighted sequences (which mini-

mizes vascular artifacts) results in increased signal intensity of the portal and hepatic veins. This may make it difficult to differentiate dilated intrahepatic bile ducts from portal-vein branches or to diagnose cystic diseases of the intrahepatic bile ducts. For these clinical indications, MR cholangiographic sequences or black-signal biliary fluid techniques are better suited because the luminal contents of the bile ducts and portal vein have opposing signal intensities.

The section thickness should be maintained at 5 mm with an intersection spacing of 1 to 2 mm to avoid signifi-

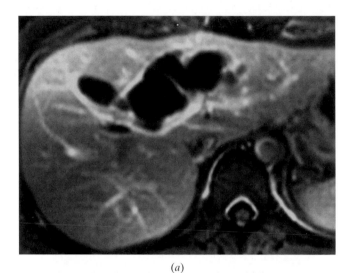

(*a*)

(*b*)

FIG. 3.5 Black- versus bright signal biliary fluid techniques. Black-signal biliary fluid. Gadolinium-enhanced T1-weighted fat-suppressed SGE image (*a*) demonstrates cystic dilatation of the intrahepatic bile ducts. Note that only the biliary fluid appears as a signal-void area, and there is optimal depiction of the bile duct walls. However, the bile duct stones are obscured with this technique because they present as signal-void areas. Bright-signal biliary fluid MR cholangiogram. Transverse heavily T2-weighted, 2D echo-train spin-echo image (*b*) in the same patient shows the intrahepatic stones (*arrows*) outlined by the bright-signal biliary fluid.

cant volume averaging. Other imaging parameters are similar to those used for examinations of the liver or pancreas. With the use of a torso multicoil array, the increased signal of the adjacent subcutaneous fat is such that fat suppression is routinely required to reduce motion artifacts.

T1-weighted sequences can be obtained using conventional spin-echo or SGE sequences. Sequences useful for demonstrating the wall of the gallbladder and bile ducts include T1-weighted fat-suppressed images with and without IV gadolinium chelates [10]. Gadolinium-enhanced T1-weighted fat-suppressed imaging is particularly well-suited for the demonstration of abnormal ductal and periductal superficial spreading tissue, as seen in ascending cholangitis or cholangiocarcinoma. Performing the acquisition during a breath-hold with SGE sequences avoids respiratory artifacts [9], which are particularly problematic after gadolinium chelate administration. In patients who are unable to breath-hold, the SGE sequences are often of limited diagnostic value. Under these circumstances, conventional spin-echo T1-weighted sequences acquired with motion compensation techniques often prove more diagnostic.

MR Cholangiography

MR cholangiographic techniques can be obtained using heavily T2-weighted gradient-echo or echo-train spin-echo sequences, and, in contrast to direct cholangiography, these techniques do not require the administration of contrast medium. Various modifications are currently under investigation, including 3D instead of 2D acquisitions and short imaging times to facilitate breath-hold techniques. Currently, there is no clear consensus regarding the optimal MR cholangiographic technique. This is due, in part, to the rapid evolution of the technology and to vendor-related differences that limit accurate comparisons of different pulse sequences.

Initial MR cholangiographic studies were performed using a heavily T2-weighted gradient-echo sequence (steady state of free precession) [12,13]. This technique may be performed as a breath-hold and acquired as a 3D data set. Two significant limitations of the gradient-echo technique exist: (1) the lack of routine visualization of the nondilated bile ducts or pancreatic duct (e.g., distal to a site of obstruction) and (2) the need for extremely long breath-holds (up to 1 minute on some MRI systems) [14–16].

Imaging approaches that have achieved greater clinical interest rely on heavily T2-weighted 2D or 3D echo-train spin-echo sequences to generate MR cholangiograms [16–20]. For these sequences, repetition times (TR) ranging from 8,000 to 12,000 msec and echo times (TE) ranging from 140 to 240 msec are commonly used. As with the gradient-echo sequence, the echo-train spin-echo sequence takes advantage of the fact that fluids with a long T2 relaxation time, such as bile, will have a very high signal intensity, whereas the surrounding liver, which has a much shorter T2 value, will generate very little signal. In addition, flowing blood will result in little or no measurable signal. This combination provides optimal contrast between the hyperintense signal of the bile and the hypointense signal of the background. The echo-train spin-echo sequence offers several advantages over the gradient-echo sequence, including (1) higher signal-to-noise and contrast-to-noise ratios that allow the use of thin sections, even for 2D imaging; (2) diminished sensitivity to both motion artifact and slow flow; (3) decreased magnetic susceptibility effects (e.g., from signal loss due to surgical clips or air in the duodenum); and (4) measurement of T2 rather than combined T2/T2* decay. In a study comparing 2D echo-train spin-echo and 3D gradient-echo sequences in 26 patients [16], the echo-train spin-echo sequence was shown to be significantly better at visualizing both the dilated and nondilated biliary tree and pancreatic duct.

Several techniques have been proposed to optimize MR cholangiography. The use of a phased-array multicoil increases the signal-to-noise ratio, thereby improving visualization of small nondilated ducts. The addition of a fat saturation technique also has become routine in order to improve conspicuity of the bile ducts that distinguishes them from the surrounding intra-abdominal fat and to decrease motion artifacts associated with the hyperintense subcutaneous fat. Use of thin sections (3 mm or less) and a high matrix size allows the acquisition of high-resolution images. MR cholangiograms (particularly for 2D acquisitions) should be acquired in the coronal, as well as the axial plane. Images acquired in the axial plane are frequently of superior diagnostic quality because they are less degraded by respiratory artifacts.

Some investigators have demonstrated the feasibility of depicting the biliary tree by using a breathing-averaged echo-train spin-echo technique. Techniques that can be used to minimize breathing-related motion artifacts include signal averaging [21,22] and respiratory gating [20]. Acquiring MR cholangiograms during quiet breathing improves the versatility of the technique: (1) Patients can be imaged regardless of their ability to breath-hold; (2) segmentation of the acquisition and the potential for serious misregistration artifact is avoided; and (3) high-resolution images with prolonged imaging times become feasible. In cooperative patients high-quality MR cholangiographic images are obtained with this technique (see Fig. 3.1).

Echo-train spin-echo sequences also can be performed in a breath-hold period lasting from 1 to 20 seconds by increasing the echo-train length. These approaches can be used as a large projectional slab (e.g., 5-cm thickness to image the major bile ducts in one data set), as a multisection acquisition, or as a thin-section

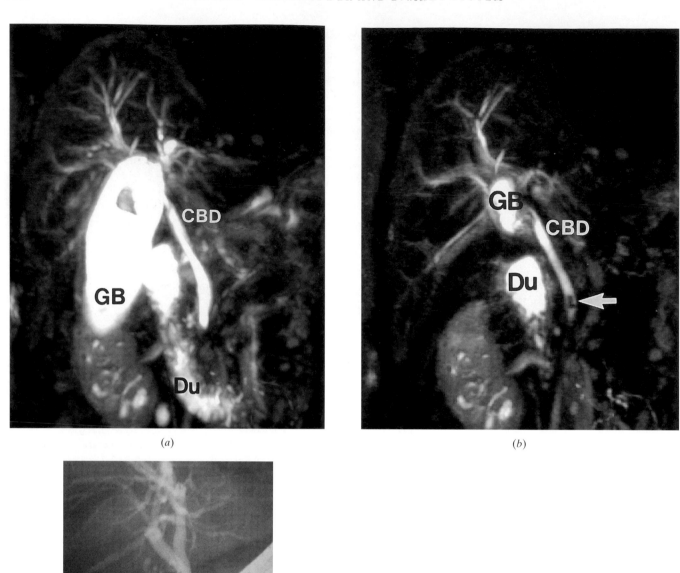

(a)

(b)

(c)

FIG. 3.6 Three-dimensional (3D) MIP reconstruction versus multiplanar reformation. A 3D MIP reconstruction MR cholangiogram (*a*) using heavily T2-weighted, 2D echo-train spin-echo images. Coronal MIP image demonstrates the biliary tree to be of normal caliber without evidence of choledocholithiasis. Incidentally, a gallstone is present. Multiplanar reformation showing a coronal reformatted image (*b*) of the same acquisition at the level of the extrahepatic bile ducts demonstrates a small signal-void focus (*arrow, b*) in the distal CBD consistent with a stone. The small CBD stone was completely obscured by the MIP format because it was surrounded by hyperintense bile. ERCP image (*c*) confirms the presence of a small distal CBD stone (*arrow, c*).

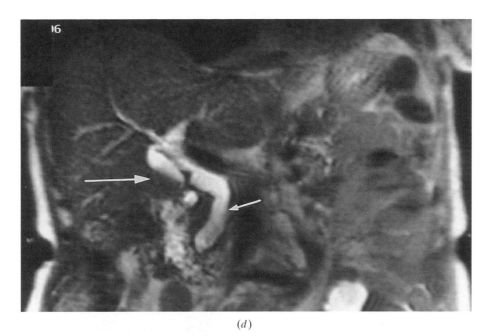

(d)

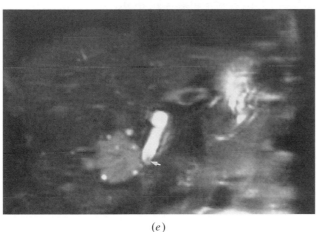

(e)

FIG. 3.6 (*Continued*) Targeted MIP reconstruction (*d*) from a set of coronal HASTE sections, and coronal single-shot T2-weighted fat-suppressed echo-train spin-echo image (*e*) in a second patient. Substantial dilation of the CBD is shown on the MIP image (*arrow, d*). Multiple calculi are visualized in the gallbladder (*long arrow, d*). However, no CBD calculus is shown on the MIP image. The coronal single-shot T2-weighted fat-suppressed echo-train spin-echo image (*e*) reveals a 5-mm CBD calculus (*arrow, e*). CBD, common bile duct; GB, gallbladder; Du, duodenum.

single-shot approach that can acquire multiple single sections in one breath-hold. The half-fourier acquisition single-shot turbo spin-echo (HASTE) sequence is one example of a thin-section single-shot technique that appears to hold considerable clinical utility because it is breathing independent and does not suffer substantially from magnetic susceptibility artifact [23] (see Fig. 3.2).

MR cholangiograms are best reviewed at a diagnostic workstation rather than on hard-copy films. Individual source images, as well as reformatted images, should be reviewed rather than relying solely on 3D reconstructed views. This avoids a number of potential pitfalls in diagnosis because much of the information obtained from the individual source images is lost when the whole volume is displayed in a maximum-intensity projection (MIP) format. For example, common bile duct (CBD) stones depicted as areas of low signal intensity may be completely obscured by the MIP format if they are surrounded by hyperintense bile (Fig. 3.6). The 3D reconstructed images, however, are better suited to providing a complete overview of the biliary tree anatomy, which is useful for treatment planning.

NORMAL ANATOMICAL STRUCTURES AND VARIANTS

Normal Anatomical Structures

Gallbladder and Cystic Duct

The gallbladder wall is usually not well-seen on T2-weighted sequences (Fig. 3.7). On T1-weighted sequences the gallbladder wall is of intermediate signal intensity, and its visibility depends largely on the signal intensity of the bile within the gallbladder (Fig. 3.8). The gallbladder wall is usually visualized following IV admin-

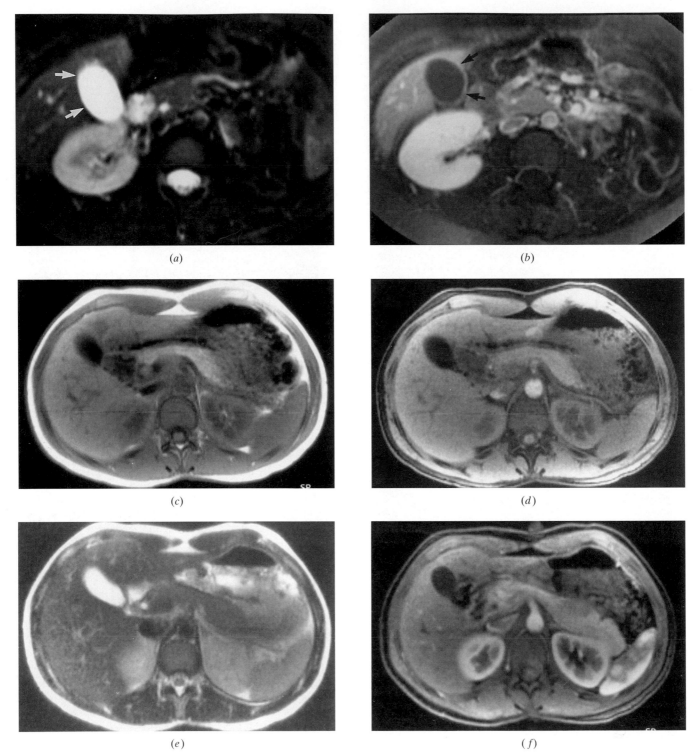

(a)

(b)

(c)

(d)

(e)

(f)

FIG. 3.7 Normal gallbladder wall. T2-weighted fat-suppressed spin-echo (*a*) and gadolinium-enhanced T1-weighted fat-suppressed spin-echo (*b*) images. The gallbladder wall (*arrows, a*) is not well-visualized on the T2-weighted image (*a*). Note that the gallbladder contents are of high signal intensity. The gallbladder wall is well-shown as a thin enhancing structure (*arrows, b*) on the gadolinium-enhanced T1-weighted fat-suppressed spin-echo image (*b*). The gallbladder wall adjacent to the liver is not clearly defined because the enhancement of gallbladder wall and liver are similar. SGE (*c*), fat-suppressed SGE (*d*), HASTE (*e*), immediate postgadolinium fat-suppressed SGE (*f*),

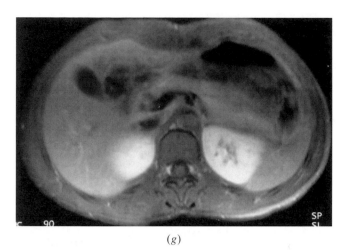

(g)

FIG. 3.7 *(Continued)* and gadolinium-enhanced T1-weighted fat-suppressed spin-echo *(g)* images in a second subject with a normal gallbladder. The bile is low in signal intensity on the T1-weighted image *(c)* and high in signal on the T2-weighted image *(d)*. The normal gallbladder wall is barely perceptible as a thin line, best shown on the gadolinium-enhanced interstitial-phase image.

istration of a gadolinium chelate, although the portion of the wall adjacent to the liver parenchyma may be obscured due to similar enhancement (see Fig. 3.7).

The gallbladder contents are uniformly hyperintense in comparison with the liver parenchyma on T2-weighted sequences (see Fig. 3.7). On T1-weighted sequences, the signal intensity of the gallbladder contents may vary from very low (water intensity) to high signal intensity, due to variations in the concentration of water, cholesterol, and bile salts [24] (see Fig. 3.8). Unconcentrated bile accumulates in the gallbladder following ingestion of a meal and demonstrates low signal intensity on T1-weighted sequences, which is consistent with the long T1 of water. With reabsorption of water and increased cholesterol and bile salt concentration, the T1 relaxation time decreases [24,25]. Therefore, the appearance of concentrated bile is usually higher than that of adjacent liver. Because concentrated bile is denser, a layering effect is frequently seen, with the hyperintense bile in the dependent position (Fig. 3.9).

The cystic duct is best depicted on the heavily T2-weighted sequences used for MR cholangiography (Fig. 3.10). The cystic duct, as well as its insertion into the common hepatic duct, is routinely seen using this technique [26].

Bile Ducts

With currently available MR cholangiographic techniques, the normal extrahepatic bile ducts, which are of high signal intensity due to the intraluminal bile, are visualized in nearly 100 percent of patients [27–29]. Occasionally, a segment of the extrahepatic bile duct may be devoid of signal (e.g., in cases of pneumobilia, in the proximity of surgical clips [see Fig. 3.3], or when motion

artifacts, often secondary to duodenal peristaltism, result in signal loss in the suprapancreatic segment of the CBD). Nondilated intrahepatic bile ducts can be followed into the outer third of the hepatic parenchyma in over 90 percent of cases with MR cholangiography [22].

On T1-weighted sequences, the signal intensity of bile in the intrahepatic bile ducts is usually low because it is not concentrated. In the CBD, however, the signal intensity is variable, depending on the concentration of the bile present in the gallbladder (see Fig. 3.8).

The major papilla is a small mucosal protrusion into the duodenum resulting from the muscles that surround the distal CBD and ventral pancreatic duct. There is considerable variation in the shape and size of the major

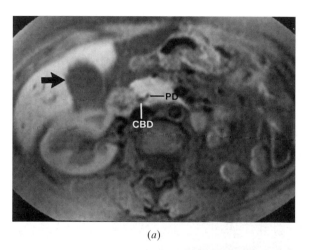

(a)

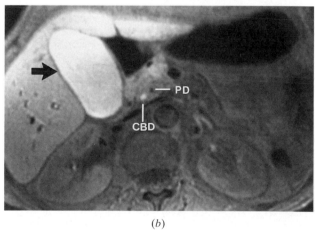

(b)

FIG. 3.8 Normal variations in signal of gallbladder bile. T1-weighted fat-suppressed spin-echo images in two patients *(a)* and *(b)*. Low signal intensity. The gallbladder contents *(arrow, a)* are hypointense similar to that of cerebrospinal fluid. The common bile duct (CBD) and pancreatic duct (PD) at the level of the pancreatic head are also of low signal intensity *(b)*. High signal intensity. The gallbladder contents *(arrow, b)*, as well as the CBD in the head of the pancreas, are markedly hyperintense, whereas the PD remains low in signal intensity. As the image is fat suppressed, the high signal intensity is not on the basis of fluid or fat composition but rather of proteinaceous composition.

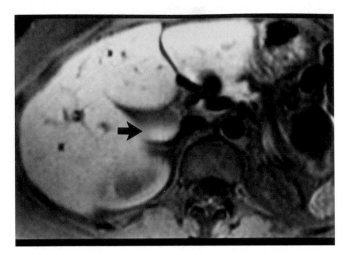

FIG. **3.9** Normal layering of gallbladder bile. T1-weighted fat-suppressed spin-echo image. There is layering of the gallbladder bile with the more concentrated, hyperintense bile (*arrow*) in a dependent location.

papilla. Along the upper aspect of the major papilla is the superior papillary fold, which often forms a hood over the papilla and may be quite prominent. The longitudinal fold extends inferiorly from the papilla. The average size of the major papilla has been reported as 15 mm in length and 7 mm in diameter [30]. The minor papilla is the termination site of the dorsal pancreatic duct and may be present proximal to the major papilla. Little has been written on the MR imaging characteristics of the normal papilla. Taourel et al. [31], using MR cholangiography, visualized the major papilla in 40 percent of cases (Fig. 3.11). The minor papilla was seen less frequently (Fig. 3.12).

Normal Variants

It is generally accepted that the presence of an aberrant right hepatic duct or an abnormal cystic duct junction places the patient at increased risk for bile duct injury during laparoscopic cholecystectomy [32]. Anatomical variants of the cystic duct that increase the risk of bile duct injury at surgery include (1) a low or medial cystic

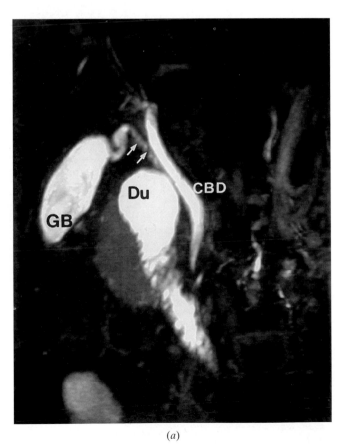

(*a*)

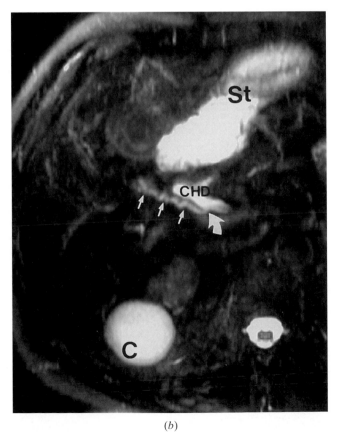

(*b*)

FIG. **3.10** Normal cystic duct anatomy. MR cholangiogram. Heavily T2-weighted, 2D echo-train spin-echo images (*a,b*). Coronal MIP image (*a*) demonstrates the cystic duct (*arrows, a*) throughout its length. Transverse MIP image (*b*) in a patient after cholecystectomy demonstrates the normal junction (*curved arrow, b*) of the cystic (*arrows, b*) and common hepatic duct. C, Renal cyst; CBD, common bile duct; CHD, common hepatic duct; Du, duodenum; GB, gallbladder; St, stomach.

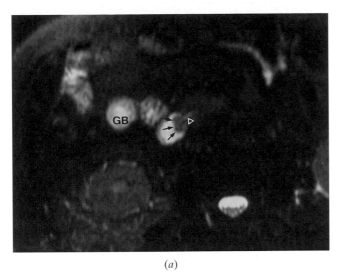

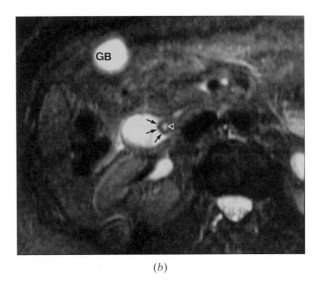

(a)   (b)

FIG. 3.11 Normal major papilla. MR cholangiogram. Heavily T2-weighted, 2D echo-train spin-echo images (a,b) The major papilla (arrows, a,b) can be seen outlined by physiologic fluid present in the duodenum. Note the ampullary portion (open arrowhead, a,b) of the CBD. The normal papilla has considerable variation in size and shape. GB, gallbladder.

duct insertion, (2) a parallel course of the cystic to the common hepatic duct, and (3) a short cystic duct. The impact of preoperative identification of these variants remains controversial [33–35]. Although the accuracy of MR cholangiography in diagnosing normal anatomical variants has not yet been established, preliminary results show that MR cholangiography can accurately detect normal anatomical variants of the biliary tree and cystic duct [26] (Figs. 3.13 and 3.14). The practical relevance of this is unclear because it is doubtful that the routine use of

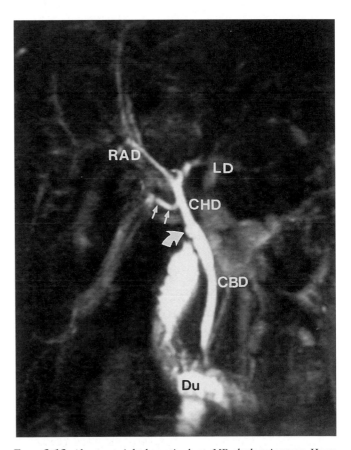

FIG. 3.13 Aberrant right hepatic duct. MR cholangiogram. Heavily T2-weighted, 2D echo-train spin-echo image. Coronal MIP image demonstrates an aberrant insertion of the posterior right hepatic duct (arrows) into the common hepatic duct (CHD). Note the normal bifurcation of the right anterior duct (RAD) and left hepatic duct (LD) at the level of the porta hepatis. Only the distal aspect of the cystic duct (curved arrow) at its junction with the CHD is imaged on this targeted MIP reconstruction. CBD, common bile duct; Du, duodenum.

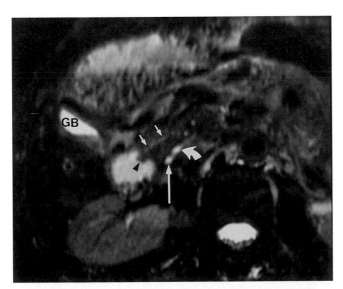

FIG. 3.12 Normal minor papilla. MR cholangiogram. Heavily T2-weighted, 2D echo-train spin-echo sequence. The dorsal pancreatic duct (arrows) can be seen entering the minor papilla (arrowhead). The ventral pancreatic duct (curved arrow) and CBD (long thin arrow) are located posteriorly. GB, gallbladder.

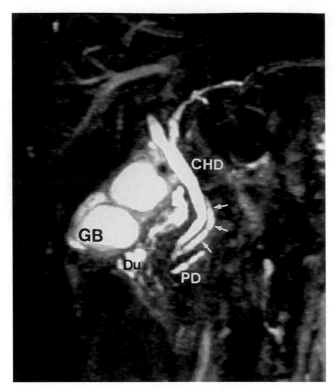

F I G . 3.14 Low cystic duct junction. MR cholangiogram. Heavily T2-weighted, 2D echo-train spin-echo sequence. Coronal MIP image shows insertion of the cystic duct (*arrows*) into the common hepatic duct (CHD) just above the level of the ampulla. Du, duodenum; GB, gallbladder; PD, pancreatic duct.

MR cholangiography can be advocated prior to every laparoscopic cholecystectomy. MR cholangiography might prove useful, however, in patients presenting with additional risk factors for bile duct injury such as obesity, cholecystitis, prior abdominal surgery, or undergoing complicated biliary reconstruction [32].

Bilioenteric Anastomosis

After a roux-en-Y or other bilioenteric anastomosis, ERCP may be very difficult technically to perform. In such instances, MR cholangiography may be particularly useful in demonstrating the diameter and morphology of the bile ducts proximal to the anastomosis.

■ DISEASE OF THE GALLBLADDER

Gallstone Disease

Cholelithiasis is diagnosed with a high degree of accuracy using ultrasound. Therefore, MRI currently plays no role in the detection of gallstones. In a recent study, MR cho-

langiography correctly predicted the presence of solitary or multiple gallstones in approximately 80 percent of patients [29]. Breath-hold or breathing-independent echo-train spin-echo (e.g., HASTE) obtained in the transverse plane demonstrates cholelithiasis with a high degree of accuracy. Because gallstones frequently are encountered incidentally, it is important to be familiar with their MRI characteristics. During the initial development of nonoperative therapies for cholelithiasis, it was hoped that MRI could be used to predict gallstone composition. The advent of laparoscopic cholecystectomy, however, obviated this need since therapeutic options are no longer based on the chemical composition of stones.

Gallstones generally present as signal-void areas on both T1- and T2-weighted images acquired at high field-strengths (Fig. 3.15). MR cholangiographic sequences are particularly effective at demonstrating small calculi due to the contrast generated between the high-signal-intensity bile and the low-signal-intensity calculi. The breathing-independent nature of the HASTE sequence also renders this technique very effective at demonstrating small calculi (see Fig. 3.15). Occasionally, areas of high signal intensity will be present in gallstones on T1- and T2-weighted sequences, or, less commonly, the stones will appear largely hyperintense on T1-weighted sequences (Fig. 3.16) [36–39]. Baron et al. [39] have shown, using spectroscopy and chemical analysis of gallstones, that the increased signal intensity on T1-weighted sequences does not correlate with areas of high lipid content. The exact cause has yet to be elucidated. However, the presence of protein macromolecules with shorter T1-relaxation times may account for this.

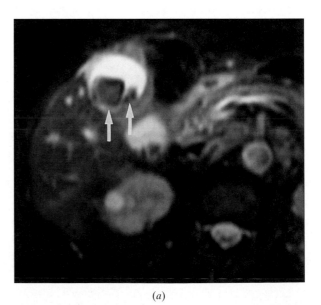

(*a*)

F I G . 3.15 Gallstones, T2-weighted sequence. Hypointense gallstone. T2-weighted fat-suppressed spin-echo image shows two gallstones (*arrows, a*) of low signal intensity in contrast to the hyperintense bile. Mixed-signal gallstone. MR cholangiogram.

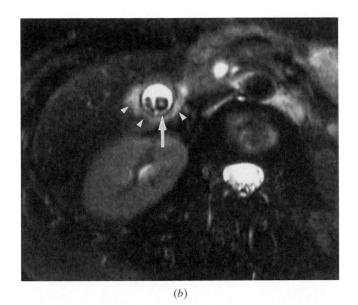

(b)

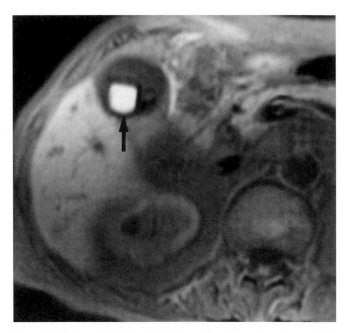

FIG. 3.16 Hyperintense gallstone, T1-weighted sequence. T1-weighted fat-suppressed spin-echo image demonstrates a gallstone (*arrow*) of uniform high signal intensity centrally with a signal-void peripheral rim.

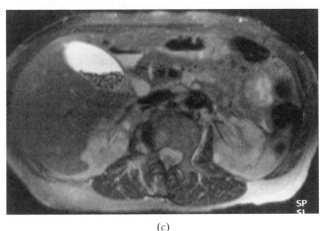

(c)

FIG. 3.15 (*Continued*) Heavily T2-weighted 2D echo-train spin-echo image (*b*) in a second patient shows a gallstone (*arrow, b*) with a hypointense rim and a hyperintense center. Inflammatory changes are noted around the gallbladder (*arrowheads, b*) in this patient with acute cholecystitis. HASTE image (*c*) in a third patient demonstrates multiple tiny nearly signal-void calculi in the gallbladder.

Because the entire cystic duct as well as its insertion into the common hepatic duct can be seen in the majority of patients with MR cholangiography, cystic duct stones may be depicted in addition to gallstones (Figs. 3.17 and 3.18).

Acute Cholecystitis

Acute cholecystitis is caused by obstruction of the cystic duct by calculus disease in 95 percent of patients and is most commonly diagnosed with ultrasound. Morphological criteria used to diagnose acute cholecystitis on ultrasound include the presence of gallstones and thickening of the gallbladder wall. In addition, the region of pain can be accurately localized with the ultrasound transducer (sonographic Murphy's sign). The presence of all these

ultrasound findings indicates a high probability of acute cholecystitis. Occasionally, however, one or more of these signs are absent. Under these circumstances, the diagnosis of acute cholecystitis, especially acalculous cholecystitis, remains challenging. The high sensitivity of gadolinium-enhanced, fat-suppressed images to inflammatory changes make this an optimal MRI technique for assessing patients in whom a diagnosis of acute cholecystitis is suspected but for whom findings at sonography are equivocal [40].

Morphological criteria in the diagnosis of acute cho-

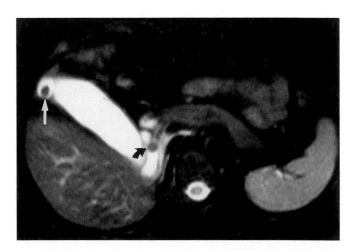

FIG. 3.17 Cystic duct stone and gallstone. T2-weighted fat-suppressed spin-echo image shows a stone (*curved arrow*) in the cystic duct, as well as a stone (*arrow*) in the phrygian cap of the gallbladder.

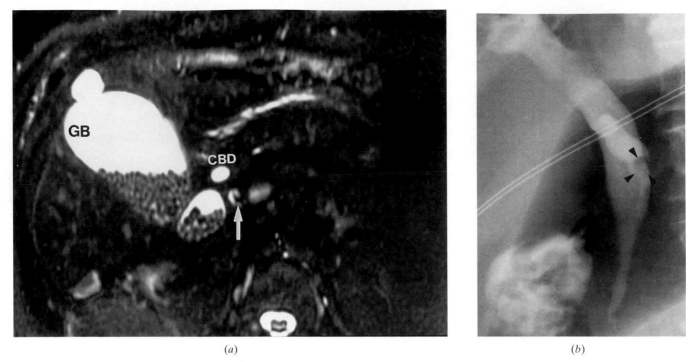

(a)   (b)

F IG . 3.18 Cystic duct stone and microlithiasis. MR cholangiogram. Heavily T2-weighted 2D echo-train spin-echo image. There are numerous tiny stones in the gallbladder (GB) and in the gallbladder infundibulum. In addition, a small stone (*arrow, a*) is present in the cystic duct that can be seen coursing posterior to the common bile duct (CBD). ERCP image (*b*) confirms the presence of a cystic duct stone (arrowheads, b). An inflammatory stricture of the CBD is also present. (Reprinted with permission from Reinhold C, Bret PM: MR cholangiopancreatography. Abdom Imaging 21:105–116, 1996)

lecystitis with MRI are similar to those described for ultrasound. A combination of T2-weighted and gadolinium-enhanced T1-weighted sequences can demonstrate the presence of gallstones, gallbladder wall thickening, pericholecystic fluid, and occasionally intramural abscesses [41] (Fig. 3.19). However, in addition to these morpholog-

ical criteria, MRI can also provide ancillary information on the vascularization of the gallbladder wall.

In patients with acute cholecystitis, the gallbladder wall and adjacent tissues demonstrate increased enhancement on gadolinium-enhanced fat-suppressed images (Fig. 3.20). This enhancement is frequently most

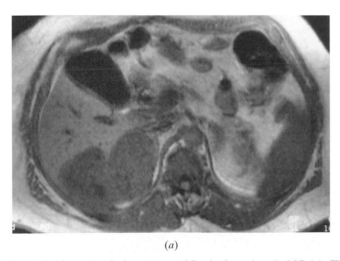

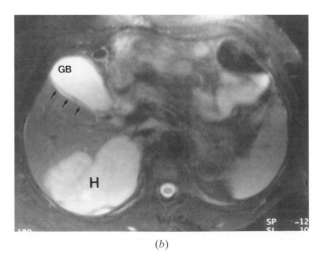

(a)   (b)

F IG . 3.19 Acute cholecystitis, mildly thickened wall. SGE (*a*), T2-weighted fat-suppressed echo-train spin-echo (*b*), immediate (*c*) and 90-second (*d*) postgadolinium SGE images. The gallbladder wall is mildly thickened (4 mm). Increased signal intensity (*arrows, b*) is apparent on the T2-weighted image (*b*). There is a giant hemangioma (H) (*b*) in the posterior segment of the liver.

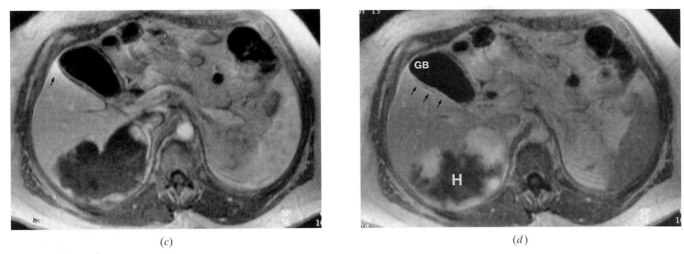

(c)   (d)

F IG. 3.19 (*Continued*) Transient increased enhancement of liver parenchyma adjacent to the gallbladder (*arrow, c*) is shown on the immediate postgadolinium SGE image (*c*). Increased enhancement of the gallbladder wall (*arrows, d*) is shown on the interstitial-phase gadolinium-enhanced SGE image. Note also the centripedal enhancement of the hemangioma. GB, gallbladder.

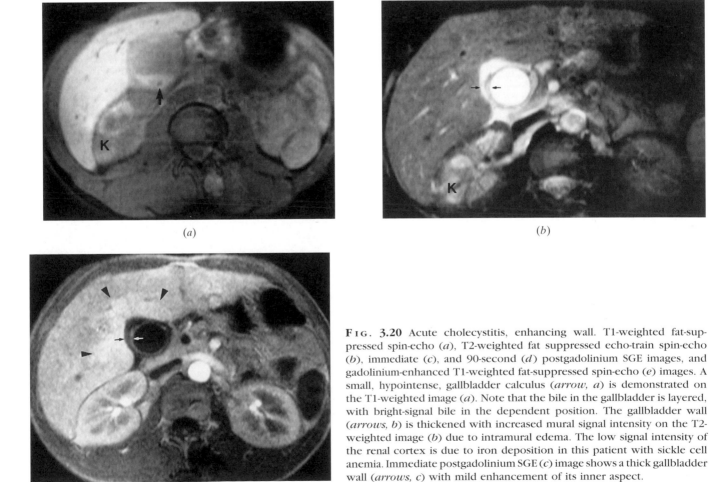

(a)   (b)

(c)

F IG. 3.20 Acute cholecystitis, enhancing wall. T1-weighted fat-suppressed spin-echo (*a*), T2-weighted fat suppressed echo-train spin-echo (*b*), immediate (*c*), and 90-second (*d*) postgadolinium SGE images, and gadolinium-enhanced T1-weighted fat-suppressed spin-echo (*e*) images. A small, hypointense, gallbladder calculus (*arrow, a*) is demonstrated on the T1-weighted image (*a*). Note that the bile in the gallbladder is layered, with bright-signal bile in the dependent position. The gallbladder wall (*arrows, b*) is thickened with increased mural signal intensity on the T2-weighted image (*b*) due to intramural edema. The low signal intensity of the renal cortex is due to iron deposition in this patient with sickle cell anemia. Immediate postgadolinium SGE (*c*) image shows a thick gallbladder wall (*arrows, c*) with mild enhancement of its inner aspect.

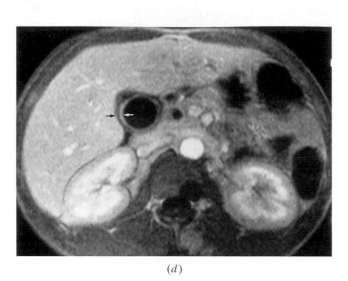

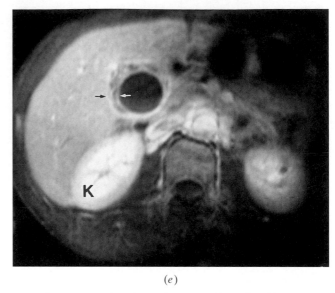

(d)

(e)

FIG. 3.20 (*Continued*) Transient increased enhancement of the liver parenchyma (*arrowheads, c*) adjacent to the gallbladder is noted, which reflects hyperemic inflammatory changes due to the close proximity to the inflamed gallbladder wall. Resolution of the transient increased hepatic enhancement and progressive enhancement of the gallbladder wall (arrows, d) are noted on the 90-second postgadolinium SGE image (*d*). Gadolinium-enhanced T1-weighted fat-suppressed spin-echo image (*e*) shows enhancement of the gallbladder wall (*arrows, e*). Note linear areas of enhancing tissue within the wall. K, kidney.

pronounced along the inner layers of the gallbladder wall on images acquired immediately after gadolinium administration and progresses to involve the entire thickness of the wall on more delayed images. In a recent study, the percentage of contrast enhancement of the gallbladder wall was shown to correlate well with the presence of acute cholecystitis and was more accurate than wall thickness in distinguishing acute from chronic cholecystitis and gallbladder malignancy [42]. All patients with an 80 percent or greater contrast enhancement of

the gallbladder wall were subsequently shown to have acute cholecystitis. These findings, although promising, must be validated in larger controlled clinical trials because an enhancing thickened gallbladder wall may be seen with other disease entities (see Fig. 3.24). An important ancillary finding was the presence of transient increased enhancement of pericholecystic hepatic parenchyma on capillary-phase images observed in 70 percent of patients with acute cholecystitis (Fig. 3.21) [42]. This reflects a hyperemic response in the liver due to the

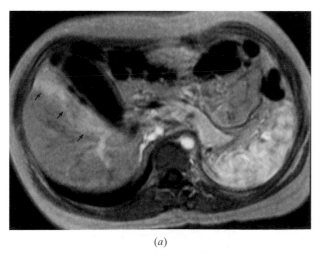

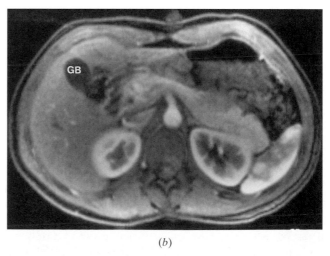

(a)

(b)

FIG. 3.21 Transient hyperemic enhancement of the liver secondary to acute cholecystitis. Immediate postgadolinium SGE image (*a*) in a patient with acute cholecystitis demonstrates increased enhancement of the liver adjacent to the gallbladder, which resolves within 1 minute of contrast administration. Immediate postgadolinium fat-suppressed SGE image (*b*) in a normal subject for comparison, demonstrates homogeneous enhancement of the liver.

adjacent inflammation of the gallbladder. On T2-weighted images, periportal high signal intensity may be observed in the setting of acute cholecystitis. However, this is a nonspecific appearance observed in a variety of biliary, liver, and pancreatic diseases [43].

Acute acalculus cholecystitis is typically observed in sick patients in the intensive care setting. An uncommon cause of acute acalculus chemical cholecystitis occurs secondary to hepatic arterial chemoembolization (Fig. 3.22).

Pathophysiologically, it has been demonstrated that the water content of bile in the gallbladder is higher in acute cholecystitis than in either chronic cholecystitis or normal states [44]. It might be expected that the signal intensity of gallbladder bile on T1-weighted sequences would decrease in patients with acute cholecystitis, thereby assisting in the differential diagnosis of gallbladder disease [45,46]. However, the higher water content is frequently offset by a higher protein content, which results in T1 shortening of the gallbladder bile. An in vitro study performed on bile obtained from surgical specimens did not demonstrate a clear correlation between signal intensity of bile and the presence of acute cholecystitis [25] (see Fig. 3.21b). Furthermore, results obtained at low field strengths may not be applicable at field strengths of 1.0 T or greater because of lower T1-dependent contrast discrimination.

Hemorrhagic Cholecystitis

An unusual form of acute cholecystitis is hemorrhagic cholecystitis. Unlike nonhemorrhagic acute cholecystitis, a larger percentage of these patients have acalculus cholecystitis. MRI is accurate in demonstrating this entity due to the varying signal intensity of blood breakdown products. The age of acute hemorrhagic cholecystitis may be predicted based on the signal intensities of the fluid present due to the predictable signal intensity of specific blood breakdown products (Fig. 3.23).

Chronic Cholecystitis

Chronic cholecystitis appears as a small, irregularly shaped gallbladder with a thickened, mildly enhancing wall on gadolinium-enhanced fat-suppressed images (Fig. 3.24). A distinguishing feature between acute and chronic cholecystitis on MR images is the degree of mural and pericholecystic tissue enhancement. The degree and extent of enhancement reflects the severity of the inflammatory process. The gallbladder wall may calcify in the setting of chronic cholecystitis, which can result in the appearance of a porcelain gallbladder. Porcelain gallbladders are at increased risk of undergoing malignant change. Calcifications are usually signal-void on MR images, such that gadolinium-enhanced fat-suppressed images are sensitive for the detection of nodular soft tissue associated with the calcifications that would imply the

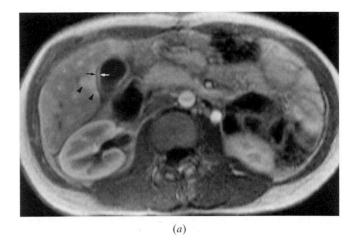

(a)

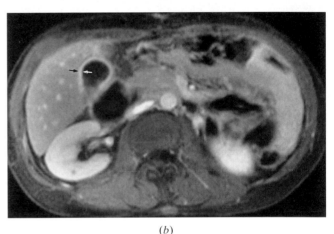

(b)

F IG. 3.22 Chemoembolization-induced acute cholecystitis. Immediate (*a*) and 90-second (*b*) postgadolinium SGE images. Transient pericholecystic enhancement of the liver parenchyma (*arrowheads, a*) is noted on the immediate postgadolinium SGE image (*a*), which has faded by 90 seconds (*b*). There is progressive enhancement of the thickened gallbladder wall (*arrows, a,b*) from (*a*) to (*b*).

presence of gallbladder cancer. A uniform wall less than 4 mm in thickness shown on MR images excludes the presence of malignancy (Fig. 3.25).

Increased Gallbladder Wall Thickness

Gallbladder wall thickening may be seen in a variety of hepatic, biliary, and pancreatic diseases. Increased thickness of the gallbladder wall may be seen uncommonly in acute hepatitis (Fig. 3.26), cirrhosis with hypoproteinemia, and pancreatitis. Increased enhancement of the gallbladder wall may also be observed due to inflammatory disease in surrounding tissues or organs. Transient increased enhancement of the adjacent hepatic parenchyma is lacking in these causes of gallbladder thickening. However, studies are lacking that demonstrate the specificity of hyperemic enhancement of the liver to distinguish acute cholecystitis from gallbladder

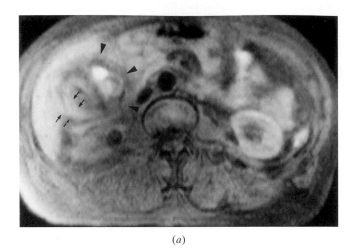

(a)

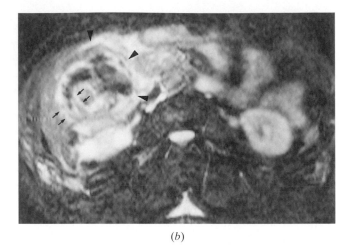

(b)

FIG. 3.23 Hemorrhagic cholecystitis. T1-weighted fat-suppressed spin-echo (*a*), T2-weighted fat-suppressed echo-train spin-echo (*b*), and interstitial-phase gadolinium-enhanced SGE (*c*) images. On the T1-weighted fat-suppressed spin-echo image (*a*) areas of high signal intensity consistent with hemorrhage are noted within the substantially thickened gallbladder wall (*small arrows, a*) and pericholecystic collection (*arrowheads, a*). On the T2-weighted image (*b*), the thickened gallbladder wall is also shown (*small arrows, b*) and contains areas of high and low signal intensity. Anteromedial to the gallbladder, the large complex pericholecystic fluid collection (*arrowheads, b*) is predominantly of low signal intensity, which in combination with the high signal intensity on the T1-weighted image is consistent with intracellular methemoglobin. The delayed postgadolinium SGE image (*c*) shows to better advantage the thick gallbladder wall (*small arrows, c*) and hemorrhagic pericholecystic fluid collection (*arrowheads, c*). Incidentally, a calculus (*long arrow, c*) is present in the right renal collecting system.

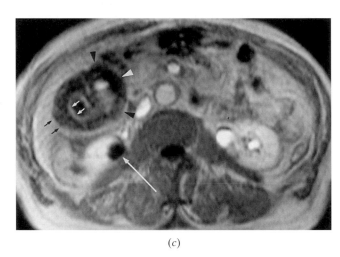

(c)

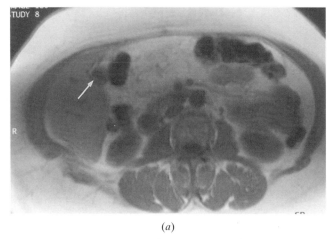

(a)

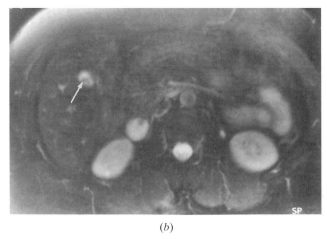

(b)

FIG. 3.24 Chronic cholecystitis. SGE (*a*), T2-weighted fat-suppressed spin-echo (*b*), immediate postgadolinium SGE (*c*), and 90-second postgadolinium fat-suppressed SGE (*d*) images. The gallbladder is shrunken and irregular in shape, and the wall is noted to be, in part, high in signal intensity on the precontrast T1-weighted image (*arrow, a*). On the T2-weighted image (*b*), the gallbladder wall is poorly defined, and low-signal-intensity cholelithiasis is present (*arrow, b*).

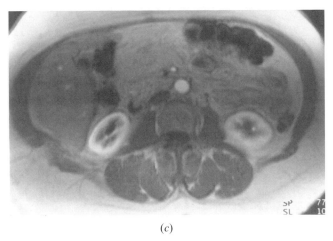

(c)

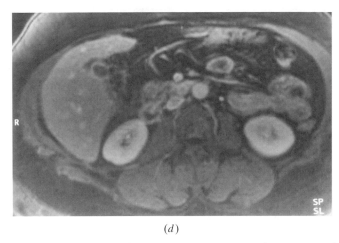

(d)

F I G . 3.24 (*Continued*) The gallbladder wall enhances moderately on the immediate postgadolinium SGE image (*c*), and no increased enhancement is noted in the adjacent liver parenchyma. On the 90-second postgadolinium fat-suppressed SGE image (*d*) the gallbladder wall is well-visualized and measures approximately 4 mm in thickness.

wall inflammation related to disease extrinsic to the gallbladder wall.

Gallbladder Polyps

Gallbladder polyps are small, typically 1-cm masses that arise from the gallbladder wall. The majority are cholesterol polyps and do not have malignant potential. Polyps are typically low to intermediate in signal intensity on T1- and T2-weighted images and enhance moderately with gadolinium, with enhancement most intense on images obtained between 1 and 2 minutes after contrast administration (Fig. 3.27). Distinction from calculi can be made readily on the basis of gadolinium enhancement, and may be further facilitated if the polyp is located on the nondependent surface of the gallbladder wall, as

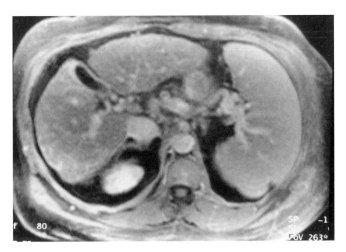

F I G . 3.25 Porcelain gallbladder. A CT imaging study (not shown) demonstrated diffuse calcification of the gallbladder wall. The interstitial-phase gadolinium-enhanced SGE image demonstrates uniform enhancement of a smooth 4-mm thick gallbladder wall, which excludes superimposed malignancy.

calculi generally layer on the dependent surface or float horizontally within the gallbladder.

Gallbladder Carcinoma

Gallbladder carcinoma is a rare neoplasm more commonly seen in females than in males [47]. Tumors occur in elderly patients (>60 years of age). There is a strong association with calculous disease because approximately 75 percent of patients have gallstones. The 5-year survival rate is poor because most cases present with advanced disease. The most common cell type is adenocarcinoma. MRI findings in cases of gallbladder carcinoma are similar to those reported with CT imaging [47]. Gallbladder carcinoma is characterized on imaging studies by a mass either filling or replacing the gallbladder (frequently centered around gallstones) or by a mass protruding into the gallbladder lumen [47,48] (Fig. 3.28). Tumor invasion of the adjacent liver, duodenum, and pancreas is a frequent occurrence (see Fig. 3.28).

Focal or diffuse thickening of the gallbladder wall greater than 1 cm is highly suggestive of the diagnosis [47]. On T2-weighted sequences, the tumor is usually of increased signal intensity relative to the liver with poorly delineated contours. On T1-weighted sequences gallbladder carcinoma is either iso- or hypointense relative to the adjacent liver [48,49]. Differentiation of gallbladder carcinoma from neoplastic processes with secondary involvement of the gallbladder and inflammatory disease processes may be difficult because of overlap in signal characteristics and enhancement patterns. In particular, superimposed infection or perforation of gallbladder carcinoma can be indistinguishable from severe acute cholecystitis (Fig. 3.29).

Extension of tumor to the liver, intrahepatic bile ducts, duodenum, or pancreas, as well as the presence of nodal metastases in the hepatoduodenal ligament usually

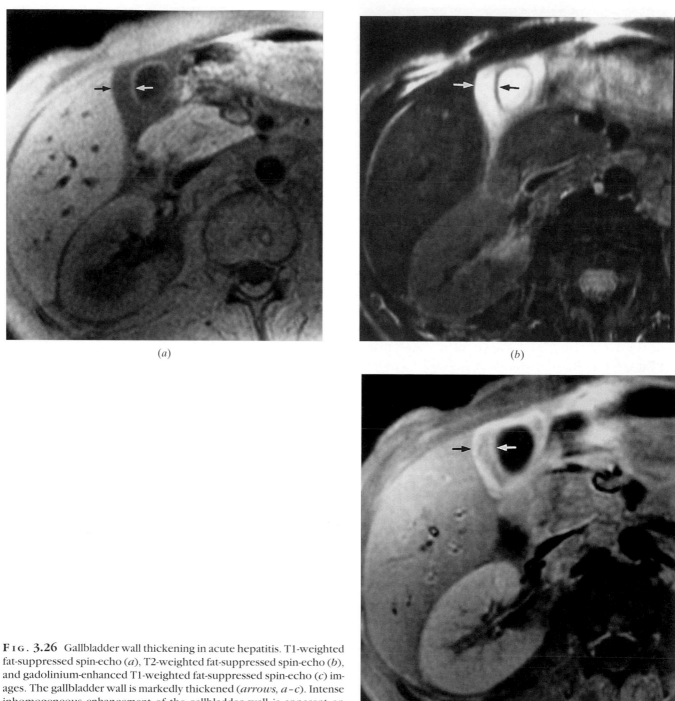

(a)

(b)

(c)

Fig. 3.26 Gallbladder wall thickening in acute hepatitis. T1-weighted fat-suppressed spin-echo (*a*), T2-weighted fat-suppressed spin-echo (*b*), and gadolinium-enhanced T1-weighted fat-suppressed spin-echo (*c*) images. The gallbladder wall is markedly thickened (*arrows, a–c*). Intense inhomogeneous enhancement of the gallbladder wall is apparent on the gadolinium-enhanced fat-suppressed image (*c*).

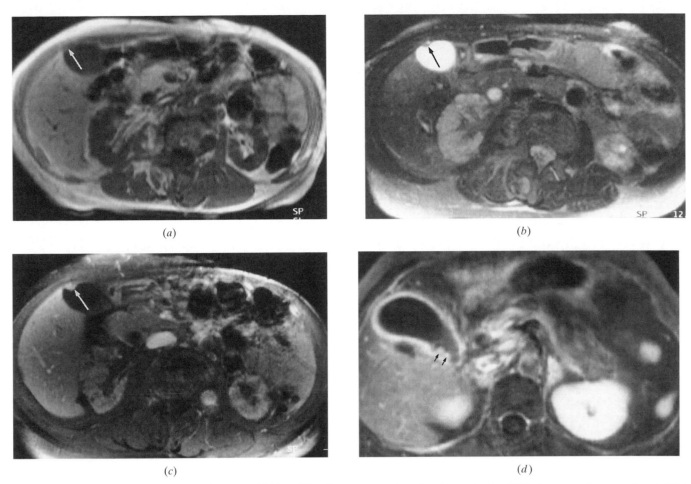

(a)

(b)

(c)

(d)

FIG. 3.27 Gallbladder polyp. SGE (*a*), breath hold T2-weighted echo-train spin-echo (*b*), and interstitial-phase gadolinium-enhanced fat-suppressed SGE (*c*) images. A 1-cm polyp is present on the nondependent surface of the gallbladder. The polyp is low in signal intensity on the T1-weighted image (*arrow, a*) and difficult to discern in the background of low-signal bile. The polyp is low in signal intensity on the T2-weighted image (*arrow, b*) and can be distinguished from high-signal-intensity bile. Relatively intense and uniform enhancement of the polyp is appreciated on the interstitial-phase gadolinium-enhanced fat-suppressed SGE image (*arrow, c*). The enhancement and location on the nondependent surface of the gallbladder distinguish the polyp from a calculus. Gadolinium-enhanced T1-weighted fat-suppressed spin-echo image (*d*) in a second patient who has coexistent acute acalculus cholecystitis demonstrates two small enhancing polyps (*arrow, d*). Note the substantial enhancement of the acutely inflamed gallbladder wall.

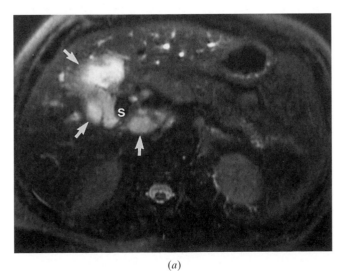

(a)

FIG. 3.28 Gallbladder carcinoma. Heavily T2-weighted 2D echo-train spin-echo (*a*), immediate postgadolinium SGE (*b*), gadolinium-enhanced spin-echo (*c*) image, axial multiplanar reformation (*d*) of heavily T2-weighted 2D echo-train spin-echo, and late gadolinium enhanced spin-echo (*e, f*) images.

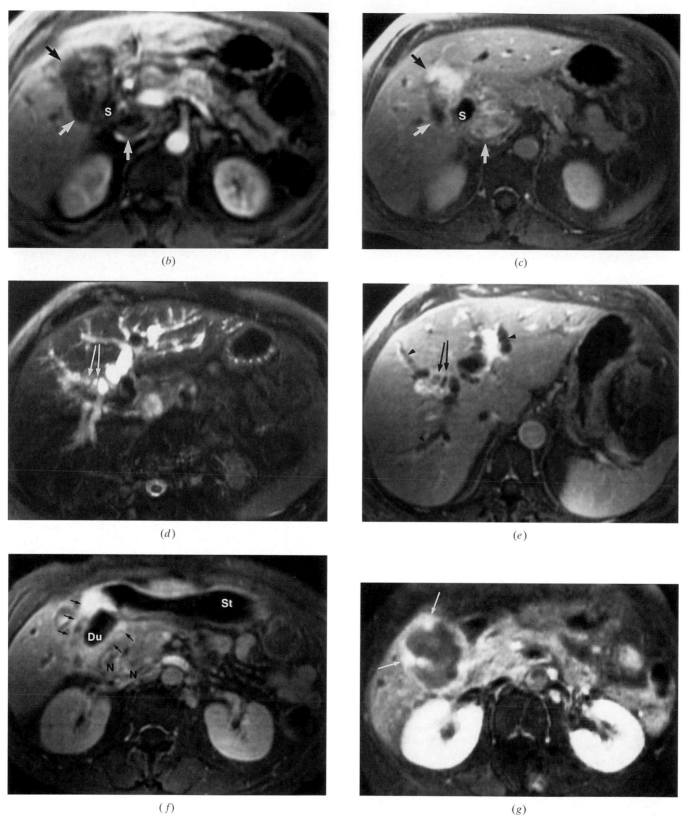

(b)

(c)

(d)

(e)

(f)

(g)

F IG . 3.28 (*Continued*) There is a large infiltrative mass (*arrows, a*) in the gallbladder fossa that partially surrounds a hypointense gallstone (S) (*a*) and invades the liver and porta hepatis. The gallbladder carcinoma (*arrows, a*) is hyperintense on the T2-weighted image (*a*) with some regions of the tumor showing markedly increased signal intensity. The carcinoma enhances mildly on the immediate postgadolinium image (*b*) and shows variable enhancement on the delayed image (*c*).Transverse multiplanar reformation shows the tumor encasing and obstructing the bile ducts (*arrows, d*). Tumor extension along the bile ducts (*arrows, e*) is well shown on the delayed postgadolinium image. Contrast this appearance with that of the uninvolved bile ducts (*arrowheads, e*). A more caudal section shows the invasion of the distal antrum and duodenal wall (*arrows, f*). Metastatic peripancreatic nodes (N) with central necrosis are also present. Du, duodenum; St, stomach. Gadolinium-enhanced T1-weighted fat-suppressed spin-echo image (*g*) in a second patient with gallbladder cancer demonstrates irregular nodular thickening of the gallbladder wall (*arrows, g*).

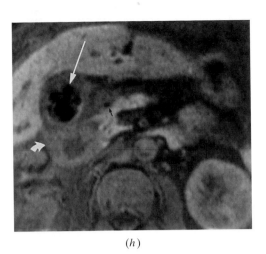

(h)

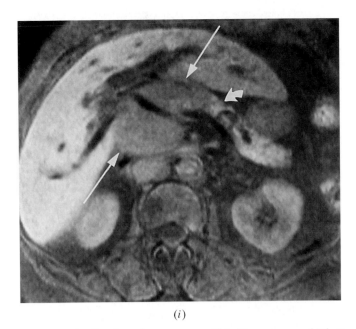

(i)

Fig. 3.28 (*Continued*) T1-weighted fat-suppressed spin-echo (*h,i*) images in a third patient demonstrate gallbladder cancer, which is intermediate in signal intensity and infiltrates along the duodenal wall (*curved arrow, h*) and head of the pancreas encasing the gastroduodenal artery (*short arrow, h*). Signal-void calculi are present within the gallbladder (*long arrow, h*). On a more superior tomographic section (*i*) a large tumor mass is present in the porta hepatis (*long arrows, i*). Distinction between intermediate-signal tumor and high-signal-intensity pancreas (*curved arrow, i*) is readily appreciated.

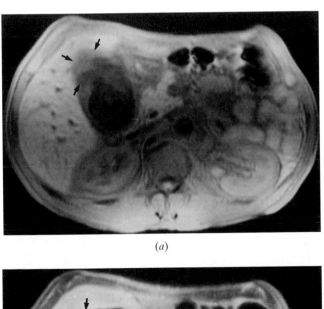

(a)

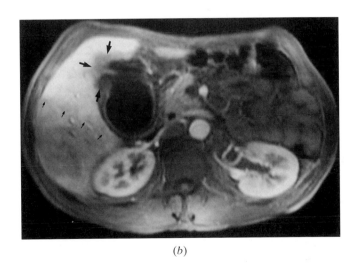

(b)

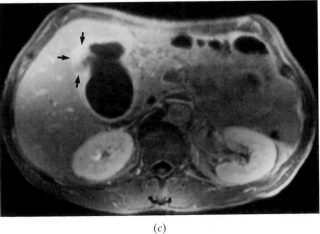

(c)

Fig. 3.29 Gallbladder carcinoma and acute cholecystitis. Fat-suppressed SGE (*a*), immediate postgadolinium fat-suppressed SGE (*b*), and interstitial-phase gadolinium-enhanced SGE (*c*) images. An irregular 4-cm mass (*arrows, a–c*) of mixed signal intensity is present within the anterolateral wall of the gallbladder. In addition, the gallbladder wall is diffusely thickened due to coexisting acute cholecystitis, with transient enhancement (*small arrows, b*) of the pericholecystic liver parenchyma on the immediate postgadolinium fat-suppressed SGE image (*b*). Note the overlap in signal intensity between portions of the tumor and the inflamed gallbladder wall on the various images.

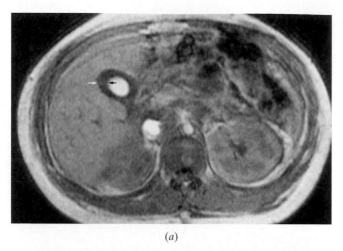

(a)

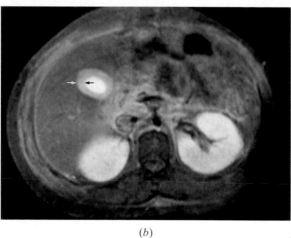

(b)

FIG. 3.30 Burkitt lymphoma of the gallbladder. SGE (a) and gadolinium-enhanced T1-weighted fat-suppressed spin-echo (b) images. There is diffuse thickening of the gallbladder wall (arrows, a,b) due to infiltration by lymphoma. Note the uniform enhancement of the wall after contrast administration (b), which is less than that observed for acute cholecystitis.

precludes surgical resection. Direct hepatic invasion or distant liver metastases are well-shown on T2-weighted or gadolinium-enhanced images and tend to possess a signal intensity similar to that of the primary tumor [48]. Tumor-spread along the bile ducts can be seen on gadolinium-enhanced images acquired approximately 1 to 5 minutes after gadolinium, and the use of fat suppression increases the conspicuity of tumor. Extension of tumor into the pancreas can be diagnosed on T1-weighted fat-suppressed images prior to and after gadolinium administration. T1-weighted images without fat saturation provide good signal contrast between fatty tissue and the tumor. Persistence of a fat plane between the tumor and surrounding structures (e.g., the duodenum) excludes invasion. Similarly, invasion of the hepatoduodenal ligament is better demonstrated with MRI than with CT im-

aging, especially on T1-weighted sequences without fat suppression [48], or on gadlinium enhanced fat suppressed images. MR cholangiographic sequences may prove useful in demonstrating extension of the tumor to the intrahepatic bile ducts and are optimal for diagnosing the presence of concomitant gallstone disease.

Metastases to the Gallbladder

A variety of neoplastic disease can metastasize to the gallbladder. Among the most common primary malignancies are breast carcinoma, melanoma, and lymphoma. Malignant involvement is more commonly focal with breast cancer and melanoma, whereas diffuse mural involvement is more common with lymphoma (Fig. 3.30).

■ DISEASE OF THE BILE DUCTS

Presence and Location of Bile Duct Obstruction

Ultrasound and CT imaging are highly accurate in diagnosing the presence and location of bile duct obstruction, and until recently MRI has played a limited role in this clinical setting [50]. The advent of MR cholangiography has generated new interest in evaluating the biliary tree with MRI in patients with suspected bile duct obstruction. In its current state of development MR cholangiography can diagnose the presence of bile duct obstruction in 91 to 100 percent of cases and can determine the level of obstruction in 85 to 100 percent of cases [14,20,22,27,51]. The bile ducts distal to the site of obstruction are routinely identified, including the distance from the site of obstruction to the ampulla. This anatomic information is important for adequate treatment planning. MR cholangiography depicts the intrahepatic bile ducts more consistently than ERCP, particularly in cases of complete or high-grade obstruction. Indeed, underfilling of the intrahepatic bile ducts often occurs with ERCP in these situations. In addition, the risk of sepsis, inherent to direct cholangiography in an obstructed system, is obviated by MR cholangiography.

The weaker signal observed at the periphery of the bile ducts due to associated volume averaging may lead to underestimation of the duct caliber by MR cholangiography. This phenomenon can be further compounded by the presence of motion artifact. These limitations may explain, in part, the discrepancy between the observed caliber of ducts measured at MR cholangiography and ERCP. Another important factor contributing to observed differences in ductal caliber is that distention of the ducts is inevitable at ERCP during filling with contrast, particularly in postcholecystectomy or obstructed patients, whereas at MR cholangiography the ducts are examined in their true physiologic state. Bile duct obstruction is diagnosed with MR cholangiography if the maximal diameter of the extrahepatic bile duct (measured on coronal source images) exceeds 7 mm in patients with their gallbladders in place, and 10 mm in patients who have undergone a cholecystectomy.

Benign Causes of Bile Duct Obstruction

Choledocholithiasis

Since the advent of laparoscopic cholecystectomy, there has been renewed interest in the preoperative diagnosis of choledocholithiasis. Despite technical advances in recent years, the diagnostic accuracy of ultrasound and CT imaging in diagnosing choledocholithiasis remains low, with modest sensitivities reported in most series [52–60]. Consequently, ERCP remains the modality of choice for establishing the diagnosis of CBD stones. In addition, ERCP has the added advantage of allowing therapeutic intervention at the time of initial diagnosis. However, significant complications occur in about 10 percent of patients after sphincterotomy, with an overall mortality of 1.5 percent [61]. Furthermore, the sensitivity and specificity of ERCP in the diagnosis of CBD stones is only 90 percent and 96 percent, respectively [62]. MR cholangiographic techniques are ideally suited for detecting CBD stones because the heavily T2-weighted images depict calculi as signal-void areas against a background of high-signal-intensity bile (Fig. 3.31, 3.32). Therefore, for some clinical indications, MR cholangiography, whose accuracy in preliminary studies appears to be comparable to that of ERCP, may be performed if sonography or CT imaging is negative. This is true, for example, of patients

for whom ERCP is unsuccessful, such as patients with surgical bypass procedures (Billroth II anastomosis, hepatojejunostomy), patients with acute pancreatitis who are at higher risk of complications from ERCP, and patients with a low clinical suspicion for CBD stones. However, the accuracy of MRCP in diagnosing choledocholithiasis in this subgroup of patients has not been fully evaluated.

Data available on the accuracy of MR cholangiography in the diagnosis of CBD stones is still preliminary. Using a 3D gradient-echo sequence, Ishizaki et al. [15] correctly diagnosed all six cases of choledocholithiasis in 20 patients presenting with obstructive jaundice. In a nonblinded, retrospective review of 10 patients with known choledocholithiasis, we were able to demonstrate the stones in all 10 patients using a 2D echo-train spin-echo sequence [19]. More recently, using 2D echo-train spin-echo and a torso phased-array multicoil, we achieved a sensitivity of 90 percent, a specificity of 100 percent, and an overall accuracy of 97 percent for the detection of choledocholithiasis in a population of 110 patients being investigated for biliary obstruction [63]. These results are superior to those we obtained in a previous study (sensitivity 81 percent and specificity 98 percent for diagnosing choledocholithiasis), in which the examinations were performed in the body coil and with lower resolution imaging parameters [27]. Using a 3D echo-train spin-echo technique, Laghi et al. [64] obtained an 89 percent sensitivity and a 100 percent specificity in the diagnosis of choledocholithiasis in a group of 40 patients with a 45 percent prevalence of choledocholithiasis.

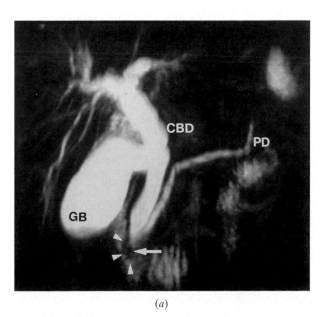

(a)

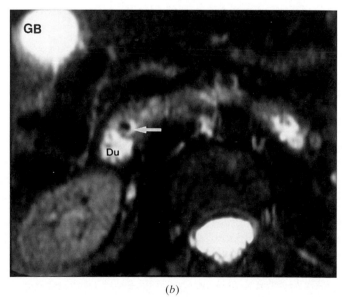

(b)

F IG. 3.31 Choledocholithiasis. MR cholangiogram. Coronal MIP reconstruction (a) of a set of heavily T2-weighted 2D echo-train spin-echo sections, and transverse source heavily T2-weighted 2D echo-train spin-echo (b) images. There is moderate dilatation of the common bile duct (CBD) (a) down to the ampulla and mild dilatation of the pancreatic duct (PD) (a).

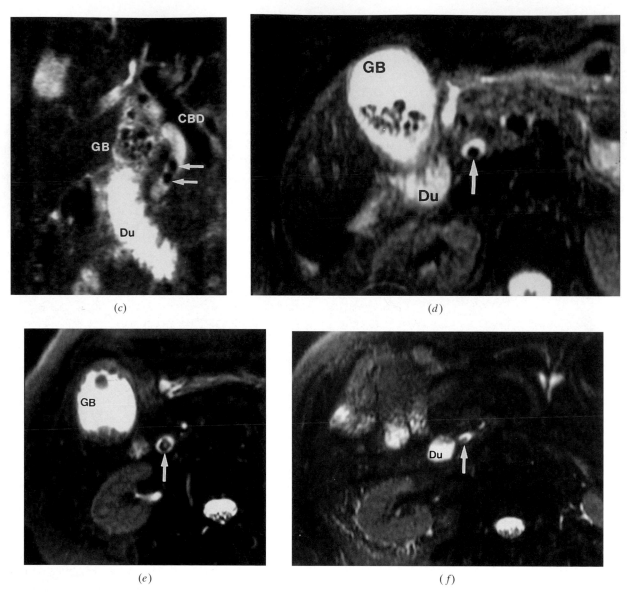

FIG. 3.31 (*Continued*) The ampullary region (*arrowheads, a*) appears prominent, and there is a suggestion of a small signal-void area (*arrow, a*) that could represent a stone. Source image (*b*) through the distal CBD clearly confirms the presence of a 5-mm stone (*arrow, b*).Coronal multiplanar reformation (*c*) of a set of heavily T2-weighted 2D echo-train spin-echo sections, and heavily T2-weighted 2D echo-train spin-echo (*d*) images in a second patient. The multiplanar reformation image (*c*) demonstrates two stones (*arrows, c*) in the distal common bile duct (CBD) (*c*), which is mildly dilated. Multiple stones are present in the gallbladder. Transverse source image (*d*), shows the CBD stone in a dependent position. Heavily T2-weighted 2D echo-train spin-echo image (*e*) in a third patient. A 6-mm quadrangular stone (*arrow, e*) is visualized in a mildly dilated CBD. There is associated cholelithiasis. Heavily T2-weighted 2D echo-train spin-echo image (*f*) in a fourth patient without CBD dilatation, a 3-mm stone (*arrow, f*) is well-visualized. Du, duodenum; GB, gallbladder. (Parts *a* and *b* are reprinted with permission from Reinhold C, Bret PM: MR cholangiopancreatography. Abdom Imaging 21:105–116, 1996)

A number of pitfalls must be avoided when diagnosing choledocholithiasis on MR cholangiography. Surgical clips in the right upper quadrant may obscure a portion of the extrahepatic bile duct due to associated signal-void artifacts. Furthermore, it must be emphasized that the signal within the biliary tree is generated by the long T2 of bile and that the presence of pneumobilia, hematobilia, protein plugs, or calculi will result in T2 shorten-ing. Therefore, a signal-void defect within the bile duct is not specific for calculi. Axial MRI sections often allow the differentiation of pneumobilia, which floats anterior to bile, from choledocholithiasis, which lies in the dependent portion of the bile duct lumen [65] (Fig. 3.33). The posterosuperior pancreaticoduodenal artery and vein run alongside the CBD and frequently cross it along its inferior aspect. Because vessels appear as signal-void foci

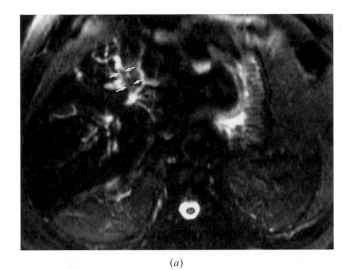

(*a*)

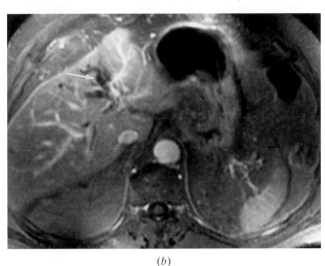

(*b*)

F IG . 3.32 Intrahepatic bile-duct stones. Transverse multiplanar reformation (*a*) of a set of heavily T2-weighted 2D echo-train spin-echo sections, and gadolinium-enhanced T1-weighted fat-suppressed spin-echo (*b*) images. The transverse multiplanar reformation image (*a*) depicts three stones (*arrows, a*) in the medial segment of the left lobe resulting in mild obstruction. Compare the size of the dilated intrahepatic ducts in the medial segment with the normal ducts in the right lobe. The gadolinium enhanced T1-weighted fat-suppressed spin-echo image (*b*) confirms the absence of an obstructing mass lesion. Note the low signal intensity of the dilated bile ducts (*arrow, b*) that obscures the visualization of the hypointense stones.

on MR cholangiographic sequences, care must be taken not to mistake these for calculi (Fig. 3.34). The vascular nature of these signal voids can usually be confirmed by their tubular appearance on adjacent sections.

Ampullary Stenosis

Ampullary stenosis most frequently occurs in the context of choledocholithiasis as a sequela of stone passage. MR

degree of dilatation of the biliary tree is usually moderate but can be severe. The absence of substantial dilatation of the pancreatic duct and the inability to demonstrate an obstructive lesion usually permit distinction from malignant disease with MRI [66]. The combination of MR

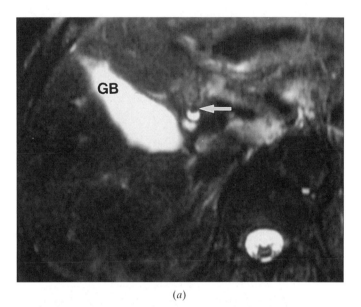

(*a*)

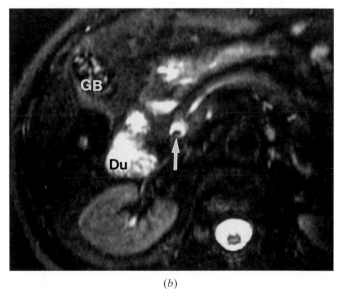

(*b*)

F IG . 3.33 Pneumobilia versus calculi. Heavily T2-weighted 2D echo-train spin-echo (*a*) image shows a signal-void area (*arrow, a*) anteriorly in the nondependent position of the common hepatic duct consistent with pneumobilia. ERCP with endoscopic sphincterotomy performed immediately prior to the MR cholangiogram showed no stones, but resulted in extensive pneumobilia postsphincterotomy. Heavily T2-weighted 2D echo-train spin-echo (*b*) image in a second patient demonstrates calculi, which, as opposed to pneumobilia, lie in the dependent position (*arrow, b*) of the bile ducts. Numerous gallstones are also present in this patient. Du, duodenum; GB, gallbladder.

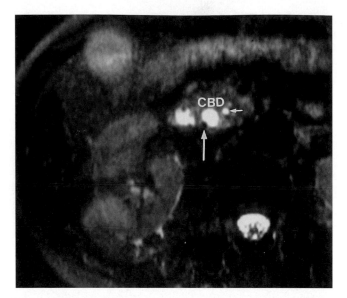

FIG. 3.34 Vessels mimicking calculi. Heavily T2-weighted 2D echo-train spin-echo image demonstrates a small signal-void focus (*arrow*) along the right posterolateral aspect of the common bile duct (CBD). On serial sections (not shown), this was demonstrated to be a vessel due to its tubular nature. The pancreatic duct (*small arrow*) is identified to the left of the CBD.

cholangiography, noncontrast T1-weighted fat-suppressed imaging, and immediate postgadolinium SGE are an effective approach to demonstrate periampullary tumors (Fig. 3.35). Nevertheless, small periampullary cancers are at times difficult to exclude, and ERCP with endoscopic biopsy may be necessary to establish this diagnosis. Furthermore, in the acute setting, ampullary stenosis may be associated with edema of the ampulla (Fig. 3.36), and in some instances progressive fibrotic changes lead to enlargement of the ampulla (Fig. 3.37). Follow-up ERCP and biopsy may be necessary to exclude an ampullary tumor under these circumstances.

Bile duct obstruction due to ampullary stenosis also must be differentiated from postcholecystectomy CBD dilatation. Therefore, it is somewhat misleading to diagnose bile duct obstruction solely on the basis of CBD diameter measurements, so associated relevant clinical symptomatology and laboratory abnormalities are usually required before endoscopic sphincterotomy is indicated. ERCP has the added advantage over MR cholangiopancreatography in that it can diagnose delayed emptying of the bile ducts, thereby providing both functional and anatomic information.

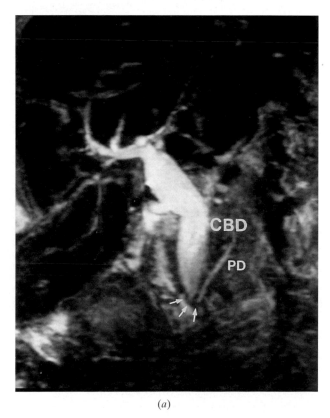

(a)

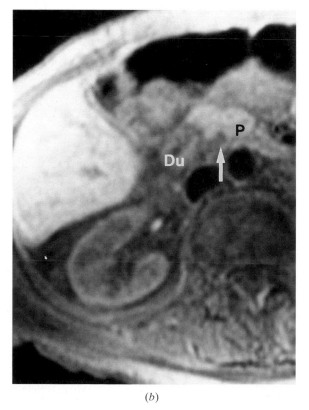

(b)

FIG. 3.35 Ampullary stenosis. Coronal MIP reconstruction (*a*) of a set of heavily T2-weighted 2D echo-train spin-echo sections and T1-weighted fat-suppressed spin-echo (*b*) images. Coronal MIP reconstruction demonstrates mild intra- and moderate extrahepatic bile duct dilatation. The common bile duct (CBD) (*a*) can be followed to the ampulla (*arrows, a*) where it is seen to taper. No mass is identified. There is no associated dilatation of the pancreatic duct (PD) (*a*). On the T1-weighted fat-suppressed spin-echo image (*b*) the distal CBD (*arrow, b*) at the level of the ampulla is surrounded by the hyperintense signal of the pancreas (P) (*b*) confirming the absence of an obstructing mass. Du, duodenum.

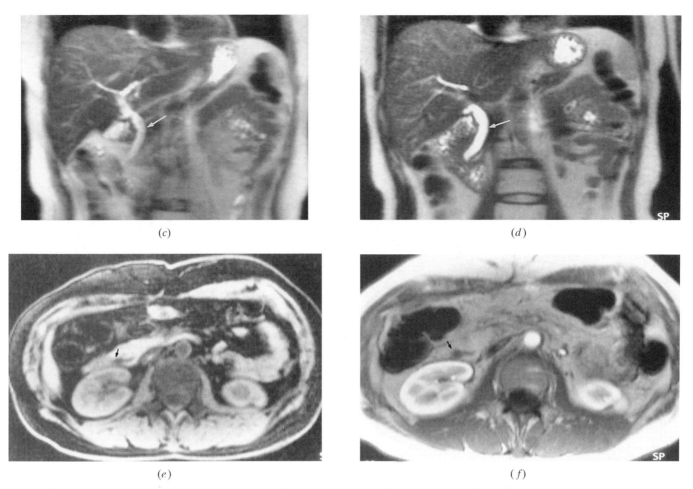

(c)   (d)

(e)   (f)

FIG. 3.35 (*Continued*) A 3D MIP reconstruction (*c*) of a set of coronal HASTE sections, coronal HASTE source image (*d*), fat-suppressed SGE (*e*), and immediate postgadolinium SGE (*f*) images in a second patient. The MR cholangiographic images (*c,d*) demonstrate a moderately dilated CBD (*arrow, c,d*) with no evidence of calculi. The source image (*d*) most reliably excludes calculi. Fat-suppressed SGE image (*e*) reveals normal high signal intensity of the pancreas at the level of the ampulla (*arrow, e*) with no evidence of a mass. This is confirmed with the immediate postgadolinium SGE image (*f*) which shows normal enhancement of the pancreas at the level of the ampulla (*arrow, f*) with no evidence of a tumor.

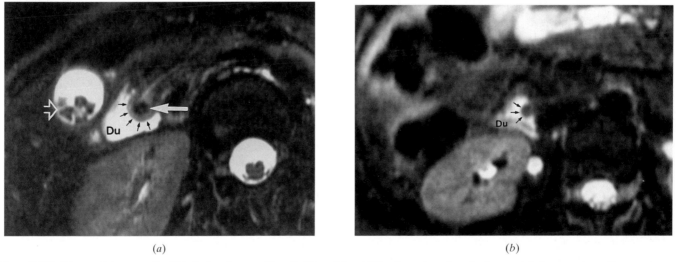

(a)   (b)

FIG. 3.36 Edema of the ampulla. MR cholangiogram. Heavily T2-weighted 2D echo-train spin-echo image (*a*) shows a stone (*large arrow, a*) impacted in an enlarged, edematous ampulla (*small arrows, a*). Note the multiple-faceted gallstones (*open arrow, a*). Heavily T2-weighted 2D echo-train spin-echo image (*b*) in a second patient with ampullary edema from a passed stone. Mild dilatation of the CBD that tapers toward the ampulla is present (not shown). The ampulla (*arrows, b*) is bulging, creating a mass effect on the duodenum. At endoscopy, an edematous enlarged ampulla was found. Du, duodenum. (Part *a* reprinted with permission from Reinhold C, Bret PM: Current status of MR cholangiopancreatography (perspective). AJR Am J Roentgenol 166:1285–1295, 1996)

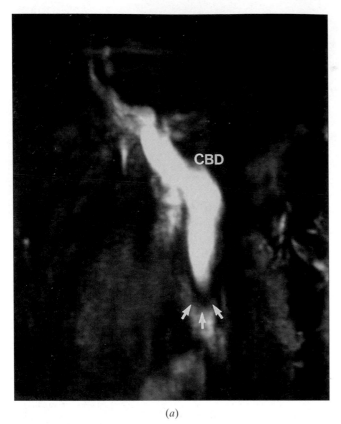

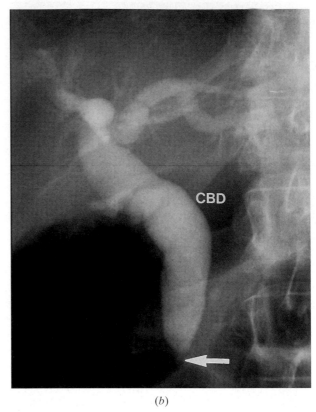

(a)   (b)

F IG . 3.37 Ampullitis. Coronal MIP reconstruction (a) of a set of heavily T2-weighted 2D echo-train spin-echo sections and ERCP (b) images. Coronal MIP reconstruction image (a) shows moderate bile duct dilatation of the CBD (a) down to the level of the ampulla (arrows, a), which is enlarged and hypointense. Differential diagnosis includes ampullitis and ampullary carcinoma. ERCP image (b) shows dilated bile ducts down to the level of the ampulla (arrow, b). At endoscopy, the ampulla was enlarged and edematous. Endoscopic biopsy performed after endoscopic sphincterotomy confirmed the diagnosis of ampullitis with fibrosis. (Reprinted with permission from Reinhold C, Bret PM: Current status of MR cholangiopancreatography (perspective). AJR Am J Roentgenol 166:1285–1295, 1996)

Sclerosing Cholangitis

Primary sclerosing cholangitis may occur in isolation, but 70 percent of patients have inflammatory bowel disease, most commonly ulcerative colitis [67]. Secondary sclerosing cholangitis is seen in the context of preexisting biliary disease such as prior surgery, biliary stones, prior infection, or following hepatic arterial FUDR chemotherapy [68,69]. Sclerosing cholangitis may produce severe damage to the liver parenchyma and progress to end-stage cirrhosis. The fibrotic disease process involves the intra- and extrahepatic biliary system [67,69–71]. Enlarged portal lymph nodes are not uncommon. The hepatic parenchyma may be normal, even in patients with liver failure and portal hypertension. Unlike primary biliary cirrhosis, which predominates in women, approximately 70 percent of patients with sclerosing cholangitis are male.

The imaging appearance of sclerosing cholangitis is characterized by dilated segments of the biliary tree interspersed with narrowed segments resulting in a beaded and stenotic appearance [72,73]. Bile duct walls also are thickened, usually on the order of 3 to 4 mm

[73,74]. One role of imaging in the evaluation of sclerosing cholangitis is to generate a detailed map of the biliary tree anatomy, including the depiction of strictures that are multifocal and involve both the extra- and intrahepatic bile ducts (Fig. 3.38). ERCP is often limited by the multiplicity of the bile duct strictures and the difficulty in opacifying the ducts proximal to a high-grade stenosis. The abnormalities of the bile duct caliber can be diagnosed with MR cholangiographic sequences, but the accuracy of this technique for demonstrating these changes has not been established. Display in 3D format may facilitate demonstration of strictures and beading. Visualization of the duct wall is best shown on breath-hold fat-suppressed SGE images acquired 1 minute after gadolinium administration. Because the inflammatory process is mild, intense enhancement is not usually present [66] (Fig. 3.39).

The most important differential diagnosis of sclerosing cholangitis is cholangiocarcinoma. Bile duct wall thickening and dilation are features of cholangiocarcinoma. These entities may be distinguished on the basis

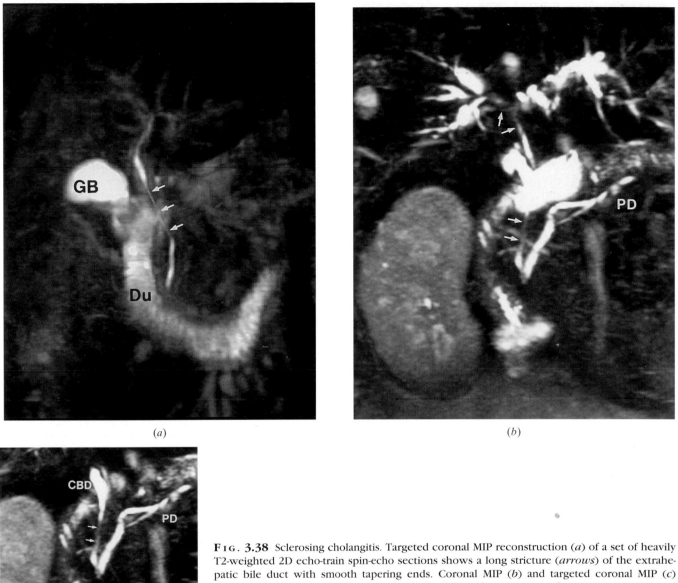

(a)

(b)

(c)

F IG . 3.38 Sclerosing cholangitis. Targeted coronal MIP reconstruction (*a*) of a set of heavily T2-weighted 2D echo-train spin-echo sections shows a long stricture (*arrows*) of the extrahepatic bile duct with smooth tapering ends. Coronal MIP (*b*) and targeted coronal MIP (*c*) reconstructions of a set of heavily T2-weighted 2D echo-train spin-echo sections in a second patient. Coronal MIP image (*b*) demonstrates similar appearing strictures (*arrows, b*) involving the common bile duct, as well as the common hepatic duct, with extension into the right and left main ducts. Note the beaded appearance of the intrahepatic bile ducts. This coronal MIP image provides an overview of the intra-and extra-hepatic bile ducts. The targeted MIP reconstruction (*c*) shows to better advantage the distal common bile duct (CBD) stricture (*arrows, c*). Du, duodenum; GB, gallbladder; PD, pancreatic duct.

of the degree of dilation of the biliary tree: severe in malignant disease and mild to moderate in benign disease [75]. Wall thickness in benign disease usually does not exceed 5 mm (Fig. 3.40), whereas the wall frequently exceeds 5 mm in malignant disease [74]. Although MR cholangiography can be used to detect areas of dominant stricture formation, dilatation, or both, the low spatial resolution of current MR cholangiographic techniques limits detailed analysis of the stricture morphology, especially in the setting of a cholangiocarcinoma complicating sclerosing cholangitis.

Also to be considered in the differential diagnosis is infective cholangitis. Most frequently, the clinical picture permits distinction between sclerosing cholangitis and infective cholangitis. However, overlap does exist. The most reliable distinction on MR images between these

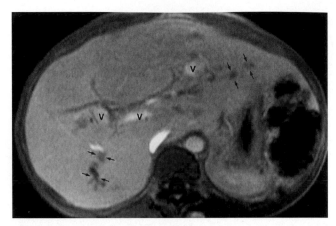

FIG. 3.39 Sclerosing cholangitis. Interstitial-phase gadolinium-enhanced fat suppressed SGE image demonstrates a beaded appearance of the intrahepatic bile ducts (*arrows*), particularly in the left lobe and posterior segment of the right lobe. No significant enhancement is present of the bile duct wall. Note that the portal-vein branches (V) are opacified, facilitating their differentiation from dilated intrahepatic bile ducts.

two entities is that duct wall enhancement is considerably greater on gadolinium-enhanced fat-suppressed SGE images with infective cholangitis.

Cystic Diseases of the Bile Ducts

Caroli's disease, choledochal cysts, and choledochocele are conditions that result from dilation of various parts of the biliary tree. In Caroli's disease, the distal intrahepatic bile ducts are dilated and follow a segmental distribution. These cystic expansions are demonstrated as continuous with the biliary tree, which permits their diagnosis on tomographic images. MR cholangiography with 3D display likely is an accurate method for demonstrating Caroli's disease because the luminal contents of the bile ducts appear hyperintense in contrast to the portal vein, which usually appears as signal-void. Cystic expansions of the intrahepatic biliary tree are shown as oval-shaped structures in continuity with the biliary tree that are nearly signal-void on black-bile techniques and high in signal intensity on bright-bile or MR cholangiographic techniques (Fig. 3.41).

Choledochal cysts have a variety of appearances, but most typically appear as uniform dilation of the extrahe-

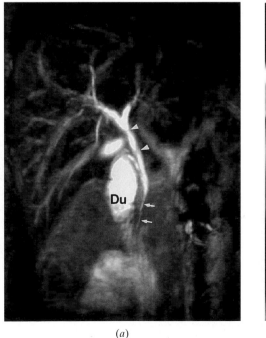

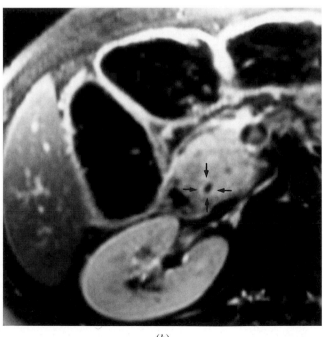

(a)   (b)

FIG. 3.40 Sclerosing cholangitis. Coronal MIP reconstruction (*a*) of a set of heavily T2-weighted 2D echo-train spin-echo sections and gadolinium-enhanced T1-weighted fat-suppressed spin-echo (*b*) images. The coronal MIP image demonstrates a smooth stricture (*arrows, a*) with tapering ends of the distal CBD resulting in mild obstruction. No abnormalities are seen of the intrahepatic bile ducts. The apparent areas of narrowing (*arrowheads, a*) of the common hepatic duct represent artifacts of the MIP reconstruction (misregistration artifact associated with patient motion) and were not present on the source images (not shown). Transverse gadolinium-enhanced T1-weighted fat-suppressed spin-echo image (*b*) through the head of the pancreas at the level of the stricture shows the narrowed lumen of the CBD. The wall of the CBD is slightly thickened (3 mm) and demonstrates mild enhancement (*arrows, b*). Du, duodenum.

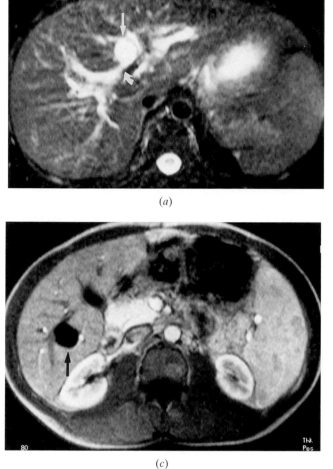

(a)

(b)

(c)

FIG. 3.41 Caroli's disease. T2-weighted fat-suppressed spin-echo (*a*), and immediate postgadolinium SGE (*b,c*) images. Cystic intrahepatic duct ectasia (*arrow, a–c*) is present in the left (*a,b*) and right (*c*) lobes of the liver. Differentiation from a liver cyst is assisted by the demonstration of continuity with a mildly dilated bile duct (*curved arrow, a,b*) entering the cystic space. Note the improved differentiation of the bile ducts from the portal-vein branches on the gadolinium-enhanced SGE images (*b,c*), compared with the T2-weighted fat-suppressed spin-echo image (*a*). Gradient-moment nulling on the T2-weighted image has resulted in high signal of the portal-vein branches, which are difficult to distinguish from dilated intrahepatic bile ducts on this image in isolation.

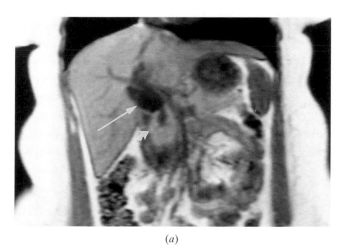

(a)

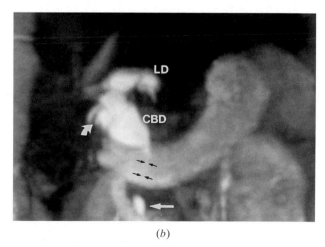

(b)

FIG. 3.42 Choledochal cyst. Coronal SGE (*a*), and coronal MIP reconstruction (*b*) of a set of heavily T2-weighted 2D echo-train spin-echo sections. Cystic expansion of the CBD (*long arrow, a*) above the head of the pancreas (*curved arrow, a*) is appreciated on the black-signal bile SGE image (*a*). The left hepatic duct (LD) (*b*) and upper CBD (*b*) are dilated in a fusiform fashion and are shown as high-signal-intensity structures on the coronal MIP image (*b*). A saccular dilatation of the distal CBD (*arrow, b*), as well as of the cystic duct (*curved arrow, b*) at its insertion into the common hepatic duct, is present. The mid-CBD (*small arrows, b*), although not well-depicted on the MIP format, was shown to be of small caliber on the individual source images (not shown).

patic bile ducts [76–78]. An increased incidence of cholangiocarcinoma is associated with choledochal cysts [78]. Direct coronal imaging demonstrates a dilated tubular structure that follows the expected course of the common bile duct [76]. MR cholangiography has been shown in isolated cases to accurately diagnose these entities (Fig. 3.42). However, at present, series reports have not been described. In addition, MR cholangiography can diagnose the presence of biliary calculi and stricture formation that frequently complicate cystic diseases of the bile ducts [79] (Fig. 3.43).

Choledochoceles are cystic expansions of the distal CBD as it enters into the duodenum. The choledochocele

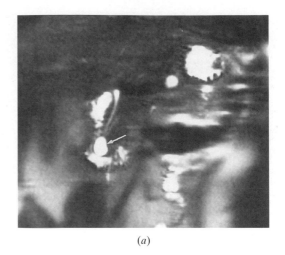

(a)

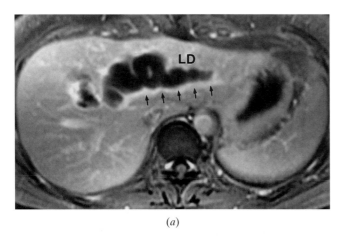

(a)

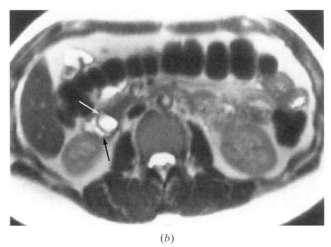

(b)

FIG. 3.44 Choledochocele. Coronal fat-suppressed HASTE (*a*) and transverse HASTE (*b*) images. Cystic expansion of the distal CBD (*arrow, a*) forming a choledochocele is appreciated on the coronal image (*a*). The transverse image demonstrates that the choledochocele (*white arrow, a,b*) bulges into the duodenum (*black arrow, b*).

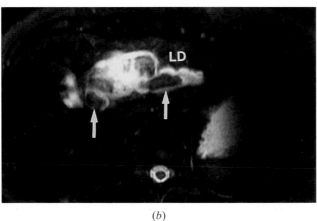

(b)

FIG. 3.43 Choledochal cyst. Patient with previous choledochojejunostomy for saccular dilatation of the common bile duct. Gadolinium-enhanced T1-weighted fat-suppressed spin-echo (*a*) and heavily T2-weighted 2D echo-train spin-echo (*b*) images. The cystic dilatation of the left hepatic duct (LD) (*a,b*) is well demonstrated on the black-signal bile T1-weighted image (*a*). There is no thickening or abnormal enhancement of the bile duct wall to suggest the presence of a superimposed cholangiocarcinoma. The apparent thickening of the inferior wall represents the portal vein (*arrows, a*) coursing along the left hepatic duct. The MR cholangiographic image (*b*) shows multiple stones (*arrows, b*) in the dilated left hepatic duct, which could not be visualized on the black-bile image (*a*).

bulges into the duodenum and creates a "cobra-head" appearance on cholangiographic images (Fig. 3.44).

Infective Cholangitis

Infective cholangitis, also termed ascending cholangitis, results from infection of the biliary tree secondary to gastrointestinal organisms. Most frequently, these infections occur from direct extension from the gastrointestinal tract resulting in an ascending cholangitis. Duct wall thickening and ductal dilatation are imaging features. The presence of substantial enhancement of the duct walls and intrahepatic abscess collections on gadolinium-enhanced images confirm the diagnosis (Fig. 3.45). Infective cholangitis not uncommonly results in recurrent liver infections (Fig. 3.46). Thrombosis of the portal vein is a common associated finding (Fig. 3.47) that aids in the

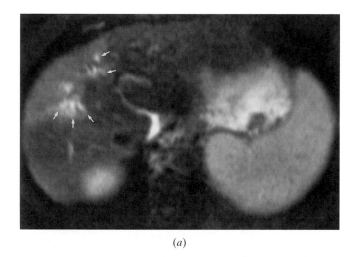

(a)

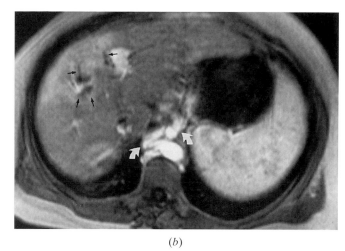

(b)

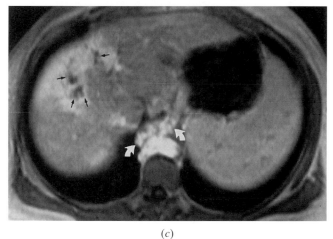

(c)

FIG. 3.45 Infective cholangitis. T2-weighted fat-suppressed spin-echo (*a*), immediate (*b*), and 90-second (*c*) postgadolinium SGE images. The periphery of the anterior segment of the right lobe and the medial segment of the left lobe are high in signal intensity on the T2-weighted image (*a*) and demonstrate increased enhancement on the postgadolinium images (*b,c*), reflecting active inflammation of the liver parenchyma. The bile ducts (*arrows, a–c*) of these segments are dilated and show increased mural enhancement better appreciated on the interstitial-phase image (*c*). Note the presence of splenomegaly with multiple small hypointense foci consistent with Gamna-Gandy bodies (*a–c*). In addition, esophageal varices (*curved arrows, b,c*) are seen on the postgadolinium images (*b,c*).

distinction of infective cholangitis from sclerosing cholangitis, in which this occurrence is uncommon.

Bile Duct Injuries

Reported rates of bile duct injury during cholecystectomy have increased in the laparoscopic era, and ERCP is currently the procedure of choice for detecting bile leaks, bile duct injuries, or both. MRI and MR cholangiography can demonstrate a fluid collection in the gallbladder bed, but it cannot determine whether or not the duct is actually leaking. The management of bile leaks needs to be tailored to the type of leak present, taking into account the existing anatomy, the cause of the leak, and the leak site [80]. This information is readily available by mapping the biliary tree anatomy with MR cholangiography. MR cholangiography probably has little role to play in the management of simple leaks, but may be useful in evaluating more complex leaks, such as one or more excluded hepatic segments in the setting of complete transection of an aberrant right intrahepatic duct. Whereas a common pitfall of ERCP is to overlook the unopacified or excluded bile duct, MR cholangiography can readily diagnose the

presence and associated dilatation of the excluded bile duct usually draining the right posterior hepatic segments (Fig. 3.48).

Malignant Causes of Bile Duct Obstruction

Cholangiocarcinoma

In the western population, cholangiocarcinoma is associated most commonly with ulcerative colitis, often with preexisting sclerosing cholangitis [81]. Other associations include aniline dye exposure, liver fluke infestation, and choledochal cyst. Cholangiocarcinoma occurs in older patients (>60 years of age). Tumor histology is usually mucus-secreting adenocarcinoma. The presenting features are jaundice and weight loss in more than 75 percent of patients. Tumors are classified as central or peripheral in location. Central tumors refer to lesions arising from main hepatic ducts (i.e., common hepatic duct [CHD] or CBD), whereas peripheral tumors arise from peripheral intrahepatic branches [82–86]. Cholangiocarcinoma occurs most frequently (in about 50 percent of cases) at

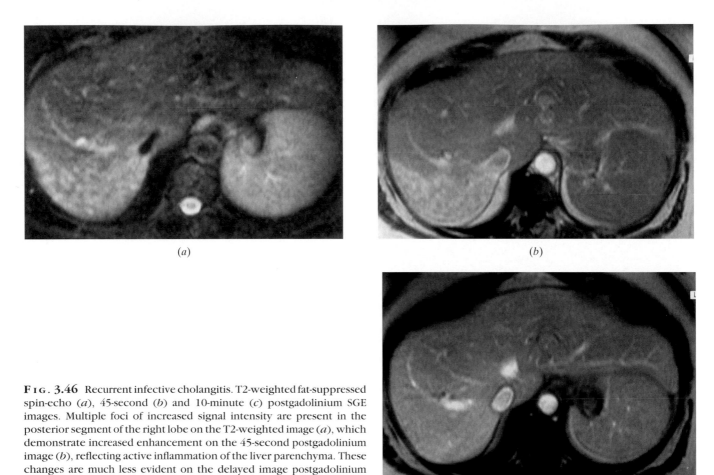

FIG. 3.46 Recurrent infective cholangitis. T2-weighted fat-suppressed spin-echo (*a*), 45-second (*b*) and 10-minute (*c*) postgadolinium SGE images. Multiple foci of increased signal intensity are present in the posterior segment of the right lobe on the T2-weighted image (*a*), which demonstrate increased enhancement on the 45-second postgadolinium image (*b*), reflecting active inflammation of the liver parenchyma. These changes are much less evident on the delayed image postgadolinium administration (*c*).

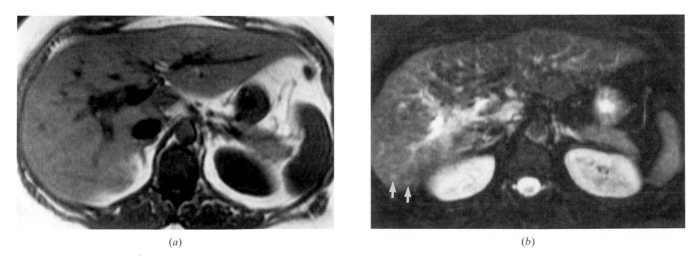

FIG. 3.47 Infective cholangitis with portal-vein thrombosis. SGE (*a*), T2-weighted fat-suppressed spin-echo (*b*), immediate (*c*), and 45-second (*d,e*) postgadolinium SGE images. The signal intensity of the liver is uniform on the precontrast T1-weighted image (*a*). Small hyperintense lesions (*arrows, b*) in the posterior segment of the right lobe of the liver are consistent with foci of infection on the T2-weighted image (*b*).

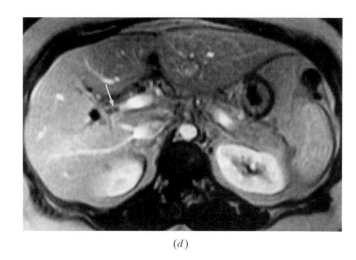

(d)

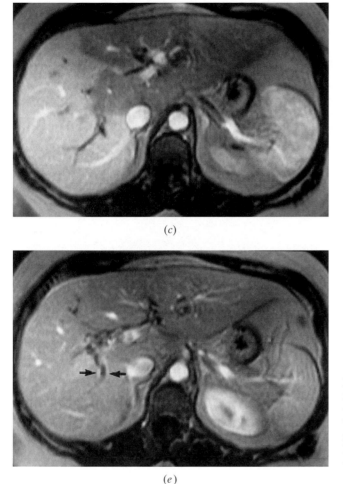

(c)

(e)

FIG. **3.47** (*Continued*) Transient increased enhancement of the right lobe of the liver on the immediate postgadolinium SGE image (*c*) is present due to thrombosis of the right portal vein. Nearly signal-void thrombus (*arrow, d*) is appreciated obstructing a high-signal gadolinium-containing main portal vein on the 45-second image (*d*). Increased enhancement of biliary duct walls is also appreciated on the 45-second postgadolinium SGE images (*arrow, e*).

the junction of the right and left hepatic ducts and are termed *Klatskin tumors* [82]. The CHD and CBD are next in frequency followed by intrahepatic peripheral tumors. Because peripheral tumors do not cause significant impairment in overall liver function, they tend to present later as large intrahepatic focal mass lesions [83].

The presence of high-grade obstruction of the biliary tree and a bile duct wall thickness greater than 5 mm are findings on CT images consistent with cholangiocarcinoma [74]. These features also have been observed with MRI [9,66]. In some cases, however, the thickening of the bile duct walls may not exceed 5 mm. An important ancillary finding is the presence of high-grade intrahepatic ductal dilatation. Therefore, in patients with segments of bile duct measuring less than 5 mm in thickness but with associated high-grade biliary obstruction, the possibility of cholangiocarcinoma should be entertained (Fig. 3.49). On gadolinium-enhanced fat-suppressed MR images, cholangiocarcinomas usually enhance to a moderate degree, with progressive enhancement from the capillary to the interstitial or portal venous phase (Fig. 3.50). The pattern of enhancement reflects the hypovas-

cular, desmoplastic composition of the majority of cholangiocarcinomas. The enhancement of the tumor permits better delineation of intrahepatic tumor extension than on CT images [9,66]. In some instances the pattern of enhancement may permit differentiation from hepatocellular carcinoma, which can mimic the imaging appearance of cholangiocarcinoma. Hepatocellular carcinomas typically are hypervascular, enhance intensely on immediate postgadolinium images, and fade over time (Fig. 3.51). Ductal tumors, which arise in the intrapancreatic portion of the CBD, are well-delineated on fat-suppressed images as low-signal-intensity masses surrounded by the high signal intensity of the pancreatic head (Fig. 3.52). (Peripheral [intrahepatic] tumors are described in greater detail in Chapter 2 on the Liver.)

Most cholangiocarcinomas are unresectable at the time of initial diagnosis and can be treated only with palliative biliary drainage. The role of imaging, in addition to establishing the diagnosis of cholangiocarcinoma, is to determine the presence of tumor extension, especially along the intrahepatic bile ducts, and to determine the best approach for palliative drainage in cases of non-

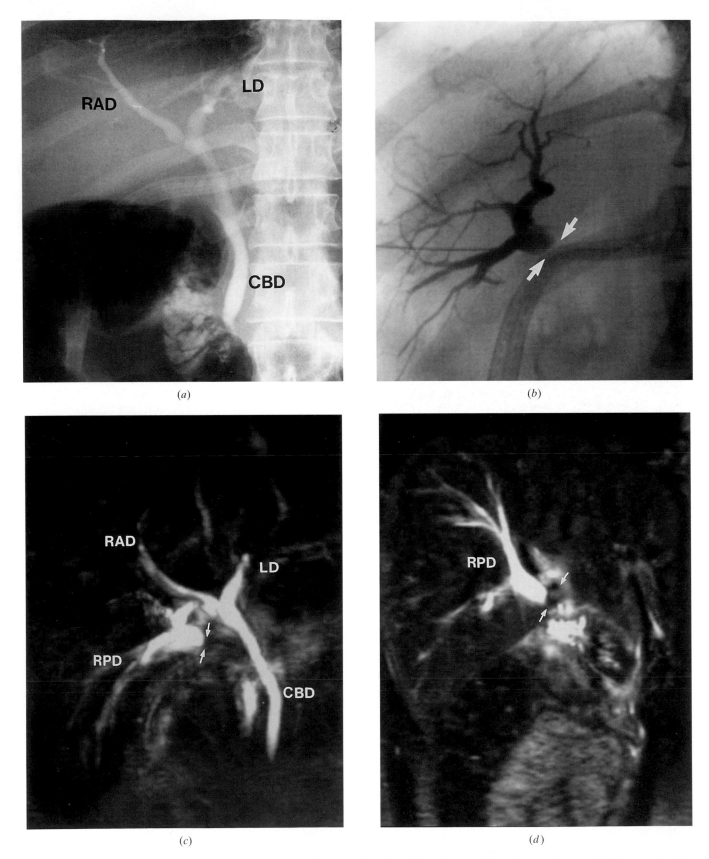

FIG. 3.48 Excluded biliary segment. ERCP (*a*), percutaneous transhepatic cholangiogram (*b*), and targeted coronal MIP reconstruction (*c*) of a set of heavily T2-weighted 2D echo-train spin-echo sections. ERCP image (*a*) shows a normal left hepatic duct (LD) (*a*) joining the right anterior hepatic duct (RAD) (*a*). No filling is seen of the right posterior hepatic duct raising the possibility of an excluded segment. Percutaneous transhepatic cholangiogram image (*b*) shows complete obstruction (*arrows, b*) of the right posterior hepatic duct. Targeted coronal MIP reconstruction image (*c*) demonstrates the obstructed (*arrows, c*) aberrant right posterior hepatic duct (RPD) (*c*), in addition to providing a complete overview of the biliary tree. CBD, common bile duct. Coronal oblique multiplanar reformation (*d*) of a set of heavily T2-weighted 2D echo-train spin-echo sections in a second patient. There is obstruction of the (RPD) (*d*) by a clip (*arrows, d*) placed across the duct at the time of laparoscopic cholecystectomy. The RPD was mistaken for the cystic duct at the time of surgery due to its aberrant insertion into the common hepatic duct (not shown).

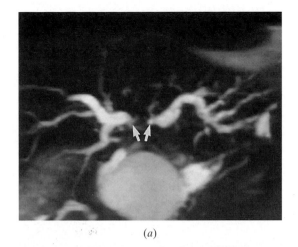

(a)

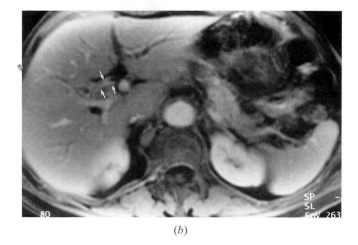

(b)

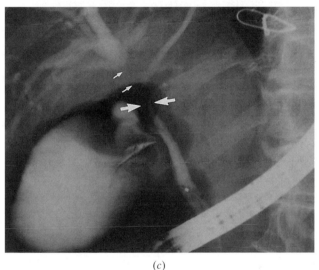

(c)

FIG. 3.49 Klatskin tumor. Transverse MIP reconstruction (*a*) of a set of heavily T2-weighted 2D echo-train spin-echo sections, interstitial-phase gadolinium-enhanced fat-suppressed SGE (*b*) and ERCP (*c*) images. There is obstruction of the right and left main hepatic ducts at the level of the porta hepatis (*arrows, a*). Gadolinium-enhanced fat-suppressed SGE image (*b*) demonstrates a mass (*small arrows, b*) measuring 4 mm in maximal thickness, extending into the right main hepatic duct. ERCP (*c*) confirms the obstruction (*arrows, c*) at the level of the porta hepatis, and the extension of the tumor into the right main hepatic duct (*small arrows, c*). Note underfilling of the left hepatic ducts.

resectable tumors [87]. Both ERCP and transhepatic cholangiography are of limited value in tumors that extend beyond the porta hepatis, due to incomplete opacification of the bile ducts proximal to the lesion, particularly when multiple stenoses isolate the intrahepatic bile duct segments. In addition, both techniques result in opacification of poorly drained bile ducts, which exposes the patient to increased risks of septic complications. MR cholangiography in this clinical setting can provide a detailed map of the biliary tree anatomy (Fig. 3.53). The 3D MIP reconstructions, which simulate the images obtained at direct contrast cholangiography, greatly facilitate identification of the various intrahepatic bile duct segments. In addition, the combination of axial-targeted MIP reconstructions (at the bile duct bifurcation) and interstitial-phase gadolinium-enhanced fat-suppressed SGE permit identification of tumor-spread along the intrahepatic bile ducts (Fig. 3.54). Superficial tumor-spread on gadolinium-enhanced SGE is demonstrated by increased thickness (>2 mm) of the bile duct walls and increased enhancement. It should be noted that after biliary stent placement, distinction between inflammatory ductal changes and superficial spreading tumor may not be feasible. Complete tumor staging, which documents involvement of the liver, portal nodes, or the portal vein, can often be obtained from the combination of MR cholangiography and conventional MR sequences [9]. An uncommon appearance for advanced cholangiocarcinomas is demonstration of intraperitoneal spread of tumor (Fig. 3.55).

Periampullary Carcinoma

Tumors that arise in the region of the ampulla are termed periampullary carcinomas and include carcinomas arising from the ampulla, duodenum, and distal CBD. Patients usually present with obstruction of both the CBD and the pancreatic ducts. Presentation is similar to that of pancreatic ductal adenocarcinoma. The prognosis, however, of periampullary carcinoma is much better than that of pancreatic cancer, with an 85 percent 5-year survival for localized lesions following Whipple surgery, and 10 to 25 percent for more infiltrative tumors [88]. Patients

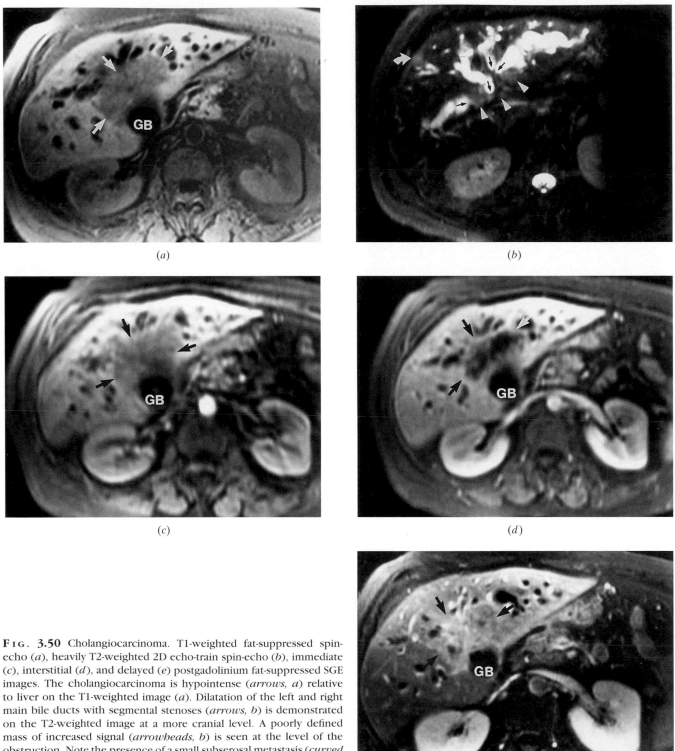

F IG . 3.50 Cholangiocarcinoma. T1-weighted fat-suppressed spin-echo (*a*), heavily T2-weighted 2D echo-train spin-echo (*b*), immediate (*c*), interstitial (*d*), and delayed (*e*) postgadolinium fat-suppressed SGE images. The cholangiocarcinoma is hypointense (*arrows, a*) relative to liver on the T1-weighted image (*a*). Dilatation of the left and right main bile ducts with segmental stenoses (*arrows, b*) is demonstrated on the T2-weighted image at a more cranial level. A poorly defined mass of increased signal (*arrowheads, b*) is seen at the level of the obstruction. Note the presence of a small subserosal metastasis (*curved arrow, b*) of similar signal intensity. Progressive enhancement of the tumor (*arrows, c–e*) is demonstrated on the serial gadolinium-enhanced SGE images. GB, gallbladder.

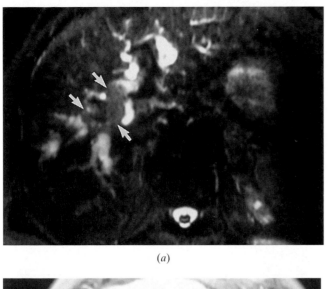

(a)

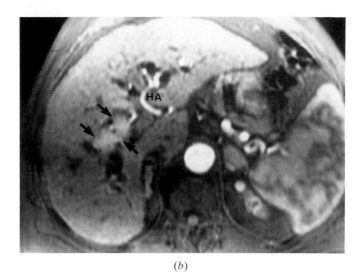

(b)

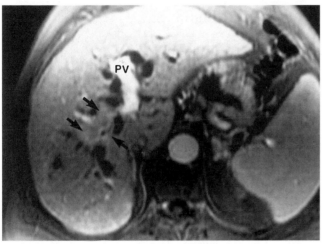

(c)

FIG. 3.51 Hepatocellular carcinoma mimicking cholangiocarcinoma. Transverse multiplanar reformation (a) of a set of heavily T2-weighted 2D echo-train spin-echo sections, immediate (b), and interstitial-phase gadolinium-enhanced fat-suppressed SGE images. A mass (arrows, a–c) is present largely within the right main hepatic duct, which results in proximal obstruction. Note that the obstructed ducts are hyperintense on the bright-signal bile MR cholangiogram (a), and hypointense on the black-signal bile SGE images (b,c). Diffuse heterogeneous enhancement of the mass (arrows) is present on the immediate postgadolinium image (b), which partially washes out on the interstitial-phase image (c). HA, hepatic artery; PV, portal vein.

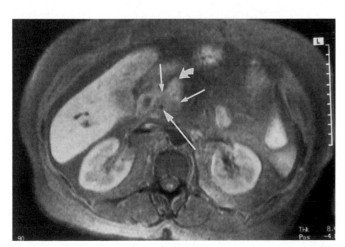

FIG. 3.52 Intrapancreatic cholangiocarcinoma. T1-weighted fat-suppressed spin-echo image demonstrates a low-signal-intensity tumor mass (arrows) surrounding the signal-void CBD (long arrow) in the head of the pancreas. Note the good contrast resolution between low-signal-intensity tumor and high-signal-intensity pancreas (curved arrow).

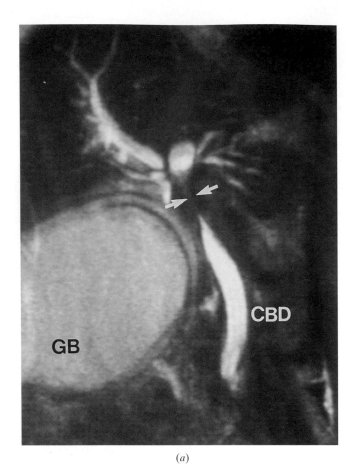

(a)

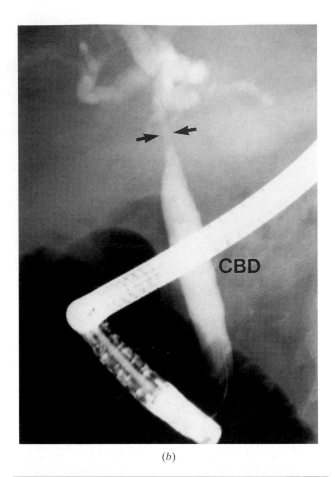

(b)

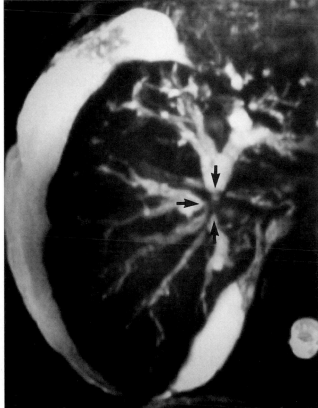

(c)

FIG. 3.53 Cholangiocarcinoma. Coronal targeted MIP reconstruction (*a*) of a set of heavily T2-weighted 2D echo-train spin-echo sections, ERCP (*b*) and transverse-targeted MIP reconstruction (*c*). The coronal targeted MIP reconstruction (*a*) shows a stricture (*arrows, a*) at the level of the common hepatic duct and porta hepatis. The bile ducts proximal and distal to the site of obstruction are well-seen. The gallbladder is distended. ERCP image (*b*) confirms the presence of a stricture (*arrows, b*), but because of underfilling, does not allow detailed assessment of tumor extension along the intrahepatic bile ducts. The transverse MIP reconstruction of the porta hepatis shows to better advantage the segmental extension of the cholangiocarcinoma (*arrows, c*). Ascites is also present. GB, gallbladder; CBD, common bile duct. (Reprinted with permission from Reinhold C, Bret PM: Current status of MR cholangiopancreatography (perspective). AJR Am J Roentgenol 166:1285–1295, 1996)

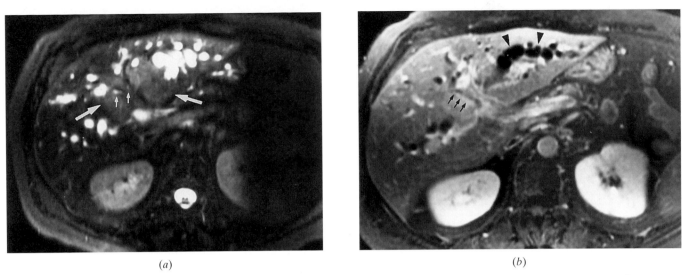

(a)   *(b)*

F IG . 3.54 Cholangiocarcinoma. Transverse multiplanar reformation (*a*) of a set of heavily T2-weighted 2D echo-train spin-echo sections and gadolinium-enhanced T1-weighted spin-echo (*b*) images. The transverse multiplanar reformation demonstrates an infiltrative mass (*arrows, a*) at the level of the porta hepatis encasing the bile ducts (*small arrows, a*). The gadolinium-enhanced T1-weighted spin-echo image (*b*) shows to better advantage the tumor spread along the bile ducts (*small arrows, b*). Compare this appearance with the uninvolved bile ducts whose walls (*arrowheads, b*) are almost imperceptible.

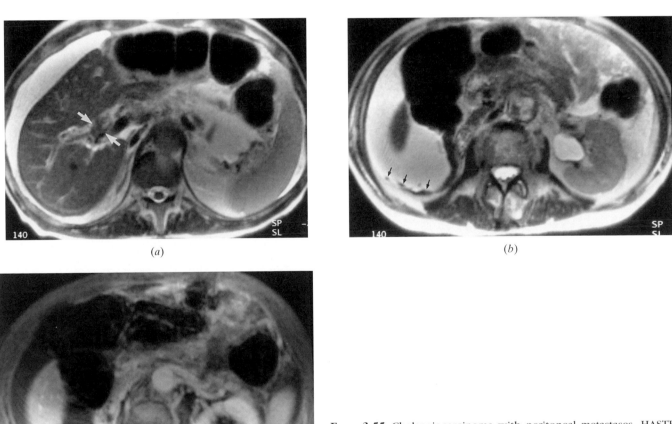

(a)   *(b)*

F IG . 3.55 Cholangiocarcinoma with peritoneal metastases. HASTE (*a,b*) and interstitial-phase gadolinium-enhanced fat-suppressed SGE (*c*) images. There is a mass (*arrows, a*) at the level of the porta hepatis. Note the ascites surrounding the liver. On a more caudal section (*b*), peritoneal implants (*arrows, b*) are present, which demonstrate enhancement (*arrows, c*) on the gadolinium-enhanced image.

(c)

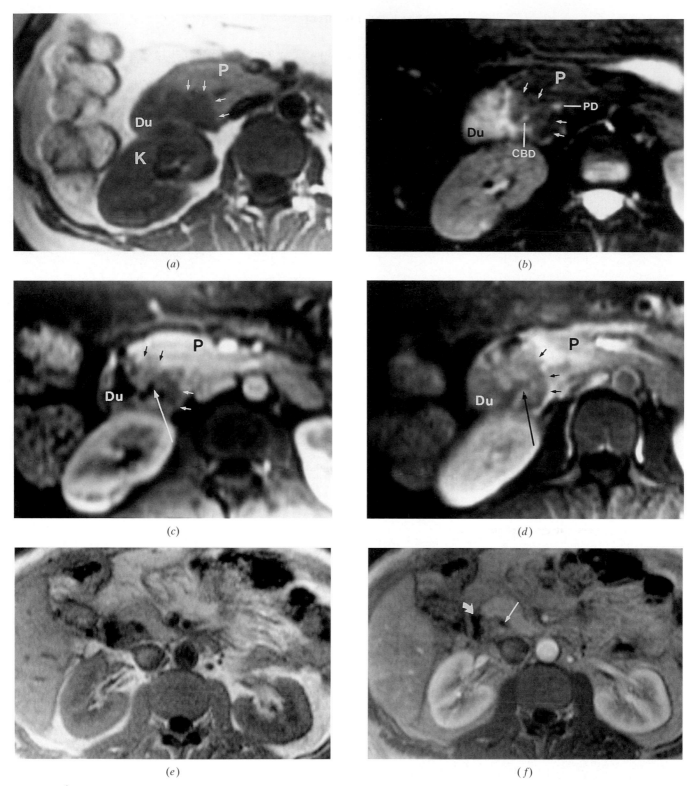

FIG. 3.56 Ampullary carcinoma. T1-weighted spin-echo (*a*), T2-weighted fat-suppressed spin-echo (*b*), immediate (*c*), and delayed (*d*) postgadolinium SGE images. There is a mass (*arrows, a*) at the level of the ampulla that is hypointense to the high-signal-intensity normal pancreas on the T1-weighted image. A fat plane is seen separating the tumor from the right kidney (K) (*a*). The mass is isointense to the pancreas (P) (*b*) on the T2-weighted image (*b*). Note the mass effect on the duodenum (Du) (*b*). The common bile duct (CBD) (*b*) is encased by the tumor, whereas the pancreatic duct (PD) (*b*) at this level is spared. The tumor (*arrows, c*) enhances to a lesser degree than the background normal pancreas on the immediate postgadolinium SGE image (*c*). An ulceration (*long thin arrow, c*) is present within the tumor mass. Decreased conspicuity between the tumor and the pancreas is noted on the delayed postgadolinium SGE image (*d*). An enhancing rim (*arrows, d*) is present around the tumor, which may represent compressed pancreatic tissue. SGE (*e*) and immediate postgadolinium SGE (*f*) images in a second patient demonstrate a 2.5-cm ampullary cancer that surrounds the distal CBD (*arrow, f*) and protrudes into the duodenum (*curved arrow, f*). There is good contrast between higher signal pancreas and low-signal tumor on both images. A CT imaging study performed 1 month prior (not shown) did not demonstrate the tumor.

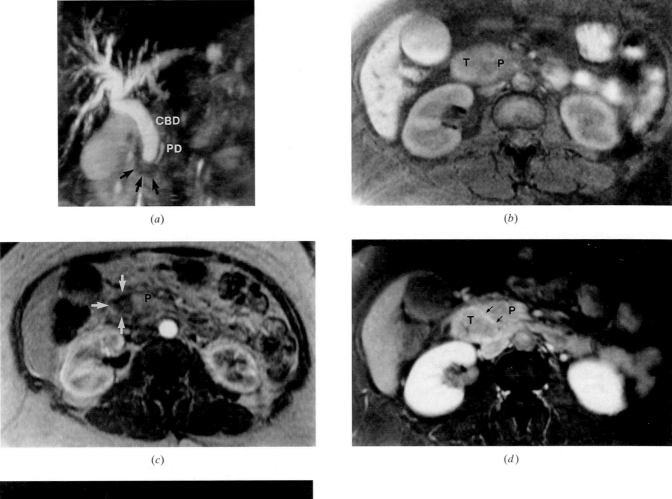

(a)

(b)

(c)

(d)

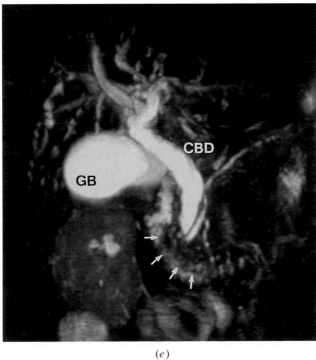

(e)

FIG. 3.57 Ampullary carcinoma. Coronal MIP reconstruction (*a*) of a set of heavily T2-weighted 2D echo-train spin-echo sections, T1-weighted fat-suppressed spin-echo (*b*), immediate postgadolinium SGE (*c*), and delayed postgadolinium fat-suppressed spin-echo (*d*) images. There is a mass (*arrows, a*) at the level of the ampulla, resulting in marked dilatation of the intra- and extrahepatic bile ducts. Dilatation of the pancreatic duct is also present. On the T1-weighted fat-suppressed spin-echo image (*b*) the tumor (T) (*b*) is not visualized against the abnormal low signal intensity (hypointense relative to the liver) of the background pancreas (P) (*b*). The pancreas is hypointense due to chronic pancreatitis caused by pancreatic duct obstruction. The tumor demonstrates heterogeneous diminished enhancement (*arrows, c*) relative to the background pancreas on the immediate postgadolinium SGE image (*c*) and shows an enhancing rim (*arrows, d*) on the more delayed gadolinium-enhanced fat suppressed SGE image (*d*). CBD, common bile duct; GB, gallbladder; PD, pancreatic duct. Coronal MIP reconstruction (*e*) of a set of heavily T2-weighted 2D echo-train spin-echo sections in a second patient demonstrates an ampullary cancer (*small arrows, e*) that obstructs the CBD.

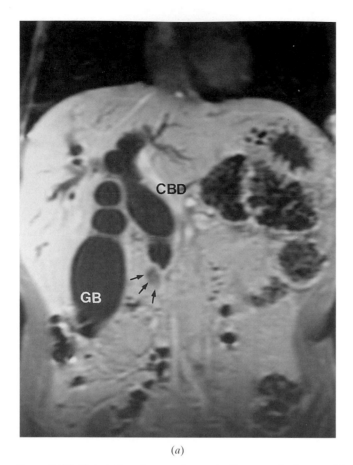

(a)

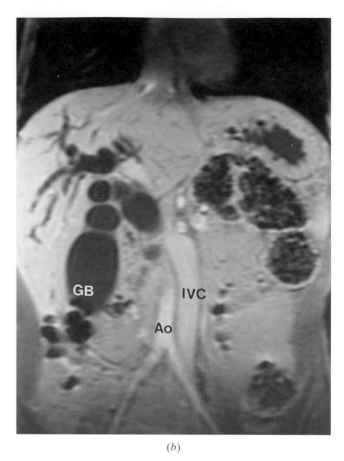

(b)

F I G . 3.58 Metastatic adenocarcinoma to the ampulla. Interstitial-phase gadolinium-enhanced fat-suppressed SGE images (*a,b*). There is an extrinsic mass (*arrows, a,b*) at the level of the ampulla resulting in bile duct obstruction. A more posterior section shows the presence of a left-sided inferior vena cava (IVC). Ao, aorta; CBD, common bile duct; GB, gallbladder.

with ulcerative colitis and Gardner's syndrome are at increased risk of developing periampullary carcinomas. Periampullary tumors can range in size from millimeters to larger than 10 centimeters. Symptoms will depend on the proximity of the origin of the tumor to the ampulla. Tumors close to the origin of the ampulla present earlier with signs of obstruction.

Periampullary tumors may be visualized on T1-weighted fat-suppressed images as a low-signal-intensity mass in the region of the ampulla. However, obstruction of the pancreatic duct eventually results in chronic pancreatitis that appears as generalized diminished signal intensity of the pancreas on T1-weighted fat-suppressed images. In the presence of chronic pancreatitis these tumors are poorly shown on T1-weighted fat-suppressed images. Diminished heterogeneous enhancement occurs in a background of higher signal-enhanced pancreatic parenchyma on immediate postgadolinium-enhanced SGE images (Figs. 3.56 and 3.57). This appearance is not substantially affected by the presence of chronic pancreatitis. A recent report has described that ampullary carcinomas are best visualized on immediate postgadolinium

SGE images, which reflects the fact that these tumors are more hypovascular than background pancreatic tissue [89].

Ampullary carcinomas, especially when intraductal, remain a challenge for MR cholangiography performed in isolation [27]. In contrast, ERCP provides an endoscopic view of the ampulla in all cases and allows for biopsy of suspicious lesions. Although future refinements in technique may allow for improved visualization of the ampulla at MR cholangiography, the major papilla is currently visible in only 40 percent of patients [26]. Therefore, precontrast T1-weighted fat-suppressed SGE and immediate postgadolinium SGE images should be used in combination with MR cholangiography in patients suspected of having biliary obstruction caused by tumor.

Metastases to the Ampulla

In rare instances tumors may metastasize to the ampulla resulting in CBD obstruction. The appearance of metastatic disease may resemble primary tumors of the ampulla (Fig. 3.58).

FUTURE DIRECTIONS

Further refinements of MR cholangiographic techniques hold the promise of supplanting the majority of diagnostic ERCP studies and replacing ultrasound and CT imaging for the investigation of CBD pathology. The clinical applications of contrast agents excreted in the bile has yet to be determined, but they may play a role both for the investigation of hepatocellular function and for biliary tract morphology.

CONCLUSION

The widespread availability of MR cholangiography has increased the role of MRI in the investigation of biliary tract disease. Currently the combination of MR cholangiography, precontrast fat-suppressed SGE, immediate postgadolinium SGE and interstitial-phase gadolinium-enhanced fat-suppressed SGE is an effective, comprehensive imaging approach for the investigation of the full range of biliary tract diseases.

REFERENCES

1. Lenriot J, Le Neel J, Hay J, Jaeck D, Millat, B, Fagniez P: Cholangio-pancréatographie rétrograde et sphinctérotomie endoscopique pour lithiase biliaire. Gastoenterol Clin Biol 17:244–250, 1993.
2. Assouline Y, Liguory C, Ink O, Fritsch J, Choury A, Lefebvre J, Pelletier G, Buffet C, Etienne J: R_sultats actuels de la sphinct_rotomie endoscopique pour lithiase de la voie biliaire prinicpale. Gastoenterol Clin Biol 17:251–258, 1993.
3. Hamm B, Staks T, Muhler A, Bollow M, Taupitz M, Frenzel T, Wolf KJ, Weinmann HJ, Lange L: Phase I clinical evaluation of Gd-EOB-DTPA as a hepatobiliary MR contrast agent: Safety, pharmacokinetics, and MR imaging. Radiology 195:785–792, 1995.
4. Vogl TJ, Hamm B, Schnell B, McMahon C, Branding G, Lissner J, Wolf KJ: Mn-DPDP enhancement patterns of hepatocellular lesions on MR images. Magn Reson Imaging 3:51–58, 1993.
5. Liou J, Lee JK, Borrello JA, Brown JJ: Differentiation of hepatomas from nonhepatomatous masses: Use of MnDPDP-enhanced MR images. Magn Reson Imaging 12:71–79, 1994.
6. Lim KO, Stark DD, Leese PT, Pfefferbaum A, Rocklage SM, Quay SC: Hepatobiliary MR imaging: First human experience with MnDPDP. Radiology 178:79–82, 1991.
7. Bernardino ME, Young SW, Lee JK, Weinreb JC: Hepatic MR imaging with Mn-DPDP: Safety, image quality, and sensitivity. Radiology 183:53–58, 1992.
8. Schuhmann-Giampieri G, Schmitt-Willich H, Press WR, Negishi C, Weinmann HJ, Speck U: Preclinical evaluation of Gd-EOB-DTPA as a contrast agent in MR imaging of the hepatobiliary system. Radiology 183:59–64, 1992.
9. Low RN, Sigeti JS, Francis IR, Weinman D, Bower B, Shimakawa A, Foo TK: Evaluation of malignant biliary obstruction: Efficacy of fast multiplanar spoiled gradient-recalled MR imaging vs. spin-echo MR imaging, CT, and cholangiography. AJR Am J Roentgenol 162:315–323, 1994.
10. Semelka RC, Shoenut JP, Greenberg HM, Mickflickier AB: The liver. In: Semelka RC, Shoenut JP (eds.). MRI of the Abdomen with CT Correlation. New York: Raven Press, pp. 13–41, 1993.
11. Reinhold C, Bret PM, Rohoman L, Denton T: Value of flow compensation in postcontrast T1-weighted spin-echo pulse sequences of the liver (abstract). J Mag Reson Imaging 4(P):43, 1994.
12. Wallner BK, Schumacher KA, Weidenmaier W, Friedrich JM: Dilated biliary tract: Evaluation with MR cholangiography with a T2-weighted contrast-enhanced fast sequence. Radiology 181:805–808, 1991.
13. Morimoto K, Shimoi M, Shirakawa T, Aoki Y, Choi S, Miyata Y, Hara K: Biliary obstruction: Evaluation with three-dimensional MR cholangiography. Radiology 183:578–580, 1992.
14. Hall-Craggs MA, Allen CM, Owens CM, Theis BA, Donald JJ, Paley M, Wilkinson ID, Chong WK, Hatfield ARW, Lees WR, Russell RCG: MR cholangiography: Clinical evaluation in 40 cases. Radiology 189:423–427, 1993.
15. Ishizaki Y, Wakayama T, Okada Y, Kobayashi T: Magnetic resonance cholangiography for evaluation of obstructive jaundice. Am J Gastroenterol 88:2072–2077, 1993.
16. Reinhold C, Guibaud L, Genin G, Bret PM: MR cholangiopancreatography: Comparison between two-dimensional fast spin-echo and three-dimensional gradient-echo pulse sequences. J Mag Reson Imaging 4:379–384, 1995.
17. Outwater EK: MR cholangiography with a fast-spin echo sequence (abstract). J Mag Reson Imaging 3(P):131, 1993.
18. Takehara Y, Ichijo K, Tooyama N, Kodaira N, Yamamoto H, Tatami M, Saito M, Watahiki H, Takahashi M: Breath-hold MR cholangio-pancreatography with a long-echo-train fast spin-echo sequence and a surface coil in chronic pancreatitits. Radiology 192:73–78, 1994.
19. Guibaud L, Bret PM, Reinhold C, Atri M, Barkun ANG: Diagnosis of choledocholithiasis: Value of MR cholangiography. AJR Am J Roentgenol 163:847–850, 1994.
20. Barish MA, Yucel EK, Soto JA, Chuttani R, Ferrucci JT: MR cholangiopancreatography: Efficacy of three-dimensional turbo spin-echo technique. AJR Am J Roentgenol 165:295–300, 1995.
21. Reinhold C, Bret PM, Guibaud L, Barkun A, Genin G, Atri M: Magnetic resonance cholangiopancreatography (MRCP): Potential clinical applications. Radiographics 16:309–320, 1996.
22. Macaulay SE, Schulte SJ, Sekijima JH, Obregon RG, Simon HE, Rohrmann CA, Jr, Freeny PC, Schmiedl UP: Evaluation of a non-breath-hold MR cholangiography technique. Radiology 196:227–232, 1995.
23. Miyazaki T, Yamashita Y, Tsuchigame T, Yamamoto H, Urata J, Takahasi M. MR cholangiopancreatography using HASTE (half-fourier acquisition single-shot turbo spin-echo) sequences. Am J Roetgen 166:1297–1303, 1996.
24. Demas BE, Hricak H, Moseley M, Wall SD, Moon K, Goldberg HI, Margulis AR: Gallbladder bile: An experimental study in dogs using MR imaging and proton MR spectroscopy. Radiology 157:453–455, 1985.
25. Loflin TG, Simeone JF, Mueller PR, Saini S, Stark DD, Butch RJ, Brady TJ, Ferrucci JT Jr: Gallbaldder bile in cholecystitis: In vitro MR evaluation. Radiology 157:457–459, 1985.
26. Taourel P, Bret PM, Reinhold C, Barkun AN, Atri M: MR cholangiography of anatomical variants of the biliary tree. Radiology 199:521–527, 1996.
27. Guibaud L, Bret PM, Reinhold C, Atri M, Barkun AN: Bile duct obstruction and choledocholithiasis: Diagnosis with MR cholangiography. Radiology 197:109–115, 1995.
28. Reinhold C, Bret PM: MR cholangiopancreatography. Abdom Imaging 21:105–116, 1996.
29. Reuther G, Kiefer B, Tuchmann A: Cholangiography before biliary surgery: Single-shot MR cholangiography versus intravenous cholangiography. Radiology 198:561–566, 1996.
30. Sterling JA: The common channel for bile and pancreatic ducts. Surg Gynecol Obstet 98:420–424, 1954.
31. Taourel P, Reinhold C, Bret PM, Barkun AN, Atri M: Biliary and

pancreatic ductal anatomy: Normal findings and variants demonstrated with MR cholangiopancreatography (abstract). RSNA 197(P):502, 1995.

32. Strasberg SM, Hertl M, Soper NJ: An analysis of the problem of biliary surgery during laparoscopic cholecystectomy. J Am Coll Surg 180:101–125, 1995.

33. Barkun JS, Fried GM, Barkun AN, Sigman HH, Hinchey EJ, Garzon J, Wexler MJ, Meakins JL: Cholecystectomy without operative cholangiography. Implications for common bile duct injury and retained common bile duct stones. Ann Surg 218(3):371–377, 1993.

34. Sackier JM, Berci G, Phillips E, Carroll B, Shapiro S, Paz-Partlow M: The role of cholangiography in laparoscopic cholecystectomy. Arch Surg 126(8):1021–1025, 1991.

35. Soper NJ, Brunt LM: The case for routine operative cholangiography during laparoscopic cholecystectomy. Surg Clin North Am 74:953–959, 1994.

36. Moeser PM Julian, Karstaedt N, Sterchi M: Unusual presentation of cholelithiasis on T1-weighted MR imaging. J Comput Assist Tomogr 12:150–152, 1988.

37. Moon KL Jr, Hricak H, Margulis AR, et al: Nuclear magnetic resonance imaging characteristics of gallstones in vitro. Radiology 148:753–756, 1983.

38. Moriyasu F, Ban N, Nishida O, et al: Central signals of gallstones in magnetic resonance imaging. Am J Gastroenterol 82:139–142, 1987.

39. Baron RL, Shuman WP, Lee SP, Rohrmann CA Jr, Golden RN, Richards TL, Richardson ML, Nelson JA: MR appearance of gallstones in vitro at 1.5 T: Correlation with chemical composition. AJR Am J Roentgenol 153:497–502, 1989.

40. Semelka RC, Shoenut JP, Mickflickier AB: The gallbladder and biliary tree. In: Semelka RC, Shoenut JP (eds.). MRI of the Abdomen with CT Correlation. New York: Raven Press, pp. 43–52, 1993.

41. Weissleder R, Stark DD, Compton CC, Simeone JF, Ferrucci JT: Cholecystitis: Diagnosis by MR imaging. Magn Reson Imaging 6:345–348, 1988.

42. Loud PA, Semelka RC, Kettritz U, Brown JJ, Reinhold C: MRI of acute cholecystitis: Comparison with the normal gallbladder and other entities. Magn Reson Imaging 14(4):349–355, 1996.

43. Matsui O, Kadoya M, Takashima T, Kameyama T, Yoshikawa J, Tamura S: Intrahepatic periportal abnormal intensity on MR images: An indication of various hepatobiliary diseases. Radiology 17:335–338, 1989.

44. Svanik J, Thornell E, Zettergren L: Gallbladder function in experimental cholecystitis. Surgery 89:500–506, 1981.

45. McCarthy S, Hricak H, Cohen M, Fisher MR, Winkler ML, Filly RA, Margulis AR: Cholecystitis: Detection with MR imaging. Radiology 158:333–336, 1986.

46. Pu Y, Yamamoto F, Igimi H, Shilpakar SK, Kojima T, Yamamoto S, Luo D: A comparative study usefulness of magnetic resonance imaging in the diagnosis of acute cholecystitis. J Gastroenterol 29:192–198, 1994.

47. Rooholamini SA, Tehrani NS, Razavi MK, Au AH, Hansen GC, Ostrzega N, Verma RC: Imaging of gallbladder carcinoma. Radiographics 14:291–306, 1994.

48. Sagoh T, Itoh K, Togashi K, Shibata T, Minami S, Noma S, Yamashita K, Nishimura K, Asato R, Mori K, Nishikawa T, Kakano Y, Konishi J: Gallbladder carcinoma: Evaluation with MR imaging. Radiology 174:131–136, 1990.

49. Rossman MD, Friedman AC, Radecki PD, Caroline DF: MR imaging of gallbladder carcinoma. AJR Am J Roentgenol 148:143–144, 1987.

50. Dooms GC, Fisher MR, Higgins CB, Hricak H, Goldberg HI, Margulis AR: MR imaging of the dilated biliary tract. Radiology 158:337–341, 1986.

51. Laubenberger J, Büchert M, Schneider B, Blum U, Hennig J, Langer M: Breath-hold projection magnetic resonance-cholangio-pancreatography (MRCP): A new method for examination of the bile and pancreatic ducts. Magn Reson Med 33:18–23, 1995.

52. Panasen P, Partanen K, Pikkarainen P, Alhava E, Pirinen A, Janatuinen E: Ultrasonography, CT, and ERCP in the diagnosis of choledochal stones. Acta Radiol 33:53–56, 1992.

53. Rigauts H, Marchal G, Van Steenbergen W, Ponette W: Comparison of ultrasound and ERCP in the detection of the cause of obstructive biliary disease. Rofo Fortschr Geb Rontgenstr Neuen Bildgeb Verfahr 156:252–257, 1992.

54. O'Connor HJ, Hamilton I, Ellis WR, Watters J, Lintott DJ, Axon AT: Ultrasound detection of choledocholithiasis: Prospective comparison with ERCP in the postcholecystectomy patient. Gastrointest Radiol 11:161–164, 1986.

55. Cronan JJ: US diagnosis of choledocholithiasis: A reappraisal. Radiology 161:133–134, 1986.

56. Stott MA, Farrand PA, Guyer PB, Dewbury KC, Browning JJ, Sutton R: Ultrasound of the common bile duct in patients undergoing cholecystectomy. J Clin Ultrasound 19:73–76, 1991.

57. Wermke W, Schultz HJ: Sonographic diagnosis of bile duct calculi: Results of a prospective study of 222 cases of choledocholithiasis. Ultraschall Med 8:116–120, 1987.

58. Dong B, Chen M: Improved sonographic visualization of choledocholithiasis. J Clin Ultrasound 15:185–190, 1987.

59. Baron RL: Common bile duct stones: Reassessment of criteria for CT diagnosis. Radiology 162:419–424, 1987.

60. Todua FI, Karmazanovskii GG, Vikhorev AV, Todua FI, Karmazanovskii GG, Vikhorev AV: Computerized tomography of the mechanical jaundice in the involvement of the distal region of the common bile duct. Vestn Rentgenol Radio 2:15–22, 1991.

61. Cotton PB, Lehman G, Vennes J, Geenen JE, Russell RCG, Meyers WC, Liguory C, Nicki N: Endoscopic sphincterotomy complications and their management: An attempt at consensus. Gastrointest Endosc 37(3):383–393, 1991.

62. Frey CF, Burbige EJ, Meinke WB, Pullos TG, Wong HN, Hickman DM, Belber J: Endoscopic retrograde cholangiopancreatography. Am J Surg 144(1):109–114, 1982.

63. Reinhold C, Taourel P, Bret PM, Barkun A, Atri M: MR Cholangiography of choledocholithiasis by using a multicoil array and high-resolution imaging parameters (abstract). Radiology 197(P):342, 1995.

64. Laghi A, Catalano C, Broglia L, Messina A, Scipioni A, Pavone P, Passariello R: Optimized 3D MR cholangiography in the evaluation of bile duct stones: Superiority over endoscopic retrograde cholangiopancreatography (abstract). Int Soc Magn Reson Med 3(P):1446, 1995.

65. Reinhold C, Bret PM. Current status of MR cholangiopancreatography (perspective). AJR Am J Roentgenol 166:1285–1295, 1996.

66. Semelka RC, Shoenut JP, Kroeker MA, Hricak H, Minuk GY, Yaffe CS, Micflikier AB: Bile duct disease: Prospective comparison of ERCP, CT, and fat suppression MRI. Gastrointest Radiol 17:347–352, 1992.

67. LaRusso NF, Wiesner RH, Ludwig J, MacCarty RL: Current concepts. Primary sclerosing cholangitis. N Engl J Med 310:899–903, 1984.

68. Shea WJ, Jr., Demas BE, Goldberg HI, Hohn DC, Ferrell LD, Kerlan RK: Sclerosing cholangitis associated with hepatic arterial FUDR chemotherapy: Radiographic-histologic correlation. AJR Am J Roentgenol 146:717–721, 1986.

69. Wiesner RH, LaRusso NF: Clinicopathologic features of the syndrome of primary sclerosing cholangitis. Gastroenterology 79:200–206, 1980.

70. Chapman RW, Arborgh BA, Rhodes JM, Summerfield JA, Dick R, Scheuer PJ, Sherlock S: Primary sclerosing cholangitis: A review of its clinical features, cholangiography, and hepatic histology. Gut 21:870–877, 1980.

71. Schwartz SI: Primary sclerosing cholangitis: A disease revisited. Surg Clin North Am 53:1161–1167, 1973.

72. Majoie CB, Reeders JW, Sanders JB, Huibregtse K, Jansen PL: Pri-

mary sclerosing cholangitis: A modified classification of cholangiographic findings. AJR Am J Roentgenol 157:495–497, 1991.

73. Teefey SA, Baron RL, Rohrmann CA, Shuman WP, Freeny PC: Sclerosing cholangitis: CT findings. Radiology 169:635–639, 1988.

74. Schulte SJ, Baron RL, Teefey SA, Rohrmann CA, Jr., Freeny PC, Shuman WP, Foster MA: CT of the extrahepatic bile ducts: Wall thickness and contrast enhancement in normal and abnormal ducts. AJR Am J Roentgenol 154:79–85, 1990.

75. Baron RL, Stanley RJ, Lee JK, Koehler RE, Levitt RG: Computed tomographic features of biliary obstruction. AJT Am J Roentgenol 140:1173–1178, 1983.

76. Shanley DJ, Gagliardi JA, Daum-Kowalski R: Choledochal cyst complicating pregnancy: Antepartum diagnosis with MRI. Abdom Imaging 19:61–63, 1994.

77. Rattner DW, Schapiro RH, Warshaw AL: Abnormalities of the pancreatic and biliary ducts in adult patients with choledochal cysts. Arch Surg 118:1068–1073, 1983.

78. Pollack M, Shirkhoda A, Charnsangavej C: Computed tomography of choledochocele. J Comput Assist Tomogr 9:360–362, 1985.

79. Rizzo RJ, Szucs RA Turner MA: Congenital abnormalities of the pancreas and biliary tree in adults. Radiographics 15:49–68., 1995.

80. Bismuth H: Postoperative strictures of the biliary tract. In Blumgart LH (ed.). The Biliary Tract. New York: Churchill-Livingston, pp. 209–218, 1983.

81. MacCarty RL, LaRusso NF, May GR, Bender CE, Wiesner RH, King JE, Coffey RJ: Cholangiocarcinoma complicating primary sclerosing cholangitis: Cholangiographic appearances. Radiology 156:43–46, 1985.

82. Carr DH, Hadjis NS, Banks LM, Hemingway AP, Blumgart LH: Computed tomography of hilar cholangiocarcinoma: A new sign. AJR Am J Roentgenol 145:53–56, 1985.

83. Hamrick-Turner J, Abbitt PL, Ros PR: Intrahepatic cholangiocarcinoma: MR appearance. AJR Am J Roentgenol 158:77–79, 1992.

84. Thorsen MK, Quiroz F, Lawson TL, Smith DF, Foley WD, Stewart ET: Primary biliary carcinoma: CT evaluation. Radiology 152:479–483, 1984.

85. Engels JT, Balfe DM, Lee JK: Biliary carcinoma: CT evaluation of extrahepatic spread. Radiology 172:35–40, 1989.

86. Dooms GC, Kerlan RK, Jr., Hricak H, Wall SD, Margulis AR: Cholangiocarcinoma: Imaging by MR. Radiology 159: 89–94, 1986.

87. Adson MA, Farnell MB: Hepatobiliary cancer—surgical considerations. Mayo Clin Proc 56:686–699, 1981.

88. Yamaguchi K, Enjoji M: Carcinoma of the ampulla of Vater: A clinicopathologic study and pathologic staging of 109 cases of carcinoma and 5 cases of adenoma. Cancer 59:506–515, 1987.

89. Semelka RC, Kelekis NL, John G, Ascher SM, Burdeny DA, Siegelman ES: Ampullary Carcinoma: Demonstration by Current MR Techniques. J Mag Reson Imaging 7:153–156, 1977.

PANCREAS

R. C. SEMELKA, M.D., N. L. KELEKIS, M.D., AND S. M. ASCHER, M.D.

NORMAL ANATOMY

The anatomic divisions of the pancreas include the head, neck, uncinate process, body, and tail. The pancreas often resembles a field hockey stick in shape. The tail is located in the region of the splenic hilum, and the body is oriented in an oblique fashion extending to the right of midline. The neck of the pancreas passes anterior to the portal vein and curves posteriorly and inferiorly to form the head of the pancreas. The uncinate process is a medial triangle-shaped extension of the head of the pancreas. The uncinate process lies posterior to the superior mesenteric vein. The anatomic relationship of the head of the pancreas includes the second portion of the duodenum laterally, the gastroduodenal artery anteriorly, the inferior vena cava posterolaterally, the third portion of the duodenum posteroinferiorly, and the superior mesenteric vessels medially. Considerable variation in the size of the head of the pancreas occurs.

The splenic vein lies along the posterior surface of the body and tail of the pancreas. This constant relationship is an important landmark for the identification of the pancreatic body. The left adrenal gland is seated posterior to the splenic vein. The tail of the pancreas often drapes over the left kidney and terminates in the splenic hilum. The tail may be folded anteriorly over the body of the pancreas. The stomach lies anterior to the pancreas and is separated from it by parietal peritoneum and the lesser sac. The transverse mesocolon forms the inferior boundary of the lesser sac and is formed by the fusion of parietal peritoneal leaves that cover the anterior surface of the pancreas. The lesser sac and transverse mesocolon are common pathways for fluid tracking and accumulation in acute pancreatitis.

The outer surface of the pancreas may vary in appearance from smooth to lobulated. In elderly patients fatty replacement of the pancreas occurs frequently as a normal degenerative process and results in a feathery, lobulated appearance. The pancreas does not have a serosal covering, which accounts for the extensive dissemination of fluid in pancreatitis and the early spread of pancreatic ductal cancer into retroperitoneal fat.

The pancreatic duct measures 1 to 2 mm in diameter in normal subjects. The normal pancreatic head should measure 2 to 2.5 cm in diameter, with the remainder of the gland approximately 1 to 2 cm thick. The main pancreatic duct extends from the tail of the pancreas through the head and empties via the sphincter of Oddi into the second part of the duodenum. The main duct is termed the *Duct of Wirsung.* A smaller accessory duct, the *Duct of Santorini*, extends from the body of the pancreas through the neck and enters separately into the duodenum in a more proximal location.

The pancreas performs two distinct functions involving two specific cell types: exocrine function performed by acinar cells and endocrine function performed by islet cells. The major hormones released by the pancreas are insulin and glucagon.

MRI TECHNIQUE

New MRI techniques that limit artifacts in the abdomen have increased the role of MRI to detect and characterize pancreatic disease. Breath-hold spoiled gradient-echo (SGE) techniques, fat-suppression techniques, and dynamic administration of gadolinium chelate have resulted in image quality of the pancreas sufficient to detect and characterize focal pancreatic mass lesions smaller than 1 cm in diameter, and to evaluate diffuse pancreatic disease [1–4]. The recent implementation of MR cholangiopancreatography (MRCP) has permitted good demonstration of the biliary and pancreatic ducts to assess ductal obstruction, dilatation, and abnormal duct pathways [5–7]. The combination of tissue-imaging sequences and MRCP provides comprehensive information to evaluate the full range of pancreatic disease.

MRI of the pancreas is optimal at high field (≥ 1.0 T) due to a good signal-to-noise (S/N) ratio, which facilitates breath-hold imaging, and increased fat-water frequency shift, which facilitates chemically selective excitation-spoiling fat suppression. T1-weighted chemically selective fat suppression and T1-weighted breath-hold SGE are effective techniques for imaging pancreatic parenchyma. The normal pancreas is high in signal intensity (SI) on T1-weighted fat-suppressed images due to the presence of aqueous protein in the acini of the pancreas [1]. Normal pancreas is well-shown using this technique (Fig. 4.1) [8,9]. In elderly patients the signal intensity of the pancreas may diminish and be lower than that of liver [2]. This may reflect changes of fibrosis secondary to the aging process.

Our standard MR protocol includes T1-weighted fat-suppressed imaging (either SGE or spin-echo), SGE, and postgadolinium imaging in the capillary phase (immediate postcontrast) and interstitial phase (1 to 10 minutes postcontrast) [4]. T2-weighted echo-train spin-echo sequences such as T2-weighted half-fourier acquisition snapshot turbo spin-echo (HASTE) provide a sharp anatomic display of the common bile duct (CBD) on coronal plane images and of the pancreatic duct on transverse plane images. T2-weighted fat-suppressed images are useful for demonstrating liver metastases and islet-cell tumors. T2-weighted images also provide information on the complexity of the fluid in pancreatic pseudocysts,

which may reflect the presence of complications such as necrotic debris or infection. Regarding gadolinium enhancement, the pancreas demonstrates a uniform capillary blush on immediate postcontrast images, which renders it higher in signal intensity than liver and adjacent fat (Fig. 4.2) [4]. By 1 minute after contrast the pancreas becomes approximately isointense with fat, and beyond 2 minutes the pancreas is lower in signal intensity than background fat (Fig. 4.3). Pancreatic head is readily distinguished from duodenum on immediate postgadolinium images because the pancreas is rendered substantially higher in signal intensity (see Fig. 4.3).

The characteristic high signal intensity of normal pancreas on precontrast T1-weighted fat-suppressed images is useful in circumstances of abnormalities of position. Following left nephrectomy, the tail of the pancreas falls into the renal fossa, which can simulate recurrent disease on CT examination. Normal pancreas can be readily distinguished by its high signal intensity (Fig. 4.4).

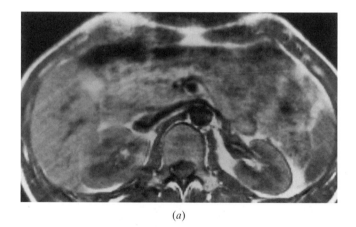

(a)

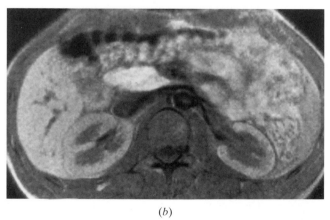

(b)

FIG. 4.1 Normal head of pancreas. T1 spin-echo (T1-SE) (*a*) and T1-weighted fat-suppressed spin-echo (*b*) images. The normal pancreatic head is poorly visualized on the T1-SE image (*a*) due to ghosting artifact and minimal signal difference between pancreas and background tissue. On the T1-weighted fat-suppressed image (*b*), the head is clearly visualized due to minimal-phase artifact and good conspicuity of high signal-intensity pancreatic tissue.

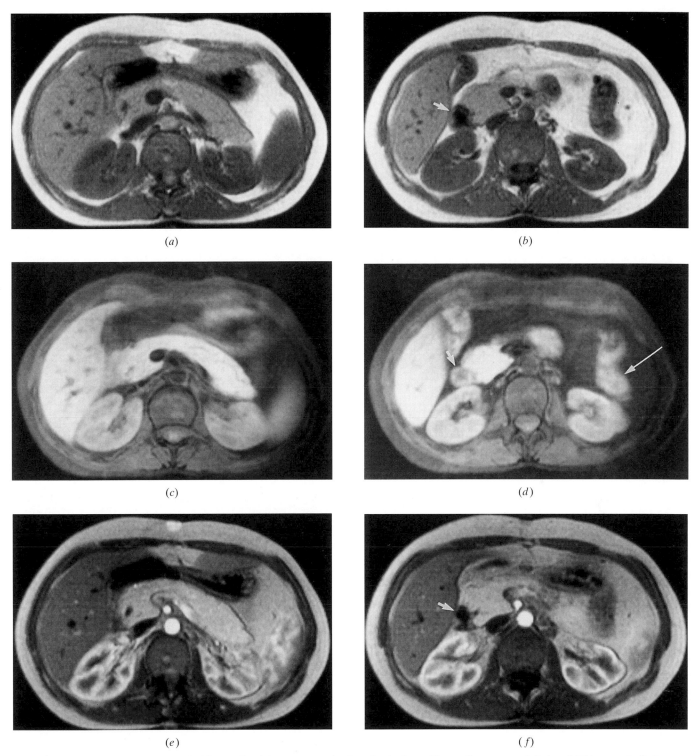

FIG. 4.2 Normal pancreas. SGE (*a,b*), T1-weighted fat-suppressed spin-echo (*c,d*), and immediate postgadolinium SGE images (*e,f*). Images of the pancreatic body (*a,c,e*) and head (*b,d,f*) illustrate the appearance of normal pancreas. Lack of breathing artifact renders the pancreas well-shown on precontrast SGE images (*a,b*). The normal pancreas is high in signal intensity on precontrast T1-weighted fat-suppressed images (*c,d*) due to the presence of aqueous protein in the acini of the pancreas. A uniform capillary blush is apparent on the immediate postgadolinium images (*e,f*). The head of the pancreas is clearly distinguishable from duodenum (*arrow b,d,f*). Small bowel has a feathery appearance and is moderate in signal intensity on T1-weighted fat-suppressed images (*long arrow, d*), which is clearly different from the homogeneous or marbled high signal intensity of the pancreas.

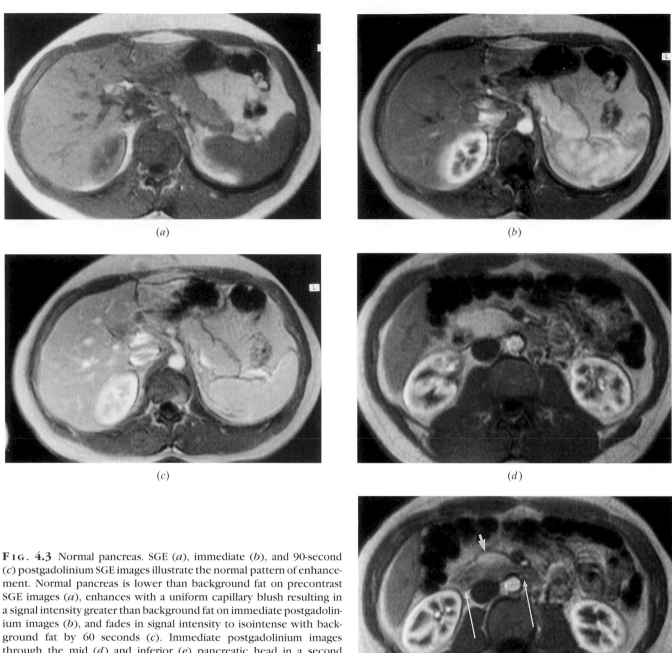

FIG. 4.3 Normal pancreas. SGE (*a*), immediate (*b*), and 90-second (*c*) postgadolinium SGE images illustrate the normal pattern of enhancement. Normal pancreas is lower than background fat on precontrast SGE images (*a*), enhances with a uniform capillary blush resulting in a signal intensity greater than background fat on immediate postgadolinium images (*b*), and fades in signal intensity to isointense with background fat by 60 seconds (*c*). Immediate postgadolinium images through the mid (*d*) and inferior (*e*) pancreatic head in a second patient. Enhancement of the pancreas is more intense than that of normal bowel on immediate postgadolinium images. The most inferior aspect of the pancreatic head (*small arrow, e*) can be distinguished from lesser enhancing adjacent duodenum (*long arrows, e*).

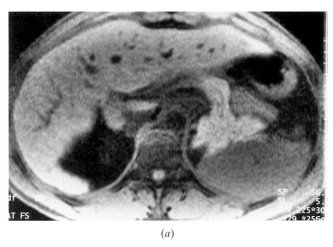
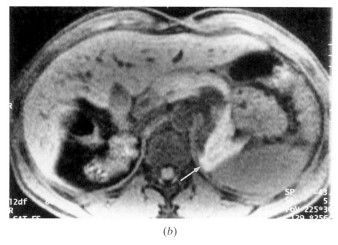

(a)   (b)

F IG . 4.4 Pancreatic tail sitting in left renal fossa following left nephrectomy. Noncontrast T1-weighted fat suppressed SGE images (a,b) demonstrate normal high-signal-intensity pancreas situated in the right renal fossa (arrow, b).

DEVELOPMENTAL ANOMALIES

Pancreas divisum is the most clinically important and common major anatomic variant. This anomaly results from the failure of embryological fusion of the head and body of the pancreas. These portions of the pancreas have separate ductal systems: the head drained by the Duct of Wirsung and the body by the Duct of Santorini. The incidence of this anomaly varies between 1.3 to 6.7 percent of the population [10]. A recent study described 108 patients who underwent both endoscopic retrograde cholangiopancreatography (ERCP) and MRCP and reported exact correlation between these modalities for the detection and exclusion of pancreas divisum [6]. On MRCP images, separate entries of the ducts of Santorini and Wirsung may be consistently shown due to the good conspicuity of the linear high-signal-intensity tubular structures (Fig. 4.5). Variations in pancreas divisum are also shown, which include the dominant dorsal duct syndrome (see Fig. 4.5).

Pancreas divisum, on occasion, results in recurrent acute pancreatitis. It is believed that there is partial obstruction to the passage of pancreatic exocrine secretions from the dorsal pancreas through the narrow orifice at the duodenum, which may result in leakage of secretions into the pancreatic tissue causing pancreatitis. The pancreas may appear normal in signal intensity on T1-weighted fat-suppressed images and gadolinium SGE images because the attacks of recurrent acute pancreatitis are often mild, and changes of chronic pancreatitis usually do not develop.

Annular pancreas is a more uncommon congenital anomaly in which pancreatic tissue surrounds the second portion of the duodenum in an annular fashion. Patients may present with duodenal obstruction. On MR images, pancreatic tissue is identified encasing the duodenum.

T1-weighted fat-suppressed images are particularly effective at demonstrating this entity due to the high signal intensity of pancreatic tissue, which is readily distinguished from the lower signal intensity of adjacent tissue and duodenum [11].

Congenital absence of the dorsal pancreatic anlage is a congenital anomaly usually identified as an incidental finding. The head of the pancreas terminates with a rounded contour, unlike surgical or posttraumatic absence of the distal pancreas which has more squared-off or irregular terminations (Fig. 4.6).

CONGENITAL DISEASE

Cystic Fibrosis
Cystic fibrosis is a dysfunction of exocrine glands characterized by chronic bronchopulmonary infections, malabsorption secondary to pancreatic insufficiency, and an increased sweat-sodium concentration. MRI has been shown to demonstrate pancreas changes in patients with cystic fibrosis [12,13]. The lack of ionization radiation may be of value in this young patient population. Three basic patterns of pancreatic abnormalities have been described: pancreatic enlargement with complete fatty replacement, atrophic pancreas with partial fatty replacement, and diffusely atrophic pancreas without fatty replacement [12,13]. Fatty replacement is high in signal intensity on T1-weighted images. The fatty nature of this tissue is confirmed by demonstrating loss of signal intensity on T1-weighted fat-suppressed images (Fig. 4.7).

Primary Hemochromatosis
Primary hemochromatosis is a hereditary disease in which iron is deposited in organ parenchyma. The liver, pancreas, and heart are primarily affected. Iron deposi-

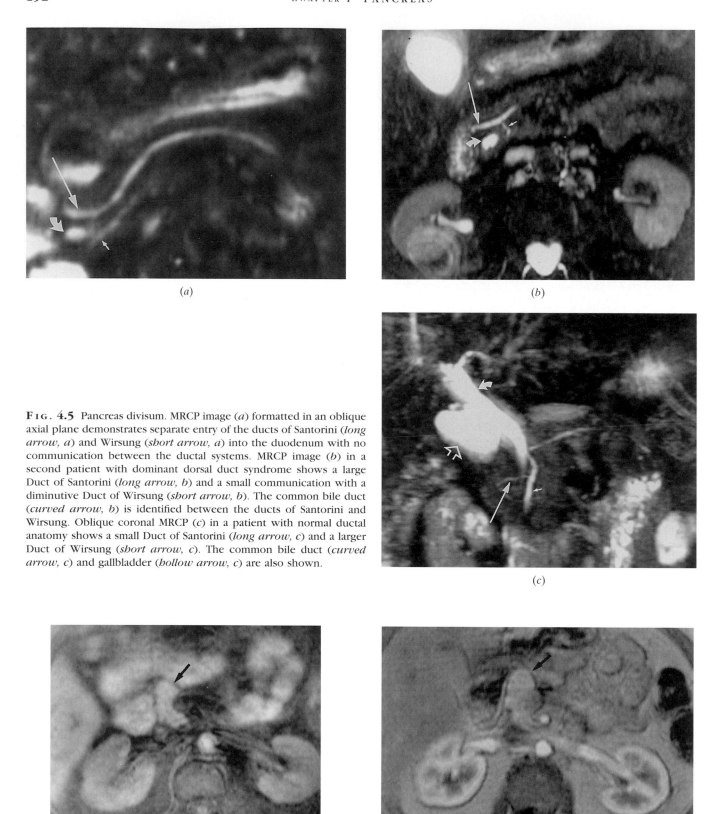

FIG. 4.5 Pancreas divisum. MRCP image (*a*) formatted in an oblique axial plane demonstrates separate entry of the ducts of Santorini (*long arrow, a*) and Wirsung (*short arrow, a*) into the duodenum with no communication between the ductal systems. MRCP image (*b*) in a second patient with dominant dorsal duct syndrome shows a large Duct of Santorini (*long arrow, b*) and a small communication with a diminutive Duct of Wirsung (*short arrow, b*). The common bile duct (*curved arrow, b*) is identified between the ducts of Santorini and Wirsung. Oblique coronal MRCP (*c*) in a patient with normal ductal anatomy shows a small Duct of Santorini (*long arrow, c*) and a larger Duct of Wirsung (*short arrow, c*). The common bile duct (*curved arrow, c*) and gallbladder (*hollow arrow, c*) are also shown.

(a)

(b)

(c)

(a)

(b)

FIG. 4.6 Absence of the dorsal pancreas anlage. T1-weighted fat-suppressed spin-echo (*a*) and immediate postgadolinium SGE (*b*) images. A normal-appearing head of the pancreas is apparent. The pancreas terminates with a rounded contour (*arrow, a,b*) at the level of the pancreatic neck.

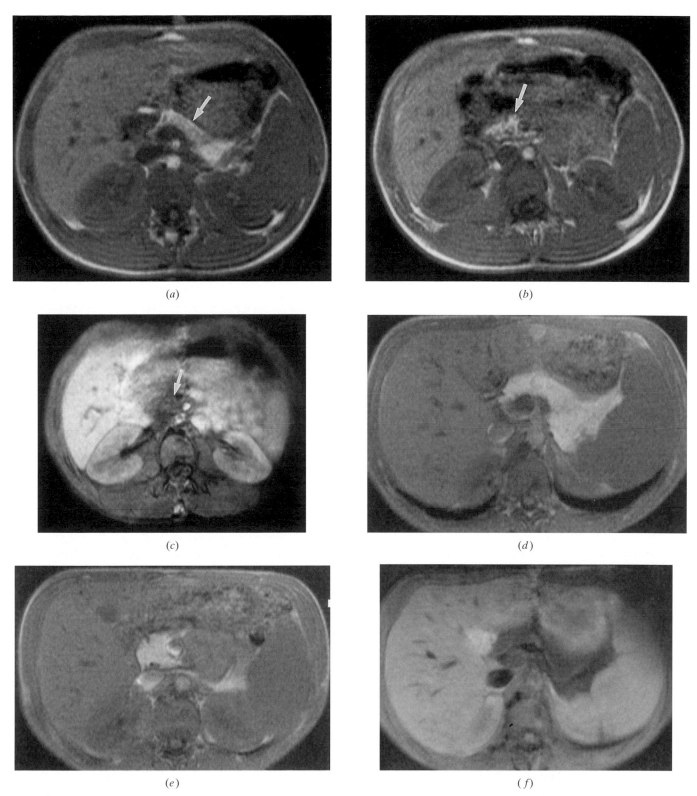

FIG. 4.7 Pancreas in cystic fibrosis. SGE images of the body (*a*) and head (*b*) of the pancreas and T1-weighted fat-suppressed spin-echo image (*c*) through the pancreatic head. The pancreas is high in signal intensity and atrophic on SGE images (*arrow, a, b*) and suppresses on fat-suppressed images (*arrow, c*). These findings are consistent with an atrophic, fatty, replaced pancreas. SGE images of the body (*d*) and head (*e*), T1-weighted fat-suppressed spin-echo images of the body (*f*) and head (*g*) and gated T1-SE image (*h*) of the lungs in a second patient.

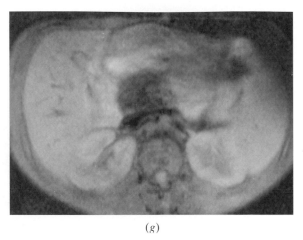

(g)

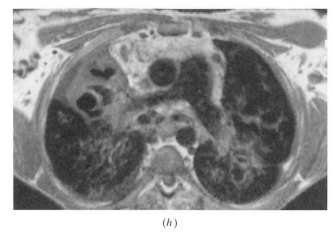

(h)

FIG. 4.7 (*Continued*) The pancreas is high in signal intensity and enlarged on the SGE images (*d,e*) and suppresses on fat-suppressed images (*f,g*). These findings are consistent with an enlarged fatty replaced pancreas. Extensive pulmonary fibrosis is present (*h*), a finding consistent with cystic fibrosis.

tion results in a loss of signal intensity that is more pronounced on T2- or T2*-weighted sequences (Fig. 4.8), but in severe deposition a loss of signal intensity is also apparent on T1-weighted images. Iron deposition in primary hemochromatosis is most substantial in the liver. Deposition of iron in the pancreas tends to occur late in the course of disease after liver damage is irreversible [14,15].

Von Hippel-Lindau Disease
Von Hippel-Lindau disease is an autosomal dominant condition with variable presentation. This condition is characterized by central nervous system (CNS) hemangioblastomas and retinal angiomas. A variety of other mass lesions may occur in other organ systems. Patients with von Hippel-Lindau may develop pancreatic cysts, islet-

cell tumors, or microcystic adenoma. In one series, cysts were the most common pancreatic lesions and were present in 19 of 52 patients in whom no other pancreatic lesions were present (Fig. 4.9) [16].

MASS LESIONS

Adenocarcinoma
Pancreatic ductal adenocarcinoma accounts for 95 percent of the malignant tumors of the pancreas. Pancreatic adenocarcinoma is the fourth most common cause of cancer death in the United States [17]. The lesion is more common in males and blacks [18]. The age range for tumor occurrence is the fourth through eighth decade, with tumor incidence peaking in the eighth decade [19].

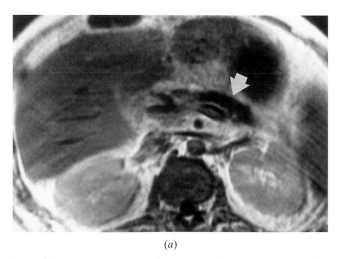

(a)

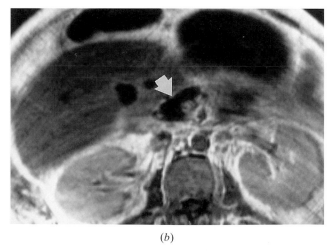

(b)

FIG. 4.8 Iron deposition in the pancreas from primary hemochromatosis. T1-SE images through the body (*a*) and head (*b*) of the pancreas. The pancreas (*arrow, a,b*) is signal-void on T1-weighted images due to the susceptibility effect of iron. The liver is a transplanted liver and therefore has not sustained iron deposition.

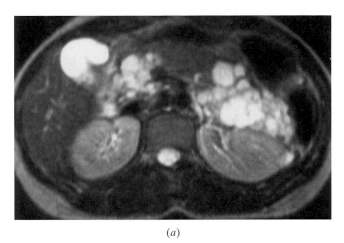

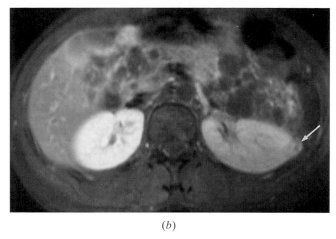

(a) (b)

FIG. 4.9 Pancreatic cysts in von Hippel-Lindau disease. T2-weighted echo-train spin-echo (*a*) and gadolinium-enhanced T1-weighted fat-suppressed spin-echo (*b*) images. Multiple pancreatic cysts are scattered throughout the pancreas, which are high in signal intensity on T2-weighted images (*a*) and low in signal intensity on gadolinium-enhanced images (*b*). Thick septations are present between many of the clustered cysts. A small renal cancer is identified in the left kidney (*arrow, b*).

The tumor has a poor prognosis, with a 5-year survival of 5 percent [18]. Approximately 60 percent of pancreatic adenocarcinomas occur in the head, 15 percent in the body, and 5 percent in the tail, with 20 percent having a diffuse involvement [20]. Tumors in the head of the pancreas are in close relation to CBD. They tend to present smaller in size than tumors in the body or tail due to the development of jaundice secondary to obstruction of the CBD. Painless jaundice is the classical presenting feature of pancreatic cancer occurring in the head.

Pancreatic cancer usually presents late when the disease is advanced. At initial investigation 65 percent of patients have advanced local disease or distant metastases; 21 percent have localized disease with spread to regional lymph nodes; and only 14 percent have tumor confined to the pancreas [21]. The most common sites of metastases, in order of decreasing frequency, are liver, regional lymph nodes, peritoneum, and lungs [20]. The rich lymphatic supply and lack of a capsule account for the early spread of cancer to regional lymph nodes. The nodal groups involved include parapancreatic, para-aortic, paracaval, paraportal, and celiac. Calcification rarely occurs in pancreatic cancer, although the tumor can occur in a pancreas containing calcification.

Pancreatic cancer arising in the head of the pancreas causes abrupt obstruction of the CBD and pancreatic duct [22]. This appearance on MRCP studies results in the "double duct sign," which was originally described on ERCP (Fig. 4.10). Enlargement of the head of the pancreas with dilatation of the CBD and pancreatic duct and atrophy of the body and tail of the pancreas are a common appearance for pancreatic cancer. Enlargement of the head of the pancreas with obstruction of both ducts is not unique to pancreatic cancer, and this appearance also may be observed uncommonly in patients with focal

pancreatitis. Other secondary features that assist in the diagnosis of pancreatic cancer include the presence of lymphadenopathy, encasement of the celiac axis or superior mesenteric artery, and liver metastases [20,23]. On tomographic images, vascular encasement is observed as a loss of the fat plane around vessels [24]. Liver metastases are the only absolute indication of malignancy as lymphadenopathy, and vascular encasement may rarely occur in inflammatory disease. As liver metastases are not common at initial presentation, the most useful imaging feature for the diagnosis of pancreatic cancer is the demonstration of a definable focal mass within the pancreatic parenchyma.

Detection of cancer is best performed by noncontrast T1-weighted fat-suppressed images and immediate postgadolinium SGE images (Fig. 4.11) [1,4,25,26]. Normal pancreatic tissue is well-delineated from tumors, and tumor margins are well-shown using these sequences in all regions of the pancreas. Conventional spin-echo images are generally limited in the detection of pancreatic cancer [27]. Tumors are generally minimally hypointense relative to pancreas on T2-weighted images and are therefore difficult to visualize. A recent study compared single-phase spiral CT imaging with MRI including noncontrast T1-weighted fat-suppressed spin-echo and immediate postgadolinium SGE for the detection or exclusion of pancreatic cancer in 16 patients with findings indeterminate for cancer on spiral CT imaging [26]. Immediate postgadolinium SGE was found to be the most sensitive approach to detect pancreatic cancer, particularly in the head of the pancreas. Both immediate postgadolinium SGE and T1-weighted fat-suppressed spin-echo imaging performed well at excluding cancer, and both were significantly superior to spiral CT imaging (Fig. 4.12). These findings are similar to those reported by Gabata et al.

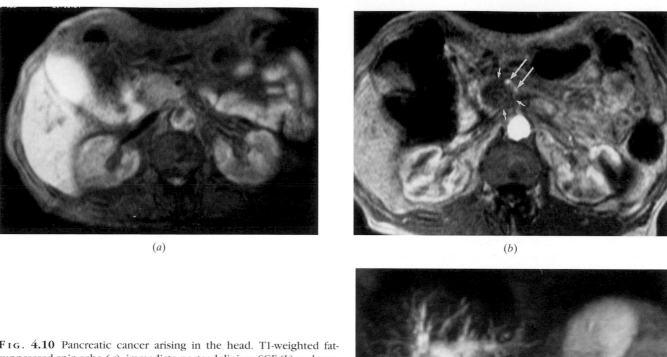

(a)   (b)

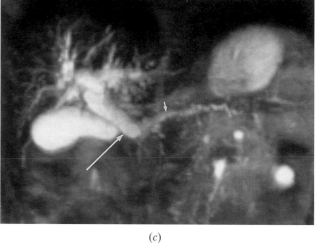

(c)

FIG. 4.10 Pancreatic cancer arising in the head. T1-weighted fat-suppressed spin-echo (*a*), immediate postgadolinium SGE (*b*) and non-breath-hold 3D MIP MRCP (*c*) images. A 3.5-cm cancer arises from the head of the pancreas. The tumor is low in signal intensity on the T1-weighted fat-suppressed spin-echo image (*a*) and cannot be distinguished from adjacent pancreas, which is also low in signal intensity. On the immediate postcontrast image (*b*) the tumor is well-shown as a low-signal-intensity mass (*small arrows, b*) and is closely applied to the superior mesenteric vein SMV and superior mesenteric artery SMA (*arrows, b*). The MRCP image (*c*) demonstrates obstruction of the CBD (*long arrow, c*) and pancreatic duct (*small arrow, c*) creating the "double duct" sign.

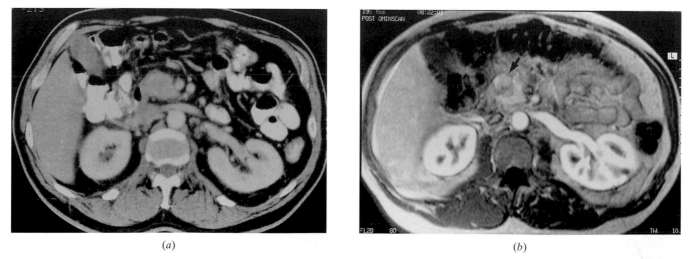

(a)   (b)

FIG. 4.11 Small pancreatic cancer arising in the head. Dynamic contrast-enhanced CT (*a*) and immediate postgadolinium SGE (*b*) images. The nonorgan-deforming cancer is not apparent on the CT image (*a*). On the immediate postgadolinium image (*b*), a heterogeneous low-signal-intensity tumor (*arrow, b*) is identified in the head of the pancreas, clearly demarcated from uniform enhancing pancreatic tissue.

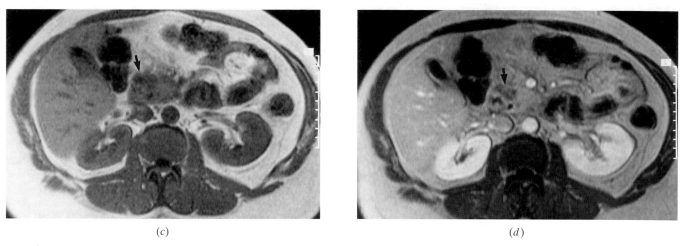

(c)   *(d)*

F IG . 4.11 (*Continued*)   SGE (*c*) and 45-second postgadolinium (*d*) SGE images in a second patient. A 2-cm pancreatic cancer is present that is minimally lower in signal intensity than pancreas on the precontrast image (*c*) and enhances substantially less than pancreas on the early postgadolinium image (*arrow, d*).

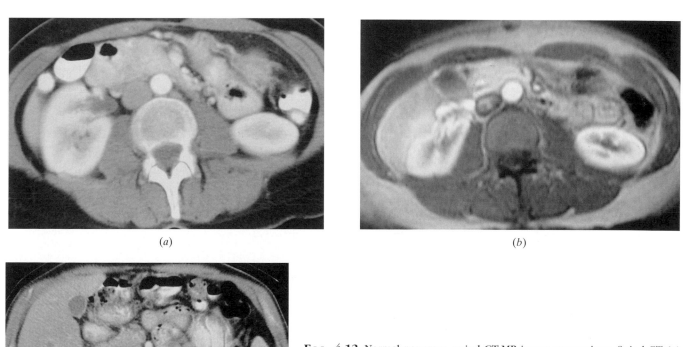

(a)   *(b)*

F IG . 4.12 Normal pancreas, spiral CT-MR image comparison. Spiral CT (*a*) and immediate postgadolinium SGE (*b*) images. The head of the pancreas appears large and heterogeneous on the spiral CT image (*a*), which was considered indeterminate for pancreatic cancer. On the immediate postgadolinium SGE image (*b*), the head of the pancreas enhances in a normal uniform pattern which excludes the presence of cancer. Spiral CT (*c*), T1-weighted fat-suppressed spin-echo (*d*) and immediate postgadolinium SGE (*c*) images in a second patient. The head of the pancreas appears large with a bulbous contour of the uncinate process, findings which were considered inconclusive for pancreatic cancer.

(c)

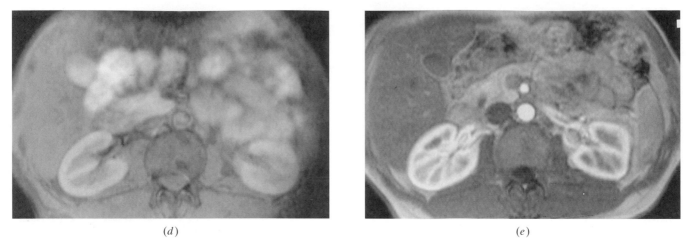

(d) *(e)*

FIG. 4.12 (*Continued*)   Normal high signal intensity on the precontrast T1-weighted fat-suppressed spin-echo image (*d*) and uniform moderately intense enhancement on the immediate postgadolinium SGE image (*e*) exclude the presence of cancer.

[25], who compared these MR techniques to dynamic contrast-enhanced CT imaging.

Pancreatic cancers enhance to a lesser extent than normal pancreatic tissue on early postcontrast images due to their desmoplastic, fibrotic composition [25]. It is therefore critical to exploit this difference in vascularity in contrast-enhanced studies by imaging in the dynamic capillary phase of enhancement (Fig. 4.13) [25,26]. Thin image section thickness is also helpful, but 8-mm thick sections may be sufficiently thin to detect even small (<1-cm) cancers due to the high contrast resolution on SGE images. An adequate signal-to-noise ratio may be achieved with section thickness of 5 mm by using a phased-array surface coil. SGE acquired as a three-dimensional (3D) technique may maintain a sufficient signal-to-noise ratio with even thinner section thickness (3 to

4 mm). Although pancreatic cancers are lower in signal intensity than pancreas on immediate postgadolinium (capillary-phase) images, the appearance of cancers on >1-minute postgadolinium (interstitial-phase) images is variable [25]. The enhancement of cancer relative to pancreas reflects the volume of extracellular space and venous drainage of cancers compared to pancreatic tissue. In general, however, pancreatic tumors, particularly if they are large, tend to remain low in signal intensity on later images (Fig. 4.14), whereas smaller tumors may range from hypointense to hyperintense.

Pancreatic cancers appear as low signal-intensity masses on T1-weighted fat-suppressed images and are clearly separated from normal pancreatic tissue, which is high in signal intensity [4,25,26]. Pancreatic tissue distal to pancreatic cancer often is lower in signal intensity

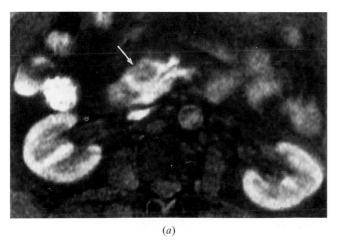
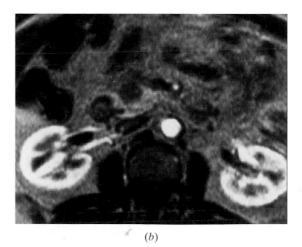

(a) *(b)*

FIG. 4.13   Small pancreatic cancer arising in the head. T1-weighted fat-suppressed spin-echo (*a*), immediate postgadolinium SGE (*b*), and interstitial-phase gadolinium-enhanced T1-weighted fat-suppressed spin-echo (*c*) images. A small nonorgan-deforming cancer is present in the head of the pancreas (*arrow, a*).

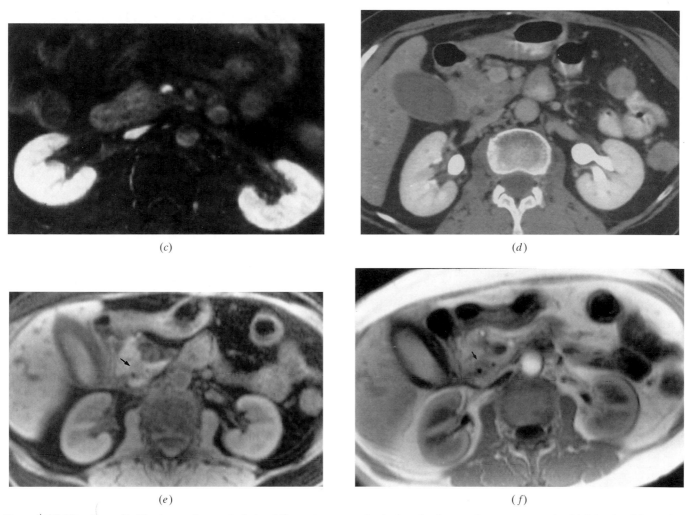

(c) *(d)*

(e) *(f)*

FIG. 4.13 *(Continued)* The tumor does not obstruct the main pancreatic duct, so background pancreas remains high in signal intensity on T1-weighted fat-suppressed images *(a)*. The immediate postgadolinium SGE image *(b)* demonstrates normal capillary enhancement of the pancreas with minimal enhancement of the cancer. The interstitial-phase gadolinium enhanced T1-weighted fat-suppressed image demonstrates minimally higher signal intensity of the tumor compared to the background pancreas reflecting a greater accumulation of gadolinium. Spiral CT *(d)*, fat-suppressed SGE *(e)*, and immediate postgadolinium SGE *(f)* images in a second patient. The pancreatic cancer is not visualized on the spiral CT image *(d)*. On the T1-weighted, fat-suppressed image, the tumor is low in signal intensity *(arrow, e)* relative to background pancreas. On the immediate postgadolinium image *(f)* the tumor *(arrow, f)* enhances less than background pancreas.

than normal pancreatic tissue [25,26]. This is due to the development of chronic pancreatitis secondary to obstruction of the pancreatic duct, which results in decrease of proteinaceous fluid content [25,28]. In these cases, depiction of cancer is poor on noncontrast T1-weighted fat-suppressed images [25,26]. However, immediate postgadolinium SGE images are able to define the size and extent of cancers that obstruct the pancreatic duct [25,26]. Demonstration of a thin rim of greater enhancing pancreatic tissue is commonly observed in pancreatic cancer, particularly those arising in the head, which is a feature that helps to establish the focal nature of the disease process (Fig. 4.15). These tumors appear as low-signal-

intensity mass lesions in a background of slightly greater enhancing chronically inflamed pancreas. Tumors are usually large when they cause changes of distal chronic pancreatitis, and in this setting diagnosis is not problematic. Uninvolved pancreatic parenchyma in pancreatic tail cancers usually is normal and high in signal intensity on T1-weighted fat-suppressed images (Fig. 4.16). This differs from the circumstance of pancreatic head cancer and reflects the fact that chronic pancreatitis occurs distally and not proximally to cancer.

Local extension of cancer and lymphovascular involvement is well-demonstrated on nonsuppressed T1-weighted images [29,30]. Low-signal-intensity tumor is

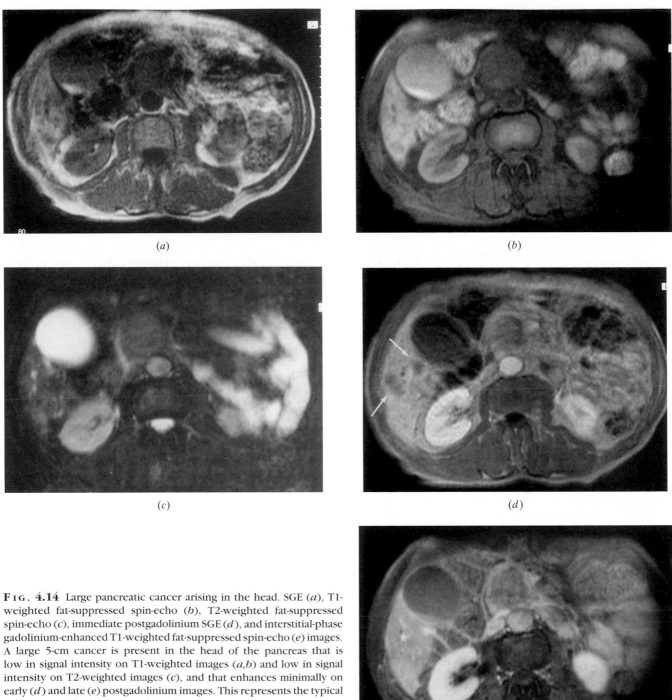

(a)   *(b)*

(c)   *(d)*

(e)

Fig. 4.14 Large pancreatic cancer arising in the head. SGE (*a*), T1-weighted fat-suppressed spin-echo (*b*), T2-weighted fat-suppressed spin-echo (*c*), immediate postgadolinium SGE (*d*), and interstitial-phase gadolinium-enhanced T1-weighted fat-suppressed spin-echo (*e*) images. A large 5-cm cancer is present in the head of the pancreas that is low in signal intensity on T1-weighted images (*a,b*) and low in signal intensity on T2-weighted images (*c*), and that enhances minimally on early (*d*) and late (*e*) postgadolinium images. This represents the typical appearance of a large pancreatic ductal cancer. Liver metastases are present, and are most clearly defined on immediate postgadolinium images as focal low-signal-intensity masses with irregular rim enhancement (*arrows, d*).

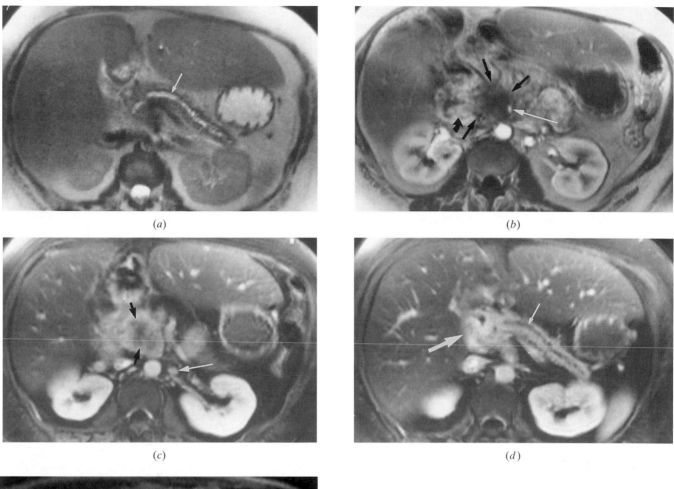

(a) (b)

(c) (d)

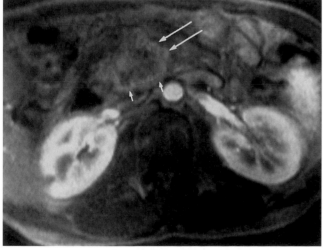

(e)

Fig. 4.15 Pancreatic cancer arising in the head. Half-fourier single-shot turbo spin-echo (HASTE) (*a*), immediate postgadolinium SGE (*b*), and 2-minute gadolinium-enhanced fat-suppressed SGE (*c,d*) images. A large 4-cm tumor is present in the head of the pancreas that results in obstruction of the pancreatic duct (*arrow, a, d*). The tumor is markedly low in signal intensity on the immediate postgadolinium image (*short arrows, b*), and encasement of the SMA is shown (*thin arrow, b*). Adjacent duodenum is thick-walled, which is consistent with invasion (*curved arrow, b*). The tumor shows diminished central enhancement on the interstitial-phase fat-suppressed SGE image (*arrows, c*). Small periaortic lymph nodes are identified (*long arrows, c*). Tumor extension into the porta hepatis is present (*large arrow, d*). Immediate postgadolinium SGE image (*e*) in a second patient shows a 4-cm low-signal-intensity tumor in the head of the pancreas. A thin rim of enhancing pancreatic tissue is present (*small arrows, e*). Close approximation of the tumor to superior mesenteric vessels (*thin arrows, e*) is defined.

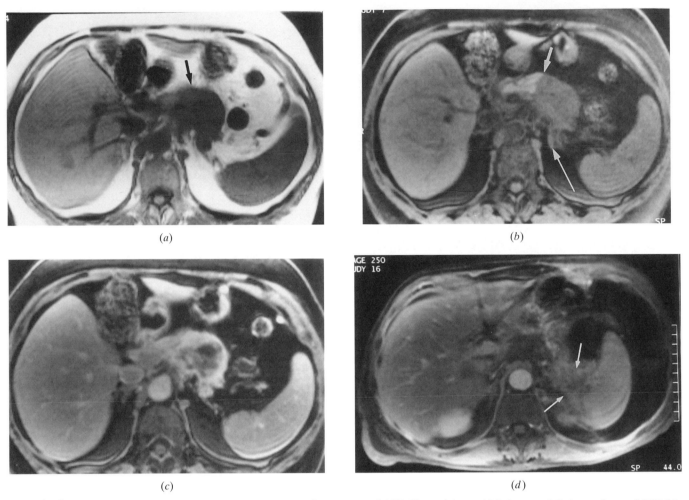

(a)   (b)

(c)   (d)

FIG. 4.16 Pancreatic cancer arising from the tail. SGE (*a*), fat-suppressed SGE (*b*), and interstitial-phase gadolinium-enhanced SGE (*c*) images. A large pancreatic tail cancer is present that has encased the splenic vein. The tumor is low in signal intensity on the T1-weighted image (*arrow, a*). Demarcation of tumor from uninvolved pancreas (*arrow, b*) is clearly shown on the precontrast T1-weighted fat-suppressed image (*b*). The left adrenal is involved (*long arrow, b*). Heterogeneous enhancement with central low signal intensity is apparent on the interstitial-phase image (*c*). Interstitial-phase gadolinium-enhanced SGE image (*d*) in a second patient demonstrates a pancreatic tail cancer (*arrows, d*) that invades the splenic hilum.

well-shown in a background of high-signal-intensity fat. Gadolinium-enhanced fat-suppressed SGE images, acquired in the interstitial phase of enhancement (1 to 10 minutes postcontrast), demonstrate intermediate-signal-intensity tumor tissue extension into low-signal-intensity-suppressed fat (Fig. 4.17). In comparison, noncontrast T1-weighted fat-suppressed images generally show minimal-signal-intensity difference between tumor, which is low in signal intensity, and suppressed background fat [25]. Invasion of adjacent organs is well-shown on a combination of sequences including T1-weighted images and interstitial-phase gadolinium-enhanced fat-suppressed T1-weighted images (Fig. 4.18).

Vascular encasement may be shown using a variety of sequences. T1-weighted spin-echo imaging has been

reported to be superior to dynamic contrast-enhanced CT imaging for the determination of vascular encasement [29]. Vascular patency may be evaluated by either a flow-sensitive gradient-echo technique [31] or by dynamic gadolinium-enhanced SGE [4,32]. Gadolinium-enhanced SGE generates reproducible, good image quality. Immediate postgadolinium SGE images are useful for evaluating arterial patency, and immediate and 45-second postgadolinium SGE images for evaluating venous patency (Fig. 4.19).

Lymph nodes are well-shown on T2-weighted fat-suppressed spin-echo and interstitial-phase gadolinium-enhanced fat-suppressed T1-weighted images. Lymph nodes are moderately high in signal intensity in a background of low-signal-intensity suppressed fat using both

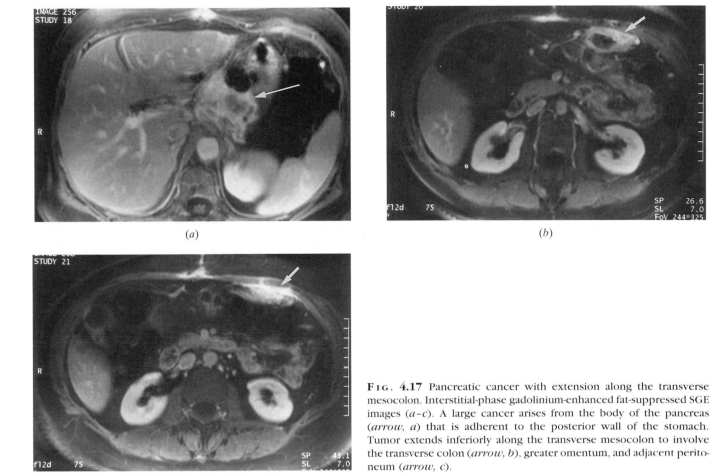

(a)

(b)

(c)

FIG. 4.17 Pancreatic cancer with extension along the transverse mesocolon. Interstitial-phase gadolinium-enhanced fat-suppressed SGE images (a–c). A large cancer arises from the body of the pancreas (arrow, a) that is adherent to the posterior wall of the stomach. Tumor extends inferiorly along the transverse mesocolon to involve the transverse colon (arrow, b), greater omentum, and adjacent peritoneum (arrow, c).

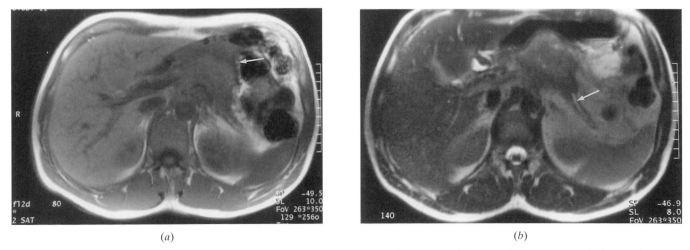

(a)

(b)

FIG. 4.18 Pancreatic cancer arising from the body. SGE (a), HASTE (b), immediate postgadolinium SGE (c), interstitial-phase gadolinium-enhanced T1-weighted fat-suppressed SGE (d,e), and coronal interstitial-phase gadolinium-enhanced T1-weighted fat-suppressed SGE (f) images. A large cancer is present arising from the body of the pancreas (arrow, a) that invades the posterior wall of the stomach.

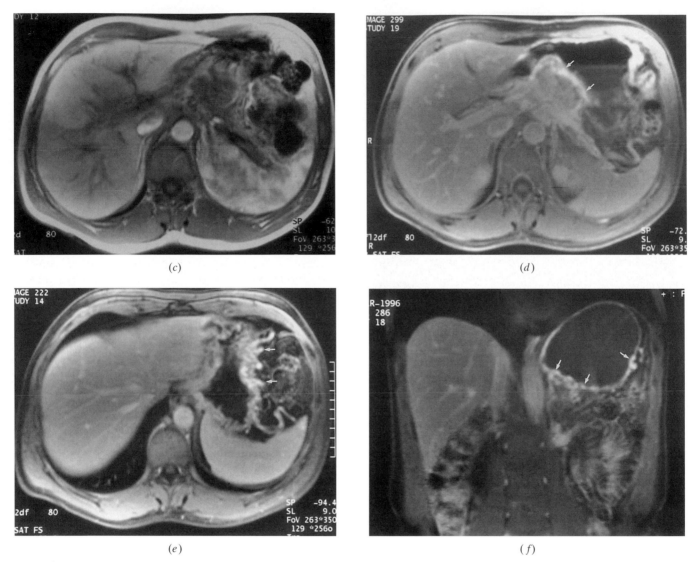

(c)

(d)

(e)

(f)

FIG. 4.18 (*Continued*) Atrophy of the pancreatic tail with ductal dilatation (*arrow, b*) is well-shown on the HASTE image (*b*). Heterogeneous minimal enhancement of the tumor is present on the immediate postgadolinium SGE image (*c*). Improved demonstration of the stomach wall invasion was achieved by gastric distention with orally administered water on the interstitial-phase fat-suppressed SGE image (*small arrows, d*). Multiple varices along the greater curvature of the stomach are present due to thrombosis of the splenic vein. Varices are well-shown on gadolinium-enhanced T1-weighted fat-suppressed SGE images as high-signal-intensity tubular structures (*arrows, e, f*).

of these techniques (Fig. 4.20). T2-weighted fat-suppressed imaging is particularly useful for the evaluation of lymph nodes in close approximation to the liver due to the signal-intensity difference between moderately high-signal-intensity nodes and moderately low-signal-intensity liver. Lymph nodes are also conspicuous on nonsuppressed T1-weighted images as low-signal-intensity focal masses in a background of high-signal-intensity fat [30].

Liver metastases from pancreatic cancers are generally irregular in shape and are low in signal intensity on conventional or fat-suppressed T1-weighted images, minimally hyperintense on T2-weighted images, and demonstrate irregular rim enhancement on immediate

postcontrast SGE images (Fig. 4.21). The low-signal-intensity centers of metastatic lesions reflect the desmoplastic nature of the primary cancer [1]. The hypovascular nature of these metastases permits the distinction between these lesions and cysts and hemangiomas, even when lesions are 1 cm in diameter. Transient ill-defined increased perilesional hepatic parenchymal enhancement may be observed on immediate postgadolinium images. This may reflect hepatic parenchymal vasculitis induced by mucin elaborated by these tumors. A similar appearance is more commonly observed for colon cancer metastases.

The best use of MRI for the investigation of pancreatic

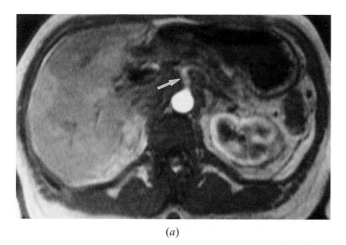

(a)

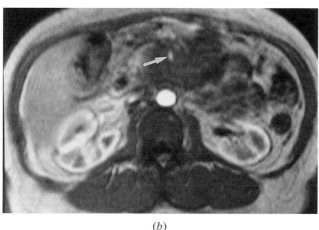

(b)

FIG. 4.19 Pancreatic cancer with local extension and vascular encasement. Immediate postgadolinium SGE images from superior (a) and 2 cm more caudal (b) locations. Low-signal-intensity tumor is present encasing the celiac axis (*arrow, a*) and SMA (*arrow, b*). Tumor local extension is well-defined as low-signal-intensity tissue in a background of high-signal-intensity fat. High-signal-intensity gadolinium-enhanced vessels are conspicuous within the low-signal-intensity tumor.

cancers includes examining patients with diminished renal function or iodine contrast allergy, detecting small nonorgan-deforming cancers (due to the high contrast resolution of precontrast T1-weighted fat-suppressed imaging and immediate postgadolinium SGE images), determining tumor location for imaging guided biopsy, evaluating vascular involvement, and detecting and characterizing associated liver lesions. MRI may be particularly valuable in patients who have an enlarged pancreatic head with no definition of a mass on CT images. Because surgery remains the main therapeutic treatment of patients with pancreatic cancer [18], earlier detection of potentially curable disease may result in improved patient survival.

Islet-Cell Tumors

Islet-cell tumors are of neuroendocrine origin, and the great majority arise from the pancreas. These tumors are relatively rare with a reported incidence of fewer than 1 per 100,000 [33]. Islet-cell tumors may be hormonally functional or nonfunctional [33]. The histology of islet-cell tumors includes gastrinoma, insulinoma, glucagonoma, VIPoma, somatostatinoma, and ACTHoma, with the last three tumors being extremely rare. Although insulinomas are reported as the most common islet-cell tumor, in our experience gastrinomas are more frequently encountered.

Hormonally functional tumors tend to present when they are small in size due to symptoms related to the hormones secreted by the tumors. Nonfunctional tumors account for approximately 15 percent of islet-cell tumors and tend to present with symptoms due to large tumor mass or metastatic disease [34]. Insulinomas are most commonly benign tumors; gastrinomas are malignant in approximately 50 percent of cases; and the great majority of the rarer islet-cell tumors are malignant. The liver is the most common organ for metastatic spread. There is also a particular propensity for splenic metastases.

In the MRI investigation for islet-cell tumors, precontrast T1-weighted fat-suppressed images, immediate postgadolinium SGE images, and T2-weighted fat-suppressed images or breath-hold T2-weighted images are useful [1,35–38]. Tumors are low in signal intensity on T1-weighted fat-suppressed images; demonstrate homogeneous, ring, or diffuse heterogeneous enhancement on immediate postgadolinium SGE; and are high in signal

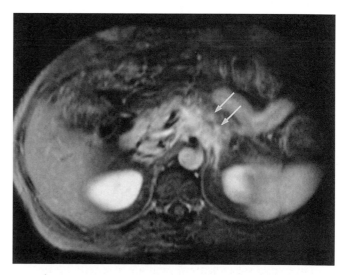

FIG. 4.20 Peripancreatic lymph nodes. Gadolinium-enhanced T1-weighted fat-suppressed spin-echo image demonstrates a pancreatic cancer arising from the body of the pancreas. Several involved peripancreatic nodes smaller than 1 cm (*arrows*) are shown as small, enhancing rounded structures.

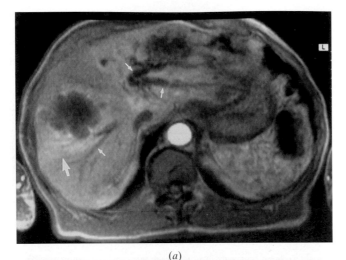

(a)

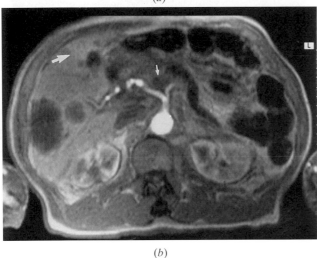

(b)

F I G . 4.21 Liver metastases from pancreatic cancer. Immediate postgadolinium SGE images from upper (*a*) and mid (*b*) hepatic levels. Multiple irregular hepatic metastases are present that possess rim enhancement. Ill-defined perilesional enhancement (*arrow, a,b*) is apparent surrounding several metastases. Substantial intrahepatic bile duct dilatation is also identified (*small arrows, a*) secondary to CBD obstruction by the pancreatic head cancer. Low-signal-intensity tissue (*small arrows, b*) surrounds the celiac axis, a finding consistent with tumor involvement.

intensity on T2-weighted fat-suppressed spin-echo images (Fig. 4.22). In rare instances, islet-cell tumors may be very desmoplastic, appear low in signal intensity on T2-weighted images, and demonstrate negligible contrast enhancement (Fig. 4.23). In these cases, the tumors may mimic the appearance of pancreatic ductal adenocarcinoma. Large, noninsulinoma, islet-cell tumors not uncommonly contain regions of necrosis [39].

The features that distinguish the majority of islet-cell tumors from ductal adenocarcinomas include high signal intensity on T2-weighted images, increased homogeneous enhancement on immediate postgadolinium im-

ages, and hypervascular liver metastases [37]. Because islet-cell tumors rarely obstruct the pancreatic duct, T1-weighted fat-suppressed images almost always show high signal intensity of background pancreas rendering good depiction of low-signal-intensity tumors in the majority of cases [36,37]. Lack of pancreatic ductal obstruction is a feature differentiating islet-cell tumor from pancreatic cancer, as also is lack of vascular encasement.

Gastrinomas

Gastrinomas secrete gastrin, which causes elevated acid production by the gastric mucosa with resultant peptic ulcer disease. This clinical picture is termed the *Zollinger-Ellison syndrome*. Ulcers located in the postbulbar region of the duodenum or in the jejunum, particularly if multiple, suggest the diagnosis of a gastrinoma. Esophagitis is not infrequently observed in these patients.

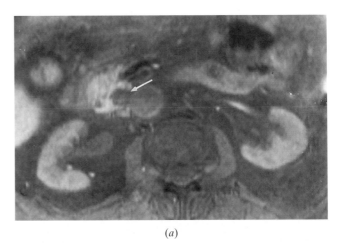

(a)

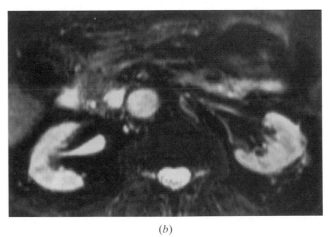

(b)

F I G . 4.22 Islet cell tumor, gastrinoma. T1-weighted fat-suppressed spin-echo (*a*) and T2-weighted fat-suppressed spin-echo (*b*) images. Islet-cell tumors (*arrow, a*) are usually low in signal intensity in a background of high-signal-intensity pancreas on T1-weighted fat-suppressed images (*a*), and high in signal intensity on T2-weighted images (*b*). The uncinate process is a common location for gastrinomas.

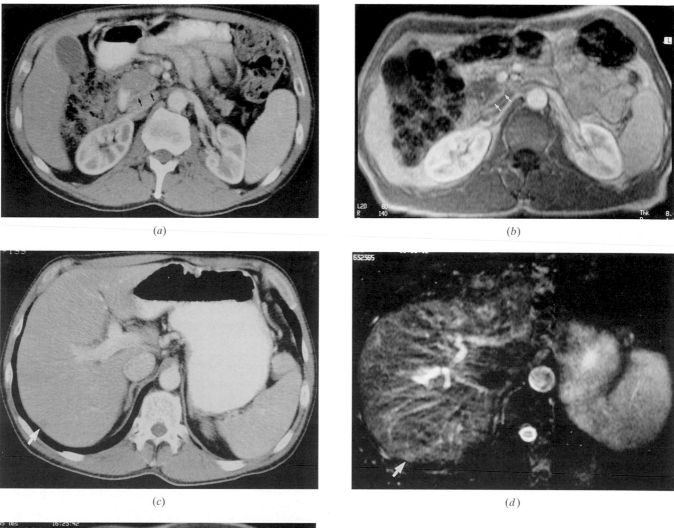

(a)   (b)

(c)   (d)

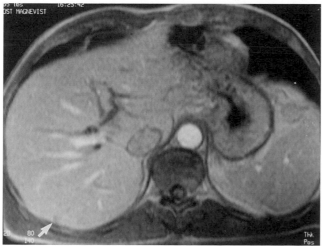

(e)

FIG. 4.23 Hypovascular islet-cell tumor with liver metastases. Spiral CT (*a*) and immediate postgadolinium SGE (*b*) images. Low-attenuation/signal-intensity tumor is well-shown in the head of the pancreas on both spiral CT (*a*) and MR (*b*) images. A thin rim of greater enhancing normal pancreas is noted posterior to the tumor (*small arrows, a,b*). On a higher tomographic section, an ill-defined low-density lesion is noted in the liver on spiral CT image (*arrow, c*) that was considered indeterminate. On the T2-weighted fat-suppressed spin-echo image (*d*), the liver lesion is noted to be low in signal intensity (*arrow, d*), which is not consistent with cyst or hemangioma and is compatible with a hypovascular metastasis. On the 45-second postgadolinium SGE images (*e*), the lesion enhances in a diminished fashion with faint peripheral rim enhancement (*arrow, e*) consistent with a hypovascular metastasis. A cyst would appear nearly signal-void, which is comparable in appearance to the dilated biliary ducts on the postgadolinium image (*e*). The hypovascular nature of this primary tumor is uncommon for islet-cell tumors.

Gastrinomas occur most frequently in the region of the head of the pancreas including pancreatic head, duodenum, stomach, and lymph nodes in a territory termed the *gastrinoma triangle* [23]. The anatomical boundaries of the triangle are the porta hepatis as the superior point of the triangle and the second and third parts of the duodenum forming the base. They may be located throughout the pancreas. Although gastrinomas are usually solitary, multiple gastrinomas are not uncommon. When they are multiple, tumors are commonly located throughout the pancreas including the body and tail [35].

Gastrinomas are not as frequently hypervascular as insulinomas. Mean size at presentation is 4 cm [39]. CT imaging is able to detect gastrinomas reliably when the tumors measure more than 3 cm in diameter, but performs less well in the detection of smaller tumors [40]. Conventional spin-echo MRI also has been limited in the detection of gastrinomas [41,42]. However, MRI, using current techniques, is very effective at detecting tumors <1 cm in diameter.

Gastrinomas are low in signal intensity on T1-weighted fat-suppressed images and high in signal intensity on T2-weighted fat-suppressed images, demonstrating peripheral ring-like enhancement on immediate postgadolinium SGE images (Fig. 4.24). These imaging features are observed in the primary lesion and in hepatic metastases. Central low signal intensity on postgadolinium images reflects central hypovascularity. Occasionally, lesions will be cystic. The enhancing rim of the primary tumor varies substantially in thickness, with the thickness of the rim reflecting the degree of hypervascularity of the tumor. If the enhancing rim is thin, it may appear nearly imperceptible due to similar enhancement of the surrounding pancreatic parenchyma. Gastrinomas not infrequently occur outside the pancreas, and fat-suppressed T2-weighted images are particularly effective at detecting these high-signal-intensity tumors in the background of suppressed fat (Fig. 4.25). Multiple gastrinomas may be scattered throughout the pancreas and frequently are small. T2-weighted breathing-independent HASTE may be effective at demonstrating these tumors because breathing-averaged T2-weighted sequences may result

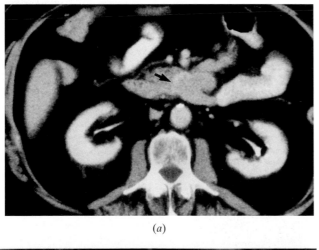

(a)

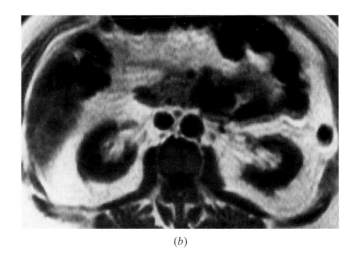

(b)

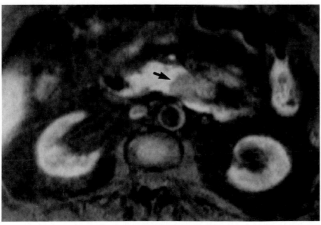

(c)

FIG. 4.24 Gastrinoma. Dynamic contrast-enhanced CT (*a*), SGE (*b*), and T1-weighted fat-suppressed spin-echo (*c*) images. A 2-cm gastrinoma is present arising from the uncinate process of the pancreas (*a–c*). The tumor is most conspicuous on the T1-weighted fat-suppressed spin-echo image (*arrow, c*), and was not identified on the CT examination prospectively. An enhancing rim (*arrow, a*) is apparent on the CT image.

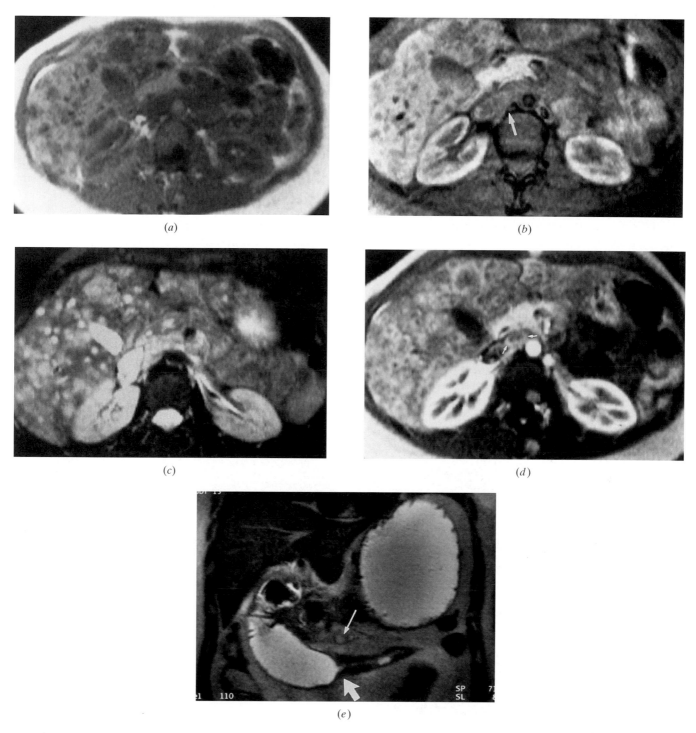

(a)

(b)

(c)

(d)

(e)

Fig. 4.25 Extrapancreatic gastrinoma. SGE (*a*), T1-weighted fat-suppressed spin-echo (*b*), T2-weighted fat-suppressed spin-echo (*c*), and immediate postgadolinium SGE (*d*) images. T1-weighted images (*a,b*) demonstrate an extrapancreatic gastrinoma located posterior to the head of the pancreas with multiple liver metastases smaller than 1.5 cm with similar low signal intensity. The primary tumor (*arrow, b*) is more clearly visible on the T1-weighted fat-suppressed image (*b*) due to the good signal difference between pancreas and tumor. On the T2-weighted fat-suppressed image (*c*), multiple high-signal-intensity foci are present throughout the primary tumor with an identical appearance to the well-defined-high-signal-intensity liver metastases. On the immediate postgadolinium image (*d*), multiple ring-enhancing lesions are apparent in both the primary tumor (*arrow, d*) and the liver metastases. Coronal HASTE (*e*), fat-suppressed HASTE (*f*), and 90-second postgadolinium fat-suppressed SGE (*g*) images in a second patient demonstrate a gastrinoma (*arrow, e–g*) superior to the fourth portion of the duodenum.

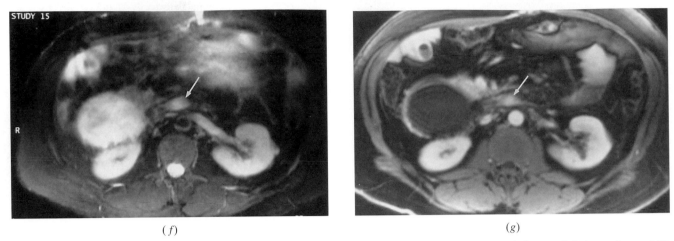

(f)

(g)

FIG. 4.25 (*Continued*) The mass is uniformly high in signal intensity on T2-weighted and interstitial-phase gadolinium-enhanced T1-weighted (*f*) images. Stricturing of the fourth part of the duodenum (*large arrow, e*) reflects peptic ulcer disease in Zollinger-Ellison syndrome. Two prior CT imaging examinations were reported as negative.

in blurring which masks the presence of these tumors (Fig. 4.26).

Gastrointestinal findings that may be observed in gastrinomas include gastric wall hypertrophy with intense mural enhancement on early postgadolinium SGE images (Fig. 4.27), increased esophageal enhancement, and abnormal enhancement or thickness of proximal small bowel (see Fig. 4.25). These features reflect the inflammatory changes of peptic ulcer disease and gastric hyperplasia due to the effects of gastrin.

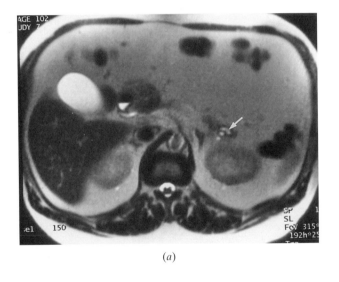

(a)

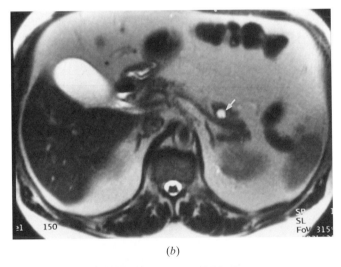

(b)

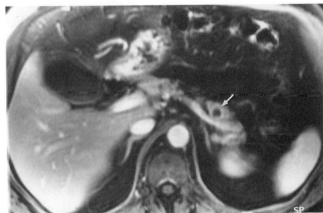

(c)

FIG. 4.26 Multiple gastrinomas. HASTE (*a,b*), and interstitial-phase gadolinium enhanced fat-suppressed SGE (*c*) images demonstrate multiple high-signal-intensity gastrinomas smaller than 1 cm in the tail of the pancreas. The absence of breathing artifact on the HASTE images has resulted in good resolution of the small tumors (*arrows, a,b*). Ring enhancement is apparent on the largest, 8-mm, tumor (*arrow, c*).

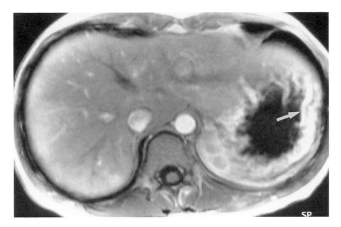

FIG. 4.27 Gastric-wall hyperplasia. Immediate postgadolinium SGE image demonstrates intense enhancement of the prominent gastric rugal folds (*arrow*).

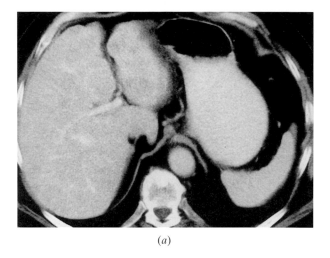

(*a*)

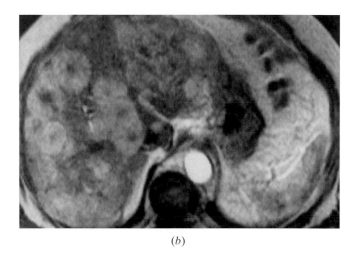

(*b*)

Islet-cell tumor metastases to the liver in general are well-shown on MR images. Gastrinoma metastases frequently are relatively uniform in size and shape [37]. These metastases are generally hypervascular and possess uniform intense rim enhancement on immediate postgadolinium SGE images. Unlike pancreatic cancer liver metastases, ill-defined perilesional enhancement is not observed for gastrinoma metastases, despite the substantial hepatic arterial blood supply of these tumors. Typically, lesions are very high in signal intensity on T2-weighted fat-suppressed images and have well-defined margins. This T2-weighted appearance may be confused with hemangiomas that have a similar appearance. Islet-cell liver metastases are differentiated from hemangiomas by their enhancement patterns. Islet-cell metastases have uniform ring enhancement on immediate postgadolinium images that fades with time [28], whereas hemangiomas have discontinuous rim enhancement on immediate postgadolinium images with centripetal progression of enhancement. (For a discussion on hemangiomas see Chapter 2 on the Liver.) These appearances are better shown on MR than CT images due to the higher sensitivity of MRI to contrast enhancement, faster delivery of a compact bolus of intravenous contrast, and greater imaging temporal resolution [28]. The peripheral enhancing rim may be thin or thick, resulting in differences in the degree of vascularity. Occasionally, thick rim enhancement may have a peripheral-based spoke-wheel enhancement. Centripetal enhancement of gastrinoma metastases may occur on serial postgadolinium images. Peripheral washout is commonly observed for hypervascular gastrinoma metastases (Fig. 4.28).

Insulinomas

Insulinomas are common islet-cell tumors and are frequently functional. Tumors present when they are small in size (<2 cm) due to the severity of the symptomatology [39]. Patients present with signs and symptoms of hypo-

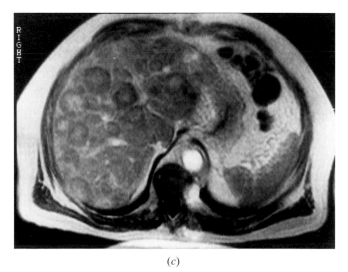

(*c*)

FIG. 4.28 Liver metastases from gastrinomas. Dynamic contrast-enhanced CT (*a*), immediate (*b*), and 10-minute (*c*) postgadolinium SGE images. Metastases are poorly visualized on the CT image (*a*). On the immediate postgadolinium SGE image (*b*) multiple metastases of similar size are identified with uniform intense rim enhancement. Peripheral washout is well-shown on the 10-minute postcontrast image (*c*).

glycemia. Insulinomas are usually very vascular. Angiography has been reported as superior to CT imaging in detecting these tumors due to their small size and increased vascularity [43].

Insulinomas are low in signal intensity on T1-weighted images and high in signal intensity on T2-weighted images. Insulinomas are well-shown on T1-weighted fat-suppressed images (Fig. 4.29) [36]. Small insulinomas typically enhance homogeneously on immediate postgadolinium SGE images (Fig. 4.30) [37]. Larger tumors, which measure more than 2 cm in diameter, often show ring enhancement. Liver metastases from insulinomas typically have peripheral ring-like enhancement, although small metastases tend to enhance homogeneously. Enhancement of small metastases frequently

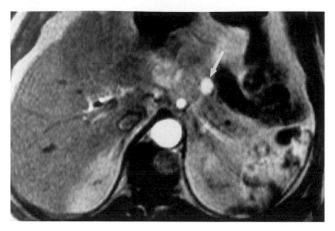

F I G. 4.30 Insulinoma. Immediate postgadolinium SGE image demonstrates a 1.2-cm uniformly enhancing insulinoma (*arrow*) arising from the body of the pancreas.

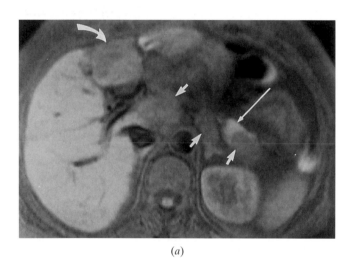

(*a*)

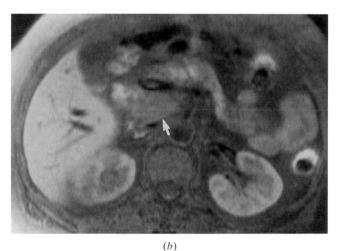

(*b*)

F I G. 4.29 Multiple malignant insulinomas. T1-weighted fat-suppressed spin-echo images from cranial (*a*) and more caudal (*b*) locations. Multiple low-signal-intensity insulinomas (*arrows, a,b*) ranging in diameter from 1 to 5 cm are present throughout the pancreas. Intervening pancreatic tissue is noted to be normal in signal intensity (*long arrow, a*). Liver metastases are also present (*curved arrow, a*).

occurs transiently in the capillary phase of enhancement and fades on images acquired at 1 minute after injection.

Glucagonoma, Somatostatinoma, VIPoma, and ACTHoma

These islet-cell tumors are considerably rarer than insulinomas or gastrinomas. They are almost always malignant, with liver metastases present at the time of diagnosis [33,38,39,44–47]. Tumors are large and heterogeneous on MR images [44–47]. They are usually low in signal intensity on T1-weighted fat-suppressed images and high in signal intensity on T2-weighted fat-suppressed images, enhancing heterogeneously on postgadolinium images (Fig. 4.31) [38]. Liver metastases are generally heterogeneous in size and shape, unlike gastrinoma metastases, which are typically more uniform (Fig. 4.32) [37]. Metastases possess irregular peripheral rims of intense enhancement on immediate postgadolinium SGE images (Fig. 4.33). Peripheral spoke-wheel enhancement may be observed in liver metastases on immediate postgadolinium images (see Fig. 4.31). Hypervascular liver metastases are best shown on immediate postgadolinium SGE images, which are superior to spiral CT images for this determination [38]. Splenic metastases are not uncommon (see Fig. 4.32).

Microcystic Adenoma

Microcystic adenoma is a benign serous fluid-containing neoplasm characterized by multiple tiny cysts [48]. This tumor frequently occurs in older patients and has an increased association with von Hippel-Lindau disease [16,48]. The tumor occasionally contains a central scar. Tumors range in size from 1 to 12 cm with an average diameter at presentation of 5 cm. The lesion has either a smooth or nodular contour. On MR images the tumors are well-defined and do not demonstrate invasion of fat

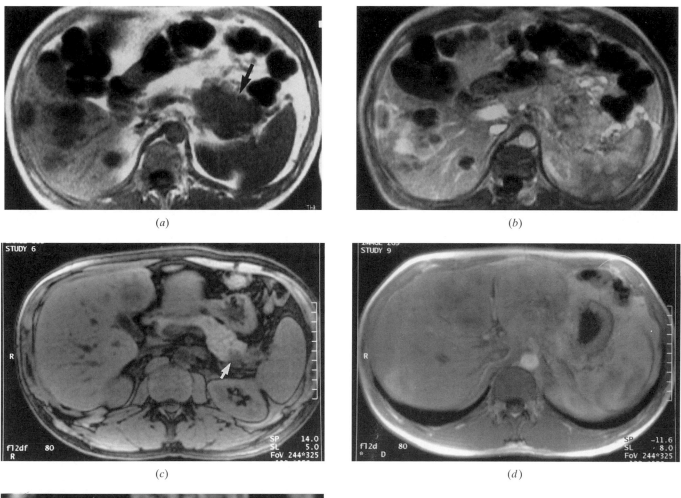

(a)

(b)

(c)

(d)

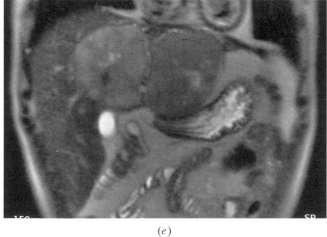

(e)

FIG. 4.31 Glucagonoma. SGE (*a*) and immediate postgadolinium SGE (*b*) images. A 6-cm tumor (*arrow, a*) arises from the tail of the pancreas (*a*). Multiple liver metastases are present that are low in signal intensity on the precontrast T1-weighted image (*a*). On the immediate postgadolinium SGE image (*b*), the primary tumor enhances heterogeneously. Intense ring enhancement is present in many of the liver metastases reflecting hypervascularity. Fat-suppressed SGE (*c*), coronal HASTE (*d*), and immediate postgadolinium SGE (*e*) images in a patient with VIPoma. A 2-cm tumor arises from the tail of the pancreas (*arrow, c*) that appears low in signal intensity on the T1-weighted image. Multiple metastases are present that are moderately low-signal intensity on the T1-weighted image (*c*), moderately high-signal intensity on the T2-weighted image (*d*), and enhance in a moderately intense peripheral spoke-wheel type radial fashion on the immediate postgadolinium SGE image (*e*).

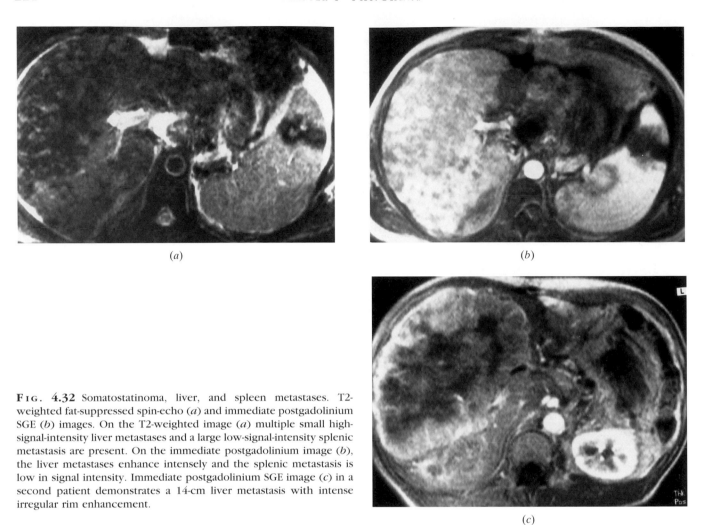

F IG. 4.32 Somatostatinoma, liver, and spleen metastases. T2-weighted fat-suppressed spin-echo (*a*) and immediate postgadolinium SGE (*b*) images. On the T2-weighted image (*a*) multiple small high-signal-intensity liver metastases and a large low-signal-intensity splenic metastasis are present. On the immediate postgadolinium image (*b*), the liver metastases enhance intensely and the splenic metastasis is low in signal intensity. Immediate postgadolinium SGE image (*c*) in a second patient demonstrates a 14-cm liver metastasis with intense irregular rim enhancement.

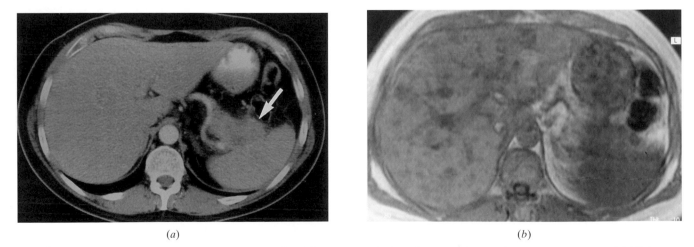

F IG. 4.33 ACTHoma. Spiral CT (*a*), SGE (*b*), T2-weighted fat-suppressed spin-echo (*c*), and immediate postgadolinium SGE (*d*) images. A 4-cm ACTHoma is present in the tail of the pancreas, which is shown on all images (*arrow, a*). Direct extension of the primary tumor into the spleen is most clearly shown on the immediate postgadolinium SGE image (*arrows, d*).

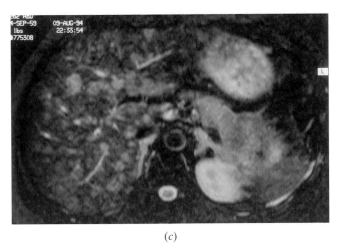

(c)

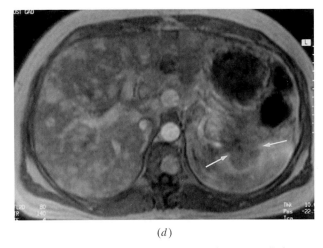

(d)

FIG. 4.33 (*Continued*) Multiple liver metastases are present, which are poorly seen on the spiral CT image (*a*), but are well-shown on the MR images (*b-d*). Liver metastases are most conspicuous on the immediate postgadolinium SGE image (*d*). (Reproduced with permission from Kelekis NL, Semelka RC, Molina PL, Doerr ME: ACTH-secreting islet cell tumor: Appearances on dynamic gadolinium-enhanced MRI. Magn Reson Imaging 13:641–644, 1995)

or adjacent organs [49]. On T2-weighted images the small cysts and intervening septations may be well-shown as a cluster of small grape-like high-signal-intensity cysts. This appearance is more clearly shown on breath-hold or breathing independent sequences such as HASTE, because the thin septations blur during a longer duration nonbreath-hold sequence (Fig. 4.34). Cystic pancreatic masses that contain cysts measuring less than 1 cm in diameter most likely represent microcystic adenomas. Cysts that measure between 1 and 2 cm in diameter may be observed in either microcystic or macrocystic adenoma, and cysts larger than 2 cm are observed for macrocystic adenoma/adenocarcinoma. Uncommonly serous neoplasms may have cysts larger than 2 cm in diameter [49]. Relatively thin uniform septations and ab-

sence of invasion of adjacent organs are features that distinguish this benign tumor from macrocystic tumors (Fig. 4.35). Tumor septations usually enhance minimally with gadolinium on early or late postcontrast images, although moderate enhancement or early postcontrast images may occur. Delayed enhancement of the central scar may occasionally be observed [1].

Macrocystic Adenoma/Adenocarcinoma

Macrocystic adenoma/adenocarcinoma are mucin-containing tumors that are malignant or have malignant potential [48–51]. These tumors occur more frequently in females (6 to 1), and approximately 50 percent occur in patients between the ages of 40 and 60 years [52]. These tumors usually are located in the body and tail of the

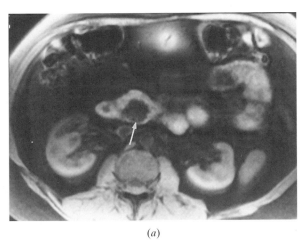

(a)

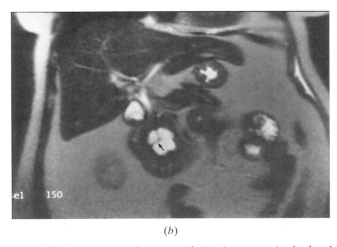

(b)

FIG. 4.34 Microcystic adenoma. T1-weighted fat-suppressed SGE (*a*) and HASTE (*b*) images. A 3-cm mass lesion is present in the head of the pancreas. The lesion is well-defined and low in signal intensity (*arrow, a*) in a background of high-signal-intensity pancreas on the T1-weighted fat-suppressed SGE image (*a*). On the breathing-independent T2-weighted image (*b*), definition of fine septations (*small arrow, b*) within the cystic mass show that the cysts are microcysts measuring less than 1 cm in diameter.

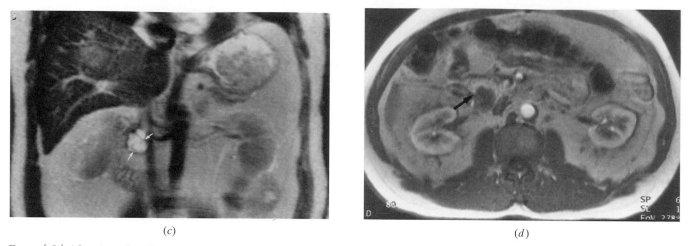

(c)   (d)

FIG. 4.34 (*Continued*)   The microcystic adenoma is high in signal intensity on the T2-weighted image due to the high fluid content. HASTE (*c*) and immediate postgadolinium SGE (*d*) images in a second patient demonstrate a 3-cm microcystic cystadenoma in the head of the pancreas. Fine septations are apparent on the HASTE image (*arrows, c*), and the tumor is sharply demarcated from normal enhancing pancreas on the immediate postgadolinium image (*arrow, d*).

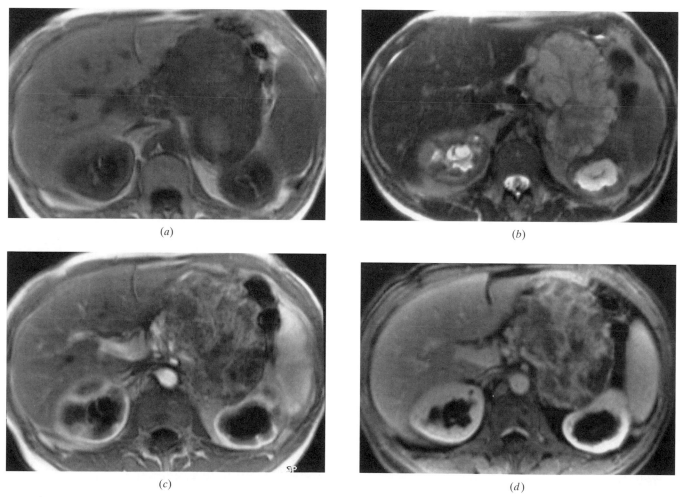

(a)   (b)

(c)   (d)

FIG. 4.35 Serous cystadenoma with macrocysts. SGE (*a*), HASTE (*b*), immediate postgadolinium SGE (*c*), and 90-second postgadolinium fat-suppressed SGE (*d*) images. A 10-cm mass arises from the tail of the pancreas. The tumor is mildly hypointense with regions of hyperintensity on precontrast T1-weighted images (*a*). Multiple septations are present throughout the mass, well shown on the breathing independent T2-weighted image (*b*). Some of the cysts measure >2 cm. Moderately intense enhancement of the septations is present on immediate (*c*) and 90-second (*d*) postcontrast images.

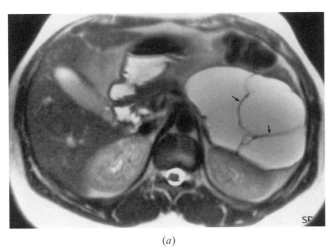
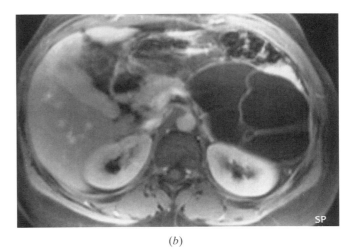

(a)   (b)

FIG. 4.36 Macrocystic adenoma. HASTE (*a*) and 90-second postgadolinium fat-suppressed SGE (*b*) images. A well-defined cystic mass arises from the body and tail of the pancreas that is low in signal intensity on the T1-weighted image (not shown) and high in signal intensity on the T2-weighted image (*a*), and that demonstrates enhancement of septations on the postgadolinium SGE image (*b*). No evidence of tumor nodules, invasion of adjacent tissue, or liver metastases is appreciated. The uniform thickness of the septations is clearly defined on the breathing-independent HASTE image (*arrows, a*). Cystic spaces are irregular in shape and measure larger than 2 cm in diameter, which is consistent with a macrocystic adenoma.

pancreas. They are large (mean diameter of 10 cm), multiloculated, and encapsulated [50,51]. There is a great propensity for invasion of local organs and tissues.

On gadolinium-enhanced T1-weighted fat-suppressed images, large, irregular cystic spaces separated by thick septa are demonstrated [1]. Macrocystic adenomas are well-defined and show no evidence of metastases or invasion of adjacent tissues (Fig. 4.36). Low-grade malignant tumors may be very large, but may not show evidence of metastases or local invasion (Fig. 4.36). Macrocystic adenocarcinoma may be very locally aggressive malignancies with extensive invasion of adjacent tissues and organs (Fig. 4.37). Absence of demonstration of tumor invasion into surrounding tissue does not, however, exclude malignancy. The higher inherent soft-tissue contrast of MRI compared to CT imaging results in superior differentiation between microcystic and macrocystic adenomas because of sharp definition of cysts that permits evaluation of cyst size and margins [50]. Macrocysts within these tumor are generally larger than 2 cm in diameter and irregular in shape. Breath-hold T2-weighted images are particularly effective at defining the cysts.

Mucin produced by these tumors may result in high signal intensity on T1- and T2-weighted images of the primary tumor and liver metastases. Liver metastases are generally hypervascular and have intense ring enhancement on immediate gadolinium images. Metastases are commonly cystic and may contain mucin, which results in mixed low and high signal intensity on T1- and T2-weighted images (Fig. 4.38).

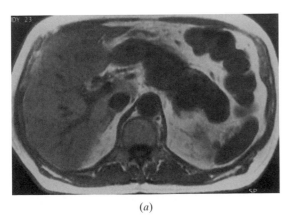
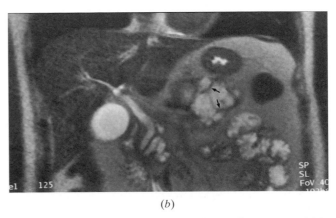

(a)   (b)

FIG. 4.37 Macrocystic adenoma with carcinoma in situ. SGE (*a*), coronal HASTE (*b*), and 90-second postgadolinium fat-suppressed SGE (*c*) images. A multicystic mass involves the entire body and tail of the pancreas (*a–c*). Septations are well-defined on the breathing-independent T2-weighted image (*arrows, b*).

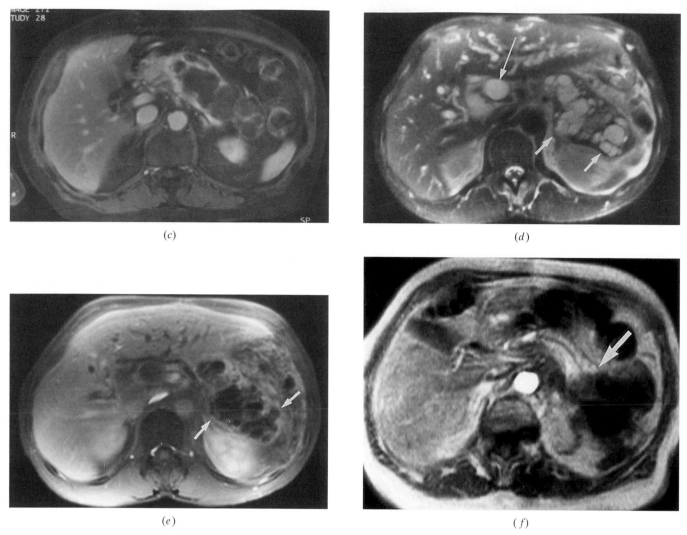

(c)

(d)

(e)

(f)

Fig. 4.37 (*Continued*)   The slight irregularity of the septations and the extent of tumor are features compatible with malignant changes. HASTE (*d*) and 90-second postgadolinium fat-suppressed SGE (*e*) in a second patient demonstrate a macrocystic adenocarcinoma in the body and tail (*arrows, d,e*). Dilatation of the CBD (*long arrow, d*) and intrahepatic biliary tree are also present. Macrocystic adenocarcinoma. Immediate postgadolinium SGE image (*f*) in a third patient demonstrates a tumor arising from the tail of the pancreas (*arrow*) that contains thick septations and multiple large cysts. The tumor is locally aggressive and invades into the splenic hilum (not shown).

Solid and Papillary Epithelial Neoplasm

These rare tumors have low-grade malignant potential, and occur most frequently in females between 20 and 30 years of age [53]. A previous report describing the MRI appearance of solid and papillary epithelial neoplasms found that all tumors were well-demarcated lesions that contained central high signal intensity on T1-weighted images [53]. This central high signal intensity represented hemorrhagic necrosis. The presence of overt hemorrhage may be related to tumor size because smaller tumors may appear heterogeneous but not overtly hemorrhagic (Fig. 4.39)

Lymphoma

Non-Hodgkin's lymphoma may involve peripancreatic lymph nodes or may directly invade the pancreas [54]. Intermediate-signal-intensity peripancreatic lymph nodes are distinguished from high-signal-intensity-pancreas on T1-weighted fat-suppressed images. Invasion of the pancreas is shown by loss of the normal high signal

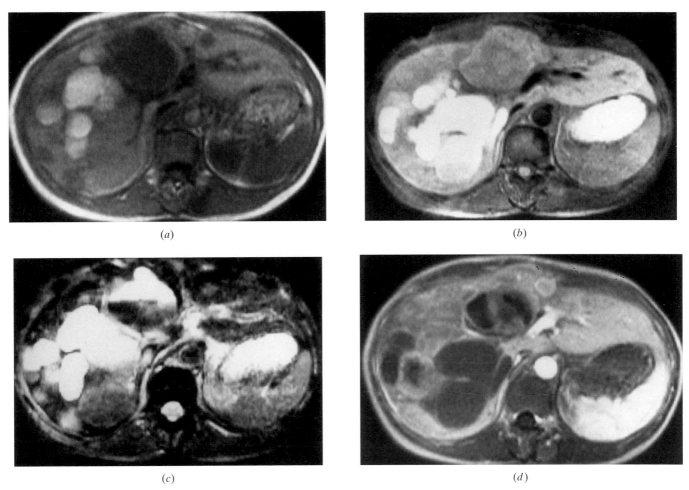

                    (a)   (b)

                    (c)   (d)

F IG . 4.38 Macrocystic adenocarcinoma liver metastases. SGE (a), T1-weighted fat-suppressed spin-echo (b), T2-weighted fat-suppressed spin-echo (c) and immediate postgadolinium SGE (d) images. Multiple metastases are present throughout the liver that are mixed in low and high signal intensities on T1-weighted (a,b) and T2-weighted (c) images. This appearance is consistent with the presence of mucin in these tumors. On the immediate postgadolinium image (d), enhancement of the walls of the cysts is appreciated.

intensity of the pancreas on T1-weighted fat-suppressed images (Fig. 4.40).

Metastases

Metastases may involve peripancreatic lymph nodes or invade the pancreas. Primary malignancies include gastrointestinal, kidney, breast, lung, prostate, and melanoma. A recent report described the MRI appearance of renal cancer metastases to the pancreas. Diffuse micronodular, multifocal, and solitary metastatic deposits were described [55]. Metastases were low in signal intensity on T1-weighted images and high in signal intensity on T2-weighted images. Small metastases (<1 cm in diameter)

enhanced uniformly on immediate postgadolinium SGE images, and larger metastases enhanced in a ring fashion (Fig. 4.41). This appearance is analogous to the appearance of hypervascular metastases to the liver and reflects the pathophysiology of parasitization of host blood supply by metastatic disease. Renal cancer metastases resemble the appearance of islet-cell tumors. Clinical history of renal cancer, even if remote, is essential to obtain in order to establish the correct diagnosis.

Melanoma metastases may be high in signal intensity on T1-weighted images due to the paramagnetic properties of melanin (Fig. 4.42) [1]. Metastatic deposits tend to be focal, well-defined masses.

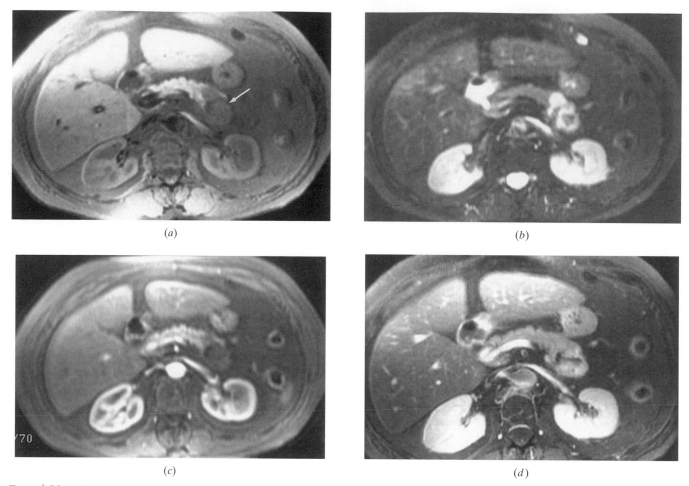

(a)   (b)

(c)   (d)

FIG. 4.39 Solid and papillary epithelial neoplasm. Fat-suppressed SGE (*a*), T2-weighted fat-suppressed spin-echo (*b*), immediate postgadolinium SGE (*c*), and interstitial-phase gadolinium-enhanced T1-weighted fat-suppressed spin-echo (*d*) images. A 4-cm tumor mass arises from the tail of the pancreas that is low in signal intensity on the T1-weighted image (*arrow, a*), heterogeneous on the T2-weighted image (*b*), enhances negligibly on the immediate postgadolinium SGE image (*c*), and shows heterogeneous enhancement on the interstitial-phase image (*d*).

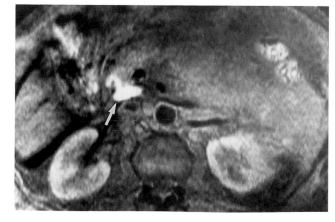

FIG. 4.40 Lymphoma. T1-weighted fat-suppressed spin-echo image demonstrates replacement of the majority of the pancreas with intermediate-signal ill-defined lymphomatous tissue. The ventral portion of the pancreatic head is spared (*arrow*). (Reproduced with permission from Semelka RC, Shoenut JP, Kroeker MA, Micflikier AB. The Pancreas. In: Semelka RC, Shoenut JP. MRI of the abdomen with CT correlation. Raven Press. New York NY, p. 59–76, 1993.)

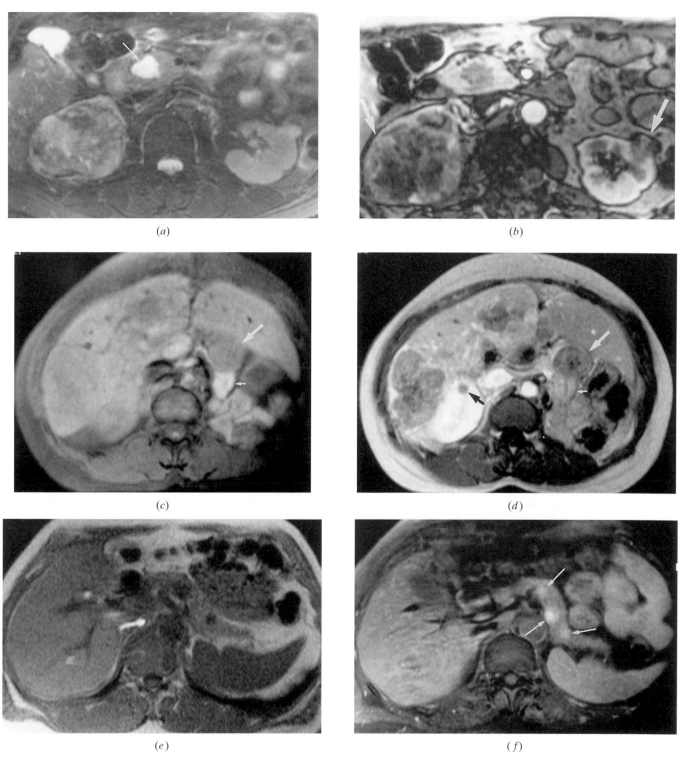

(a)

(b)

(c)

(d)

(e)

(f)

FIG. 4.41 Pancreatic metastases from renal cancer. T2-weighted fat-suppressed echo-train spin-echo (a) and immediate postgadolinium SGE (b) images demonstrate a solitary metastasis in the head of the pancreas. This lesion is high in signal intensity on the T2-weighted image (arrow, a) and demonstrates predominantly peripheral enhancement on the immediate postgadolinium image (b). Bilateral renal cell cancers are also identified (large arrows, b). T1-weighted fat-suppressed spin-echo (c) and immediate postgadolinium SGE (d) images in a second patient demonstrate a 3-cm mass in the distal body of the pancreas (arrow, c,d). The uninvolved tail of the pancreas has a normal high signal intensity (small arrow, c,d). Multiple liver metastases are present that demonstrate predominant rim enhancement on the immediate postgadolinium image (d). Multiple renal cancers are present (black arrow, d). SGE (e) and gadolinium-enhanced T1-weighted fat-suppressed spin-echo (f) images of the body of the pancreas, and immediate postgadolinium SGE image (g) of the head of the pancreas in a third patient.

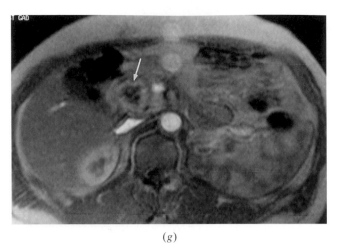

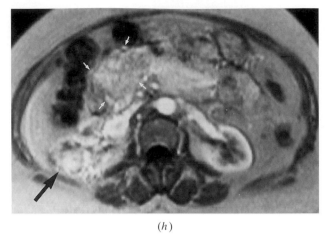

(g)   (h)

FIG. **4.41** (*Continued*) Three metastases are present in the body of the pancreas (*arrows, f*) that are low in signal intensity on the precontrast SGE image (*e*) and enhance uniformly and with moderate intensity on the interstitial-phase gadolinium-enhanced image (*f*). A larger 3-cm metastasis is present in the head of the pancreas that demonstrates rim enhancement (*arrow, g*). An immediate postgadolinium SGE image (*h*) in a fourth patient demonstrates multiple micronodular metastases to the pancreas smaller than 5 mm, which enhance uniformly and intensely on the immediate postgadolinium image (*small arrows, h*). The renal cancer is also shown (*arrow, h*). (Reproduced with permission from [55])

INFLAMMATORY DISEASE

Pancreatitis

Pancreatitis occurs secondary to chronic alcoholism, gallstones, hypercalcemia, hyperlipoproteinemia, blunt abdominal trauma, penetrating peptic ulcer disease, viral infections (most frequently Epstein-Barr), and certain drugs [56]. Predisposition may also be inherited as an autosomal dominant trait [57].

    Acute Pancreatitis. Acute pancreatitis arises in the majority of cases from excessive alcohol intake or gall-

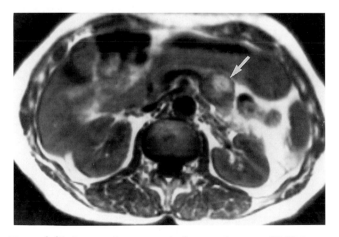

FIG. **4.42** Pancreatic metastasis from melanoma. T1-SE image demonstrates a high-signal-intensity mass in the tail of the pancreas (*arrow*). The high signal intensity of the mass is due to the paramagnetic effect of melanin. (Reproduced with permission from [1])

stone disease [56]. Alcohol-related acute pancreatitis most frequently results in acute recurrent pancreatitis, whereas gallstone-related pancreatitis typically results in a single attack. The passage of biliary sludge may also cause acute pancreatitis [58]. At least 95 percent of patients with acute pancreatitis experience severe midepigastric pain that radiates to the back. Nausea and vomiting occur in 75 to 85 percent of patients, and fever occurs in approximately 50 percent.

    Acute pancreatitis results from the exudation of fluid containing activated proteolytic enzymes into the interstitium of the pancreas and leakage of this fluid into surrounding tissue. Trypsin is suspected to be the primary enzyme involved in the coagulative necrosis.

    The signal-intensity features of the pancreas in uncomplicated mild acute pancreatitis resemble those of normal pancreatic tissue. The pancreas is high in signal intensity on precontrast T1-weighted fat-suppressed images and enhances in a normal uniform fashion on immediate postgadolinium images reflecting a normal capillary blush (Fig. 4.43). The diagnosis of acute pancreatitis on MR images relies on the presence of morphological changes [1]. Morphologically, the pancreas shows either focal or diffuse enlargement, which may be subtle. Peripancreatic fluid is well-shown on noncontrast or immediate postgadolinium SGE images and appears as low signal-intensity strands of fluid or fluid collections in a background of high-signal-intensity fat. MRI is sensitive for the detection of subtle changes of acute pancreatitis, particularly minor peripancreatic inflammatory changes. CT imaging examinations appear normal in 15 to 30 percent of patients with clinical acute pancreatitis [59]. The sensitivity of MRI may exceed that of CT imaging, sug-

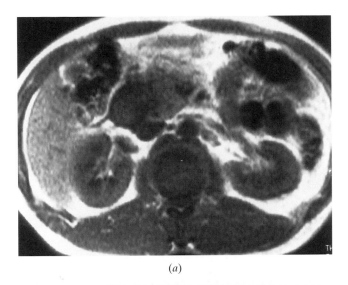

(a)

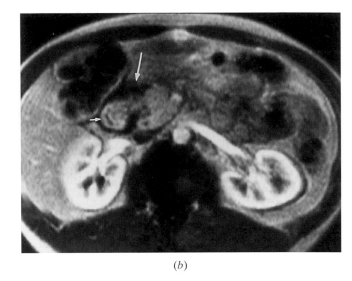

(b)

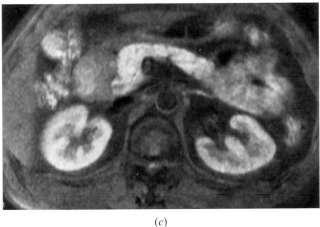

(c)

F IG . 4.43 Mild acute pancreatitis. SGE (a) and immediate postgadolinium SGE (b) images of the head of the pancreas, and a T1-weighted
fat-suppressed spin-echo image (c) of the body of the pancreas. On
the precontrast T1-weighted image (a), ill-defined low-signal-intensity
reticular strands surround a slightly enlarged pancreatic head, a finding
consistent with peripancreatic fluid. On the immediate postgadolinium
image (b), signal-void fluid (arrow, b) surrounds the head of the pancreas and duodenum (small arrow, b). The body of the pancreas is
normal and high in signal intensity on the T1-weighted fat-suppressed
image (c), reflecting a normal content of aqueous protein in the pancreatic acini consistent with mild pancreatitis. (Reproduced with permission from Semelka RC, Shoenut JP, Kroeker MA, Micflikier AB: The
Pancreas. In: Semelka RC, Shoenut JP. MRI of the abdomen with CT
correlation. Raven Press. New York NY, p. 59–76, 1993.)

gesting a role for MRI in the evaluation of patients with
suspected acute pancreatitis and negative CT imaging
examination. As the extent of pancreatitis becomes more
severe, the pancreas develops a heterogeneous appearance on precontrast T1-weighted fat-suppressed images
and enhances in a more heterogeneous, diminished fashion on immediate postgadolinium images (Fig. 4.44).

Percentage of pancreatic necrosis has been considered an important prognostic indicator in patients with
acute pancreatitis [60,61]. Dynamic gadolinium-enhanced
SGE images may be useful for this determination because
MRI is very sensitive for the demonstration of the presence or absence of gadolinium enhancement. Saifuddin
et al. [62] described comparable results for dynamic contrast-enhanced CT images and immediate postgadolinium SGE images for determining the presence of pancreatic necrosis. Complications of acute pancreatitis such as
hemorrhage, pseudocyst formation, or abscess are well-
examined by MRI. Hemorrhagic fluid collections are high
in signal intensity on T1-weighted fat-suppressed images,
and depiction of hemorrhage is superior on MR images

compared to CT images (Fig. 4.45). Simple pseudocysts
are low in signal intensity or signal-void in a background
of normal-signal-intensity pancreatic tissue on both SGE
and T1-weighted fat-suppressed images (Fig. 4.46). Extrapancreatic pseudocysts are well-shown on breath-hold
SGE images due to high contrast with high-signal-intensity fat. Image acquisition in multiple planes permits determination of pseudocyst location in relation to various
organs and structures (Fig. 4.47). Simple pseudocysts are
relatively homogeneous and high in signal intensity on
T2-weighted images. Pseudocysts complicated by necrotic debris, hemorrhage, or infection are heterogeneous
in signal intensity on T2-weighted images [62]. Proteinaceous fluid tends to layer in a gradation of concentration
with low-signal-intensity concentrated proteinaceous
material in the dependent portion of the cyst. Necrotic
material may appear as irregularly shaped regions of low
signal intensity in the pseudocyst. This information may
provide both therapeutic and prognostic information because pseudocysts that contain necrotic material may not
respond to simple percutaneous drainage and thus re-

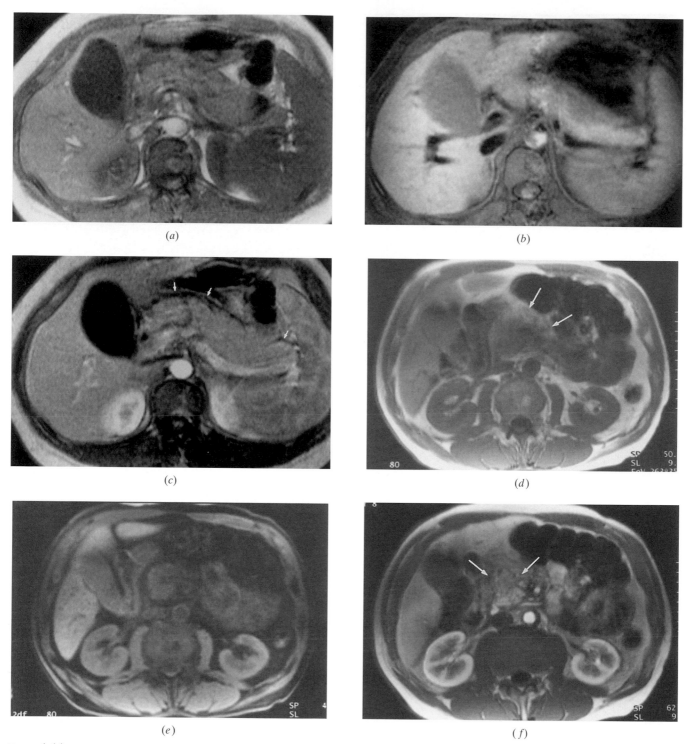

(a)   *(b)*

(c)   *(d)*

(e)   *(f)*

F IG. 4.44 Moderately severe acute pancreatitis. SGE (*a*), T1-weighted fat-suppressed spin-echo (*b*), and immediate postgadolinium SGE (*c*) images. The pancreas is diffusely enlarged (*a–c*). The signal intensity of the pancreas is heterogeneous on the T1-weighted fat-suppressed image (*b*), which suggests a decrease in the proteinaceous fluid content within the acini of the pancreas. Signal-void fluid is shown surrounding the body and tail of the pancreas on the immediate postgadolinium image (*arrows, c*). The intensity of pancreatic enhancement is less than normal for pancreas on the capillary-phase image (*c*). SGE (*d*), T1-weighted fat-suppressed SGE (*e*), and immediate postgadolinium SGE (*f*) images in a second patient. Peripancreatic fluid is well-shown as low-signal-intensity stranding in the high-signal-intensity fat on the SGE image (*arrows, d*). The anterior portion of the head of the pancreas is lower in signal intensity on the precontrast fat-suppressed image (*e*) and enhances less (*arrows, f*) on immediate postgadolinium images (*f*), reflecting more severe changes of pancreatitis. Relative sparing of either anterior or posterior portions of the head of the pancreas is not uncommon due to separate pancreatic ductal systems. Despite the focal nature of the diminished enhancement of the dorsal head of the pancreas, there is lobular architecture similar to that of the ventral pancreatic head. A pancreatic neoplasm would not exhibit lobular architecture.

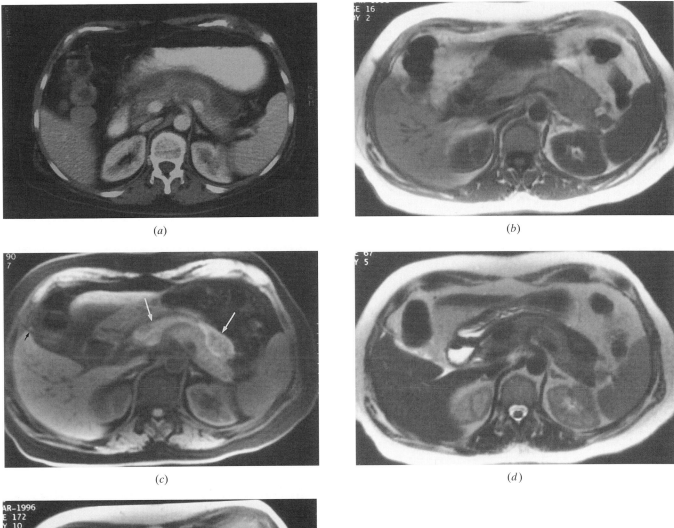

(a)

(b)

(c)

(d)

(e)

FIG. 4.45 Hemorrhagic pancreatitis. Contrast-enhanced spiral CT (a), SGE (b), fat-suppressed SGE (c), HASTE (d), and immediate postgadolinium SGE (e). The CT image demonstrates an enlarged pancreas with free fluid along its anterior margin, findings consistent with acute pancreatitis. On the SGE image (b), the fluid collections are noted to be hyperintense, which is accentuated on the fat-suppressed image (arrows, c). The fluid is low in signal on the T2-weighted image (d), and therefore possesses the signal characteristics of intracellular methemoglobin in acute blood. The pancreas enhances relatively uniformly on the immediate postgadolinium image, reflecting the absence of pancreatic necrosis (e). A collapsed acutely inflamed gallbladder (arrow, e) is present, in which a cholecystostomy catheter was placed (small arrow, c,e).

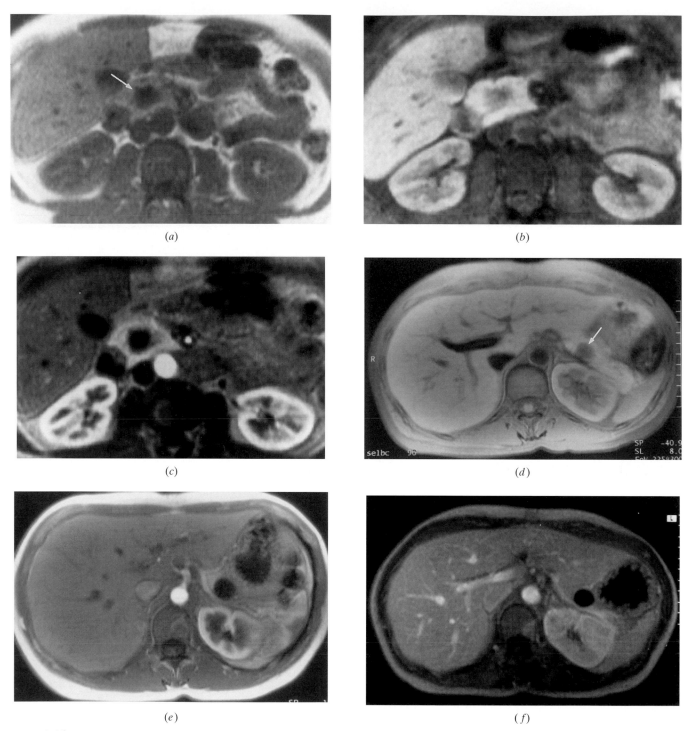

(a)

(b)

(c)

(d)

(e)

(f)

F I G . 4.46 Pseudocyst in acute pancreatitis. SGE (*a*), T1-weighted fat-suppressed spin-echo (*b*), and immediate postgadolinium SGE (*c*) images. A low-signal-intensity pseudocyst is present in the head of the pancreas (*arrow, a*) (*a–c*). The pancreas has a normal high signal intensity on the T1-weighted fat-suppressed image (*b*), and there is normal uniform enhancement of the pancreas on the immediate postgadolinium image (*c*). These imaging features are consistent with a pseudocyst in the setting of acute pancreatitis because the background pancreas has normal signal intensity features. The lesion did not change in size and shape on delayed images excluding a poorly vascularized tumor. T1-weighted fat-suppressed SGE (*d*), immediate (*e*), and 90-second (*f*) postgadolinium SGE images in a second patient.

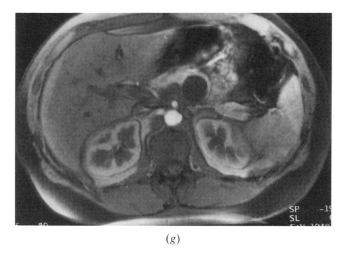

(g)

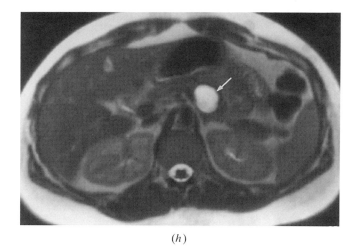

(h)

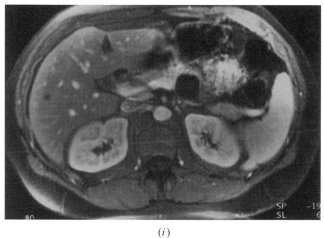

(i)

FIG. 4.46 (Continued) A low-signal-intensity lesion is present in the tail of the pancreas (arrow, d) with normal signal intensity surrounding the pancreas on the T1-weighted fat-suppressed image. The lesion is signal-void on early (e) and late (f) postgadolinium images, which is consistent with a pseudocyst. Fat-suppressed SGE (g), HASTE (h), and immediate postgadolinium fat-suppressed SGE (i) images in a third patient with a simple pseudocyst. A 3.5-cm sharply marginated pseudocyst is present in the body of the pancreas that is signal-void in a background of high-signal-intensity pancreas on fat-suppressed SGE (g) and uniformly high in signal intensity on the T2-weighted image (arrow, h), and that does not enhance and remains sharply defined on the immediate postgadolinium image (i).

quire open debridement. Breathing independent T2-weighted sequences such as HASTE may be of particular value in evaluating these pseudocyst collections as many patients are very debilitated and unable to cooperate with breath-holding instructions.

Chronic Pancreatitis. Chronic pancreatitis is acquired either as a disease process distinct from acute pancreatitis or as a complication of repeated attacks of acute pancreatitis. There is a strong association between alcoholism and development of chronic pancreatitis [63,64]. Obstruction of the pancreatic duct from various causes, including pancreatic ductal cancer, results in chronic pancreatitis [64]. Acute pancreatitis secondary to gallstone disease rarely results in chronic pancreatitis. Chronic pancreatitis is associated with decreased endocrine as well as exocrine function [63,64]. Patients with chronic pancreatitis have an increased risk of developing pancreatic cancer [65].

An analysis of patients with chronic pancreatitis imaged on current generation contrast-enhanced CT images showed the following features: 66 percent had dilation of the main pancreatic duct, 54 percent had parenchymal atrophy, 50 percent had pancreatic calcifications, 34 percent had pseudocysts, 32 percent had focal pancreatic enlargement, 29 percent had biliary ductal dilatation, and 16 percent had densities in peripancreatic fat or fascia. No abnormalities were present in 7 percent of patients [66]. Calcification, which is the pathognomonic feature of chronic pancreatitis on CT images, is a late phenomenon following development of fibrosis and is observed in only half of these patients. CT imaging, therefore, is not sensitive for detecting early changes of chronic pancreatitis. Focal chronic pancreatitis may be difficult to distinguish from adenocarcinoma in the head of the pancreas because both entities may cause focal enlargement, obstruction of the common bile duct and pancreatic duct, atrophy of the tail of the pancreas, and obliteration of the fat plane around the superior mesenteric artery (SMA) [67–68].

MRI may perform better than CT imaging at detecting changes of chronic pancreatitis in that MRI detects not only morphological findings, but also the presence of fibrosis. Because fibrosis is a precursor to the develop-

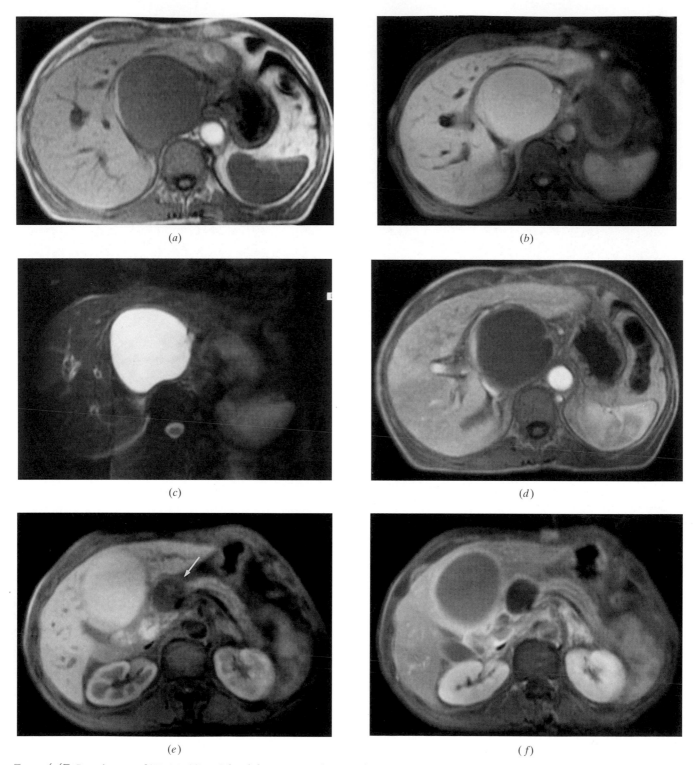

FIG. 4.47 Pseudocysts. SGE (*a*), T1-weighted fat-suppressed spin-echo (*b*), T2-weighted fat-suppressed echo-train spin-echo (*c*), and immediate postgadolinium SGE (*d*) images obtained superior to the pancreas, T1-weighted fat-suppressed spin-echo (*e*) and gadolinium-enhanced T1-weighted fat-suppressed spin-echo (*f*) images at the level of the body of the pancreas, coronal gadolinium-enhanced SGE images from midhepatic (*g*) and more anterior (*h*) locations, and sagittal-plane (*i*) SGE images. An 8-cm pseudocyst is present in the region of the porta hepatis that is mildly high in signal intensity on T1-weighted images (*a,b*) and high in signal intensity on the T2-weighted image (*b*). The mild, high signal intensity on T1-weighted images is more conspicuous with fat suppression (*b*) and consistent with dilute blood or protein. The homogeneous signal intensity on T2-weighted images suggests that the fluid, although proteinaceous, is not complicated by infection or cellular debris.

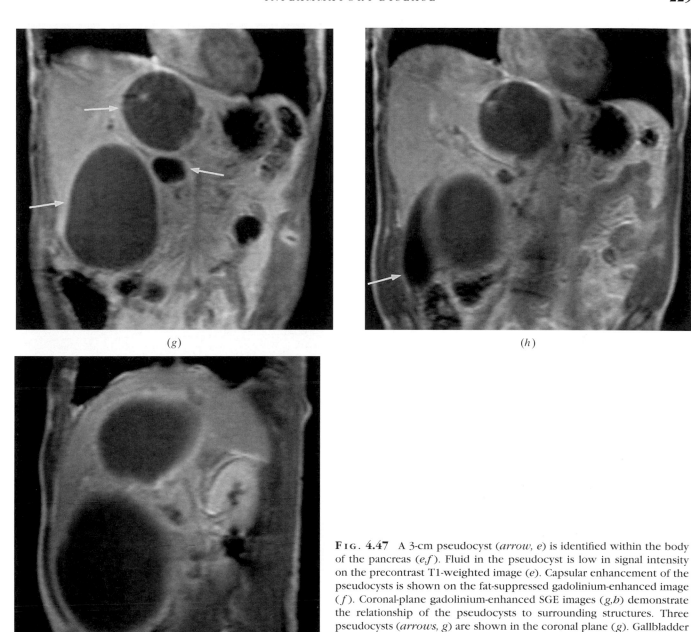

(g)

(h)

(i)

FIG. 4.47 A 3-cm pseudocyst (*arrow, e*) is identified within the body of the pancreas (*e,f*). Fluid in the pseudocyst is low in signal intensity on the precontrast T1-weighted image (*e*). Capsular enhancement of the pseudocysts is shown on the fat-suppressed gadolinium-enhanced image (*f*). Coronal-plane gadolinium-enhanced SGE images (*g,h*) demonstrate the relationship of the pseudocysts to surrounding structures. Three pseudocysts (*arrows, g*) are shown in the coronal plane (*g*). Gallbladder (*arrow, h*) is displaced laterally by the large pseudocyst in the porta hepatis. The sagittal plane image (*i*) demonstrates the anteroposterior orientation of the pseudocysts to other structures.

ment of calcification, MRI may be able to detect chronic pancreatitis at an earlier stage than CT imaging. Fibrosis is shown by a diminished signal intensity on T1-weighted fat-suppressed images and diminished heterogeneous enhancement on immediate postgadolinium SGE images [70]. Low signal intensity on T1-weighted fat-suppressed images reflects loss of the aqueous protein in the acini of the pancreas. Diminished enhancement on capillary-phase images reflects disruption of the normal capillary bed and replacement with less vascularized granulation tissue. A study that described MRI findings in 13 patients with chronic calcifying pancreatitis and 9 patients with acute recurrent pancreatitis demonstrated differences between these groups on T1-weighted fat-suppressed images and immediate postgadolinium SGE images. All patients with pancreatic calcifications on CT examination had a diminished-signal-intensity pancreas on T1-weighted fat-suppressed images and an abnormally low percentage of contrast enhancement on immediate postgadolinium SGE images (Fig. 4.48). Patients with acute recurrent pancreatitis had signal-intensity features of the pancreas comparable to those of normal pancreas.

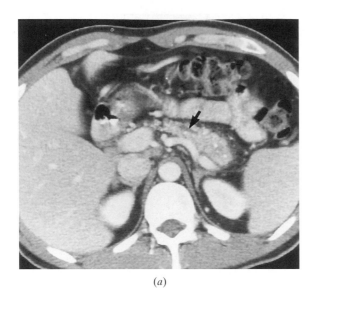

(a)

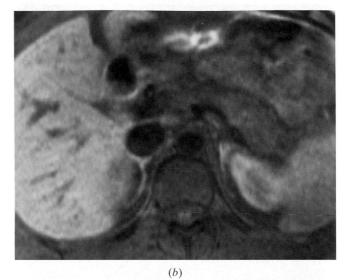

(b)

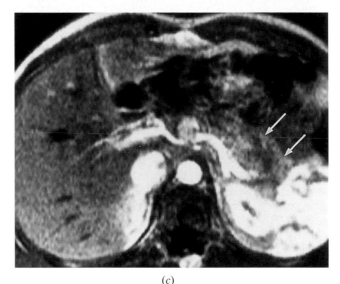

(c)

FIG. 4.48 Chronic pancreatitis. Contrast-enhanced CT (*a*) T1-weighted fat-suppressed spin-echo (*b*) and immediate postgadolinium SGE (*c*) images. The CT image demonstrates pancreatic calcifications, which is diagnostic for chronic pancreatitis. Mild pancreatic ductal dilatation (*arrow, a*) and mild pancreatic enlargement are also present. The pancreas is low in signal intensity on the T1-weighted fat-suppressed image, which is consistent with loss of aqueous protein in the acini. The immediate postgadolinium SGE image demonstrates heterogeneous diminished enhancement of the pancreas (*arrows, c*) reflecting replacement of the normal capillary bed with lesser vascularized fibrotic tissue. (Reproduced with permission from [4])

Focal enlargement of the head of the pancreas with chronic pancreatitis may be difficult to distinguish from cancer on CT images. On MR images these two entities may be distinguished. Both entities result in low signal intensity of the enlarged region of pancreas on noncontrast T1-weighted fat-suppressed and T2-weighted images. On immediate postgadolinium images, focal pancreatitis shows heterogeneous enhancement with the presence of signal-void cysts and calcifications and without evidence of a definable, minimally enhanced mass lesion. Demonstration of a definable, marginated mass lesion suggests the diagnosis of tumor. Diffuse low signal intensity of the entire pancreas, including the area of focal enlargement, on T1-weighted fat-suppressed and immediate postgadolinium SGE images is typical for chronic pancreatitis (Fig. 4.49). Pancreatic pseudocysts

occur with an incidence of 10 percent in patients with chronic pancreatitis [64]. Small pseudocysts and cysts are well-shown on gadolinium-enhanced T1-weighted fat-suppressed images as nearly signal-void oval structures (Fig. 4.50). Pseudocysts are generally high in signal intensity on T2-weighted images, but signal intensity varies considerably based on the presence of blood, protein, infection, and debris.

Necrotizing Granulomatous Pancreatitis. A variety of rare inflammatory conditions may affect the pancreas. Inflammatory diseases may appear as ill-defined focal masses that show irregular infiltration of pancreatic tissue (Fig. 4.51). Differentiation between malignant and inflammatory diseases may not, however, be reliably made on imaging studies.

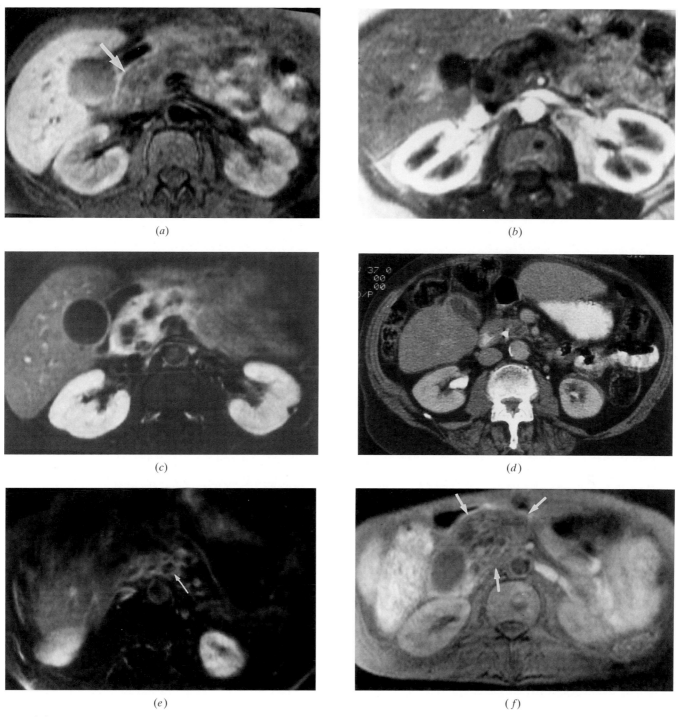

(a) (b)

(c) (d)

(e) (f)

F IG. 4.49 Chronic pancreatitis with focal enlargement of the head of the pancreas. T1-weighted fat-suppressed spin-echo (a), immediate postgadolinium SGE (b), and gadolinium-enhanced T1-weighted fat-suppressed spin-echo (c) images. The head of the pancreas is enlarged (*arrow, a*). The pancreas is diffusely low in signal intensity on the precontrast T1-weighted fat-suppressed image (a). The pancreas shows diffuse diminished enhancement on the immediate postgadolinium image (b). The lack of definition of a focal mass lesion on the immediate postgadolinium image is the most important observation that excludes tumor. On the interstitial-phase gadolinium-enhanced image (c), signal-void foci are identified that represent cysts, pseudocysts, dilated pancreatic duct and calcifications. Dynamic contrast-enhanced CT (d) and gadolinium-enhanced T1-weighted fat-suppressed spin-echo (e) images in a second patient. The head of the pancreas is enlarged on the CT image (d), and was considered to represent cancer.

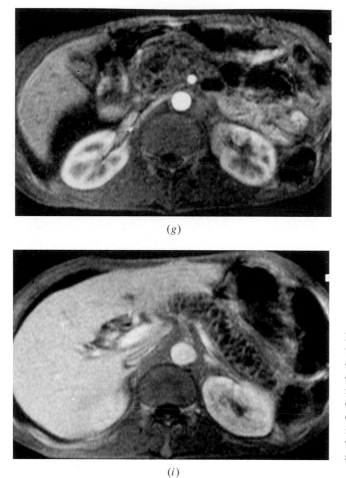

(g)

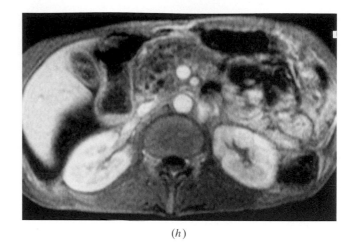

(h)

(i)

FIG. 4.49 (*Continued*)   On the MR images (*e*) multiple small signal-void cysts and pseudocysts (*arrow, e*) are shown with no demonstration of a poorly enhancing mass lesion. T1-weighted fat-suppressed spin-echo (*f*), immediate (*g*), and 90-second (*h*) postgadolinium SGE images in a third patient demonstrate enlargement of the pancreatic head (*arrow, f*). The head enhances in a diminished fashion on immediate (*g*) and 90-second (*h*) postgadolinium images with no definition of a mass lesion. Multiple small signal-void foci represent calcifications. The 90-second postgadolinium image (*i*) demonstrates that signal-void foci are also present throughout the body and tail.

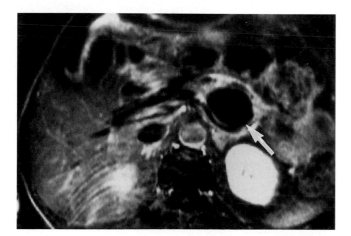

FIG. 4.50   Chronic pancreatitis with pseudocyst. Gadolinium-enlarged T1-weighted fat-suppressed spin-echo image demonstrates a large pseudocyst (*arrow*) arising from the body of the pancreas.

Trauma.   Traumatic injury of the pancreas may result in a spectrum of abnormalities from mild contusion to transection. Stenosis of the pancreatic duct with distal ductal dilatation may be observed as a sequela of trauma. A combination of tissue imaging sequences and MR pancreatography can facilitate this diagnosis by the demonstration of ductal dilatation and changes of chronic pancreatitis of the pancreas distal to the stenosis (Fig. 4.52).

Pancreatic Transplants

Dynamic gadolinium-enhanced MRI has been employed to assess rejection of pancreatic transplants [71,72]. Percentage of enhancement in six normal grafts was 98 + 23 percent within the first minute compared to 42 + 20 percent in six dysfunctional grafts [70]. MR angiography

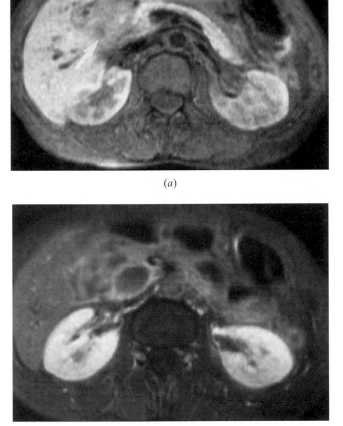

(a)

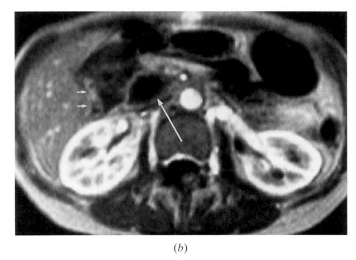

(b)

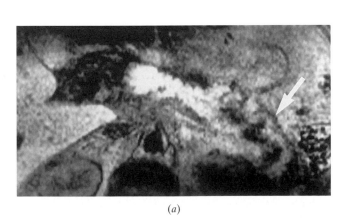

(c)

FIG. 4.51 Necrotizing granulomatous pancreatitis. T1-weighted fat-suppressed spin-echo (*a*), immediate postgadolinium SGE (*b*), and gadolinium-enhanced T1-weighted fat-suppressed spin-echo (*c*) images. A heterogeneous low-signal-intensity mass is present, arising from the lateral aspect of the head of the pancreas (*arrow, a*). The remainder of the pancreas is normal and moderately high in signal intensity on T1-weighted fat-suppressed spin-echo images (*a*). The lesion enhances in a heterogeneous minimal fashion on immediate postgadolinium SGE images (*b*). The duodenum (*small arrows, b*) is displaced laterally by the mass. The mass contains a cystic component (*thin arrow, b*). Heterogeneous enhancement of the mass is also present on the interstitial-phase gadolinium-enhanced T1-weighted fat-suppressed image (*c*).

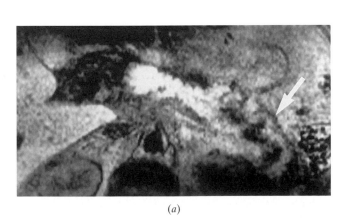

(a)

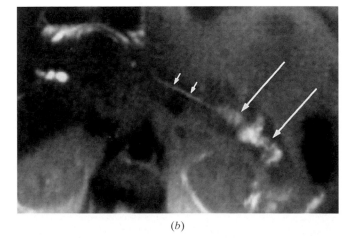

(b)

FIG. 4.52 Posttraumatic stenosis of the pancreatic duct. Fat-suppressed SGE (*a*), HASTE (*b*), immediate (*c*) and 90-second (*d*) postgadolinium fat-suppressed SGE images in a woman who had undergone abdominal trauma 6 years earlier. A transition is noted in the body of the pancreas between normal-appearing proximal pancreas and abnormal-appearing distal pancreas containing an irregularly dilated pancreatic duct.

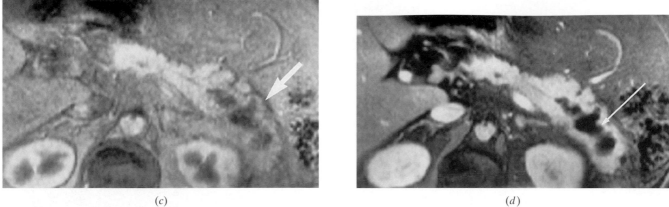

(c)   (d)

F I G . 4.52 (*Continued*) On the precontrast, fat-suppressed image (*a*) the distal pancreas (*arrow, a*) is noted to be low in signal intensity consistent with changes of chronic pancreatitis. On the HASTE image (*b*) a transition is well-shown between normal caliber pancreatic duct (*small arrows, b*) and abnormally expanded distal pancreatic duct (*long arrows, b*). The distal pancreas is noted to enhance minimally on the immediate postgadolinium image (*arrow, c*). Enhancement of the pancreas is more uniform on the interstitial phase image (*d*), with clear definition of the irregularly dilated pancreatic duct (*long arrow, e*).

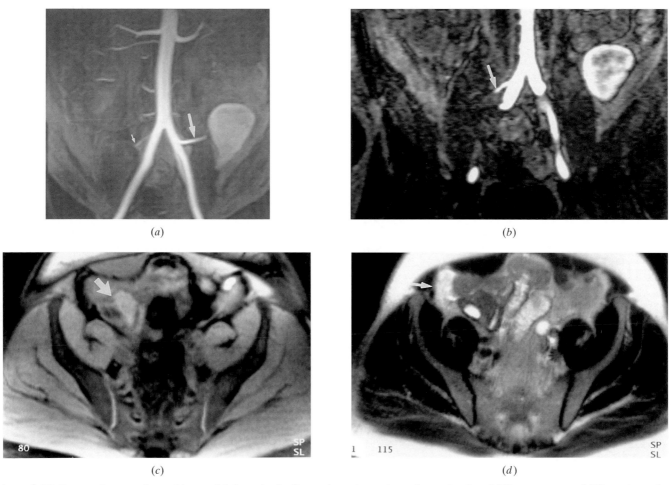

(a)   (b)

(c)   (d)

F I G . 4.53 Pancreatic transplant with arterial thrombosis. Coronal maximum-intensity projection (MIP) reconstructed MR angiography (MRA) (*a*) source image (*b*) from a set of 2-mm thin coronal sections acquired immediately after gadolinium injection with a 3D fast imaging with steady state precession (FISP) breath-hold sequence, fat-suppressed SGE (*c*), and HASTE (*d*) images. The MIP reconstruction MRA image demonstrates a normal artery (*arrow, a*) feeding the renal transplant in the left pelvis and an occluded artery (*small arrow, a*) feeding the pancreas transplant in the right pelvis. In order to establish the diagnosis of occlusion, examination of the source images is essential; occlusion is confirmed on the source image (*arrow, b*) as abrupt termination of the contrast-enhanced vascular lumen. The transplant is identified in the right side of the pelvis on T1-weighted (*arrow, c*) and T2-weighted (*d*) images. Inflammatory fluid (*arrow, d*) is noted adjacent to the pancreas transplant.

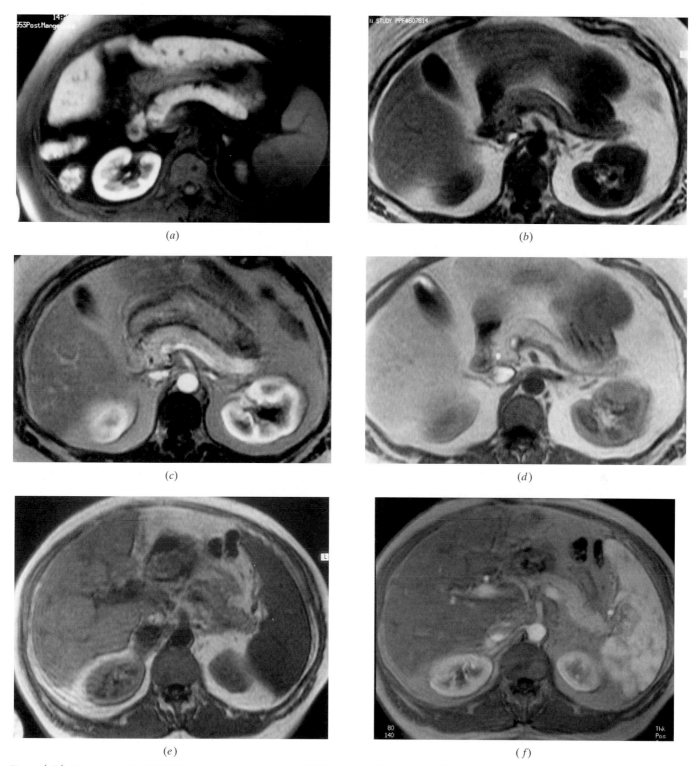

(a)

(b)

(c)

(d)

(e)

(f)

FIG. 4.54 Manganese (Mn)-DPDP-enhanced pancreas. Mn-DPDP-enhanced T1-weighted fat-suppressed spin-echo image (a) demonstrates uniform enhancement of the pancreas. Intense renal cortical enhancement is also identified. SGE (b), immediate postgadolinium SGE (c), and Mn-DPDP-enhanced SGE (d) images in a second patient demonstrate that the pancreas enhances greater with gadolinium than with Mn-DPDP.

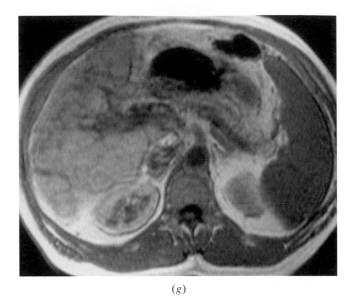

(g)

FIG. 4.54 (*Continued*)   The pancreas is higher in signal intensity relative to background fat on the gadolinium-enhanced image (*c*) and lower than background fat on the Mn-DPDP-enhanced image (*d*). SGE (*e*), immediate postgadolinium SGE (*f*), and Mn-DPDP enhanced SGE (*g*) in a third patient demonstrate the same findings.

also has been employed to detect acute vascular compromise, with high sensitivity and specificity (Fig. 4.53) [71].

FUTURE DIRECTIONS

The role of new contrast agents, such as manganese (Mn)-DPDP, to evaluate disease of the pancreas is currently under investigation. Normal pancreas enhances with Mn-DPDP and focal lesions do not. The degree of enhancement is less than with gadolinium, but the duration of enhancement is longer (Fig. 4.54) [72]. New tissue-specific pancreatic agents are also under development [74].

CONCLUSION

MRI is sensitive and specific in the evaluation of pancreatic disease. MRI is sensitive for pancreatic disease in the following settings: (1) T1-weighted fat-suppressed and dynamic gadolinium-enhanced SGE imaging for the detection of chronic pancreatitis, ductal adenocarcinoma, and islet-cell tumors; (2) T2-weighted fat-suppressed imaging and T2-weighted breath-hold imaging for the detection of islet-cell tumors; and (3) precontrast breath-hold SGE imaging for the detection of acute pancreatitis. Relatively specific morphologic and signal-intensity features permit characterization of acute pancreatitis, chronic pancreatitis, ductal adenocarcinoma, insulinoma,

gastrinoma, glucagonoma, microcystic cystadenoma, macrocystic cystadenoma, and solid and papillary epithelial neoplasm. MRI is effective as a problem-solving modality, because it is able to distinguish chronic pancreatitis from normal pancreas, and chronic pancreatitis with focal enlargement from pancreatic cancer in the majority of cases.

CT imaging remains the first-line imaging modality in the evaluation of pancreatic disease because of greater machine accessibility and familiarity with this modality. MRI studies should be considered in the following settings: (1) patients with elevated serum creatinine, allergy to iodine contrast, or other contraindications for iodine contrast administration; (2) patients with prior CT imaging who have focal enlargement of the pancreas with no definable mass; (3) patients in whom clinical history is worrisome for malignancy and findings on CT imaging are equivocal or difficult to interpret; and (4) situations requiring distinction between chronic pancreatitis with focal enlargement and pancreatic cancer. Patients with biochemical evidence of islet-cell tumors should be examined by MRI as the first-line imaging modality because of the high sensitivity of current MRI techniques for detecting the presence of islet-cell tumors and determining the presence of metastatic disease.

REFERENCES

1. Semelka RC, Ascher SM: MRI of the pancreas—state of the art. Radiology 188:593–602, 1993.
2. Winston CB, Mitchell DG, Outwater EK, Ehrlich SM: Pancreatic signal intensity on T1-weighted fat satuation MR images: Clinical correlation. J Magn Reson Imaging 5:267–271, 1995.
3. Mitchell DG, Vinitski S, Saponaro S, Tasciyan T, Burk DL Jr, Rifkin MD: Liver and pancreas: Improved spin-echo T1 contrast by shorter echo time and fat suppression at 1.5 T. Radiology 178:67–71, 1991.
4. Semelka RC, Kroeker MA, Shoenut JP, Kroeker R, Yaffe CS, Micflikier AB: Pancreatic disease: Prospective comparison of CT, ERCP, and 1.5 T MR imaging with dynamic gadolinium enhancement and fat suppression. Radiology 181:785–791, 1991.
5. Takehara Y, Ichijo K, Tooyama N, et al: Breath-hold MR cholangio-pancreatography with a long-echo-time fast spin-echo sequence and a surface coil in chronic pancreatitis. Radiology 192:73–78, 1994.
6. Bret PM, Reinhold C, Taourel P, Guibaud L, Atri M, Barkun AN: Pancreas divisum: Evaluation with MR cholangiopancreatography. Radiology 199:99–103, 1996.
7. Soto JA, Barish MA, Yucel EK, et al: Pancreatic duct: MR cholangio-pancreatography with a three-dimensional fast spin-echo technique. Radiology 196:459–464, 1995.
8. Semelka RC, Simm FC, Recht M, Deimling M, Lenz G, Laub GA: MRI of the pancreas at high field strength—a comparison of six sequences. J Comput Assist Tomogr 15(6):966–971, 1991.
9. Mitchell DG, Winston CB, Outwater EK, Ehrlich SM: Delineation of pancreas with MR imaging: Multiobserver comparison of five pulse sequences. J Magn Reson Imag 5:193–199, 1995.
10. Delhaye M, Engelholm, Cremer M: Pancreas divisum: Congenital anatomic variant or anomaly? Contribution of endoscopic retrograde dorsal pancreatography. Gastroenterology 89:951–958, 1985.

11. Deasi MB, Mitchell DG, Munoz SJ: Asymptomatic annular pancreas: Detection by magnetic resonance imaging. Magn Reson Imaging 12:683–685, 1994.

12. Tham RTOTA, Heyerman HGM, Falke THM, et al: Cystic fibrosis: MR imaging of the pancreas. Radiology 179:183–186, 1991.

13. Ferroi F, Bova D, Campodonico F, et al: Cystic fibrosis: MR assessment of pancreatic damage. Radiology 198:875–879, 1996.

14. Siegelman ES, Mitchell DG, Outwater E, Munoz SJ, Rubin R: Idiopathic hemochromatosis: MR imaging findings in cirrhotic and precirrhotic patients. Radiology 188:637–641, 1993.

15. Siegelman ES, Mitchell DG, Semelka RC: Abdominal iron deposition: Metabolism, MR findings, and clinical importance. Radiology 199:13–22, 1996.

16. Hough DM, Stephens DH, Johnson CD, Binkovitz LA: Pancreatic lesions in von Hippel-Lindau disease: Prevalence, clinical significance, and CT findings. AJR Am J Roentgenol 162:1091–1094, 1994.

17. Boring CC, Squires TS, Tong T: Cancer statistics, 1991. CA Cancer J Clin 41:19–51, 1991.

18. Warshaw AL, Fernández-del Castillo C: Pancreatic carcinoma. New Eng J Med 326:455–465, 1992.

19. Moossa AR: Pancreatic cancer: Approach to diagnosis, selection for surgery and choice of operation. Cancer 50:2689–2698, 1982.

20. Clark LR, Jaffe MH, Choyke PL, Grant EG, Zeman RK: Pancreatic imaging. Radiol Clin North Am 23:489–501, 1985.

21. Cubilla AL, Fitzgerald PJ: Cancer of the pancreas (nonendocrine): A suggested morphologic clarification. Semin Oncol 6:285–297, 1979.

22. Baron RL, Stanley RJ, Lee JKT, Koehler RE, Levitt RG: Computed tomographic features of biliary obstruction. AJR Am J Roentgenol 140:1173–1178, 1983.

23. Wittenberg J, Simeone JF, Ferrucci JT Jr, Mueller PR, van Sonnenberg E, Neff CC: Non-focal enlargement in pancreatic carcinoma. Radiology 144:131–135, 1982.

24. Megibow AJ, Bosniak MA, Ambos MA, Beranbaum ER: Thickening of the celiac axis and/or superior mesenteric artery: A sign of pancreatic carcinoma on computed tomography. Radiology 141:449–453, 1981.

25. Gabata T, Matsui O, Kadoya M, et al: Small pancreatic adenocarcinomas: Efficacy of MR imaging with fat suppression and gadolinium enhancement. Radiology 193:683–688, 1994.

26. Semelka RC, Kelekis NL, Molina PL, Scharp T, Calvo B: Pancreatic masses with inconclusive findings on spiral CR. Is there a role for MRI? J Magn Reson Imaging 6:585–588, 1996.

27. Steiner E, Stark DD, Hahn PF, et al: Imaging of pancreatic neoplasms: Comparison of MR and CT. AJR Am J Roentgenol 152:487–491, 1989.

28. Sarles H, Sahel J: Pathology of chronic calcifying pancreatitis. Am J Gastroenterol 66:117–139, 1976.

29. Vellet AD, Romano W, Bach DB, Passi RB, Taves DH, Munk PL: Adenocarcinoma of the pancreatic ducts: Comparative evaluation with CT and MR imaging at 1.5 T. Radiology 183:87–95, 1992.

30. Pavone P, Occhiato R, Michelini O, et al: Magnetic resonance imaging of pancreatic carcinoma. Eur Radiol 1:124–130, 1991.

31. Patt R, Zeman RK, Nauta R, Ascher SM, Wooley P, Silverman P: Vascular encasement by pancreatobiliary neoplasms: Assessment with dynamic CT, spin-echo MR imaging, and gradient-echo MR imaging. Radiology 181(p):259, 1991.

32. McFarland EG, Kaufman JA, Saini S, et al: Preoperative staging of cancer of the pancreas: Value of MR angiography versus conventional angiography in detecting portal venous invasion. AJR Am J Roentgenol 166:37–43, 1996.

33. Mozell E, Stenzel P, Woltering EA, Rösch J, O'Dorisio TM: Functional endocrine tumors of the pancreas: Clinical presentation, diagnosis, and treatment. Curr Probl Surg 27:304–385, 1990.

34. Thompson NW, Eckhauser FE, Vinik AI, Lloyd RV, Fiddian-Green RD, Strodel WE: Cystic neuroendocrine neoplasms of the pancreas and liver. Ann Surg 199:158–164, 1984.

35. Mitchell DG, Cruvella M, Eschelman DJ, Miettinen MM, Vernick JJ: MRI of pancreatic gastrinomas. J Comput Assist Tomogr 16:583–585, 1992.

36. Kraus BB, Ros PR: Insulinoma: Diagnosis with fat-suppressed MR imaging. AJR Am J Roentgenol 162:69–70, 1994.

37. Semelka RC, Cummings M, Shoenut JP, Yaffe CS, Kroeker MA, Greenberg HM: Islet cell tumors: A comparison of detection by dynamic contrast-enhanced CT and MR imaging with dynamic gadolinium enhancement and fat suppression. Radiology 186:799–802, 1993.

38. Kelekis NL, Semelka RC, Molina PL, Doerr ME: ACTH-secreting islet cell tumor: Appearances on dynamic gadolinium-enhanced MRI. Magn Reson Imaging 13:641–644, 1995.

39. Buetow PC, Parrino TV, Buck JL, et al: Islet cell tumors of the pancreas: pathologic-imaging correlation among six, necrosis and cysts, calcification, malignant behavior, and functional status. AJR Am J Roentgenol 165:1175–1179, 1995.

40. Wank SA, Doppman JL, Miller DL, et al: Prospective study of the ability of computed axial tomography to localize gastrinomas in patients with Zollinger-Ellison syndrome. Gastroenterology 92:905–12, 1987.

41. Frucht H, Doppman JL, Norten JA, et al: Gastrinomas comparison of MR imaging with CT, angiography, and US. Radiology 171:713–717, 1989.

42. Muller MF, Meyenberger C, Bertschinger P, Schaer R, Marincek B: Pancreatic tumors: Evaluation with endoscopic US, CT, and MR imaging. Radiology 190:745–751, 1994.

43. Galiber AK, Reading CC, Charboneau JW, et al: Localization of pancreatic insulinoma: Comparison of pre- and intraoperative US with CT and angiography. Radiology 166:405–408, 1988.

44. Tjon A, Tham RTO, Jansen JBMJ, Falke THM, et al: MR, CT, and ultrasound findings of metastatic vipoma in pancreas. J Comput Assist Tomogr 13(1):142–144, 1989.

45. Carlson B, Johnson CD, Stephens DH, Ward EM, Kvois LK: MRI of pancreatic islet cell carcinoma. J Comput Assist Tomogr 17:735–740, 1993.

46. Tjon A, Tham RTO, Jansen JBMJ, Falke THM, Lamers CBMW: Imaging features of somatostatinoma: MR, CT, US, and angiography. J Comp Assist Tomogr 18:427–431, 1994.

47. Doppman JL, Nieman LK, Cutler GB Jr, et al: Adrenocorticotripic hormone-secreting islet cell tumors: Are they always malignant? Radiology 190:59–64, 1994.

48. Ros PR, Hamrick-Turner JE, Chiechi MV, Ross LH., Gallego P, Burton SS: Cystic masses of the pancreas. Radiographics 12:673–686, 1992.

49. Lewandrowski K, Warshaw A, Compton C: Macrocystic serous cystadenoma of the pancreas: A morphologic variant differing from microcystic adenoma. Hum Pathol 23:871–875, 1992.

50. Minami M, Itai Y, Ohtomo K, Yoshida H, Yoshikawa K, Iio M: Cystic neoplasms of the pancreas: Comparison of MR imaging with CT. Radiology 171:53–56, 1989.

51. Friedman AC, Liechtenstein JE, Dachman AH: Cystic neoplasms of the pancreas: Radiological-pathological correlation. Radiology 149:45–50, 1983.

52. Compagno J, Oertel JE: Mucinous cystic neoplasms of the pancreas with overt and latent malignancy (cystadenocarcinoma and cystadenoma): A clinicopathologic study of 41 cases. Am J Clin Pathol 69:573–580, 1978.

53. Ohtomo K, Furai S, Oneone M, Okada Y, Kusano S, Uchiyama G: Solid and papillary epithelial neoplasm of the pancreas: MR imaging and pathologic correlation. Radiology 184:567–570, 1992.

54. Zeman RK, Schiebler M, Clark LR, et al: The clinical and imaging spectrum of pancreaticoduodenal lymph node enlargement. AJR Am J Roentgenol 144:1223–1227, 1985.

55. Kelekis NL, Semelka RC, Siegelman ES: MRI of pancreatic metastases from renal cancer. J Comp Assist Tomogr 20:249–253, 1996.

56. Steinberg W, Tenner S: Acute pancreatitis. N Engl J Med 1198–1210, 1994.

57. Kattwinkel J, Lapey A, DiSant'Agnese PA, Edwards WA, Jufty MP: Hereditary pancreatitis: Three new kindreds and a critical review of the literature. Pediatrics 51:5–69, 1973.

58. Lee SP, Nicholls JF, Park HZ: Biliary sludge as a cause of acute pancreatitis. N Engl J Med 326:589–593, 1992.

59. Balthazar E: CT diagnosis and staging of acute pancreatitis. Radiol Clin North Am 27:19–37, 1989.

60. Balthazar EJ, Robinson DL, Megibow AJ, Ranson JHC: Acute pancreatitis: Value of CT in establishing prognosis. Radiology 174:331–336, 1990.

61. Johnson CD, Stephens DH, Sarr MG: CT of acute pancreatitis: Correlation between lack of contrast enhancement and pancreatic necrosis. AJR Am J Roentgenol 156:93, 1991.

62. Saifuddin A, Ward J, Ridgway J, Chalriners AG: Comparison of MR and CT scanning in severe acute pancreatitis: initial experiences. Clin Radiol 48:111–116, 1993.

63. Bank S: Chronic pancreatitis: clinical features and medical management. Am J Gastroenterol 81:153–167, 1986.

64. Steer ML, Waxman I, Freedman S: Chronic pancreatitis. N Eng J Med 332:1482–1490, 1995.

65. Lowenfels AB, Maisonneuve P, Cavallini G, et al: Pancreatitis and the risk of pancreatic cancer. N Eng J Med 328:1433–1437, 1993.

66. Luetmer PH, Stephens DH, Ward EM: Chronic pancreatitis reassessment with current CT. Radiology 171:353–357, 1989.

67. Aranha GV, Prinz RA, Freeark RJ, Greenlee HB: The spectrum of biliary tract obstruction from chronic pancreatitis. Arch Surg 119:595–600, 1984.

68. Lammer J, Herlinger H, Zalaudek G, Hofler H: Pseudotumorous pancreatitis. Gastrointest Radiol 10:59–67, 1985.

69. Sostre CF, Flournoy JG, Bova JG, Goldstein HM, Schenker S: Pancreatic phlegmon: Clinical features and course. Dig Dis Sci 30:918–927, 1985.

70. Semelka RC, Shoenut JP, Kroeker MA, Micflikier AB: Chronic pancreatitis: MR imaging features before and after administration of gadopentetate dimeglumine. J Mag Reson Imaging 3:79–82, 1993.

71. del Pilar Fernandez M, Bernardino ME, Neylan JF, Olson RA: Diagnosis of pancreatic transplant dysfunction: Value of gadopentatate dimeglumine-enhanced MR imaging. AJR Am J Roentgenol 156:1171–1176, 1991.

72. Krebs TL, Daly B, Wong JJ, Chow CC, Bartlett ST: Vascular complications of pancreatic transplantation: MR evaluation. Radiology 196:793–798, 1995.

73. Kettritz U, Warshauer DM, Brown ED, Schlund JF, Eisenberg LB, Semelka RC: Enhancement of the normal pancreas: Comparison of manganese-DPDP and gadolinium chelate. Eur Radiol 6:14–18, 1996.

74. Reiner P, Weissleder R, Shen T, Knoefel WT, Brady TJ: Pancreatic receptors: Initial feasibility studies with a targeted contrast agent for MR imaging. Radiology 193:527–531, 1994.

CHAPTER 5

SPLEEN

N. L. KELEKIS, M.D., D. A. BURDENY, M.D., AND R. C. SEMELKA, M.D.

NORMAL ANATOMY

The spleen, located posteriorly in the left upper quadrant of the abdomen, is typically crescent-shaped, with the lateral border convex conforming to the abdominal wall and left hemidiaphragm and the medial border concave conforming to the stomach and left kidney. The splenic hilum is directed anteromedially, and the splenic artery and vein enter the spleen at this location. The splenic vein follows a relatively straight course along the posterior surface of the body and tail of the pancreas. The splenic artery is slightly superior to the vein and is often tortuous. The spleen is suspended by diaphragmatic attachments and by the splenorenal and splenocolic ligament. These commonly dilate in the presence of portal hypertension. Isolated dilatation of these vessels is seen in the presence of splenic vein thrombosis.

The spleen is composed of white and red pulp. The red pulp is further divided into two components based on blood circulation or pathways. One pathway involves the passage of blood cells through a filtration process in the splenic chords, which is termed the open circulation and is functionally slow. The other pathway is a direct passage through capillaries in the splenic sinuses to the splenic vein, which is termed the closed circulation and is functionally rapid [1].

MRI TECHNIQUE

Our standard MRI protocol includes breath-hold T1-weighted SGE, T2-weighted imaging (usually fat-sup-

pressed echo-train spin-echo), and immediate and delayed postgadolinium SGE, with the delayed images often acquired with fat suppression. Normal splenic parenchyma is invariably low in signal intensity on T1-weighted images and usually high in signal intensity on T2 weighted images (Fig. 5.1). Signal intensity on T2-weighted images of the spleen varies and not uncommonly is relatively low. This is usually secondary to prior blood transfusions, which result in iron deposition in the reticuloendothelial system (RES) of the spleen (Fig. 5.2). The signal intensity of most forms of benign and malignant disease processes parallels the pattern of low signal intensity on T1-weighted images and high signal intensity on T2-weighted images. As a result, noncontrast MR images are limited in the detection of splenic disease. Differences in blood supply of spleen and diseased tissue permit detection of abnormalities on immediate postgadolinium images.

Immediate postgadolinium breath-hold T1-weighted spoiled gradient-echo (SGE) sequences demonstrate the different circulations in the normal spleen as regions of transient higher and lower contrast enhancement, usually in an arciform or serpiginous pattern [2–5]. This appears as an alternating pattern of high-signal (closed circulation) and low-signal (open circulation) stroma. Variations of this pattern occur such as central low and peripheral high signal intensity. This variegated pattern becomes homogeneous and high in signal intensity within 1 minute after contrast. Three variations in splenic enhancement patterns have been described in spleen not infiltrated by disease on immediate postgadolinium images [4]. The most common (79% of patients) is serpiginous

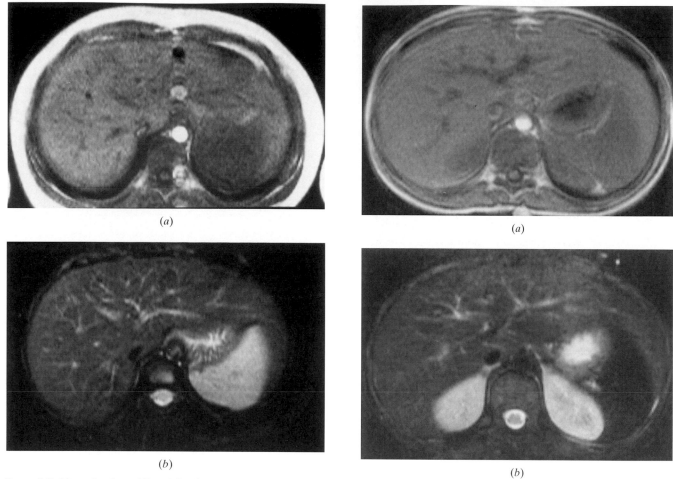

FIG. 5.1 Normal spleen. T1-weighted SGE (*a*) and T2-weighted fat-suppressed spin-echo (*b*) images. Normal spleen is low in signal intensity on T1-weighted images (*a*) and high in signal intensity on T2-weighted images (*b*). Liver is higher in signal intensity on T1-weighted images and lower in signal intensity on T2-weighted images than spleen, which results in a clear distinction between the elongated lateral segment of the liver and the adjacent spleen.

FIG. 5.2 Iron deposition in the spleen. T1-weighted SGE (*a*) and T2-weighted fat-suppressed spin-echo (*b*) images. Signal intensity of the spleen is only slightly lower than normal on the T1-weighted image (*a*), which is consistent with mild iron deposition in the RES. Signal intensity of the spleen is noted to be nearly signal-void on the T2-weighted image (*b*), with low signal intensity also noted of liver and bone marrow due to iron deposition in the RES in these organs.

enhancement, termed *arciform*. This pattern has been observed in all normal spleens in nondiseased patients and in some spleens of patients with inflammatory or neoplastic disease (Fig. 5.3). The second most common pattern (16% of patients) is homogeneous high-signal-intensity enhancement (Fig. 5.4). This has been observed in patients with inflammatory or neoplastic diseases, hepatic focal fatty infiltration, or hepatic enzyme abnormalities. A nonspecific immune response may be responsible for this pattern of enhancement. This appearance may represent the conversion of a mixture of slow and fast channels to only fast channels, reflecting a mechanism to increase transit of immune system cells. The third pattern is uniform low signal intensity (5% of patients) (Fig. 5.5). This was found in all patients who had undergone multiple recent blood transfusions. The T2-shorten-

ing effects from hemosiderin deposition in the RES supersede the T1-shortening effects of gadolinium [6,7].

Superparamagnetic iron oxide particles are selectively taken up by the RES and have been used to evaluate the spleen. These particles diminish the signal intensity of the normal spleen on T2-weighted sequences, whereas tumors remain unchanged in signal characteristics [8,9]. Superparamagnetic iron oxide crystals embedded in a starch matrix (magnetic starch microspheres [MSM], Nycomed Imaging, Oslo, Norway) have been studied in animal models, and have been shown to increase conspicuity of both focal and diffuse splenic lesions [10]. Normal spleen diminishes in signal on T2-weighted or T2*-weighted images, whereas focal or diffuse disease retains signal, which renders disease conspicuous by being relatively high in signal intensity.

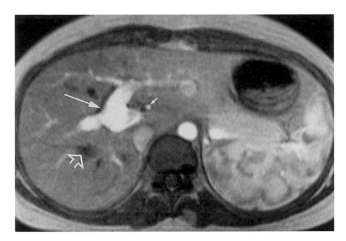

FIG. 5.3 Arciform enhancement in the normal spleen. Note the serpiginous, tubular bands of low signal intensity throughout the splenic parenchyma. Contrast identified in portal vein (*long arrow*), hepatic arteries (*short arrow*), and lack of contrast in hepatic veins (*hollow arrow*) defines the capillary phase of enhancement.

DISEASE ENTITIES

Normal Variants and Congenital Disease
Accessory spleens are common and may occur in up to 40 percent of individuals [11,12]. They are clinically important insofar as they must be differentiated from other mass lesions. In patients with hypersplenism, identification of accessory spleens is critical prior to splenectomy to avoid accessory spleen hypertrophy and recur-

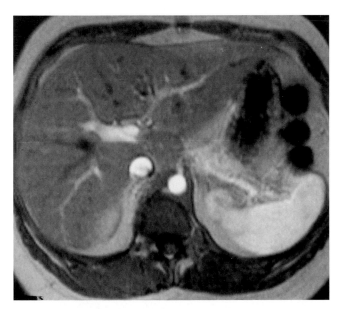

FIG. 5.4 Homogeneous intense splenic enhancement. The spleen is noted to enhance intensely and uniformly in the capillary phase of enhancement. Contrast in hepatic arteries and portal veins, and no contrast in hepatic veins demonstrate that the image was acquired in the capillary phase of enhancement.

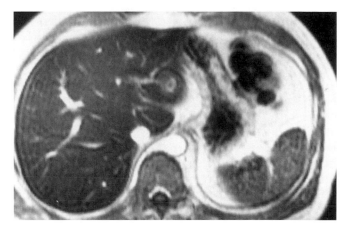

FIG. 5.5 Homogeneous low-signal-intensity splenic enhancement. The spleen is low in signal intensity on immediate postgadolinium images due to the predominate T2-shortening effects of iron in the spleen.

rence [11,12]. Accessory spleens parallel the signal intensity of the spleen on all MRI sequences, including their enhancement on immediate postgadolinium images (Fig. 5.6). Splenules may also be confidently characterized in the patient who has undergone repeated blood transfusions because they will be nearly signal-void on T2- or T2*-weighted sequences due to iron deposition within the RES of the splenules. This effect also may be achieved with the use of iron oxide particles [13].

Asplenia and Polysplenia
Asplenia and polysplenia are congenital syndromes characterized by abdominal situs and cardiovascular abnormalities. Asplenia tends to have more severe cardiac involvement and hence a poorer prognosis [14]. In cardiac MRI studies in which cardiovascular anomalies raise the possibility asplenia or polysplenia syndromes, a limited abdominal MRI should be performed at the same time to evaluate abdominal situs, abdominal vessels, and the presence and number of spleens.

Gaucher's Disease
Gaucher's disease is a multisystem hereditary disease caused by deficient glucocerebrosidase activity. Glucocerebroside, a glycolipid, accumulates in organ macrophages [15]. The abdominal manifestations of Gaucher's disease in a population of 46 patients have been described using conventional spin-echo techniques [15]. All patients had hepatosplenomegaly. Splenic nodules of variable signal intensity were present in 14 patients (30%). Fifteen patients (33%) had splenic infarcts with or without associated subcapsular fluid collections, and 4 patients (9%) had both infarcts and nodules. Focal areas of abnormal signal intensity were noted in the livers of 9 patients (20%).

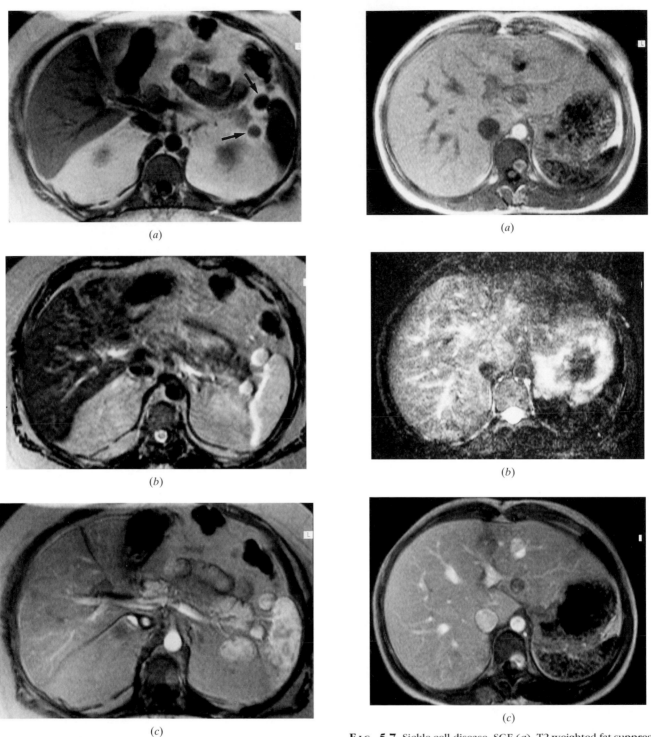

(a)

(b)

(c)

(a)

(b)

(c)

FIG. 5.6 Splenules. SGE (a), T2-weighted spin-echo (b), and immediate postgadolinium SGE (c) images. Two splenules are identified (arrows, a) that parallel the signal intensity of the spleen. They are low in signal intensity on T1-weighted images (a), high in signal intensity on T2-weighted images (b), and enhance intensely on immediate postgadolinium images (c). The splenules show heterogeneous enhancement on immediate postcontrast images, which suggests that they have architecture similar to that of the spleen.

FIG. 5.7 Sickle-cell disease. SGE (a), T2-weighted fat-suppressed spin-echo (b), and immediate postgadolinium SGE (c) images. The spleen is noted to be small and low in signal intensity on all MR images (a–c) and is nearly signal-void on T2-weighted fat-suppressed spin-echo (b) images. On the precontrast SGE image (a), multiple 1-cm signal-void foci are noted in the small low-signal-intensity spleen. These foci are better demarcated after contrast administration (c) due to minimal enhancement of surrounding splenic parenchyma.

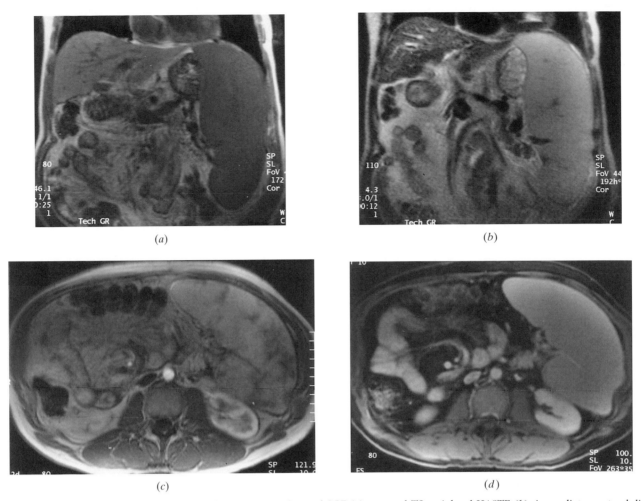

(a)

(b)

(c)

(d)

FIG. 5.8 Splenomegaly secondary to portal hypertension. Coronal SGE (*a*), coronal T2-weighted HASTE (*b*), immediate postgadolinium SGE (*c*), and 90-second postgadolinium fat-suppressed SGE (*d*) images. Massive splenomegaly is demonstrated on all MR images. No focal lesions are present on precontrast T1- (*a*) or T2-weighted images (*b*). The presence of arciform enhancement on immediate postgadolinium SGE images (*c*) excludes the presence of malignant disease. At 90 seconds the spleen becomes homogeneous in signal (*d*).

Sickle-Cell Disease

The manifestations of sickle-cell anemia vary and depend on whether the patient is homozygous or heterozygous for the hemoglobinopathy. In patients with homozygous disease the spleen is nearly signal-void due to the sequela of iron deposition from blood transfusions coupled with microscopic perivascular and parenchymal calcifications [16]. This decrease in signal intensity was found to be diffuse in most patients with signal-void foci due to calcifications and/or foci of greater iron deposition (Fig. 5.7). Hyperintense focal lesions on proton density images may occur and are believed to represent infarcts.

Splenomegaly

Splenomegaly may be observed in a number of disease states including venous congestion (portal hypertension), leukemia, lymphoma, metastases, and various infections. In North America the most common cause of splenomegaly is secondary to portal hypertension. On immediate postgadolinium images demonstration of arciform or uniform high-signal-intensity enhancement is consistent with portal hypertension and excludes the presence of malignant disease (Fig. 5.8).

MASS LESIONS

Benign Masses

Cysts

Cysts are the most common of the benign splenic lesions. Three types of nonneoplastic cysts exist: posttraumatic or pseudocyst, epidermoid cysts, and hydatid cysts [17]. Most splenic cysts are posttraumatic in origin. They are not lined by epithelium, and thus are pseudocysts. Epidermoid cysts are true cysts discovered in childhood or early adulthood that may have trabecutations or sep-

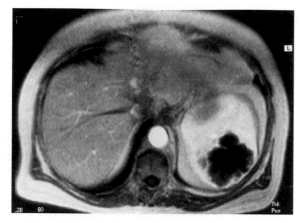

FIG. 5.9 Epidermoid cyst. Immediate postgadolinium SGE image demonstrates a signal-void cystic lesion with peripheral septations.

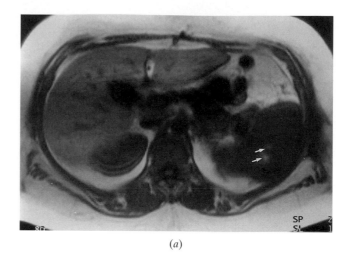

(a)

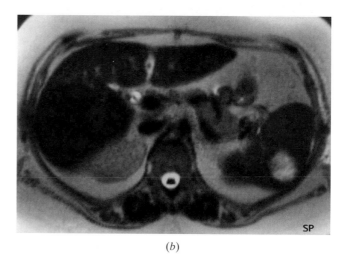

(b)

tations in their walls with occasional peripheral calcification [17,18] (Fig. 5.9). Hydatid, or echinococcal cysts, are rare. They are characterized by extensive wall calcification. The MRI features of cysts include sharp lesion margination, low signal intensity on T1-weighted images, and very high signal intensity on T2-weighted images. Cysts complicated by protein or hemorrhage may have regions of high signal intensity on T1-weighted images, regions of mixed signal intensity on T2-weighted images, or both. Cysts do not enhance on postgadolinium images. Pseudocysts may be complicated by hemorrhage particularly early in their evolution, and thus may contain foci of high signal intensity on precontrast T1-weighted images (Fig. 5.10).

Hemangiomas

Hemangiomas are the most common of the benign splenic neoplasms [19,20]. Lesions may be single or multiple. Splenic hemangiomas are mildly low to isointense on T1-weighted images and mildly to moderately hyperintense on T2-weighted images similar to hepatic hemangiomas. Hemangiomas are minimally hypointense to isointense with background spleen on T1-weighted images due to the relatively low signal intensity of spleen on these images, and minimally hyperintense relative to spleen on T2-weighted images due to the moderately high signal intensity of spleen on T2-weighted images. Three patterns of contrast enhancement are observed: (1) immediate homogeneous enhancement with persistent enhancement on delayed images, (2) peripheral enhancement with progression to uniform enhancement on delayed images (Fig. 5.11), and (3) peripheral enhancement with centripetal progression but persistent lack of enhancement of central scar. These patterns are similar to those observed for hemangiomas. However, unlike hepatic hemangiomas, splenic hemangiomas generally do not demonstrate well-defined nodules on early post-

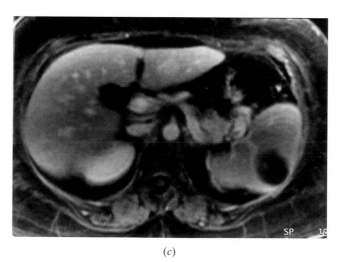

(c)

FIG. 5.10 Pseudocyst. SGE (a), HASTE (b), and 90-second postgadolinium fat-suppressed SGE (c) images. High-signal-intensity foci are identified in the cyst on the precontrast SGE image (*arrows, a*), a finding consistent with hemorrhage. Slight heterogeneity of the cyst on the T2-weighted image (b) also reflects the presence of blood degradation products. The cyst is sharply demarcated after gadolinium administration (c). The foci of blood remain high in signal intensity on postgadolinium images.

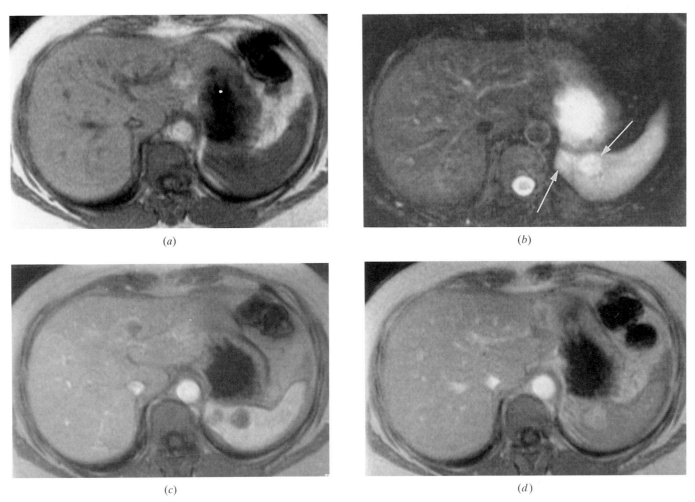

(a) (b)

(c) (d)

FIG. 5.11 Hemangiomas. SGE (a), T2 fat-suppressed spin-echo (b), 45-second (c), and 10-minute (d) postgadolinium SGE images. Two small, less than 1.5-cm hemangiomas are present that are minimally hypointense on T1-weighted images (a) and moderately hyperintense on T2-weighted images (arrows, b). Peripheral nodules are present on early postgadolinium images (c), and enhancement progresses to uniform high-signal-intensity by 10 minutes (d).

gadolinium images. This may, in part, reflect the blood supply from the background organ. Uniform high signal on immediate postgadolinium SGE images is a common appearance for small (<1.5-cm) hemangiomas, as it is with hepatic hemangiomas.

Hamartomas

Hamartomas are rare and tend to be single, spherical, and predominantly solid. They are most likely to occur in the midportion of the spleen, arising from the anterior or posterior aspect of the convex surface. These tumors are mildly low to isointense on T1-weighted images and moderately high in signal intensity on T2-weighted images [20–22]. They frequently are moderately heterogeneous due, in part, to the presence of cystic spaces of varying size. If the composition of fibrous tissue is substantial, hamartomas may have regions of low signal intensity on T2-weighted images [22]. They enhance on

immediate postgadolinium SGE images in an intense diffuse heterogeneous fashion [20,22] (Fig. 5.12). Diffuse enhancement on immediate postgadolinium images is generally observed in tumors that are native to the organ in which they occur. Lesion size and enhancement pattern may mimic a more aggressive lesion. Lesions may also resemble normal splenic parenchyma (Fig. 5.13). Enhancement becomes homogeneous on more delayed images with signal intensity slightly greater than in background spleen. The early diffuse heterogeneous enhancement permits distinction from hemangiomas [20].

Malignant Masses

Lymphoma and Other Hematologic Malignancies

Hodgkin's and non-Hodgkin's lymphomas often involve the spleen [23–25]. Lymphomatous deposits in the spleen frequently parallel the signal intensity of splenic paren-

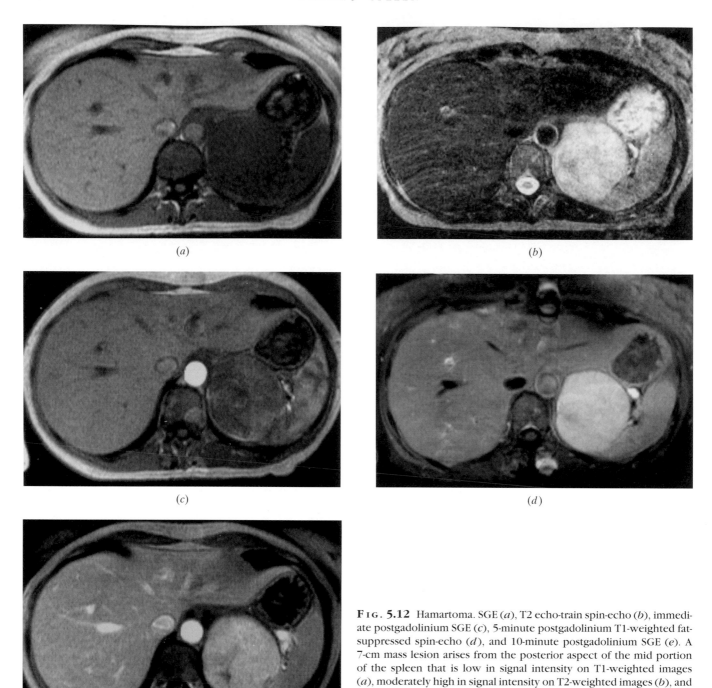

(a)

(b)

(c)

(d)

(e)

FIG. 5.12 Hamartoma. SGE (*a*), T2 echo-train spin-echo (*b*), immediate postgadolinium SGE (*c*), 5-minute postgadolinium T1-weighted fat-suppressed spin-echo (*d*), and 10-minute postgadolinium SGE (*e*). A 7-cm mass lesion arises from the posterior aspect of the mid portion of the spleen that is low in signal intensity on T1-weighted images (*a*), moderately high in signal intensity on T2-weighted images (*b*), and that demonstrates diffuse heterogeneous enhancement on immediate postgadolinium SGE images (*c*). On more delayed images (*d,e*) enhancement becomes more homogeneous and is greater than that of background spleen.

chyma on T1- and T2-weighted images. Therefore, conventional unenhanced spin-echo MRI has had only limited success in imaging lymphomatous involvement of the spleen [24]. Immediate postgadolinium SGE images, however, surpass CT images for the evaluation of lymphoma [4]. This is explained by the higher sensitivity of MRI for gadolinium and its ability to acquire images

of the entire spleen in a rapid fashion following a compact bolus of contrast.

Splenic involvement may have various appearances on immediate postgadolinium images. Diffuse involvement may appear as large, irregularly enhancing regions of high and low signal intensity (Fig. 5.14), in contrast to the uniform bands that characterize normal arciform

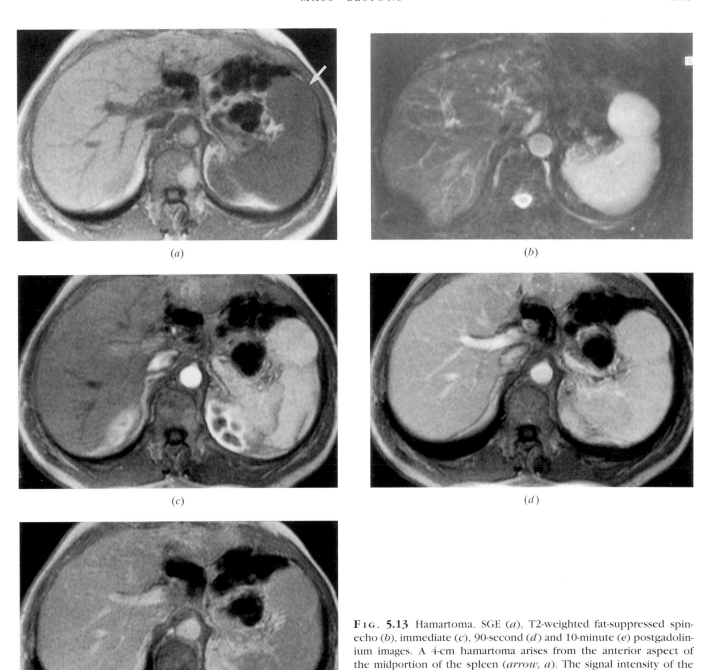

(a)

(b)

(c)

(d)

(e)

Fig. 5.13 Hamartoma. SGE (*a*), T2-weighted fat-suppressed spin-echo (*b*), immediate (*c*), 90-second (*d*) and 10-minute (*e*) postgadolinium images. A 4-cm hamartoma arises from the anterior aspect of the midportion of the spleen (*arrow, a*). The signal intensity of the hamartoma is very similar to that of background spleen on all imaging sequences. A cleavage plane from spleen is noted on the T2-weighted image (*b*). On the immediate postgadolinium image (*c*) the tumor has intense, uniform enhancement, which is different from the arciform enhancement of the normal splenic parenchyma.

enhancement. Multifocal disease is also common, appearing as focal low-signal-intensity mass lesions scattered throughout the spleen [4]. Focal lesions may occur in a background of arciform-enhancing spleen or in a background of uniformly enhancing spleen. Focal involvement appears as spherical lesions in distinction to the wavy tubular pattern of arciform enhancement of

uninvolved spleen. Focal lymphomatous deposits may be low in signal intensity compared to background spleen on T2-weighted images (Fig. 5.15), which is a feature distinguishing lymphomas from metastases, which are rarely low in signal intensity and usually isointense to hyperintense. Although splenomegaly is most often present, lymphoma may involve normal-sized spleens (Fig.

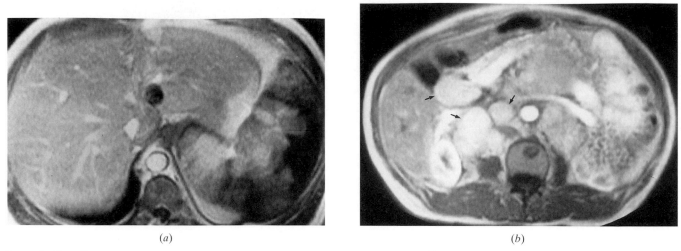

(a)   (b)

FIG. 5.14 Diffuse infiltration with lymphoma. Immediate postgadolinium SGE image (*a*) demonstrates irregular regions of high and low signal intensity in the spleen in this patient with non-Hodgkin's lymphoma. Irregular enhancement is observed in the setting of diffuse infiltration. Immediate post gadolinium SGE image (*b*) in a second patient with non-Hodgkin's lymphoma demonstrates irregular enhancement of the spleen consistent with diffuse infiltration. Enhancing lymph nodes (*arrows, b*) are also noted.

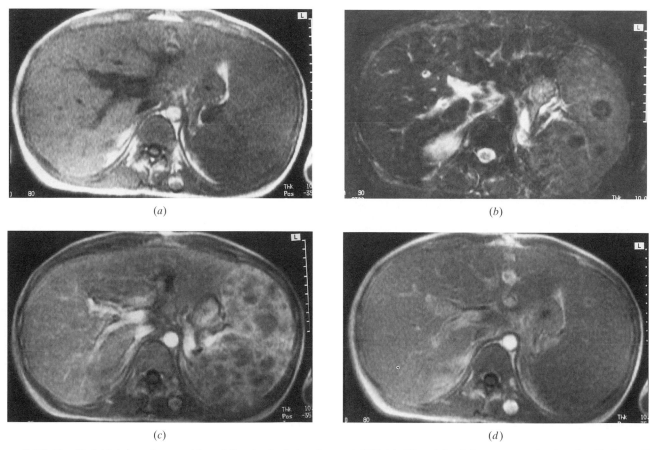

(a)   (b)

(c)   (d)

FIG. 5.15 Non-Hodgkin's lymphoma with multifocal splenic involvement. SGE (*a*), T2-weighted fat-suppressed spin-echo (*b*), immediate (*c*), and 2-minute (*d*) postgadolinium images. Splenomegaly is present. Lesions are not apparent on the precontrast SGE image. Several low-signal-intensity focal mass lesions are identified on T2-weighted images, an appearance that is not uncommon for lymphoma but rare for other malignant tumors. Multiple focal masses are most clearly demonstrated on immediate postgadolinium images (*c*). Lymphomatous foci become isointense with background spleen by 2 minutes after contrast (*d*).

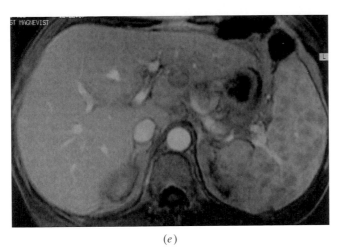

(e)

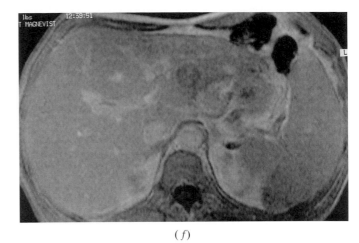

(f)

FIG. 5.15 (*Continued*) Immediate (*e*) and 90-second (*f*) postgadolinium SGE images in a second patient. Multiple low-signal-intensity masses are identified on the immediate postgadolinium image (*e*). Lesions become isointense with background spleen by 90 seconds.

5.16). Lymphoma also may appear as a large mass involving spleen and contiguous organs such as stomach, adrenal, or kidney. Bulky lymphadenopathy is frequently, but not invariably, present. It is critical to acquire SGE images within the first 30 seconds after contrast administration because foci of lymphoma equilibrate early, becoming isointense with normal splenic tissue within 2 minutes and frequently earlier [2,4]. A rare appearance is that of a solitary mass involving the spleen which may also show relatively internal diffuse heterogeneous enhancement on immediate postgadolinium SGE images (Fig. 5.17). This appearance may mimic that of splenic hamartomas. The presence of symptoms and signs of systemic disease may suggest the diagnosis of lymphoma.

Superparamagnetic particles also improve the accuracy of diagnosing splenic lymphoma [9,10]. These particles are selectively taken up by the RES cells and cause a decrease in signal intensity. By contrast, superparamagnetic particles are not taken up by malignant cells. Therefore, splenic lymphoma remains hyperintense compared to the normal spleen, improving tumor-spleen contrast [9,10].

Chronic lymphocytic leukemia frequently involves the spleen and may result in massive splenomegaly. Focal deposits are more infiltrative and less well-defined than lymphoma. Deposits are well shown after gadolinium administration and appear as irregular hypointense masses on early postcontrast images (Fig. 5.18). Malignancies related to leukemia, such as angioimmunoblastic lymphadenopathy with dysproteinemia, have a similar appearance, with irregular regions of low signal intensity within the spleen on immediate postgadolinium images (Fig. 5.19). Lymphadenopathy is frequently present.

Metastases

Splenic metastases may be found in up to 50 percent of patients with advanced malignant disease [26]. Islet-cell tumors, malignant melanoma, breast carcinoma, and lung carcinoma are the primary tumors that most commonly metastasize to the spleen, with islet-cell tumors having a propensity to involve the spleen. Metastases tend to be in the form of nodules or aggregates of tumor, and they are particularly prone to disrupt the normal splenic architecture. Splenic metastases often are occult on conventional spin-echo imaging [25]. One notable exception is melanoma because its paramagnetic properties may result in a mixed population of high- and low-signal-intensity lesions on both T1- and T2-weighted images. Lesion detection is improved by acquiring immediate postgadolinium SGE images [2,4] (Fig. 5.20). Metastases are lower in signal intensity than normal splenic tissue on these images [2,4,20]. Images must be acquired within the first 30 seconds after gadolinium administration because me-

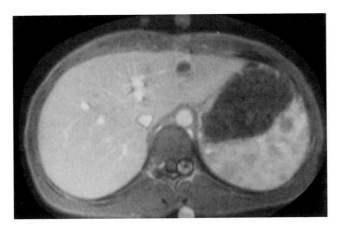

FIG. 5.16 Hodgkin's lymphoma. Immediate postgadolinium image demonstrated multiple low-signal-intensity masses within a normal sized spleen. Lesions are present in a background of arciform enhancing spleen.

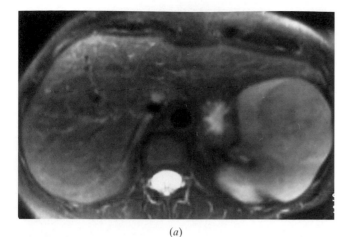

(a)

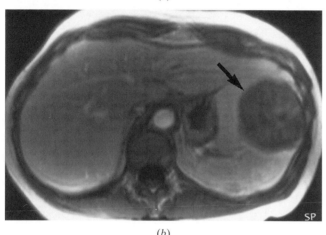

(b)

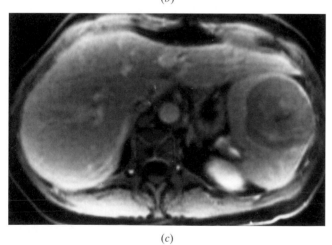

(c)

FIG. 5.17 Splenic lymphoma presenting as a solitary mass. T2-weighted fat-suppressed echo-train spin-echo (a), immediate postgadolinium SGE (b), and 90-second postgadolinium fat-suppressed SGE (c) images. A 6-cm solitary mass arises from the spleen which is mildly heterogeneous and hyperintense on the T2 weighted image (a). The mass enhances moderately in a diffuse heterogeneous fashion on the immediate postgadolinium image (arrow, b) with slightly increased signal intensity by 90 seconds postcontrast (c). The appearance resembles a hamartoma. The patient presented with systemic symotoms which is a picture more in keeping with lymphoma than hamartoma. The patient did not have retroperitoneal adenopathy, which is another uncommon feature of splenic lymphoma.

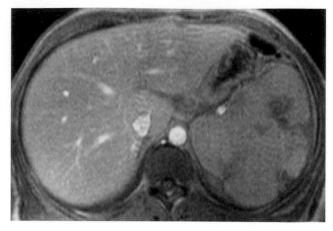

FIG. 5.18 Chronic lymphocytic leukemia. The spleen is noted to be massively enlarged and contains irregularly marginated focal low-signal-intensity masses on 45-second postgadolinium SGE image.

tastases rapidly equilibrate with splenic parenchyma. Image acquisition with superparamagnetic iron oxide particles renders metastases higher in signal intensity than normal spleen [8,10]. An attractive feature of iron oxide particles is that the imaging window is longer (60 minutes) than for gadolinium (<1 minute) [8–10].

Direct Tumor Invasion

Direct tumor invasion is most commonly observed with pancreatic cancers including ductal adenocarcinoma, islet-cell tumor, and macrocystic cystadenocarcinoma (Fig. 5.21). Direct extension from tumors of gastric, colonic, renal and adrenal origin, in a decreasing order of frequency, are also observed. Lymphoma has a particular propensity to involve the spleen in continuity with other organs.

Angiosarcoma

Angiosarcoma is rare, but it represents the most common primary nonlymphoid malignant tumor of the spleen. Tumors may be single or multiple and demonstrate an aggressive growth pattern. Rupture is not uncommon, and hemorrhage is a frequent finding. Angiosarcomas commonly demonstrate a variety of signal intensities on T1-weighted images due to the varying ages of blood products [27]. Tumors are usually very vascular and enhance intensely with gadolinium [27].

Infection

Viral infection may result in splenomegaly. The three most common viruses to involve the spleen are Epstein-Barr, varicella, and cytomegalovirus. Nonviral infectious agents that involve the spleen in patients with normal immune status include histoplasmosis, tuberculosis, and echinococcosis [28]. These infectious agents are observed

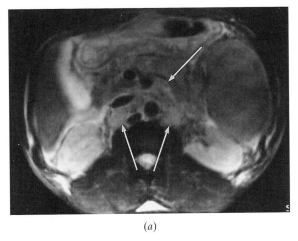

(a)

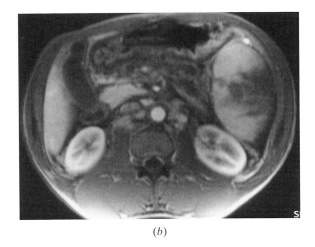

(b)

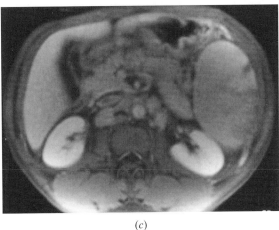

(c)

FIG. 5.19 Angioimmunoblastic lymphadenopathy with dysproteinemia. T2-weighted fat-suppressed spin-echo (*a*), immediate postgadolinium SGE (*b*), and 90-second postgadolinium fat-suppressed SGE (*c*) images. The spleen is noted to be markedly enlarged. Lymphadenopathy is moderately high in signal intensity on T2-weighted images and is conspicuous due to the suppression of fat signal intensity (*arrows, a*). Mild enhancement of lymph nodes is noted on immediate postgadolinium SGE (*b*). Lymph nodes enhance more intensely in the interstitial phase and are more clearly defined by the suppression of fat signal intensity. Splenic involvement is demonstrated by irregular, poorly marginated, large regions of diminished enhancement on the immediate postgadolinium image (*b*). Enhancement of the spleen is more uniform by 90 seconds after contrast (*c*), and signal intensity is mildly heterogeneous on the T2-weighted image (*a*).

in immunocompromised patients with an even greater frequency (Fig. 5.22). In the immunocompromised patient, the most common hepatosplenic infection is fungal infection with *Candida albicans* [29,30]. Patients with acute myelogeneous leukemia are at particular risk for developing this infection. Multiorgan involvement is common. The gastrointestinal tract is almost invariably involved, and although esophageal disease is well-shown on MR images, involvement of the intestines is frequently not visible. Esophageal candidiasis is common and rarely associated with hepatosplenic candidiasis, whereas small intestine candidiasis is more frequently associated with this infection. Lesions are most commonly observed in the spleen and liver, whereas renal disease is somewhat uncommon. MR images can demonstrate lesions in the acute phase, subacute treated phase, and chronic healed phase [29,31]. Lesions in each of these phases have distinctive MRI appearances. These varying appearances are more distinct for liver lesions. (For an in-depth discussion, see Chapter 2 on the Liver.) Acute lesions are generally more apparent in the spleen than in the liver, whereas the reverse is true for subacute-treated and chronic-healed lesions. In the acute phase, hepatosplenic candidiasis results in small (<1-cm) well-defined ab-

scesses in the spleen and liver. They are well-shown on T2-weighted fat-suppressed images as high-signal-intensity rounded foci (Fig. 5.23). Lesions also may be visible on postgadolinium images, but they usually are not visualized on precontrast SGE images. MRI has been shown to be superior to contrast-enhanced CT imaging for the detection of fungal microabscesses [29]. MRI should be used routinely in the investigation of hepatosplenic candidiasis because patient survival depends on swift pharmacologic intervention with antifungal agents.

The MRI appearance of bacterial (pyogenic) abscesses has not been well-described in the literature. Bacterial abscesses tend to be larger than fungal lesions, and due to the high protein content, they should be of mixed high signal intensity on T2-weighted images and should have substantial perilesional enhancement on gadolinium-enhanced images.

Sarcoidosis

Lesions of sarcoidosis are small (<1 cm) and hypovascular. Due to their hypovascularity, the lesions are low in signal intensity on T1- and T2-weighted images and enhance on gadolinium-enhanced images in a minimal and delayed fashion [32] (Fig. 5.24). Low signal intensity

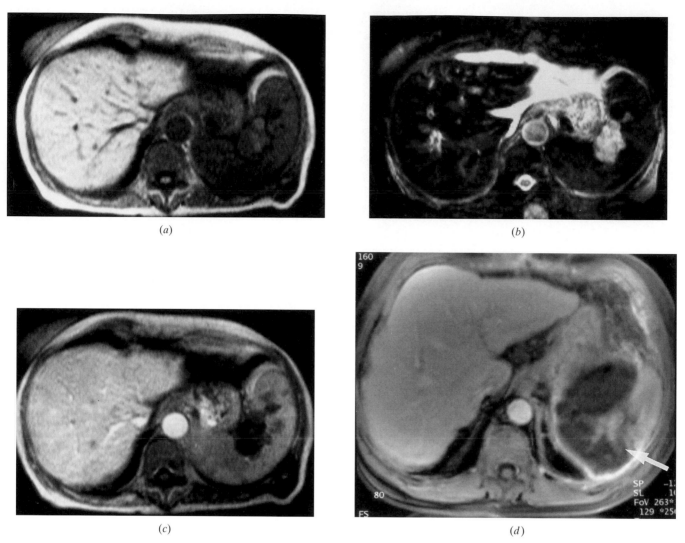

(a)

(b)

(c)

(d)

F IG . 5.20 Splenic metastases. SGE (*a*), T2-weighted fat-suppressed spin-echo (*b*) and immediate postgadolinium SGE (*c*) images in a woman with endometrial cancer. Metastases are noted throughout the spleen that are mixed hypointense and isointense on T1-weighted images (*a*), mixed isointense and hyperintense on T2-weighted images (*b*), and low in signal intensity on immediate postgadolinium images (*c*). Note that metastases are best shown on the immediate postgadolinium image. The largest metastasis is distinctly demonstrated on the T2-weighted image (*b*). However, the smaller lesions are poorly shown, despite the presence of iron deposition. Ascites is also present, and is low in signal intensity on pre- and postcontrast T1-weighted images and high in signal intensity on T2- weighted images. Transverse 90 second postgadolinium fat-suppressed SGE image (*d*) in a second patient demonstrates an expansile destructive lesion (*arrow, d*) in the posterior aspect of the spleen associated with a large subcapsular fluid collection.

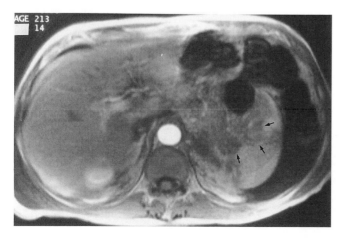

F IG . 5.21 Direct tumor invasion. Immediate postgadolinium SGE image demonstrates invasion of the splenic hilum by a large infiltrative pancreatic ductal adenocarcinoma (*arrows*).

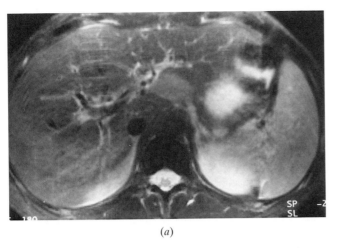

(a)

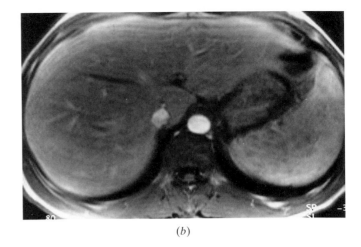

(b)

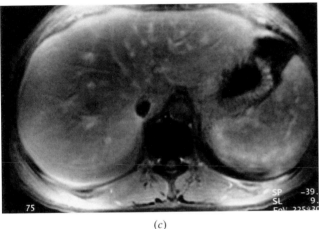

(c)

FIG. 5.22 Hepatosplenorenal histoplasmosis. T2-weighted fat-suppressed echo-train spin-echo (a), immediate postgadolinium SGE (b), and 90-second postgadolinium fat-suppressed SGE (c) images in a patient with human immunodeficiency virus (HIV) infection. Multiple lesions smaller than 1 cm are demonstrated in the liver, spleen, and kidneys. Lesions are poorly visualized on T2-weighted images as small minimally hyperintense lesions (a). On immediate postgadolinium images lesions appear low in signal intensity (b). By 90 seconds after gadolinium, lesions enhance more than background tissue (arrows, c)

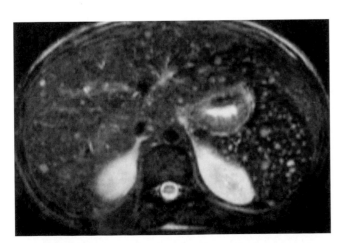

FIG. 5.23 Hepatosplenic candidiasis. T2-weighted fat-suppressed echo-train spin-echo image demonstrates multiple, well-defined, high-signal-intensity candidiasis abscesses smaller than 1 cm in the liver and spleen.

on T2-weighted images is a feature distinguishing between these lesions and acute infective lesions.

Gamna-Gandy Bodies

Foci of iron deposition occur commonly in patients with cirrhosis and portal hypertension due to microhemorrhages in the splenic parenchyma. On occasion, such foci are observed in patients receiving blood transfusions [33,34]. Lesions vary in size but are generally smaller than 1 cm. Lesions are signal-void on all pulse sequences [33,34] (Fig. 5.25). Susceptibility artifact is demonstrated on gradient-echo images as blooming artifact, and this artifact is pathognomonic for this entity.

Trauma

The spleen is the most commonly ruptured abdominal organ in the setting of trauma. Injury to the spleen may take several forms: subcapsular hematoma, contusion, laceration, and devascularization/infarct. Subcapsular or intraparenchymal hematoma secondary to contusion or laceration demonstrates a time course of changes in signal intensity due to the paramagnetic properties of the degradation products of hemoglobin. Subacute hemor-

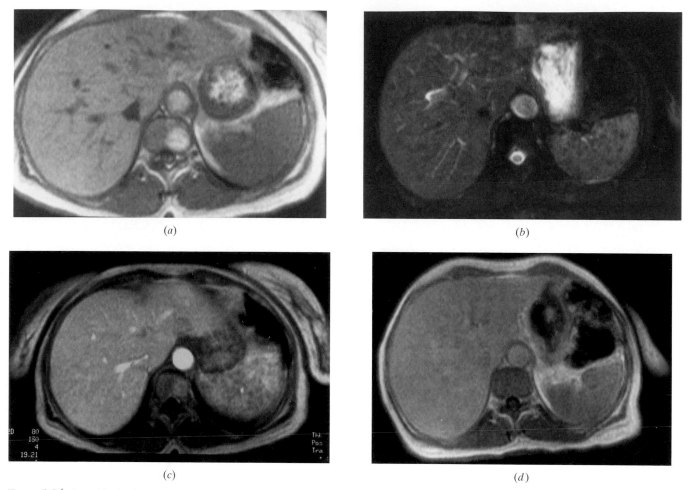

(a)

(b)

(c)

(d)

FIG. 5.24 Sarcoidosis. SGE (*a*), T2-weighted fat-suppressed spin-echo (*b*), immediate (*c*), and 10-minute (*d*) postgadolinium images. Multiple sarcoidosis granulomas smaller than 1 cm are present in the spleen. Lesions are mildly hypointense to isointense on T1-weighted images (*a*), moderately hypointense on T2-weighted images (*b*), and hypointense on immediate postgadolinium images (*c*), gradually enhancing to near isointensity on delayed postgadolinium images (*d*). Hypointensity on T2-weighted images distinguish these lesions from those of infectious etiologies. (Reproduced with permission from reference 32.)

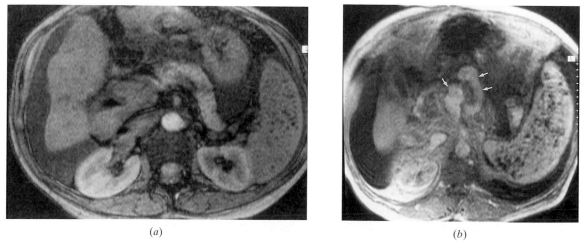

(a)

(b)

FIG. 5.25 Gamna-Gandy bodies of the spleen. Precontrast SGE image (*a*) in one patient and immediate postgadolinium SGE image (*b*) in a second patient. Both patients have cirrhosis with portal hypertension. Gamna-Gandy bodies are small signal-void foci that cause susceptibility artifact in the spleen. Note that both patients possess an irregular liver contour due to cirrhosis and have ascites due to portal hypertension. Varices are evident in the second patient on the immediate postgadolinium image (*arrows, b*).

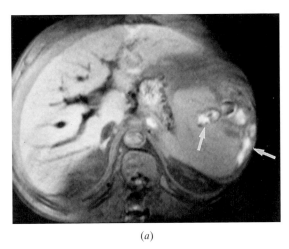

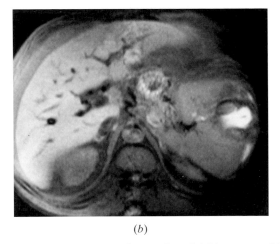

(a)   (b)

F I G . 5.26 Splenic laceration. T1-weighted fat-suppressed spin-echo images from adjacent cranial (*a*) and caudal (*b*) tomographic sections. Mixed, predominantly high-signal-intensity fluid is present in an intraparenchymal and subcapsular location (*arrows, a*) in the spleen, which represents subacute blood.

rhage is particularly conspicuous because of its distinctive high signal intensity on T1- and T2-weighted images (Fig. 5.26). Traumatic injury of the spleen, especially devascularization, is well-shown on immediate postgadolinium SGE images. Areas of devascularization are nearly signal-void compared to the high signal intensity of vascularized tissue.

Infarcts

Splenic infarcts are a common occurrence in the setting of arterial emboli. Infarcts appear as peripheral wedge-shaped defects that are most clearly defined on 1 to 5-minute postgadolinium images as low-signal-intensity regions (Fig. 5.27).

Subcapsular Fluid Collections

Multiple causes for subcapsular fluid collections exist, the most common being sequela to trauma. Enhancement

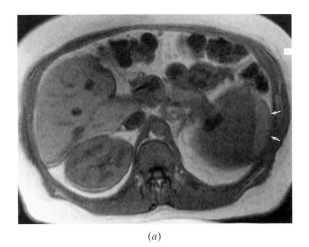

(a)

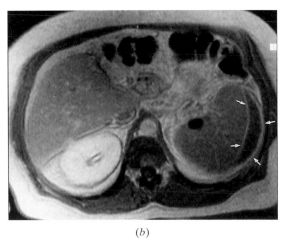

(b)

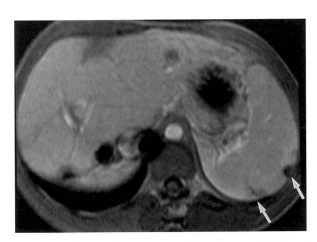

F I G . 5.27 Splenic infarcts. On the 1-minute postgadolinium image, peripheral wedge-shaped defects are noted in the spleen (*arrows*) secondary to infarcts.

F I G . 5.28 Subcapsular fluid collection secondary to pancreatitis. SGE (*a*) and 90-second postgadolinium SGE (*b*) images. A subcapsular fluid collection is present that is slightly high in signal intensity on the T1-weighted image, a finding consistent with the presence of blood or protein (*arrows, a*). Enhancement of the capsule and surface of the spleen on the postgadolinium image (*arrows, b*) confirms the subcapsular location of the fluid collection.

of the capsule and surface of the spleen may be observed on postgadolinium images, which confirms the location of these fluid collections (Fig. 5.28).

CONCLUSION

MRI of the spleen is a robust technique and surpasses CT imaging in many clinical settings. The major indication for MRI is the investigation of hepatosplenic candidiasis. Other circumstances in which MRI may be of value include the detection of malignant lesions (metastases or lymphoma), infections, and the characterization of lesions such as hemangiomas or hamartomas. MRI should be considered in patients with elevated serum creatinine or those with allergy to iodinated contrast material for the investigation of possible splenic disease. MRI is useful as further investigation of patients with splenomegaly demonstrated on CT images to determine if underlying tumor infiltration is present. The future of superparamagnetic iron oxide particles for evaluating the spleen will depend on their efficacy, cost, and patient tolerance, as well as their performance compared with dynamic gadolinium-enhanced MRI.

REFERENCES

1. Weiss L: The red pulp of the spleen: Structural basis of blood flow. Clin Haematol 12:375–393, 1983.
2. Mirowitz SA, Brown JJ, Lee JKT, Heiken JP: Dynamic gadolinium-enhanced MR imaging of the normal spleen: Normal enhancement patterns and evaluation of splenic lesions. Radiology 179:681–686, 1991.
3. Mirowitz SA, Gutierrez E, Lee JKT, Brown JJ, et al: Normal abdominal enhancement patterns with dynamic gadolinium-enhanced MR imaging. Radiology 180:637–640, 1991.
4. Semelka RC, Shoenut JP, Lawrence PH, Greenberg HM, Madden TP, Kroeker MA: Spleen: Dynamic enhancement patterns on gradient-echo MR images enhanced with gadopentetate dimeglumine. Radiology, 185:479–482, 1992.
5. Hamed MM, Hamm B, Ibrahim ME, Taupitz M, et al: Dynamic MR imaging of the abdomen with gadopentate dimeglumine: Normal enhancement patterns of liver, spleen, stomach, and pancreas. AJR Am J Roentgenol 158:303–307, 1992.
6. Siegelman ES, Mitchell DG, Rubin R, et al: Parenchymal versus reticuloendothelial iron overload in the liver: Distinction with MR imaging. Radiology 179:361–366, 1991.
7. Siegelman ES, Mitchel DG, Semelka RC: Abdominal iron deposition: Metabolism, MR findings, and clinical importance. Radiology 199:13–22, 1996.
8. Weissleder R, Hahn PF, Stark DD, Elizondo G, et al: Superparamagnetic iron oxide: Enhanced detection of focal splenic tumors with MR imaging. Radiology 169:399–403, 1988.
9. Weissleder R, Elizondo G, Stark DD, Hahn PF, et al: The diagnosis of splenic lymphoma by MR imaging: Value of superparamagnetic iron oxide. AJR Am J Roentgenol 152:175–180, 1989.
10. Kreft BP, Tanimoto A, Leffler S, Finn JP, Oksendal AN, Stark DD: Contrast-enhanced MR imaging of diffuse and focal splenic disease with use of magnetic starch microspheres. J Magn Reson Imaging 4:373–379, 1994.
11. Ambriz P, Munoz R, Quintanar E, Sigler L, et al: Accessory spleen compromising response to splenectomy for idiopathic thrombocytopenic purpura. Radiology 155:793–796, 1985.
12. Beahrs JR, Stephens DH: Enlarged accessory spleens: CT appearance in post splenectomy patients. AJR Am J Roentgenol 141:483–486, 1981.
13. Storm BL, Abbitt PL, Allen DA, Ros PR: Splenosis: Superparamagnetic iron oxide-enhanced MR imaging. AJR Am J Roentgenol 159:333–335, 1992.
14. Elliott LP: Summation of roentgenologic findings in entities presenting with cyanosis and decreased vascularity. In Elliot LP (ed.). Cardiac Imaging in Infants, Children, and Adults. New York: Lippincott, pp. 00, 1991.
15. Hill SC, Damaska BM, Ling A, Patterson K, et al: Gaucher disease: Abdominal MR imaging findings in 46 patients. Radiology 184:561–566, 1992.
16. Adler DD, Glazer GM, Aisen AM: MRI of the spleen: Normal appearance and findings in sickle-cell anemia. AJR Am J Roentgenol 147:843–845, 1986.
17. Urrutia M, Mergo PJ, Ros LH, Torres GM, Ros PR: Cystic masses of the spleen: Radiologic-pathologic correlation. Radiographics 16:107–129, 1996.
18. Shirkhoda A, Freeman J, Armin AR, Cacciarelli AA, Morden R: Imaging features of splenic epidermoid cyst with pathologic correlation. Abdom Imaging 20:449–451, 1995.
19. Disler DG, Chew FS: Splenic hemangioma. AJR Am J Roentgenol 157:44, 1991.
20. Ramani M, Reinhold C, Semelka RC, Siegelman ES, Liang L, Ascher SM, Brown JJ, Eisen RN, Bret PM. Splenic hemangiomas and hamartomas: MR imaging characteristics of 28 lesions. Radiology 202:166–172, 1997.
21. Ohtomo K, Fukuda H, Mori K, Minami M, et al: CT and MR appearances of splenic hamartoma. J Comput Assist Tomogr, 16:425–428, 1992.
22. Pinto PO, Avidago P, Garcia H, Aves FC, Marques C: Splenic hamartoma: a case report. Eur Radiol 5:93–95, 1995.
23. Bragg DG, Colby TV, Ward JH: New concepts in the non-Hodgkin lymphoma: Radiologic implications. Radiology 159:289–304, 1986.
24. Castellino RA: Hodgkin disease: Practical concepts for the diagnostic radiologist. Radiology 159:305–310, 1986.
25. Hahn PF, Weissleder R, Stark DD, et al: MR imaging of focal splenic tumors. AJR Am J Roentgenol 150:823–827, 1988.
26. Hirst AEJ, Bullock WJ: Metastatic carcinoma of the spleen. Am J Med Sci 223:414–417, 1952.
27. Rabushka LS, Kawashima A, Fishman EK: Imaging of the spleen: CT with supplemental MR examination. Radiographics 14:307–332, 1994.
28. Senturk H, Kocer N, Papila C, Uras C, Dogusoy G: Primary macronodular hepatosplenic tuberculosis: Two cases with US, CT, and MR findings. Eur Radiol 5:451–455, 1995.
29. Semelka RC, Shoenut JP, Greenberg HM, Bow EJ: Detection of acute and treated lesions of hepatosplenic candidiasis: Comparison of dynamic contrast-enhanced CT and MR imaging. J Magn Reson Imaging 2:341–345, 1992.
30. Cho J-S, Kim EE, Varma DGK, Wallace S: MR imaging of hepatosplenic candidiasis superimposed on hemochromatosis. J Comput Assist Tomogr 14:774–776, 1990.
31. Kelekis N, Semelka RC, Burdeny DA: Dark ring sign: Finding in patients with fungal liver lesions undergoing treatment with antifungal antibiotics. Magn Reson Imaging 14:615–618, 1996.
32. Warshauer DM, Semelka RC, Ascher SM: Nodular sarcoidosis of the liver and spleen: Appearance on MR images. J Magn Reson Imaging 4:553–557, 1994.
33. Sagoh T, Hoh K, Togashi K, et al: Gamna-Gandy bodies of the spleen: Evaluation with MR imaging. Radiology 172:685–687, 1989.
34. Minami M, Itai Y, Ohtomo K, et al. Siderotic nodules in the spleen: MR imaging of portal hypertension. Radiology 172:681–684, 1989.

CHAPTER 6

GASTROINTESTINAL TRACT

S. M. ASCHER, M.D., R. C. SEMELKA, M.D., AND N. L. KELEKIS, M.D.

The widespread availability of breath-hold SGE sequences, fat-suppressed T1-weighted sequences, and single-shot echo-train T2-weighted sequences, coupled with the use of intravenous gadolinium chelates, makes routine imaging of the gastrointestinal tract feasible. These techniques arrest bowel motion, remove competing high signal of intra-abdominal fat, expand the dynamic range of abdominal tissue signal intensities, decrease susceptibility artifacts, and distinguish between intraluminal bowel contents and bowel wall [1]. The role of oral contrast agents remains controversial.

Current applications of gastrointestinal MRI include (1) distinguishing type and severity of inflammatory bowel disease (IBD) [1–6]; (2) identifying enteric abscesses and fistulae [7,8]; (3) preoperative staging of malignant neoplasms, especially rectal carcinoma [5,9,10]; and (4) differentiating postoperative and radiation therapy changes from recurrent carcinoma [11–16].

■ THE ESOPHAGUS

NORMAL ANATOMY

The esophagus is composed of three layers: an inner circular muscle layer, an outer longitudinal muscle layer, and a squamous epithelial lining. The lack of a serosal surface explains the rapid spread of esophageal cancer into adjacent mediastinal fat. The esophagus lies posterior to the trachea in the neck. As it enters the thoracic inlet, the esophagus courses toward the left to reside in the posterior mediastinum. The esophagus then enters the abdomen via the diaphragmatic esophageal hiatus and lies immediately anterior to the aorta. The normal esophageal wall thickness is 3 mm. On tomographic images the esophagus tends to be collapsed, although a small amount of air in the lumen is not abnormal.

MRI TECHNIQUE

Techniques useful for MRI of the esophagus include fat saturation, gadolinium enhancement, and cardiac gating (Fig. 6.1). T1-weighted ECG-gated fat-suppressed spin-echo imaging performs adequately, particularly for imaging the esophagus posterior to the heart. The esophagus near the gastroesophageal junction may be well-visualized using spoiled gradient-echo (SGE) and fat-suppressed SGE pre- and postintravenous gadolinium administration. Some investigators have found the use of oral agents especially formulated for the esophagus, such as gadopentetate dimeglumine-barium paste, also to be beneficial [17].

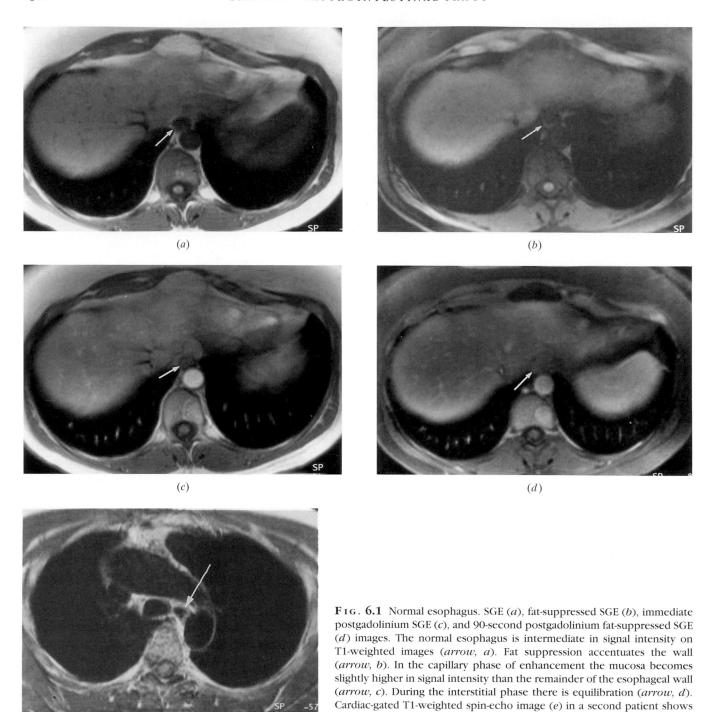

F IG . 6.1 Normal esophagus. SGE (*a*), fat-suppressed SGE (*b*), immediate postgadolinium SGE (*c*), and 90-second postgadolinium fat-suppressed SGE (*d*) images. The normal esophagus is intermediate in signal intensity on T1-weighted images (*arrow, a*). Fat suppression accentuates the wall (*arrow, b*). In the capillary phase of enhancement the mucosa becomes slightly higher in signal intensity than the remainder of the esophageal wall (*arrow, c*). During the interstitial phase there is equilibration (*arrow, d*). Cardiac-gated T1-weighted spin-echo image (*e*) in a second patient shows a small amount of air in the lumen of a normal esophagus (*arrow, e*).

CONGENITAL LESIONS

Duplication Cysts

Gastrointestinal duplication cysts may occur throughout the alimentary tube. The cysts occur in or adjacent to the wall of a portion of the gastrointestinal tract, and although they are lined by mucosa, it may not be the same as that of the involved segment. Duplication cysts usually are discovered in childhood or infancy if they cause mass effect and/or infection secondary to intestinal stasis when they communicate with bowel [18]. Alternatively, patients may present with peptic ulcers or pancreatitis if the cysts contain gastric or pancreatic mucosa, respectively. In the esophagus they tend to be small, ovoid, fluid-filled structures in the lower one-third of the esophagus. Cysts have variable signal intensity on T1-weighted images, depending on the concentration of mucin or protein within them. Duplication cysts are generally high in signal intensity on T2-weighted images [19]. The cyst wall enhances after intravenous gadolinium administration, whereas the fluid-filled lumen does not enhance and may appear to be signal-void. The degree of mucosal enhancement may assist the diagnosis: gastric mucosa enhances to a greater degree than other gastrointestinal tract mucosa.

MASS LESIONS

Benign Masses

Leiomyomas

Leiomyomas are the most common benign tumors of the esophagus and arise from the circular smooth muscle layer. They occur in the distal esophagus and may be single or multiple [20,21]. On MRI, esophageal leiomyomas present as small, oval masses and may be pedunculated. Leiomyomas typically enhance greater than adjacent bowel in a uniform manner (Fig. 6.2).

Varices

Varices develop in the setting of portal hypertension or splenic-vein thrombosis. They occur along the lower esophagus, the stomach, and other locations with portosystemic communications. Varices can be demonstrated as signal-void tubular structures on spin-echo images, high-signal-intensity structures on 2D time-of-flight (TOF) MR angiography (MRA), or enhancing serpiginous structures on dynamic 2D or 3D gadolinium-enhanced SGE or fat-suppressed SGE images (Fig. 6.3).

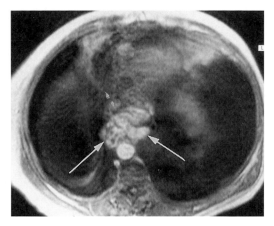

F I G. 6.3 Esophageal varices. Transverse 45-second postgadolinium SGE image in a patient with portal hypertension. Enhancing serpiginous tubular structures (*arrows*) in the lower esophagus are consistent with varices.

Malignant Masses

Squamous-cell carcinoma accounts for 95 percent of primary esophageal malignancies, with adenocarcinoma accounting for the remaining 5 percent.

The etiology of squamous-cell carcinoma is unknown, but there is an association with alcohol consumption and tobacco use [22]. It occurs more commonly in males (3 to 1) and African-Americans [23]. Primary adenocarcinoma of the esophagus may arise de novo in Barrett esophagus, or it may arise in the stomach and cross the gastroesophageal junction to involve the distal esophagus and simulate achalasia [24]. It is more common in Caucasian males. Tumors that commonly metastasize to the esophagus include breast and lung cancer and melanoma.

Gadolinium-enhanced fat-suppressed SGE technique delineates primary tumors of the distal esophagus well, whereas cardiac gating is necessary to image midesophageal cancers posterior to the heart (Fig. 6.4) [25]. Squamous-cell cancers (see Fig. 6.4) and adenocarcinomas (Fig. 6.5) appear similar on MR images. Predisposing factors or tumor location may aid in making this distinction. Some investigators have reported encouraging results with the addition of oral contrast agents [17]. The success of MRI in staging esophageal cancer varies. Moderate accuracies (75 to 100%) have been reported for detecting pericardial, aortic, and tracheobronchial invasion with conventional unenhanced spin-echo technique [26–29]. However, the detection of mediastinal extension and tumor-laden normal-sized lymph nodes, both of which occur early in the disease process, remain problematic. The combined use of fat suppression and intravenous gadolinium may improve identification of mediastinal involvement. The presence of multiple (i.e., >5) paraesophageal normal sized lymph nodes is worrisome for tumor involvement. A comprehensive exam for stag-

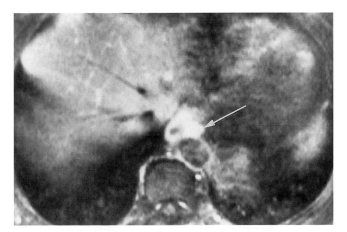

F I G. 6.2 Esophageal leiomyoma. Gadolinium-enhanced T1-weighted fat-suppressed spin-echo image shows a 2-cm leiomyoma (*arrow*) arising from the lateral aspect of the distal esophagus. Leiomyomas are the most common benign tumors of the esophagus. (Reprinted with permission from Shoenut JP, Semelka RC, Silverman R, Yaffe CS, Mickflikier AB: The gastrointestinal tract. In Semelka RC, Shoenut JP (eds.). MRI of the Abdomen with CT Correlation. New York: Raven Press, pp. 119–143, 1993)

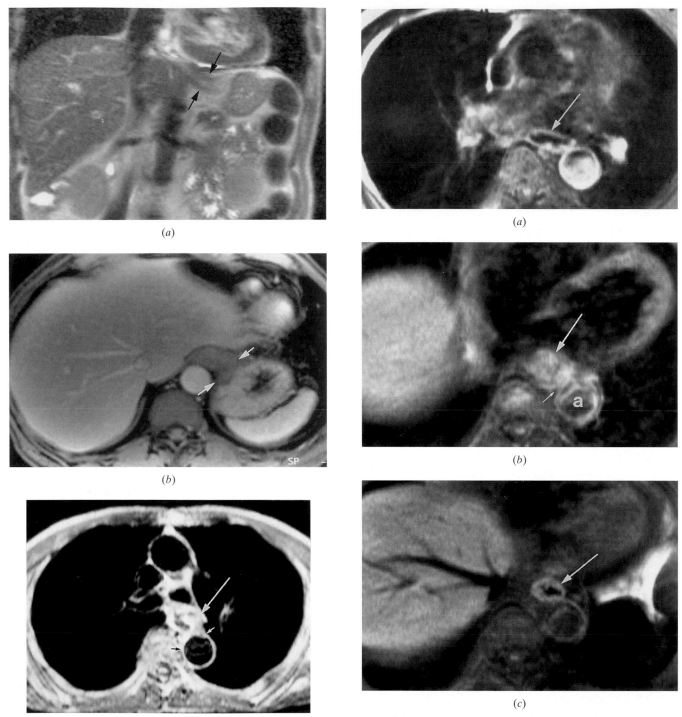

(a)

(b)

(c)

(a)

(b)

(c)

FIG. 6.4 Esophageal squamous-cell carcinoma. Coronal HASTE (a), and 45-second postgadolinium fat-suppressed SGE (b) images. Increased thickness of the distal esophagus is present on the precontrast image (arrows, a). The squamous-cell carcinoma of the distal esophagus is clearly defined, and tumor is shown to extend to the gastroesophageal junction (arrows, b). Lack of extension into the stomach is well-shown by demonstration of normal enhancing higher-signal gastric mucosa. Gadolinium-enhanced gated T1-weighted spin-echo image (c) in a second patient with squamous-cell carcinoma of the midesophagus. A 2 cm-cancer (arrow, c) is present that shows heterogeneous extension into the aortic wall (small arrows, c).

FIG. 6.5 Esophageal adenocarcinoma. Gadolinium-enhanced T1-weighted fat-suppressed (a,b) and T1-weighted fat-suppressed (c) spin-echo images in a patient with esophageal adenocarcinoma. Above the tumor at the level of the midthorax, the esophagus has a normal-appearing thin wall (arrow, a). More inferiorly at the level of the mitral valve, a 2.5-cm tumor (long arrow, b) is identified in the esophagus. Note the interface of the tumor with the descending aorta ("a",b) is less than 90° (short arrow, b). Below the tumor the esophagus once again has a normal thin wall (arrow, c). (Reprinted with permission from Shoenut JP, Semelka RC, Silverman R, Yaffe CS, Mickflikier AB: The gastrointestinal tract. In Semelka RC, Shoenut JP (eds.). MRI of the Abdomen with CT Correlation. New York: Raven Press, pp. 119–143, 1993)

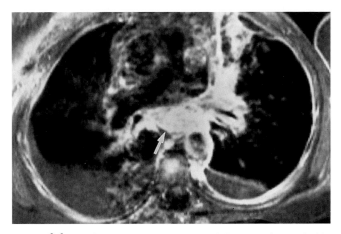

FIG. 6.6 Esophageal metastases. Gadolinium-enhanced T1-weighted fat-suppressed image in a woman with metastatic breast carcinoma. Enhancing tumor (*arrow*) encases the esophagus and extends along the left hilum and left mediastinum and invades the chest wall. (Reprinted with permission from Shoenut JP, Semelka RC, Silverman R, Yaffe CS, Mickflikier AB: The gastrointestinal tract. In Semelka RC, Shoenut JP (eds.). MRI of the Abdomen with CT Correlation. New York: Raven Press, pp. 119–143, 1993)

ing patients with esophageal carcinoma should include a metastatic survey of the liver. Metastases to the esophagus may be indistinguishable from a primary esophageal tumor; history helps to establish the diagnosis (Fig. 6.6).

INFLAMMATORY AND INFECTIOUS DISORDERS

Reflux Esophagitis
Twenty percent of the North American population experience reflux esophagitis ("heartburn"), and many seek medical attention [30,31]. The enormity of this problem is underscored by the recent boom in over-the-counter sales of antacids and H2-blockers. Reflux esophagitis may result from several disease entities and/or their treatments: hiatal hernia, achalasia, and scleroderma. Hiatal hernia is the most common condition predisposed to reflux esophagitis. (For a more complete discussion of hiatal hernia see Chapter 7 on the Peritonal Cavity.) Achalasia is a primary esophageal disorder. There is failure

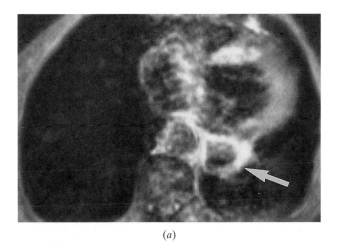

(*a*)

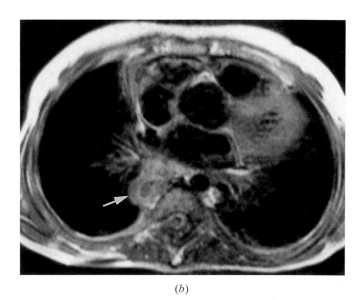

(*b*)

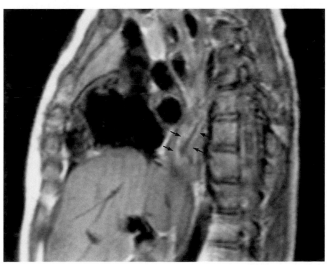

(*c*)

FIG. 6.7 Reflux esophagitis. Gadolinium-enhanced T1-weighted fat-suppressed spin-echo (*a*), gadolinium-enhanced gated transverse (*b*), and sagittal (*c*) T1-weighted spin-echo images in two different patients (*a*) and (*b,c*) with reflux esophagitis. In a patient with achalasia (*a*), balloon dilation for achalasia predisposes to reflux esophagitis. The esophagus appears dilated, and the wall is thickened with increased mural enhancement. The esophagus in a second patient with reflux esophagitis due to hiatal hernia shows increased thickness of the esophageal wall (*arrow, b*) and increased signal intensity of the mucosa. The superior extent of inflamed mucosa (*small arrows, c*) is well-shown on the sagittal image (*c*).

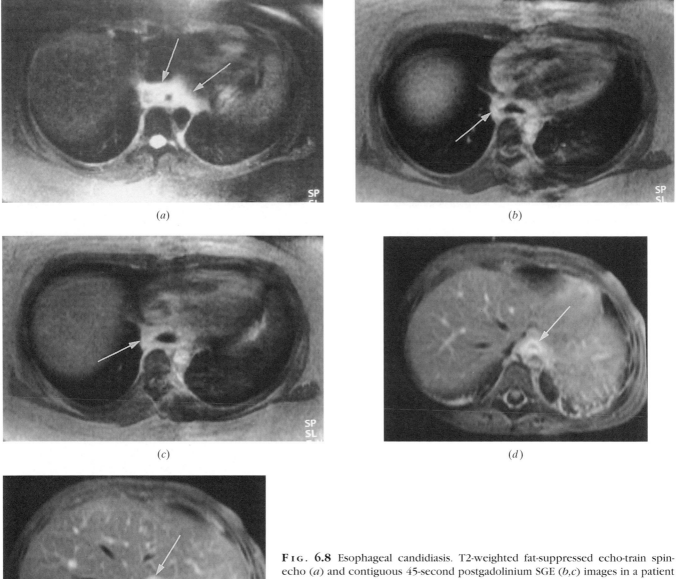

FIG. 6.8 Esophageal candidiasis. T2-weighted fat-suppressed echo-train spin-echo (*a*) and contiguous 45-second postgadolinium SGE (*b,c*) images in a patient with AIDS. The high signal intensity on the T2-weighted images reflects both the fungal plaques that coat the esophagus as well as the underlying inflamed wall (*arrows, a*). Following contrast, the thickened esophageal wall enhances (*arrow, b,c*). Gadolinium-enhanced T1-weighted fat-suppressed spin-echo images (*d,e*) in a second immunocompromised patient with acute myelogenous leukemia on chemotherapy. Capillary leakage associated with inflammation leads to marked mucosal enhancement (*arrow, d,e*) in this patient with *Candida albicans* esophageal invasion.

of relaxation of the lower esophageal sphincter (LES) coupled with nonperistaltic esophageal contractions. Balloon dilation of the LES is the mainstay of treatment and may lead to reflux esophagitis. When scleroderma involves the esophagus, the stomach and esophagus function as one cavity permitting substantial reflux of gastric contents. In all of these conditions, MRI demonstrates a thickened esophageal wall, and after the administration of gadolinium, the inflamed wall shows marked enhancement (Fig. 6.7).

Radiation Esophagitis

Patients undergoing radiation therapy are at risk of developing secondary esophageal changes. In the early period, 4 to 6 weeks after treatment, mucosal edema may be seen. Later, 6 to 8 months after treatment, strictures may develop.

Corrosive Esophagitis

Ingestion of caustic material produces esophagitis, which is most injurious after ingestion of strongly alkaline agents. These substances cause a liquefactive necrosis that penetrates the entire esophageal wall instantly. Acute changes include edema and ulceration. Stricture formation occurs later, and there is a strong association between corrosive stricture and the development of carcinoma.

Infectious Disease

Esophageal infection by *Candida albicans*, cytomegalovirus (CMV), and herpes simplex virus (HSV) is increasing. This reflects the large numbers of immunocompromised patients. Bone marrow transplant, chemotherapy, acquired immunodeficiency syndrome (AIDS), administration of exogenous steroids, and blood dyscrasias allow *Candida albicans*, a fungus that may be present normally in the esophagus, to invade it. Infection is diffuse with white-colored plaques coating the mucosa. The mucosa becomes friable and ulceration results. MRI demonstrates a high-signal-intensity thickened esophageal wall on T2-weighted images. Hyperemia and capillary leakage account for the marked enhancement after intravenous gadolinium injection (Fig. 6.8).

■ THE STOMACH

NORMAL ANATOMY

The stomach serves two important functions: it is a reservoir for ingested foods and a mixer for the mechanical and chemical breakdown of foodstuffs. Although the stomach is typically J-shaped and resides in the posterior aspect of the left upper quadrant, its position varies with degree of distention and body habitus. The stomach has four anatomic components: cardia, fundus, body, and antrum. The antrum ends at the pylorus, a narrow channel that connects the stomach to the duodenum. The stomach's curved morphology also gives rise to a greater (caudal) and lesser (cephalic) curvature in addition to anterior and posterior walls. Four distinct layers comprise the stomach: mucosa, submucosa, muscularis, and serosa. Subdivisions exist within each layer. The muscularis propria has three different muscle groups: inner oblique, middle circular, and outer longitudinal, and the mucosa is composed of distinct endocrine and exocrine cells.

MRI TECHNIQUE

Imaging the stomach requires optimal distention and arrest of respiratory motion and peristalsis. Some investigators have advocated the use of glucagon to accomplish these goals. However, up to 30 percent of patients may experience one or more side effects including nausea, diaphoresis, and hypotension [32]. Having patients fast prior to imaging can eliminate peristalsis but does not lead to adequate distention. Air has been used to expand the stomach, but at high field strengths this results in marked susceptibility artifact. For most purposes, water is an acceptable oral contrast agent.

A recommended imaging protocol includes (1) T1-weighted fat-suppressed SGE imaging before and after intravenous gadolinium, (2) unenhanced T1-weighted SGE imaging, and (3) single shot T2-weighted echo-train spin-echo (e.g., half-fourier single-shot turbo spin-echo (HASTE)) imaging (Fig. 6.9). The SGE and HASTE se-

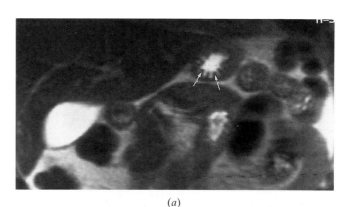

(a)

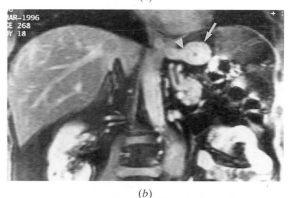

(b)

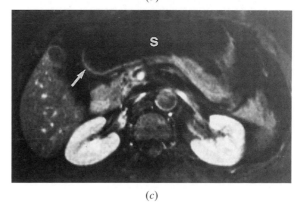

(c)

FIG. 6.9 Normal stomach. Coronal HASTE (*a*), coronal (*b*), and transverse (*c*) interstitial-phase gadolinium-enhanced fat-suppressed SGE images in three different patients with a normal stomach. HASTE is well-suited for imaging the rugal folds (*arrows, a*). Following intravenous contrast the stomach wall shows marked enhancement (*arrow, b,c*). The normal gastroesophageal junction (*arrowhead, b*) is frequently well-defined by imaging in transverse and coronal planes. Optimal stomach ("*s*",*c*) distention was obtained after ingestion of a negative oral contrast agent. Gastric distention can also be achieved with water.

quences benefit from gastric distention with water. Out-of-phase T1-weighted fat-suppressed SGE imaging is helpful for the evaluation of carcinoma. Gastric mucosa enhances more intensely than other bowel mucosa after intravenous gadolinium [33]. This observation may be exploited for diagnosing gastric mucosa-lined duplication cyst or Meckel's diverticulum.

CONGENITAL LESIONS

Congenital lesions of the stomach are rare, except for hypertrophic pyloric stenosis. The diagnosis is usually a clinical one with ultrasound reserved for equivocal cases. Gastric duplication cysts account for less than 4 percent of duplications of the gastrointestinal tract. They occur along the greater curvature and are more common in females. Occasionally, gastric duplication cysts calcify and in 15 percent the cysts communicate with the gastric lumen. Although gastric duplication cysts are uncommon, they are important to recognize because 35 percent of these patients will have other congenital anomalies [34]. Pancreatic rests occur throughout the alimentary tract, but are most common along the greater curvature or posterior antral wall of the stomach. They are submucosal in location, and half may have a small umbilication, a rudimentary ductal opening.

MASS LESIONS

Benign Masses

Polyps

Gastric polyps may be hyperplastic, adenomatous, or hamartomatous. They may be isolated findings or associated with a polyposis syndrome. Eighty percent of gastric polyps are hyperplastic and benign, whereas 20 percent are adenomatous. Of the latter group, approximately one-third contain a focus of adenocarcinoma [35]. Malignant potential is related to size: Up to 46 percent of adenomas larger than 2 cm harbor carcinoma [36]. Both hyperplastic and adenomatous polyps are found in patients with chronic atrophic gastritis and Gardner's and Familial polyposis syndromes, conditions associated with an increased incidence of malignancy. (For a more complete discussion on polyposis syndromes see the section on the Large Intestine later in this chapter.) Although most polyps are asymptomatic, anemia related to chronic blood loss, iron deficiency, or malabsorption of vitamin B_{12}, may be present. Hamartomas may be an incidental finding or can occur in patients with Peutz-Jeghers syndrome. Hamartomas have no malignant potential.

Benign polyps are masses that are isointense with the gastric wall on unenhanced MR images. Adequate distention of the stomach is mandatory in order to distinguish a polyp from a prominent rugal fold. Benign polyp enhancement is usually isointense to slightly hyperintense compared to normal gastric mucosa (Fig. 6.10). However, in polyps complicated by invasive adenocarcinoma, abnormal enhancement and disruption of the underlying gastric wall may be present.

Leiomyomas

Leiomyomas are the most common benign nonepithelial tumors of the stomach. They arise from the smooth muscle of the gastric wall. They may grow inward and mimic a polyp, or extend to the serosa and present as an exophytic mass. When large, the overlying gastric mucosa may ulcerate, leading to gastrointestinal bleeding. The other mesenchymal gastric wall elements also may give rise to benign neoplasms: fibromas, hemangiomas, lipomas, and neurogenic tumors. In the absence of ulceration these tumors are indistinguishable from each other on MRI, except for lipomas. Similar to fatty lesions elsewhere

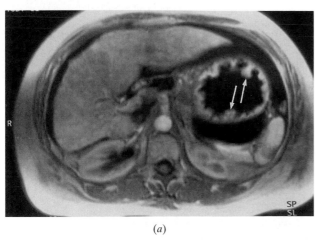
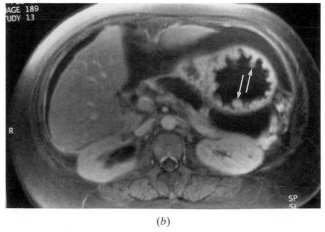

(a)   (b)

FIG. 6.10 Gastric polyps. Immediate postgadolinium SGE (*a*) and 90-second postgadolinium fat-suppressed SGE (*b*) images in a patient with Gardner's syndrome demonstrate multiple enhancing gastric polyps (*arrows, a,b*). The polyps possess intense enhancement.

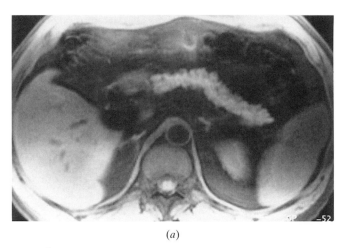
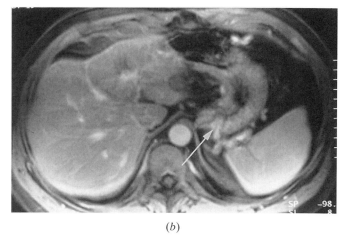

(a)   (b)

FIG. 6.11 Gastric varices. Fat-suppressed SGE (a) and 90-second postgadolinium fat-suppressed SGE (b) images. No splenic vein is identified posterior to the pancreas (a). Following intravenous gadolinium (b) administration, gastric varices enhance. These veins are part of the portosystemic circulation that is recruited to provide alternative venous channels in the presence of splenic vein thrombosis. A prominent varix is identified in the gastric wall (arrow, b).

in the body, lipomas will be high in signal intensity on T1-weighted images and decrease in signal intensity on fat-suppressed images.

Varices

Portal hypertension and splenic vein thrombosis lead to gastric varices. Varices restricted to the short gastric veins along the greater curvature of the stomach should raise the suspicion of splenic-vein thrombosis (Fig. 6.11).

Malignant Masses

Adenocarcinoma

The incidence of gastric adenocarcinoma is on the decline. At present, 22,800 Americans are diagnosed with gastric cancer each year [37]. Males are affected twice as often as females. Predisposing conditions include atrophic gastritis, pernicious anemia, adenomatous polyps, dietary nitrates, and being Japanese [38,39]. The tumors predilect the body and antrum and may be ulcerating, polypoid, or scirrhous. The scirrhous morphology spreads superficially to involve the entire organ, and the result is a rigid aperistaltic viscus referred to as *linitis plastica*. Gastric cancer may spread hematogenously to the liver and lung, contiguously to adjacent organs, lymphatically to regional and remote lymph nodes, and/or intraperitoneally to the abdominal lining, mesentery, and serosa. The overall prognosis is poor. A TNM system is used for staging (Table 6.1).

Early in the disease, symptoms are vague and include dyspepsia and anorexia preceding weight loss. Later, vomiting and hematemesis may occur in association with a palpable epigastric mass and anemia.

Table 6.1 TNM Staging for Cancer of the Stomach

T—Primary tumor

Tx	Primary tumor cannot be assessed
T0	No evidence of primary tumor
Tis	Preinvasive carcinoma (carcinoma in situ)
T1	Tumor limited to the mucosa or mucosa and submucosa regardless of extent and location
T2	Tumor with deep infiltration occupying not more than one-half of one region
T3	Tumor with deep infiltration occupying more than one-half but not more than of one region
T4	Tumor with deep infiltration occupying more than one-half but not more than one region or extending to neighboring structures

N—Regional lymph nodes

Nx	Regional lymph nodes cannot be assessed
N0	No evidence of regional lymph node metastasis
N1	Metastasis in lymph node(s) within 3 cm of the primary tumor along the greater or lesser curvatures
N2	Evidence of lymph node metastasis more than 3 cm from the primary tumor including those along the left gastric, splenic, celiac, and common hepatic arteries
N3	Evidence of involvement of the para-aortic and hepatoduodenal lymph nodes and/or other intra-abdominal lymph nodes

M—Metastases

Mx	Distant metastases cannot be assessed
M0	No distant metastases
M1	Distant metastases

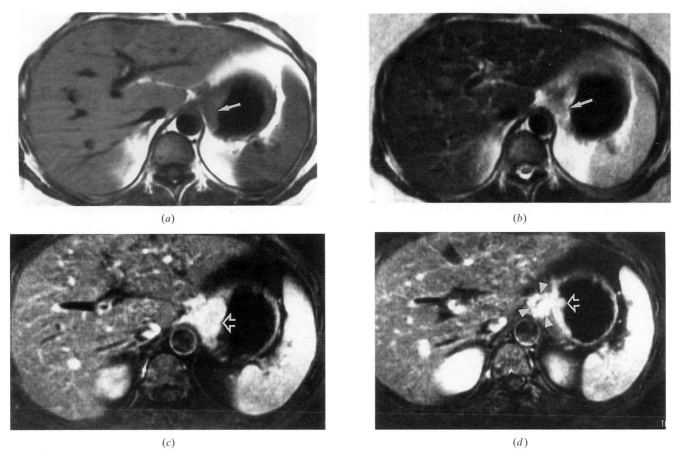

F I G . 6.12 Gastric adenocarcinoma, cardia. T1-weighted (*a*), T2-weighted (*b*), and gadolinium-enhanced T1-weighted fat-suppressed spin-echo (*c,d*) images in a patient with gastric cancer. The stomach has been distended with negative oral contrast agent. Gastric adenocarcinoma causes wall thickening medially, which is intermediate in signal intensity on the T1-weighted image (*arrow, a*) and heterogeneous and slightly hyperintense on the T2-weighted image (*arrow, b*). After intravenous gadolinium administration, the tumor (*open arrows, c,d*) enhances more than the normal stomach. The distal esophagus is also abnormally thickened with increased enhancement (*arrowheads, d*), which is consistent with spread across the gastroesophageal junction.

The goals of MRI in patients with gastric cancer is to demonstrate the primary tumor, assess the depth of invasion, and detect extra gastric disease. Adequate distention is necessary for surveying the gastric wall. On T1-weighted sequences, gastric adenocarcinoma is isointense to normal stomach and may be apparent as focal wall thickening. On T2-weighted images, tumors usually are slightly higher in signal intensity than adjacent normal stomach [40]. Tumors enhance heterogeneously after gadolinium administration, and often enhance greater than adjacent gastric mucosa. Tumors that originate in the cardia (Fig. 6.12), body, antrum (Fig. 6.13), and pylorus (Fig. 6.14) are all well-shown. Scirrhous carcinoma (linitis plastica) tends to be lower in signal intensity than normal adjacent stomach on T2-weighted images due to its desmoplastic nature. Linitis plastica enhances only modestly after intravenous contrast (Fig. 6.15). In contradistinction, the other morphologic types of gastric carcinoma enhance more intensely with intravenous gadolin-

ium. Gadolinium-enhanced fat-suppressed SGE imaging aids in identification of transmural spread. Gadolinium enhanced out-of-phase T1-weighted SGE imaging has been described for detecting extraserosal spread [41]. Irregularity or loss of the low-signal-intensity phase-cancellation band that normally surrounds the stomach implies extraserosal spread. However, if the stomach abuts other organs such as the liver, this phase-cancellation artifact will not be present, and tumor penetration using this approach cannot be established at these interfaces. In vitro work with resected gastric cancer specimens at high field strength has demonstrated mucosal, submucosal, and muscle invasion [40].

The metastatic workup for gastric adenocarcinoma includes a survey of the remainder of the abdomen and pelvis. Peritoneal implants and regional lymph nodes are best identified on gadolinium-enhanced fat-suppressed SGE images. The metastases enhance conspicuously against the background of low-signal-intensity fat. Detec-

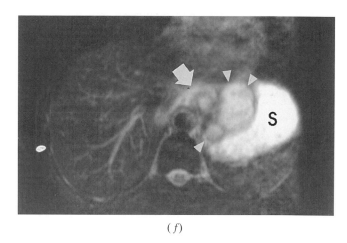

(e)

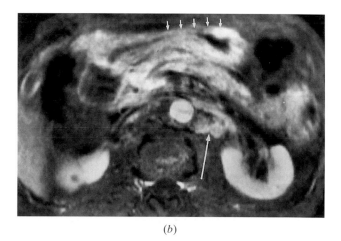

(f)

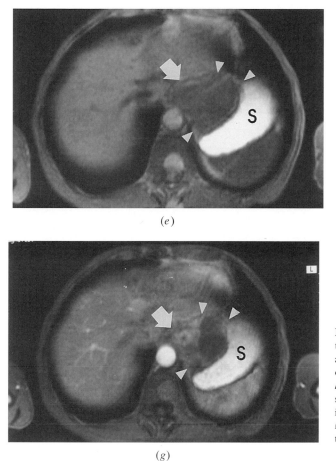

(g)

FIG. **6.12** (*Continued*) SGE (*e*), T2-weighted fat-suppressed echo-train spin-echo (*f*), and immediate postgadolinium SGE (*g*) images in a second patient. The stomach (*s,e,f,g*) has been distended with a positive oral contrast agent. A large tumor in the cardia of the stomach (*arrowheads, e,f,g*) causes mass effect upon the lumen. The cancer is low in signal intensity on the T1-weighted image (*e*), heterogeneous and high in signal intensity on the T2-weighted image (*f*), and enhances heterogeneously after intravenous contrast (*g*). Note that the tumor also involves the distal esophagus (*large arrow, e,f,g*).

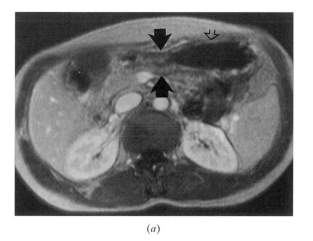

(a)

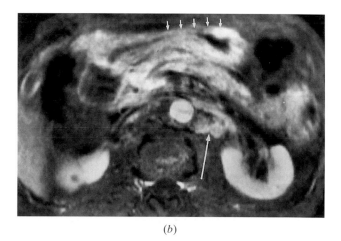

(b)

FIG. **6.13** Gastric adenocarcinoma, antrum. Transverse 45-second postgadolinium SGE image (*a*) demonstrates thickening and increased enhancement of the antrum secondary to gastric carcinoma (*solid arrows, a*). The remaining normal stomach has a thin wall (*open arrow, a*). Gadolinium-enhanced T1-weighted fat-suppressed spin-echo image (*b*) in a second patient shows circumferential involvement of the body and antrum of the stomach (*short arrows, b*). Enhancing left para-aortic lymphadenopathy is also present (*long arrow, b*).

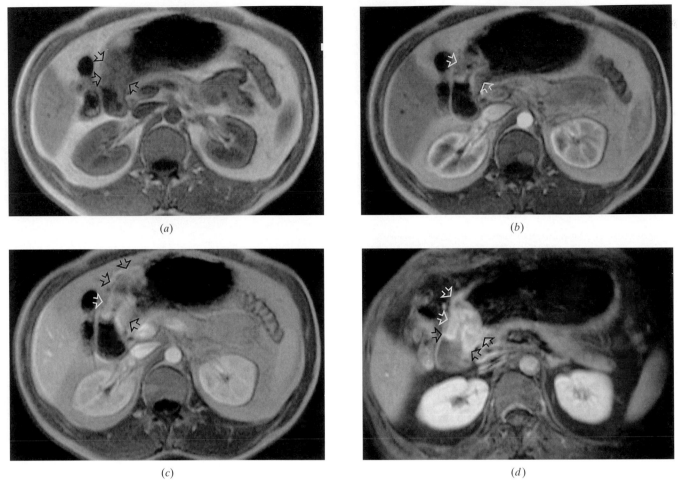

(a)   *(b)*

(c)   *(d)*

F IG. 6.14 Gastric adenocarcinoma, pylorus. SGE (*a*), 1-second (*b*), 45-second (*c*) postgadolinium SGE, and interstitial-phase gadolinium-enhanced T1-weighted fat-suppressed spin-echo (*d*) images. A circumferential pyloric channel adenocarcinoma with duodenal extension (*arrows, a–d*) is present. The tumor enhances heterogeneously (*b*) and increases in signal intensity on the 3-minute interstitial-phase image (*d*). This reflects accumulation of contrast in the interstitial space of the tumor.

tion of hepatic involvement is facilitated by T2-weighted fat-suppressed sequences and dynamic SGE techniques. This combined approach is superior to conventional CT imaging [42].

Leiomyosarcoma

Leiomyosarcomas are hypervascular neoplasms. They most commonly arise in the stomach where they differ from adenocarcinoma and lymphoma in that they have a large exophytic component. Central necrosis is common. Spread is via direct extension and hematogenous metastases. High-grade leiomyosarcomas are heterogeneous and high in signal on T2-weighted and gadolinium-enhanced fat-suppressed SGE images because of their increased vascularity (Fig. 6.16). During the capillary phase of imaging, they show marked enhancement that persists throughout the interstitial phase. The necrotic portions of the tumor remain signal-void on postcontrast images.

Dynamic contrast-enhanced T1-weighted imaging also detects hepatic metastases. The hypervascular lesions show early ring or uniform enhancement, which rapidly becomes isointense with normal hepatic parenchyma. Low-grade tumors enhance only minimally (Fig. 6.17).

Kaposi's Sarcoma

Kaposi's sarcoma usually is observed in patients with AIDS. It has both cutaneous and gastrointestinal manifestations. Although approximately 50 percent of patients with AIDS-related Kaposi's sarcoma will have gastrointestinal lesions at autopsy, most patients are asymptomatic. In rare instances, gastrointestinal Kaposi's sarcoma may cause obstruction, intussusception, or hemorrhage. The stomach is the most common site of gut involvement, but lesions may occur throughout the gastrointestinal tract. Kaposi's sarcoma should be considered in an AIDS patient who has gastrointestinal lesions in concert with

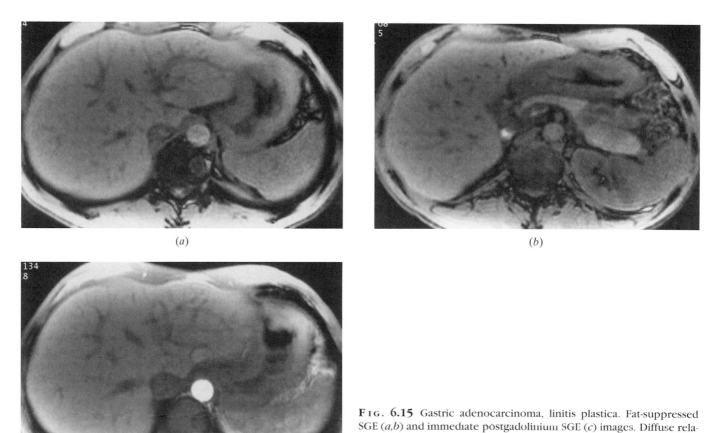

(a)

(b)

(c)

FIG. 6.15 Gastric adenocarcinoma, linitis plastica. Fat-suppressed SGE (*a,b*) and immediate postgadolinium SGE (*c*) images. Diffuse relatively homogeneous gastric wall thickening is present (*a,b*). Minimal enhancement is appreciated on the immediate postgadolinium SGE image (*c*).

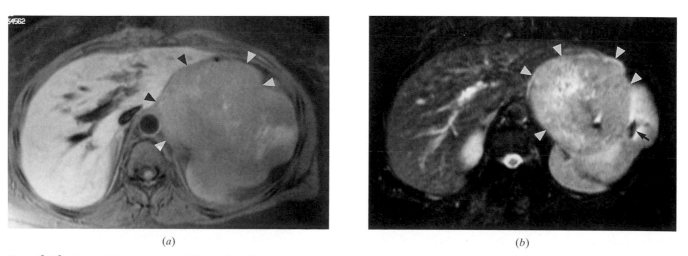

(a)

(b)

FIG. 6.16 Gastric leiomyosarcoma. T1-weighted fat-suppressed spin-echo (*a*), T2-weighted fat-suppressed spin-echo (*b*), 45-second postgadolinium SGE (*c*), and gadolinium-enhanced fat-suppressed spin-echo (*d*) images. A large exophytic gastric leiomyosarcoma arises from the lesser curvature (*arrowheads, a,b,c,d*) and is contiguous with the spleen. The tumor is heterogeneous and high in signal intensity on the T2-weighted image (*b*) and enhances intensely (*c,d*).

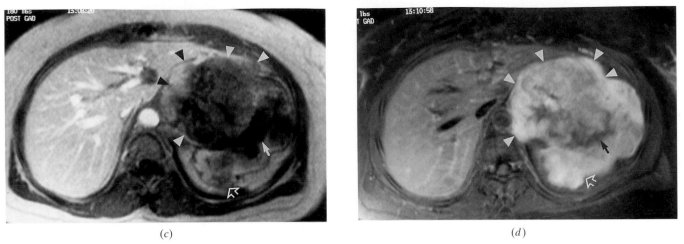

(c)   *(d)*

FIG. 6.16 (*Continued*) Enhancing tumor extends adjacent to the spleen (*open arrow, c,d*). Signal-void areas within the tumor are consistent with necrosis. Air within the lumen is also signal-void (*solid arrow, b,c,d*).

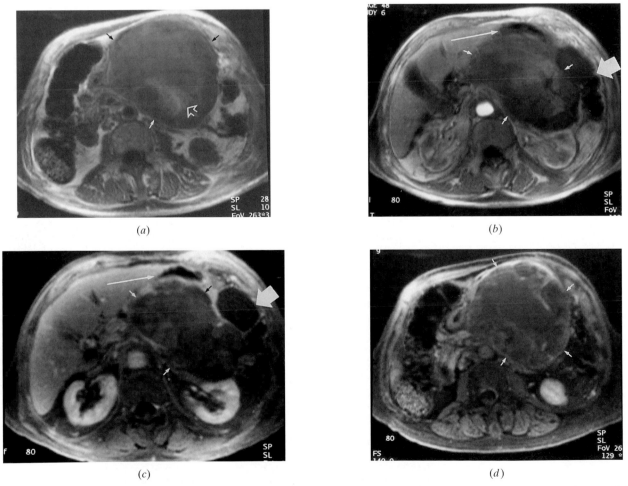

(a)   *(b)*

(c)   *(d)*

FIG. 6.17 Gastric leiomyosarcoma, low grade. Transverse SGE (*a*), immediate postgadolinium SGE (*b*), and 90-second postgadolinium fat-suppressed SGE (*c,d*) images in a low-grade leiomyosarcoma (*short arrows, a–d*). On the precontrast image, high signal within the tumor represents hemorrhage (*open arrow, a*). Low-grade leiomyosarcomas enhance minimally after intravenous contrast. The tumor causes mass effect upon the remaining stomach (*long arrow, b,c*) and the adjacent colon (*large arrow, b,c*).

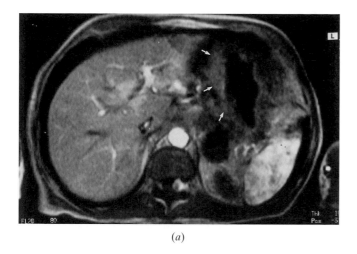

(a)

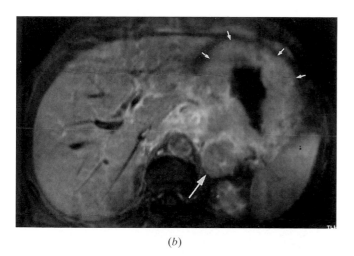

(b)

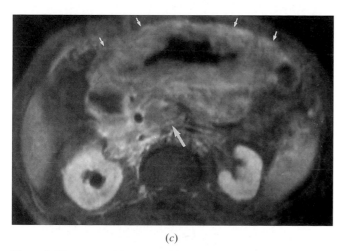

(c)

F I G . **6.18** Non-Hodgkin's lymphoma of the stomach. Immediate postgadolinium SGE (*a*) and gadolinium-enhanced T1-weighted fat-suppressed spin-echo (*b,c*) images. There is diffuse circumferential lymphomatous infiltration of the stomach wall (*short arrows, a,b,c*). Lymphoma extends to the left adrenal gland (*long arrow, b*). At a lower tomographic section, prominent retroperitoneal lymphadenopathy is present (*arrow, c*), which is commonly observed in the setting of gastric lymphoma.

bulky retroperitoneal lymphadenopathy, hepatic and splenic lesions, and infiltration of the psoas or abdominal wall [43].

Lymphoma

Primary gastric lymphoma is rare. Hodgkin's and non-Hodgkin's lymphomas are more commonly observed in the context of widespread disease. In fact, the stomach is the most common site of extranodal involvement in non-Hodgkin lymphoma. Infiltration of the gastric wall by tumor cells results in diffuse mural thickening [44,45]. Non-Hodgkin's lymphoma preserves gastric distensibility, whereas Hodgkin's lymphoma mimics scirrhous adenocarcinoma: a desmoplastic reaction predominates, leading to a noncompliant aperistaltic viscus. Diffuse gastric wall thickening is best seen on HASTE and gadolinium-enhanced fat-suppressed SGE images (Fig. 6.18). Involved regional lymph nodes also can be identified with these techniques.

Metastases

Metastases to the stomach occur by direct extension as well as by hematogenous or lymphatic spread. Specifically, colon carcinoma arising in the transverse colon invades the stomach via the gastrocolic ligament, whereas pancreatic carcinoma invades the posterior wall of the gastric body and antrum via the transverse mesocolon. Lung and breast carcinoma and melanoma are the most common primary malignancies that result in hematogenous gastric metastases (Fig. 6.19), although metastases from other malignancies may occur. Breast cancer metastases are noteworthy in that submucosal involvement may be indistinguishable from scirrhous carcinoma.

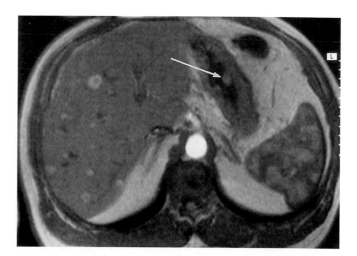

F I G . **6.19** Melanoma metastasis to the stomach. Immediate postgadolinium SGE image in a patient with metastatic melanoma. Malignant melanoma metastasizes hematogenously, and in this patient multiple liver metastases and a gastric metastasis (*long arrow*) are identified. The metastases are high in signal on this T1-weighted image due to the paramagnetic properties of melanin.

INFLAMMATORY AND INFECTIOUS DISORDERS

Ulcers

Benign gastric ulcers most commonly occur along the lesser curvature. Three types have been described. Type I ulcers are found in patients with normal or low gastric output and are associated with antral gastritis and *Helicobacter pylori* in gastric aspirate cultures. Type II ulcers occur in the prepyloric region and are associated with duodenal ulcers. Type III ulcers usually occur in the antrum and are found in patients taking nonsteroidal anti-inflammatory medications. Barium studies and endoscopy are still the mainstays of diagnosis.

Other inflammatory conditions that may involve the stomach include Crohn's disease, tuberculosis, and sarcoidosis. Hypertrophy of the rugal folds may be seen with AIDS-related hypertrophic gastritis, Zollinger-El-lison syndrome, and Menetrier disease [46]. The use of the HASTE technique coupled with adequate distention permits detection of rugal thickening. The hyperemia and capillary leakage that accompanies inflammation is highlighted on T1-weighted fat-suppressed SGE images: the inflamed tissue demonstrates early marked enhancement, which persists as the contrast pools in the interstitium (Fig. 6.20).

The Postoperative Stomach

A spectrum of surgical procedures involves the stomach. These procedures may be categorized as drainage with or without partial gastric resection, antireflux operations, gastroplasty, resection, and feeding gastrostomy. Familiarity with the exact surgical procedure performed aids radiologic investigation. The HASTE technique allows visualization of stomach changes following surgery, such as bowel anastamoses (Fig. 6.21).

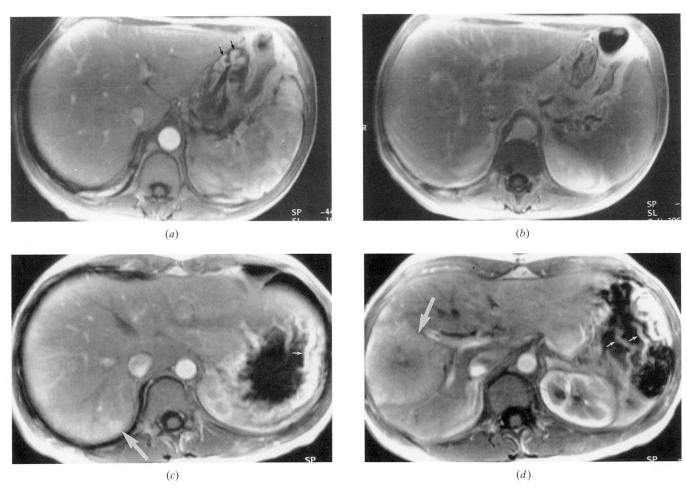

(a)

(b)

(c)

(d)

F IG . 6.20 Hypertrophic gastritis. Immediate (*a*) and 45-second (*b*) postgadolinium SGE images in a patient with AIDS. Thickening of the gastric rugae with marked mucosal enhancement (*arrows, a*) secondary to hypertrophic gastritis is present. Hypertrophic gastritis is not uncommon in patients with HIV infection. Immediate postgadolinium SGE images (*c,d*) in a second patient with Zollinger-Ellison syndrome. Intense enhancement and increased thickness of gastric rugae are appreciated (*small arrows, c,d*). Hypervascular liver metastases are also present (*large arrow, c,d*).

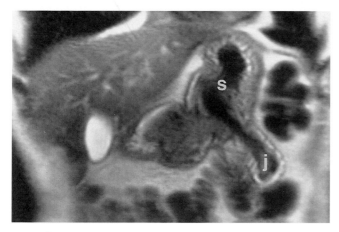

F I G. **6.21** Gastrojejunostomy. Coronal T2-weighted HASTE image shows the side-to-end anastomosis of the stomach (*s*) to the jejunum (*j*) in this patient status postgastrointestinal bypass surgery.

■ THE SMALL INTESTINE

NORMAL ANATOMY

The small bowel measures approximately 20 to 22 feet from the ligament of Treitz to the ileocecal valve. Its mucosal folds, termed *valvulae conniventes*, increase its surface area and aid digestion and resorption. The duodenum is in continuation with the pylorus. It extends in a C shape to curve around the pancreatic head to end at the duodenal-jejunal flexure. The duodenum is divided into four parts: bulb and descending, horizontal, and ascending segments. The bulb is the only intraperitoneal portion of the duodenum and is the most mobile. The second portion is in close proximity to the head of the pancreas, and both the pancreatic and common bile duct enter its posteromedial aspect. The mesenteric small intestine begins at the jejunum. The jejunum occupies the superior and left abdomen, whereas the ileum occupies the inferior and right abdomen. Their mesenteric attachment gives rise to two distinct borders: the concave or mesenteric border and the convex or antimesenteric border. In addition to differences in location, the ileum has a narrower lumen with fewer mucosal folds and a greater number of mesenteric arcades. Normal bowel wall thickness should not exceed 3 or 4 mm.

MRI TECHNIQUE

Previously, MRI had a limited role in assessing the small bowel because of poor intrinsic contrast resolution and motion artifacts caused by peristalsis. Several oral contrast agents that improve contrast resolution are commercially available for bowel opacification, and they are dis-

cussed at the end of this chapter. The combination of breathing-independent HASTE images and pre- and post-contrast fat-suppressed SGE images is an effective approach for imaging the bowel (Fig. 6.22). Fasting at least 5 hours prior to the exam or an antiperistaltic drug will decrease blurring artifact. Ingested water coupled with the HASTE technique provides high-quality images of the small bowel (see Fig. 6.22). Images should be obtained in the axial and coronal planes. Unenhanced SGE images with and without fat suppression followed by gadolinium-enhanced T1-weighted fat-suppressed SGE images are necessary for a comprehensive exam. Normal bowel on unenhanced images has a feathery appearance because of the valvulae conniventes, and after intravenous gadolinium enhances in a moderate and uniform fashion (see Fig. 6.22). Small bowel enhances less than the gastric wall (see Fig. 6.22). The administration of intravenous gadolinium permits evaluation of the bowel wall and assessment of lymphadenopathy, associated peritoneal disease, and accompaning fistula if present.

CONGENITAL LESIONS

Malrotation

Malrotation is a spectrum of conditions resulting from the failure of the duodenojejunal and cecocolic segments to rotate and become fixed. The most common form, nonrotation, is readily apparent on tomographic images, demonstrated by the lack of passage of the third and fourth part of the duodenum anterior to the aorta. The other types of malrotation occur less frequently and include incomplete rotation, reversed rotation, and anomalous fixation or fusion of the mesenteries.

Diverticulum

Small bowel diverticula may occur commonly in the duodenum. Multiple small bowel diverticula may be associated with intestinal bacterial overgrowth and resultant metabolic complications. Diverticula may be demonstrated on MR images as air or air fluid-containing structures that arise from the bowel (Fig. 6.23). Change in size of the diverticulum may be observed between sequences in an MRI examination reflecting contraction and expansion.

Meckel's Diverticulum

A Meckel's diverticulum is a remnant of the omphalomesenteric duct (vitelline duct). Normally, this duct is obliterated by the fifth week of gestation. Meckel's diverticulum is common with a prevalence of about 2 percent in the general population. It occurs within 25 cm of the ileocecal valve along the antimesenteric border. Most patients with Meckel's diverticulum are asymptomatic. If the diverticulum contains gastric mucosa, ulceration and bleeding

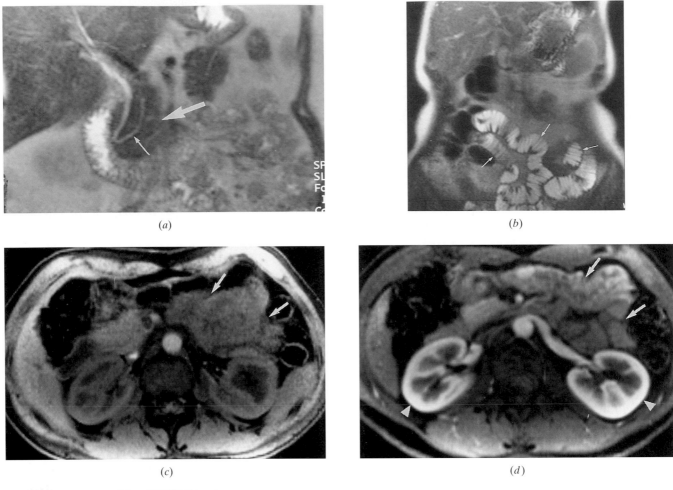

(a)

(b)

(c)

(d)

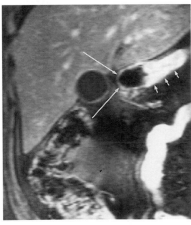

(e)

FIG. 6.22 Normal small bowel. Coronal HASTE (*a,b*) images of the normal small intestine in two different patients. The valvulae conniventes of the C loop of the duodenum (*a*) and of multiple loops of jejunum and ileum are well-shown as low-signal-intensity bands on the HASTE image (*arrows, b*) and stand out in relief against the high-signal-intensity intraluminal contents and moderately high-signal-intensity fat. Normal head of pancreas (*large arrow, a*), and common bile duct (*thin arrow, a*) are demonstrated. Fat-suppressed SGE (*c*) and immediate postgadolinium T1-weighted fat-suppressed SGE (*d*) images in a third patient with normal small bowel. On the precontrast fat-suppressed SGE image (*b*), the normal small bowel has a feathery appearance (*arrows, b*). Immediately after intravenous contrast the walls of the small intestine (*arrows, c*) show modest enhancement. In contradistinction, the renal cortex shows marked enhancement (*arrowheads, c*). The renal cortex can be used as an internal standard to judge the severity of inflammatory bowel disease because severe disease enhances comparably to renal cortex. Coronal 90-second postgadolinium fat-suppressed SGE image (*e*) in a fourth patient demonstrates the pyloroduodenal junction. The collapsed pylorus (*short arrows*) and air-filled duodenal bulb (*long arrows*) enhance after intravenous gadolinium.

may result. Alternatively, intussusception and inflammation may occur irrespective of the type of the mucosa present. The mainstay of diagnosis has been 99m Tc-pertechnetate scintigraphy and enteroclysis. MRI, like scintigraphy, exploits the presence of gastric mucosa in making the diagnosis. Because gastric mucosa enhances more than any other segment of bowel, a gastric-lined

Meckel's diverticulum will demonstrate marked enhancement on immediate (capillary-phase) and interstitial-phase postgadolinium images (Fig. 6.24) [47,48].

Atresia and Stenosis
Congenital atresia and stenosis are the result of intestinal ischemia in utero. They occur with equal frequency in the

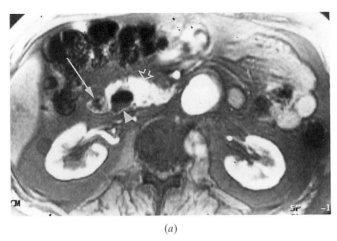 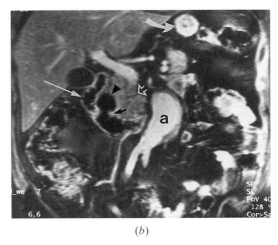

(a)   *(b)*

FIG. 6.23 Duodenal diverticulum. Transverse immediate (*a*), and coronal 90-second (*b*) postgadolinium fat-suppressed SGE images. An air and fluid containing diverticulum (*arrowhead, a,b*) is interposed between the duodenum (*long arrow, a,b*) and the head of the pancreas (*open arrow, a,b*). On the coronal image, a neck (*short arrow, b*) connecting the diverticulum to the duodenum is well-shown, which confirms that the lesion represents a diverticulum and not a cystic mass in the head of the pancreas. Duodenal diverticula are common and usually incidental findings. The normal gastric wall (*curved arrow, b*) enhances more intensely than normal small bowel. An abdominal aortic aneurysm ("*a*",*a,b*) is also present.

jejunum and ileum and less commonly in the duodenum. Twenty-five percent of cases will have a synchronous gastrointestinal anomaly. Barium studies are the most common means of diagnosis, although T2-weighted HASTE images can highlight the atretic/stenotic segment and proximal obstruction (Fig. 6.25).

Choledochocele
Choledochocele is a congenital anomaly characterized by cystic dilation of the distal common bile duct in the region of the papilla. Clinically, it may be associated with

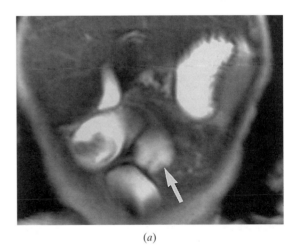

(a)

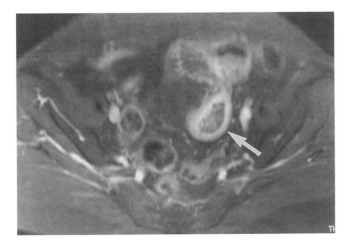

FIG. 6.24 Meckel's diverticulum. Gadolinium-enhanced T1-weighted fat-suppressed spin-echo image in a patient with lower gastrointestinal bleeding. A teardrop-shaped Meckel's diverticulum (*arrow*) extends from a loop of mildly dilated ileum. The inner wall of the diverticulum enhances to a greater extent than adjacent small bowel and colon. This allows detection of the diverticulum, and the degree of enhancement is consistent with the presence of gastric mucosa.

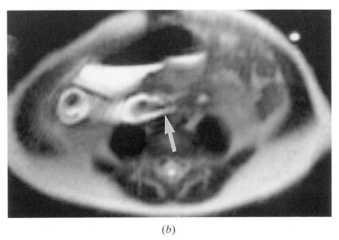

(b)

FIG. 6.25 Congenital stenosis, duodenum. Coronal (*a*) and transverse (*b*) HASTE images. The coronal image demonstrates dilation of the third part of the duodenum (*arrow, a*). The duodenum is noted to narrow (*arrow, b*) at the crossing of the superior mesenteric artery on the transverse image (*b*).

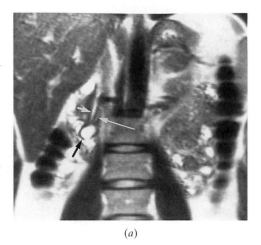

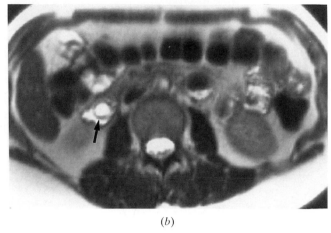

(a)   (b)

FIG. 6.26 Choledochocele. Coronal (a), and transverse (b) HASTE images in a patient with recurrent bouts of pancreatitis. A high-signal-intensity choledochocele (*black arrow, a,b*) protrudes into the duodenum. The HASTE image clearly defines the cystic nature of the lesion, which excludes an ampullary tumor, and demonstrates the relationship to the common bile duct (*small arrow, a*) and the pancreatic duct (*long arrow, a*).

abdominal pain, bleeding, jaundice, and pancreatitis. The diverticulum can contain calculi. On imaging examinations these may appear as polypoid masses indistinguishable from papillary edema or carcinoma. When large enough, they can protrude into the duodenum and even occlude it. MR cholangiopancreatography (MRCP) (see Chapter 3 on the Gallbladder and Biliary System) and HASTE images facilitate establishing the correct diagnosis (Fig. 6.26).

MASS LESIONS

Benign Masses

Polyps
Benign polyps are infrequently symptomatic and are usually incidental findings at autopsy. Clinically evident polyps present with pain, obstruction, or bleeding. Polyps are the most common lead points for intussusception in adults. Adenomatous polyps account for approximately 25 percent of small bowel tumors and may be tubular or villous. Isolated small bowel adenoma predilects the ileum. However, multiple duodenal adenomas predominate in the setting of Gardner's and Familial polyposis syndromes. Small bowel hamartomas occur commonly in Peutz-Jeghers syndrome and rarely in juvenile polyposis syndromes.

Similar to polyps elsewhere in the gastrointestinal tract, small bowel polyps appear as enhancing masses on gadolinium-enhanced fat-suppressed SGE images (Fig. 6.27). On HASTE images polyps appear as rounded low-signal-intensity masses (see Fig. 6.27). The polyps originate from the wall of a small bowel segment and protrude into the lumen. Although it may not be possible to exclude a focus of carcinoma within the polyp, extraserosal extension of a polyp is compatible with malignant degeneration.

Leiomyomas
The frequency of small bowel leiomyoma is comparable to that of adenoma. Leiomyomas are smooth-muscle lesions that originate in the submucosa or subserosa. Depending on their location, they may protrude into the lumen or produce a mass effect on adjacent bowel. They are usually solitary lesions. As leiomyomas enlarge, they undergo central necrosis and bleeding. On MRI the submucosal lesions may be indistinguishable from polyps. Uniform enhancement greater than that of adjacent bowel is observed on postgadolinium images (Fig. 6.28).

Lipomas
These fatty tumors are found preferentially in the duodenum or ileum. Like leiomyomas, they may ulcerate and bleed. Lipomas are high in signal intensity on T1-weighted images and will have signal intensity comparable to intra-abdominal fat on T2-weighted images. On T1-weighted fat-suppressed images these lesions will show a characteristic loss of signal intensity.

Varices
Duodenal varices may be seen in isolation or in conjunction with portal vein obstruction. They may be life-threatening when actively bleeding, but they are amenable to sclerotherapy. SGE or fat-suppressed SGE images obtained between 30 and 90 seconds after gadolinium demonstrate the varices as thin tubular structures within the bowel wall (Fig. 6.29).

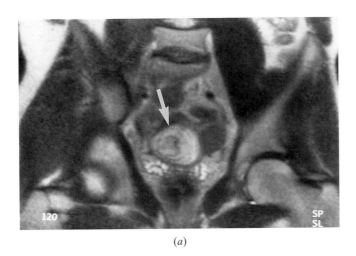

(a)

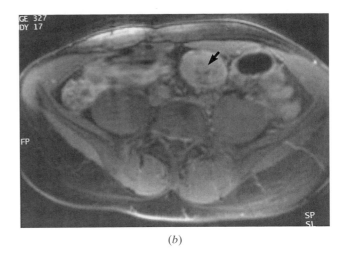

(b)

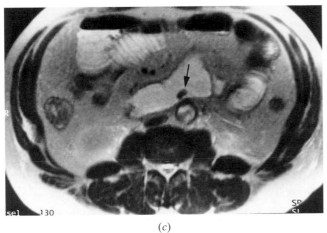

(c)

FIG. 6.27 Small bowel polyps. HASTE (*a*) and gadolinium-enhanced fat-suppressed SGE (*b*) images of a hamartoma in Peutz-Jeghers syndrome. A bowel-within-bowel appearance (*arrow, a*) is identified on the HASTE image (*a*) in the proximal jejunum due to intussusception. The intussusception is caused by a hamartomatous polyp that has acted as a lead point. The hamartoma is shown as a 1-cm uniformly enhancing mass (*arrow, b*) on the gadolinium-enhanced fat-suppressed SGE image (*b*). HASTE image (*c*) in a second patient demonstrates a 1-cm polyp (*arrow, c*) within a slightly dilated loop of duodenum.

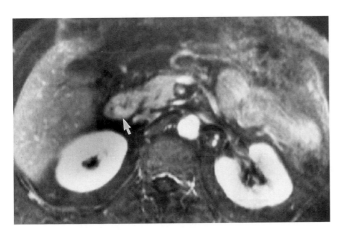

FIG. 6.28 Duodenal leiomyoma. Gadolinium-enhanced T1-weighted fat-suppressed spin-echo image shows a uniformly enhancing mass (*arrow*) protruding into the duodenum. When intraluminal, leiomyomas are indistinguishable from polyps. (Reprinted with permission from Shoenut JP, Semelka RC, Silverman R, Yaffe CS, Mickflikier AB: The gastrointestinal tract. In Semelka RC, Shoenut JP (eds.). MRI of the Abdomen with CT Correlation. New York: Raven Press, pp. 119–143, 1993)

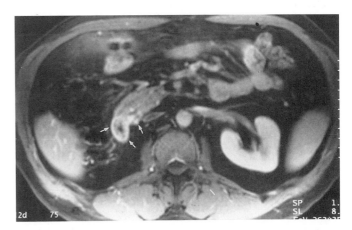

FIG. 6.29 Periduodenal and duodenal varices. Transverse 90-second postgadolinium fat-suppressed SGE image in a patient with splenic vein thrombosis. Periduodenal and duodenal varices are clearly shown as thin enhancing tubular structures adjacent to and within the wall of the duodenum. Venous blood is rerouted to periduodenal and duodenal varices as one of the collateral pathways in the setting of splenic vein thrombosis.

Malignant Masses

Adenocarcinomas

Small bowel tumors account for only 1 percent of all gastrointestinal malignancies, and half are adenocarcinomas [28]. The most common site for small bowel adenocarcinoma is the duodenum. This tumor frequently occurs in close proximity to the ampulla and as a result may cause obstructive jaundice [49]. Other symptoms, regardless of location, include intestinal obstruction, chronic blood loss, or both. Patients usually are asymptomatic early in the course of their disease. Hence presentation is often late with advanced disease [28]. MRI has played only an ancillary role in the evaluation of small bowel tumors. The combined use of HASTE and gadolinium-enhanced fat-suppressed SGE imaging has resulted in reproducible high image quality for the evaluation of small bowel neoplasms, which may increase the role of MRI [50]. Duodenal neoplasms are particularly well-shown due to the relatively fixed position of the duodenum in the anterior pararenal space. Tumors enhance in a heterogeneous moderate fashion on interstitial-phase gadolinium-enhanced images (Fig. 6.30). HASTE images provide information about the tumor itself and can be performed simultaneously as on a MR cholangiopancreatogram to evaluate the biliary tree. Dynamic gadolinium-enhanced SGE images also may be used to survey the liver for metastatic disease, whereas delayed postcontrast fat-suppressed SGE images may be obtained to determine the presence of lymphadenopathy and intraperitoneal spread.

Leiomyosarcomas

The ileum is the second most common site in the gastrointestinal tract for leiomyosarcomas. As in the stomach, these tumors tend to be large and ulcerating. Gadolinium-enhanced SGE or fat-suppressed SGE images demonstrate heterogeneous and substantial enhancement of the primary tumor (Fig. 6.31). Local or intraperitoneal recurrence is not uncommon after surgical resection (Fig. 6.32). MRI is particularly effective at detecting liver metastases because these tend to be hypervascular and often are small.

Lymphomas

Primary small intestinal lymphomas arise from mural lymphoid tissue. The terminal ileum is the most common

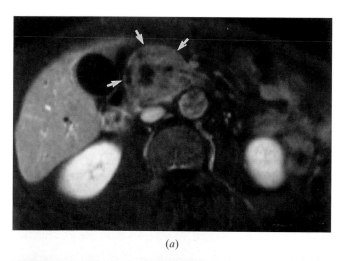

(a)

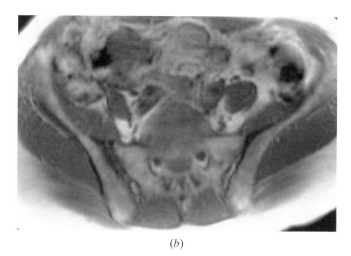

(b)

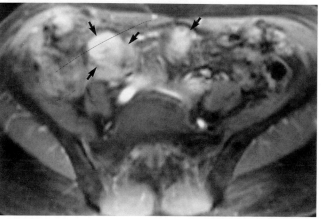

(c)

FIG. 6.30 Small bowel adenocarcinoma. Gadolinium-enhanced T1-weighted fat-suppressed spin-echo (a), SGE (b), and postgadolinium T1-weighted fat-suppressed spin-echo (c) images in two different patients (a) and (b,c) with small bowel adenocarcinoma. In the first patient (a) the size and extent of a large duodenal tumor (arrows, a) is well-shown on the gadolinium-enhanced fat-suppressed image. In the second patient (b,c), the neoplasm is difficult to identify on the precontrast SGE image (b) because it is isointense with background bowel. On the gadolinium-enhanced fat-suppressed SGE image (c), the distal jejunal tumors are conspicuous (arrows, c) because they are higher in signal intensity and heterogeneous compared to background bowel.

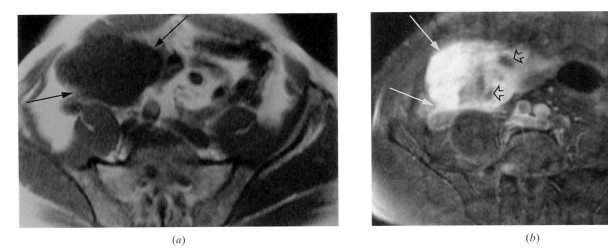

(a)   (b)

F IG. 6.31 Small intestine leiomyosarcoma. SGE (*a*) and gadolinium-enhanced T1-weighted fat-suppressed spin-echo (*b*) images. A large exophytic mass (*arrows, a*) arises from the ileum. Lack of proximal bowel obstruction is consistent with its eccentric origin. The tumor's large size coupled with intense enhancement (*arrows, b*) and regions of necrosis (*open arrows, b*) are typical features of leiomyosarcomas.

site affected, which reflects the relatively greater amount of lymphoid tissue present in this segment compared to the duodenum and jejunum [51]. The most frequent histologies to involve the small bowel are poorly differen-

tiated lymphocytic and diffuse histiocytic lymphomas [52]. Different morphologic types of small intestine lymphoma are recognized: polypoid, infiltrating, and exoenteric. The exophytic component of the exoenteric

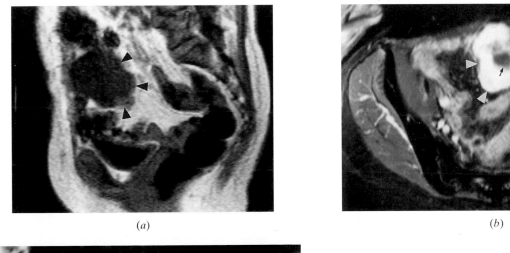

(a)   (b)

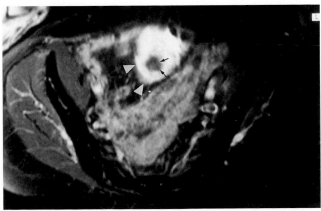

(c)

F IG. 6.32 Recurrent small intestine leiomyosarcoma. Sagittal SGE (*a*) and gadolinium-enhanced T1-weighted fat-suppressed spin-echo (*b,c*) images in a patient with previous surgical resection for leiomyosarcoma. Recurrent leiomyosarcoma exhibits features similar to those of the primary tumor: large size, exophytic growth, hypervascularity, and central necrosis. The eccentric location of the tumor (*arrowheads, a–c*) is seen on all imaging planes. Marked enhancement following intravenous contrast reflects hypervascularity. Necrosis often accompanies these large tumors (*short arrows, b,c*). Note the susceptibility artifact (*long arrow, b*) associated with surgical clips from prior resection.

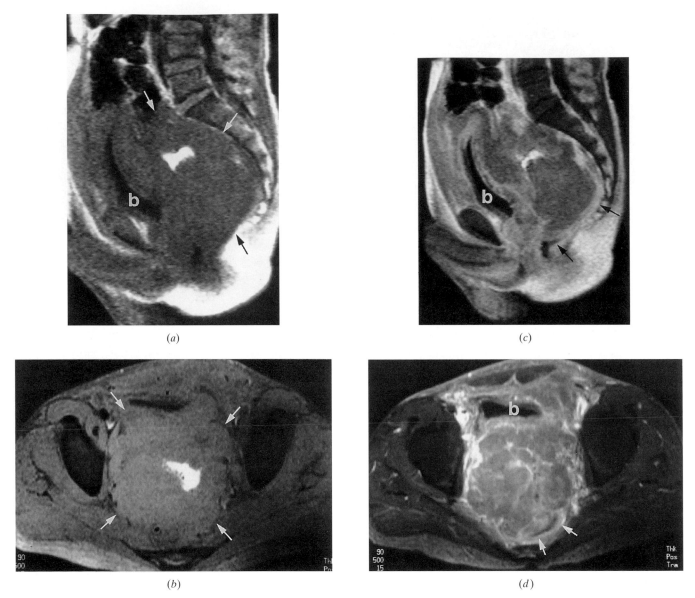

FIG. 6.33 Small intestine lymphoma. Sagittal SGE (*a*), T1-weighted fat-suppressed spin-echo (*b*), sagittal 45-second postgadolinium SGE (*c*), and gadolinium-enhanced T1-weighted fat-suppressed spin-echo (*d*) images in a patient with diffuse lymphomatous infiltration of the distal jejunum and ileum. A large pelvic mass (*arrows, a,b*) is seen on precontrast images. Following intravenous gadolinium, minimal enhancement of the mass is present on early postgadolinium images (*c*), and heterogeneous slightly greater enhancement is present on the interstitial-phase image (*d*). Minimal enhancement on early postgadolinium images with slight increase and heterogeneous enhancement on more delayed images is common for lymphoma in general. The relationship of the mass to adjacent structures can be assessed by imaging in multiple planes. The rectum (*arrows, c,d*) is displaced and compressed by the tumor. Despite extensive disease, there is no proximal small bowel obstruction, a characteristic finding with small intestine lymphoma. High signal intensity within the pelvic mass is consistent with hemorrhage "*b*",*a,c*, bladder.

form is prone to ulceration and fistulization. Twenty percent of cases have multiple lesions, and more than one morphology may coexist. A distinguishing feature of small bowel lymphoma is the preservation of distensibility despite bulky disease. Bowel obstruction is uncommon. Secondary extranodal small intestine involvement is present in up to 50 percent of patients with advanced lymphoma. The MRI features of small intestine lymphoma include moderately enhancing thickened loops of bowel, and large tumor masses that invest the bowel but do not result in obstruction (Fig. 6.33). The presence of splenic lesions and mesenteric and retroperitoneal lymphadenopathy supports the diagnosis.

Carcinoids

Carcinoids are the most common primary neoplasm of the small bowel. These are neuroendocrine tumors that occur in the distal ileum, in which location they are almost always malignant. Men and women are affected with equal frequency. Most patients present with tumor-re-

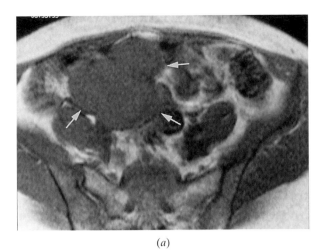

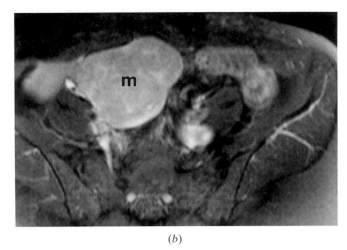

(a)   (b)

FIG. 6.34 Ileal carcinoid. SGE (*a*) and gadolinium-enhanced T1-weighted fat-suppressed spin-echo (*b*) images. The carcinoid tumor (*arrows, a*) causes asymmetric bowel wall thickening, is isointense with bowel on the T1-weighted image (*a*), and enhances heterogeneously and moderately intensely on gadolinium-enhanced interstitial-phase images (*b*).

lated symptoms: bleeding and bowel obstruction or intussusception. Particular to ileal carcinoids are regional mesenteric metastases and vascular sclerosis. The primary tumor may be quite small with the accompanying lymphadenopathy and desmoplastic reaction in the root of the mesentery presenting as the only visible manifestation of disease. However, when large enough, the primary tumor causes asymmetric bowel wall thickening and enhances heterogeneously, ranging from minimal to moderate in intensity following intravenous gadolinium (Fig. 6.34). The characteristic desmoplastic changes in the mesentery and retroperitoneum that occur in response to the secretion of serotonin and tryptophan are low in signal on both T1- and T2-weighted images and show negligible enhancement after contrast. Liver metastases are responsible for the "carcinoid syndrome," which is characterized by vasomotor instability, intestinal hypo-

motility, and bronchoconstriction [53]. Liver metastases are often hypervascular and high in signal intensity on T2-weighted images, possessing intense ring enhancement on immediate postgadolinium SGE images. Occasionally carcinoid liver metastases are hypovascular paralleling to the desmoplastic nature of the primary tumor. In this circumstance they will appear nearly isointense with liver on T2-weighted images and demonstrate faint ring enhancement on immediate postgadolinium SGE images.

Metastases

Metastases to the small bowel occur most frequently via serosal seeding or by direct extension along the mesentery. Ovarian and gastric carcinomas favor the former method of spread, whereas pancreatic carcinomas favor the latter. Tumor may extend directly from other organs

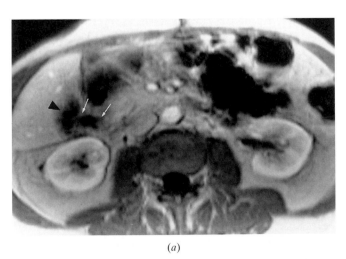

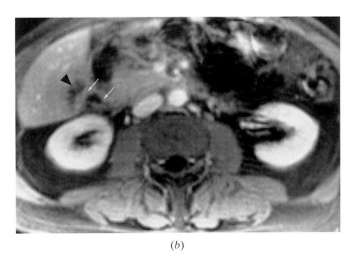

(a)   (b)

FIG. 6.35 Liver metastasis to liver and duodenum. Immediate postgadolinium SGE (*a*) and 90-second postgadolinium fat-suppressed SGE (*b*) images in a patient with colon cancer metastasis to liver and duodenum. A peripheral hepatic metastasis (*arrowhead, a,b*) transgresses the liver capsule to directly invade the adjacent duodenum (*arrows, a,b*).

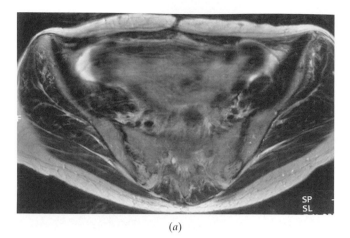

(a)

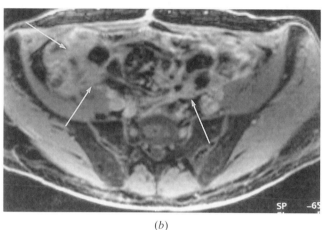

(b)

FIG. 6.36 Ovarian carcinoma metastases to the peritoneal and serosal surfaces. Transverse 512-resolution T2-weighted echo-train spin-echo (a) and 90-second postgadolinium fat-suppressed SGE (b) images highlight the improvement in disease detection afforded by breath-hold gadolinium-enhanced fat-suppressed SGE. On the high-resolution T2-weighted image, bowel motion degrades image quality; no metastatic disease can be identified. On the gadolinium-enhanced fat-suppressed SGE image, the acquisition during suspended respiration avoids breathing artifact and minimizes bowel motion. Enhancement of irregularly thickened tissue along the peritoneum and serosal surface of bowel (arrows, b) is consistent with widespread metastatic disease.

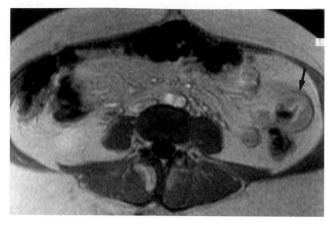

FIG. 6.37 Hematogenous metastases. Transverse 45-second postgadolinium SGE image demonstrates an eccentric mural tumor in the midjejunum (arrow). This tumor was a hematogenous metastasis from uterine leiomyosarcoma.

and tissues (Fig. 6.35). On gadolinium-enhanced fat-suppressed SGE images, metastases are high in signal intensity in contrast to the low signal intensity of intra-abdominal fat. Malignant peritoneal tissue enhances moderately to substantially on interstitial-phase gadolinium-enhanced images and appears as nodular or irregularly thickened peritoneal or serosal tissue (Fig. 6.36). Gadolinium-enhanced fat-suppressed imaging has been shown to be particularly useful, and in some cases superior to CT imaging in detecting small tumor nodules [54]. Although hematogenous dissemination is the least common method of spread, this is not a rare entity due to the large numbers of patients with breast and lung carcinomas. Metastases lodge on the antimesenteric border

of the small bowel and may be visualized as mural-bowel masses (Fig. 6.37). They also may act as lead points for intussusception.

INFLAMMATORY, INFECTIOUS, AND DIFFUSE DISORDERS

Inflammatory Bowel Disease
Crohn's disease and ulcerative colitis are the most common forms of inflammatory bowel disease (IBD). MRI findings correlate well with clinical evaluation, endoscopy, and histologic findings. It is a robust technique capable of diagnosing type, evaluating severity, and monitoring response to treatment in patients with IBD [1–4].

Crohn's Disease
In North America Crohn's disease is the most common inflammatory condition to affect the small bowel. The incidence is greatest in the second and third decades of life, and males are affected more frequently than females. Crohn's disease occurs in families and has an increased incidence in Jews. The etiology is not well-understood, but is likely multifactorial: genetic, autoimmune, and infectious [55]. Crohn's disease usually presents in young adults, but can occur after 50 years of age. Symptoms include nonbloody diarrhea, abdominal pain, weight loss, and fever. Patients with Crohn's disease have an increased incidence of colon cancer.

Involvement of the terminal ileum occurs in approximately 70 percent of patients, with isolated terminal ileal involvement present in 30 percent and terminal ileal and cecal disease present in 40 percent of the total. Five percent of patients will manifest Crohn's disease in the duodenum or jejunum. Twenty to thirty percent will have isolated colon involvement [56].

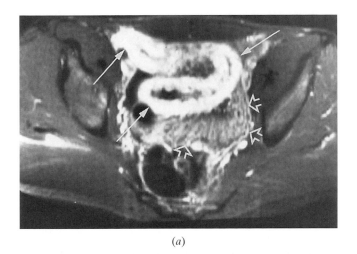

(a)

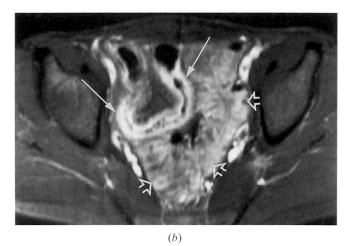

(b)

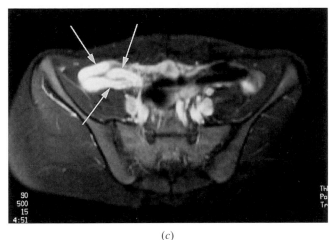

(c)

FIG. 6.38 Severe Crohn's disease. Gadolinium-enhanced T1-weighted fat-suppressed spin-echo images (*a–c*) in three patients with severe Crohn's disease. A thickened loop of substantially enhancing ileum (*arrows, a*) with associated mesenteric inflammation (*open arrows, a*) are characteristic findings for Crohn's disease. In the second patient (*b*), similar findings of a thickened, intensely enhancing loop of ileum (*arrows, b*) with associated mesenteric inflammation (*open arrow, b*) are identified. In the third patient (*c*), multiple thickened loops of intensely enhancing ileus are present (*arrows, c*).

Crohn's disease is a transmural process characterized by noncaseating granulomas. Prominent lymph follicles, lymphangiectasia, and submucosal edema are also noted. Grossly, apthous ulcers are the earliest manifestations. In time, the ulcers extend transmurally, often beyond the intestinal serosa to become sinus tracts or fistulae. In addition, strictures, abscesses, and inflammatory lymph nodes may complicate the disease. Patients are usually treated medically. Surgery is reserved for complicated cases, but anastomotic recurrence is common.

Crohn's disease is well-examined by MRI. Severe disease is characterized by wall thickness more than 1 cm, length of involvement more than 15 cm, and mural enhancement more than 100 percent (Fig. 6.38). Mild disease results in subtle findings that may only be appreciated on gadolinium-enhanced fat-suppressed images (Fig. 6.39). Multiplanar imaging provides comprehensive information on disease extent and complications (Fig. 6.40). HASTE and gadolinium-enhanced T1-weighted fat-suppressed SGE images demonstrate characteristic findings: transmural involvement, skip lesions, and mesenteric inflammatory changes. The transmural bowel pro-

cess is circumferential but asymmetric, and routinely involves the terminal ileum and cecum. Identification of rectal sparing, sinus tracts, fistulae, abscesses, or strictures support the diagnosis of Crohn's disease. The mesenteric changes include inflammatory standing, a function of dilated vasa rectae and sinus tracts, reactive lymphadenopathy, and abundant ("creeping") fat. Some investigators have reported promising results when imaging patients with Crohn's disease after oral administration of perflurooctylbromide (perflubron) [57].

Good correlation has been reported between MRI findings and disease activity [2,4,5]. In contradistinction, barium studies have limited correlation with symptomatology or response to therapy. Moreover, the potential harm of radiation exposure from serial barium examinations in pregnant women and patients of reproductive age is not insignificant [56]. MRI may be the modality of choice to examine for the presence of Crohn's disease in patients with contraindication to barium examinations or CT imaging. Pregnant patients are one example (Fig. 6.41).

The MRI criteria of mild, moderate, and severe dis-

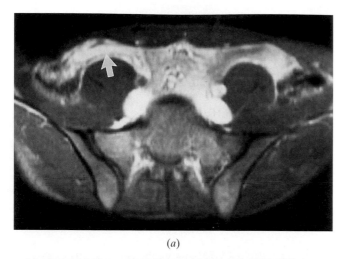

(a)

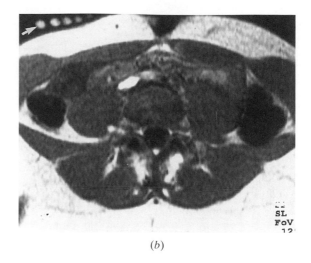

(b)

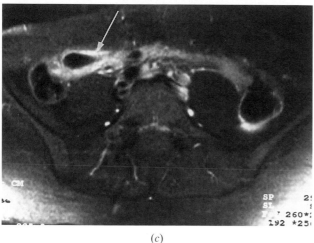

(c)

FIG. 6.39 Mild to moderate Crohn's disease. Transverse gadolinium-enhanced T1-weighted fat-suppressed image (*a*) demonstrates moderate inflammatory disease of the terminal ileum (*arrows, a*), that has a wall thickness of 5 mm, less than 10 cm of diseased bowel, and wall enhancement. SGE (*b*) and gadolinium-enhanced T1-weighted fat-suppressed spin-echo (*c*) images in a second patient with mild Crohn's disease. The unenhanced image (*b*) appears unremarkable. On the gadolinium-enhanced image, transmural enhancement is apparent with wall thickness of 5 mm, length of involved segment of less than 10 cm, and mural enhancement. This constellation of imaging findings is consistent with mild disease. Assessment of severity of disease must be determined on the nondependent bowel wall (*arrow, c*) after intravenous contrast administration. Lipid beads (*small arrow, b*) demarcate the area of patient tenderness.

ease has been described and is a function of wall thickness, length of diseased segment, and percentage of mural contrast enhancement (Table 6.2). MRI assessment is made on gadolinium-enhanced T1-weighted fat-suppressed images using the nondependent bowel surface. It is critical that the time point for determining percentage of enhancement is standardized. This establishes repro-

ducible measures of disease activity between studies in the same patient. We have used a time point of 2.5 minutes after injection. Immediate postgadolinium images reflect increased inflammatory vascularity and increased capillary blood flow. Commonly the inner half of the bowel wall enhances most intensely in this phase of enhancement in severely inflamed bowel. Later interstitial-phase images demonstrate more uniform enhancement in diseased bowel, reflecting capillary leakage and decreased venous removal in transmurally inflamed bowel. A recent pilot study found good correlation between clinical indices to measure Crohn's activity (Crohn's Disease Activity Index [CDAI] and modified Index of the International Organization for the Study of Inflammatory Bowel Disease [IOIBD]) and an MRI determinant, the MRI product (wall thickness × length of diseased segment × percentage mural enhancement [MRP]) (Fig. 6.42) [4]. This work suggests that MRI may be the best modality for evaluating the severity of Crohn's disease. It may provide complementary or confirmatory information to clinical assessment.

MRI also may have a role in the evaluation of acute

Table 6.2 Crohn's Disease Severity Criteria

Severity	Contrast Enhancement (%)	Wall Thickness (mm)	Length of Diseased Segment (cm)
Mild*	<50	<5	<5
Moderate	50–100	5–20	variable
Severe	>00	>10	>5**

*Bowel-wall thickening must be at least 4 mm, and one of the other 2 criteria must be satisfied.
**Typically >10 cm of affected bowel.
Reprinted with permission from Ascher SM, Semelka RC: MRI of the gastrointestinal tract. In Higgins CB, Hricak H, Helms CA (eds.). Magnetic Resonance Imaging of the Body. New York: Raven Press, p. 677–700, 1997.

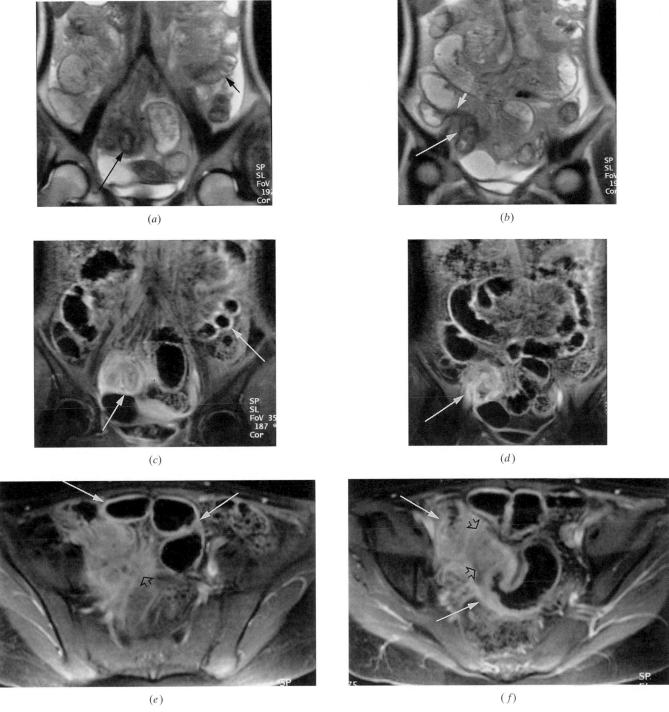

F IG . 6.40 Severe Crohn's disease. Coronal HASTE (*a,b*), coronal 90-second postgadolinium fat-suppressed SGE (*c,d*), and fat-suppressed SGE (*e,f*) images in a patient with severe disease. Coronal HASTE images from midabdominal plane (*a*) and 2 cm more anterior (*b*) demonstrate thickened loops of distal small bowel (*long arrows, a,b*). The terminal ileum is well-shown at its entry into the cecum (*small arrow, b*). Coronal gadolinium-enhanced fat-suppressed SGE images acquired from similar tomographic sections, respectively, demonstrate substantial enhancement of the thickened loops of bowel and surrounding tissues. An enhancing fistulous tract (*arrow, d*) is apparent close to the ileocecal valve. Transverse gadolinium-enhanced images demonstrate intense enhancement of multiple loops of bowel, including loops with wall thickness of 4 mm (*arrows, e*). On the more inferior tomographic section narrowing of distal ileum is apparent, which accounts for the mild dilation of more proximal loops (*arrows, e*). Inflammatory mesenteric changes are evident (*hollow arrows, e,f*). Normal-appearing proximal jejunum (*small arrow, a*) is appreciated on the HASTE image.

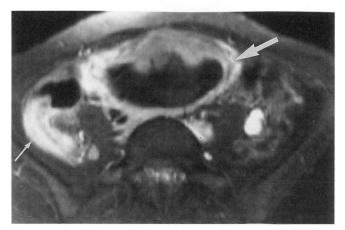

FIG. 6.41 Crohn's disease in pregnancy. Gadolinium-enhanced T1-weighted fat-suppressed spin-echo image in a patient in the second trimester of pregnancy. Thickened and intensely enhancing distal ileum is present (*arrow*). The pregnant uterus is also well-shown (*large arrow*).

exacerbations of Crohn's disease. Specifically, in patients with long-standing disease, marked enhancement of the mucosa with a thickened and minimally enhancing outer layer is suggestive of acute-on-chronic involvement (Fig. 6.43).

Ulcerative Colitis

Ulcerative colitis is an inflammatory mucosal disease that affects the large bowel and will be discussed later. Small bowel involvement ("backwash ileitis") is the sequelae of pancolonic disease. Free reflux of colon contents into

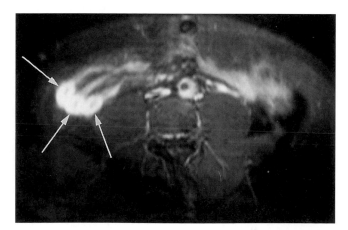

FIG. 6.42 Crohn's disease activity assessment. Gadolinium-enhanced T1-weighted fat-suppressed spin-echo image in a patient with active Crohn's disease. There is good correlation between clinical indices (CDAI, 185, [active disease >150]; modified IOIBD index, 8 [scale 1–10]) and MRI findings (*arrows*) of thickened wall, length of diseased segment, and percentage of mural enhancement (MRP, 4,664). (Reprinted with permission from Kettritz U, Isaacs K, Warshauer DM, Semelka RC: Crohn's disease: Pilot study comparing MRI of the abdomen with clinical evaluation. J Clin Gastroenterol 21:249–253, 1995)

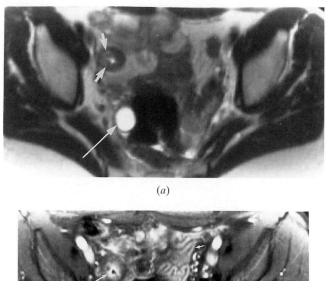

(a)

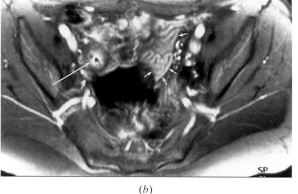

(b)

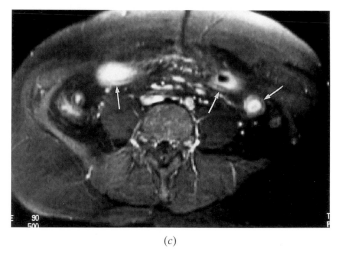

(c)

FIG. 6.43 Acute-on-chronic Crohn's disease. HASTE (*a*) and gadolinium-enhanced T1-weighted fat-suppressed spin-echo (*b*) images in a patient with long-standing disease. Increased thickness of distal ileum is present, which demonstrates increased signal intensity in the inner aspect of the wall (*arrow, a*). Acute exacerbation is characterized by intense mucosal enhancement (*long arrow, b*) with minimal enhancement of the outer wall in substantially thickened bowel. Accompanying hyperemia of the mesentery reflects the active inflammatory process (*short arrows, b*). Incidental note is made of a right adnexal cyst (*long arrow, a*) and free fluid in the pelvis. Gadolinium-enhanced T1-weighted fat-suppressed spin-echo image (*c*) in a second patient with a long history of Crohn's disease. Thickened loops of small bowel with intense enhancement of the inner wall are apparent (*arrows, c*). This appearance is that of acute mucosal exacerbation superimposed on a chronically thickened wall.

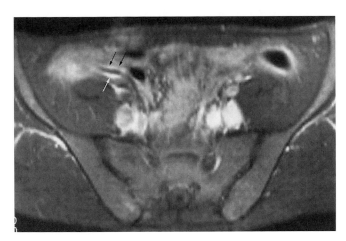

FIG. 6.44 Backwash ileitis. Gadolinium-enhanced T1-weighted fat-suppressed spin-echo image in a patient with ulcerative colitis. Pancolonic involvement with ulcerative colitis results in a patulous ileocecal valve. Reflux of colon contents into the ileum causes inflammatory changes (*arrows*). (Reprinted with permission from Shoenut JP, Semelka RC, Silverman R, Yaffe CS, Mickflikier AB: The gastrointestinal tract. In Semelka RC, Shoenut JP (eds.). MRI of the Abdomen with CT Correlation. New York: Raven Press, pp. 119-143, 1993)

the ileum via a patulous ileocecal valve is believed to be responsible [56]. The lumen of the ilium is moderately dilated, and the wall is inflamed (Fig. 6.44).

Pouchitis

A continent ileostomy ("pouch") is often fashioned for patients after total colectomy. These continent reservoirs are at risk for inflammation ("pouchitis"). This condition is more common in patients with Crohn's disease [58] for which MRI features include an enhancing and thickened pouch wall and inflammatory stranding of the "peri-pouch" fat (Fig. 6.45).

Fistulae

Fistulae are tracts connecting hollow viscera to each other and/or the skin. They result from compromise to the visceral wall and are commonly seen in the setting of infection, inflammation, neoplasia, radiation therapy, and ischemia (embolic, thrombotic, or vasoconstrictive). MRI's superior contrast and spatial resolution, in conjunction with direct image acquisition in any plane, makes it a very effective modality in the workup of fistulae. The appearance of a fistula will depend on its contents, the degree of inflammation, and the type of sequence employed. Fluid-filled tracts are high in signal intensity on T2-weighted sequences, whereas gas-filled tracts are signal-void. Fat suppression combined with intravenous gadolinium highlight the enhancing fistulous tracks amid the surrounding low-signal-intensity intra-abdominal fat. Focal discontinuity of the involved organ at the site of tract penetration is diagnostic [7,8].

Infectious Enteritis

Active inflammation may be due to a variety of bacterial, protozoal, or viral pathogens. *Yersinia enterocolitica* infection includes acute gastroenteritis, terminal ileitis, mesenteric lymphadenitis, and colitis [59]. Yersinia ileitis and Yersinia enterocolitis may mimic appendicitis and Crohn's disease, respectively. *Campylobacter jejuni* may produce diarrhea, severe gastroenteritis, or colitis [60]. *Giardia lamblia* and *Strongyloides stercoralis* are protozoa that typically involve proximal small bowel. The increasing population of immunocompromised patients has led to an increase in occurrence of infectious granulomatous disease of the bowel. Tuberculosis mycobacteria infection involves the terminal ileum. Patients may be symptomatic from the acute inflammatory response, late fibrotic stenosis, or both. *Mycobacterium avium intracellulare* favors the colon and is frequently accompanied by bulky retroperitoneal lymphadenopathy. *Cytomegalovirus* and *Cryptosporidium* are infections common in AIDS patients. In all of these inflammatory conditions, the MRI findings may be nonspecific demonstrating bowel wall thickening, increased secretions, and mesenteric edema. Gadolinium-enhanced fat-suppressed SGE imaging demonstrates bowel wall thickening and increased enhancement, and detects the presence of abscesses by the identification of encapsulated fluid collections that possess an enhancing rim. History, coupled with the segment of bowel affected, may suggest the correct diagnosis. Specifically, in a patient with AIDS, mild diarrhea with small bowel wall thickening secondary to submucosal hemorrhage is typical of *Cryptosporidium* infection, whereas severe diarrhea with thickened and mildly dilated, fluid-filled proximal small bowel involvement is typical of *Cytomegalovirus* infection [43].

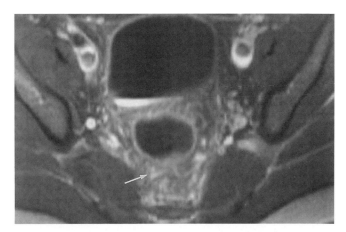

FIG. 6.45 Pouchitis. Gadolinium-enhanced T1-weighted fat-suppressed spin-echo image demonstrates slight thickening of the pouch with stranding in the surrounding fat (*arrow*).

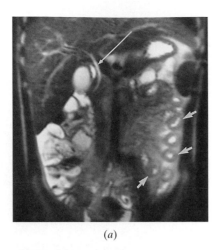

(a)

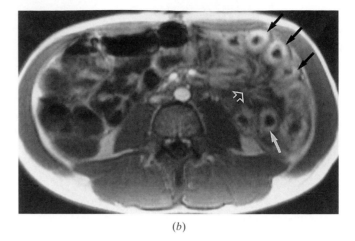

(b)

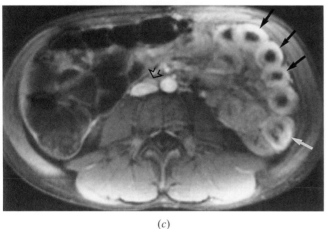

(c)

FIG. 6.46 Chemotherapy toxicity enteritis. Coronal HASTE (a), immediate postgadolinium SGE (b), and 90-second postgadolinium fat-suppressed SGE (c) images in a patient with chemotherapy toxicity enteritis. Many etiological agents may cause inflammation of the small bowel. The findings are nonspecific and include diffuse circumferential wall thickening (*short arrows, a*), marked bowel wall enhancement (*arrows, b,c*), mesenteric infiltration and hyperemia (*open arrow, b*), and lymphadenopathy (*open arrow, c*). Note the normal common bile duct on the T2-weighted HASTE image (*long arrow, a*).

Drug Toxicity

Inflammatory changes of small bowel may result from a number of etiologies. Chemotherapy toxicity is one example. Diffuse wall thickening and increased enhancement are observed (Fig. 6.46), similar in appearance to infectious causes of diffuse small bowel disease.

Pancreatitis

Small bowel changes also may occur adjacent to an active inflammatory process. Specifically, in patients with pancreatitis, small bowel wall thickening and focal ileus are seen on gadolinium-enhanced SGE images (Fig. 6.47). An MRI colon cutoff sign also may be demonstrated.

Radiation Enteritis

Radiation therapy for malignant disease may cause an enteritis with tumor doses greater than 45 Gy. The majority of cases are secondary to treatment of female genital tract malignancy. The distal jejunum and ilium are the most common sites to be affected. At histopathology, the ischemic changes of radiation damage are a small-vessel obliterative endarteritis of the intestinal wall and mesentery. Mucosal and submucosal edema develop, accompa-

nied by an inflammatory infiltrate. Early postradiotherapy complications include ulceration, necrosis, bleeding, perforation, abscess, and fistula formation. Later, progressive fibrosis leads to strictures, bowel fixation, and angulation. Varying degrees of small bowel obstruction may result. Gadolinium-enhanced fat-suppressed SGE imaging is the most effective technique for detecting the diffuse early ischemic and inflammatory changes of radiation enteritis as well as the more focal late fibrotic sequelae. Radiation changes appear as diffuse symmetric bowel wall thickening and enhancement of multiple loops of small bowel in the same region of the abdomen. This can be readily distinguished from recurrent disease, which demonstrates irregular, nodular bowel wall thickening (Fig. 6.48).

Ischemia and Hemorrhage

Ischemia and hemorrhage may occur in tandem or as isolated events. Ischemia, regardless of etiology, leads to wall edema secondary to capillary leakage. If prolonged, hemorrhagic infarction can result. The MRI findings parallel the severity of blood flow compromise. Early changes include mural thickening and increased enhancement on

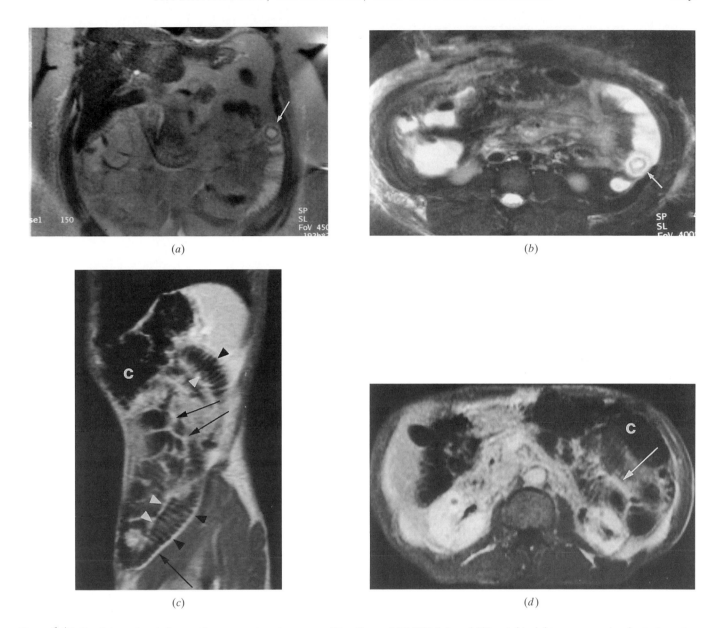

FIG. 6.47 Small intestine inflammation secondary to pancreatitis. Coronal HASTE (*a*) and T2-weighted fat-suppressed echo-train spin-echo (*b*) images demonstrate circumferential high signal intensity of the wall of the jejunum (*arrow, a,b*) secondary to edema caused by inflammatory changes induced by pancreatitis. The outer wall is high in signal intensity, whereas the inner wall is low in signal intensity, reflecting the extrinsic nature of the bowel inflammation. Sagittal (*c*) and transverse (*d*) interstitial-phase gadolinium-enhanced SGE images in a second patient demonstrate dilation (*arrowheads, c*) of small bowel with increased wall enhancement (*arrows, c,d*). The transverse colon ("*c*",*c,d*) shows a transition from normal caliber to narrowed, which is the transverse colon cutoff sign of pancreatitis.

late postcontrast images (Fig. 6.49). Increased enhancement on interstitial-phase images reflects leaky capillaries. Necrotic bowel manifests MRI findings consistent with hemorrhage, and in severe cases, portal venous gas may be observed (see Fig. 6.49). Vascular compromise or thrombosis may be well-shown on early (less than 1 minute) postgadolinium images (Fig. 6.50). Bowel wall hemorrhage from trauma or ischemia may be diagnosed by high signal intensity within the submucosa on both

T1- and T2-weighted sequences due to the presence of extracellular methemoglobin. Noncontrast T1-weighted fat-suppressed images are the most sensitive for the detection of subacute blood (Fig. 6.51).

Hypoproteinemia

Hypoproteinemia may arise from a number of causes, the most common of which are cirrhosis and malnourishment. Generalized bowel wall thickening is present,

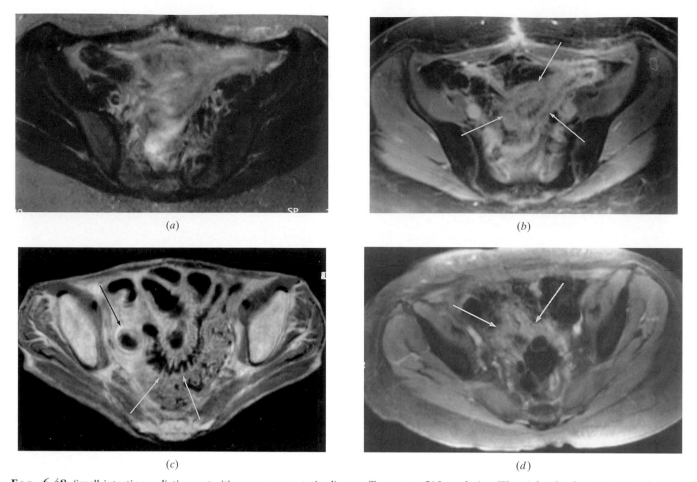

(a)   *(b)*

(c)   *(d)*

F IG . 6.48 Small intestine radiation enteritis versus metastatic disease. Transverse 512-resolution T2-weighted echo-train spin-echo (*a*), 90-second postgadolinium fat-suppressed SGE (*b*), 90-second postgadolinium SGE (*c*) images in two patients (*a,b*) and (*c*) with radiation enteritis, respectively. In the first patient, the T2-weighted echo-train spin-echo image (*a*) is degraded by blurring artifact secondary to peristalsis. Breath-hold technique coupled with gadolinium-enhanced fat-suppressed imaging at the same level highlights postradiation therapy changes of the small bowel: diffuse, symmetric wall thickening with increased enhancement (*arrows, b*). Similar changes are noted in the second patient following radiation therapy (*arrows, c*). Transverse 90-second postgadolinium fat-suppressed SGE image (*d*) in a third patient with recurrent ovarian cancer demonstrates irregular focal thickening of small bowel. Note the difference between the symmetric and uniform bowel thickening associated with radiation changes (*b,c*) and the more focal and asymmetric changes produced by metastatic disease to the small bowel (*arrows, d*).

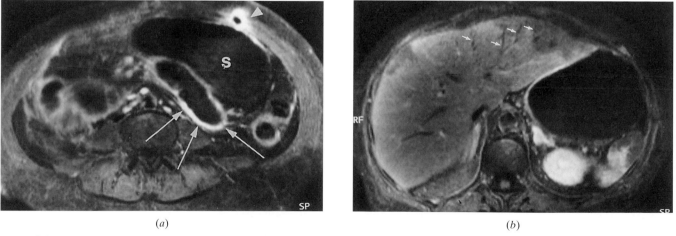

(a)   *(b)*

F IG . 6.49 Small bowel ischemia. Gadolinium-enhanced T1-weighted fat-suppressed spin-echo images (*a,b*). The patient had undergone previous small bowel resection. Increased enhancement of a loop of proximal small bowel (*arrows, a*) is present. The stomach ("s",*a*) also contains regions of increased mural enhancement. Increased enhancement results from leaky capillaries in ischemic bowel disease. Portal venous gas (*small arrows, b*) is an ominous finding suggesting bowel necrosis. Susceptibility artifact (*arrowhead, a*) is noted within the anterior abdominal wall.

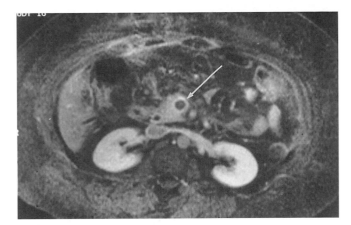

FIG. 6.50 Superior mesenteric vein (SMV) thrombosis. Transverse 90-second postgadolinium fat-suppressed SGE image demonstrates signal-void thrombus in the SMV with increased enhancement of the SMV wall (*arrow*), which was due to infection associated with thrombosis.

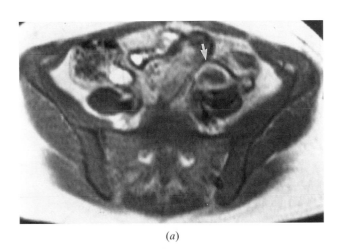

(a)

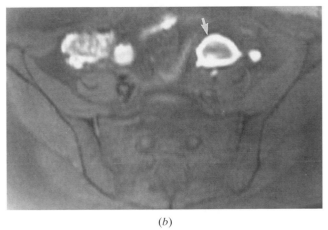

(b)

FIG. 6.51 Submucosal hemorrhage. SGE (*a*) and T1-weighted fat-suppressed spin-echo (*b*) images in a woman status posthysterectomy who had undergone vigorous intraoperative bowel retraction. Increased signal intensity in the bowel wall on the SGE image (*arrow, a*) becomes more conspicuous after fat suppression (*arrow, b*). (Reprinted with permission from Shoenut JP, Semelka RC, Silverman R, Yaffe CS, Mickflikier AB: The gastrointestinal tract. In Semelka RC, Shoenut JP (eds.). MRI of the Abdomen with CT Correlation. New York: Raven Press, pp. 119–143, 1993)

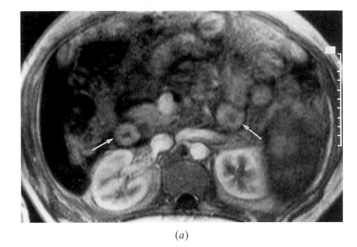

(a)

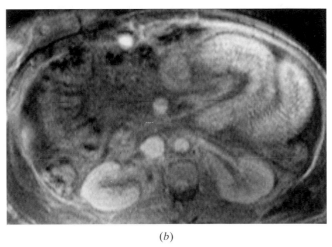

(b)

FIG. 6.52 Small bowel edema in cirrhosis. Immediate postgadolinium SGE (*a*) and 90-second postgadolinium SGE (*b*) images in two patients with cirrhosis. Ascites and diffuse thickening of multiple loops of small bowel (*arrows, a,b*) are present. Third spacing of fluid secondary to hypoproteinemia accounts for the bowel wall thickening.

which is best appreciated in the jejunum. Unlike inflammatory conditions, enhancement on gadolinium-enhanced images is negligible (Fig. 6.52).

Intussusception

The most common cause of intussusception in adults is the presence of a small bowel polyp, which acts as a lead point. The prolapsing bowel segment is referred to as the intussusceptum, and the bowel segment into which the prolapse has occurred is referred to as intussuscipiens. Intussusception is well-shown on HASTE images due to the sharp anatomic detail of this sequence. In the setting of intussusception, fluid in dilated bowel provides excellent intrinsic contrast for the bowel-within-bowel appearance (Fig. 6.53).

Graft-versus-Host Disease

Graft-versus-host disease is a complication that may occur after heterotopic bone marrow transplantation. The

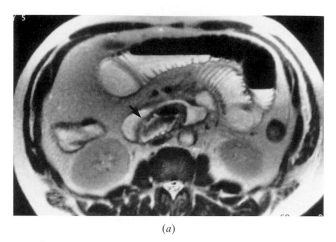

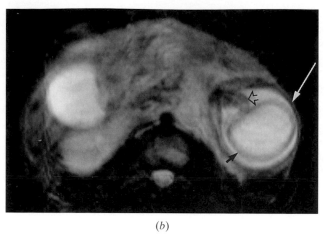

(a)   (b)

FIG. 6.53 Small bowel intussusception. HASTE (*a*) and T2-weighted fat-suppressed echo-train spin-echo (*b*) images in two different patients. In the first patient, the HASTE image (*a*) provides clear definition of the bowel-within-bowel appearance (*arrow, a*) of intussusception. In the second patient (*b*), respiratory and bowel motion degrades the majority of the peritoneal cavity. However, the dilated, relatively fixed, hypotonic loop of the intussuscipiens (*long arrow, b*) is relatively well-shown. The intussusceptum (*short arrows, a*) is clearly shown, and its mesentery (*hollow arrow, b*) is also appreciated. In this second patient adequate visualization of the intussusception occurred in this nonbreath-hold study because of the hypotonicity of the involved bowel segments.

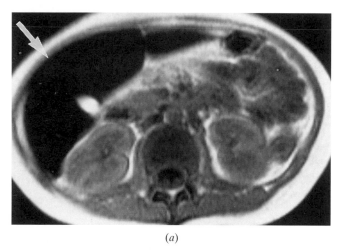

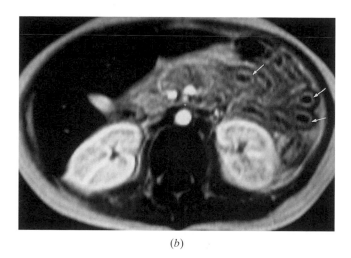

(a)   (b)

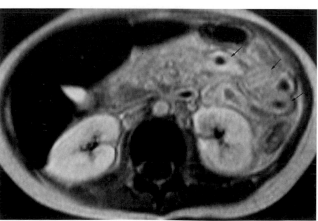

(c)

FIG. 6.54 Graft-versus-host disease. SGE (*a*), immediate (*b*), and 90-second (*c*) postgadolinium SGE images in a patient status postbone-marrow transplant. Unenhanced images suggest thickening of multiple loops of small bowel. Immediately following intravenous contrast, intense mucosal enhancement of multiple loops of small bowel (*arrows, b*) is appreciated. On the interstitial-phase image (*c*), enhancement has spread to involve the majority of the wall (*arrows, c*). This enhancement pattern reflects hyperemia and capillary leakage, respectively. The decreased signal intensity of the liver (*arrow, a*) is consistent with iron overload secondary to multiple blood transfusions. (Reprinted with permission from Ascher SM, Semelka RC: MRI of the gastrointestinal tract. In Higgins CB, Hricak H, Helms CA (eds.). Magnetic Resonance Imaging of the Body. New York: Raven Press, pp. 677–700, 1997.)

acute form involves the gastric antrum, small bowel, and colon. On MR images there is diffuse bowel wall thickening with increased enhancement of the inner wall layers (Fig. 6.54). The chronic form of graft-versus-host disease is usually associated with esophageal involvement. This desquamative esophagitis leads to webs and strictures.

THE LARGE INTESTINE

NORMAL ANATOMY

The large bowel measures approximately 4.5 feet in length and is subdivided into the appendix, cecum, ascending colon, transverse colon, descending colon, sigmoid colon, rectum, and anus. Its functions include absorption of water and electrolytes, storage of fecal matter, and secretion.

The cecum lies below the level of the ileocecal valve. It usually is located in the right lower quadrant, but it does have a mesentery and sometimes is freely mobile. This mobility predisposes the cecum to volvulus formation. The ascending and descending colon are retroperitoneal and located in the anterior pararenal space. The transverse colon is located anteriorly in the peritoneal cavity suspended by the transverse mesocolon, which originates from the peritoneal covering of the anterior surface of the pancreas. The gastrocolic ligament connects the superior surface of the transverse colon to the greater curvature of the stomach. The sigmoid colon is intraperitoneal and suspended on a mesentery, whereas the rectum is retroperitoneal and relatively fixed. The frontal and lateral surfaces of the rectum are covered with peritoneum, which is then reflected anteriorly forming the rectovaginal recess in females and the rectovesical recess in males. Below the coccyx, the rectum traverses the levator ani muscles to become the anal canal.

The colon consists of four layers: the mucosa, submucosa, muscularis, and serosa; and the bowel wall is usually less than 4 mm thick. The muscularis consists of an inner circular and an outer longitudinal layer. Thickened muscular bundles of the outer muscle layer form the taeniae coli. Because the taeniae are shorter in length than the colon, they produce the characteristic sacculations or haustra. Colonic luminal diameter is greatest in the cecum and gradually narrows distally to the level of the rectal ampulla, where it again expands.

MRI TECHNIQUE

The technique and considerations for studying the large bowel parallel those for the small bowel. Fasting at least 4 to 6 hours prior to imaging or the injection of intramuscular glucagon limit peristalsis. Even so, blurring artifact associated with the long acquisition times of T2-weighted conventional and even fast spin-echo technique precludes routine T2-weighted imaging of much of the colon. However, the HASTE technique overcomes this limitation and should be performed in the axial and coronal planes for imaging colonic disease, with the sagittal plane reserved for imaging the rectum. Gadolinium-enhanced fat-suppressed SGE imaging is particularly effective. Normal colon is thin-walled, has haustrations, and enhances minimally with gadolinium (Fig. 6.55).

The rectum deserves special mention. In contradistinction to the remainder of the large bowel, the rectum's relatively fixed position benefits from high resolution (512 matrix) T2-weighted echo-train spin-echo imaging. This is particularly useful for the evaluation of rectal carcinoma: to assess bowel wall involvement, to determine the relationship to adjacent structures, and to distinguish recurrence from fibrosis. Endorectal MRI also may be used to study the rectum. The endoluminal surface coil optimizes spatial resolution and demonstrates the rectal wall layers, anal sphincter complex, and disease processes [9,10,61,62]. The use of intraluminal contrast to distend the colon may improve detection of mucosal abnormalities [63]. The layers of the rectal wall can be visualized on gadolinium-enhanced T1-weighted fat-suppressed images, high resolution T2-weighted images, and endorectal coil T2-weighted images (see Fig. 6.55). The transition between the rectum and the anal canal can be determined by the observation that the rectum contains intraluminal air and the anal canal is collapsed (Fig. 6.56).

CONGENITAL ANOMALIES

Malrotation
Nonrotation, the most common rotational abnormality, was discussed earlier. In this condition the large bowel will occupy the left side of the abdomen.

Duplication
Colonic duplication is thought to be the result of early intrauterine vascular insult. It may be limited to a single segment of large bowel, or it can involve the entire colon (Fig. 6.57). Symptoms will depend on whether or not there is communication of the duplication with the remainder of the colon. Patients with right colon duplication are at risk for intussusception.

Anorectal Anomalies
Most cases of anorectal anomalies occur in association with other congenital malformations. MRI has been successful in evaluating these patients because it directly demonstrates the rectal pouch and sphincter muscles in

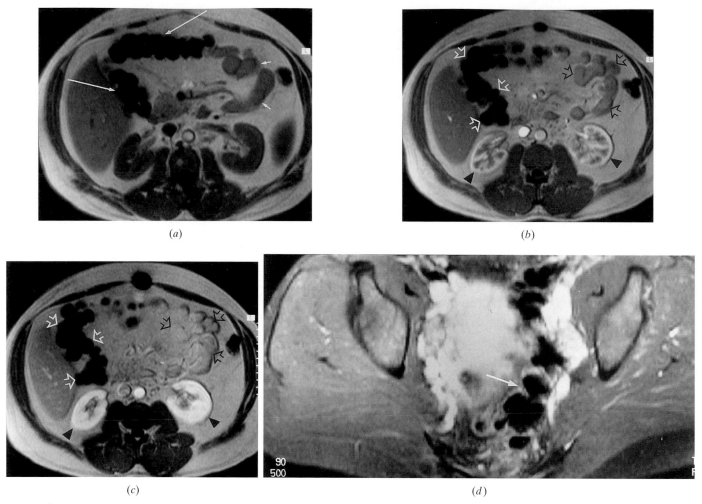

(a)

(b)

(c)

(d)

FIG. 6.55 Normal large bowel. SGE (*a*), immediate (*b*), and 90-second (*c*) postgadolinium SGE images. Air-filled colon (*long arrows, a*) and normal small bowel (*short arrows, a*) are seen on the precontrast T1-weighted image (*a*). Following intravenous gadolinium administration the walls of the large and small bowel (*open arrows, b,c*) enhance less than adjacent renal parenchyma (*arrowheads, b,c*) on capillary-phase (*b*) and interstitial-phase (*c*) images. Gadolinium-enhanced T1-weighted fat-suppressed spin-echo image (*d*) in another subject demonstrates a normal-appearing sigmoid colon that shows minimal mural enhancement, thin wall, and haustrations (*arrow, d*).

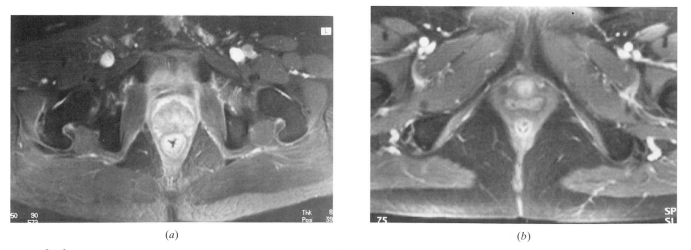

(a)

(b)

FIG. 6.56 Normal rectum and anal canal. Gadolinium-enhanced T1-weighted fat-suppressed spin-echo image (*a*) in a man highlight the different layers of the rectum (from inner layer to outer layer): high-signal-intensity mucosa, low-signal-intensity muscularis mucosa and lamina propria, high-signal-intensity submucosa, and low-signal-intensity muscularis propria. The rectum contains air within the lumen. Gadolinium-enhanced T1-weighted fat-suppressed spin-echo image (*b*) in a woman demonstrates the same enhancement features of the anal canal. Note that the anal canal is collapsed and does not contain air.

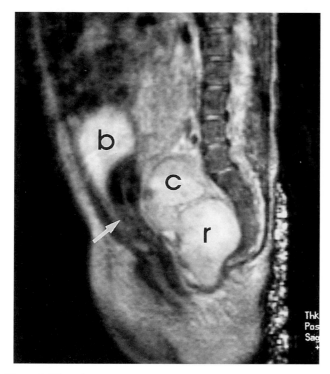

F I G . 6.57 Colonic duplication. T2-weighted spin-echo image in a patient with colonic duplication. The uterus (*arrow*) and bladder (*b*) are anteriorly displaced by two fluid-filled viscous structures that represent the rectum (*r*) and the duplication cyst (*c*).

multiple planes. This allows exact determination of the location and developmental status of the sphincter muscles as well as identification of associated anomalies of the kidneys and spine. MRI is also helpful for postoperative assessment of the neorectum and sphincteric muscles (Fig. 6.58) [64].

MASS LESIONS

Benign Masses

Polyps and Polyposis Syndromes
Colonic adenomatous polyps are the most common large bowel neoplasm. They may be tubular, tubulovillous, or villous. Of the three glandular patterns, villous adenomas, commonly found in the rectosigmoid and cecum, have the highest incidence for cancerous degeneration [36]. Multiple colonic adenomas are seen in association with Familial polyposis or Gardner's syndromes, whereas multiple colonic hamartomas may be seen in Peutz-Jeghers or juvenile polyposis syndromes.

A number of polyposis syndromes have been described. The most common are Familial polyposis, Gardner's, Peutz-Jeghers, and the juvenile polyposis syndromes. Familial polyposis syndrome is an autosomal dominant disorder characterized by multiple adenomas of the gastrointestinal tract. The adenomas predilect the

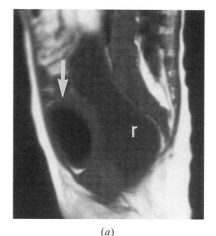

(*a*)

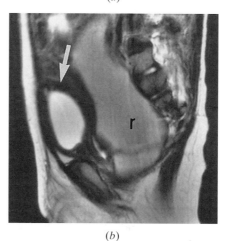

(*b*)

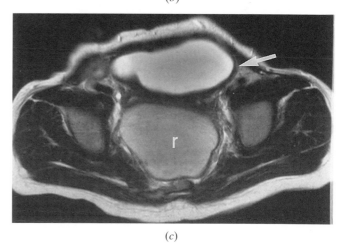

(*c*)

F I G . 6.58 Surgical repair of persistent cloaca. Sagittal T1-weighted spin-echo (*a*), sagittal T2-weighted echo-train spin-echo (*b*) and transverse T2-weighted echo-train spin-echo (*c*) images. A capacious neorectum ("*r*",a,b,c) is present. The bladder (*large arrow, a-c*) is thick walled and anteriorly displaced. Absence of the vagina is noted.

colon and rectum, and there is a 100 percent risk of malignant transformation to colorectal carcinoma. Gardner's syndrome is an autosomal dominant condition with diffuse adenomatous polyps, bony abnormalities (osteomas), and soft tissue tumors. As with Familial polyposis syndrome, the adenomas in patients with Gardner's syndrome will undergo cancerous transformation with time. These patients are also at increased risk for developing small bowel and gastric malignancies. Peutz-Jeghers syndrome is an autosomal dominant disorder with buccal mucocutaneous pigmentation and gastrointestinal hamartomas. The hamartomas favor the small bowel in 95 percent of cases, with colonic and stomach involvement in up to 25 percent. Although the hamartomas are not premalignant, up to 3 percent of patients with Peutz-Jeghers syndrome will develop adenocarcinoma of the stomach or duodenum, and 5 percent of women will have ovarian cysts or tumors. There are three distinct syndromes associated with juvenile polyps of the alimentary tract: juvenile polyposis, gastrointestinal juvenile polyposis, and the Cronkhite-Canada syndromes. Hamartomas are common to all three syndromes [65,66].

Gadolinium-enhanced fat-suppressed SGE images can demonstrate polyps, whether they occur in isolation or in association with a polyposis syndrome. The most common appearance is an enhancing sessile or pedunculated mass arising from the bowel wall and protruding into the lumen. If enhancing interstices are seen, the possibility of a villous adenoma should be raised. Similarly, extension beyond the bowel wall signifies cancerous degeneration.

Lipomas

Lipomas are the second most common benign neoplasm of the large bowel. They usually originate in the submucosa. Most are asymptomatic, although changes in bowel habits, bleeding, or both have been reported in patients with large lesions. The most common locations for co-lonic lipomas are the cecum, ascending colon, and sigmoid colon. The MRI appearance of lipomas with T1-weighted and fat-suppressed T1-weighted sequences is pathognomonic: high in signal intensity on T1-weighted images and diminished in signal intensity on fat-suppressed T1-weighted images (Fig. 6.59) [67].

Other Mesenchymal Neoplasms

Fibromas, leiomyomas, hemangiomas and neurofibromas are all rare.

Mucocele

A mucocele results from obstruction of the appendix with associated mucus distention. In most cases the obstruction is postinflammatory. However, obstruction can be due to a mucinous cystadenocarcinoma. Mucoceles are frequently asymptomatic unless they become secondarily infected or rupture. Ruptured mucoceles are accompanied by pseudomyxoma peritonei. Because of the possibility of an underlying malignancy and the risk of rupture, mucoceles should be prophylactically removed. T2-weighted HASTE images show a high-signal-intensity tubular structure in the region of the appendix. Mucoceles have a higher signal intensity than simple fluid on T1-weighted sequences owing to their protein content. In uncomplicated cases, the wall of the mucocele is thin and enhances minimally after intravenous gadolinium administration (Fig. 6.60).

Varices

Rectal varices develop in patients with portal hypertension. The incidence of hemorrhoids is not increased in these patients [68].

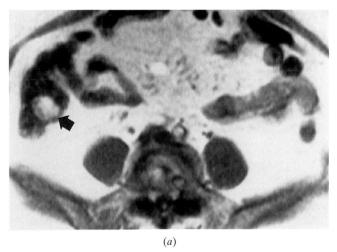
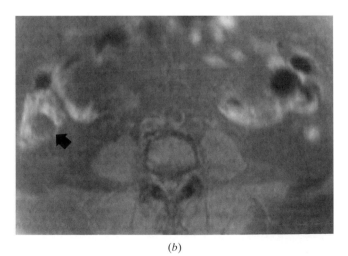

(a)   (b)

FIG. 6.59 Cecal lipoma. SGE (a) and T1-weighted fat-suppressed spin-echo (b) images. A mass in the cecum is high in signal intensity on the T1-weighted image (arrow, a) and diminishes in signal intensity on the fat-suppressed image (arrow, b). These imaging characteristics are pathognomonic for a fat containing tumor. The cecum is a common location for large bowel lipomas. (Reprinted with permission from Shoenut JP, Semelka RC, Silverman R, Yaffe CS, Mickflikier AB: Magnetic resonance imaging evaluation of the local extent of colorectal mass lesions. J Clin Gastroenterol 17:248–253, 1993)

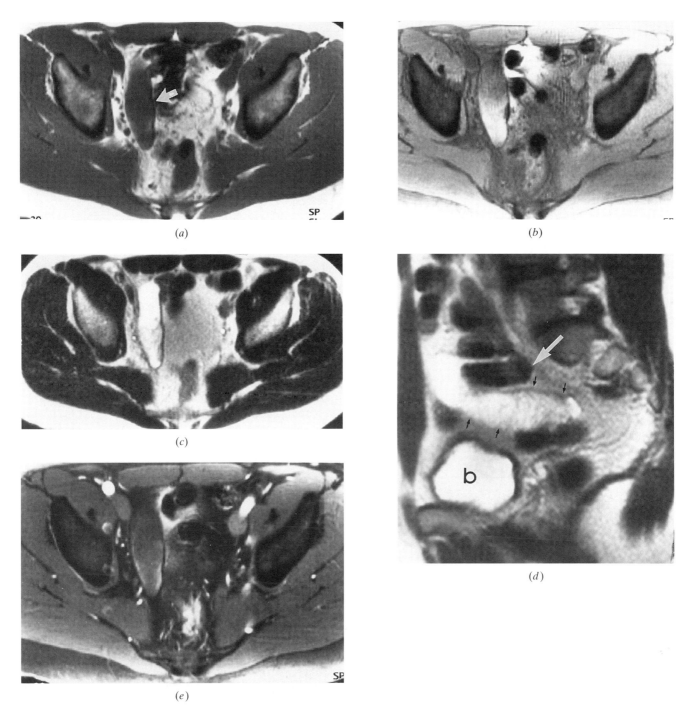

FIG. 6.60 Mucocele of the appendix. SGE (*a*), fat-suppressed SGE (*b*), HASTE (*c*), sagittal HASTE (*d*), and immediate postgadolinium fat-suppressed SGE (*e*) images. An oblong-shaped mucocele of the appendix is present (*arrow, a*) that contains high-signal-intensity material in the dependent portion of the cyst on the T1-weighted image (*a*), which is accentuated with the application of fat suppression (*b*). The mucocele is high in signal intensity on the T2-weighted image with slight heterogeneity in the dependent portion (*c*). The sagittal plane image (*d*) shows the orientation of the mucocele (*small arrows, d*) to the base of the cecum (*arrow, d*) and the relationship to the bladder (''*b*'',*d*). No appreciable enhancement of the mucocele wall is noted on the postgadolinium image (*e*), which excludes the diagnosis of abscess.

Malignant Masses

Adenocarcinoma

Adenocarcinoma of the colon is the most common gastro-intestinal tract malignancy and the second most common visceral cancer in North America. The estimated incidence in the United States is 138,000 new cases per year and the 5-year survival is 50 to 60 percent [37]. The incidence of adenocarcinoma of the colon increases with advancing age. Sporadic cancers are increased in first-degree family relatives of patients with known colorectal carcinoma. Other conditions that predispose to the development of colon cancer include Familial polyposis, Gardner's syndrome, Lynch's syndrome, ulcerative colitis, Crohn's colitis, and previous ureterosigmoidostomies. Cancers occur most often in the rectosigmoid colon, but right-sided cancers are reported to occur in increasing frequency [69]. Tumors may be polypoid, circumferential ("apple core"), or plaque-like. Symptoms reflect tumor location and morphology, with most patients reporting a combination of change in bowel habits, bleeding, pain, and weight loss. A TNM system is used for staging (Table 6.3).

Table 6.3 TNM Staging for Cancer of the Colon

T—Primary tumor	
Tx	Primary tumor cannot be assessed
T0	No evidence of primary tumor
Tis	Preinvasive carcinoma (carcinoma in situ)
T1	Tumor limited to the mucosa or mucosa and sub-mucosa
T2	Tumor with extension to muscle or muscle and serosa
T3	Tumor with extension beyond the colon to immedi-
T3a	ately contiguous structures
T3b	Tumor without fistula formation
	Tumor with fistula formation
T4	Tumor with deep infiltration occupying more than one-half but not more than one region or extending to neighboring structures
N—Regional lymph nodes	
Nx	Regional lymph nodes cannot be assessed
N0	No evidence of regional lymph node metastasis
N1	Evidence of regional lymph node involvement
N2, N3	Not applicable
N4	Evidence of involvement of juxta-regional lymph nodes
M—Metastases	
Mx	Distant metastases cannot be assessed
M0	No distant metastases
M1	Distant metastases

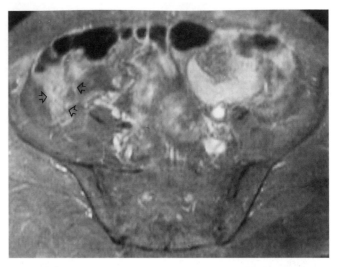

F I G. 6.61 Appendiceal adenocarcinoma. Gadolinium-enhanced T1-weighted fat-suppressed spin-echo image demonstrates heterogeneous enhancing infiltrative tumor arising from the appendix (*open arrows*).

Conventional spin-echo MRI is comparable to conventional CT imaging for overall staging of patients with colorectal carcinoma. Accuracies of approximately 80 percent have been reported for these two modalities [70,71]. Recently, investigators have shown good correlation between gadolinium-enhanced fat-suppressed MRI techniques and surgical specimens for tumor size, bowel wall involvement, peritumoral extension, and lymph node detection [5]. Malignant lymph nodes are usually not enlarged in gastrointestinal malignancies. However, the presence of more than 5 lymph nodes that measure smaller than 1 cm in a regional distribution related to the tumor correlates well with tumor involvement. All

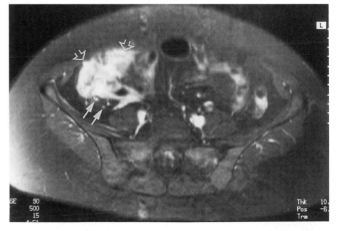

F I G. 6.62 Colonic adenocarcinoma, cecum. Gadolinium-enhanced T1-weighted fat-suppressed spin-echo image demonstrates a large heterogeneous intensely enhancing cecal carcinoma (*hollow arrow*) that extends to the anterior peritoneal wall. Multiple enhancing lymph nodes smaller than 5 mm are identified (*arrows*), which are malignant.

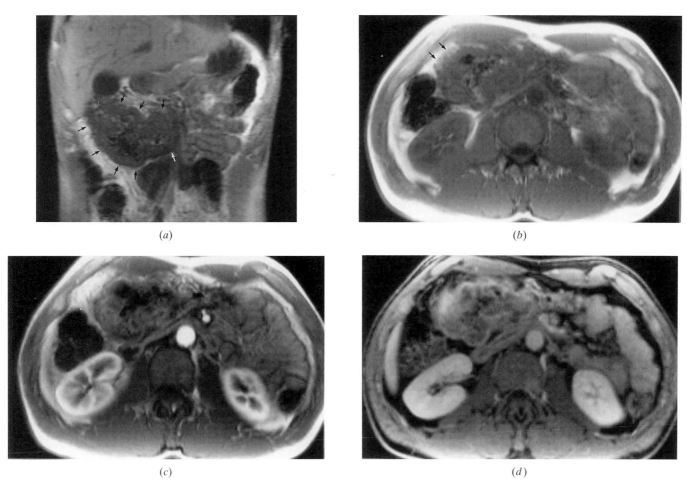

(a)   *(b)*

(c)   *(d)*

F I G . 6.63 Colon adenocarcinoma, transverse colon. Coronal SGE (*a*), SGE (*b*), immediate postgadolinium SGE (*c*), and 90-second postgadolinium fat-suppressed SGE (*d*) images. A large cancer arises from the transverse colon (*small arrows, a*). The outer margin of the bowel involved with tumor is indistinct (*small arrows, b*), a finding consistent with lymphovascular extension. The tumor is heterogeneous and moderate in signal intensity on capillary-phase (*c*) and interstitial-phase (*d*) images.

segments of the colon and the appendix may be well-examined and, in general, gadolinium-enhanced fat-suppressed SGE images result in the most reproducible image quality for the colon above the rectum (Figs. 6.61 to 6.65). Rectal cancers benefit from the combined use of gadolinium-enhanced fat-suppressed SGE and high-resolution T2-weighted echo-train spin-echo images (Fig. 6.66). Gadolinium-enhanced fat-suppressed SGE imaging also works well for imaging perirectal tumor extension, regional lymph nodes, and intraperitoneal tumor seeding. This reflects the high contrast resolution of this technique for enhancing disease (Fig. 6.67). Image acquisition of T2-weighted echo-train spin-echo or HASTE postgadolinium is a novel approach for evaluation of rectosigmoid carcinoma. Dependent, concentrated gadolinium in the bladder is low in signal intensity and can be exploited to increase the conspicuity of high-signal-intensity tumor invasion of the bladder wall (see Fig. 6.66).

Because the spatial resolution of body-coil imaging

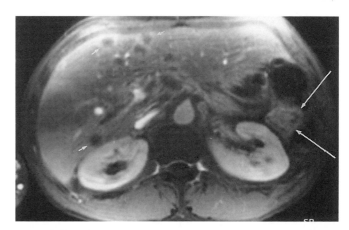

F I G . 6.64 Colon adenocarcinoma, proximal descending colon. Transverse 90-second postgadolinium SGE image demonstrates a heterogeneously enhancing tumor (*long arrows*) in the proximal descending colon with prominent enhancing strands in the surrounding mesentery consistent with lymphovascular extension. Multiple ring-enhancing liver metastases are apparent (*small arrows*).

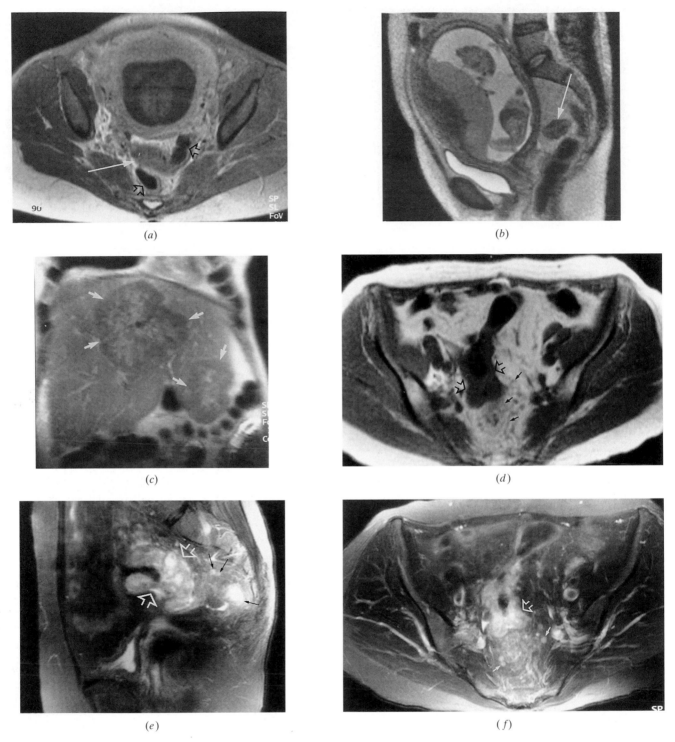

(a)

(b)

(c)

(d)

(e)

(f)

FIG. 6.65 Sigmoid adenocarcinoma. SGE (*a*), and sagittal and coronal HASTE (*b,c*), images in a pregnant patient with colon cancer. The SGE image shows air-filled colon (*hollow arrows, a*) proximal and distal to the 4-cm sigmoid cancer (*arrow, a*). The HASTE images show the primary tumor (*arrow, b*) and the liver metastases (*arrows, c*). The gravid uterus is well-imaged with the single-shot T2-weighted breathing-independent technique (*b*). SGE (*d*), sagittal T2-weighted fat-suppressed spin-echo (*e*) and gadolinium-enhanced T1-weighted fat-suppressed spin-echo (*f*) images in a second patient with advanced sigmoid adenocarcinoma. The precontrast image demonstrates abnormal thickening of the sigmoid colon (*open arrows, d*) with low-signal-intensity strands infiltrating the pericolonic fat (*arrows, d*). The primary tumor (*open arrows, e,f*) and pericolonic extension are well-shown as high-signal-intensity structures in a low-signal-intensity background on both fat-suppressed T2-weighted (*e*) and gadolinium-enhanced T1-weighted fat-suppressed (*f*) images. Multiple small regional malignant lymph nodes are identified (*small arrows, e,f*).

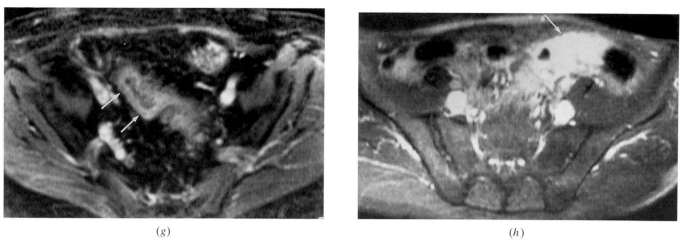

(g)　　　　　　　　　　　　　　　　(h)

FIG. 6.65 (*Continued*) Transverse 90-second postgadolinium SGE image (*g*) in a third patient demonstrates a circumferential 4-cm sigmoid colon cancer (*arrows, g*) that does not show lymphovascular extension. Gadolinium-enhanced T1-weighted fat-suppressed spin-echo image (*h*) in a fourth patient demonstrates an intensely enhancing sigmoid colon cancer (*arrow, h*) involving the anterior peritoneum.

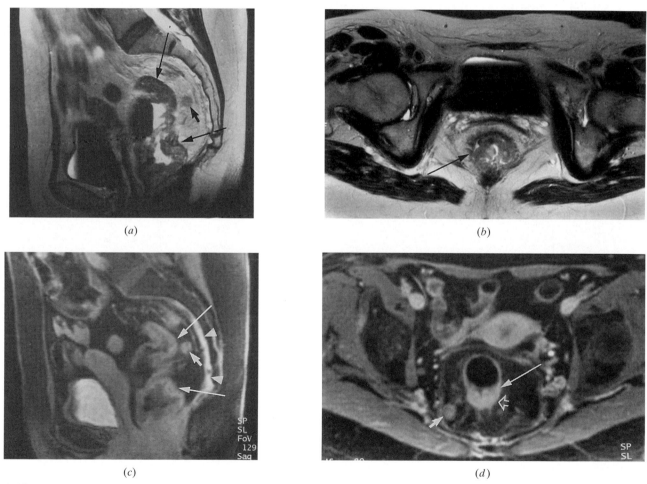

(a)　　　　　　　　　　　　　　　　(b)

(c)　　　　　　　　　　　　　　　　(d)

FIG. 6.66 Rectal adenocarcinoma. Sagittal and transverse postgadolinium high-resolution T2-weighted echo-train spin-echo (*a,b*) and sagittal and transverse postgadolinium fat-suppressed SGE (*c,d*) images in a patient with advanced colon cancer. A large rectal cancer is present (*long arrows, a,c*). The craniocaudal extent of tumor is well-shown on sagittal images (*a,c*). The tumor extends inferiorly in the rectum (*arrow, b*) to the anal verge. Lymphovascular extension with involved lymph nodes (*small arrows, a,c,d*) is present. At the superior margin the tumor is mainly posterior in location (*hollow arrow, d*). The transition from normal colon to tumor (*long arrow, d*) is clearly shown. Presacral spread of tumor is shown as enhancing tissue on the sagittal gadolinium-enhanced fat-suppressed image (*arrowheads, c*).

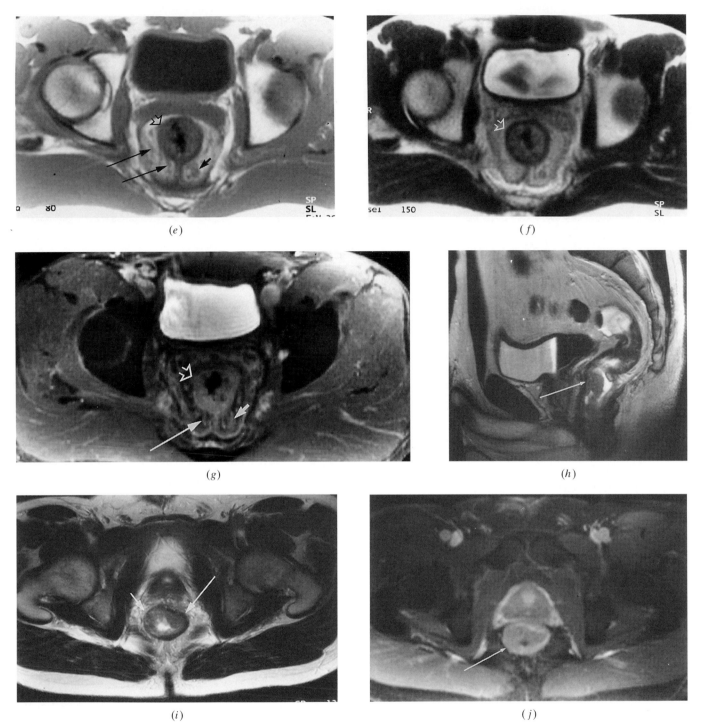

F I G . **6.66** (*Continued*) SGE (*e*), HASTE (*f*), and postgadolinium fat-suppressed SGE (*g*) images in a second patient with rectal adenocarcinoma and similar imaging findings. The rectal tumor (*hollow arrows, e,f,g*), lymphovascular extension (*long arrows, e,g*), and perirectal lymph nodes (*short arrow, e,g*) are well-shown. Sagittal and transverse postgadolinium 512 resolution T2-weighted echo-train spin-echo (*h,i*), and interstitial-phase gadolinium-enhanced fat-suppressed SGE (*j*) images in a third patient. Asymmetric tumor involvement of the rectal wall is apparent on the 512-resolution T2-weighted images (*long arrow, h,i*). Tumor penetrates the full thickness of the right aspect of the rectum (*short arrow, i,j*). This is shown by interruption of the low-signal-intensity muscular wall on the T2-weighted image (*long arrow, i*). On the gadolinium-enhanced fat-suppressed SGE image lower-signal-intensity tumor (*arrow, j*) penetrates the full thickness of the higher-signal-intensity wall. Post gadolinium T2-weighted imaging is a novel technique for assessing possible bladder invasion. Enhancing tumor is conspicuous against the low signal intensity produced by concentrated gadolinium excreted into the bladder. In this case, the bladder is spared.

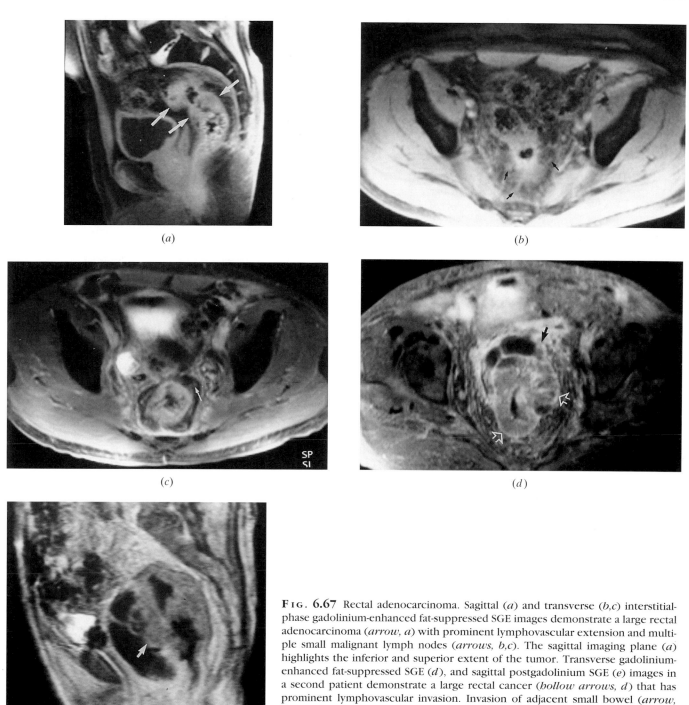

(a)

(b)

(c)

(d)

(e)

Fig. 6.67 Rectal adenocarcinoma. Sagittal (*a*) and transverse (*b,c*) interstitial-phase gadolinium-enhanced fat-suppressed SGE images demonstrate a large rectal adenocarcinoma (*arrow, a*) with prominent lymphovascular extension and multiple small malignant lymph nodes (*arrows, b,c*). The sagittal imaging plane (*a*) highlights the inferior and superior extent of the tumor. Transverse gadolinium-enhanced fat-suppressed SGE (*d*), and sagittal postgadolinium SGE (*e*) images in a second patient demonstrate a large rectal cancer (*hollow arrows, d*) that has prominent lymphovascular invasion. Invasion of adjacent small bowel (*arrow, d,e*) is shown.

limits assessment of the depth of bowel wall invasion, many groups advocate the use of surface coils. Commercially available torso phased-array, Helmholtz, and endoluminal coils boost the signal-to-noise ratio and improve spatial resolution. Image quality and anatomic detail have been found to be superior with the torso phased-array coil in comparison to the MRI system circularly polarized body coil [72]. Images acquired with the Helmholtz coil

in patients with rectal carcinoma allowed differentiation between tumors confined to the bowel wall and those infiltrating the perirectal fat [73]. The use of a phased-array coil has superseded Helmholtz coil usage due to its superior imaging properties. Of all the surface coil configurations, the endorectal coil provides the highest signal-to-noise ratio and spatial resolution of the rectum. This reflects the close proximity of the coil to the organ

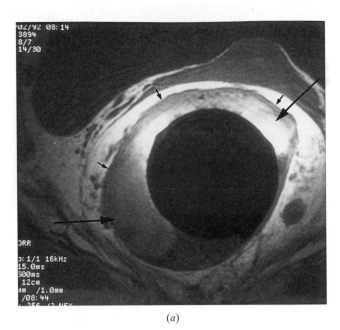
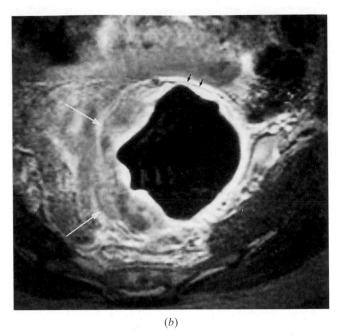

(a)   (b)

F I G . 6.68 Endorectal coil imaging of rectal cancer. Gadolinium-enhanced T1-weighted image (*a*) demonstrates a T2 rectal cancer (*long arrows, a*). Preservation of low-signal-intensity muscular wall (*short arrows, a*) along the outer margin of the tumor confirms lack of full thickness involvement. Gadolinium-enhanced T1-weighted fat-suppressed spin-echo image (*b*) in a second patient with T3 rectal cancer. Heterogeneous moderate enhancing tumor (*long arrows, b*) is noted to extend beyond the confines of muscularis propria (*short arrows, b*). [Courtesy of Rahel A. Huch Böni].

being imaged. Endorectal coil imaging permits differenti-ation of the anatomic layers of the rectal wall on T2-weighted fat-suppressed images [10]. Local staging of rectal carcinoma also benefits from endorectal coil im-aging (Fig. 6.68) [9,10].

Recurrence rates for rectosigmoid carcinoma, which are reported to range from 8 to 50 percent, are a function of the stage of the primary tumor at initial presentation [12]. Tumors tend to recur locally, and curative surgery is feasible. The sagittal imaging plane facilitates MRI de-tection of recurrent rectal carcinoma. Using T1-weighted, T2-weighted, and gadolinium-enhanced T1-weighted se-quences, one study reported a 93.3 percent accuracy in detecting recurrent disease [12]. Others have shown that MRI outperforms conventional CT imaging and is more specific than transrectal ultrasound for identifying recur-rent tumor [11,13,14,15]. Specifically, MRI correctly diag-nosed recurrent rectal carcinoma in 83.2 percent of pa-tients versus transrectal ultrasound, which diagnosed recurrence in only 41.6 percent [16].

Recurrent tumor tends to be low in signal intensity on T1-weighted images and enhances moderately after intravenous gadolinium (Fig. 6.69) [6,11,70,71,74]. On T2-weighted images, recurrent tumor usually is moderately high in signal intensity. This may be difficult to appreciate on echo-train spin-echo sequences since the surrounding fat is also moderately high in signal intensity on these sequences (see Fig. 6.69). Caution must be exercised in

interpreting images in patients with possible recurrent disease on echo-train spin-echo sequences; tumor ap-pears lower in signal intensity compared to its appear-ance on conventional spin-echo sequences. This reflects the relatively high signal intensity of fat on echo-train spin-echo sequences. Demonstration of sacral invasion is well-shown on T2-weighted fat-suppressed echo-train spin-echo and gadolinium-enhanced T1-weighted fat-suppressed images. Marrow is low in signal intensity on both of these sequences, particularly in the setting of postradiation fatty replacement, which is often present in these patients, and tumor extension is conspicuous due to its high signal intensity (Fig. 6.70). In the assessment of sacral involvement, imaging in the sagittal plane is essential for visualizing invasion of the cortex of the sacrum. In selected cases, oblique coronal images (fol-lowing the angulation of the sacrum) are helpful (see Fig. 6.70). Recurrent tumor often has a nodular configuration. Recurrent rectosigmoid cancer and posttreatment (surgi-cal and/or radiation) fibrosis frequently coexist (Fig. 6.71).

Postradiation fibrosis in patients more than 1 year after therapy often demonstrates low signal intensity in the surgical bed on T1- and T2-weighted images and may show negligible enhancement after intravenous gadolin-ium administration [6,11,69,70,74] (Fig. 6.72). Enhance-ment of fibrosis with gadolinium, particularly on fat-sup-pressed images, often persists for 1.5 to 2 years after

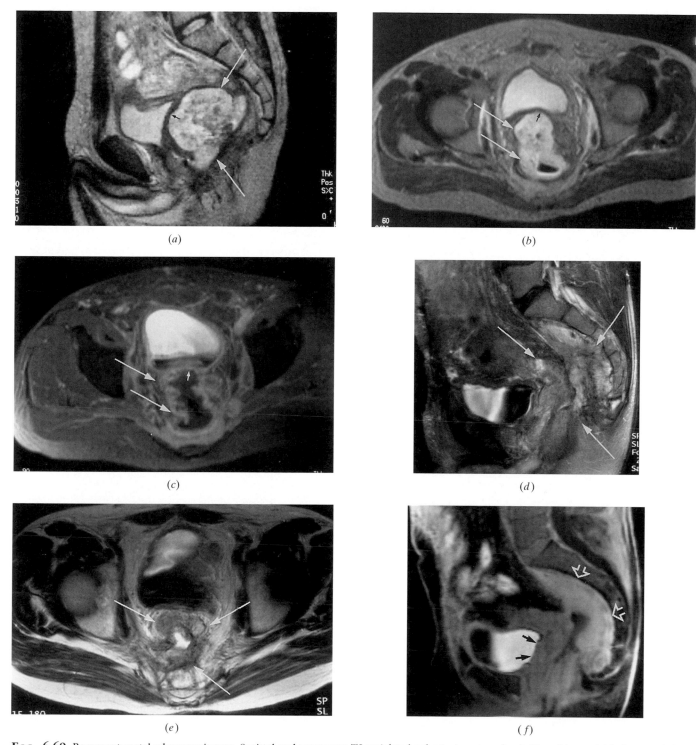

(a)

(b)

(c)

(d)

(e)

(f)

FIG. 6.69 Recurrent rectal adenocarcinoma. Sagittal and transverse T2-weighted echo-train spin-echo (*a,b*) and interstitial-phase gadolinium-enhanced T1-weighted fat-suppressed spin-echo (*c*) images. A large heterogeneous mass occupies the rectal fossa, a finding consistent with recurrence. Recurrent tumors are usually moderately high in signal intensity on T2-weighted images (*long arrows, a,b*) and enhance moderately after intravenous contrast (*long arrows, c*). Central necrosis is well-shown on the gadolinium-enhanced T1-weighted fat-suppressed image. The tumor is contiguous with the bladder wall (*short arrow, a–c*), but the low signal intensity of the bladder wall on the T2-weighted images shows that the bladder wall is not invaded. Sagittal and transverse postgadolinium 512-resolution T2-weighted echo-train spin-echo (*d,e*), and sagittal and transverse interstitial-phase gadolinium-enhanced fat-suppressed SGE (*f,g*) images in a second patient with recurrent rectal tumor. The 512-resolution T2-weighted images show a large heterogeneous tumor in the rectal bed (*arrows, d,e*). Low-signal-intensity urine reflects concentrated gadolinium dependently.

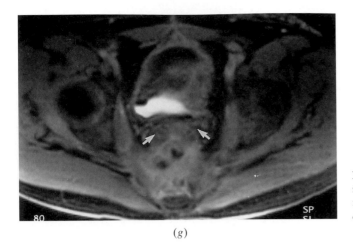

(g)

FIG. 6.69 (*Continued*) The contrast-enhanced fat-suppressed SGE images (*f,g*) demonstrate extensive recurrent disease involving the rectal fossa, rectovesical space (*arrows f,g*), presacral space (*open arrows, f*), and sciatic foramina.

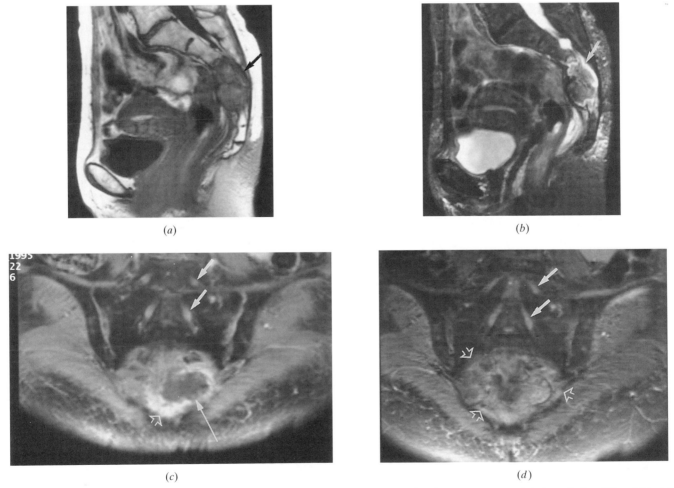

(a)

(b)

(c)

(d)

FIG. 6.70 Recurrent rectal adenocarcinoma invading sacrum. Sagittal T1-weighted SGE (*a*), sagittal 512-resolution T2-weighted fat-suppressed echo-train spin-echo (*b*), and oblique coronal postgadolinium fat-suppressed SGE (*c,d*) images. A large recurrent tumor mass invades the sacrum and is intermediate in signal intensity on the T1-weighted image (*arrow, a*) and heterogeneously high in signal intensity on the T2-weighted image (*arrow, b*). After contrast the tumor enhances heterogeneously (*open arrows, c, d*) and contains an area of central necrosis (*long arrow, c*). S1 and S2 sacral segments are not involved, and uninvolved S1 and S2 nerve roots are shown (*short arrows, c,d*). Sparing of the upper two sacral segments is a finding on which surgeons used to base surgical resection. At surgery the upper margin of the tumor involved S3, sparing the S2 sacral segment.

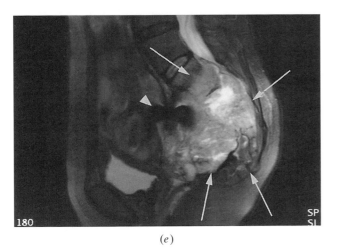

(e)

FIG. 6.70 (Continued) Sagittal 512-resolution T2-weighted echo-train spin-echo image (e) in a second patient demonstrates sacral invasion by a large recurrent rectal adenocarcinoma (arrows, e). This tumor involves the entire sacrum and precludes surgical resection attempt. Surgical clip from prior resection produces a signal-void susceptibility artifact (arrowhead, e).

therapy, which is longer than the period of time that fibrosis is high in signal intensity on T2-weighted images. Fibrosis often has a plaque-like appearance in morphology. Unfortunately, the imaging features of postradiation changes, especially in patients receiving doses in excess of 45 Gy, may not always follow a predictable time course, and overlap in signal behavior between recurrent tumor and post treatment fibrosis exists [75]. On echo-train spin-echo images, the high signal intensity of fat admixed with fibrous tissue may simulate recurrence (Fig. 6.73). Although the T2-weighted signal intensity of fibrosis usually decreases 1 year after radiation, granulation

tissue may show persistent high signal intensity up to 3 years after therapy, particularly if intervening inflammation or infection has developed. Persistent increased signal intensity is most pronounced on gadolinium-enhanced T1-weighted fat-suppressed images. Finally, recurrent tumor may mimic radiation fibrosis when desmoplastic features predominate [6,11,70–72]. Clinical history will often aid radiologic diagnosis: elevation of CEA levels, onset of presacral pain, or both are harbingers of recurrence irrespective of imaging features.

Squamous-Cell Carcinoma

Squamous-cell cancer occurs in the anal canal, and its imaging characteristics resemble those of adenocarcinoma. Evaluation of local and distant spread is aided by gadolinium-enhanced fat-suppressed SGE images.

Lymphoma

Lymphoma can involve the colon, usually as part of widespread disease in elderly patients, whereas primary large bowel lymphoma is most often seen in patients with human immunodeficiency virus (HIV) infection or chronic ulcerative colitis [76,77]. Non-Hodgkin's lymphoma is the most common histology, and the cecum is the most common site of involvement. The MRI appearance includes isolated or multiple enhancing masses. Alternatively, diffuse nodularity with wall thickening may be seen after intravenous gadolinium administration (Fig. 6.74) [44,45]. Coexistent lymphadenopathy and splenic lesions aid diagnosis.

Carcinoid Tumors

Carcinoid tumors are most frequently diagnosed in the rectum. A retrospective report of 170 carcinoid tumors

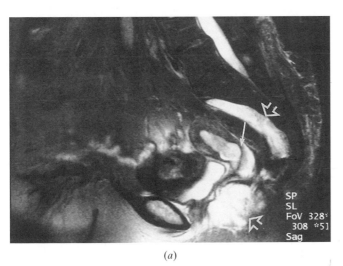

(a)

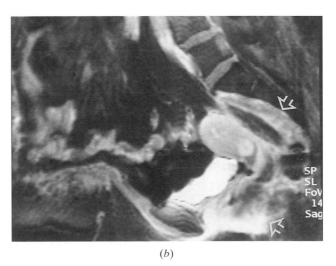

(b)

FIG. 6.71 Recurrent rectal adenocarcinoma and postradiation therapy changes. Sagittal postgadolinium 512-resolution T2-weighted fat-suppressed echo-train spin-echo (a) and sagittal interstitial-phase gadolinium-enhanced fat-suppressed SGE (b) images in a woman status postradiotherapy for rectal adenocarcinoma. Recurrent tumor is high in signal intensity on the T2-weighted fat-suppressed image and enhances following gadolinium administration (open arrows, a,b). Cervical stenosis (arrow, a) secondary to radiation therapy causes widening of the proximal endocervical and endometrial canal.

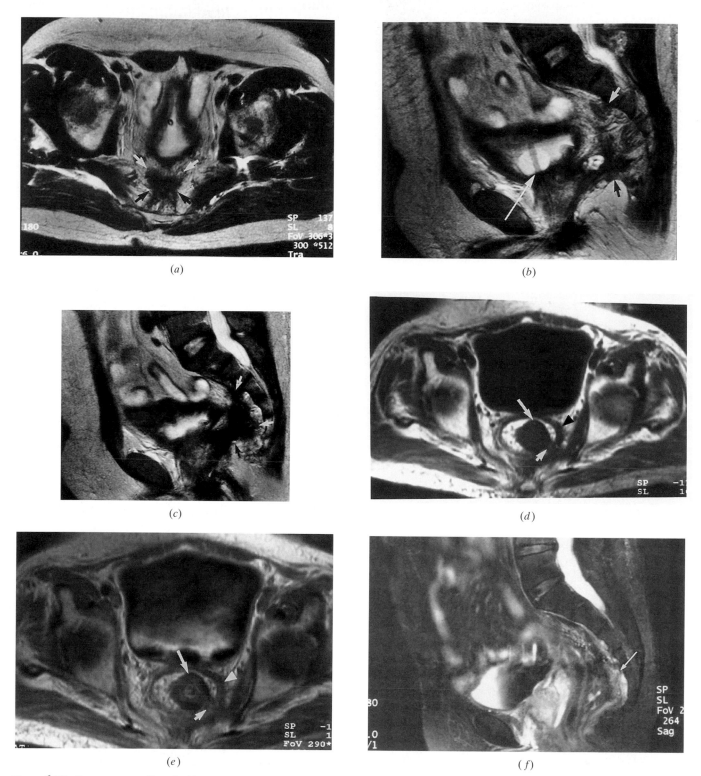

FIG. 6.72 Posttreatment fibrosis. Transverse (*a*) and sagittal (*b,c*) 512-resolution T2-weighted echo-train spin-echo images demonstrate low signal intensity in the surgical bed (*arrows, a–c*) consistent with fibrosis. Fibrosis has a plaque-like morphology, whereas recurrence tends to be more nodular. A Foley catheter is in place (*long arrow, b*). SGE (*d*) and postgadolinium SGE (*e*) images in a second patient show thickening of the rectal wall (*long arrow, d,e*) and perirectal tissue (*arrowhead, d,e*). Prominent perirectal strands are also present (*short arrow, d,e*). Negligible enhancement is consistent with perirectal fibrosis. The perirectal halo of fibrotic tissue is a common finding following radiation therapy for rectal cancer.

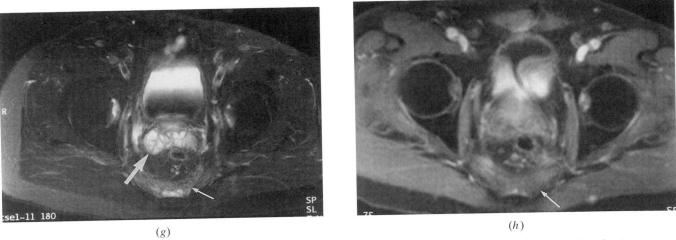

(g) (h)

F IG . 6.72 (*Continued*) Sagittal (*f*) and transverse (*g*) 512-resolution T2-weighted fat-suppressed echo-train spin-echo images and interstitial-phase gadolinium-enhanced fat-suppressed SGE (*h*) images in a third patient demonstrate plate-like tissue in the presacral space that is low in signal intensity on T2-weighted images (*arrow, f,g*) and does not enhance substantially following gadolinium administration (*arrow, h*). Normal seminal vesicles have a cluster-of-grapes appearance (*large arrow, g*) on T2-weighted images, which permits distinction from recurrent tumor.

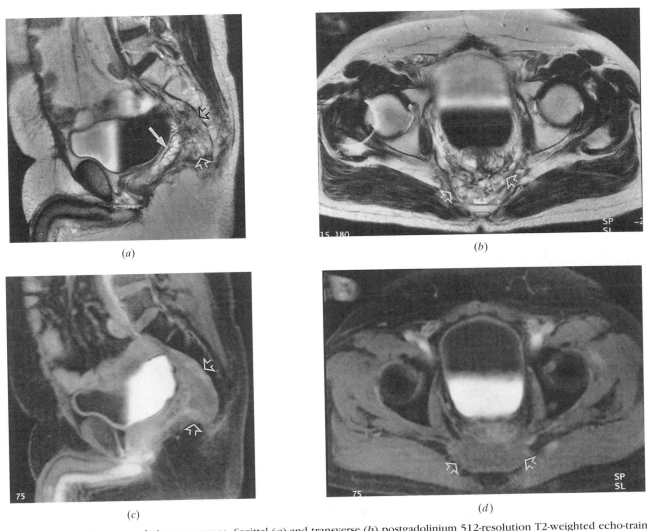

(a) (b)

(c) (d)

F IG . 6.73 Radiation fibrosis simulating recurrence. Sagittal (*a*) and transverse (*b*) postgadolinium 512-resolution T2-weighted echo-train spin-echo, and sagittal (*c*) and transverse (*d*) interstitial-phase gadolinium-enhanced fat-suppressed SGE images in a patient 1.5 years after treatment for rectal cancer. Heterogeneous, bulky high-signal-intensity tissue occupies the rectal fossa (*open arrows, a,b*), on the T2-weighted echo-train spin-echo images worrisome for recurrent disease. Other diagnostic possibilities include granulation tissue associated with radiation, inflammation, or infection. The heterogeneity is misleading because it reflects low-signal-intensity fibrotic tissue interspersed with high-signal-intensity fat, a consequence of the echo-train spin-echo technique. Minimal enhancement on the gadolinium-enhanced fat-suppressed SGE is consistent with fibrosis (*open arrows, c,d*). The seminal vesicles are distinguished from tissue in the rectal bed by the normal high-signal-intensity and grape-like morphology on the T2-weighted image (*arrow, a*).

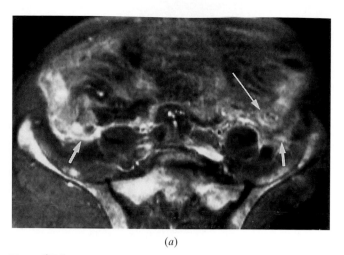

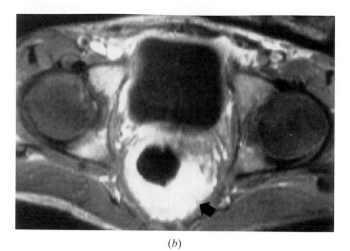

(a)   (b)

F I G . 6.74 Colonic lymphoma. Gadolinium-enhanced T1-weighted fat-suppressed spin-echo images (a,b) in two patients with lymphoma. In the first patient with Burkitt's lymphoma (a), there is enhancing soft tissue in both paracolic gutters (arrows, a), thickening of the descending colon (long arrow, a), and ill-defined stranding in the mesentery. Note the diffuse enhancing bone marrow involvement. The second patient (b) has HIV infection and a primary rectal lymphoma (arrow, b). Human immunodeficiency virus (HIV) patients are at risk for developing primary large-bowel lymphoma. (Reprinted with permission from Shoenut JP, Semelka RC, Silverman R, Yaffe CS, Mickflikier AB: The gastrointestinal tract. In Semelka RC, Shoenut JP (eds.). MRI of the Abdomen with CT Correlation. New York: Raven Press, pp. 119–143, 1993)

found that 94 (55%) were primary rectal lesions. Larger tumors were associated with metastatic disease and poor survival [78]. The imaging features of carcinoid tumors have been discussed elsewhere. As with other rectal diseases, direct sagittal plane imaging is useful. Liver metastases are best studied with dynamic gadolinium-enhanced SGE technique.

Melanoma

Primary colonic melanoma is rare and carries a poor prognosis [79]. Owing to the paramagnetic effects of mel-

anin, the lesion can have a characteristic high signal intensity on T1-weighted images and demonstrate ring enhancement after gadolinium administration (Fig. 6.75).

Metastases

Metastases to the large bowel result from direct extension. Ovarian and cervix cancer commonly spread in this manner. Colorectal involvement is well-seen on postgadolinium fat-suppressed T1-weighted images [54] (Fig. 6.76).

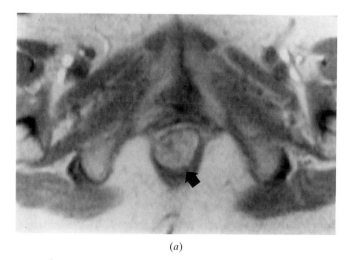

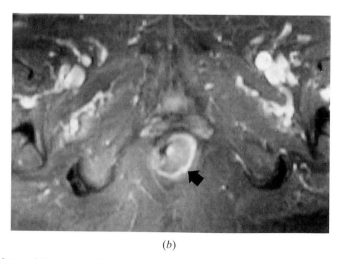

(a)   (b)

F I G . 6.75 Anorectal malignant melanoma. SGE (a) and gadolinium-enhanced T1-weighted fat-suppressed spin-echo (b) images in a patient with melanoma. Melanoma may be bright on T1-weighted sequences (arrow, a) owing to the paramagnetic properties of melanin. Rim enhancement is apparent following contrast and allows accurate determination of mural extent (arrow, b) (Reprinted with permission from Shoenut JP, Semelka RC, Silverman R, Yaffe CS, Mickflikier AB: The gastrointestinal tract. In Semelka RC, Shoenut JP (eds.). MRI of the Abdomen with CT Correlation. New York: Raven Press, pp. 119–143, 1993)

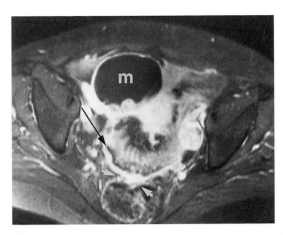

FIG. 6.76 Ovarian carcinoma metastatic to colon. Gadolinium-enhanced T1-weighted fat-suppressed spin-echo image in a patient with metastatic ovarian carcinoma. A complex cystic mass (*m*) encases the sigmoid colon (*long arrow*) and invades the rectum (*short arrows*). Tumor extension is clearly defined as enhancing tissue in a background of suppressed fat. (Reprinted with permission from Shoenut JP, Semelka RC, Silverman R, Yaffe CS, Mickflikier AB: The gastrointestinal tract. In Semelka RC, Shoenut JP (eds.). MRI of the Abdomen with CT Correlation. New York: Raven Press, pp. 119–143, 1993)

INFLAMMATORY AND INFECTIOUS DISORDERS

Ulcerative Colitis

Ulcerative colitis is an inflammatory disease of the large bowel. It has a predictable distribution: Disease begins in the rectum and spreads proximally in a contiguous fashion to involve part or all of the colon. The incidence of ulcerative colitis is greatest in the second, third, and fourth decades of life. There is a Caucasian, Jewish, and female predominance, and a positive family history is reported in up to 25 percent of cases [80]. The cause is unknown, but similar to Crohn's disease, a multifactorial etiology has been postulated. Ulcerative colitis is variable in presentation, but symptoms tend to be indolent with intermittent diarrhea and rectal bleeding. Patients with ulcerative colitis are at risk for developing toxic megacolon, which may be the presenting feature. Chronic ulcerative colitis is associated with a substantially increased risk of colon cancer.

Ulcerative colitis is a mucosal disease. Mucosal ulcers result from the coalescence of microabscesses in the crypts of Lieberkuhn. In chronic cases the colon shortens, the walls thicken, and the result is an ahaustral segment. This appearance has been likened to that of a "lead pipe."

The MRI appearance of ulcerative colitis reflects the underlying physiology: (1) rectal involvement progressing in a retrograde fashion to involve a variable amount of colon and (2) submucosal sparing (Fig. 6.77). The latter is especially well seen on gadolinium-enhanced fat-suppressed SGE images showing marked mu-cosal enhancement and negligible submucosal enhancement. Comparable to other inflammatory processes, the vasa rectae are prominent. Submucosal sparing is pronounced in long-standing disease because of submucosal edema and lymphangiectasia [1,2,3,6]. Toxic megacolon, unlike acute exacerbation and chronic indolent ulcerative colitis, is a transmural process. The bowel is dilated, and the entire bowel wall enhances after intravenous contrast administration. Patients are prostrate with debilitating bloody diarrhea, fever, leukocytosis, and abdominal pain.

Crohn's Colitis

Isolated colon involvement is noted in about a quarter of cases. When Crohn's colitis is limited to the anorectal region, differentiation from ulcerative colitis may be difficult [56]. Crohn's colitis also may present with toxic megacolon (Fig. 6.78). Crohn's colitis is distinguished from ulcerative colitis by the following features: (1) persistence of colonic redundancy and haustrations in pancolonic disease and (2) transmural enhancement, which at times may show the most intense enhancement in the submucosal layer, a layer that is spared in ulcerative colitis (Fig. 6.79).

Diverticulitis

Diverticula occur throughout the colon and tend to be most numerous in the sigmoid colon (Fig. 6.80). Inflamed diverticula favor the left colon, whereas diverticula, which undergo hemorrhage, tend to occur in the right colon. Several studies have shown cross-sectional imaging to be equivalent to, and in some cases superior to, barium enema in the evaluation of diverticulitis [81,82]. Bowel wall thickening and diverticular abscesses are well-seen on gadolinium-enhanced fat-suppressed SGE images combined with HASTE images (Fig. 6.81). Similarly, sinus tracts and fistulas can be identified with this technique. On unenhanced T1-weighted SGE images, inflammatory changes appear as low-signal-intensity curvilinear strands located within the high signal intensity of the pericolonic fat. Sinus tracts, fistulas, and abscess walls enhance and are well shown in a background of suppressed fat on gadolinium-enhanced fat-suppressed SGE images. It is frequently difficult to distinguish a perforated colon cancer from diverticulitis, and the two may coexist (Fig. 6.82).

Appendicitis

Diagnostic imaging in cases of appendicitis is typically reserved for unusual presentations. Although CT imaging and ultrasound have surpassed barium enema in the workup of appendicitis [83,84], MRI has several features that make it an attractive alternative. Specifically MRI has high contrast resolution for inflammatory processes and does not involve ionizing radiation. The latter is not insignificant because appendicitis is most common in children

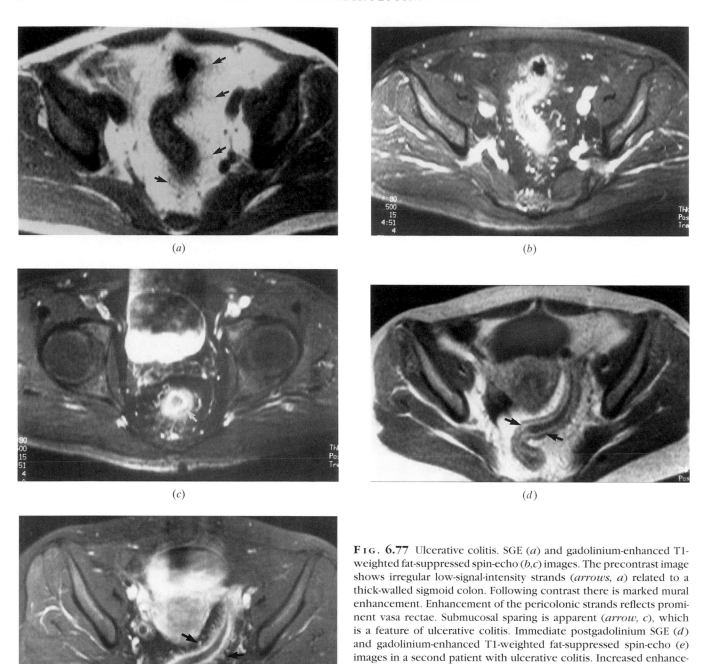

(a)

(b)

(c)

(d)

(e)

F I G . 6.77 Ulcerative colitis. SGE (a) and gadolinium-enhanced T1-weighted fat-suppressed spin-echo (b,c) images. The precontrast image shows irregular low-signal-intensity strands (*arrows, a*) related to a thick-walled sigmoid colon. Following contrast there is marked mural enhancement. Enhancement of the pericolonic strands reflects prominent vasa rectae. Submucosal sparing is apparent (*arrow, c*), which is a feature of ulcerative colitis. Immediate postgadolinium SGE (d) and gadolinium-enhanced T1-weighted fat-suppressed spin-echo (e) images in a second patient with ulcerative colitis. Increased enhancement on the immediate postgadolinium image (d) reflects increased capillary blood flow observed in severe disease. On the interstitial-phase image (e), there is marked mucosal enhancement with prominent vasa rectae (*short arrows, e*) and submucosal sparing (*long arrows, e*).

and young adults of reproductive age. On gadolinium-enhanced T1-weighted fat-suppressed images the inflamed appendix and surrounding tissues show marked enhancement. Inflammatory stranding in the surrounding fat is well-seen on unenhanced T1-weighted SGE images. In cases complicated by a periappendiceal abscess, the abscess rim will show enhancement after intravenous contrast administration, whereas the cavity remains signal-void (Fig. 6.83).

Abscess

Abscess formation is often a complication of gastrointestinal or biliary surgery, diverticulitis, appendicitis, or in-

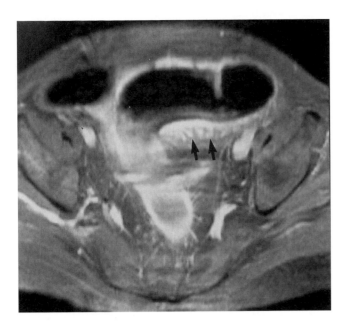

FIG. 6.78 Crohn's disease presenting as toxic megacolon. Gadolinium-enhanced T1-weighted fat-suppressed spin-echo image in a patient with toxic megacolon. Dilation and full thickness involvement characterize toxic megacolon, a complication of inflammatory bowel disease (IBD). Note the prominent vasa rectae (*arrows*), a common finding in the setting of bowel inflammation. (Reprinted with permission from Shoenut JP, Semelka RC, Silverman R, Yaffe CS, Mickflikier AB: Magnetic resonance imaging in inflammatory bowel disease. J Clin Gastroenterol 17:73–78, 1993)

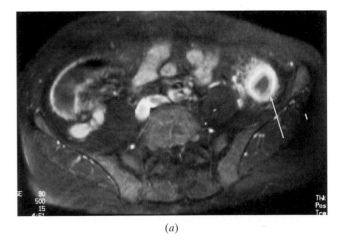

(*a*)

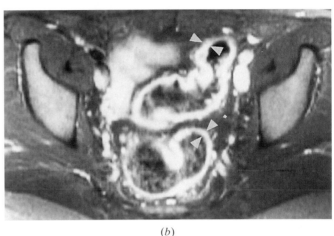

(*b*)

FIG. 6.79 Crohn's colitis. Gadolinium-enhanced T1-weighted fat-suppressed spin-echo image (*a*) demonstrates transmural enhancement with greater enhancement of the submucosa (*arrow, a*) than the other bowel-wall layers, which is diagnostic of Crohn's disease and excludes the diagnosis of ulcerative colitis. In a second patient with Crohn's colitis, gadolinium-enhanced T1-weighted fat-suppressed spin-echo image (*b*) shows full thickness enhancement of the sigmoid colon (*arrowheads, b*). The distribution of colon involvement is compatible with ulcerative colitis. However, the colon has remained redundant with persistence of haustrations despite severe disease. These findings combined with transmural enhancement are consistent with Crohn's colitis. Note the enhancing pericolonic inflammation in both patients. (Reprinted with permission from Shoenut JP, Semelka RC, Magro CM, Silverman R, Yaffe CS, Mickflikier AB: Comparison of magnetic resonance imaging and endoscopy in distinguishing the type and severity of inflammatory bowel diseases. J Clin Gastroenterol 19:31–35, 1994)

flammatory bowel disease (IBD). CT imaging and ultrasound are the mainstay of diagnosis and have the added advantage of ease of percutaneous drainage capabilities. For MRI to compete effectively with these modalities, automatic table motion, MRI-compatible needle and drainage equipment, and ultrafast imaging techniques must be in common usage. A fluid collection with an enhancing rim is compatible with an abscess. This is best shown on gadolinium-enhanced fat-suppressed SGE sequences. The presence of signal-void air within the collection confirms the diagnosis (Fig. 6.84) [85]. The role of oral or rectal contrast to distinguish bowel from abscess is not firmly established. Most abscesses can be confidently differentiated from bowel with gadolinium-enhanced fat-suppressed SGE and HASTE images acquired in two planes. This approach demonstrates the oval shape of abscesses and permits their distinction from adjacent tubular bowel. Enhancement of periabscess tissues on immediate postgadolinium fat-suppressed SGE images confirms the inflammatory nature of the fluid collections (Fig. 6.85). In patients with a contraindication to iodinated intravenous contrast (allergy and/or diminished renal function), MRI should be considered for the evaluation of abscess. MRI also may be effective as a method to follow therapeutic interventions (Fig. 6.86).

Colonic Fistulas

MRI is an effective imaging modality for evaluating colonic fistulas [7,8,86–88]. In particular, the multiplanar imaging capability of MRI has been shown to be useful for surgical planning for perirectal/perianal fistulas. The relationship of fistulas to the levator ani muscle is well shown on a combination of transverse, coronal, and sagittal plane images. T1-weighted images, T2-weighted im-

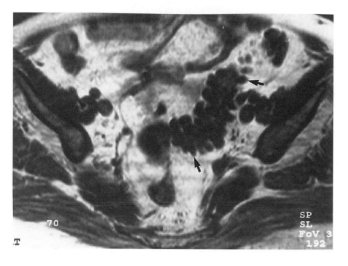

F IG . 6.80 Diverticulosis. SGE image demonstrates multiple signal void sacculations arising from the sigmoid colon consistent with diverticulosis. Diverticula are common and often incidental findings. Complication of diverticula include diverticulitis and frank abscess. (Reprinted with permission from Ascher SM, Semelka RC: MRI of the gastrointestinal tract. In: Higgins CB, Hricak H, Helms CA (eds.). Magnetic Resonance Imaging of the Body, Raven Press, pp. 677–700, 1997.)

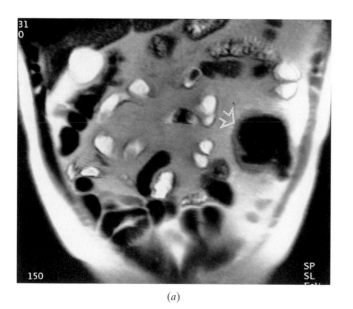

(a)

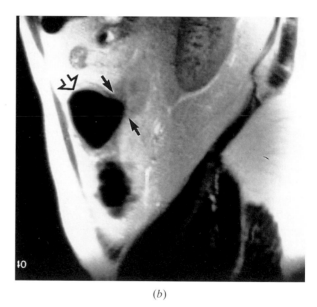

(b)

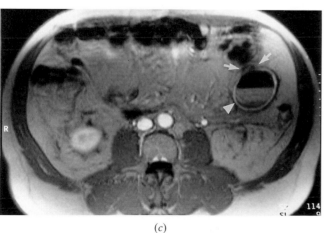

(c)

F IG . 6.81 Diverticular abscess. Coronal (a) and sagittal (b) HASTE, and immediate postgadolinium SGE (c) images. An air and fluid containing fluid collection (*open arrow, a,b*) originates from the descending colon (*solid arrows, b,c*), a finding consistent with a diverticular abscess. On the immediate postgadolinium image the inner wall of the abscess (*arrowhead, c*) enhances. An air/fluid level is apparent on the transverse image (c).

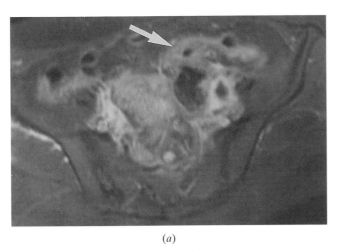
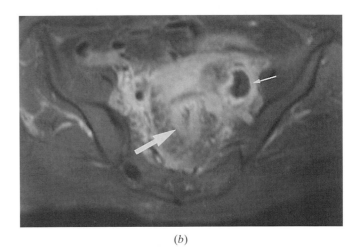

(a)   (b)

F IG . 6.82 Colon cancer with coexistent diverticulitis. Gadolinium-enhanced T1-weighted fat-suppressed spin-echo images (a,b) demonstrate a heterogeneously enhancing thickened segment of sigmoid colon (*large arrows, a,b*) with an adjoining abscess (*thin arrow, b*) features that were considered compatible with diverticulitis. Colon cancer was found in conjunction with diverticulitis at surgery.

ages and gadolinium-enhanced T1-weighted fat-suppressed images all provide good contrast between fistulas and surrounding tissues (Fig. 6.87).

Infectious Colitis

Pseudomembranous colitis occurs in the setting of antibiotic use. The infectious organism most frequently implicated is *Clostridium difficile* [89]. The severity of the disease varies from mild to life-threatening. MRI shows thickening of the affected large bowel with marked enhancement (Fig. 6.88). Typhlitis occurs in neutropenic patients, usually leukemics. The cecum and ascending colon are the segments most commonly affected. MRI findings are nonspecific in patients with infectious colitis and generally demonstrate increased wall thickness and enhancement. Other infectious agents that target the colon include *Shigella, Salmonella, Escherichia coli*, amebiasis, and cholera.

Patients with AIDS are prone to cytomegalovirus colitis. Bowel wall thickening secondary to submucosal hemorrhage is the most characteristic finding. *Mycobacterium avium intracellulare* also affects the large bowel and produces wall thickening (Fig. 6.89) [43]. Patients with AIDS frequently develop proctitis. Opportunistic infection leads to rectal wall thickening and stranding in the perirectal space. Occasionally frank perirectal abscesses occur. Gadolinium-enhanced fat-suppressed SGE images highlight bowel wall thickening and abscess formation. Unenhanced SGE imaging is effective for showing perirectal stranding, which appears low in signal intensity in a background of high-signal-intensity fat. Patients with severe colitis may develop chronic wasting.

Radiation Enteritis

The rectum is the most susceptible segment of large bowel to develop radiation enteritis. This reflects its fixed position in the radiation port. In one study, the T1- and T2-weighted MRI features of the rectum in 42 patients with a status of postpelvic radiation therapy were graded with respect to wall thickness and signal intensity of the muscular layers and submucosa. All grades of tissue change were seen in the rectum regardless of the time from start of therapy. MRI had excellent sensitivity for depicting abnormalities, but specificity was limited [75]. This underscores the need for interpreting MRI examinations in the light of clinical history. The routine use of intravenous gadolinium in combination with fat suppression is effective for evaluating postradiation changes. High-resolution T2-weighted images demonstrate the findings of submucosal edema in acute radiation proctocolitis well (Fig. 6.90).

Intraluminal Contrast Agents

The goals of intraluminal contrast agent use are twofold: (1) reliable differentiation of bowel from adjacent structures and (2) better delineation of bowel wall processes. Oral contrast agents fall into two major categories: positive (signal intensity increasing) and negative (signal intensity decreasing) agents. Positive agents shorten T1-relaxation time, whereas negative agents either shorten T2-relaxation time or rely on immobile protons to decrease intraluminal signal intensity. Biphasic intraluminal agents are formulated to produce high signal intensity on T1-weighted images and low signal intensity on T2-weighted images [90].

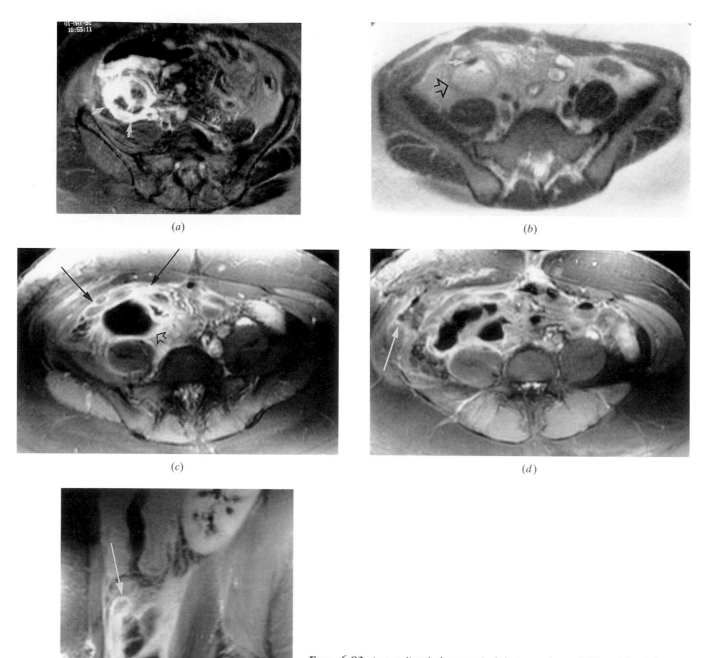

(a)

(b)

(c)

(d)

(e)

FIG. 6.83 Appendiceal abscess. Gadolinium-enhanced T1-weighted fat-suppressed spin-echo image (*a*) demonstrates a low-signal-intensity appendiceal abscess with a prominent enhancing rim (*arrow, a*). HASTE (*b*), transverse (*c,d*), and sagittal (*e*) postgadolinium fat-suppressed SGE images in a second patient. A large multiloculated appendiceal abscess is present (*hollow arrow, b,c,e*). Air within the abscess is signal-void (*arrow, b*) on the T2-weighted image. Following gadolinium administration (*c,d,e*) the abscess rim enhances (*open arrow, c,e*), and extensive enhancement of periabscess tissue is present (*long arrows, c,d,e*).

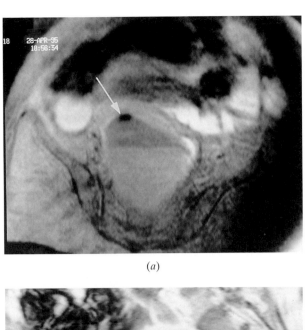

(a)

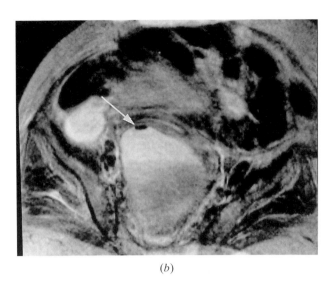

(b)

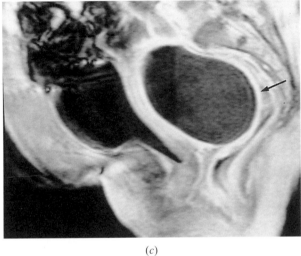

(c)

FIG. 6.84 Pouch of Douglas abscess. T1-weighted fat-suppressed spin-echo (a), T2-weighted echo-train spin-echo (b) and sagittal 45-second postgadolinium SGE (c) images. An 8-cm pouch of Douglas abscess is present that contains a focus of air that is signal-void on T1-weighted (a) and T2-weighted (b) images (arrow, a,b). The abscess has a thick, enhancing rim (arrow, c) on the early postgadolinium image (c) with increased enhancement of surrounding tissue. Note the layering of debris on all the MR images (a–c).

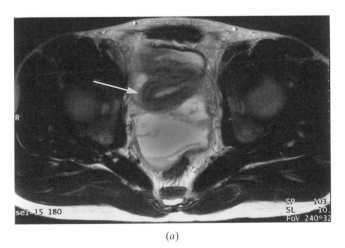

(a)

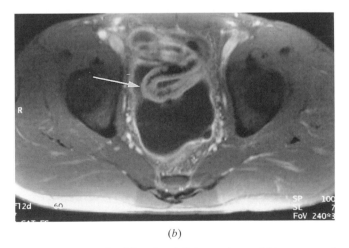

(b)

FIG. 6.85 Midabdominal and pelvic abscesses. Transverse 512-resolution echo-train spin-echo (a) and gadolinium-enhanced fat-suppressed SGE (b) images through the pelvis, and sagittal 512-resolution echo-train spin-echo (c) and sagittal gadolinium-enhanced fat-suppressed SGE (d) images through the pelvis and midabdomen. An 8-cm, irregular, oval-shaped abscess is present in the recto vesicle space that demonstrates dependent layering of low-signal-intensity debris on the T2-weighted image (a) and substantial enhancement of the abscess wall (b). Inflammatory thickening of a loop of ileum (arrow, a) abutting the abscess is identified.

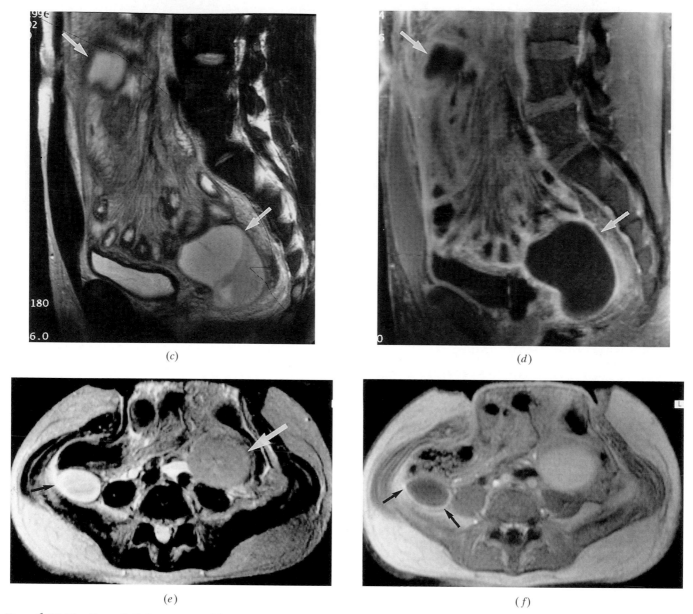

(c)   *(d)*

(e)   *(f)*

FIG. 6.85 (*Continued*) Enhancement of the serosal surface of the bowel is appreciated (*arrow, b*). The sagittal plane images demonstrate the pelvic and the midabdominal abscesses (*arrows, c,d*). Layering of low-signal-intensity material in the dependent portion of the pelvic abscess is shown on the T2-weighted image (*c*). Enhancement of the abscess wall and increased enhancement of multiple loops of small bowel are noted on the gadolinium-enhanced fat-suppressed SGE image (*d*). Transverse 512-resolution T2-weighted echo-train spin-echo (*e*) and immediate postgadolinium SGE (*f*) images in a second patient. This patient with chronic renal failure had undergone multiple abdominal surgical procedures for bowel ischemia and has a large anterior abdominal wall dehiscence with exposed peritoneal lining. A retrocecal abscess collection is present (*arrows, e,f*) that is high in signal intensity on the T2-weighted image and demonstrates ring enhancement on the immediate postgadolinium image. A chronically failed renal transplant is also identifiable (*large arrow, e*).

Positive Intraluminal Contrast Agents

Oral manganese, which occurs naturally in green tea and blueberry juice, shortens T1- and T2-relaxation times [91,92]. Both foodstuffs have been used successfully to opacify the gastrointestinal tract. Manganese chloride is a commercially available oral agent, LumenHance™

(Bracco; Princeton, New Jersey) that is combined with a polymer to produce a biphasic agent. Clinical trials with this agent show promise [93].

Ferric ammonium citrate (FAC) is the principal ingredient in the over-the-counter product, Gerritol (Beecham; Bristol, Tennessee). It effectively marks the proximal small bowel (Fig. 6.91), but image quality is degraded

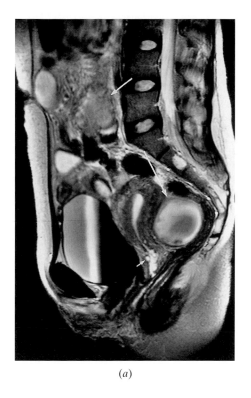

(a)

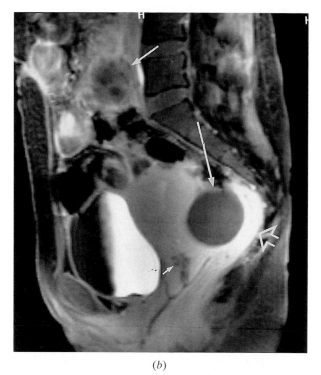

(b)

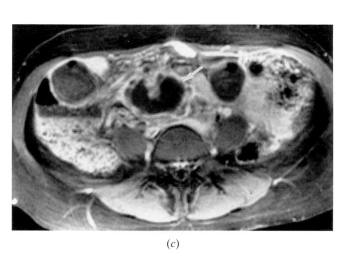

(c)

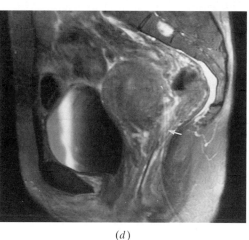

(d)

FIG. 6.86 Pelvic abscess, pre- and post catheter drainage. Sagittal 512-resolution T2-weighted echo-train spin-echo (*a*), sagittal interstitial-phase gadolinium-enhanced fat-suppressed SGE (*b*), and transverse interstitial-phase gadolinium-enhanced fat-suppressed SGE (*c*) images. The sagittal images demonstrate a 5-cm abscess in the pouch of Douglas (*long arrow, a,b*), and a smaller midabdominal abscess (*short arrow, a,b*). On the T2-weighted image, heterogeneous signal is present in the dependent portion, which is a common finding in abscesses. On the postgadolinium images, substantial enhancement of the abscess wall and the adjacent rectum (*hollow arrow, b*) is present. Multiple Nabothian cysts are present in the cervix (*small arrow, a,b*). The transverse gadolinium-enhanced fat-suppressed image through the midabdomen demonstrates a 4-cm abscess (*arrow, c*) with enhancement of the abscess wall and the periabscess tissue. Sagittal 512-resolution T2-weighted echo-train spin-echo image (*d*) and transverse interstitial-phase gadolinium-enhanced fat-suppressed SGE (*e*) images obtained 1 week after transrectal placement of a drainage catheter demonstrate substantial resolution of the pelvic abscess. The drainage catheter is identified as a signal-void tube (*arrow, d,e*). The degree of inflammatory reaction has also substantially diminished, but persistent enhancing tissue around the catheter is visualized (*e*).

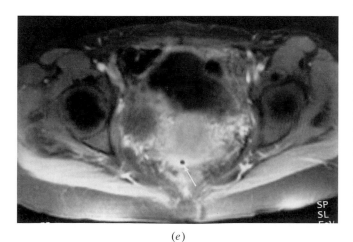

(e)

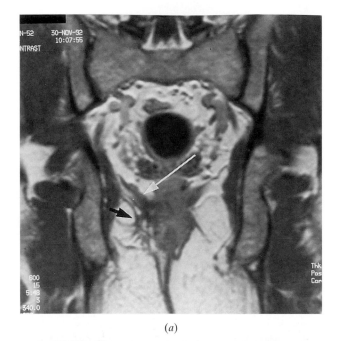

(a)

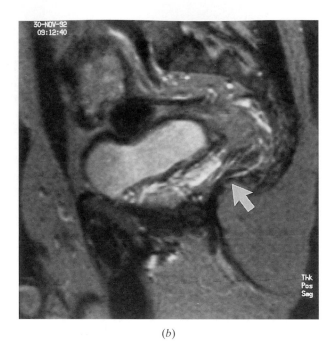

(b)

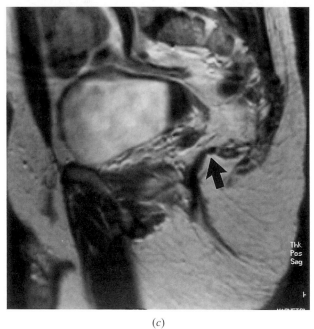

(c)

FIG. 6.87 Periabscess fistula. Coronal T1-weighted spin-echo (a), sagittal T2-weighted spin-echo (b), and gadolinium-enhanced T1-weighted spin-echo (c) images. A complex fistula (arrow, a) is present in a left perianal location that extends to the levator ani muscle (long arrow, a). The fistula is low in signal on T1-weighted (arrow, a), T2-weighted (arrow, b), and postgadolinium (arrow, c) images, reflecting the chronic fibrotic nature of the fistulas.

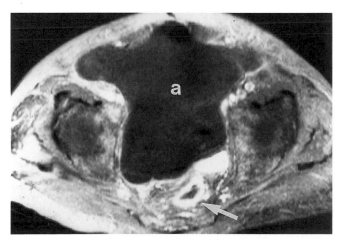

FIG. 6.88 Pseudomembranous colitis. Gadolinium-enhanced T1-weighted fat-suppressed spin-echo image in a patient on a prolonged course of oral antibiotics. The rectosigmoid is thick walled, and transmural enhancement is apparent (arrow). This is nonspecific for severe bowel inflammation. Clinical history and laboratory results establish the diagnosis of pseudomembranous colitis. Note the large volume of ascites (''a''). (Reprinted with permission from Shoenut JP, Semelka RC, Silverman R, Yaffe CS, Mickflikier AB: The gastrointestinal tract. In Semelka RC, Shoenut JP (eds.). MRI of the Abdomen with CT Correlation. New York: Raven Press, pp. 119–143, 1993)

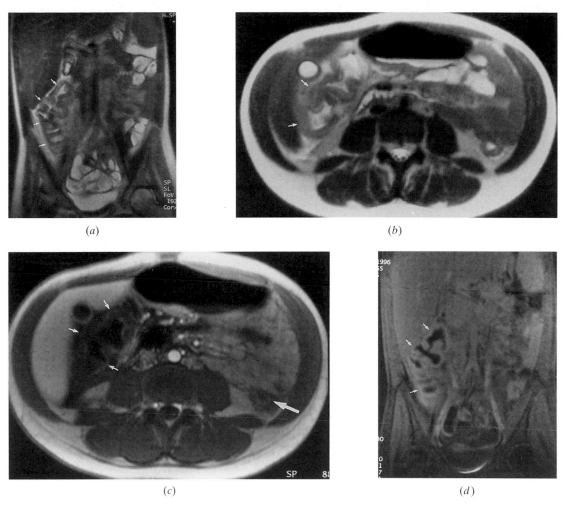

(a) (b)

(c) (d)

F IG. 6.89 *Mycobacterium avium intracellulare* (MAI) colitis. Coronal (*a*), and transverse (*b*) HASTE, immediate postgadolinium SGE (*c*), and coronal 90-second postgadolinium fat-suppressed SGE (*d*) images in a patient with Mycobacterium avium intracellulare colitis. HASTE images (*a,b*) demonstrate marked wall thickening of the ascending colon (*small arrows, a,b*) with relative sparing of the descending colon. The mucosal surface enhances on the immediate postgadolinium image (*small arrows, c*) with negligible enhancement of the thickened outer wall. Less severe involvement is also seen of the descending colon (*arrow, c*). Enhancement of the wall increases and becomes more uniform (*small arrows, d*) on interstitial-phase images reflecting capillary leakage.

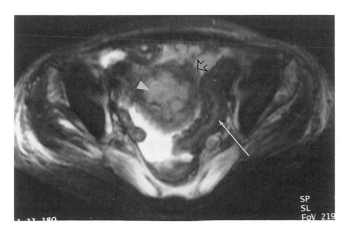

F IG. 6.90 Radiation enteritis. Transverse 512-resolution T2-weighted echo-train spin-echo image in a patient following radiation therapy. The sigmoid colon is thick-walled with marked submucosal edema (*arrow*). The circumferential and symmetric nature of the bowel-wall changes are suggestive of radiation enteritis. Note the thick-walled bladder (*open arrow*) and its heterogeneous contents (*arrowhead*), findings consistent with hemorrhagic cystitis, another sequela of radiation therapy. Free pelvic fluid is also present.

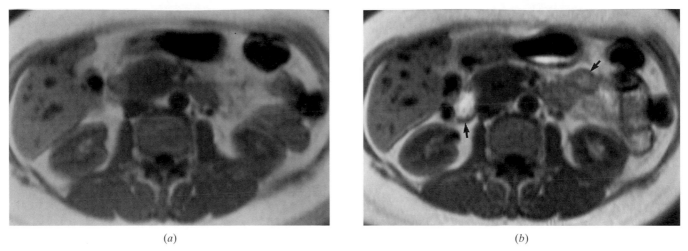

(a)   (b)

FIG. 6.91 Positive oral contrast agent. SGE images before (*a*) and after ingestion of ferric ammonium citrate (FAC) (*b*). Oral contrast causes high signal intensity within the bowel (*arrows, b*). The bowel loops are readily distinguished from the adjacent pancreas following oral contrast administration. Note that FAC not only marks the bowel, but distends it as well.

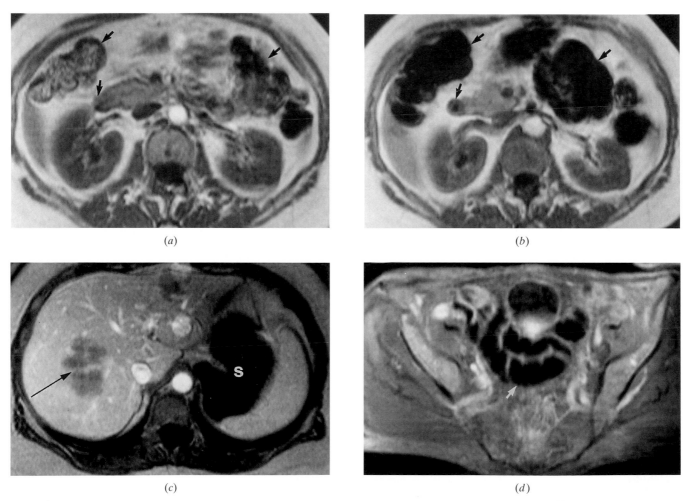

(a)   (b)

(c)   (d)

FIG. 6.92 Negative oral contrast agent. SGE images before (*a*) and after (*b*) perflouroocytlbromide (PFOB) ingestion, gadolinium-enhanced SGE image after PFOB ingestion (*c*), and gadolinium-enhanced T1-weighted fat-suppressed spin-echo image after PFOB ingestion (*d*) in three different patients. In the first patient (*a,b*), bowel contents are heterogeneous before PFOB intake (*arrows, a*), but following ingestion of PFOB, they become nearly signal-void (*arrows, b*). PFOB is signal-void in the stomach (''s'',*c*) of a woman with hepatic metastases (*arrow, c*) from cervical carcinoma. In a third patient (*d*) distal small bowel is signal-void (*arrow, d*) following PFOB administration. Oral agents distend the bowel, which may aid detection of mucosal abnormalities.

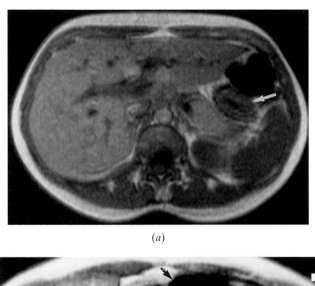

(a)

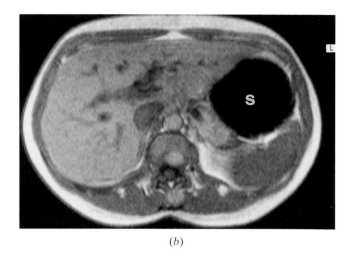

(b)

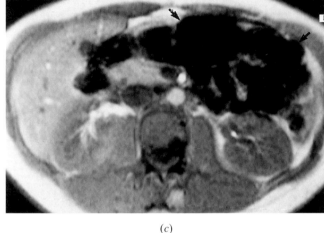

(c)

FIG. 6.93 Negative oral contrast agent. SGE before (*a*) and after (*b,c*) oral magnetic particle (OMP) ingestion. Prior to OMP ingestion, the stomach is collapsed with apparent wall thickening. Once distended with oral contrast, the stomach wall is barely perceptible. Similarly, the small and large bowel are distended and marked by OMP (*arrows, c*). Susceptibility artifact is visualized in many of the loops of bowel (*c*).

distally secondary to induced peristalsis [94,95]. Specifically designed oral FAC preparations for MRI have been tested. Oral magnetic resonance (OMR), Oncomembrane (Seattle, Washington) is a commercial formulation of FAC that can opacify bowel. Gastrointestinal side effects were reported in 22 percent of patients at the recommended dose [96]. In another study, ferric iron admixed with phytate was found to be an effective and well-tolerated intraluminal contrast agent [97].

Gadopentetate dimeglumine, Magnevist™ (Shering AG; Berlin, Germany), shortens T1- and T2-relaxation times with the T1 effects predominating. It may be mixed with mannitol to lessen dilutional effects during bowel transit, or it may be mixed with barium paste for use in the esophagus. Both preparations are tolerated by patients and effectively mark the bowel and demonstrate mucosal abnormalities [98]. Currently, this agent is available only in Europe.

Negative Intraluminal Contrast Agents

Perflouroocytlbromide (PFOB) perflubron, Imagent GI™ (Alliance Pharmaceutical; San Diego, California), is a neg-

ative oral contrast agent without hydrogen atoms (Fig. 6.92). One study showed that PFOB performed better when glucagon was given to decrease peristalsis and prolong transit time, whereas another study showed no significant difference in motion artifact irrespective of glucagon administration [99,100]. Overall patient tolerance is good, although some patients complain of an oily taste, rectal incontinence, or both up to three hours after ingestion.

Superparamagnetic particles are negative contrast agents that diminish intraluminal signal intensity by exploiting T2* effects. Oral magnetic particles (OMP) (WIN 39996; Nycomed; Oslo, Norway), a suspension of paramagnetic ferrite crystals adsorbed to a polymer, cellulose and starch, effectively marks the bowel when given in the appropriate dose (Fig. 6.93) [101]. The agent is well-tolerated, but susceptibility effects degrade image quality on gradient-echo sequences [102,103]. A suspension of salinized iron oxide particles (Ferumoxsil™, formerly AMI-121™, known in Europe as Lumirem™, Advanced Magnetics Inc., Boston, Massachusetts; Laboratoire, Guerbet SA, Aulnay-Sousbois, France) is another preparation shown to increase diagnostic confidence in the evaluation of gynecologic disease [104]. Other investigators have found it to be efficacious in the abdomen and to have good patient tolerance [105,106].

Barium sulfate at high concentrations has negative oral contrast agent properties [107]. Its safety record is established and it can be administered orally or rectally. In an effort to improve its signal-diminishing properties and palatability, barium sulfate has been combined with other negative oral agents with some success [108].

Clay-containing substances found in over-the-counter products such as Kaopectate™, and kaolin-pectate (Upjohn; Kalamazoo, Michigan) produce diamagnetic shortening of T1- and T2-relaxation times in aqueous solutions. Although these substances are effective at decreasing intraluminal signal intensity, patient compliance is limited by their lack of palatability.

Several investigators have reported success with using air as an intraluminal negative contrast agent [108–112]. Susceptibility artifacts predominate at high field strength and preclude the use of oral or rectal administration of air.

Other Intraluminal Agents

A host of over-the-counter foodstuffs have been tested as potential intraluminal contrast agents. They are usually high in signal intensity on both T1- and T2-weighted sequences, a reflection of their lipid components and/or paramagnetic trace elements and/or fluid states. They are well-suited for opacifying the proximal gastrointestinal tract, but dilutional effects limit their usefulness distally [113,114].

CONCLUSION

Breath-hold scanning techniques as well as reproducible chemically selective excitation-spoiling fat suppression, single-shot T2-weighted echo-train spin-echo and routine usage of intravenous gadolinium have all contributed to the emergence of gastrointestinal MRI. MRI is well-established for the investigation of primary or recurrent rectal carcinomas. Current imaging technique renders MRI comparable to CT imaging for the investigation of colonic, small bowel, and gastric malignancies. The superior ability of MRI to evaluate liver metastases may render MRI preferable to CT imaging in the investigation of these malignancies. Inflammatory bowel disease and abscesses are extremely well shown on MR images due to the high sensitivity of gadolinium-enhanced fat-suppressed SGE procedures for the detection of inflammatory enhancement. MRI should be considered in the investigation of these entities in patients with contraindications to iodinated contrast or CT examination.

FUTURE DIRECTIONS

Future directions include the use of oral contrast agents described earlier, new intravenous agents, and new imaging techniques. Regarding intravenous agents, iron oxide particle agents have been used for MR lymphography in experimental models [115]. This agent is taken up by normal lymphoid tissue and hyperplastic lymph nodes, which decrease uniformly in signal intensity on T2-weighted images, whereas nodes involved with malignant disease retain signal intensity. This agent may increase the specificity of detecting the presence of malignant involvement in normal-sized (<1 cm) lymph nodes, a circumstance that is observed with gastrointestinal malignancies. Future imaging directions include real-time, dynamic alimentary track imaging (MRI upper GI), 3D intraluminal display (MRI endoscopy), and therapeutic interventions.

REFERENCES

1. Semelka RC, Shoenut JP, Silverman R, Kroeker MA, Yaffe CS, Micflikier AB: Bowel disease: Prospective comparison of CT and 1.5 T pre- and postcontrast MR imaging with T1-weighted fat-suppressed and breath-hold FLASH sequences. J Magn Reson Imaging 1:625–632, 1991.
2. Shoenut JP, Semelka RC, Silverman R, Yaffe CS, Mickflikier AB: Magnetic resonance imaging in inflammatory bowel disease. J Clin Gastroenterol 17:73–78, 1993.
3. Shoenut JP, Semelka RC, Magro CM, Silverman R, Yaffe CS, Mickflikier AB: Comparison of magnetic resonance imaging and endoscopy in distinguishing the type and severity of inflammatory bowel diseases. J Clin Gastroenterol 19:31–35, 1994.
4. Kettritz U, Isaacs K, Warshauer DM, Semelka RC: Crohn's disease: Pilot study comparing MRI of the abdomen with clinical evaluation. J Clin Gastroenterol 21:249–253, 1995.
5. Shoenut JP, Semelka RC, Silverman R, Yaffe CS, Mickflikier AB: Magnetic resonance imaging evaluation of the local extent of colorectal mass lesions. J Clin Gastroenterol 17:248–253, 1993.
6. Shoenut JP, Semelka RC, Silverman R, Yaffe CS, Mickflikier AB: The gastrointestinal tract. In Semelka RC, Shoenut JP (eds.). MRI of the Abdomen with CT Correlation. New York: Raven Press, pp. 119–143, 1993.
7. Outwater E, Schiebler ML: Pelvic fistulas: Findings on MR images. AJR Am J Roentgenol 160:327–330, 1993.
8. Semelka RC, Hricak H, Kim B, et al: Pelvic fistulas: Appearances on MR images. Abdom Imaging 22:91–95, 1997.
9. Chan TW, Kressel HY, Milestone B, Tomachefski J, Schnall M, Rosato E, Daly J: Rectal carcinoma: Staging at MR imaging with endorectal surface coil. Radiology 181:461–467, 1991.
10. Schnall MD, Furth EE, Rosato F: Rectal tumor stage: Correlation of endorectal MR imaging and pathologic findings. Radiology 190:709–714, 1994.
11. de Lange EE, Fechner RE, Wanebo HJ: Suspected recurrent rectosigmoid carcinoma after abdominoperineal resection: MR imaging and histopathologic correlation. Radiology 170:323–328, 1989.
12. Balzini L, Ceglia E, D'Ippolito G, et al: Local recurrence of rectosigmoid cancer: What about the choice of MRI for diagnosis? Gastrointest Radiol 15:338–342, 1990.

13. Gomberg JS, Friedman AC, Radecki PD, Grumbach K, Caroline DF: MRI differentiation of recurrent colorectal carcinoma from postoperative fibrosis. Gastroint Radiol 11:361–363, 1986.

14. Krestin GP, Steibrich W, Friedman G: Recurrent rectal cancer: Diagnosis with MR versus CT. Radiology 168:307–311, 1988.

15. Pema PJ, Bennett WF, Bova JG, Warman P: CT vs MRI in diagnosis of recurrent rectosigmoid carcinoma. J Comput Assist Tomogr 18:256–261, 1994.

16. Waizer A, Powsner E, Russo I, et al: Prospective comparative study of magnetic resonance imaging versus transrectal ultrasound for preoperative staging and follow-up of rectal cancer. Dis Colon Rectum 34:1068–1072, 1991.

17. Pavone P, Cardone G.P, Cisterno S, Di Girolamo M, et al: Gadopentetate dimeglumine-barium paste for opacification of the esophageal lumen on MR images. AJR Am J Roentgenol 159:762–764, 1992.

18. Macpherson RI: Gastrointestinal tract duplications: Clinical, pathologic, etiologic and radiologic considerations. Radiographics, 13:1063–1080, 1993.

19. Rafal RB, Markisz JA: Magnetic resonance imaging of an esophageal duplication cyst. Am J Gastroenterol 86:1809–1811, 1991.

20. American Joint Committee: Clinical staging systems for cancer of the esophagus. Cancer 25:50–57, 1975.

21. Habrey K, Winnfield AL: Multiple leiomyomas of the esophagus. Am J Dig Dis 19:678–680, 1974.

22. Winbeck M, Berges W: Oesophageal lesions in the alcoholic. Clin Gastroenterol 10:375–388, 1981.

23. Maram ES, Kurland LT, Ludwig J, Brian DD: Esophageal carcinoma in Olmstead county, Minnesota, 1935–1971. Mayo Clin Proc 52:24–27, 1977.

24. Kahrihas PJ, Kishk SM, Helm JF, Dodds WJ, et al: Comparison of pseudoachalasia and achalasia. Am J Med 82:439–446, 1987.

25. Templeton PA, Kui M, White CS, Krasna MJ: Use of gadolinium-enhanced MR imaging to evaluate for airway invasion in patients with esophageal carcinoma. Radiology 193(P):311, 1994.

26. Halvorsen RA, Herfkins RJ, Wolfe WG, et al: Comparison of magnetic resonance to computed tomography for staging esophageal carcinoma. American Roentgen Ray Society Proceedings, p. 133, 1987.

27. Quint LE, Glazer GM, Orringer MGB: Esophageal imaging by MR and CT: Study of normal anatomy and neoplasms. Radiology 156:727–731, 1985.

28. Trenker SW, Halvorsen RA, Thompson WM: Neoplasms of the upper gastrointestinal tract. Radiol Clin North Am 32:15–24, 1994.

29. Halvorsen RA, Thompson WM: Primary neoplasms of the hollow organs of the gastrointestinal tract. Cancer 67:188–189, 1991.

30. Nebel OT, Fornes MF, Castell DO: Symptomatic gastro-esophageal reflux: Incidence and precipating factors. Am J Dig Dis 21:953–956, 1976.

31. Behar J, Sheahan MB, Biancani P, Spiro HM, Storer EH: Medical and surgical management of reflux esophagitis. N Engl J Med 293:263–268, 1975.

32. Chernish SM, Maglinte DDT: Glucagon: Common untoward reactions—review and recommendations. Radiology 177:145–146, 1990.

33. Hamed MM, Hamm B, Ibrahim ME, Taupitz M, Mahfouz AE: Dynamic MR imaging of the abdomen with gadopentetate dimeglumine: Normal enhancement pattern of liver, spleen, stomach, and pancreas. AJR Am J Roentgenol 158:303–307, 1992.

34. Scholz FJ, Vincent ME: The stomach. In: Putnam CE, Ravin CE (eds.). Textbook of Diagnostic Imaging. Philadelphia: Saunders, pp. 778–807, 1988.

35. Nakamura T, Nakano G: Histopathological classification and malignant change in gastric polyps. J Clin Pathol 38:754–764, 1985.

36. Eisenberg RL: Single filling defects in the colon. In Eisenberg RL (ed.). Gastrointestinal Radiology. Philadelphia: Lippincott, pp. 681–710, 1983.

37. Wingo PA, Tong T, Bolden S: Cancer statistics, 1995. CA Cancer J Clin 45(1):8–30, 1995.

38. Haenszel W, Kurihara M: Studies of Japanese migrants: 1. Mortality from cancer and other disease among Japanese in the United States. J Natl Cancer Inst 40:43–68, 1968.

39. Coggon D, Acheson ED: The geography of cancer of the stomach. Br Med Bull 40:335–341, 1984.

40. Auh Yh, Lim T-H, Lee DH, Young YK, et al: In vitro MR imaging of the resected stomach with a 4.7-T Super conducting magnet. Radiology 191:129–134, 1994.

41. Matushita M, Oi H, Murakami T, et al: Extraserosal invasion in advanced gastric cancer: Evaluation with MR imaging. Radiology 192:87–91, 1994.

42. Semelka RC, Shoenut JP, Kroeker MA, et al: Focal liver disease: Comparison of dynamic contrast-enhanced CT and T2-weighted fat-suppressed, FLASH, and dynamic gadolinium-enhanced MR imaging at 1.5 T. Radiology 184:687–694, 1992.

43. Jeffrey RB: Abdominal imaging in the immunocompromised patient. Radiol Clin North Am 30:579–596, 1992.

44. Chou CK, Chen LT, Sheu RS, Yang CW, et al: MRI manifestations of gastrointestinal lymphoma. Abdom Imaging 19:495–500, 1994.

45. Chou CK, Chen LT, Sheu RS, Wang ML, et al: MRI manisfestations of gastrointestinal wall thickening. Abdom Imaging 19:389–394, 1994.

46. Radin R: HIV infection: Analysis in 259 consecutive patients with abnormal abdominal CT findings. Radiology 197:712–722, 1995.

47. MacKey WC, Dineen P: A fifty year experience with Meckel's diverticulum. Surg Gynecol Obstet 156:56–64, 1983.

48. Chew FS, Zambuto DA: Meckel's diverticulum. AJR Am J Roentgenol 159:982, 1992.

49. Teplick SK, Glick SN, Keller MS: The duodedenum. In Putnam CE, Ravin CE (eds.): Textbook of Diagnostic Imaging. Philadelphia: Saunders, pp. 808–846, 1988.

50. Semelka RC, John G, Kelekis NL, Burdeny DA, Ascher SM: Small bowel neoplastic disease: Demonstration by MRI. J Mag Reson Imaging. In press.

51. Al-Mondhiry H: Primary lymphomas of the intestine: East-west contrast. Am J Hematol 22:89–105, 1986.

52. Martin RG: Malignant tumors of the small intestine. Surg Clin North Am 66:779–785, 1986.

53. Rubesin SE, Gilchrist AM, Bronner M, Saul SH, et al: Non-Hodgkin lymphoma of the small intestine. Radiographics 10:985–998, 1990.

54. Semelka RC, Lawrence PH, Shoenut JP, Heywood M, et al: Primary malignant ovarian disease: Prospective comparison of contrast enhanced CT and pre- and post intravenous Gd-DPTA enhanced fat-suppressed and breath hold MRI with histological correlation. J Magn Reson Imaging 3:99–106, 1993.

55. Brahme F, Linstrom C, Wenckert A: Crohn's disease in a defined population. Gastroenterology 69:342–351, 1975.

56. Goldberg HI, Caruthers B Jr, Nelson JA, Singleton JW: Radiographic findings of the national cooperative Crohn's disease study. Gastroenterol 77:925, 1979.

57. Anderson CM, Brown JJ, Balfe DM, Heiken JP, et al: MR imaging of Crohn disease: Use of perflubron as a gastrointestinal contrast agent. J Magn Reson Imaging 4:491–496, 1994.

58. Deutsch AA, McLeod RS, Cullen J, Cohen Z: Results of the pelvic-pouch procedure in patients with Crohn's disease. Dis Colon Rectum 34:475–477, 1991.

59. Gutmann LT: Yersinia enterocolitica and Yersinia pseudotuberculosis. In Gorbach SI (ed.). Infectious Diarrhea. Boston: Blackwell Scientific, p.65, 1986.

60. Lambert ME, Schofield PF, Ironside AG, Mandal BK: Campylobacter colitis. Br Med J 1:857–859, 1979.

61. Hussain SM, Stoker J, Lameris JS: Anal sphincter complex: Endoanal MR imaging of normal anatomy. Radiology 197:671–677, 1995.

62. Stoker J, Hussain SM, van Kempen D, Elevelt AJ, Lameris JS: Endoanal coil MR imaging in anal fistulas. AJR Am J Roentgenol 166:360–362, 1996.

63. Okizuka HO, Sugimura K, Ishida T: Preoperative local staging of rectal carcinoma with MR imaging and a rectal balloon. J Magn Reson Imaging 3:329–335, 1993.

64. Sato YS, Pringle KC, Bergman RA, Yuh WT, et al: Congenital anorectal anomalies: MR imaging. Radiology 168:157–162, 1988.

65. Eisenberg RL: Multiple filling defects in the colon. In Eisenberg RL (ed.): Gastrointestinal Radiology. Philadelphia: Lippincott, pp. 711–739, 1983.

66. Eisenberg RL: Solitary filling defects in the jejunum and ileum. In Eisenberg RL (ed.): Gastrointestinal Radiology. Philadelphia: Lippincott, pp. 492–504, 1983.

67. Younathan CM, Ros PR, Burton SS: MR imaging of colonic lipoma. J Comput Assist Tomogr 15:492–494, 1991.

68. Bernstein WC: What are hemorrhoids and what is their relationship to the portal venous system? Dis Colon Rectum 26:829–834, 1983.

69. Kee F, Wilson RH, Gilliland R, Sloan JM, et al: Changing site distribution of colorectal cancer. Br Med J 305:158, 1992.

70. Butch RJ, Stark DD, Wittenberg J, et al: Staging rectal cancer by MRI and CT. AJR Am J Roentgenol 146:1155–1160, 1996.

71. Thoeni RF: Colorectal cancer: Cross-sectional imaging for staging of primary tumor and detection of local recurrence. AJR Am J Roentgenol 156:909–915, 1991.

72. Smith RC, Reinhold C, McCauley TR, et al: Multicoil high-resolution fast spin-echo MR imaging of the female pelvis. Radiology 184:671–675, 1992.

73. De Lange EE, Gechner RE, Edge SB, Spaulding CA: Preoperative staging of rectal carcinoma with MR imaging: Surgical and histopathologic correlation. Radiology 176:623–628, 1990.

74. Ito K, Kato T, Tadokoro M, et al: Recurrent rectal cancer and scar: Differentiation with PET and MR imaging. Radiology 182:549–552, 1992.

75. Sugimura K, Carrington BM, Quivey JM, Hricak H: Postirradiation changes in the pelvis: Assessment with MR imaging. Radiology 175:805–813, 1990.

76. Bartolo D, Goepel JR, Parsons MA: Rectal malignant lymphoma in chronic ulcerative colitis. Gut 23:164–168, 1982.

77. Dragosics B, Bauer P, Radaasziewicz T: Primary gastrointestinal non-Hodgkin's lymphomas. Cancer 55:1060–1073, 1985.

78. Jetmore AB, Ray JE, Gathright BJ, McMullen KM, et al: Rectal carcinoids: The most frequent carcinoid tumor. Dis Colon Rectum 35:717–725, 1992.

79. Pack GT, Oropeza R: A comparative study of melanoma and epidermoid carcinoma of the anal canal. Dis Colon Rectum 10:161–176, 1967.

80. Acheson ED: The distribution of ulcerative colitis and regional enteritis in United States veterans with particular reference to the Jewish religion. Gut 1:291–293, 1960.

81. Hulnick DH, Megibow AJ, Balthazar EJ, Naidich DP, Bosniak MA: Computed tomgraphy in the evaluation of diverticulitis. Radiology; 152:491–495, 1984.

82. Cho KC, Morehouse HT, Alterman DD, Thornhill BA: Sigmoid diverticulitis: Diagnostic role of CT—comparison with barium enema studies. Radiology 170:111–115, 1990.

83. Balthazar E, Megibow AJ, Siegal SE, Birnbaum BA: Appendicitis: Prospective evaluation with high-resolution CT. Radiology 180:21–24, 1991.

84. Jeffrey RB, Laing FC, Townsend RR: Acute appendicitis: Sonographic criteria based on 250 cases. Radiology 167:327–329, 1988.

85. Semelka RC, John G, Kelekis NL, Burdeny DA, Ascher SM: Bowel

86. Luniss PJ, Armstrong P, Barker PG, Reznek RH, Phillips RKS: Magnetic resonance imaging of anal fistulae. Lancet 340:394–396, 1992.

87. Barker PG, Luniss PJ, Armstrong P, Reznek RH, Cottam K, Phillips RK: Magnetic resonance imaging of fistula-in-ano: Technique, interpretation and accuracy. Clin Radicl 49:7–13, 1994.

88. Myhr GE, Myrvold HE, Nilsen G, Thoresen JE, Rinck PA: Perianal fistulas: Use of MR imaging for diagnosis. Radiology 191:545–549, 1994.

89. Larson H, Price AB, Honour P: Clostridium difficile and the etiology of pseudomembranous colitis. Lancet 1:1063–1066, 1978.

90. Tammo HPR, Davis MA, Ros PR: Intraluminal contrast agents for MR imaging of the abdomen and pelvis. J Magn Reson Imaging 4:291–300, 1994.

91. Satoh S, Munechika H, Ri K, Hishida T, Nagasawa O: Green tea as a positive enhancement agent for MR imaging of the gastrointestinal tract (abstract). Radiology 189(P):133, 1993.

92. Hiraishi K, Narabayashi I, Fujita O, Yamamoto K, et al: Blueberry juice: Preliminary evaluation as an oral contrast agent in gastrointestinal MR imaging. Radiology 194:119–123, 1995.

93. Bernardino ME, Weinreb JC, Mitchell DG: Fast MR imaging of the bowel with a manganese chloride T1/T2 contrast agent (abstract). Radiology 189(P):203, 1993.

94. Wesbey GE, Brasch RC, Goldberg HI, Engelstad BL: Dilute oral iron solutions as gastrointestinal contrast agents for magnetic resonance imaging: Initial clinical experience. Magn Reson Imaging 3:57–66, 1985.

95. Li KCP, Tart RP, Storm B, Rolfes R, Ang P, Ros PR: MRI contrast agents: Comparative study of five potential agents in humans. Proceedings of the Annual Meeting of the Annual Meeting of the Society of Magnetic Resonance in Medicine p. 791, 1989.

96. Patten RM, Lo SK, Phillips JJ: Positive bowel contrast agent for MR imaging of the abdomen: Phase 2 and 3 clinical trials. Radiology 189:277–283, 1993.

97. Unger EC, Fritz TA, Palestrant D, Meakem TJ, et al: Preliminary evaluation of iron phytate (inositol hexaphosphate) as a gastrointestinal MR contrast agent. J Magn Reson Imaging 3:119–124, 1993.

98. Kaminsky S, Laniado M, Gogoll M, et al: Gadopentetate dimeglumine as a bowel contrast agent: Safety and efficacy. Radiology 178:503–508, 1991.

99. Brown JJ, Duncan JR, Heiken JP, et al: Perfluorocytlbromide as a gastrointestinal contrast agent for MR imaging: Use with and without glucagon. Radiology 181:455–460, 1991.

100. Mattrey RF, Tramber MA, Brown JJ, Young SW, et al: Perflubron as an oral contrast agent for MRI imaging: Results of a phase III clinical trial. Radiology 191:841–848, 1994.

101. Rubin DL, Muller HH, Sidhu MK, Young SW, et al: Liquid oral magnetic particles as a gastrointestinal contrast agent for MR imaging: Efficacy in vivo. J Magn Reson Imaging 3:113–118, 1993.

102. Oksendal AN, Jacobsen TF, Gundersen HG, Rinck PA, Rummeny E, et al: Superparamagnetic particles as an oral contrast agent in abdominal magnetic resonance imaging. Invest Radiol 26:67–70, 1991.

103. Boudghene FP, Bach-Ganso T, Grange JD, Lame S, et al: Contribution of oral magnetic particles in MR imaging of the abdomen with spin-echo and gradient-echo sequences. J Magn Reson Imaging 3:107–112, 1993.

104. Haldermann-Heusler RC, Wight E, Marincek BM: Oral superparamagnetic contrast agent (ferumoxsil): Tolerance and efficacy in MR imaging of gynecologic diseases. J Magn Reson Imaging 4:385–391, 1995.

105. Ros PR, Green AM, Bernadino ME, Harms SE, Unger P, Hahn PF:

Safety and efficacy of superparamagnetic iron oxide: Summary of multicenter phase II/III clinical trials. (abstract). Radiology 181(P):93, 1991.

106. Torres GM, Ros PR, Burton SS, Barreda R, Erquiaga E: Retroperitoneal MR imaging before and after oral administration of superparamagnetic iron oxide contrast material (abstract). Radiology 177(P):358, 1990.

107. Langmo L, Ros PR, Torres GM, Erquiaga E: Comparison of MR imaging after barium administration with CT in pelvic disease. J Mag Reson Imaging 2:89–91, 1992.

108. Liebig T, Stoupis C, Ros PR, Ballinger JR, Briggs RW: A potentially artifact-free oral contrast agent for gastrointestinal MRI. Magn Reson Med 30:646–649, 1993.

109. Weinreb JC, Maravilla KR, Redman HC, Nunnally R: Improved MR imaging of the upper abdomen with glucagon and gas. J Comput Assist Tomogr 8:835–838, 1984.

110. Zerhouni EA, Brennecke CM, Fishman EK, Zimmer R, Soulen RL: Development of gaseous contrast agents for MRI of the abdomen and pelvis. (abstract). In Proceedings of the 34th Annual Meeting of the Association of University Radiologists. Reston, Association of University Radiologists, 516, 1986.

111. Jenkins JPR, Braganza JM, Hickey DS, Isherwood I, Machin M: Quantitative tissue characterization in pancreatic disease using magnetic resonance imaging. Br J Radiol 60:33–341, 1987.

112. Chou C, Liu G, Chen L, Jaw T: Retrograde air insufflation in MRI: A technical note. Abdom Imaging 18:211–214, 1993.

113. Bisset GS III: Evaluation of potential practical oral contrast agents for pediatric magnetic resonance imaging: Preliminary observations. Pediatr Radiol 20:61–66, 1989.

114. Balzarini L, Aime S, Barbero L, Ceglia E, et al: Magnetic resonance imaging of the gastrointestinal tract: Investigation of baby milk as a low cost contrast medium. Eur J Radiol 15:171–174, 1992.

115. Guimaraes R, Clemont O, Bittoun J, Carnot F, Frija G: MR lymphadenopathy with superparamagnetic iron manoparticles in rats: Pathologic basis for contrast enhancement. AJR Am J Roentgenol 162:201–207, 1994.

CHAPTER 7

PERITONEAL CAVITY

S. M. ASCHER, M.D. AND R. C. SEMELKA, M.D.

NORMAL ANATOMY

Peritoneum lines the peritoneal cavity and envelopes the abdominal and pelvic viscera. Peritoneal folds within the cavity, termed *ligaments*, provide physical support for the organs and serve to protect nutrient vessels. The more important folds are given specific names. *Mesentery* are the peritoneal folds that connect the small intestine and sigmoid colon to the posterior abdominal wall. The *greater omentum* extends from the greater curvature of the stomach to lie anterior in the abdomen and reflects back onto the transverse colon; it forms a protective drape over the abdominal contents. The *lesser omentum* or *gastrohepatic ligament* joins the lesser curvature of the stomach to the liver. Its medial free edge is called the *gastroduodenal ligament*, through which runs the portal vein, hepatic artery, and common bile duct. The *transverse mesocolon* extends from the pancreas to the transverse colon. In addition to providing support and protection, these peritoneal ligaments divide the cavity up into subspaces that interconnect and effect the spread and localization of disease.

The transverse mesocolon separates the peritoneal cavity into *supra-* and *inframesocolic spaces*. The supramesocolic compartment can be further divided into right and left peritoneal spaces. The right peritoneal space includes the right perihepatic space and the lesser sac, demarcated anteriorly by the lesser omentum. These spaces communicate via the *epiploic foramen* (foramen of Winslow), which is bounded by the *gastroduodenal ligament* of the lesser omentum. The right perihepatic space consists of a subphrenic space and a subhepatic space and is partially divided by the right coronary ligament. The posterior aspect of the right subhepatic space encloses a recess between the liver and kidney called the *hepatorenal fossa* (Morrison's pouch). This space commonly accumulates fluid in the setting of gallbladder, second portion of duodenum, liver, or ascending colon disease. The lesser sac is a potential space that distends in the presence of certain disease processes, especially pancreatitis. Malignant disease tends to affect the lesser sac and greater peritoneal cavity proportionally. Benign disease, except for pancreatitis, primarily affects the greater peritoneal cavity [1,2].

The left peritoneal space can be divided into anterior and posterior perihepatic spaces, and anterior and posterior subphrenic spaces. The perihepatic spaces tend to be involved with diseases affecting the left lobe of the liver and stomach, whereas the anterior subphrenic space may also be affected by disease of the splenic flexure. The posterior subphrenic space is most commonly involved in disease of the spleen.

The inframesocolic compartment of the peritoneal cavity is divided into a small right space and a larger infracolic space. The right side is limited inferiorly by the junction of the distal small bowel mesentery with the cecum, whereas the left infracolic space opens to the pelvis.

The *paracolic gutters* are located lateral to the peritoneal attachment of the ascending and descending colon. The right paracolic gutter is continuous with the right perihepatic space. On the left side, however, the *phrenicocolic ligament* forms a partial barrier between the paracolic gutter and the left subphrenic space. The pelvis is the most dependent portion of the peritoneal cavity in both the erect and recumbent positions. Therefore, both benign and malignant fluid preferentially pool in this location [3,4]. The pelvic cavity consists of the lateral paravesical spaces and the midline rectovaginal space in women (pouch of Douglas or cul de sac), and rectovesical space in men.

The peritoneal reflections are conduits for intraperitoneal fluid, which flows along the path of least resistance. Specifically, flow along the right paracolic gutter and into the pelvis is relatively unimpeded. Greater resistance to flow occurs along the left paracolic gutter, and flow across midline is impeded by the falciform ligament [5].

MRI TECHNIQUE

Techniques that minimize motion and maximize spatial and contrast resolution are well suited for imaging peritoneal disease. The multiplanar capabilities of MRI are also useful. Breathing-independent single shot T2-weighted echo-train spin-echo [e.g., half-fourier single-shot turbo spin-echo (HASTE)] and fat-suppressed spoiled gradient-echo (SGE) techniques, which can acquire 21 sections in a 20-second breath-hold are the major advances that allow superior peritoneal cavity evaluation. Our standard MRI protocol includes breath-hold T1-weighted SGE, T2-weighted imaging (HASTE), and immediate and delayed postgadolinium SGE techniques, with the delayed images acquired with fat suppression. This approach can be modified for the disease being studied.

For fibrotic processes, the T1-weighted SGE technique maximizes contrast resolution between the high-signal intraperitoneal fat and the low-signal diseased tissue, whereas, for inflammatory and neoplastic conditions, the routine use of the gadolinium-enhanced T1-weighted fat-suppressed SGE technique facilitates peritoneal evaluation. Unlike the liver, which mandates imaging during the capillary phase of enhancement, these peritoneal processes are best studied during the interstitial phase (2 to 10 minutes after injection) when leaky capillaries allow contrast to pool in the interstitium. This time course allows for dynamic scanning of a target organ (e.g., the liver) during the capillary phase and a survey of the peritoneum during the interstitial phase. This is particularly advantageous in conditions that simultaneously affect the solid viscera and peritoneum, such as ovarian, colorectal, and pancreatic carcinoma.

DISEASE ENTITIES

Normal Variants and Congenital Disease

Congenital variation of the peritoneal reflections are rare. They usually are related to malrotation of the bowel or situs anomalies during gestation [6]. Lymphangiomas are congenital malformations caused by disruption of the normal communication between lymphatic tissue and lymphatic channels. They usually are multiloculated cysts containing serous or chylous fluid, but may be complicated by hemorrhage. The imaging characteristics reflect the cyst contents; lymphangiomas with high protein content are high in signal intensity on T1-weighted images [7].

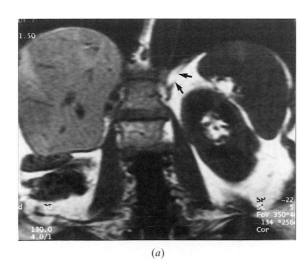

(a)

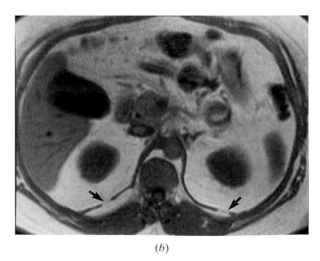

(b)

FIG. 7.1 Bochdalek's hernia. Coronal breath-hold T1-weighted SGE image (*a*) shows the discontinuity of the posterior diaphragm (*arrows*).

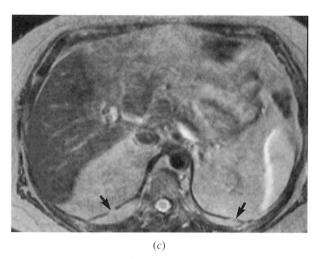

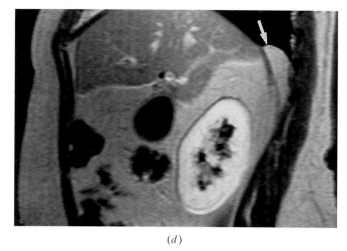

(c)   (d)

F IG. 7.1 (*Continued*) The rent in the diaphragm allows fat and/or viscera to migrate superiorly into the chest. SGE (*b*), T2 spin-echo (T2-SE) (*c*), and sagittal 90-second postgadolinium SGE (*d*) images demonstrate rents in the diaphragm bilaterally (*arrows, b,c*) and herniation of fat into the pleural space (*arrow, d*).

Hernias

Bochdalek's hernia is a common congenital diaphragmatic hernia that occurs in the left posterolateral aspect of the pleuroperitoneal canal [8]. MRI shows the discontinuity of the diaphragm in multiple planes (Fig. 7.1). Sliding hiatal hernias result from a weakened or torn phrenoesophageal membrane. The gastroesophageal junction is above the esophageal hiatus of the diaphragm (Fig. 7.2). Gastroesophagography is the most common means of demonstrating these hernias, but they also can be seen on MR images acquired during a breath-hold. Multiplanar MRI also is able to identify abdominal wall hernias and their contents, and this may be helpful in obese patients where physical exam is hampered. Inguinal hernias are the result of a persistent *processus vaginalis*, that portion

of the abdominal peritoneum that enters the deep inguinal ring. At birth, the open processus vaginalis communicates with the peritoneal cavity; it normally closes during infancy. If, however, the processus remains patent, abdominal viscera may protrude into it forming an *inguinal hernia* [9] (Fig. 7.3). *Spigelian hernia* is a rare hernia of the anterior abdominal wall caused by a defect in the aponeurosis between the transversus and the rectus muscle. The peritoneal sac herniates through the rent of the aponeurosis and dissects laterally (Fig. 7.3). *Paraumbilical hernia* arises near the umbilicus and protrudes through the linea alba (Fig. 7.4). Although they may be congenital, paraumbilical hernias are more common in obese and multiparous women; diastasis of the recti abdomini is the common underlying factor [9].

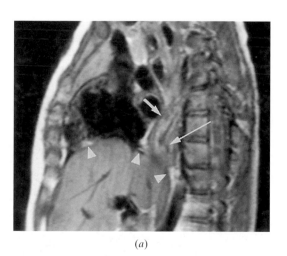

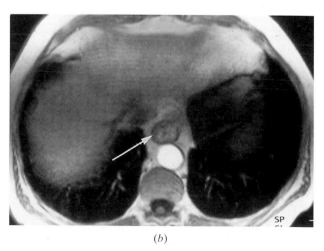

(a)   (b)

F IG. 7.2 Hiatal hernia. Sagittal T1-weighted SGE image (*a*) in a patient with heartburn. The gastroesophageal junction (*long arrow, a*) is above the diaphragm (*arrowheads, a*), which is diagnostic of a hiatal hernia. Thickening of the esophageal wall (*short arrow, a*) is consistent with reflux esophagitis.

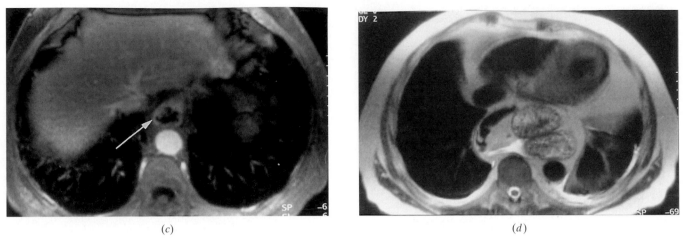

(c)   (d)

FIG. 7.2 (*Continued*) Immediate postgadolinium SGE (*b*), and 90-second postgadolinium SGE imaging in a second patient demonstrate stomach in the lower mediastinum (*arrows, b,c*). Gastric rugae are well-shown on the gadolinium-enhanced fat-suppressed image (*c*). HASTE image (*d*) in a third patient shows a large hiatal hernia with surrounding herniated fat.

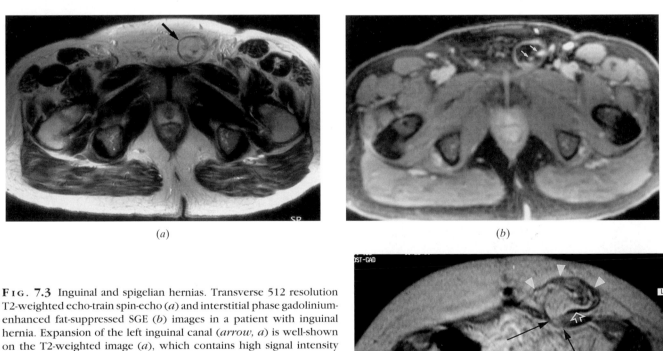

(a)   (b)

FIG. 7.3 Inguinal and spigelian hernias. Transverse 512 resolution T2-weighted echo-train spin-echo (*a*) and interstitial phase gadolinium-enhanced fat-suppressed SGE (*b*) images in a patient with inguinal hernia. Expansion of the left inguinal canal (*arrow, a*) is well-shown on the T2-weighted image (*a*), which contains high signal intensity tissue with an appearance identical to surrounding fat. Fat within the expanded inguinal canal diminishes in signal intensity on the fat suppressed image and enhancing testicular vessels are well seen (*arrows, b*). Gadolinium-enhanced T1-weighted SGE image (*c*) in a second patient with spigelian hernia. A bowel-containing hernia sac (*arrowheads, c*) protrudes through a defect in the aponeurosis between the transversus and rectus muscles (*solid arrows, c*). The lateral margin of the hernia sac is the intact external oblique muscle and fascia (*open arrow, c*).

(c)

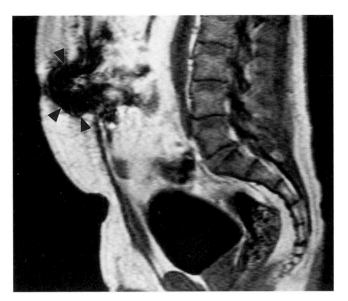

FIG. 7.4 Paraumbilical hernia. Sagittal T1-weighted SGE image shows signal-void air-containing bowel (*arrowheads*) in the subcutaneous tissues in a patient with a paraumbilical hernia.

Mass Lesions

Benign Masses

Cysts and Pseudocysts

Mesenteric cysts most commonly occur in the small bowel mesentery. Their etiology is not well-understood. Although most mesenteric cysts are incidental findings, they can be symptomatic. They may produce chronic or acute pain if complicated by rupture, hemorrhage, torsion, or bowel obstruction. The cysts tend to be singular and thin-walled, and may contain septae. Their contents are usually serous or chylous fluid, though in complicated cases, blood and/or other proteinaceous fluid predominates [10,11]. The cyst contents affect the MRI appearance. Simple cysts will be round, well-marginated, low in signal intensity on T1-weighted images, and high in signal intensity on T2-weighted images (Fig. 7.5). Cysts complicated by protein or hemorrhage will have higher signal intensity on T1-weighted images and/or heterogeneous signal intensity on T2-weighted images. Following

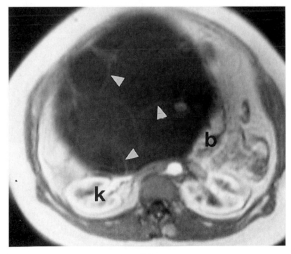

(a)

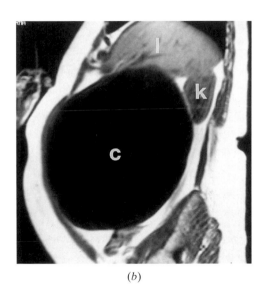

(b)

(c)

FIG. 7.5 Mesenteric cyst. Coronal T1-weighted turbo-SGE (*a*), sagittal T1-weighted SGE (*b*), and immediate postgadolinium fat-suppressed SGE (*c*) images. A large septated cystic mass ("*c*",*a,b*) arising from the small bowel mesentery causes mass effect upon the adjacent bowel ("*b*",*a,c*), left kidney ("*k*",*b,c*) and liver ("*l*",*a,b*). Cysts that are low in signal intensity on T1-weighted images (*a,b*) and high in signal intensity on T2-weighted images (not shown) are consistent with serous fluid. Immediately after intravenous gadolinium administration (capillary phase) the septae traversing the cyst enhance (*arrowheads, c*). These imaging characteristics are consistent with an uncomplicated mesenteric cyst.

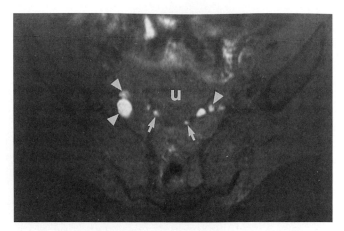

FIG. 7.6 Endometriosis. Axial T1-weighted fat-suppressed spin-echo image demonstrates high-signal-intensity foci of ovarian endometriomas (*arrowheads*) and smaller endometriosis implants adherent to the uterine serosa (*arrows*). T1-weighted fat-suppressed spin-echo or SGE technique is the most sensitive and specific sequence for detecting the blood product-laden deposits of endometriosis. (Reprinted with permission from Ascher SM, Agrawal R, Bis KG, Brown E, et al: Endometriosis: Appearance and detection with conventional, fat-suppressed, and contrast-enhanced fat-suppressed spin-echo techniques. J Magn Reson Imaging 5:251–257, 1995)

contrast administration, the cyst wall and septae, if present, will enhance (see Fig. 7.5).

Peritoneal pseudocysts are created when fluid released from functioning ovaries is trapped by peritoneal adhesions. Peritoneal pseudocysts are not true cysts since their walls are formed by the surrounding anatomic structures. In uncomplicated cases they are low in signal intensity on T1-weighted images and very high in signal intensity on T2-weighted images. Contrast-enhanced T1-weighted images surpass CT imaging and ultrasound by showing that the lesions are not encapsulated by a true wall, and by defining the relationship of the pseudocyst to other organs and tissue by direct multiplanar imaging [12]. These findings are more apparent on gadolinium-enhanced fat-suppressed images.

Lipomas and Pseudotumoral Lipomatosis

Lipomas are benign tumors that rarely involve the peritoneal cavity. Their imaging features parallel those of lipomas elsewhere in the body and are comparable to those of surrounding fat. These lesions are high in signal intensity on nonsuppressed T1-weighted images. Because fat signal varies considerably on T2-weighted images depending upon the sequence employed, comparison of the signal intensity of the lesion should be made to that of adjacent fat. T1-weighted fat-suppressed SGE images will show loss of the tumor's signal intensity in comparison to nonfat-suppressed images, thereby definitively characterizing their fatty nature.

Mesenteric pseudotumoral lipomatosis is proliferation of the mesenteric fat with associated mass effect upon adjacent structures. It may be idiopathic, or it can be associated with steroid use, Cushing's syndrome, or obesity. Cross sectional imaging is helpful in excluding a discrete tumor and for identifying either diffuse or focal prominent normal mesenteric fat. The signal characteristics of this entity mimic those of benign lipomas [13].

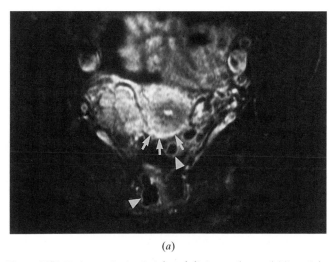

(a)

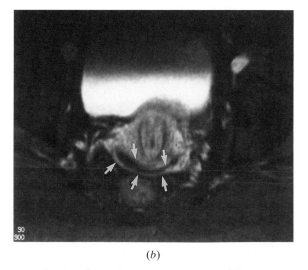

(b)

FIG. 7.7 Endometriosis. Axial gadolinium-enhanced T1-weighted fat-suppressed spin-echo (*a,b*) images from two different patients. Following intravenous contrast, there is moderate enhancement of the endometriosis implants in the first patient (*arrows, a*) in the cul de sac. The bowel wall enhances to a lesser extent (*arrowheads, a*). The high-signal-intensity contents within the bowel lumen reflect a rescaling phenomena associated with fat suppression. In contradistinction, there is no increased enhancement of the peritoneum lining the cul de sac in the second patient (*arrows, b*) who also had pelvic pain. At laparoscopy, endometriosis was present in patient *a*, but absent in patient *b*. Intravenous gadolinium may help detect certain populations of endometriosis implants.

Endometriosis

Endometrial foci outside the lining of the uterus are termed *endometriosis*. It most commonly affects the ovaries, but may occur elsewhere in the abdominopelvic cavity and even the thorax. The pathogenesis of endometriosis remains controversial. It likely is related to induction and/or transplantation of endometrial cells into the abdominal cavity [14]. Endometriomas have variable signal intensity but are commonly high in signal intensity on T1-weighted images and heterogeneously high in signal intensity on T2-weighted images [15]. Protein and blood breakdown products tend to demonstrate a gradation of signal intensity on T2-weighted images, which has been termed *shading* [15]. Recent work has shown that T1-weighted fat-suppressed imaging is the most sensitive MRI technique for identifying endometriomas (Fig. 7.6) [16]. Unfortunately, detecting small peritoneal endometriosis implants remains problematic [17], although contrast-enhanced fat-suppressed imaging has met with mixed results (Fig. 7.7).

Desmoids

Desmoids occur in patients with Gardner's syndrome who have undergone bowel resection [18,19]. These tumors are extremely fibrous and can vary substantially in size. They are locally aggressive and may recur after surgical removal. Desmoids have variable morphology: well circumscribed (Fig. 7.8) or irregular borders (Fig. 7.9). Chronically formed tumors are low in signal intensity on T1- and T2-weighted images and enhance only minimally following intravenous gadolinium chelate (see Fig.

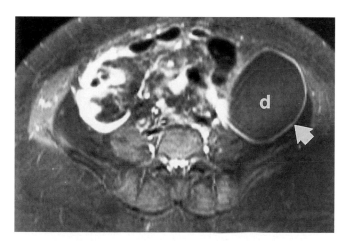

F IG . 7.8 Desmoid tumor. Axial gadolinium-enhanced T1-weighted fat-suppressed spin-echo image in a woman with Gardner's syndrome and intra-abdominal desmoid tumor. The desmoid tumor (*d*) exhibits minimal enhancement confirming its fibrous nature. Mural enhancement is apparent (*arrow*) and, on the basis of this image, the tumor could be mistaken for a cyst. T2-weighted images would distinguish the two: a desmoid tumor would remain low in signal intensity, whereas a cyst would demonstrate high signal intensity.

7.8). In the acute phase, tumors may have regions of high signal intensity on T2-weighted images that also show heterogeneous increased enhancement (see Fig. 7.9).

Malignant Mass

Mesothelioma

Mesothelioma is a tumor most often associated with asbestos exposure. Although it typically involves the pleura, the peritoneum is involved in up to 40 percent of cases [20]. Peritoneal mesothelioma spreads along serosal surfaces and may directly invade solid and hollow viscera. Early in the disease small nodules may be seen. Later, these may coalesce to form large confluent masses, the classic "omental cake." Alternatively, a desmoplastic effect with straightening and encasement of vessels and bowel has been described. This stellate morphology is most commonly seen with mesenteric mesotheliomas [21,22,23]. The MRI appearance of mesothelioma is nonspecific, but a solid peritoneal mass seen in the setting of synchronous pleural disease should suggest the correct diagnosis.

Metastases

Metastatic tumors that involve the peritoneum most commonly arise from the ovary, colon, stomach, pancreas, and lymph tissue [20,24]. Dissemination occurs by several routes: direct spread, intraperitoneal seeding, hematogenous emboli, and lymphatic dissemination [4,25].

Direct Spread. Tumors that have full-thickness penetration commonly spread along visceral peritoneal surfaces to involve adjacent structures [20,26,27]. This direct extension is facilitated by the ligaments that interconnect the various organs.

Intraperitoneal Seeding. Intraperitoneal seeding of tumor follows pathways of least resistance. The most commonly affected areas are the rectovesical/rectovaginal fossa, sigmoid mesocolon, right paracolic gutter, and the small bowel mesentery near the ileocecal valve [4,28]. Ovarian cancer most frequently spreads in this manner, followed by colon, stomach, and pancreatic carcinoma. Contrast-enhanced T1-weighted fat-suppressed technique is the best method for demonstrating peritoneal disease: Both the enhancing discrete metastatic implants and the diffusely thickened involved peritoneal surfaces stand out in relief against the low signal intensity of the suppressed intraperitoneal fat (Figs. 7.10 to 7.13) [20,29]. Moreover, recent advances in breath-hold T1-weighted fat-suppressed SGE imaging can eliminate ghosting and blurring artifacts, further increasing the conspicuity of small implants. Gadolinium-enhanced breath-hold fat-suppressed SGE combined with breathing independent

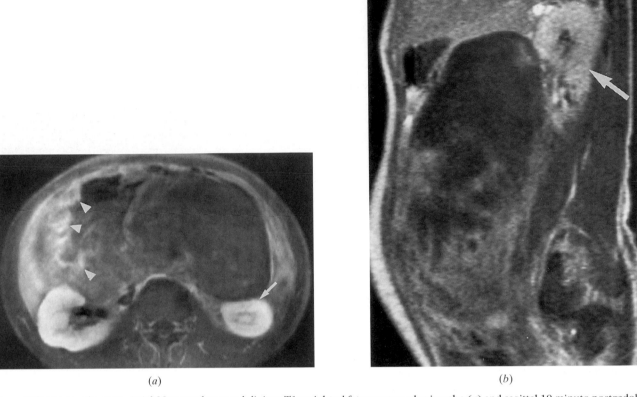

(a)   (b)

F I G . 7.9 Desmoid tumor. Axial 90-second postgadolinium T1-weighted fat-suppressed spin-echo (*a*) and sagittal 10-minute postgadolinium SGE (*b*) images in a woman with Gardner's syndrome and intra-abdominal desmoid tumor. The right aspect of the mass enhances (*arrowheads*) more than the left aspect. The greater enhancement on the right reflects active disease. This large desmoid produces a mass effect on the kidneys (*arrows, a,b*). Imaging in the sagittal plane helps define the craniocaudad extent of the tumor.

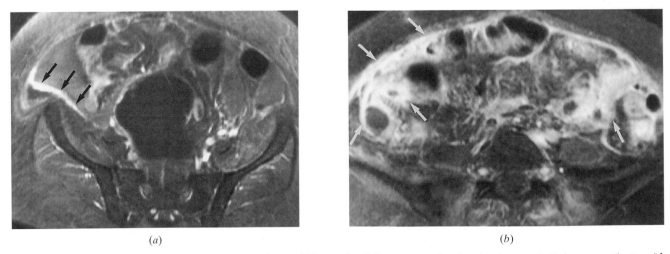

(a)   (b)

F I G . 7.10 Peritoneal metastases. Axial gadolinium-enhanced T1-weighted fat-suppressed spin-echo images (*a,b*) in two patients with ovarian carcinoma. Gadolinium-enhanced T1-weighted fat-suppressed images highlight peritoneal metastases. The discrete metastatic deposits (*arrows, a*) and the diffusely thickened involved peritoneal and serosal surfaces (*arrows, b*) show marked enhancement following gadolinium administration. The enhancing metastases are well-shown in the background of low-signal-intensity intra-abdominal fat.

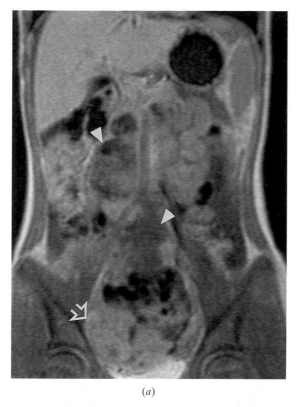

(a)

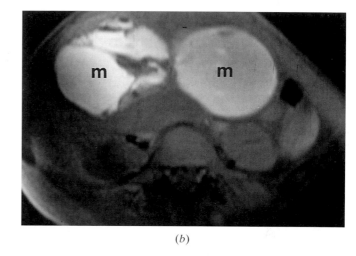

(b)

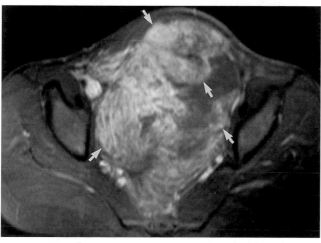

(c)

FIG. 7.11 Metastatic immature teratoma. Coronal T1-weighted turbo SGE (*a*), axial T1-weighted fat-suppressed spin-echo (*b*), and axial gadolinium-enhanced T1-weighted fat-suppressed SGE (*c*) images in a patient with metastatic immature teratoma. The primary tumor (*open arrow, a*) originates in the ovary and has spread to the peritoneal cavity (*arrowheads, a*). The unenhanced fat-suppressed image highlights the non-lipomatous metastases (*m* in image *b*). After the administration of intravenous gadolinium, the metastases that coat the peritoneal and serosal surfaces enhance substantially (*arrows, c*).

HASTE imaging may be the most sensitive approach for detecting peritoneal metastases (Figs. 7.13 and 7.14). These MRI techniques have been shown to be equal to and, in some cases, superior to contrast-enhanced CT imaging [29,30]. Some investigators also suggest introducing a negative bowel contrast agent via a nasogastric tube or an enema tip prior to imaging to increase lesion detection. Using this technique, they describe the MRI appearance of peritoneal carcinomatosis as linear or nodular seeding along the small intestine, and transverse and sigmoid colon; stellate, plaque-like, and bulky tumors in the mesentery and greater omentum; and focal thickening along the right paracolic gutter [31,32]. Although the use of intraluminal air has been described, at 1.5 T the susceptibility effects of air outweigh the advantages. For this purpose, instilling water may be an acceptable alternative. Peritoneal metastases in close approximation to the liver are also well-shown on T2-weighted fat-suppressed echo-train spin-echo images because both the fat and liver are relatively low in signal

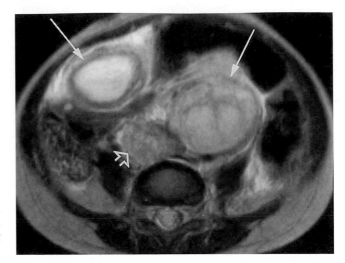

FIG. 7.12 Metastatic yolk sac tumor. Axial 512-resolution T2-weighted echo-train spin-echo image in a patient with metastatic yolk-sac tumor. Ovarian yolk-sac tumors spread to the peritoneum (*solid arrows*), omentum, and retroperitoneal lymph nodes (*open arrow*).

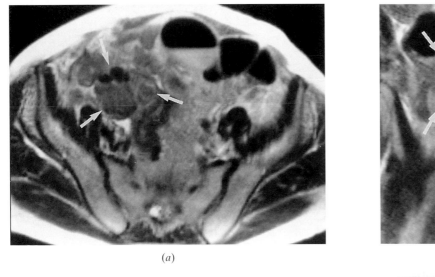

(*a*)

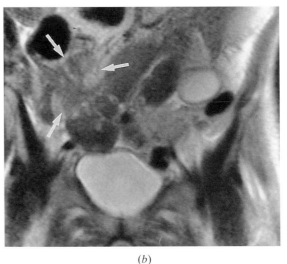

(*b*)

FIG. 7.13 Metastatic pancreatic adenocarcinoma. Axial (*a*) and coronal (*b*) T2-weighted HASTE, and axial T1-weighted fat-suppressed SGE (*c*) images in a patient with metastatic carcinoma. The HASTE images show a mass in the right lower quadrant (*arrows, a,b*). Following intravenous contrast the serosal and peritoneal metastases enhance (*long arrows, c*). Incidental note is made of an enhancing bone metastasis in the left ilium (*arrows, c*). Note that while the fat adjacent to the torso phased-array coil is high in signal intensity, the intra-abdominal and marrow fat has been successfully suppressed.

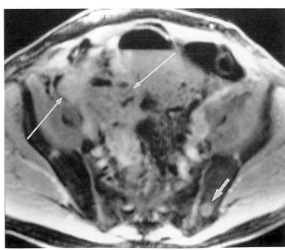

(*c*)

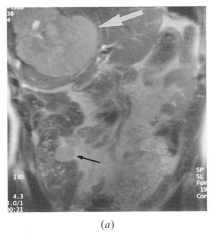

(a)

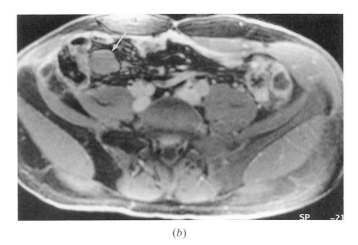

(b)

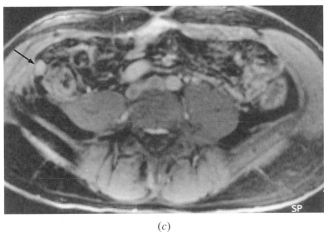

(c)

FIG. 7.14 Peritoneal metastases from synovial sarcoma. Coronal HASTE (a) and interstitial-phase gadolinium-enhanced T1-weighted fat-suppressed SGE (b,c) images. The coronal HASTE image demonstrates a large subcapsular liver metastasis (*large arrow, a*) and a 2-cm peritoneal metastasis (*small arrow, a*) medial to the ascending colon. The gadolinium-enhanced fat-suppressed image demonstrates moderate uniform enhancement of this metastatic deposit (*arrow, b*). On a higher tomographic section through the pelvis a 6-mm moderately enhancing metastatic deposit is well-shown (*arrow, c*).

intensity rendering moderately high-signal-intensity peritoneal metastases conspicuous (Fig. 7.15). As breathing artifact is less problematic in the pelvis, peritoneal metastases also may be well-shown using echo-train spin-echo imaging. The sagittal plane is particularly effective at showing implants along the bladder surface (Fig. 7.16).

Omental metastases frequently coexist in patients with peritoneal metastases. Four morphologic patterns of omental involvement have been described: rounded, cake-like, ill-defined, and stellate [22,33]. Irrespective of contour, these masses enhance after intravenous gadolinium administration (Fig. 7.17). Negative oral contrast

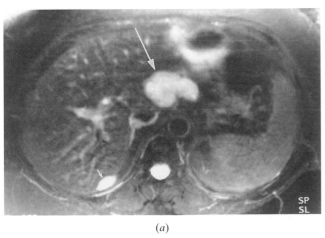

(a)

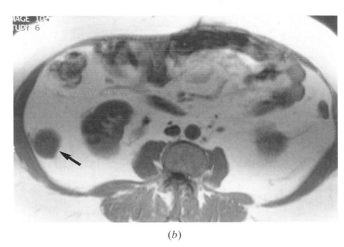

(b)

FIG. 7.15 Peritoneal metastases from ovarian cancer. T2-weighted fat-suppressed echo-train spin-echo (a) and SGE (b) images of the liver and interstitial-phase gadolinium-enhanced fat-suppressed SGE image in coronal (c) and transverse (d) planes of the midabdomen. A lobulated 4-cm peritoneal implant along the gastrohepatic ligament is moderately high in signal intensity (*arrow, a*) and contrasts well with moderately low-signal-intensity liver.

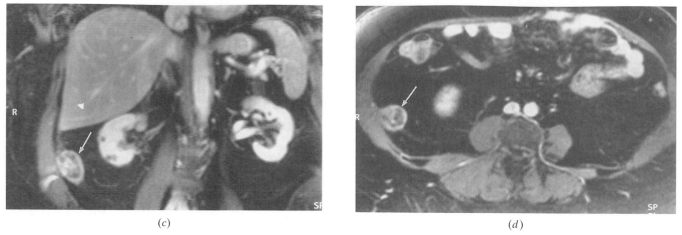

(c)   *(d)*

F I G . 7.15 (*Continued*)   A subcapsular liver metastasis is also present (*small arrow, a*) that demonstrates a characteristic biconvex lens shape indicating its subcapsular location. SGE image through the midabdomen shows a 2-cm low-signal-intensity peritoneal metastasis (*arrow, b*) that contrasts well with high-signal-intensity fat. Gadolinium-enhanced fat-suppressed SGE images demonstrate heterogenous speckled enhancement of the mass (*arrow, c,d*).

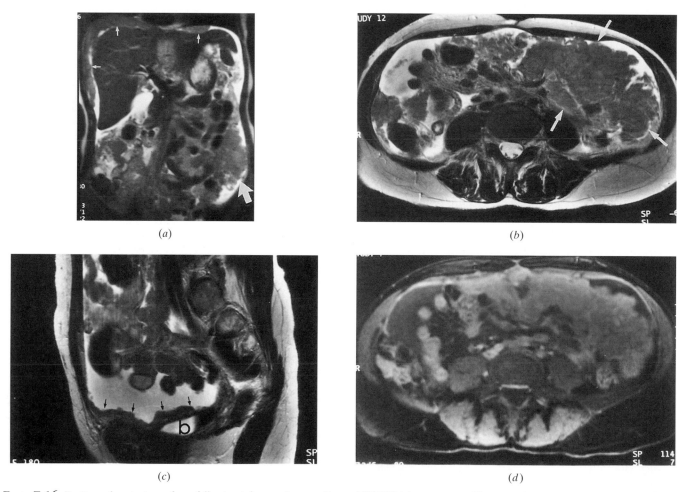

(a)   *(b)*

(c)   *(d)*

F I G . 7.16   Peritoneal metastases from fallopian tube carcinoma. Coronal HASTE (*a*), transverse (*b*), sagittal (*c*) 512-resolution T2-weighted echo-train spin-echo, and interstitial-phase gadolinium-enhanced SGE (*d*) images. Extensive peritoneal-based metastases are present that appear intermediate in signal intensity on T2-weighted images (*a–c*). The coronal image demonstrates an irregular layer of metastatic deposit measuring up to 2 cm in thickness along the diaphragmatic surface and the liver capsule (*small arrows, a*). Bulky peritoneal metastases are present in the left lower abdomen (*large arrow, a*) and in the pelvis. The transverse high-resolution T2-weighted image demonstrates extensive bulky peritoneal metastases (*arrows, b*). Peritoneal seeding along the peritoneal reflection over the bladder ("*b*,"*c*) is well-shown on the sagittal plane image (*small arrows, c*). Heterogeneous and moderate enhancement of the metastases is shown on the gadolinium-enhanced fat-suppressed SGE image obtained at the midabdomen level (*d*).

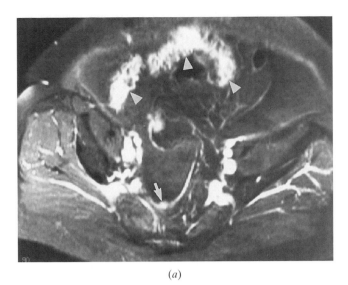

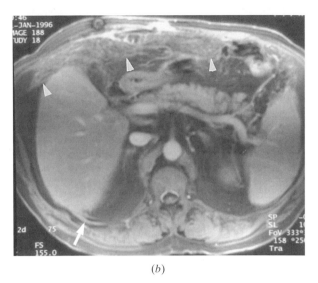

(a)   (b)

Fig. 7.17 Omental metastases. Axial gadolinium-enhanced T1-weighted fat-suppressed spin-echo images in a patient with metastatic ovarian carcinoma (a) and metastatic leiomyosarcoma (b). The enhancing "omental cake" (arrowheads, a,b) is characteristic of metastatic ovarian carcinoma, but also may be seen with other malignant diseases. Enhancing peritoneal tumor deposits (arrow, a,b) are rendered very conspicuous with suppression of background fat. MRI is superior to CT imaging in detecting small peritoneal-based disease.

agents may serve to increase lesion conspicuity by marking the bowel.

Pseudomyxoma peritonei results from rupture of an ovarian or appendiceal mucinous cystadenoma or cystadenocarcinoma. The gelatinous deposits coat the peritoneal surfaces and characteristically indent and scallop the liver margin (Fig. 7.18) [34,35]. Septae are also common [20].

Hematogenous Emboli. Melanoma, breast carcinoma, and lung carcinoma all metastasize hematogenously. Tumor emboli course via the mesenteric arteries

to the antimesenteric border of the bowel. Once lodged, tumor cells establish themselves and become intramural bowel nodules [24]. Gadolinium-enhanced T1-weighted fat-suppressed SGE imaging is currently the best MRI technique for detecting these metastases.

Lymphatic Dissemination. Lymphoma spreads via the lymphatics [36]. The presence of mesenteric disease is more typical of non-Hodgkin's lymphoma than other malignancies. The morphology of involved lymph nodes is variable. They may form large confluent masses that encircle the splanchnic vessels, the "sandwich sign."

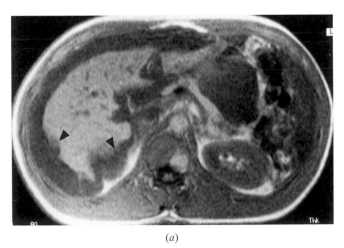

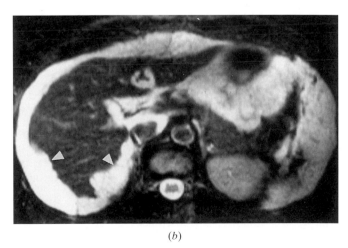

(a)   (b)

Fig. 7.18 Pseudomyxoma peritonei. SGE (a), T2-weighted fat-suppressed echo-train spin-echo (b), immediate (c) interstitial-phase (d) postgadolinium SGE, and coronal precontrast SGE (e) and 5-minute postgadolinium SGE (f) images in a patient with pseudomyxoma peritonei secondary to rupture of an appendiceal mucinous cystadenocarcinoma. On the precontrast T1-weighted SGE (a) and T2-weighted fat-suppressed echo-train spin-echo (b) images the gelatinous material surrounding the liver has regions in which the signal intensity resembles that of simple ascites.

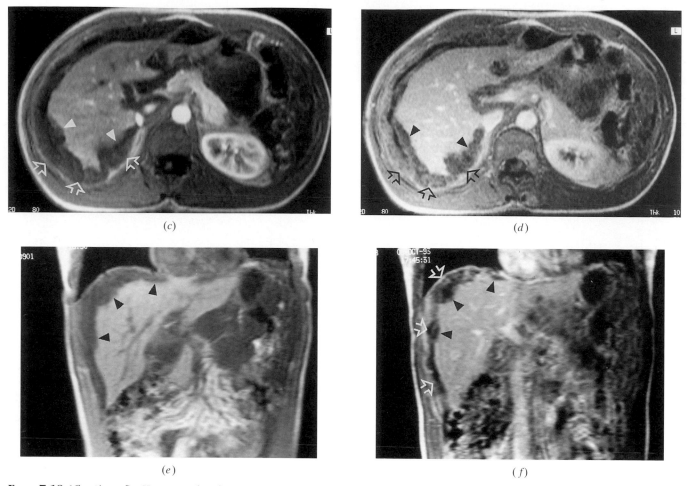

F IG . 7.18 (*Continued*)   However, the characteristic scalloping of the liver margin (*arrowheads, a–f*) coupled with the enhancement of the material (*open arrows, c,d,f*) filling the abdomen establishes the correct diagnosis. Free fluid within the abdomen does not enhance. Coronal images (*e,f*) provide a global view of the disease extent and demonstrate subdiaphragmatic disease well.

Alternatively, a profusion of small, nonpathologically enlarged lymph nodes may predominate [37,38,39]. Whereas the former pattern suggests the diagnosis of lymphoma, the latter is nonspecific. MRI has the advantage over other cross-sectional modalities in that the signal intensity of the mesenteric lymph nodes on T2-weighted images and the degree of contrast enhancement reflect their biological activity: tissue that is low in signal intensity on T2-weighted images with minimal contrast enhancement suggests fibrosis rather than recurrent or persistent disease. Evaluation of degree of contrast enhancement is aided by using T1-weighted fat-suppressed techniques. Various MRI techniques are effective at demonstrating mesenteric lymph nodes. Precontrast T1-weighted fat-suppressed spin-echo images show distinction between intermediate-signal-intensity mesenteric lymph nodes and high-signal-intensity pancreas (Fig. 7.19), and sagittal plane images may help distinguish rounded lymph nodes from tubular bowel loops (see Fig. 7.19).

Carcinoid Tumors

Mesenteric carcinoid tumor is due to a metastasis from a carcinoid tumor of the small bowel and has a characteristic appearance [40]. The release of 5-hydroxytryptophan and serotonin secreted by the tumor incites a desmoplastic reaction. The result is an irregular soft tissue mass in the root of the mesentery with associated radiating soft tissue strands [41,42]. Calcification may be present in up to 70 percent of tumors. Conventional or gradient-echo T1-weighted images are well-suited for imaging these tumors. The tumors stand out as low-signal-intensity masses against the high-signal-intensity mesenteric fat (Fig. 7.20). Short duration echo-train spin-echo sequences such as HASTE also demonstrate low-signal-intensity tissue in a background of high-signal-intensity fat (see Fig. 7.20). Fat-suppressed images reduce the contrast between the fibrotic tumor and fat. The desmoplastic nature of this tumor results in negligible enhancement with gadolinium (see Fig. 7.20).

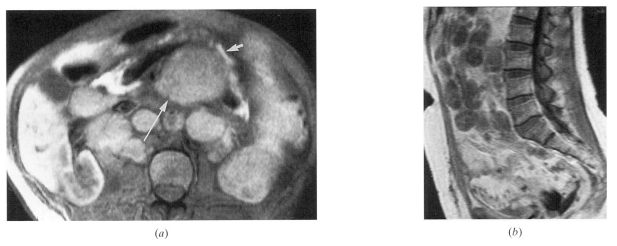

(a)   *(b)*

F I G . 7.19 Mesenteric adenopathy. T1-weighted fat-suppressed spin-echo image (*a*) demonstrates an intermediate-signal-intensity lymph node (*long arrow*) that is clearly distinguished from high-signal-intensity pancreas (*short arrow*). Sagittal plane SGE image (*b*) in a second patient demonstrates multiple rounded lymph nodes in the mesentery.

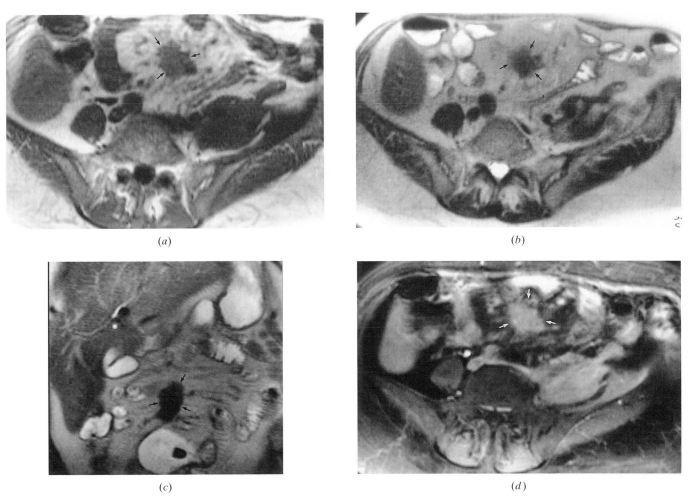

(a)   *(b)*

(c)   *(d)*

F I G . 7.20 Carcinoid tumor metastasis. SGE (*a*), T2-weighted HASTE (*b*), coronal T2-weighted HASTE (*c*), and 90-second postgadolinium fat-suppressed SGE (*d*) images in a patient with a carcinoid tumor of the small bowel. Breath-hold T1-weighted SGE images are well-suited for imaging the low-signal-intensity metastasis in the root of the small bowel mesentery (*arrows, a*); the radiating strands are highlighted by the surrounding high signal intensity of the intra-abdominal fat. The desmoplastic nature of these tumors is emphasized by its low signal intensity on T2-weighted images (*arrows, b,c*) and only modest enhancement after intravenous contrast (*arrows, d*).

INTRAPERITONEAL FLUID AND INFLAMMATION

Ascites

Ascites results from either overproduction, impaired resorption, or leakage of fluid. It is a common manifestation of many diseases: cirrhosis, obstruction (venous or lymphatic), inflammation, low albumin states, cancer, and trauma. The signal intensity of the fluid, a function of its protein content, coupled with its distribution, can suggest the underlying etiology. Simple transudates are low in signal intensity on T1-weighted sequences and very high in signal intensity on T2-weighted images (Fig. 7.21), whereas exudates, blood, and enteric contents will have higher signal intensity on T1-weighted images and more variable signal intensity on T2-weighted images [1,43,44,45]. Benign processes favor the greater sac, whereas malignant fluid tends to involve the greater and lesser sac proportionally [1,2], though exceptions are common. In simple ascites small and large bowel tend to float to the anterior abdomen in a central location (Fig. 7.22). Malignant or inflammatory ascites tends to tether bowel in different locations depending on the distribution of the disease process. Breathing-independent HASTE imaging is effective at evaluating the distribution and presence of ascites in uncooperative patients and young children (Fig. 7.23). Multiplanar imaging facilitates the evaluation of ascites distribution within various abdominal compartments (Fig. 7.24).

Cirrhosis

Portal venous hypertension in patients with cirrhosis is a frequent cause of ascites. These patients also may suffer from low protein states, which exacerbate fluid accumu-

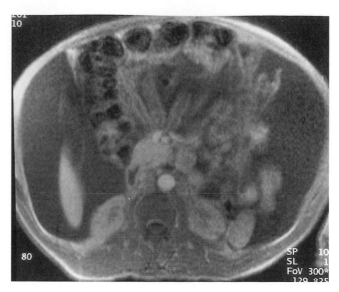

F I G . 7.22 Benign ascites. SGE image demonstrates that small and large bowels have floated anteriorly in a central location. This confirms that ascites is simple because no tethering of bowel from malignant or inflammatory adhesions has occurred.

lation. Ascites associated with hepatic cirrhosis is a transudate, with low signal intensity on T1-weighted and high signal intensity on T2-weighted sequences (Fig. 7.25).

Pancreatitis

Extrapancreatic fluid in patients with pancreatitis collects preferentially in the lesser sac [1]. The enzyme-laden fluid also may dissect into the abdominal cavity and retroperitoneum. Not infrequently, fluid tracks along tissue planes to localize subcapsularly in the liver, spleen, or both. Precontrast T1-weighted fat-suppressed SGE imaging is particularly effective at demonstrating the presence of blood in hemorrhagic pancreatitic ascites.

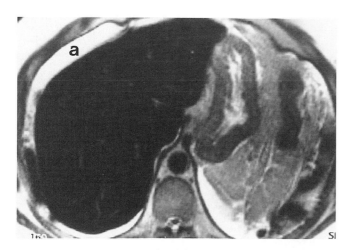

F I G . 7.21 Ascites. T2-weighted HASTE image in a patient with simple transudative ascites. High-signal-intensity ascites (*a*) surrounds the abdominal viscera. The liver is low in signal intensity secondary to iron overload from multiple transfusions.

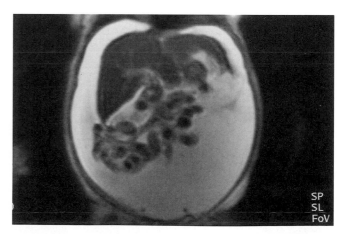

F I G . 7.23 Ascites in a neonate. Coronal HASTE image clearly shows the liver and centrally lying bowel. The central position of the bowel reflects the simple nature of ascites.

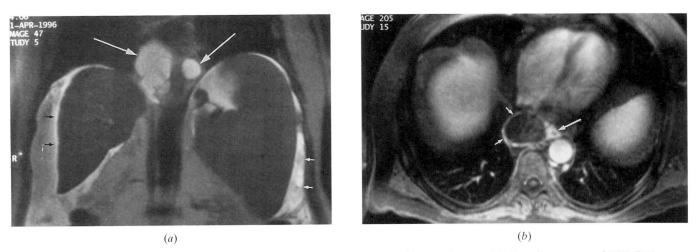

(a)   (b)

F IG. 7.24 Mediastinal extension of ascites. Coronal HASTE (*a*) and transverse 45-second postgadolinium fat-suppressed SGE (*b*) images. On the coronal image, ascites is noted along the surfaces of the liver and enlarged spleen (*small arrow, a*), and mediastinal extension of the fluid is apparent (*long arrows, a*). On the gadolinium enhanced transverse image the encapsulated collection of ascites is shown (*small arrow, b*) and close approximation to the esophagus (*long arrow, b*) is apparent.

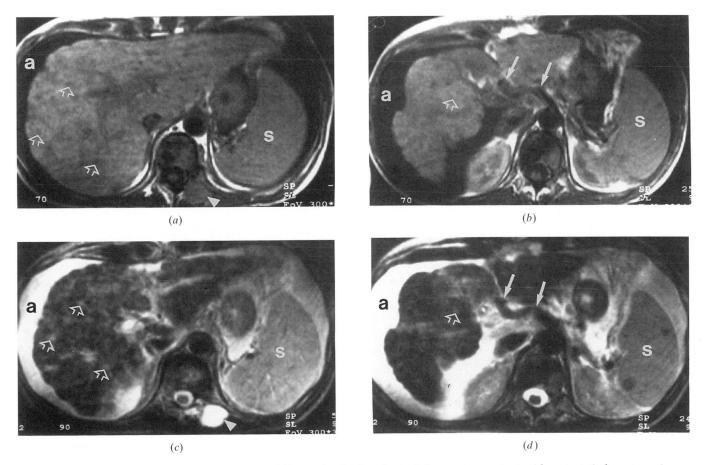

(a)   (b)

(c)   (d)

F IG. 7.25 Ascites. T1-weighted spin-echo (*a,b*) and T2-weighted spin-echo (*c,d*) images in a patient with metastatic breast carcinoma. Cirrhosis is secondary to chemotherapy-treated diffuse liver metastases (*open arrows, a–d*) and has resulted in ascites ("*a*",*a–d*). The changes of cirrhosis include a shrunken nodular liver with associated dilatations of the hepatic artery (*arrows, b,d*) and an enlarged spleen ("*s*",*a–d*). Note the metastasis in the left paraspinal muscle (*arrowheads, a,c*) and spleen. Metastases are distinguished from regenerating nodules as metastases are high signal intensity on T2-weighted images, whereas regenerating nodules are low in signal intensity.

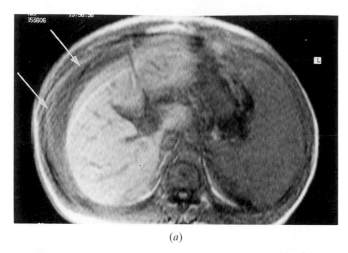

(a)

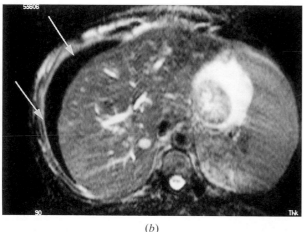

(b)

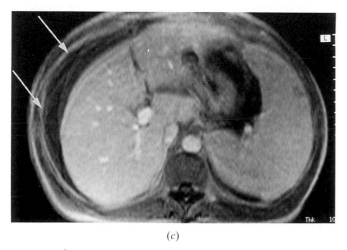

(c)

FIG. 7.26 Intraperitoneal acute blood. SGE (*a*), T2-weighted fat-suppressed spin-echo (*b*), and 1-minute postgadolinium SGE (*c*) images in a patient status postpercutaneous liver biopsy. Fluid (*arrows, a–c*) surrounding the liver exhibits the signal characteristics of acute blood (deoxyhemoglobin): isointense or low signal intensity on T1-weighted images and low signal intensity on T2-weighted images.

Intraperitoneal Blood

Intraperitoneal blood most frequently occurs in the setting of trauma. MRI can readily distinguish blood from ascites. Acute blood, in the form of *deoxyhemoglobin*, is low in signal intensity on T2-weighted images (Fig. 7.26). In contradistinction, subacute blood, in the form of *extracellular methemoglobin*, is high in signal intensity on T1- and T2-weighted images (Fig. 7.27). Fat suppression accentuates this finding. Hematomas also may demonstrate heterogeneity related to hemoglobin breakdown products admixed with blood. Not infrequently, a high-signal-intensity rim surrounding a low-signal-intensity center is seen with subacute hematomas (Fig. 7.28). These imaging characteristics represent extracellular methemoglobin encircling the retracting clot [46]. As hematomas age, a low-signal-intensity rim develops around the hematoma on both T1- and T2-weighted sequences. This rim corresponds to hemosiderin and/or fibrosis.

Intraperitoneal Bile

Free intraperitoneal bile is usually the result of surgery [47]. When present in small amounts, it is clinically occult. However, in the setting of duct injury, bile leakage may result in a biloma or bile peritonitis [47]. Free bile preferentially collects in the right upper quadrant where it incites an inflammatory reaction. A biloma results if the bile is walled off by a pseudocapsule and adhesions. The signal intensity of a biloma is variable and mimics that of the gallbladder. Bilomas may be low, intermediate, or high in signal intensity on T1-weighted images. They are high in signal intensity on T2-weighted images.

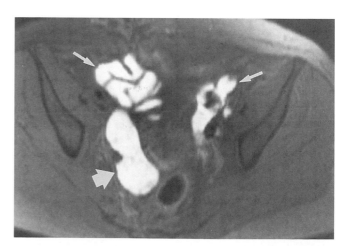

FIG. 7.27 Intraperitoneal blood. T1-weighted fat-suppressed spin-echo image in a woman 1 week after hysterectomy. There is a high-signal-intensity collection in the right pelvis consistent with subacute blood (*large arrow*). T1-weighted fat suppression is particularly sensitive for the detection of blood, but extracellular methemoglobin must be distinguished from the high signal intensity of the proteinaceous intraluminal bowel contents (*small arrows*).

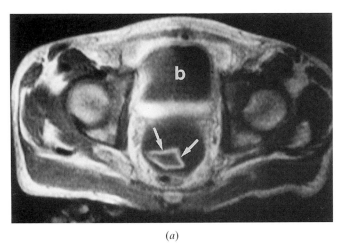

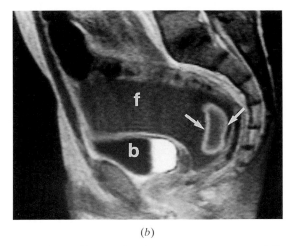

(a)   (b)

F I G . 7.28 Pelvic hematoma. Axial (*a*) and sagittal (*b*) interstitial-phase gadolinium-enhanced T1-weighted SGE images in a patient following splenic injury. Subacute hematomas may have a low-signal-intensity core with a high-signal-intensity surrounding rim (*arrows, a,b*) on T1-weighted images. These imaging characteristics reflect the retracting clot surrounded by extracellular methemoglobin. *b*, bladder; *f*, free pelvic fluid.

Intraperitoneal Urine

Bladder rupture leads to extravasation of urine. The location of the free urine is a function of whether the dome or the bladder base is injured. If the base is compromised, urine collects extraperitoneally, whereas injury to the dome results in intraperitoneal urine, also known as urine ascites. On unenhanced images, the signal intensity of urine ascites is nonspecific. Contrast administration establishes the diagnosis as high-signal-intensity gadolinium chelate in urine pools in the peritoneal cavity.

Vascular Disease

Thrombosis of the superior mesenteric vein may occur in the setting of inflammatory or infectious processes in

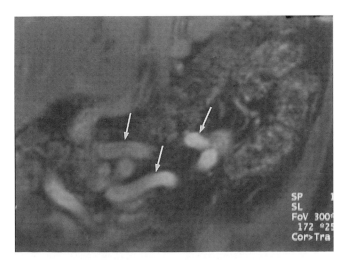

F I G . 7.29 Enlarged collateral of the superior mesenteric vein. Coronal 90-second postgadolinium fat-suppressed SGE image demonstrates an enlarged tortuous collateral vessel of the superior mesenteric vein (*arrows*).

the splanchnic circulation. (For further discussion see Portal Venous Thrombosis subsection in Chapter 2 on the Liver.) Vascular abnormalities in general are well-shown on early postgadolinium fat-suppressed SGE images (Fig. 7.29).

INFLAMMATION

Mesenteric Panniculitis

Mesenteric panniculitis, mesenteric lipofibromatosis, mesenteric lipodystrophy, and sclerosing mesenteritis are a spectrum of conditions that cause fibrofatty thickening of the mesentery with various degrees of fat necrosis, chronic inflammation, and fibrosis [48,49]. Although the etiology of mesenteric panniculitis is unclear, ischemia and autoimmune processes have been implicated as well as pancreatitis, infection, surgery, and foreign bodies [49,50,51]. The changes in the mesentery may be focal or diffuse. When diffuse, the mesenteric fat is traversed by low-signal-intensity strands on T1-weighted images [51] (Fig. 7.30). In the focal form, heterogeneous nodular masses of fat necrosis are noted. They exhibit varying amounts of fat, fluid, calcification, and soft tissue [51,52]. A variety of inflammatory or infectious etiologies may result in inflammation of the mesentery that can appear as retractile mesenteritis (see Fig. 7.30).

Peritonitis

Peritonitis may be caused by a variety of infectious or noninfectious causes, many of which relate to perforation of the bowel. Peritonitis appears as diffuse increased enhancement of the peritoneum and mesentery, and is most clearly defined on interstitial phase gadolinium-

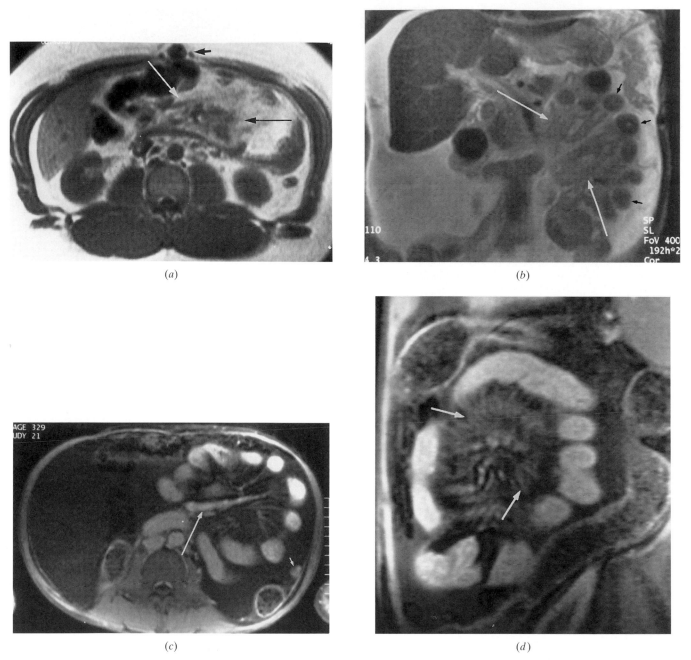

F I G . 7.30 Mesenteric lipodystrophy and tuberculous peritonitis. SGE (*a*) demonstrates low-signal-intensity stranding in the fat of the mesentery (*long arrows, a*) consistent with mesenteric lipodystrophy. A small ventral hernia is also present (*arrow, a*). Coronal HASTE (*b*), transverse (*c*), and sagittal (*d*) interstitial phase fat suppressed SGE images in a second patient with tuberculous peritonitis. A large volume of ascites is present. Multiple loops of thickened small bowel are appreciated (*short arrows, b*). The mesentery is infiltrated and intermediate in signal intensity (*long arrows, b*) on the T2-weighted image (*b*). The mesenteric vessels are closely bundled (*long arrow, c*) reflecting adherence of the vessels to each other secondary to the inflammatory process. Terminal branches of the mesenteric vessels (*arrows, d*) fan out to the thickened loops of small bowel creating a spoke-wheel type pattern on the sagittal image. Increased enhancement and mild increased thickness of the peritoneum with peritoneal-based nodules (*small arrow, c*) is also appreciated. This appearance is that of retractile mesenteritis, which can be caused by a number of etiologies including tuberculosis.

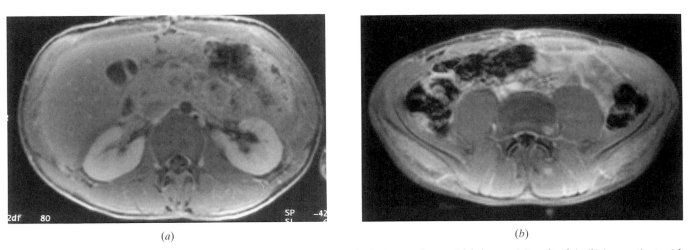

(a)   (b)

F I G . 7.31 Chemical peritonitis. Interstitial-phase gadolinium-enhanced SGE images from midabdomen (*a*) and pelvis (*b*) in a patient with chemical peritonitis secondary to intraperitoneal administration of chemotherapeutic agents. Diffuse increased enhancement is present of peritoneal, mesenteric, and serosal surfaces, which has resulted in adherence of bowel loops to each other and linear enhancing strands in the mesentery. Bowel loops and mesenteric planes are ill-defined due to the generalized inflammatory process.

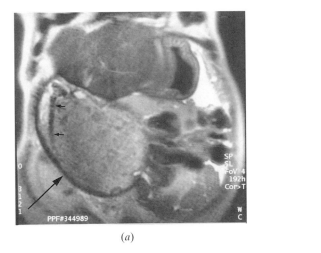

(a)

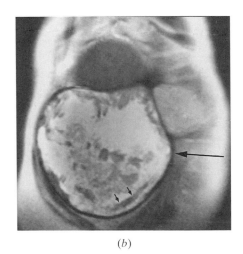

(b)

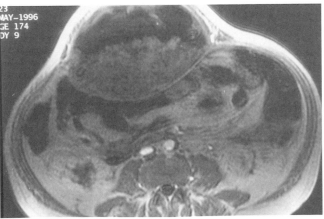

(c)

F I G . 7.32 Pseudocyst surrounding a peritoneal catheter (cocoon). Coronal HASTE image from adjacent planes (*a,b; b* is more anterior) and 90-second postgadolinium SGE (*c*) image. A 14-cm encapsulated debris-containing pseudocyst is present in the midabdomen, immediately beneath the liver. A low-signal-intensity pseudocapsule surrounds the lesion (*long arrows, a,b*). The peritoneal catheter is identified within the cocoon (*small arrows, a,b*). A substantial volume of particulate debris is present (*a–c*), which is shown to layer on the transverse gadolinium-enhanced SGE image (*c*). Outside CT imaging study had been interpreted as demonstrating a hepatocellular carcinoma (HCC).

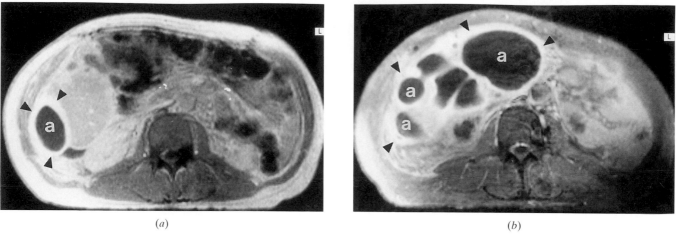

(a)   (b)

FIG. 7.33 Intra-abdominal abscess. Interstitial-phase gadolinium-enhanced T1-weighted SGE (*a*) and interstitial-phase gadolinium-enhanced T1-weighted fat-suppressed spin-echo (*b*) images in a patient with clinical suspicion of an abscess. Multiple loculated abscess collections are present along the liver capsule and in the right midabdomen ("*a*",*a,b*). The thick enhancing rims (*arrowheads, a,b*) are characteristic of the reactive inflammatory capsules associated with abscesses.

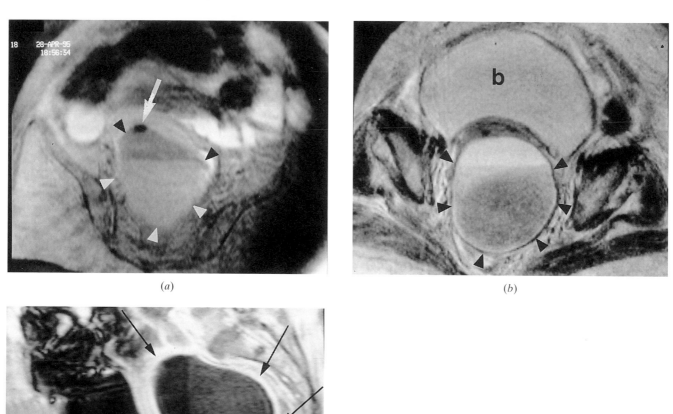

(a)   (b)

FIG. 7.34 Pelvic abscess. T1-weighted fat-suppressed spin-echo (*a*), T2-weighted fat-suppressed spin-echo (*b*), and sagittal gadolinium-enhanced T1-weighted fat-suppressed SGE (*c*) images in a patient with fever and an elevated white blood cell count. A complex fluid collection (*arrowheads, a,b*) is demonstrated in the pelvis. The variable signal intensity on the T1-weighted images reflects its protein content (*a,c*). On the T2-weighted image (*b*), low-signal-intensity debris layers in the dependent portion of the abscess. A focus of signal-void air is present (*arrow, a*), which confirms that the complex fluid collection is an abscess. Following contrast administration the wall of the abscess enhances substantially (*arrows, c*). (bladder = *b,b,c*).

(c)

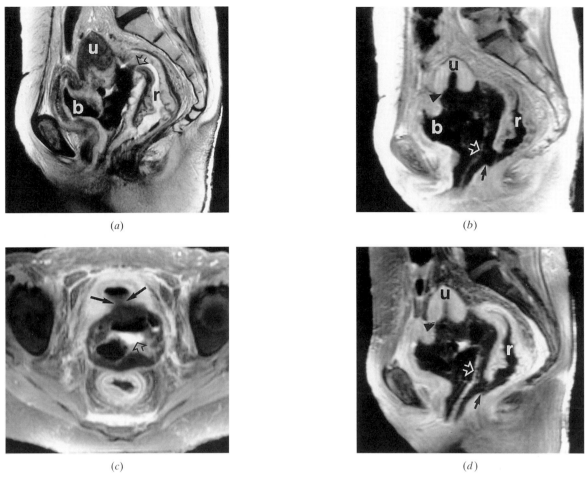

(a)

(b)

(c)

(d)

FIG. 7.35 Pelvic abscess and fistulas. Sagittal T2-weighted echo-train spin-echo (*a*), sagittal gadolinium-enhanced T1-weighted SGE (*b*), axial (*c*) and sagittal (*d*) gadolinium-enhanced T1-weighted fat-suppressed spin-echo images in a patient with cervix cancer who had undergone high dose radiation therapy. Tumor necrosis, and fistula and abscess formation are not uncommon complications of radiotherapy. A large pelvic cavity is present with communication between bladder, uterus, and rectum, which is clearly defined on the sagittal plane images (*a,b,d*). The rectal wall is substantially thickened, and submucosal edema is well-shown as high signal intensity on the T2-weighted image (*a*). The signal-void regions in the abscess cavity represent air associated with the cranial and low coupal rectal fistulas (*open arrow, a* and *solid arrow, d,* respectively) and superimposed infection. There is wide communication of the abscess cavity with the bladder. Following intravenous gadolinium administration, high- signal-intensity contrast (*open arrow, c*) exits the bladder through the large fistula (*black arrows, c*) and pools in the abscess. Portions of the uterine corpus and cervix have undergone necrosis; the uterine fundus remains. The posterior wall of the cervix and vagina (*open arrow, b,d*) is best shown on the sagittal contrast-enhanced T1-weighted fat-suppressed spin-echo image. *r*, rectum; *u*, uterine fundus; *b*, bladder.

enhanced fat-suppressed SGE images (Fig. 7.31). A localized collection of inflammatory debris may develop around tubes or catheters (e.g. CSF-peritoneal shunt or indwelling peritoneal catheters) within the peritoneal cavity, with development of a pseudocapsule. This entity is termed a cocoon (Fig. 7.32).

Abscess

Intra-abdominal abscesses are most often the sequelae of gastrointestinal or biliary surgery, diverticulitis, and Crohn's disease [53]. In the appropriate clinical setting, a focal fluid collection that demonstrates rim enhancement on gadolinium-enhanced images suggests the cor-

rect diagnosis. The addition of fat suppression and image acquisition at 2 to 10 minutes after injection (interstitial phase) can highlight the enhancement of the abscess wall and adjacent tissues (Fig. 7.33). Layering of lower-signal-intensity debris in the dependent portion of the cystic lesion on T2-weighted images is a common finding in abscesses (Fig. 7.34) When air is identified within a fluid collection, active infection and/or fistula to the bowel (Fig. 7.35) is present. The role of oral contrast agents in the examination for abscesses is unclear. However, new sequences (e.g., HASTE) in which fluid-containing bowel is well-visualized without using oral or rectal contrast are promising for distinguishing abscess from bowel. Multiplanar imaging is also effective at establishing that abscess collections are oval-shaped to distinguish them from tubular-shaped bowel [55].

FUTURE DIRECTIONS

Faster scanning times coupled with open systems and MRI compatable equipment may make routine MRI-guided percutaneous biopsies and drainages feasible, especially in patients with a contraindication to iodinated intravenous contrast [54].

CONCLUSIONS

MRI has become increasingly effective in evaluating peritoneal, omental, and mesenteric diseases. This reflects MRI's multiplanar capabilities, robust scanning techniques (breath-hold and fat-suppressed imaging), and sensitivity to intravenous contrast enhancement. The recent implementation of fat-suppressed SGE sequences, which acquire 21 sections in a 20-second breath-hold, and breathing-independent HASTE, have substantially improved the diagnostic usefulness and capability of MRI. Currently, MRI is useful for evaluating and characterizing diaphragmatic hernias, cysts, pseudocysts, endometriosis, peritoneal carcinomatosis, and intra-abdominal fluid collections.

REFERENCES

1. Cohen JM, Weinreb JC, Maravilla KP: Fluid collections in the intraperitoneal and extraperitoneal spaces: Comparison of MR and CT. Radiology 155:705–708, 1985.
2. Gore RM, Callen PW, Filly RA: Lesser sac fluid in predicting the etiology of ascites: CT findings. AJR Am J Roentgenol 139:71–74, 1982.
3. Meyers MA: The spread and localization of acute intraperitoneal effusions. Radiology 95:547–554, 1970.
4. Meyers MA: Distribution of intra-abdominal malignancy seeding dependency on dynamic of flow of ascites fluid. AJR Am J Roentgenol 119:198–206, 1973.
5. Meyers MA: Dynamic radiology of the abdomen: Normal and pathologic anatomy (2nd ed.). New York: Springer-Verlag, 1982.
6. Ruess L, Frazier AA, Sivit CJ: CT of the mesentery, omentum and peritoneum in children. Radiographics 541–542, 1995.
7. Stoupis C, Ros PR, William JL: Hemorrhagic lymphangioma mimicking hemoperitoneum: MR imaging diagnosis. J Magn Reson Imaging 3:541–542, 1993.
8. Lee GHM, Cohen AJ: CT imaging of abdominal hernias. AJR Am J Roentgenol 161:1209–1213, 1993.
9. Berger PE: Hernias of the abdominal wall and peritoneal cavity. In Franken EA Jr, Smith WL (eds.). Gastrointestinal Imaging in Pediatrics. Philadelphia: Harper & Row, pp. 446–456, 1982.
10. Vanek VW, Phillips AK: Retroperitoneal, mesenteric and omental cysts. Arch Surg 119:838–842, 1984..
11. Haney PF, Whitley NO: CT of benign cystic abdominal masses in children. AJR Am J Roentgenol 142:1279–1281, 1984.
12. Kurachi H, Murakami T, Nakamura H, et al: Imaging of peritoneal pseudocysts: Value of MR imaging compared with sonography and CT. AJR Am J Roentgenol 160:589–591, 1993.
13. Lewis VL, Shaffer HA Jr, Williamson BRJ: Pseudotumoral lipomatosis of the abdomen. J Comput Assist Tomogr 6:79–82, 1982.
14. Olive DL, Schwartz LB: Endometriosis. N Eng J Med 328:1759–1769, 1993.
15. Arrive L, Hricak H, Martin MC: Pelvic endometriosis: MR imaging. Radiology 171:687–692, 1989.
16. Sugimura K, Okizuka H, Imaoka I, Yashushi K, et al: Pelvic endometriosis: Detection and diagnosis with chemical shift MR imaging. Radiology 188:435–438, 1993.
17. Ascher SM, Agrawal R, Bis KG, Brown E, et al: Endometriosis: Appearance and detection with conventional, fat-suppressed, and contrast-enhanced fat-suppressed spin-echo techniques. J Magn Reson Imaging 5:251–257, 1995.
18. Baron RL, Lee JKT: Mesenteric desmoid tumors: Sonographic and computed-tomographic appearance. Radiology 140:777–779, 1981.
19. Magid D, Fishman EK, Jones B, Hoover HC, et al: Desmoid findings in Gardner's syndrome: Use of computed tomography. AJR Am J Roentgenol 142:1141–1145, 1984.
20. Hamrick-Turner JE, Chiechi MV, Abbitt PL, Ros PR: Neoplastic and inflammatory processes of the peritoneum, omentum, and mesentery: Diagnosis with CT. Radiographics 12:1051–1068, 1992.
21. Smith TR: Malignant peritoneal mesothelioma: Marked variability of CT findings. Abdom Imaging 19:27–29, 1994.
22. Whitley NO, Bohlman ME, Baker LP: CT patterns of mesenteric disease. J Comput Assist Tomogr 6:490–496, 1982.
23. Whitley NO, Brenner DE, Antman KH, Grant D, et al: CT of peritoneal mesothelioma: Analysis of eight cases. AJR Am J Roentgenol 138:531–535, 1982.
24. Meyers MA, McSweeney J: Secondary neoplasms of bowel. Radiology 105:1–11, 1972.
25. Daniel O: The differential diagnosis of malignant disease of the peritoneum. Br J Surg 39:147–156, 1951.
26. Meyers MA, Oliphant M, Berne AS, Feldberg MAM: The peritoneal ligaments and mesenteries: Pathways of intra-abdominal spread of disease. Radiology 163:593–604, 1987.
27. Oliphant M, Berne AS: Computed tomography of the subperitoneal space: Demonstration of direct spread of intra-abdominal disease. J Comput Assist Tomogr 6:1127–1137, 1982.
28. Semelka RC, Lawrence PH, Shoenut JP, Heywood M, et al: Primary malignant ovarian disease: Prospective comparison of contrast enhanced CT and pre- and post-intravenous Gd-DTPA enhanced fat suppress and breath hold MRI with histological correlation. J Magn Reson Imaging 3:99–106, 1993.
29. Cooper CR, Jeffrey RB, Silverman PM, Federle MP, et al: Computed tomography of omental pathology. J Comput Assist Tomogr 10:62–66, 1986.
30. Low RN, Carter WD, Saleh J, Sigeti JS: Ovarian cancer: Comparison of findings with perfluorocarbon-enhanced MR imaging, In-111-CYT-103 immunoscintigraphy, and CT. Radiology 195:391–400, 1995.
31. Chou CK, Liu GC, Chen LT, Jaw TS: MRI manifestations of peritoneal carcinomatosis. Gastrointest Radiol 17:336–338, 1992.
32. Chou CK, Liu GC, Chen LT, et al: MRI demonstration of peritoneal implants. Abdom Imaging 19:95–101, 1994.
33. Novetsky GJ, Berlin L, Epstein AJ, Lobo N, et al: Pseudomyxoma peritonei. J Comput Assist Tomogr 6:398–399, 1982.
34. Dachman AH, Lichtenstein JE, Friedman AC: Mucocele of the appendix and pseudomyxoma peritonei. AJR Am J Roentgenol 144:923–929, 1985.

35. Goffinet DR, Castellino RA, Kim H, et al: Staging laparotomies in unselected previously untreated patients with non-Hodgkin's lymphoma. Cancer 32:672–681, 1973.

36. Bernadino ME, Jing BS, Wallace S: Computed tomography of mesenteric masses. AJR Am J Roentgenol 132:33–36, 1979.

37. Levitt RG, Sagel SS, Stanley RJ: Detection of neoplastic involvement of the mesentery and omentum by computed tomography. AJR Am J Roentgenol 131:835–838, 1978.

38. Mueller PR, Ferrucci JT Jr, Harbin WP, Kirkpatrick, et al: Appearance of lymphomatous involvement of the mesentery by ultrasonography and body computed tomography: The "sandwich sign." Radiology 134:467–473, 1980.

39. Picus D, Glazer HS, Levitt RG, Husband JE: Computed tomography of abdominal carcinoid tumors. AJR Am J Roentgenol 143:581–584, 1984.

40. Pantongrag-Brown L, Buetow PC, Carr NJ, et al: Calcification and fibrosis in mesenteric carcinoid tumors: CT findings and pathologic correlation. AJR Am J Roentgenol 164:387–391, 1995.

41. Cockey BM, Fishman EK, Jones B, Siegelman SS: Computed tomography of abdominal carcinoid tumor. J Comput Assist Tomogr 10:953–962, 1985.

42. Terrier F, Revel D, Pajannen H, Richardson M, et al: MR imaging of body fluid collections. J Comput Assist Tomogr 10:953–962, 1986.

43. Walls SD, Hricak H, Baily GD, Kerlan RK Jr, et al: MR of pathologic abdominal fluid collections. J Comput Assist Tomogr 10:746–750, 1986.

44. Dooms GC, Fisher MR, Hricak H, Higgins CB: MR of intramuscular hemorrhage. J Comput Assist Tomogr 9:908–913, 1985.

45. Unger EC, Glazer HS, Lee JKT, Ling D: MRI of extracranial hematomas: Preliminary observations. AJR Am J Roentgenol 146:403–407, 1986.

46. Hahn PF, Saini S, Stark DD: Papanicolaou N, et al. Intra-abdominal hematoma: The concentric-ring sign in MR imaging. AJR Am J Roentgenol 148:115–119, 1987.

47. Zeman RK, Burrell MI: Hepatobiliary trauma. In Zeman RK, Burrell MI (eds.). Gallbladder and Bile Duct Imaging: A Clinical Radiologic Approach. New York: Churchill Livingstone, pp. 677–704, 1987.

48. Ogden WW II, Bradburn DM, Rives JD: Mesenteric panniculitis. Review of 27 cases. Ann Surg 161:864–875, 1965.

49. Bellin MF, Du LETH, Sagraty G, et al: MRI and colour-Doppler in sclerosing mesenteritis. Eur Radiol 2:373–376, 1992.

50. Gedgaudas RK, Rice RP: Radiologic evaluation of complicated pancreatitis. CRC Crit Rev Diagn Imaging 15:319–367, 1981.

51. Katz ME, Heiken JP, Glazer HS, Lee JKT: Intra-abdominal panniculitis: Clinical, radiographic, and CT features. AJR Am J Roentgenol 145:293–296, 1985.

52. Haynes JW, Brewer WH, Walsh JW: Focal fat necrosis presenting as a palpable abdominal mass: CT evaluation. J Comput Assist Tomogr 9:568–569, 1985.

53. Wang SM, Wilson SE: Subphrenic abscess: The new epidemiology. Arch Surg 112:934–936, 1977.

54. Anzai Y, Desalles AF, Black KL, Sinha S, et al: Interventional MR imaging. Radiographics 13:8971 1993.

55. Semelka RC, John G, Kelekis NL, Burdeny DA, Ascher SM: Bowel related abscesses: Demonstration by current MR techniques. J Mag Reson Imaging. In press.

ADRENAL GLANDS

R. C. SEMELKA, M.D., N. L. KELEKIS, M.D., AND
S. WORAWATTANAKUL, M.D.

NORMAL ANATOMY

The adrenal glands are paired organs that lie within the perirenal space in close proximity to the anterosuperior aspect of the kidneys. The right adrenal gland is medial to the right lobe of the liver, lateral to the right crus of the diaphragm, and posterior to the inferior vena cava (IVC). The left adrenal gland is seated posterior to the splenic vein and medial to the left crus of the diaphragm.

MRI TECHNIQUE

Techniques that have been employed to examine the adrenal glands include T2-weighted spin-echo, T2-weighted echo-train spin-echo, T2-weighted echoplanar, T1- and T2-weighted fat-suppressed spin-echo, serial postgadolinium-enhanced gradient-echo, postgadolinium T1-weighted fat-suppressed spin-echo, and out-of-phase gradient-echo imaging [1–21]. The intention of most of these techniques has been to distinguish benign from malignant disease. The approach that appears most reliable is the combined use of in-phase and out-of-phase gradient-echo techniques [9–20]. Benign adenomas have been shown to lose signal intensity on out-of-phase images due to the presence of intracytoplasmic lipid [9–20]. Metastatic lesions do not contain intracytoplasmic lipid, and therefore do not lose signal intensity on out-of-phase

images [9–20]. It is important to use out-of-phase technique without concomitant use of frequency-selective fat suppression because fat suppression will cause minimization of signal dropout [22]. The best approach is to use a spoiled gradient-echo (SGE) technique for both in-phase and out-of-phase imaging. The only variation between sequences should be the echo time (TE), with an echo time of 4.2 to 4.5 msec for in-phase imaging and echo time of 2.2 to 2.7 msec for out-of-phase imaging at 1.5 T. Use of a longer echo time (e.g., 6 to 7 msec) for out-of-phase imaging is less ideal because it introduces T2* signal loss. Overlap, however, exists between benign and malignant masses using combined in-phase and out-of-phase techniques [11–20]. This is because not all benign adrenal adenomas contain intracytoplasmic lipid [15–20], and benign masses of other etiologies (e.g., granulomatous disease) do not contain lipid.

Serial postgadolinium gradient-echo imaging may provide supplemental information to distinguish benign from malignant adrenal masses [6,7] because many metastases enhance greater and for a more prolonged period than benign adenomas. However, substantial overlap exists between metastases and adenomas [11,18]. Desmoplastic metastases enhance minimally [8], whereas normal adrenal tissue and adrenal adenomas may enhance intensely [8,18,23]. Regarding T2-weighted imaging, metastases frequently possess a longer T2 and are brighter on T2-weighted images than adenomas. Substan-

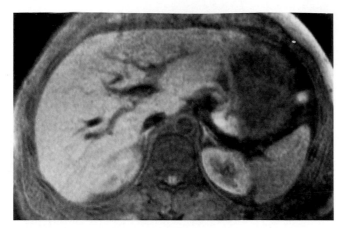

FIG. 8.1 Normal adrenals. T1 fat-suppressed spin-echo image demonstrates clear definition of the limbs of the normal adrenal glands, which appear relatively high in signal intensity in a background of suppressed fat.

tial overlap exists between benign and malignant masses using this technique [4,5,11]. Signal intensity on T2-weighted images depends on the fluid content, predominantly in the interstitial space, of the mass. Desmoplastic neoplasms have low fluid content and therefore low signal intensity, whereas some benign lesions have high fluid content and are high in signal intensity [11]. Visual perception of signal intensity on T2-weighted images is also problematic. Most adrenal masses appear at least moderately high in signal intensity on fat-suppressed T2-weighted images because the low signal intensity of fat causes rescaling of the signal intensities of abdominal organs, and most adrenal masses appear moderately low in signal intensity on echo-train spin-echo sequences due to the high signal intensity of background fat. Because no single technique is more than 95 percent accurate, a useful approach is to combine in-phase and out-of-phase

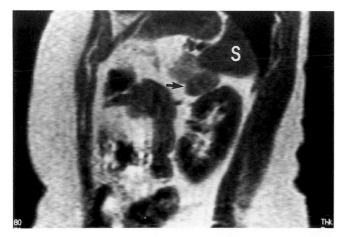

FIG. 8.2 Adrenal mass shown in the sagittal plane. Sagittal plane SGE image demonstrates an adrenal adenoma (*arrow*) that is clearly separated from kidney and spleen(s).

images with other techniques to increase the confidence of lesion characterization.

The demonstration of normal adrenal glands and small adrenal masses is well-performed with T1-weighted fat-suppressed imaging [8,12] (Fig. 8.1). The demonstration of renal corticomedullary difference on either T1-weighted fat-suppressed spin-echo images or immediate postgadolinium SGE images is helpful in distinguishing adrenal from renal tumors [13,24]. The multiplanar imaging capability of MRI is also useful for assessing large tumors in the region of the upper pole of the kidney to determine intra- or extrarenal origin by imaging in the coronal or sagittal planes [24,25]. Sagittal-plane imaging is preferred to coronal imaging [24]. The relationship between mass, kidney, and liver or spleen is shown in profile in the sagittal plane (Fig. 8.2), and en face in the coronal plane. Origin of tumor is much more clearly evaluated when the orientation between these structures is viewed in profile because partial volume effects may be observed when the organ margins are viewed en face [24].

MASS LESIONS

Diseases that affect the adrenal glands include benign and malignant tumors and adrenal hyperplasia. Because the adrenal glands perform an endocrine function, adrenal disease can be further categorized as hyperfunctioning or nonhyperfunctioning. Hyperfunctioning disease may result from adrenal hyperplasia as well as from benign and malignant tumors.

Benign Masses

Adrenal Cyst
Adrenal cysts are uncommon. Pseudocysts are the most common clinically detected cysts, and usually arise from hemorrhage into a normal adrenal gland [26]. Endothelial cysts are small lesions and are predominantly lymphogenous in origin.

The majority of adrenal cysts are low in signal intensity on T1-weighted images and high in signal intensity on T2-weighted images [12]. Because pseudocysts result from adrenal hemorrhage, variable signal intensity on T1- and T2-weighted images may be observed [27] (Fig. 8.3). Adrenal cysts are sharply marginated and signal-void on gadolinium-enhanced MR images (Fig. 8.4). Pseudocysts that contain substantial concentration of extracellular methemoglobin from subacute hemorrhage may remain slightly hyperintense on gadolinium-enhanced images. Imaging early and late after gadolinium is useful to ensure that lesions do not enhance over time, and therefore are actually cysts [11]. Hypovascular neoplasms may be nearly signal-void on early postcon-

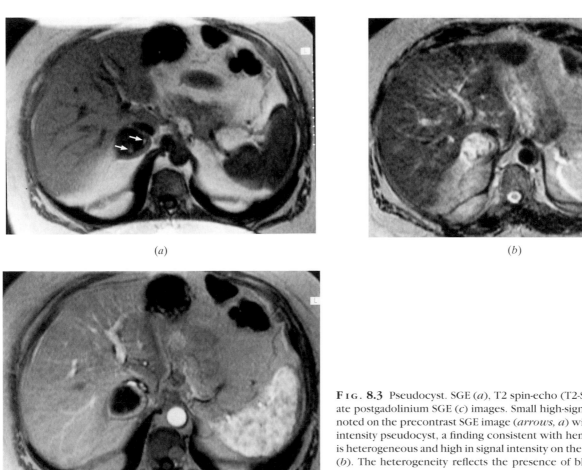

(a)

(b)

(c)

FIG. 8.3 Pseudocyst. SGE (*a*), T2 spin-echo (T2-SE) (*b*) and immediate postgadolinium SGE (*c*) images. Small high-signal-intensity foci are noted on the precontrast SGE image (*arrows, a*) within the low-signal-intensity pseudocyst, a finding consistent with hemorrhage. The mass is heterogeneous and high in signal intensity on the T2-weighted image (*b*). The heterogeneity reflects the presence of blood products. The lesion is signal-void on early (*c*) and late (not shown) postgadolinium images, which are diagnostic features for a cyst.

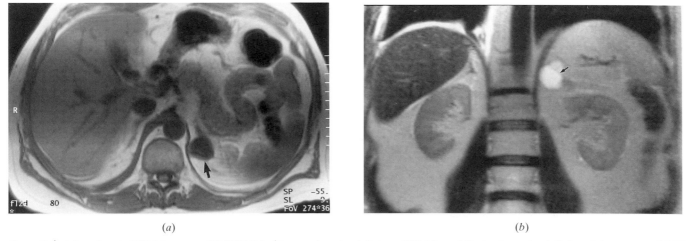

(a)

(b)

FIG. 8.4 Adrenal cyst. SGE (*a*), coronal HASTE (*b*), 45-second postgadolinium SGE (*c*), and 2-minute postgadolinium fat-suppressed SGE (*d*) images. An adrenal pseudocyst is identified arising from the left adrenal (*arrow, a*).

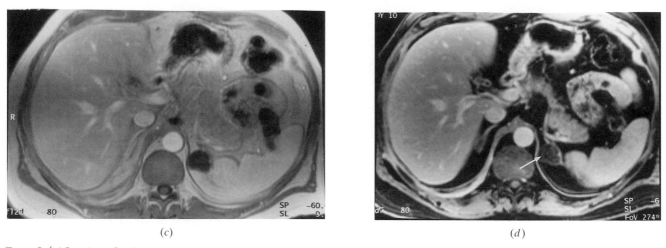

(c)

(d)

FIG. 8.4 (*Continued*) The pseudocyst is low in signal intensity on the T1-weighted image (*a*), high in signal intensity on the T2-weighted image (*b*), and does not enhance on early (*c*) or late (*d*) postgadolinium images. Thin septations are present in the pseudocyst (*arrow, b*), which are well-shown on the breathing-independent T2-weighted image (*b*) and show faint enhancement on the interstitial-phase gadolinium-enhanced fat-suppressed image (*arrow, d*).

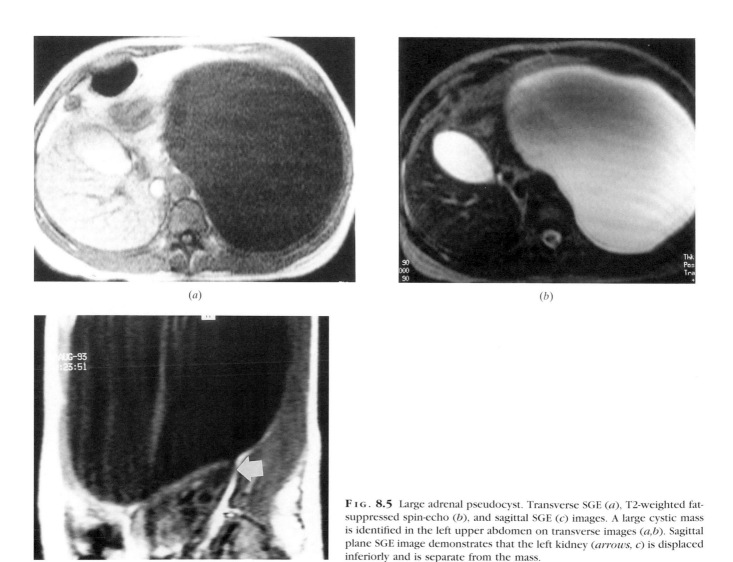

(a)

(b)

(c)

FIG. 8.5 Large adrenal pseudocyst. Transverse SGE (*a*), T2-weighted fat-suppressed spin-echo (*b*), and sagittal SGE (*c*) images. A large cystic mass is identified in the left upper abdomen on transverse images (*a,b*). Sagittal plane SGE image demonstrates that the left kidney (*arrows, c*) is displaced inferiorly and is separate from the mass.

trast images but enhance on later postgadolinium images. Pseudocysts may be large in size, and sagittal-plane imaging may be useful to demonstrate the location of the mass (Fig. 8.5).

Nonhyperfunctioning Adenoma

Adrenal adenomas are the most common adrenal masses and are most frequently nonhyperfunctioning. Incidental adenomas are reported in 2 to 8 percent of autopsies. Increased incidence has been reported in patients who are elderly, obese, hypertensive, or with primary malignancies of bladder, kidney, and endometrium.

Adenomas are oval-shaped masses and vary in diameter from 1 to 10 cm with the majority measuring smaller than 4 cm. The majority of adenomas are low in signal intensity on T2-weighted images [1–5]. Contrast enhancement on immediate postgadolinium images is variable and ranges from minimal to moderately intense [8,11,18].

Uniform enhancement of the entire lesion on immediate postgadolinium capillary-phase images is common for adenomas and rare for other entities. On serial postgadolinium images, rapid washout of contrast may be a feature more typical of benign than malignant masses [6,7]; however, variation exists [11,18]. These lesions enhance homogeneously and have regular margins on gadolinium-enhanced fat-suppressed images [8]. Small linear or rounded foci of low or high signal intensity may be present on various MR sequences representing small areas of cystic change, hemorrhage or variations of vascularity. Adenomas commonly possess a thin rim of enhancement, best appreciated on interstitial phase gadolinium enhanced images [28]. However, a thin rim of adrenal tissue may also be appreciated with small metastases, simulating this appearance. The most accurate method for demonstrating that a mass is an adenoma is to show loss of signal intensity on out-of-phase images [9–20] (Fig. 8.6).

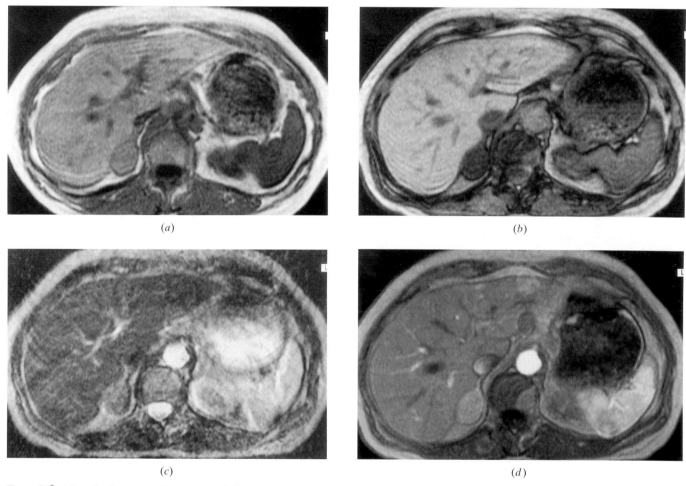

(a) *(b)*

(c) *(d)*

F IG. 8.6 Adrenal adenoma. SGE (*a*), out-of-phase SGE (*b*), T2-SE (*c*), and immediate postgadolinium SGE (*d*) images. Substantial signal-intensity drop is noted of the adrenal adenoma comparing in-phase (*a*) to out-of-phase (*b*) SGE images. The extent of signal-intensity drop is consistent with substantial intracytoplasmic lipid. The identical imaging parameters were used for these SGE images except for the echo time (TE), which was 4.5 msec for in-phase and 2.6 msec for out-of-phase images. The mass is slightly hyperintense relative to liver on T2-SE images (*c*), and considerable breathing artifact is present due to the long duration of the sequence. Immediately following contrast the adenoma enhances uniformly and intensely (*d*).

Loss of signal intensity should parallel loss of signal in marrow of the adjacent vertebral body. Caution should be exercised in using liver as the comparative organ to determine signal intensity loss because the liver may also contain fat [17,22]. The use of spleen may be problematic also because the spleen may contain iron, and T2* effect will influence signal-intensity changes, particularly if a longer echo time (e.g., 6 to 7 msec) is used for out-of-phase imaging. Renal cortex is less affected by fat or iron deposition, and may be a more accurate tissue to use as a visual comparison for signal-intensity loss. An echo-time-adjusted signal-intensity drop greater than 20 percent is diagnostic for adenomas (Fig. 8.6), while a 10 to 20 percent signal-intensity drop is suggestive of adenomas, but follow-up may be needed (Fig. 8.7). Benign lesions that do not contain intracytoplasmic lipid may

also retain signal on out-of-phase images [11,20] (Fig. 8.8). Negligible signal loss on out-of-phase images was reported in 2 of 7 resected adenomas, and both of these tumors contained minimal lipid content at histology [20]. Adenoma may contain foci of hemorrhage that appear as punctate high-signal-intensity foci on T1-weighted and /or T2-weighted images (Fig. 8.9).

Myelolipoma

Myelolipomas are rare benign tumors composed of myeloid, erythroid, and fat elements [29]. These tumors are usually small and unilateral and typically have a high fat content that gives them a pathognomonic appearance on MR images [29–35]. Occasionally, myelolipomas may be large, and in these cases direct sagittal or coronal imaging may be helpful to demonstrate the extrarenal

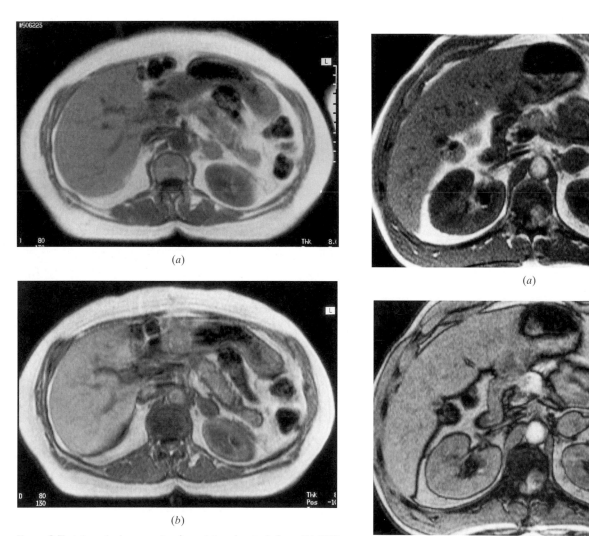

(a)

(b)

FIG. 8.7 Adrenal adenoma. In-phase (a) and out-of-phase (b) SGE images. Mild signal-intensity loss (approximately 15%) is noted from in-phase (a) to out-of-phase (b) images, which is in the low range for signal-intensity drop to diagnose an adrenal mass as an adenoma. The extent of signal-intensity drop is consistent with minimal intracytoplasmic lipid.

(a)

(b)

FIG. 8.8 Adrenal adenoma with no signal-intensity drop. In-phase (a) and out-of-phase (b) SGE images. No signal-intensity drop is noted from in-phase (a) to out-of-phase (b) images. The lack of signal-intensity drop reflects no appreciable intracytoplasmic lipid.

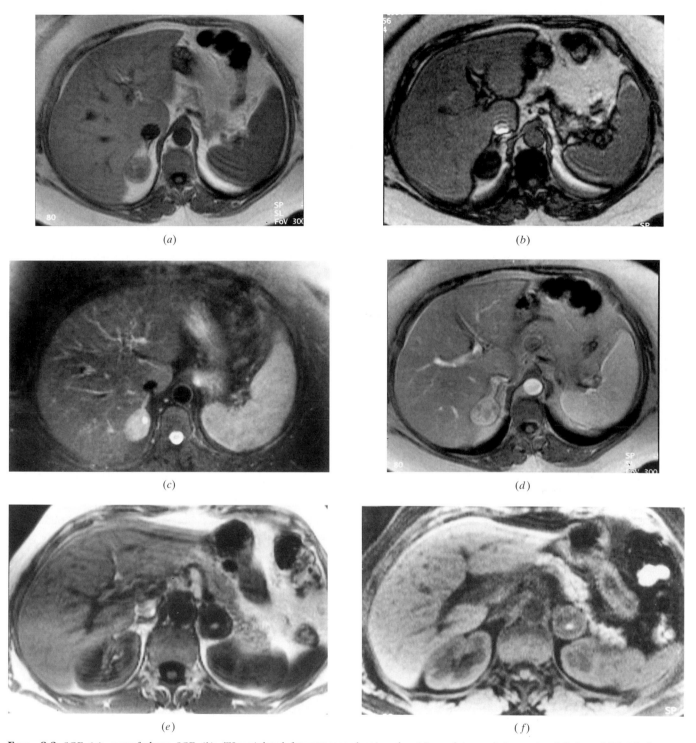

(a)

(b)

(c)

(d)

(e)

(f)

F I G . 8.9 SGE (*a*), out-of-phase SGE (*b*), T2-weighted fat-suppressed spin-echo (*c*), and immediate postgadolinium SGE (*d*) images. Substantial signal-intensity drop is present on the right adrenal adenoma comparing in-phase (*a*) to out-of-phase (*b*) SGE images. Small high-signal-intensity foci are present on T1- (*a*) and T2-weighted (*c*) images, which is consistent with hemorrhage. The adenoma enhances intensely on the immediate postgadolinium SGE image (*d*), and contains foci of diminished enhancement that correspond to punctate regions of hemorrhage. SGE (*e*), T1-weighted fat-suppressed SGE (*f*), T2-weighted fat-suppressed echo-train spin-echo (*g*), immediate postgadolinium SGE (*h*), and 2-minute postgadolinium fat-suppressed SGE (*i*) images in a second patient.

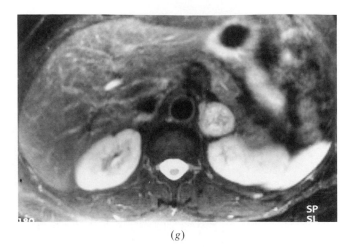

(g)

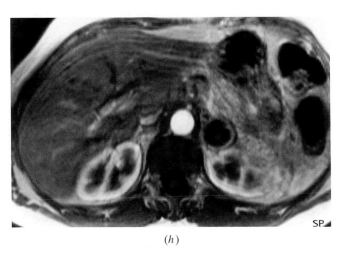

(h)

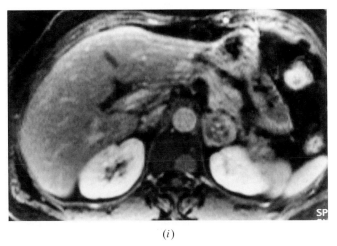

(i)

FIG. 8.9 (*Continued*) A 3-cm left adrenal adenoma is present that contains foci of high signal intensity on the T1-weighted image (*e*), which do not suppress with fat suppression (*f*). The mass is heterogeneous on the T2-weighted image (*g*) and contains multiple high-signal-intensity foci. A prominent rim of enhancement is present on the immediate postgadolinium image with minimal internal enhancement (*h*). On the interstitial-phase gadolinium-enhanced fat-suppressed image (*i*) central punctate high-signal-intensity foci are apparent.

origin of these tumors [33]. The amount of fat in these lesions may vary. On the basis of T1-weighted images alone the distinction from a hemorrhagic cyst may be difficult. The diagnosis is virtually certain if the tumor is high in signal intensity on T1-weighted images and suppresses with fat suppression [12,34,35] (Fig. 8.10). Because myelolipomas may be almost completely composed of fat, these tumors may not lose signal intensity on out-of-phase images because signal loss using this technique occurs when fat and water are of similar proportions in the same voxel.

Hemangioma

Adrenal hemangiomas tend to be large (>10 cm) and undergo central necrosis and hemorrhage [36]. Peripheral nodules are characteristic of these masses [36]. Tumors are high in signal intensity centrally on T1- and T2-weighted images due to necrosis and hemorrhage [36]. Peripheral nodules enhance intensely with gadolinium. These tumors may resemble adrenal cortical carcinomas [24].

Aldosteronoma

Aldosteronomas are rare tumors that are responsible for 75 percent of cases of primary aldosteronism (Conn's syndrome), with adrenal hyperplasia accounting for 25 percent [37]. The clinical presentation includes systemic hypertension with hypokalemia, decreased plasma renin activity, and increased plasma aldosterone. These tumors are typically small, measuring less than 3 cm in diameter with tumors commonly smaller than 1 cm. The distinction between adenoma and hyperplasia is important because patients with adenomas will respond to surgical management, whereas patients with hyperplasia are best treated medically [38]. Findings on tomographic images may result in diagnostic errors in patients who have a unilateral adenoma but in whom both adrenals have a nodular appearance. Doppman et al. [39] reported on 24 patients with primary aldosteronism in whom CT images suggested the presence of hyperplasia in 6 patients who had a unilateral aldosteronoma at surgery. T1-weighted fat-suppressed images show clear delineation of the adrenal glands and permit detection of small masses [12] (Fig. 8.11). Aldosteronomas not uncommonly contain intracytoplasmic lipid and may therefore lose signal intensity on out-of-phase images [20] (see Fig. 8.11).

Cortisol-Producing Functioning Adenoma

Functioning adrenal adenomas are responsible for approximately 20 percent of Cushing's syndrome cases. Most of these adenomas measure larger than 2 cm and are well-shown on CT and MR images [40]. Hyperfunctioning

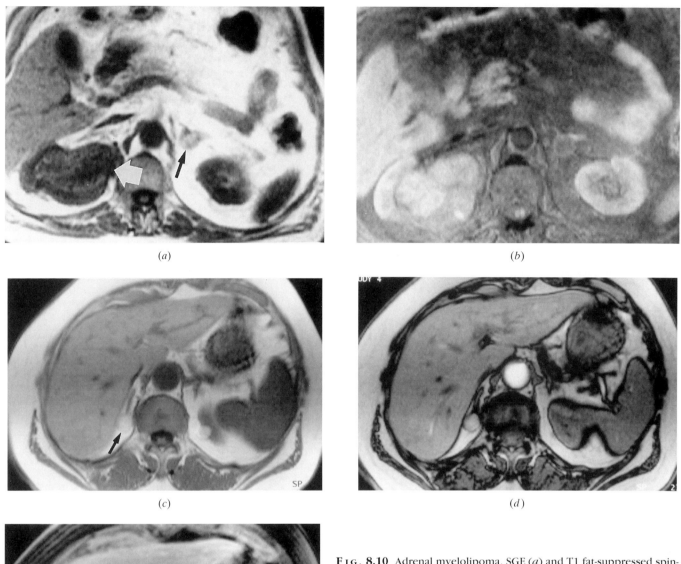

(a)

(b)

(c)

(d)

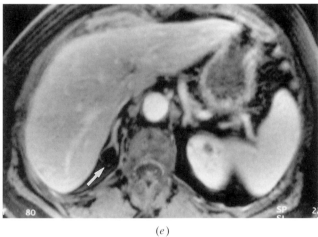

(e)

FIG. 8.10 Adrenal myelolipoma. SGE (*a*) and T1 fat-suppressed spin-echo (*b*) images. The left adrenal myelolipoma (*arrows, a*) is high in signal intensity on the SGE image and loses signal uniformly on the fat-suppressed image with a signal intensity comparable to that of background fat. A renal cancer is noted in the right kidney (*large arrow, a*). SGE (*c*), out-of-phase SGE (*d*), and interstitial phase gadolinium enhanced fat-suppressed SGE (*e*) images in a second patient. A 1.8 cm myelolipoma (*arrow, c*) is present of the right adrenal. The tumor is high in signal intensity on the in-phase SGE image because it is composed almost completely of fat. No drop in signal is present on the out-of-phase image (*d*), reflecting the near complete absence of water protons in the mass. On the fat-suppressed image the mass is near signal void (*arrow, e*) confirming that it is essentially all fat in composition.

and nonhyperfunctioning adenomas are presently not distinguishable on MR images because both have similar morphological and signal intensity features, including the tendency of both to lose signal intensity on out-of-phase images since they may contain intracytoplasmic lipid [20].

Malignant Masses

Metastases

Metastases are the most frequent malignant lesions to involve the adrenal glands. The most common primary

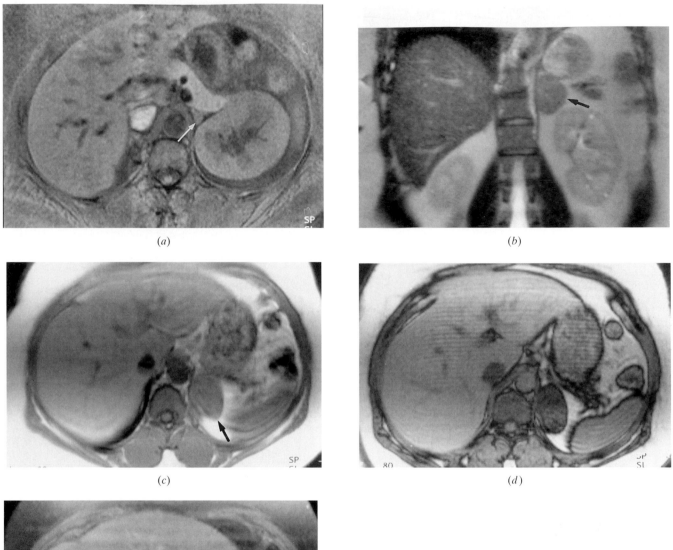

(a)

(b)

(c)

(d)

(e)

FIG. 8.11 Aldosteronoma. T1-weighted fat-suppressed spin-echo image demonstrates a 1-cm aldosteronoma arising from the medial limb of the left adrenal (*arrow*). The left kidney is enlarged due to congenital absence of the right kidney. Coronal HASTE (*b*), SGE (*c*), out-of-phase SGE (*d*), and interstitial phase gadolinium enhanced fat suppressed SGE (*e*) images in a second patient. A 3.5 cm left adrenal aldosteronoma is present (*arrow, b,c*). The mass is moderately low in signal intensity on the T2-weighted image (*b*). The mass drops in signal from in-phase (*c*) to out-of-phase (*d*) images reflecting the presence of intracytoplasmic lipid. On the post gadolinium image (*e*) the mass enhances in a relatively homogeneous fashion. This case illustrates that aldosteronomas have similar imaging findings to other benign adrenal adenomas.

tumors are lung, breast, bowel, and pancreas cancers [41]. Metastatic deposits vary in size from microscopic involvement to large tumor masses. Metastases are most frequently bilateral, but they may be unilateral. On T2-weighted images, metastases frequently are high in signal intensity [1–5]. Metastases may, however, be lower in signal intensity, particularly if the primary neoplasm is desmoplastic [4,5]. In addition, certain benign lesions have prolonged T2 values [25]. Comparison of the signal intensity of the adrenal mass to either the primary tumor or other metastatic deposits may be helpful in determining if the lesion is a metastasis because foci of tumor located in different sites frequently possess similar signal intensity [3]. Metastases frequently have irregular margins

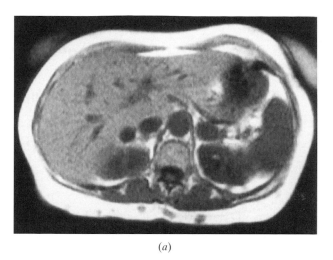

(a)

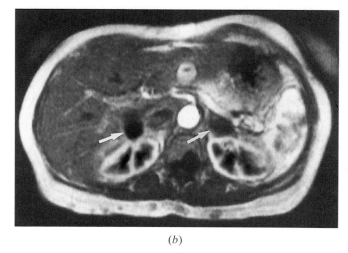

(b)

FIG. 8.12 Hypovascular adrenal metastases. SGE (a) and immediate postgadolinium SGE (b) images. These metastases are low in signal intensity on precontrast T1-weighted images (a) and enhance minimally on immediate postcontrast images (arrows, b). Minimal enhancement reflects the desmoplastic nature of these metastases. Multiple metastases are noted within the subcutaneous tissue of the patient's back.

and enhance in a heterogeneous fashion, features that are well-shown on gadolinium-enhanced T1-weighted fat-suppressed images [8]. As with other types of adrenal masses, minimal enhancement on early postgadolinium images is commonly observed (Fig. 8.12), with progressive enhancement on more delayed interstitial-phase images. Direct extension of primary tumors may occasionally be seen. This is most frequently observed in pancreatic or renal cancers. Necrosis is not uncommon in large metastatic deposits. Hemorrhage is also a feature more typical of malignant than benign masses and is better shown on MR than CT images (Fig. 8.13).

The most reliable MRI feature to suggest that an adrenal mass may represent a metastasis is the demonstration that the lesion does not lose signal on out-of-phase im-

ages [9–20] (Fig. 8.14). This approach may be most reliable in the investigation of patients with a known primary malignancy.

At this time, the accuracy of out-of-phase gradient-echo images to characterize adrenal masses is unclear. Therefore, additional T2-weighted images and postgadolinium images are useful (Fig. 8.15). CT-guided biopsies are at present not obviated in all cases by MRI examination. To obviate CT-guided biopsy, accuracy of MRI must approach 95 percent [42]. Our impression is that accuracy currently may be between 85 and 90 percent. However, not all indeterminate adrenal masses need to be biopsied. In patients with no known primary malignancy, it is considered acceptable management to serially examine adrenal masses to assess change in size. Reassessment at 3 to 6 months and 1 year is performed at many centers [43–45]. It may be sufficient to acquire only in-phase and out-of-phase SGE images on follow-up examination to reduce cost.

Pheochromocytoma

Pheochromocytomas are catecholamine-producing tumors that arise from the adrenal medulla in 90 percent of cases. The remaining 10 percent occur along the course of sympathetic ganglia, most frequently in a periaortic or paracaval location including the organ of Zückerkandl (located at the aortic bifurcation). Mediastinal and bladder-wall tumors account for 2 percent of pheochromocytomas. Tumors are frequently greater than 3 cm in diameter at presentation [46]. Pheochromocytomas are bilateral in 10 percent of cases and malignant in about 10 percent of cases. Extra-adrenal tumors are malignant in a greater percentage of cases (40%). Patients present with sustained or paroxysmal hypertension, and the great major-

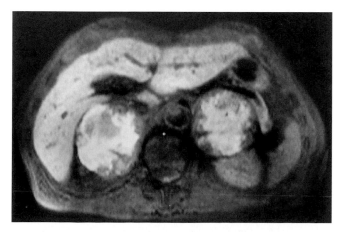

FIG. 8.13 Hemorrhagic adrenal metastases. T1-weighted fat-suppressed spin-echo image demonstrates high-signal-intensity subacute hemorrhage in bilateral adrenal metastases.

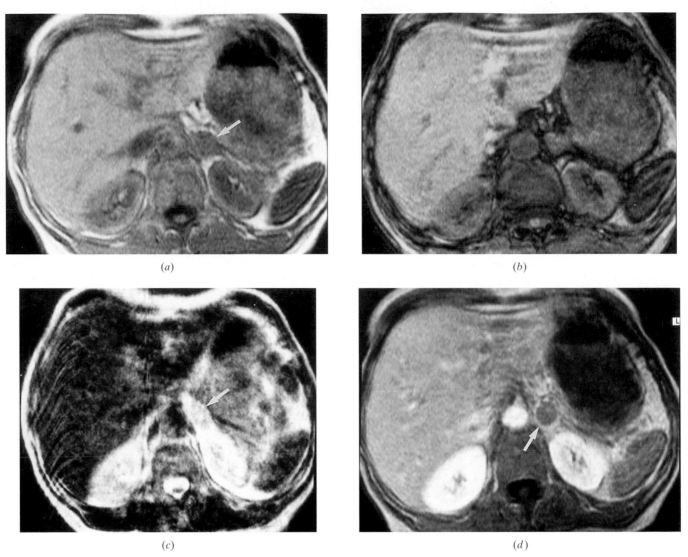

FIG. 8.14 Small left adrenal metastasis. In-phase SGE (*a*), out-of-phase SGE (*b*), T2-weighted echo-train spin-echo (*c*), and 90-second postgadolinium SGE (*d*). A 1.5-cm mass is present in the left adrenal (*arrow, a*) in a patient with primary lung cancer, which retains signal intensity from in-phase (*a*) to out-of-phase (*b*) SGE images. The mass is heterogeneous and moderately high in signal intensity on the T2-weighted image (*arrow, c*). On the 90-second postgadolinium image the mass is minimally enhanced and demonstrates a thin rim of enhancement (*arrow, d*).

ity of symptomatic patients have elevated urinary catecholamine, vanilmandelic acid (VMA), and metanephric levels. Patients with multiple endocrine neoplasia (MEN) Type 2, neurofibromatosis, von Hippel-Lindau disease, and multiple cutaneous neuromas have increased incidence of pheochromocytomas. Seventy-five percent of patients with MEN 2 have bilateral tumors, which are rarely extra-adrenal [47]. Cystic pheochromocytomas occur, and distinction from cysts may be difficult [48].

Pheochromocytomas characteristically are high in signal intensity on T2-weighted images [1] (Fig. 8.16). Although many pheochromocytomas may appear very bright (e.g., light bulbs) on T2-weighted images, a sub-

stantial number are heterogeneous and in rare instances they may have moderate signal intensity [12] (Fig. 8.17). A confounding variable is the signal intensity of background fat, which depends on the type of sequence employed. On echo-train spin-echo images masses tend to look lower in signal intensity, whereas on fat-suppressed images masses tend to appear higher in signal intensity. This reflects a signal intensity rescaling effect, depending on the signal intensity of the background fat. MRI may be the technique of choice to examine for pheochromocytomas because these lesions are most often relatively high in signal intensity on T2-weighted images independent of tumor size and location [12,49]. Therefore, small

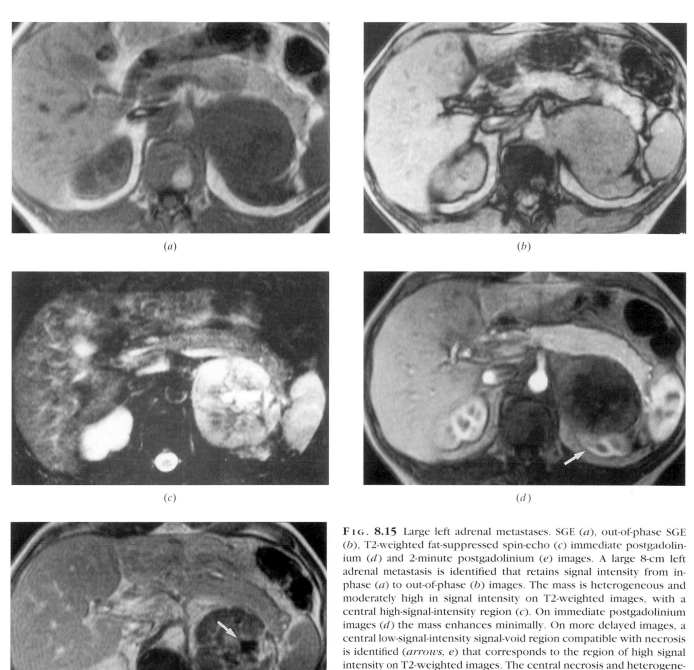

(a)

(b)

(c)

(d)

(e)

Fig. 8.15 Large left adrenal metastases. SGE (*a*), out-of-phase SGE (*b*), T2-weighted fat-suppressed spin-echo (*c*) immediate postgadolinium (*d*) and 2-minute postgadolinium (*e*) images. A large 8-cm left adrenal metastasis is identified that retains signal intensity from in-phase (*a*) to out-of-phase (*b*) images. The mass is heterogeneous and moderately high in signal intensity on T2-weighted images, with a central high-signal-intensity region (*c*). On immediate postgadolinium images (*d*) the mass enhances minimally. On more delayed images, a central low-signal-intensity signal-void region compatible with necrosis is identified (*arrows, e*) that corresponds to the region of high signal intensity on T2-weighted images. The central necrosis and heterogeneity demonstrated on T2-weighted and postgadolinium images further confirm the findings of a malignant mass on out-of-phase images. Distinction between adrenal metastasis and left kidney is best defined on the immediate postgadolinium SGE image by the demonstration of corticomedullary differentiation of the kidney (*arrow, d*).

extra-adrenal lesions are conspicuous on T2-weighted images and are usually distinguishable from other structures such as lymph nodes and bowel, which are lower in signal intensity. Cystic pheochromocytomas are as high in signal intensity as cerebrospinal fluid (CSF) on T2-weighted images [50]. Pheochromocytomas usually en-

hance minimally on immediate postgadolinium images and demonstrate substantial enhancement on later interstitial-phase images (Fig. 8.16). The early enhancement reflects few feeding vessels, and later hyperintensity reflects a large extracellular space. The large extracellular space also accounts for the high signal intensity on T2-

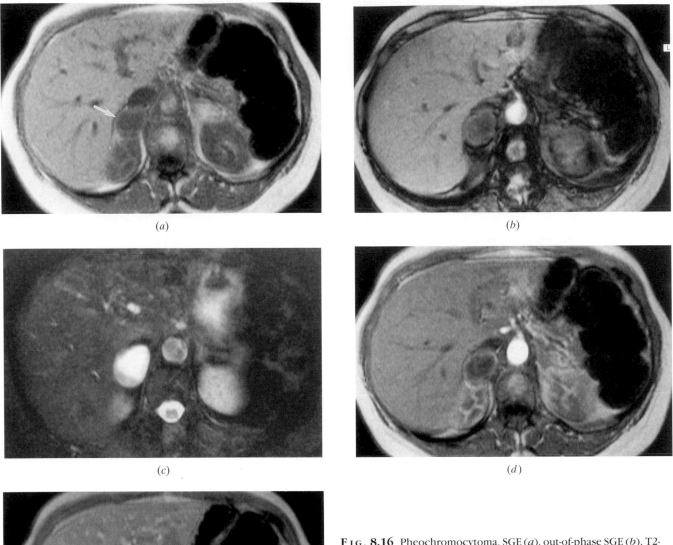

(a)

(b)

(c)

(d)

(e)

FIG. 8.16 Pheochromocytoma. SGE (*a*), out-of-phase SGE (*b*), T2-weighted fat-suppressed spin-echo (*c*), immediate postgadolinium SGE (*d*), and 2-minute postgadolinium SGE (*e*) images. A 2.5-cm pheochromocytoma arises from the right adrenal gland (*arrow, a*), which has a moderate-signal-intensity peripheral rim with a low-signal-intensity center on in-phase (*a*) and out-of-phase (*b*) SGE images. No appreciable drop of signal intensity is present on the out-of-phase image. On the T2-weighted image the mass is extremely high in signal intensity, with the peripheral rim appearing slightly low in signal intensity (*c*). On the immediate postgadolinium image the tumor rim enhances intensely with minimal central enhancement (*d*). On the more delayed image the tumor diffusely enhances in a heterogeneous fashion (*e*).

weighted images. In general, pheochromocytomas do not lose signal intensity on out-of-phase images.

Adrenal Cortical Carcinoma

Adrenal cortical carcinoma is a rare aggressive tumor. Tumors usually present when they are large, with over 90 percent of reported cases exceeding 6 cm in diameter

[24,51]. These cancers are more common in women, and tumor occurrence in patients 20 to 40 years of age is not unusual [24]. Approximately 50 percent of the tumors are hyperfunctioning, and hypercortisolism and virilization are common presentations [51]. Metastases are frequently found at presentation, with regional and para-aortic lymph nodes, lungs, and liver as common sites. Tumor

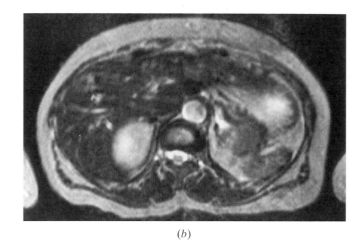

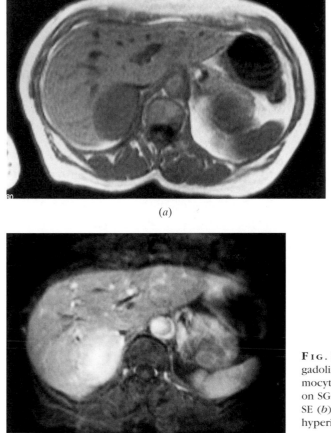

(a)

(b)

(c)

Fig. 8.17 Pheochromocytoma. SGE (*a*), T2-spin-echo (*b*), and 4-minute post-gadolinium T1-weighted fat-suppressed spin-echo (*c*) images. A 5-cm pheochromocytoma is present in the right adrenal, which is mildly low in signal intensity on SGE (*a*) and heterogeneous and moderately high in signal intensity on T2-SE (*b*). On the interstitial-phase gadolinium-enhanced image (*c*), the mass is hyperintense, reflecting accumulation of gadolinium in the large interstitial space.

thrombus into the IVC is not uncommon at presentation. Tumors are frequently necrotic and hemorrhagic.

In a recent series, MR images demonstrated central necrosis and hemorrhage in 7 of 8 adrenal cortical carcinomas [24]. Necrosis is well-shown on gadolinium-enhanced images as signal-void regions, and hemorrhage is well-shown on precontrast T1-weighted conventional or fat-suppressed images as high-signal-intensity regions (Fig. 8.18). Peripheral mural-based nodules are an unusual feature that may be observed in these tumors [24] (Fig. 8.19). Reports have described a similar appearance for adrenal hemangioma and ovarian cancer. Smaller tumors also tend to have greater enhancement of the tumor periphery than of the center, possibly reflecting their propensity to undergo central necrosis [24] (Fig. 8.20). Fat-suppressed images help delineate large tumors from adjacent pancreas and kidney. Sagittal-plane images are also useful for demonstrating that tumors do not originate from the kidney (see Fig. 8.18). On T2-weighted images, tumors have a high signal intensity, which partly reflects the frequent occurrence of central necrosis [3,24,52]. As these tumors are functional, they contain regions that

lose signal intensity on out-of-phase images [24,53,54] (Fig. 8.21). The lack of uniform loss of signal intensity helps to distinguish these tumors from adenomas.

Neuroblastoma

Neuroblastoma is one of the most common solid tumors of children younger than 5 years of age [55]. Tumors originate from neural crest and sympathetic ganglia. Neuroblastomas most commonly arise from the adrenal medulla. In older patients extra-adrenal sites increase in frequency [56]. The most common sites of metastatic disease include the skeletal system, lung, liver, and lymph nodes. Tumors are generally high in signal intensity on T2-weighted images and enhance with gadolinium. Extension into the neural canal is a feature of these tumors. MRI is particularly effective at evaluating both the primary tumor and metastases in these patients who are predominantly pediatric, due to high intrinsic soft-tissue contrast resolution, which is beneficial in patients with minimal body fat. Direct multiplanar imaging renders MRI superior to CT imaging for the demonstration of extension into the neural canal and invasion of adjacent organs

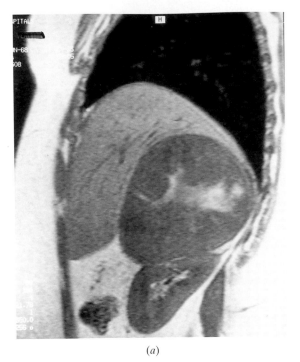

(a)

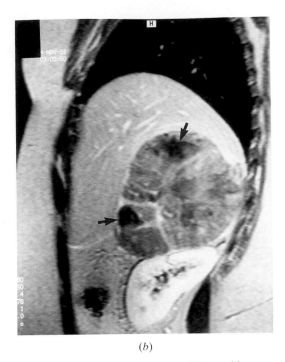

(b)

FIG. 8.18 Adrenal cortical carcinoma. Sagittal-plane SGE (a) and 90-second postgadolinium SGE (b) images in a 25-year-old woman. A 7-cm mass is identified in the right upper abdomen that indents the liver and displaces the right kidney inferiorly. The relationship of the mass to the kidney and liver are clearly defined in profile in the sagittal projection, and the mass is shown to be separate from these organs. High signal intensity is present on precontrast images, a finding consistent with central hemorrhage. The mass enhances heterogeneously following contrast administration and contains signal-void regions of necrosis (arrows, b). (Reproduced with permission from Schlund JF, Kenney PJ, Brown ED, Ascher SM, Brown JJ, Semelka RC: Adrenocortical carcinoma: MR imaging appearance with current technique. J Magn Reson Imaging 5:171–174, 1995)

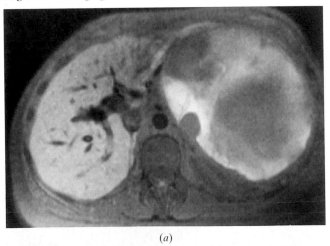

(a)

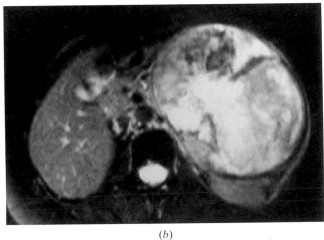

(b)

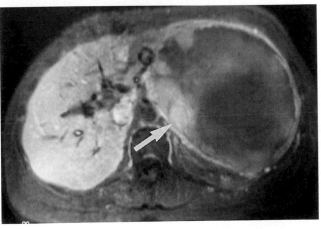

(c)

FIG. 8.19 Adrenal cortical carcinoma. T1-weighted fat-suppressed spin-echo (a), T2-weighted fat-suppressed spin-echo (b), and gadolinium-enhanced T1-weighted fat-suppressed spin-echo (c) images in a 41-year-old woman. On the precontrast T1-weighted image, central high signal intensity is present in the tumor, which is consistent with blood (a). On the T2-weighted image the tumor is heterogeneous and high in signal intensity due to the presence of central necrosis and blood products of varying age (b). Peripheral nodules enhance after contrast administration (arrow, c), and the central portion of the tumor remains largely signal-void. (Reproduced with permission from Schlund JF, Kenney PJ, Brown ED, Ascher SM, Brown JJ, Semelka RC: Adrenocortical carcinoma: MR imaging appearance with current technique. J Magn Reson Imaging 5:171–174, 1995)

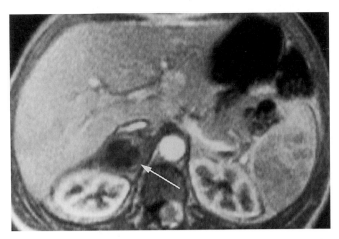

FIG. 8.20 Small adrenal cortical carcinoma. Immediate postgadolinium SGE image demonstrates a 2.5-cm right adrenal cortical carcinoma (*arrow*). Note that the tumor has an enhancing rim and is hypovascular centrally. (Reproduced with permission Semelka RC, Shoenut JP: The adrenal glands. In Semelka RC, Shoenut JP (eds.). MRI of the Abdomen with CT Correlation. New York: Raven Press, pp. 77–90, 1993.)

such as liver [55]. T2-weighted fat-suppressed spin-echo and pre- and post-contrast T1-weighted fat-suppressed spin-echo images in transverse and sagittal planes demonstrate these tumors well (Fig. 8.22). Fat-suppressed spin-echo imaging is generally recommended rather than fat-suppressed SGE techniques because patients are often too young to cooperate with breath-holding, and spin-echo imaging has a higher signal-to-noise ratio, which improves image quality in small patients.

Ganglioneuroblastoma and Ganglioneuroma

Ganglioneuroblastoma is a tumor intermediate in malignancy and cellular maturation between neuroblastoma and ganglioneuroma. Ganglioneuroma is a mature benign tumor. As with neuroblastoma, both of these tumors arise from the neural crest. Ganglioneuromas typically occur in older patients than neuroblastoma. Although all tumors may encase vessels [55], ganglioneuroblastomas and ganglioneuroma tend to be smaller and have better-defined margins (Fig. 8.23). On MR images, tumors are intermediate in signal intensity on T1-weighted images and slightly heterogeneous and high in signal intensity

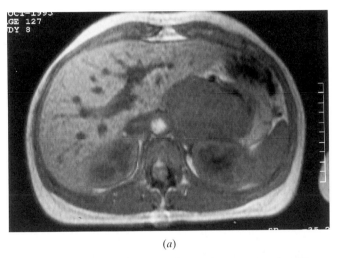

(*a*)

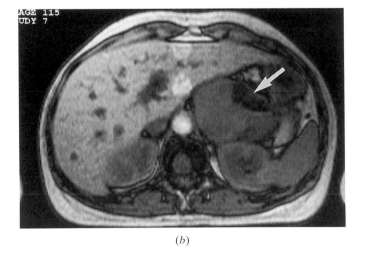

(*b*)

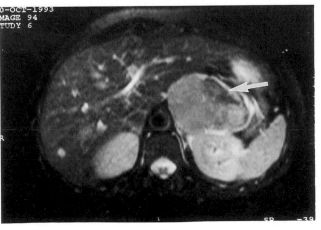

(*c*)

FIG. 8.21 Adrenal cortical carcinoma. In-phase SGE (*a*), out-of-phase SGE (*b*), and T2-weighted fat-suppressed spin-echo (*c*) images in a 37-year-old woman. On the out-of-phase image, a moderate sized region of the tumor loses signal (*arrow, b*) compared to the in-phase image, a finding consistent with fatty tissue. On the fat-suppressed T2-weighted image (*c*) the tumor is hyperintense and contains a region of low signal (*curved arrow, c*) corresponding to the region of signal drop on the out-of-phase image (*b*). Reproduced with permission from Schlund JF, Kenney PJ, Brown ED, Ascher SM, Brown JJ, Semelka RC: Adrenocortical carcinoma: MR imaging appearance with current technique. J Magn Reson Imaging 5:171–174, 1995)

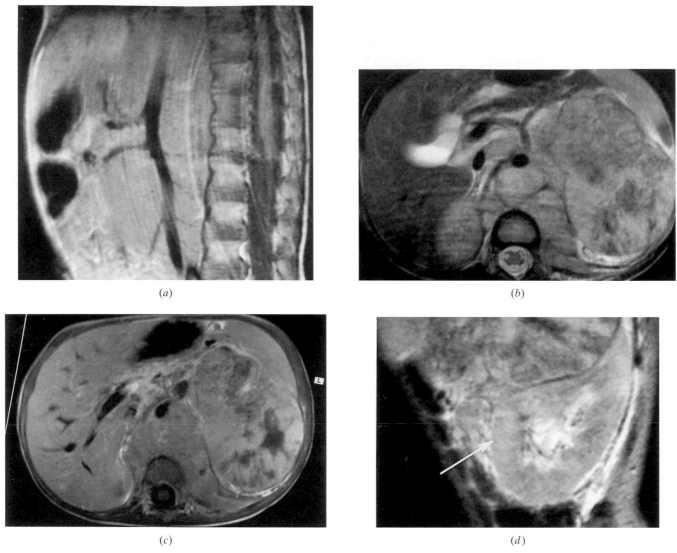

(a)   (b)

(c)   (d)

FIG. 8.22 Neuroblastoma. Sagittal-plane T1-SE (*a*), transverse T2-weighted fat-suppressed spin-echo (*b*), transverse gadolinium-enhanced T1-weighted fat-suppressed spin-echo (*c*), and sagittal gadolinium-enhanced spin-echo (*d*) images. A large abdominal mass is present in the left upper abdomen that encases the aorta and elevates it off the vertebral column (*a,b*). The mass is minimally heterogeneous and hypointense on T1-weighted images (*a*) and moderately heterogeneous and hyperintense on T2-weighted images (*b*). After gadolinium administration the mass enhances heterogeneously with regions of necrosis (*c*). The sagittal-plane image demonstrates that the mass is separate from the kidney (*arrow, d*) and displaces the kidney inferiorly.

on T2-weighted images [34]. Enhancement with gadolinium is slightly heterogeneous and moderately intense.

Lymphoma

Lymphoma occasionally involves the adrenal glands. Non-Hodgkin's lymphoma is the most frequent cell type [57,58]. Retroperitoneal lymphadenopathy is frequently an associated finding [58]. Signal intensity is intermediate on T1-weighted images and usually intermediate to minimally hyperintense on T2-weighted images. Occasionally, lymphoma may undergo necrosis, which may result in high signal intensity on T2-weighted images [59]. Gadolinium enhancement is variable but is usually minimal

on immediate postcontrast images and increases over time (Fig. 8.24), which is an enhancement pattern generally observed for lymphoma.

Hyperplasia

The majority (70%) of patients with Cushing syndrome have adrenal cortical hyperplasia secondary to an ACTH-producing pituitary microadenoma (Cushing's disease). Adrenal enlargement or hyperplasia is also identified in the context of systematic illness, acromegaly, hyperthyroidism, hypertension, diabetes, depression, and malignant disease.

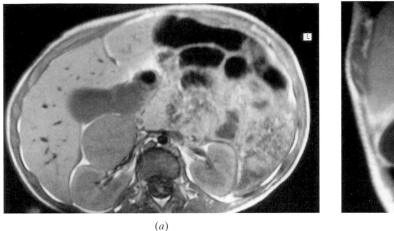
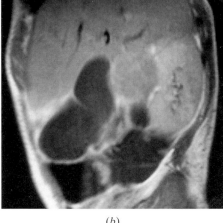

(a)   *(b)*

F IG. 8.23 Ganglioneuroblastoma. Transverse T1-SE (*a*) and sagittal postgadolinium T1-SE (*b*) images. A well-defined 3-cm extrarenal mass is identified arising anterior to the upper pole of the right kidney. On the sagittal image, the mass is shown to abut the liver and kidney with no evidence of invasion.

Adrenal hyperplasia usually involves both glands, and adreniform shape is characteristically maintained (Fig. 8.25). Unilateral adrenal enlargement may occur [34]. The adrenal glands may also appear normal in size [12]. Hyperplastic glands usually contain microscopic nodules, but macroscopic nodules (>2 cm) may be observed [12] (Fig. 8.26). Hyperplastic adrenal glands have signal-intensity appearances similar to those of normal adrenals on all MR imaging sequences [12].

Inflammatory Disease

The adrenal glands may be involved in granulomatous disease, most commonly due to tuberculosis followed by histoplasmosis and blastomycosis [60–62]. Diffuse enlargement of both adrenal glands is the most common appearance. In rare instances, massive enlargement may be seen. Slight heterogeneity of signal intensity is generally observed on T1- and T2-weighted images. Minimal heterogeneous enhancement on early postgadolinium images, which increases over time, is also common (Fig. 8.27). Signal intensity does not drop on out-of-phase images.

Adrenal Hemorrhage
Adrenal hemorrhage occurs secondary to bleeding diathesis, severe stress, and blood loss causing hypotension (surgery, childbirth, or sepsis) or trauma [55,63]. A recent

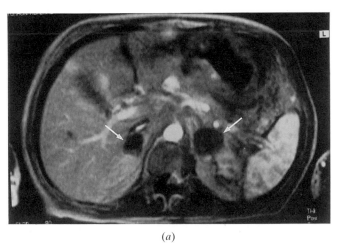
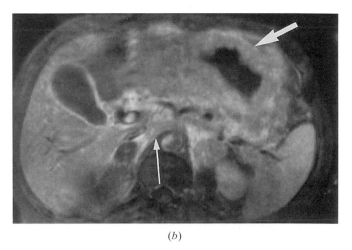

(a)   *(b)*

F IG. 8.24 Adrenal lymphoma. Immediate postgadolinium SGE (*a*) and 4-minute postgadolinium T1-weighted fat-suppressed spin-echo (*b*) images. Minimal enhancement is present of bilateral lymphomatous involvement of the adrenals on the immediate postgadolinium images (*arrows, a*). On the more delayed interstitial-phase images, mild diffuse heterogeneous enhancement is apparent (*b*). Based on the immediate postgadolinium images alone, the adrenal masses could be confused with cysts due to the hypovascularity of the tumors. Diffuse gastric wall involvement (large arrow, b) and retroperitoneal adenopathy (thin arrow, b) are also noted.

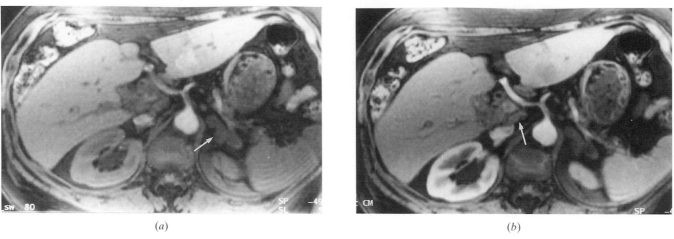

(a)   (b)

F I G . 8.25 Adrenal hyperplasia. Fat-suppressed SGE (*a*) and immediate postgadolinium fat-suppressed SGE (*b*) images. The left adrenal gland is diffusely enlarged (*arrow, a*), and the adreniform shape is maintained. The hyperplastic adrenal gland is low in signal intensity on the T1-weighted image (*a*) and enhances negligibly with gadolinium (*b*). Enlarged periportal lymph nodes are well-shown (*arrow, b*).

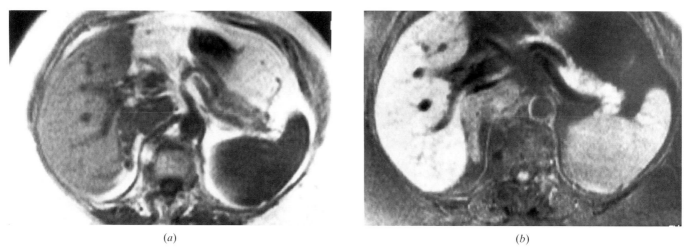

(a)   (b)

F I G . 8.26 Macronodular adrenal hyperplasia. SGE (*a*) and T1-weighted fat-suppressed spin-echo (*b*) images. The right adrenal gland is enlarged and maintains adreniform shape. A nodular contour is identified consistent with macronodules. The left adrenal was previously resected for the same disease process. (Reproduced with permission from Semelka RC, Shoenut JP: The adrenal glands. In Semelka RC, Shoenut JP (eds.). MRI of the Abdomen with CT Correlation. New York: Raven Press, pp. 77–90, 1993.)

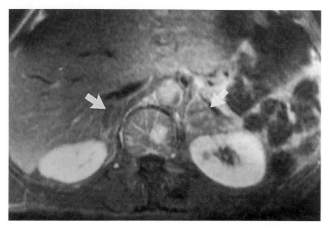

F I G . 8.27 Tuberculosis involvement of the adrenals. Gadolinium-enhanced T1-weighted fat-suppressed spin-echo image demonstrates bilateral adrenal enlargement with heterogeneous mild enhancement (*arrows*). (Reproduced with permission from Semelka RC, Shoenut JP: The adrenal glands. In Semelka RC, Shoenut JP (eds.). MRI of the Abdomen with CT Correlation. New York: Raven Press, pp. 77–90, 1993.)

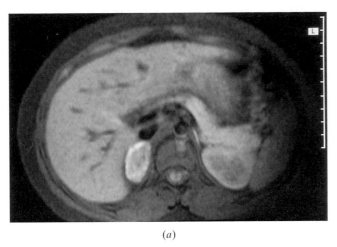
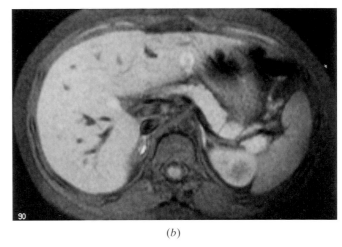

(a) *(b)*

F I G. 8.28 Adrenal hemorrhage. T1-weighted fat-suppressed spin-echo (*a*) and T1-weighted fat-suppressed spin-echo image obtained 7 weeks later (*b*). The T1-weighted fat-suppressed image acquired 1 week after abdominal trauma (*a*) demonstrates a right adrenal mass with a hyperintense peripheral rim. This appearance is classic for a subacute hematoma. Seven weeks later, the mass has diminished in size and remains high in signal intensity due to persistence of extracellular methemoglobin (*b*).

report has described the MRI appearance of adrenal hemorrhage in patients with primary antiphospholipid syndrome [64]. Acute awareness of adrenal hemorrhage on tomographic images is important in that clinical findings may be nonspecific, and fatal acute adrenal insufficiency may result [65]. MRI is very sensitive for the detection of adrenal hemorrhage and is superior to CT imaging. Subacute hemorrhage is high in signal intensity on T1-weighted images [64,66–68] and the high signal intensity is more conspicuous on fat-suppressed T1-weighted images (Fig. 8.28). Decrease in lesion size over time helps to confirm that the adrenal mass represents hemorrhage (see Fig. 8.28).

Addison's Disease

Addison's disease results from adrenal insufficiency. The tomographic appearance of the adrenal glands may assist in the diagnosis of the underlying cause [61,65,68–70]. Autoimmune disease or pituitary insufficiency is suggested by the presence of atrophic glands [55,56]. Adrenal hemorrhage may be readily diagnosed by the demonstration of high-signal-intensity substance on T1-weighted images in bilaterally enlarged glands [66–68]. Enlarged glands without hemorrhage suggest granulomatous disease [61]. Metastases may cause adrenal insufficiency, uncommonly, and the adrenal glands are massive in this setting.

FUTURE DIRECTIONS

The direction of future advance for MRI of the adrenals may include echoplanar imaging [71] and new contrast agents [72,73].

CONCLUSIONS

MRI is an effective means for evaluating adrenal pathology. The combined use of in-phase and out-of-phase SGE images is the most accurate method for distinguishing benign from malignant disease. The acquisition of other additional sequences however, is, recommended because the accuracy of this determination is between 85 and 90 percent. MRI is particularly effective at detecting pheochromocytomas. Evaluation of the primary tumor and liver metastases is useful for adrenal cortical carcinomas and neuroblastoma.

REFERENCES

1. Reining JW, Doppman JL, Dwyer AJ, Johnson AR, Knop RH: Adrenal masses differentiated by MR. Radiology 158:81–84, 1986.

2. Reinig JW, Doppman JL, Dwyer AJ, Frank J: MRI of indeterminate adrenal masses. AJR Am J Roentgenol 147:493–496, 1986.

3. Chang A, Glazer HS, Lee JKT, Ling D, Heiken JP: Adrenal gland: MR imaging. Radiology 163:123–128, 1987.

4. Baker ME, Blinder R, Spritzer C, Leight GS, Herfkens RJ, Dunnick NR: MR evaluation of adrenal masses at 1.5 T. AJR Am J Roentgenol 153:307–312, 1989.

5. Kier R, McCarthy S: MR characterization of adrenal masses: Field strength and pulse sequence considerations. Radiology 171:671–674, 1989.

6. Krestin GP, Steinbrich W, Friedmann G: Adrenal masses: Evaluation with fast gradient-echo MR imaging Gd-DTPA-enhanced dynamic studies. Radiology 171:675–680, 1989.

7. Krestin GP, Friedmann G, Fischbach R, Neufang KFR, Allolio B: Evaluation of adrenal masses in oncologic patients: Dynamic contrast-enhanced MR vs. CT. J Comput Assist Tomogr 15(1):104–110, 1991.

8. Semelka RC, Shoenut JP, Lawrence PH, Greenberg HM, Maycher B, Madden TP, Kroeker MA: Evaluation of adrenal masses with

gadolinium enhancement and fat suppressed MR imaging. J Magn Reson Imaging 3:337–343, 1993.

9. Mitchell DG, Grovello M, Matteucci T, Peterson RO, Miettinen MM: Benign adenocortical masses: Diagnosis with chemical shift MR imaging. Radiology 185:345–351, 1992.

10. Tsushima Y, Ishizaka H, Matsumoto M: Adrenal masses: Differentiation with chemical shift, fast low-angle shot MR imaging. Radiology 186:705–709, 1993.

11. Reinig JW, Stutley JE, Leonhardt CM, Spicer KM, Margolis M, Caldwell CB: Differentiation of adrenal masses with MR imaging: Comparison of techniques. Radiology 192:41–46, 1994.

12. Lee MJ, Mayo-Smith WM, Hahn PF, Goldberg MA, Boland GW, Saini S, Papanicolaou N: State-of-the-art MR imaging of the adrenal gland. Radiographics 14:1015–1029, 1994.

13. Bilbey JH, McLoughlin RF, Kurkjian PS, Wilkins GEL, Chan NHL, Schmidt N, Singer J: MR imaging of adrenal masses: Value of chemical-shift imaging for distinguishing adenomas from other tumors. AJR Am J Roentgenol 164:637–642, 1995.

14. Korobkin M, Dunnick NR: Characterization of adrenal masses. (commentary) AJR Am J Roentgenol 164:643–644, 1995.

15. Outwater EK, Siegelman ES, Huang AB, Birnbaum BA: Adrenal masses: Correlation between CT attenuation value and chemical shift ratio at MR imaging with in-phase and opposed-phase sequences. Radiology 200:749–752, 1996.

16. Mayo-Smith WW, Lee MJ, McNicholas MMJ, Hahn PF, Boland GW, Saini S: Characterization of adrenal masses (<5 cm) by use of chemical shift MR imaging: Observer performance versus quantitative measures. AJR Am J Roentgenol 165:91–95, 1995.

17. Outwater EK, Siegelman ES, Radecki PD, Piccoli CW, Mitchell DG: Distinction between benign and malignant adrenal masses: Value of T1-weighted chemical-shift MR imaging. AJR Am J Roentgenol 165:579–583, 1995.

18. Korobkin M, Lombardi TJ, Aisen AM, Francis IR, Quint LE, Dunnick NR: Characterization of adrenal masses with chemical shift and gadolinium-enhanced MR imaging. Radiology 197:411–418, 1995.

19. McNicholas MMJ, Lee MJ, Mayo-Smith WW, Hahn PF, Boland GW, Mueller PR: An imaging algorithm for the differential diagnosis of adrenal adenomas and metastases. AJR Am J Roentgenol 165:1453–1459, 1995.

20. Korobkin M, Giordano TJ, Brodeur FJ, et al: Adrenal adenomas: Relationship between histologic lipid and CT and MR findings. Radiology 200:743–747, 1996.

21. Schwartz LH, Panicek DM, Koutcher JA, Heelan RT, Bains MS, Burt M: Echoplanar MR imaging for characterization of adrenal masses in patient with malignant neoplasms: Preliminary evaluation of calculated T2 relaxation values. AJR Am J Roentgenol 164:911–915, 1995.

22. Outwater EK, Mitchell DG: Differentiation of adrenal masses with chemical shift MR imaging (letter to the editor). Radiology 193:877, 1994.

23. Small WC, Bernardino ME: Gd-DTPA adrenal gland enhancement at 1.5 T. Magn Reson Imaging 9:309–312, 1991.

24. Schlund JF, Kenney PJ, Brown ED, Ascher SM, Brown JJ, Semelka RC: Adrenocortical carcinoma: MR imaging appearance with current techniques. J Magn Reson Imaging 5:171–174, 1995.

25. Falke THM, te Strake L, Shaff MI, et al: MR imaging of the adrenals: Correlation with computed tomography. J Comput Assist Tomogr 10(2):242–253, 1986.

26. Kearny GP, Mahoney EM, Maher E, Harrison JH: Functioning and nonfunctioning cysts of the adrenal cortex and medulla. Am J Surg 134:363–368, 1977.

27. Aisen AM, Ohl DA, Chenevert TL, Perkins P, Mikesell W: MR of an adrenal pseudocyst. Magn Reson Imaging 10:997–1000, 1992.

28. Ichikawa T, Ohtomo K, Uchiyama G, Koizumi K, Monzawa S, Oba H, et al: Adrenal adenomas: Characteristic hyperintense rim sign on fat-saturated spin-echo MR images. Radiology 193:247–250, 1994.

29. Dieckmann KP, Hamm B, Pickartz H, Jonas D, Bauer HW: Adrenal myelolipoma: clinical, radiologic, and histologic features. Urology 29:1–8, 1987.

30. Palmer WE, Gerard-McFarland EL, Chew FS: Adrenal myelolipoma. AJR Am J Roentgenol 156:724, 1991.

31. Musante F, Derchi LE, Bazzochi M, et al: MR imaging of adrenal myelolipomas. JCAT 15:111–114, 1991.

32. Liessi G, Cesari S, Dell'Antoni C, Spaliviero B, Avventi P: US, CT, MR and percutaneous biopsy of adrenal myelolopomas. Eur Radiol 5:152–155, 1995.

33. Casey LR, Cohen AJ, Wile AG, Dietrich RB: Giant adrenal myelolipomas: CT and MRI findings. Abdom Imaging 19:165–167, 1994.

34. McLoughlin RF, Bilbey JH: Tumors of the adrenal gland: Findings on CT and MR imaging. AJR Am J Roentgenol 163:1413–1418, 1994.

35. Cyran KM, Kenney PJ, Memel DS, Yacoub I: Adrenal myelolipoma. AJR Am J Roentgenol 166:395–400, 1996.

36. Hamrick-Turner JE, Cranston PE, Shipkey FH: Cavernous hemangiomas of the adrenal gland: MR findings. Magnetic Resonance Imaging 12(8):1263–1267, 1994.

37. Ikeda DM, Francis IR, Glazer GM, Amendola MA, Gross MD, Aisen AM: The detection of adrenal tumors and hyperplasia in patients with primary aldosteronism: Comparison of scintigraphy, CT, and MR imaging. AJR Am J Roentgenol 153:301–306, 1989.

38. Grant CS, Carpenter P, Van Heerden JA, Hamberger B: Primary aldosteronism. Clinical management. Arch Surg 119:585–590, 1984.

39. Doppman JL, Gill JR Jr, Miller DL, et al: Distinction between hyperaldosteronism due to bilateral hyperplasia and unilateral aldosteronoma: Reliability of CT. Radiology 184:677–682, 1992.

40. Dunnick NR, Doppman JL, Gill JR, Strott CA, Keiser HR, Brennan MF: Localization of functional adrenal tumors by computed tomography and venous sampling. Radiology 142:429–433, 1982.

41. DeAtkine AB, Dunnick NR: The adrenal glands. Semin Oncol 18:131–139, 1991.

42. Silverman SG, Mueller PR, Pinkney LP, Koenker RM, Seltzer SE: Predictive value of image-guided adrenal biopsy: Analysis of results of 101 biopsies. Radiology 187:715–718, 1993.

43. Belldegrun A, Hussain S, Seltzer SE, Loughlin KR, Gittes RF, Richie JP: Incidentally discovered mass of the adrenal gland. Surg Gynecol Obstet 163:203–208, 1986.

44. Mitnick JS, Bosniak MA. Megibow AJ, Naidich DP: Nonfunctioning adrenal adenomas discovered incidentally on computed tomography. Radiology 148:495–499, 1983.

45. Herrera MF, Grant CS, van Heerden JA, Sheedy PF, Ilstrung DM: Incidentally discovered adrenal tumors: An institutional perspective. Surgery 110:1014–1021, 1991.

46. Tisnado J, Amendola MA, Konerding KF, Shirazi KK, Beachley MC: Computed tomography versus angiography in the localization of pheochromocytoma. J Comput Assist Tomogr 4:853–859, 1980.

47. Thomas JL, Bernardino ME: Pheochromocytoma in multiple endocrine adenomatosis. Efficacy of computed tomography. JAMA 245:1467–1469, 1981.

48. Bush WH, Elder JS, Crane RE, Wales LR: Cystic pheochromocytoma. Urology 25:332–334, 1985.

49. Crecelius SA, Bellah R: Pheochromocytoma of the bladder in an adolescent: Sonographic and MR imaging findings. AJR Am J Roentgenol 165:101–103, 1995.

50. Belden CJ, Powers C, Ros PR: MR demonstration of a cystic pheochromocytoma. J Magn Reson Imaging 5:778–780, 1995.

51. Henley DJ, Van Heerden JA, Grant CS, Carney JA, Carpenter PC: Adrenal cortical carcinoma—a continuing challenge. Surgery 94:926–931, 1983.

52. Smith SM, Patel SK, Turner DA, et al: Magnetic resonance imaging of adrenal cortical carcinoma. Urol Radiol 11:1–6, 1989.

53. Ferrozzi F, Bova D: CT and MR demonstration of fat within an adrenal cortical carcinoma. Abdom Imaging 20:272–274, 1995.

54. Sato N, Watanabe Y, Saga T, Mitsudo K, Dohke M, Minami K:

Adrenocortical adenoma containing a fat component CT and MR image evaluation. Abdom Imaging 20:489–490, 1995.

55. Westra SJ, Zaninovic AC, Hall TR, Kangarloo H, Boechat MI: Imaging of the adrenal gland in children. Radiographics 14:1323–1340, 1994.

56. Feinstein RS, Gatewood OMB, Fishman EK, Goldman SM, Siegelman SS: Computed tomography of adult neuroblastoma. J Comput Assist Tomogr 8:720–726, 1984.

57. Paling MR, Williamson BRJ: Adrenal involvement in non-Hodgkin lymphoma. AJR Am J Roentgenol 141:303–305, 1983.

58. Glazer HS, Lee JKT, Balfe DM, Mauro MS, Griffeth R, Sagel SS: Non-Hodgkin lymphoma: Computed tomographic demonstration of unusual extranodal involvement. Radiology 149:211–217, 1983.

59. Lee FT Jr, Thornbury JR, Grist TM, Kelcz F: MR imaging of adrenal lymphoma. Abdom Imaging 18:95–96, 1993.

60. Hauser H, Gurret JP: Miliary tuberculosis associated with adrenal enlargement CT appearance. J Comput Assist Tomogr 10:254–256, 1986.

61. Sawczuk IS, Reitelman C, Libby C, Grant D, Vita J, White RD: CT findings in Addison's disease caused by tuberculosis. Urol Radiol 8:44–45, 1986.

62. Wilson DA, Muchmore HG, Tisdal RG, Fahmy A, Pitha JV: Histoplasmosis of the adrenal glands studied by CT. Radiology 150:779–783, 1984.

63. Xarli VP, Steele AA, Davis PJ, Buescher ES, Rios CN, Garcia-Bunuel R: Adrenal hemorrhage in the adult. Medicine 57:211–221, 1987.

64. Provenzale JM, Ortel TL, Nelson RC: Adrenal hemorrhage in patients with primary antiphospholipid syndrome: Imaging findings. AJR Am J Roentgenol 165:361–364, 1995.

65. Wolverson MK, Kannegiesser H: CT of bilateral adrenal hemorrhage with acute adrenal insufficiency in the adult. AJR Am J Roentgenol 142:311–314, 1984.

66. Koch KJ, Cory DA: Simultaneous renal vein thrombosis and bilateral adrenal hemorrhage: MR demonstration. J Comput Assist Tomogr 10:681–683, 1986.

67. Brill PW, Jagannath A, Winchester P, Markisz JA, Zirinsky K: Adrenal hemorrhage and renal vein thrombosis in the newborn: MR imaging. Radiology 170:95–96, 1989.

68. Wilms G, Tits J, Vanstraelen D, Marchal G, Baert AL: Addison's disease due to bilateral post-traumatic adrenal hemorrhage: CT and MR findings. Eur Radiol 1:172–174, 1991.

69. Doppman JL, Gill JR Jr, Nienhuis AW, Earll JM, Long JA Jr: CT findings in Addison's disease. J Comput Assist Tomogr 6:757–761, 1982.

70. McMurry JF Jr, Long D, McClure R, Kotchen TA: Addison's disease with adrenal enlargement on computed tomographic scanning. Am J Med 77:365–368, 1984.

71. Schwartz LH, Panicek DM, Koutcher JA, Brown KT, Getrajdman GI, Heelan RT, et al: Adrenal masses in patients with malignancy: Prospective comparsion of echo-planar, fast spin-echo, and chemical shift MR imaging. Radiology 197:421–425, 1995.

72. Mitchell DG, Outwater EK, Matteucci T, Rubin DL, Chezmar JL, Saini S: Adrenal gland enhancement at MR imaging with Mn-DPDP. Radiology 194:783–787, 1995.

73. Weissleder T, Wang YM, Papisov M, et al: Polymeric contrast agents for MR imaging of adrenal glands. J Magn Reson Imaging 93–97, 1993.

CHAPTER 9

KIDNEYS

R. C. SEMELKA, M.D. AND N. L. KELEKIS, M.D.

NORMAL ANATOMY

The kidneys are paired organs situated in the perinephric space in the retroperitoneum. The renal parenchyma is covered by a capsule, which usually is not visible on tomographic images. The perinephric space contains bridging renal septae that extend from the kidney to the anterior and posterior (Gerota's) perinephric fascia. The anterior and posterior fascia fuse laterally to form the lateral conal fascia. Superiorly, the fascia fuse, whereas inferiorly they are open, forming a potential communication to the anterior and posterior perirenal spaces. The renal artery, vein, and ureter enter the kidney at the hilum. The kidney is composed of a cortex, medulla, and sinus. The renal sinus contains the renal collecting system, vessels, and fat.

MRI TECHNIQUE

The basic magnetic resonance imaging (MRI) examination of the kidneys involves precontrast and postgadolinium chelate T1-weighted images acquired as nonsuppressed and fat-suppressed sequences. The immediate postgadolinium images should be acquired as an immediate postgadolinium capillary-phase SGE sequence. A di-

agnostically useful protocol is as follows: (1) precontrast T1-weighted breath-hold spoiled gradient-echo (SGE), (2) precontrast breath-hold T1-weighted fat-suppressed SGE, (3) dynamic capillary-phase gadolinium-enhanced T1-weighted SGE, and (4) gadolinium-enhanced interstitial-phase T1-weighted fat-suppressed SGE (Fig. 9.1) techniques [1]. Precontrast and postcontrast image acquisition in the sagittal or coronal plane frequently is helpful in order to (1) evaluate the superior and inferior borders of renal lesions, (2) characterize lesions as cystic or solid or (3) demonstrate renal/perirenal location and extension.

MR angiography (MRA) has recently achieved diagnostically sufficient image quality to reproducibly demonstrate renal arterial disease [2,3] and may develop an important role in renal investigation (Fig. 9.2). The echotrain spin-echo (ETSE) technique may be tailored to generate an MR urogram effect, which in early reports has been shown to be effective at elucidating causes of a dilated renal collecting system [4]. Temporal changes in signal intensity (SI) of renal cortex and medulla following contrast injection provides information on renal function [5–7]. The ability to generate diverse imaging information on tissue morphology, renal vessels, collecting system, and function renders MRI a comprehensive diagnostic modality for investigating renal disease (8).

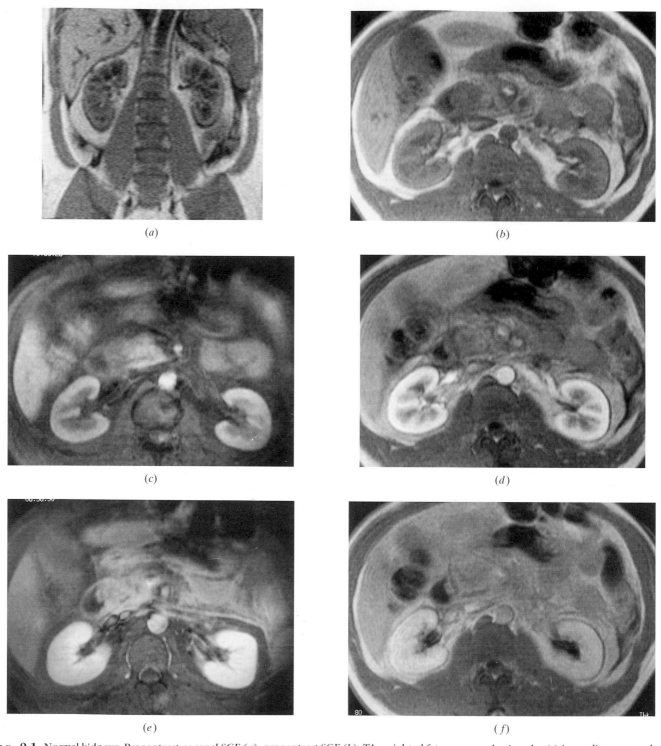

(a)

(b)

(c)

(d)

(e)

(f)

FIG. 9.1 Normal kidneys. Precontrast coronal SGE (a), precontrast SGE (b), T1-weighted fat-suppressed spin-echo (c) immediate postgadolinium SGE (d), gadolinium-enhanced T1-weighted fat-suppressed spin-echo (e), 8-minutes postgadolinium transverse (f), and 8.5-minute coronal (g) gadolinium-enhanced SGE images. Corticomedullary differentiation is shown on precontrast T1-weighted images (a–c), and on immediate postgadolinium SGE (d) images. Corticomedullary differentiation is most clearly defined on the precontrast T1-weighted fat-suppressed image (c) and the immediate postgadolinium SGE image (d). Immediate postgadolinium fat-suppressed SGE image (b) in a second patient demonstrates intense cortical enhancement and good demonstration of high-signal-intensity gadolinium-containing left renal vein.

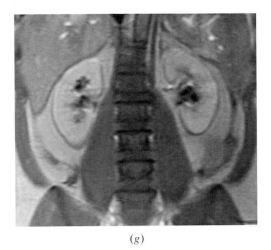

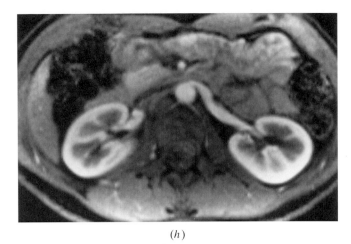

(*g*)   (*h*)

FIG. **9.1** (*Continued*)   Sharp definition of the outer renal cortex is shown due to the suppression of fat.

Gadolinium chelates are freely filtered by renal glomeruli and undergo excretion by renal tubules with no tubular reabsorption or excretion [9]. Because of this elimination pathway, gadolinium chelates are ideal for studying morphology and function of the kidneys. Gadolinium possesses the additional property of changing signal intensity based on concentration. When dilute, gadolinium enhances T1-relaxation and renders urine high in signal intensity. When concentrated, gadolinium induces magnetic susceptibility and signal intensity loss, causing urine to be low in signal intensity [5–7]. The concentrating ability of the kidneys can be evaluated by gadolinium-enhanced MRI, a property that cannot be assessed by dynamic iodine enhanced CT imaging.

NORMAL VARIANTS AND CONGENITAL ANOMALIES

Prominent columns of Bertin are frequently observed in kidneys, and it may be difficult to distinguish these from renal masses on other imaging modalities. Columns will follow the signal intensity of renal cortex on all pre- and postgadolinium images. An important observation is that on immediate postgadolinium images the column enhances to the same extent as renal cortex and follows a smooth continuous contour with cortex. On more delayed images the enhancement of the column remains isointense with cortex.

Fetal lobulation is another common normal variant. Coronal images demonstrate the undulating contour of the kidney. Immediate postgadolinium images show uniform cortical thickening, which excludes the presence of a mass (Fig. 9.3). A great variety of anomalies of the kidneys occur. The majority relate to abnormalities of renal position (including renal ascent and rotation), duplication, fusion, and agenesis. Duplication of the collecting system is a relatively common anomaly, which may on occasion be difficult to detect on transverse tomographic images. Pelvic kidney is not uncommon, and the kidney is not infrequently malformed (Fig. 9.4). The presence of intense uptake of gadolinium chelates by

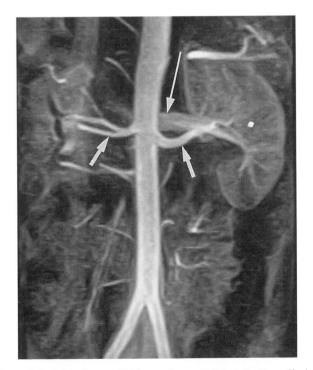

FIG. **9.2**   MRA of normal kidneys. Coronal MIP projection of bolus gadolinium enhanced 3D FISP demonstrates normal renal arteries in sharp detail (*arrows*). The left renal vein is also opacified (*long arrow*).

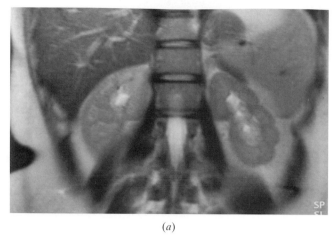

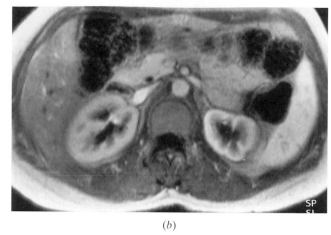

(a)   (b)

FIG. 9.3 Fetal lobulation. Coronal half Fourier single-shot turbo spin-echo (HASTE) (*a*), and transverse immediate postgadolinium SGE (*b*) images. The coronal HASTE image (*a*) demonstrates an undulating contour of the entire left kidney. The immediate postgadolinium SGE image demonstrates uniform cortical thickness, excluding the presence of a mass.

renal cortex and identification of renal corticomedullary organization allows confident diagnosis of this entity. Horseshoe kidney is the most common fusion abnormality and is readily shown on tomographic images by the fusion of the lower poles of both kidneys across the midline immediately anterior to vertebral bodies (Fig. 9.5). Crossed fused ectopy is an uncommon entity, which can be diagnosed on MR images by the identification of corticomedullary organization in the mass. Direct coronal imaging is helpful in demonstrating the fused renal moieties (Fig. 9.6).

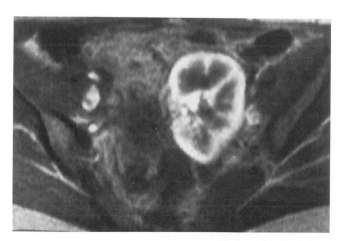

FIG. 9.4 Pelvic kidney. Immediate postgadolinium SGE image. The presence of corticomedullary differentiation identifies the pelvic mass as a kidney.

■ DISEASE OF THE RENAL PARENCHYMA

MASS LESIONS

Benign Masses

Cysts

Cysts are the most common renal mass in the adult and are usually cortical in location [10]. Cortical cysts are oval-shaped, do not enhance with gadolinium, and have a sharp margin with renal parenchyma [1,11]. Simple cysts are very low in signal intensity on T1-weighted images and very high in signal intensity on T2-weighted images. Cysts are considered simple when they contain fluid similar in composition to urine, are signal-void on T1-weighted images, and have no definable wall when they extend beyond the renal cortex [1]. Simple cysts may be observed as nearly signal-void lesions on postgadolinium images even when they measure 3 to 4 mm in diameter (Fig. 9.7). Sagittal or coronal images permit direct visualization of the superior and inferior margins of cysts.

Complicated Cysts. Cysts are considered complicated when they contain blood, septations, calcifications, or inflammatory tissue. Region of interest measurements on pre- and postgadolinium T1-weighted images are useful to ensure lack of contrast enhancement in cysts that are high in signal intensity on precontrast images.

Hemorrhagic Cyst. Hemorrhagic cysts are commonly encountered on MRI examinations. Many of these cysts are not identified as hemorrhagic on CT examina-

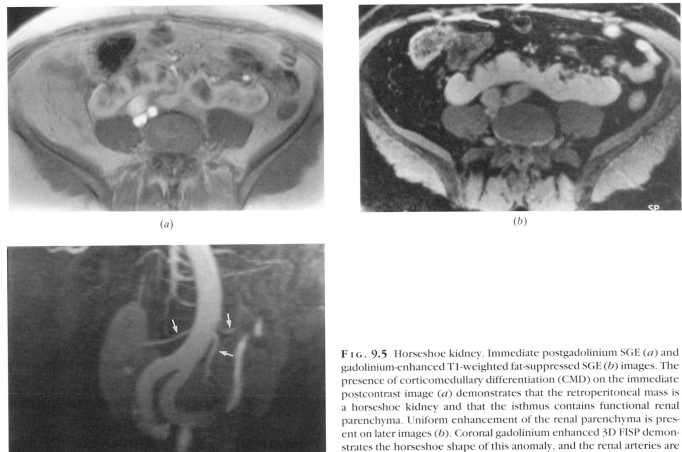

(a)

(b)

(c)

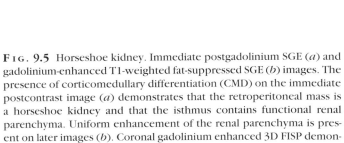

FIG. 9.5 Horseshoe kidney. Immediate postgadolinium SGE (*a*) and gadolinium-enhanced T1-weighted fat-suppressed SGE (*b*) images. The presence of corticomedullary differentiation (CMD) on the immediate postcontrast image (*a*) demonstrates that the retroperitoneal mass is a horseshoe kidney and that the isthmus contains functional renal parenchyma. Uniform enhancement of the renal parenchyma is present on later images (*b*). Coronal gadolinium enhanced 3D FISP demonstrates the horseshoe shape of this anomaly, and the renal arteries are well-displayed (*arrows, c*).

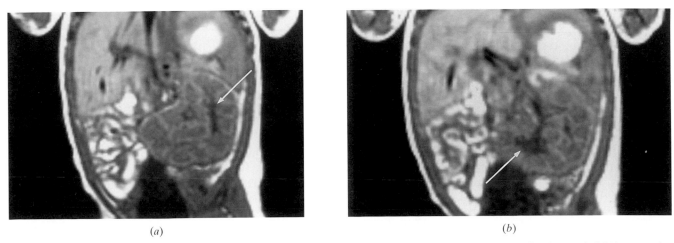

(a)

(b)

FIG. 9.6 Crossed-fused ectopy. Coronal T1-weighted spin-echo images (*a,b*) demonstrate fusion of a small inferomedial kidney to the normal-sized and positioned left kidney. Clear depiction is rendered by the definition of CMD. The collecting system of the normally positioned left kidney is normal in size (*arrow, a*), whereas the crossed-fused right kidney has a mildly dilated collecting system (*arrow, b*).

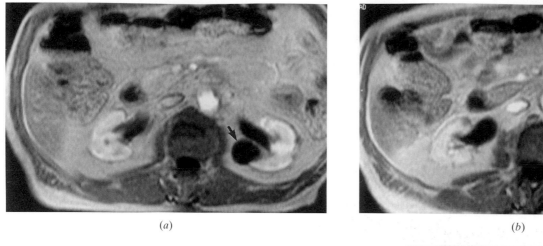

(a)   (b)

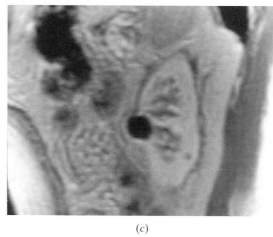

FIG. 9.7 Renal cyst. Immediate (a) and 5-minute (b) postgadolinium SGE images. A cyst is present arising from the posterior aspect of the left kidney. The cyst is signal-void, sharply marginated, and has no definable wall on the immediate postgadolinium image (arrow, a). No change in the appearance of the cyst occurs on the delayed postcontrast image (b). Sagittal 5-minute postgadolinium SGE image (c) of the left kidney in a second patient demonstrates a sharp superior and inferior margin of the renal cyst confirming that it is a simple cyst.

(c)

tions, which reflects the higher sensitivity of MRI for the detection of blood. The majority of hemorrhagic cysts are high in signal intensity on T1- and T2-weighted images because imaging studies are often acquired in the subacute phase of hemorrhage, which lasts from 1 to 26 weeks after bleeding. Observation that most hemorrhagic cysts are high signal intensity on T1- and T2-weighted images reflects the long time period in which blood is present as extracellular methemoglobin. Hemorrhagic cysts may be readily diagnosed as benign if they are homogeneously high in signal intensity on T1- and T2-weighted images or if they show a fluid-fluid level and have a smooth thin wall. Many cysts that are high in signal intensity on precontrast T1-weighted images become low in signal intensity after gadolinium administration because of rescaling of abdominal tissue signal intensities with the presence of gadolinium (Fig. 9.8). Occasionally, organizing hemorrhage contains fibrous strands that may make distinction from solid neoplasms difficult.

Relatively acute hemorrhage that contains intracellular deoxyhemoglobin or intracellular methemoglobin may pose a diagnostic problem. On T2-weighted images, these cysts may be low in signal intensity and have an appearance resembling solid neoplasms (Fig. 9.9). Due to the not uncommon occurrence of relatively acute blood in cysts, caution must be exercised in using T2-weighted information to determine whether lesions are cystic or solid. In the acutely hemorrhagic lesion, demonstrating a lack of enhancement on serial postgadolinium images acquired up to 8 to 10 minutes after contrast injection assists in demonstrating that they are cysts (see Fig. 9.9). Clinical history and follow-up MRI at 3 to 6 months also may be required.

Septated Cysts. Septations in cysts may occur as a result of various events, including fibrin strands after hemorrhage or inflammation, or close juxtaposition of two or more cysts. Demonstration that septations are thin (2 mm) and uniform, and that no enhancing nodular components are present, helps to ascertain that septated cysts are not malignant (Fig. 9.10).

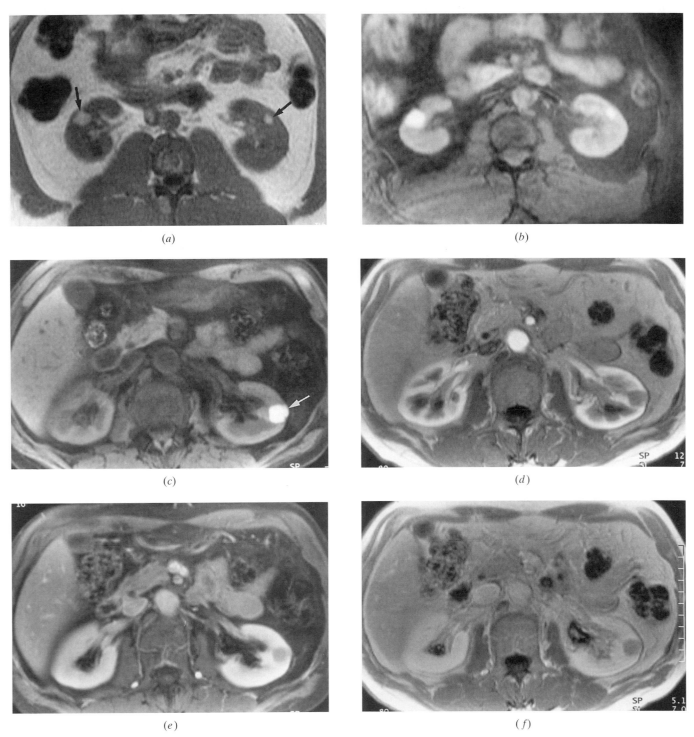

(a)

(b)

(c)

(d)

(e)

(f)

FIG. 9.8 Hemorrhagic renal cysts. Precontrast SGE (*a*) and T1-weighted fat-suppressed images. Bilateral renal cysts are apparent on the T1-weighted SGE image (*a*), which are high in signal intensity (*arrows, a*), a finding consistent with subacute blood or fat. The T1-weighted image with fat suppression (*b*) demonstrates that these lesions remain high in signal intensity, and therefore are not fat-containing. Fat suppression accentuates the high signal intensity of these cysts. Fat-suppressed SGE (*c*), immediate postgadolinium SGE (*d*), 90-second postgadolinium fat-suppressed SGE (*e*), and 5-minute postgadolinium SGE (*f*) images in a second patient. A well-defined, uniformly high-signal-intensity hemorrhagic cyst is present in the left kidney on the fat-suppressed image (*arrow, c*). The cyst does not change in size or shape and does not demonstrate internal enhancement on serial postgadolinium images. Due to the intrinsic high signal intensity of the hemorrhage, the cyst is low in signal but not signal-void on the postcontrast images.

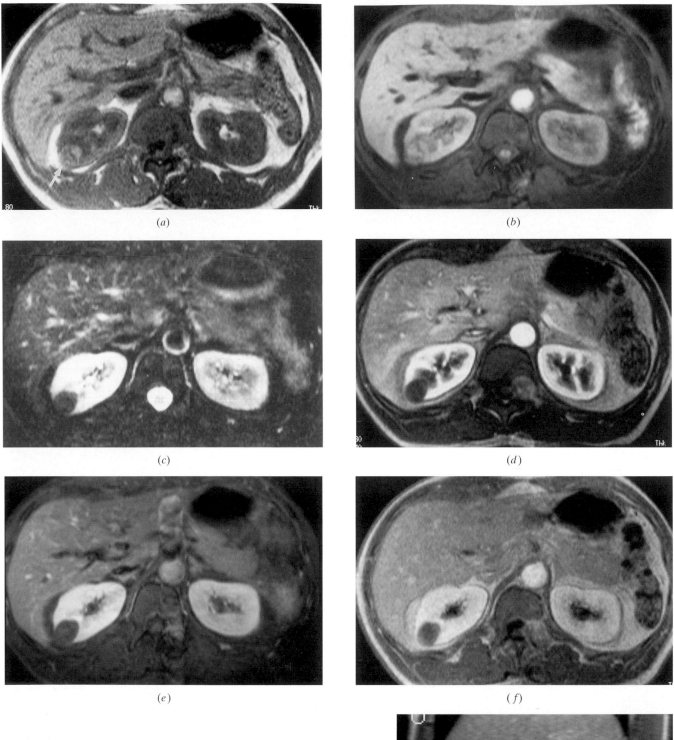

FIG. 9.9 Hemorrhagic cyst containing relatively acute blood (intracellular methemoglobin). Precontrast SGE (*a*), precontrast T1-weighted fat-suppressed spin-echo (*b*), T2-weighted fat-suppressed spin-echo (*c*), immediate postgadolinium SGE (*d*), gadolinium-enhanced T1-weighted fat-suppressed spin-echo (*e*), 8-minute transverse (*f*) and 8.5-minute sagittal (*g*) postgadolinium SGE images. A lesion is present in the right kidney (*arrow, a*), which is mixed high signal intensity on precontrast T1-weighted images (*a,b*), low in signal intensity on T2-weighted image (*c*), and low in signal intensity on early (*d*) and delayed (*e–g*) images. The low signal intensity on the T2-weighted image (*c*) may mimic a solid lesion. Although the lesion is low in signal intensity and not signal-void on postcontrast images, it is sharply marginated, has no definable wall or nodularity and does not change in size and shape between early (*d*) and late (*e–g*) postcontrast images. The postcontrast sagittal plane image demonstrates that the superior and inferior margins of the cyst (*arrow, g*) are sharply defined.

386

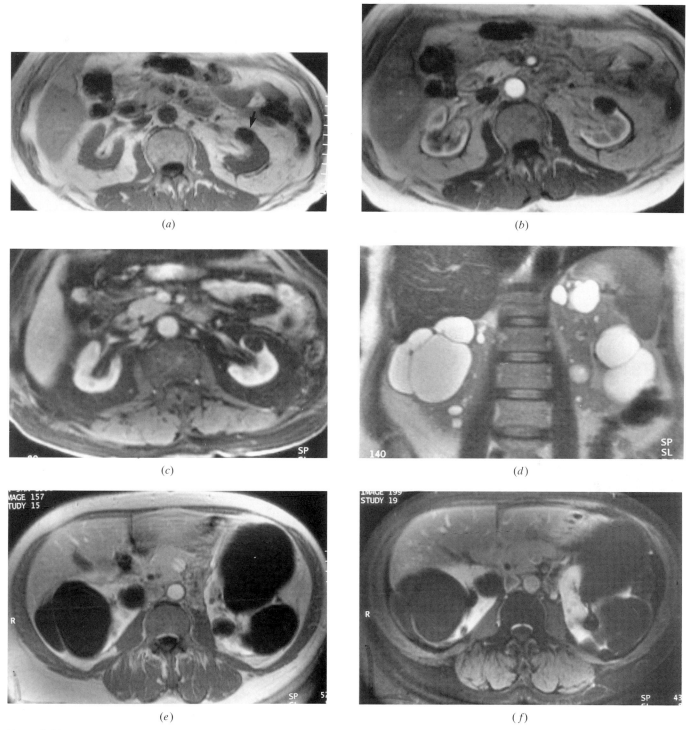

FIG. 9.10 Renal cysts. SGE (*a*), immediate postgadolinium SGE (*b*) and 90-second postgadolinium fat-suppressed SGE (*c*) images. No corticomedullary differentiation is apparent on the precontrast image consistent with diminished renal function. A renal cyst is present in the anterior cortex of the left kidney (*arrow, a*). The cyst does not enhance following contrast administration (*b*). On the 90-second postgadolinium image (*c*), thin internal septations are apparent. Coronal HASTE (*d*), immediate postgadolinium SGE (*e*), and 90-second postgadolinium fat-suppressed SGE (*f*) images in a second patient. Multiple closely grouped cysts are present in both kidneys, which create an appearance of multicystic masses (*d*). Renal parenchyma enhances normally (*e*), and the cysts do not change in size and shape on serial postgadolinium images (*e,f*) with no internal enhancement demonstrated.

Calcified Cysts. Calcium is generally signal-void on MR images. Although calcium is difficult to appreciate on MR images, the lack of signal allows clear visualization of surrounding tissue and internal morphology (Fig. 9.11) [11]. Thereby, the presence of tumor tissue is readily determined. An advantage of MRI over CT imaging and ultrasound in the evaluation of calcified cysts is that calcium does not interfere with the evaluation of adjacent soft tissue. MRI is therefore indicated for the evaluation of calcified cysts.

Inflammatory Cysts. Inflammatory cysts possess thickened walls that are frequently irregular. Cyst contents are not uncommonly moderate to high in signal intensity on T1-weighted images due to the presence of protein or subacute blood (Fig. 9.12). Cyst walls are

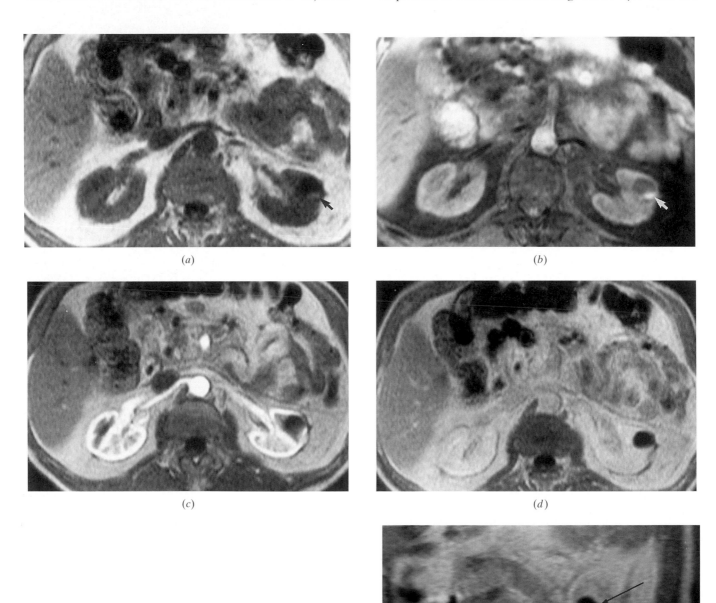

(a)   (b)

(c)   (d)

FIG. 9.11 Calcified renal cyst. Precontrast SGE (*a*), T1-fat-suppressed spin-echo (*b*), immediate (*c*) and 8-minute (*d*) postgadolinium SGE, and sagittal 8.5-minute postgadolinium SGE (*e*) images. A calcified renal cyst is present in the posterior aspect of the right kidney. A small focus of high-signal-intensity protein/blood is layered in the dependent portion of the cyst apparent on precontrast images (*arrows, a,b*). The cyst does not change in size and shape between early (*c*) and delayed (*d*) postcontrast images. The sagittal plane image demonstrates a smooth contour of the superior and inferior walls of the cyst (*arrow, e*), confirming absence of tumor tissue.

(e)

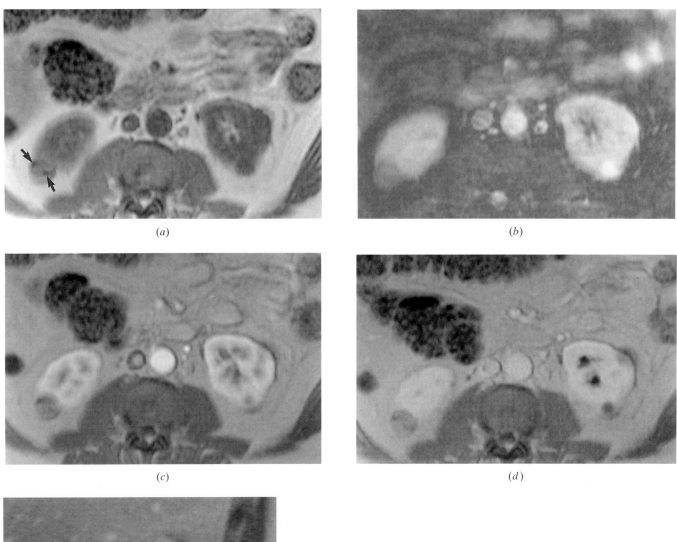

(a)

(b)

(c)

(d)

(e)

F IG . 9.12 Cyst complicated by the presence of calcification, blood and thickened wall. Precontrast SGE (*a*), T2-weighted fat-suppressed spin-echo (*b*), immediate (*c*) and 8-minute transverse (*d*), and 8.5-minute sagittal (*e*) postgadolinium SGE images. A lesion arises from the posterior aspect of the right kidney, which is mixed in signal intensity and contains signal-void calcifications (*arrows, a*) on the precontrast SGE image. The lesion is mildly low in signal intensity on the T2-weighted image (*b*), which mimics the appearance of a solid tumor. The complicated cyst remains moderate in signal intensity on postcontrast images, but it is sharply defined from adjacent cortex and does not change in size or shape between early (*c*) and late (*d,e*) images. The superior margin of the cyst is well-defined on the sagittal image (*arrow, e*).

frequently irregular and thick, and may enhance moderately with gadolinium. When infected, these cysts occasionally have a prominent perinephric component greater than that typical for cystic renal cancers. It is however often not possible to distinguish inflammatory cysts from cystic renal cancers. Surgery, therefore, likely cannot be avoided for many of these lesions. Close imaging follow-up is recommended if surgery is not initially entertained.

Parapelvic Cysts. Parapelvic cysts are pseudocysts containing urine-like fluid. They may originate secondary to prior obstruction and urine leak. They appear as oval-shaped cysts in the renal sinus (Fig. 9.13). They may be

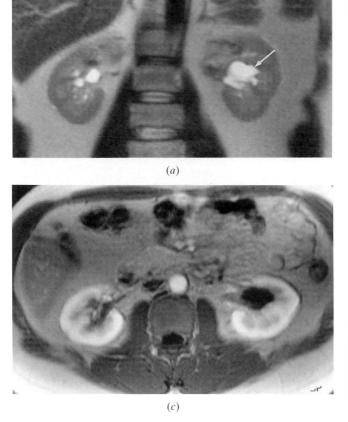

(a)

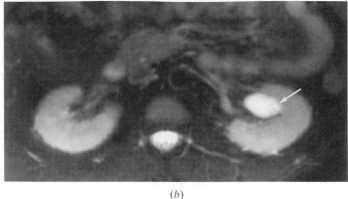

(b)

(c)

FIG. 9.13 Parapelvic cyst. Coronal HASTE (*a*), T2-weighted fat-suppressed spin-echo (*b*), and immediate postgadolinium SGE (*c*) images. An oval-shaped parapelvic cyst is present in the left renal sinus (*arrow, a,b*). The parapelvic cyst is separate from the collecting system, is high in signal intensity on T2-weighted images (*a,b*), and is signal-void and does not enhance on the postgadolinium image (*c*).

solitary or, more commonly, multiple and bilateral. At times these lesions may be difficult to distinguish from a dilated renal collecting system. Images acquired 10 to 20 minutes after gadolinium demonstrate that cystic pelvic structures represent cysts and not dilated collecting system. Gadolinium is sufficiently dilute on late postcontrast images to render urine high in signal intensity, which allows differentiation between high-signal-intensity dilute gadolinium-containing urine in the collecting system from low-signal-intensity fluid in parapelvic cysts. An MRI urogram may also demonstrate that these oval-shaped cystic lesions do not communicate with the renal collecting system.

Autosomal Dominant Polycystic Kidney Disease

Autosomal dominant polycystic kidney disease is characterized by the development of varying-sized renal cysts in both kidneys, which progress over time [12]. The disease usually becomes manifest in adult patients, which explains the alternate designation of adult polycystic kidney disease. Patients usually present late in the course of the condition with abdominal masses, hypertension, or following trauma (12). Renal failure is a late event. The disease is almost always bilateral, although unilateral disease has been described. Cysts are frequently present

in other organs including liver, spleen, and pancreas. Patients are at risk of cerebral hemorrhage from ruptured berry aneurysm.

The typical MRI appearance is that of bilaterally enlarged kidneys with multiple renal cysts of varying sizes distorting the renal architecture. Early in the course of the disease the cysts are small (Fig. 9.14). Over time,

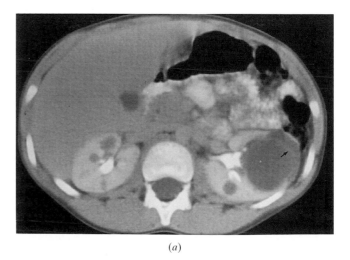

(a)

FIG. 9.14 Autosomal dominant polycystic kidney disease in the early stage of development.

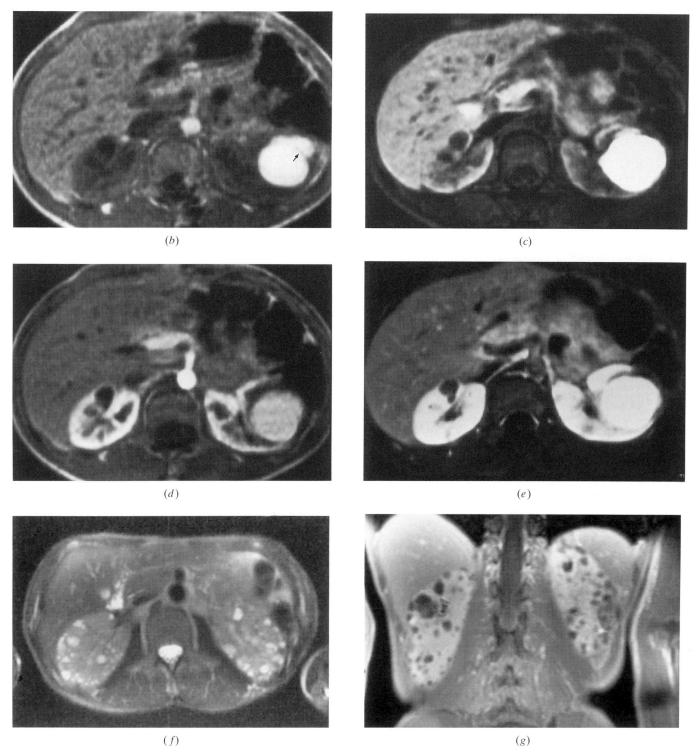

(b)

(c)

(d)

(e)

(f)

(g)

F IG . 9.14 (*Continued*) Contrast-enhanced CT (*a*), SGE (*b*), T1-weighted fat-suppressed spin-echo (*c*), immediate postgadolinium SGE (*d*) and gadolinium-enhanced T1-weighted fat-suppressed spin-echo (*e*) images. Multiple small bilateral renal cysts and a large left renal cyst are present. The majority of cysts are less than 1 cm in diameter, and the renal parenchyma is of normal thickness and not substantially distorted. These findings are consistent with early changes of autosomal dominant polycystic kidney disease. A large left renal cyst contains an internal septation on the CT image (*arrow, a*). Precontrast SGE image (*b*) shows that the cyst is high in signal intensity and contains a low-signal-intensity reticular strand (*arrow, b*). This cyst does not suppress with fat suppression (*c*) and does not enhance with gadolinium (*d*), which is consistent with subacute blood in a hemorrhagic cyst. The presence of hemorrhage is not identified on the CT image. A signal-void rim is appreciated on the postcontrast T1-FS image (*e*), which probably represents hemosiderin deposition. Fat suppressed HASTE (*f*) and coronal 90-second postgadolinium SGE image in a second patient demonstrates multiple <2 cm cysts scattered throughout the renal parenchyma consistent with early stage autosomal dominant polycystic kidney disease.

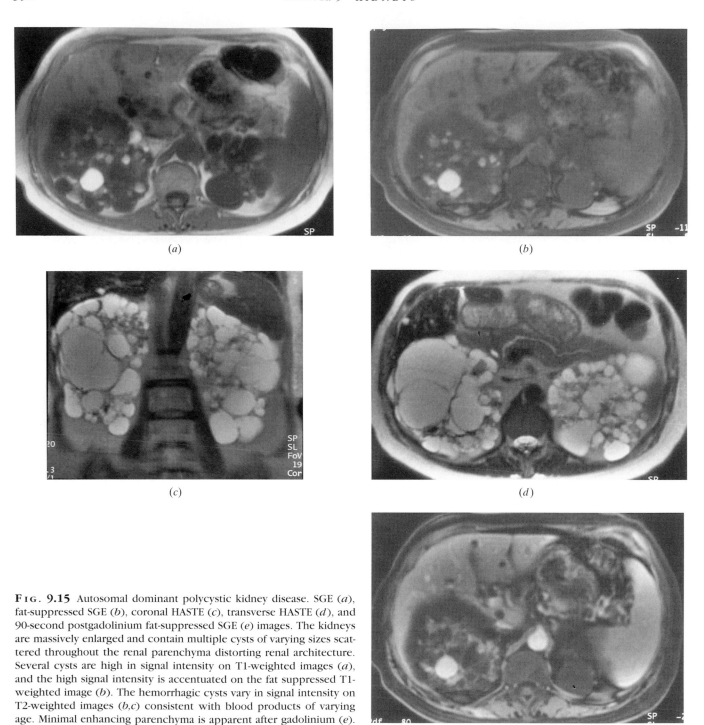

FIG. 9.15 Autosomal dominant polycystic kidney disease. SGE (*a*), fat-suppressed SGE (*b*), coronal HASTE (*c*), transverse HASTE (*d*), and 90-second postgadolinium fat-suppressed SGE (*e*) images. The kidneys are massively enlarged and contain multiple cysts of varying sizes scattered throughout the renal parenchyma distorting renal architecture. Several cysts are high in signal intensity on T1-weighted images (*a*), and the high signal intensity is accentuated on the fat suppressed T1-weighted image (*b*). The hemorrhagic cysts vary in signal intensity on T2-weighted images (*b,c*) consistent with blood products of varying age. Minimal enhancing parenchyma is apparent after gadolinium (*e*).

kidneys enlarge massively. Cysts characteristically have varying signal intensities due to the presence of blood products of differing ages [13] (Fig. 9.15). The liver is the organ in which extrarenal cysts are most commonly observed. Liver cysts range in number from solitary to numerous. Even with extensive liver involvement, cysts tend not to distort the hepatic architecture and usually are less than 2 cm in diameter.

Multicystic Dysplastic Kidney

Multicystic dysplastic kidney results from a congenital failure of fusion of the metanephrosis and ureteric bud resulting in a nonfunctional cystic renal mass. The ureter is typically atretic. Multicystic dysplastic kidney typically is large in infancy and, if left untreated, atrophies with time. The cyst wall often calcifies during the atrophic process. Multicystic dysplastic kidney may be diagnosed

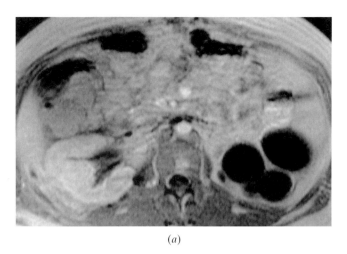 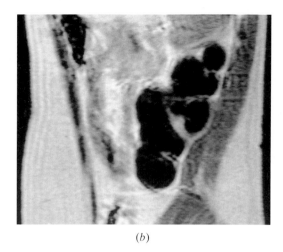

(a)   (b)

FIG. 9.16 Multicystic dysplastic kidney. Transverse 2-minute (a) and sagittal 2.5-minute (b) postgadolinium SGE images. A multicystic dysplastic kidney is present in the left renal fossa that has an cluster-of-grapes appearance with no evidence of organization into a renal collecting system, and no renal parenchyma evident.

in childhood as a large multicystic mass that has no organization into a collecting system and no evidence of normal renal parenchyma (Fig. 9.16). Lesions also may be diagnosed in utero using breathing-independent T2-weighted half Fourier single-shot turbo spin-echo (HASTE) (Fig. 9.17) images. Occasionally, a large multicystic dysplastic kidney may be observed in adolescent or adult patients.

Medullary Cystic Disease

Patients with medullary cystic disease typically present in adolescence with salt-wasting nephropathy and renal failure. On imaging studies, the renal medulla is extensively replaced by 1 to 2-cm cysts (Fig. 9.18). As renal failure progresses, smooth cortical atrophy develops.

Acquired Cystic Disease of Dialysis

Approximately 50 percent of patients on long-term hemodialysis develop multiple renal cysts [14–16]. The etiology is uncertain but may relate to ischemia or fibrosis. Kidneys are usually atrophic at the time of development of cystic disease. Cysts tend to be predominantly superficial in location in the renal cortex and tend not to expand the kidney substantially in size, in contrast to autosomal dominant cystic kidney disease in which cysts are scattered throughout the parenchyma and renal size is usually massive. Cysts generally are smaller in size than in autosomal dominant polycystic kidney disease, measuring less than 2 cm in diameter. Uncommonly, cysts may also be larger than 2 cm and/or scattered throughout renal parenchyma. Hemorrhage is frequently present in these cysts.

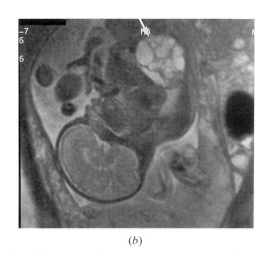

(a)   (b)

FIG. 9.17 Multicystic dysplastic kidney in fetus. Transverse (a) and sagittal (b) HASTE images of a fetus demonstrate a multicystic mass in the left renal fossa (arrow, a,b) with no evidence of organization into a renal collecting system.

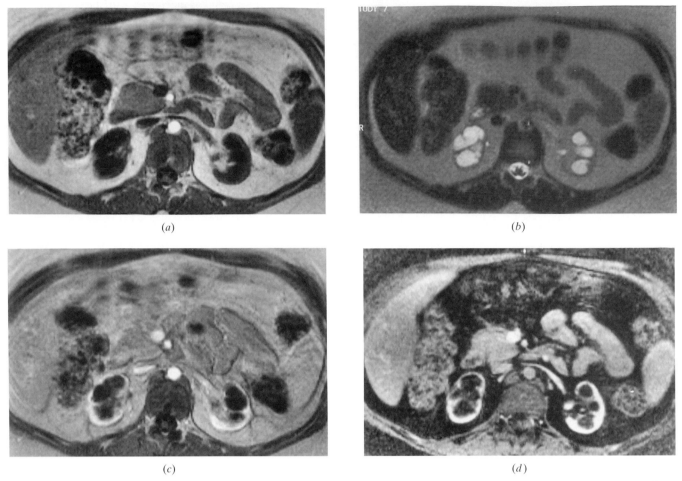

(a)   (b)

(c)   (d)

FIG. 9.18 Medullary cystic disease. SGE (a) HASTE (b), immediate postgadolinium SGE (c), and 90-second postgadolinium T1-weighted fat-suppressed SGE (d) images. Multiple cysts measuring less than 2 cm in diameter occupy the majority of the renal medulla. These simulate the appearance of corticomedullary differentiation on precontrast images (a) in this patient with chronic renal failure. The cysts are homogeneously high in signal intensity on the T2-weighted image (b). After gadolinium administration cysts in the renal medulla do not enhance and appear nearly signal-void (c,d).

On MR images multiple small cysts are scattered throughout both kidneys, mainly in a superficial renal cortical location (Fig. 9.19). Cysts are frequently high in signal intensity on precontrast T1-weighted images due to the presence of subacute blood (Fig. 9.20).

MRI is well-suited for detection of renal cancer and discrimination between nonenhancing cysts and enhancing cancers. Cysts demonstrate no evidence of enhancement and do not change in morphology on serial postcontrast images, whereas cancers and renal parenchyma will demonstrate evidence of enhancement.

Tuberous Sclerosis

Tuberous sclerosis is a neurocutaneous syndrome, part of the general category of phakomatoses with autosomal dominant inheritance, although approximately 50 percent arise from spontaneous mutation.

Patients with tuberous sclerosis have an increased incidence of renal cysts and angiomyolipomas [17,18]. Cystic disease varies considerably in extent and is usually multiple. Renal architecture is not uncommonly distorted. Cystic disease may be so extensive that the kidney disease may resemble autosomal dominant polycystic kidney disease. Angiomyolipomas are frequently multiple and bilateral (Fig. 9.21). Angiomyolipomas have a tendency to increase in size over time in patients with tuberous sclerosis [18,19].

Von Hippel-Lindau Disease

Von Hippel-Lindau disease is a neurocutaneous syndrome, part of the general category of phakomatoses with autosomal dominant inheritance. Patients with von Hippel-Lindau disease have an increased incidence of renal cysts, adenomas, and carcinoma [20]. Carcinomas

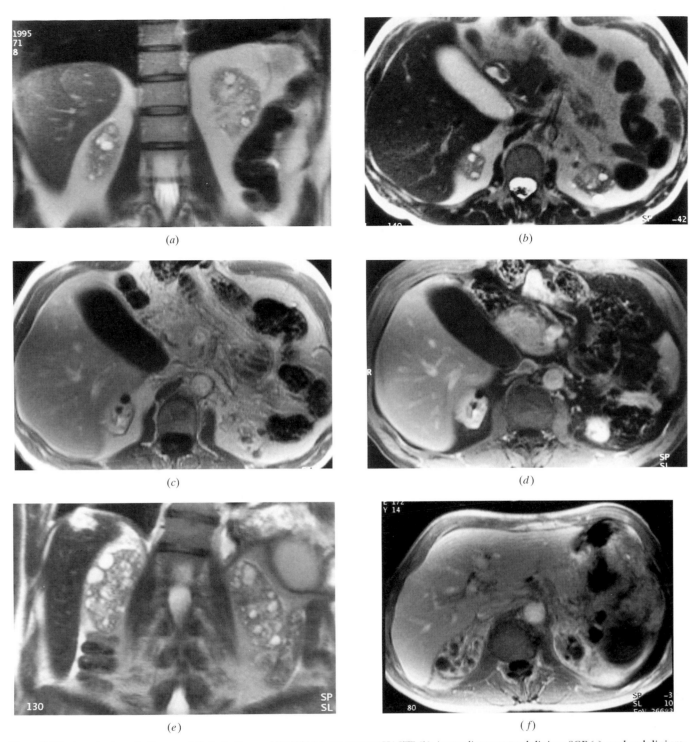

(a) *(b)*

(c) *(d)*

(e) *(f)*

F I G . 9.19 Acquired cystic disease of dialysis. Coronal HASTE (*a*), transverse HASTE (*b*), immediate postgadolinium SGE (*c*), and gadolinium-enhanced T1-weighted fat-suppressed SGE (*d*) images. Multiple cysts less than 2 cm in diameter are present in both kidneys located predominantly in a superficial cortical location. The capillary phase of enhancement (*c*) demonstrates minimal parenchymal enhancement and no corticomedullary differentiation. On the gadolinium-enhanced T1-weighted fat-suppressed spin-echo image (*c*), multiple renal cysts are well-shown in a background of moderately enhanced atrophic parenchymal tissue. Coronal HASTE (*e*) and interstitial-phase gadolinium-enhanced fat-suppressed SGE (*f*) images in a second patient on chronic hemodialysis with Alport syndrome. Multiple small cysts are scattered throughout the kidneys.

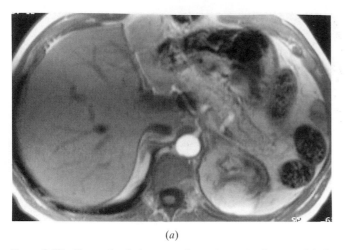

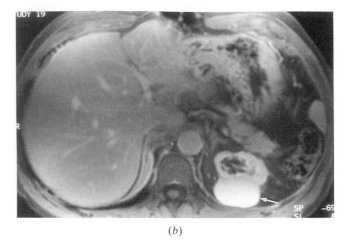

(a)   (b)

FIG. 9.20 Hemorrhagic large renal cyst in cystic disease of dialysis. Immediate postgadolinium SGE (*a*) and interstitial-phase gadolinium-enhanced fat-suppressed SGE (*b*) images demonstrate a homogeneously high-signal-intensity superficial 4-cm cyst arising from the posterior left renal cortex (*arrow, b*).

tend to be multicentric and bilateral (Fig. 9.22) [20]. T1-weighted fat-suppressed imaging with gadolinium enhancement is the most sensitive technique for detecting multiple tumors, many of which are 1 cm in diameter.

Multilocular Cystic Nephroma

Multilocular cystic nephroma is a benign lesion comprising noncommunicating cysts within a fibrous stroma. This lesion has been described as occurring most frequently in males aged 2 months to 4 years as well as adults, predominantly females, aged 40 years and older [21]. Histological differences have been described between the lesions occurring in the pediatric population (histologically cystic partially differentiated nephroblastoma)

and in the adult population (histologically cystic nephroma) [21]. In a recent MRI study, adult-type multilocular cystic nephromas were observed in males and females in their 20s and 30s in an approximately equivalent gender distribution [22]. The diagnosis of multilocular cystic nephroma on MR images requires the demonstration of a multicystic renal mass that bulges into the renal pelvis and has thick, relatively uniform, fibrous septations (Fig. 9.23) [22,23]. Septations are well-defined and relatively low in signal intensity on T2-weighted images and enhance on postgadolinium images [22]. Transverse images should be supplemented with sagittal or coronal images to demonstrate the indentation into renal pelvis. Usually cysts are low in signal intensity on T1-weighted images, but not uncommonly they are high in signal

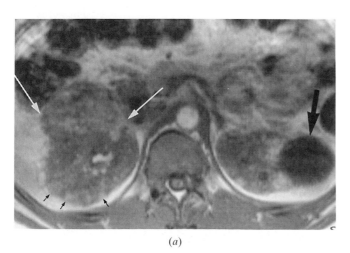

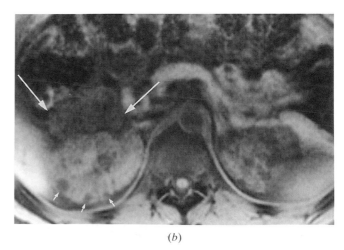

(a)   (b)

FIG. 9.21 Tuberous sclerosis. SGE (*a*), fat-suppressed SGE (*b*), HASTE (*c*), and interstitial-phase gadolinium enhanced transverse (*d*), and sagittal (*e*) fat-suppressed SGE images. Numerous varying size angiomyolipomas are present throughout both kidneys (*small arrows, a*) including a large exophytic angiomyolipoma with multiple high-signal-intensity punctuate foci of fat (*long arrows, a*).

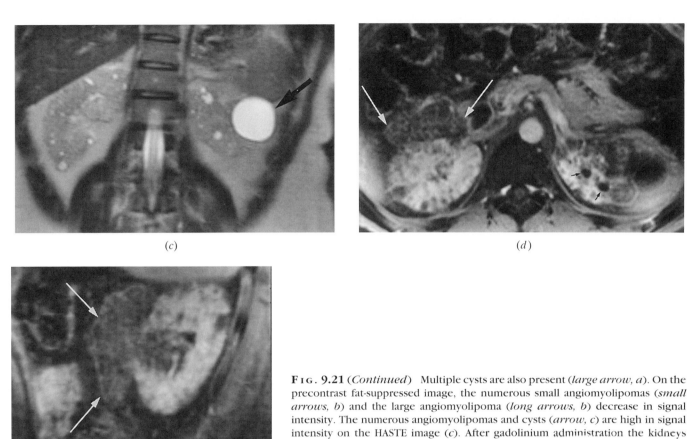

(c)

(d)

(e)

FIG. 9.21 (*Continued*) Multiple cysts are also present (*large arrow, a*). On the precontrast fat-suppressed image, the numerous small angiomyolipomas (*small arrows, b*) and the large angiomyolipoma (*long arrows, b*) decrease in signal intensity. The numerous angiomyolipomas and cysts (*arrow, c*) are high in signal intensity on the HASTE image (*c*). After gadolinium administration the kidneys are shown to be extensively replaced by angiomyolipomas and cysts (*small arrows, d*). The large exophytic angiomyolipoma (*long arrows, d,e*) is well-shown on transverse (*d*) and sagittal (*e*) postgadolinium fat-suppressed SGE images.

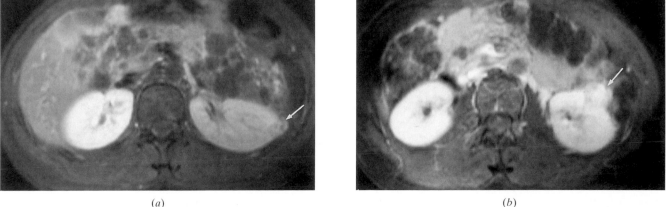

(a)

(b)

FIG. 9.22 Von Hippel-Lindau disease. Gadolinium-enhanced T1-weighted fat-suppressed spin-echo (*a,b*) images. Two small renal cancers are present in the mid (*arrow, a*) and lower (*arrow, b*) pole of the left kidney.

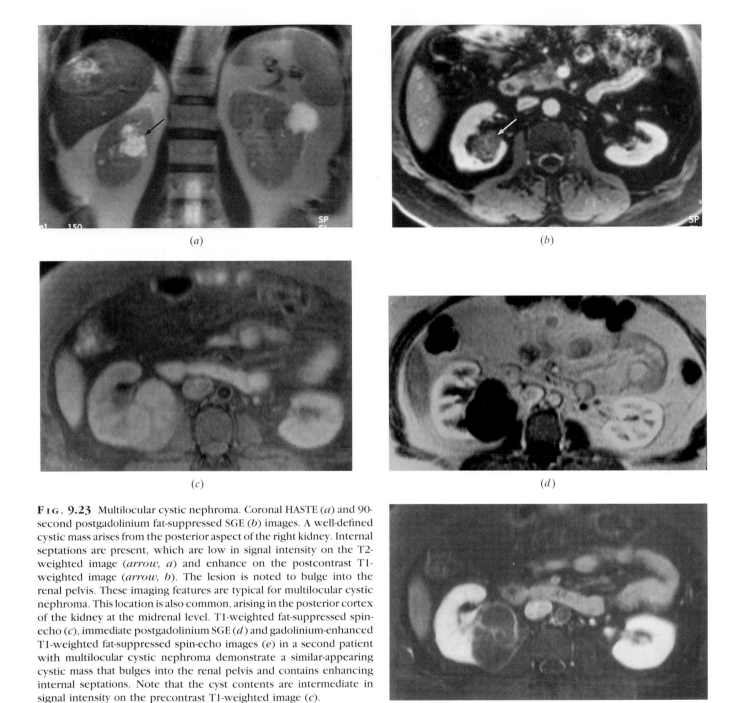

FIG. 9.23 Multilocular cystic nephroma. Coronal HASTE (*a*) and 90-second postgadolinium fat-suppressed SGE (*b*) images. A well-defined cystic mass arises from the posterior aspect of the right kidney. Internal septations are present, which are low in signal intensity on the T2-weighted image (*arrow, a*) and enhance on the postcontrast T1-weighted image (*arrow, b*). The lesion is noted to bulge into the renal pelvis. These imaging features are typical for multilocular cystic nephroma. This location is also common, arising in the posterior cortex of the kidney at the midrenal level. T1-weighted fat-suppressed spin-echo (*c*), immediate postgadolinium SGE (*d*) and gadolinium-enhanced T1-weighted fat-suppressed spin-echo images (*e*) in a second patient with multilocular cystic nephroma demonstrate a similar-appearing cystic mass that bulges into the renal pelvis and contains enhancing internal septations. Note that the cyst contents are intermediate in signal intensity on the precontrast T1-weighted image (*c*).

intensity, presumably reflecting the presence of protein-aceous material or blood (Fig. 9.24) [22,23].

Medullary Sponge Kidney

Medullary sponge kidney (MSK) is characterized by multiple cystic cavities in the papillae. Calculi are frequently present in the cystic cavities. The disease is usually bilateral, but may be unilateral or segmental. Patients present with calculi, obstruction, infection, or hematuria. Tubular ectasia is considered a precursor of MSK. On intravenous urography, tubular ectasia appears as contrast-filled tubular structures that radiate from the calyx into the papilla. A similar appearance may be appreciated on interstitial-phase gadolinium-enhanced MR images, with prominent radiating, enhancing tubular structures demonstrated in the renal papillae (Fig. 9.25).

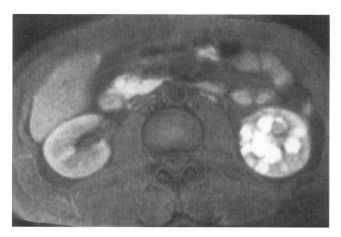

FIG. 9.24 Multilocular cystic nephroma. Precontrast T1-weighted fat-suppressed spin-echo image demonstrates a multilocular cystic nephroma in the lower pole of the left kidney. Many of the cysts are high in signal intensity compatible with either subacute blood or protein. Cysts are not uncommonly high in signal intensity on T1-weighted images in multilocular cystic nephroma.

Angiomyolipoma

Angiomyolipomas are composed of three elements: (1) blood vessels, (2) smooth muscle, and (3) fat. These tumors are virtually always benign. The fat component is usually substantial, permitting characterization on CT images and on combined T1-weighted regular and fat-suppressed images or combined T1-weighted regular and out-of-phase SGE images [24]. Although benign, these tumors may increase in size over time, with larger tumors having greater propensity to bleed [18,19,25,26]. Angiomyolipomas have a greater tendency to increase in size when they are multiple than when they are solitary [19,26]. Lesions may be detected and characterized, even when they are 1 cm in diameter, due to the high signal intensity of fat on T1-weighted images that attenuates on fat-suppressed images (Fig. 9.26). Out-of-phase images are a useful addition to an imaging protocol performed to characterize renal masses as angiomyolipomas (see Fig. 9.26). A fat-water signal-void phase-cancellation occurs at the boundary between the angiomyolipoma and the adjacent renal parenchyma [13]. When angiomyolipomas are very small (<1 cm) the phase cancellation may occupy the entire lesion and render it signal-void [27]. In a small number of cases, when muscle or vascular components predominate, distinction from renal-cell cancer may be difficult. When the diagnosis, based on imaging findings, is certain and tumors are less than 4 cm in size and asymptomatic, imaging follow-up is adequate management [25,28]. Case reports of fat within renal adenocarcinomas recently have been described [29]. At present, it is not clear if fat in renal cancer exhibits phase-cancellation on out-of-phase images or suppresses with chemically-selective techniques as observed for normal body fat and fat in angiomyolipomas.

Adenoma

Renal adenomas are benign tumors of renal cell origin and typically are small solid neoplasms [30]. The relationship of adenomas to renal-cell carcinomas is uncertain [26]. Adenomas cannot be distinguished from papillary renal-cell cancers on imaging studies [31,32]. Patients with small solid tumors may benefit from serial reassessment to detect tumor growth. Tumor growth raises the concern of malignancy [26,33–38]. It may be reasonable to follow a mass at 3 months, 6 months, 1 year, and yearly thereafter. Particularly in elderly patients, close observation likely results in the least patient morbidity [37,38].

On MR images adenomas are typically small, round masses smaller than 4 cm that are slightly hypointense on T1-weighted images, slightly hyperintense on T2-

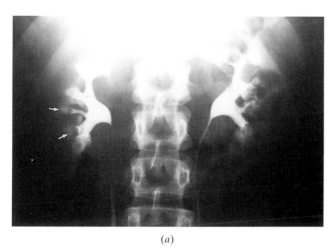

(a)

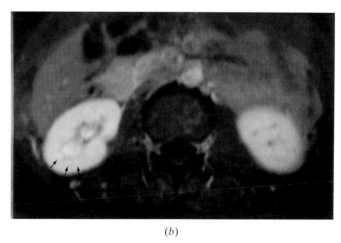

(b)

FIG. 9.25 Medullary sponge kidney. Five-minute intravenous urogram (a) and interstitial-phase gadolinium-enhanced T1-weighted fat-suppressed spin-echo (b) images. Tubular ectasia is apparent on the intravenous urogram (arrows, a). On the interstitial-phase gadolinium enhanced image (b), prominent papillary enhancement is present (arrows, b).

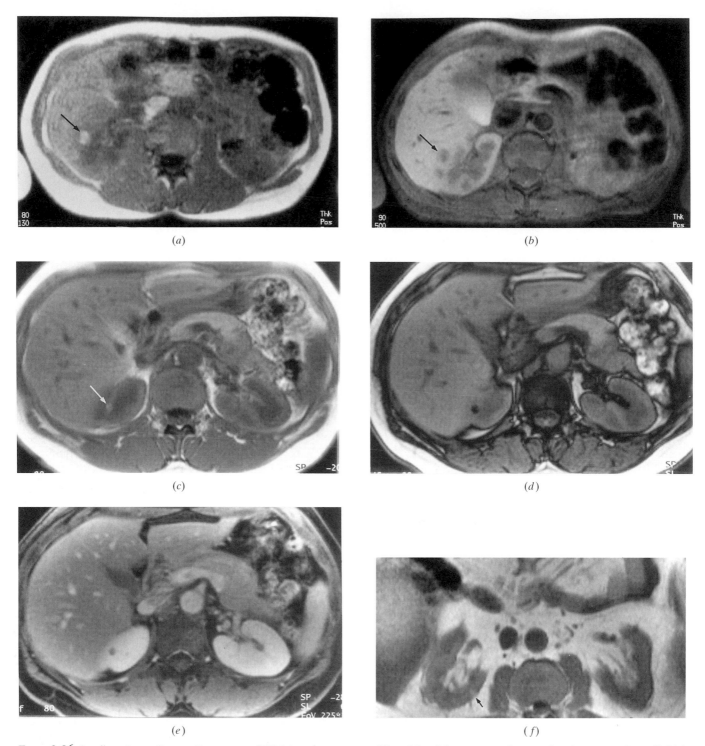

(a)

(b)

(c)

(d)

(e)

(f)

F I G . 9.26 Small angiomyolipoma. Precontrast SGE (*a*) and precontrast T1-weighted fat-suppressed spin-echo (*b*) images. A small, high-signal-intensity lesion arises from the upper pole of the right kidney on the SGE image (*arrow, a*). Fat suppression decreases the signal intensity of this lesion (*arrow, b*), confirming that it represents an angiomyolipoma. Precontrast SGE (*c*), out-of-phase SGE (*d*), and interstitial-phase gadolinium-enhanced SGE (*e*) images in a second patient demonstrate a high-signal-intensity tumor on the in-phase image (*arrow, c*) that becomes signal-void on the out-of-phase image (*d*) due to phase-cancellation artifact. The lesion is very low in signal on the postgadolinium fat-suppressed SGE image (*e*).

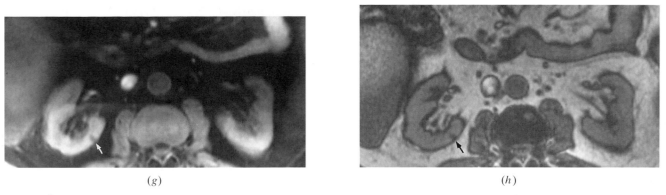

(g) (h)

F i g . 9.26 (*Continued*) SGE (*f*), fat-suppressed SGE (*g*) and out-of-phasic SGE (*h*) in a third patient. A 6 mm angiomyolipoma is present in the right kidney that is high in signal intensity on the in-phase image (*arrow, f*), suppresses to low signal intensity on the fat-suppressed image (*arrow, g*), and is signal void on the out-of-phase image (*arrow, h*).

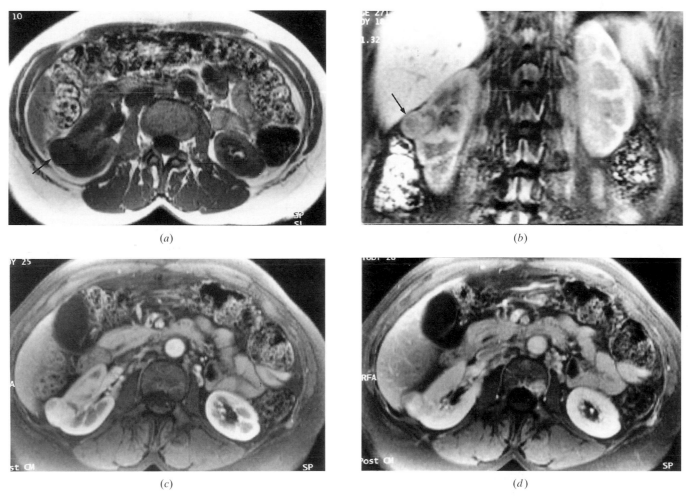

(a) (b)

(c) (d)

F i g . 9.27 Renal oncocytoma. SGE (*a*), coronal fat-suppressed SGE (*b*), immediate postgadolinium SGE (*c*), and 90-second postgadolinium fat-suppressed SGE (*d*) images. A well-defined 2-cm mass is present in the left kidney (*arrow, a,b*). The majority of the tumor enhances in a moderately intense fashion on the immediate postgadolinium image (*c*) and shows mild peripheral washout by 90 seconds (*d*). The appearance is indistinguishable from that of a small renal cancer.

weighted images, and enhance in a diffuse intense fashion on capillary-phase images [13].

Oncocytomas are a type of adenoma. These tumors demonstrate substantial central enhancement on capillary-phase images (Fig. 9.27). The characteristic early enhancement pattern is described as "spoke wheel" [13], but may not be commonly observed. In comparison, renal cancers tend to exhibit greater peripheral enhancement. A central scar also may be observed in oncocytoma. Neither pattern of enhancement nor presence of central scar may be specific enough to permit distinction from renal-cell carcinoma [32,39].

Malignant Masses

Renal-Cell Carcinoma

Renal-cell carcinoma is the most common renal neoplasm. The incidence is more than 25,000 with a mortality above 10,000 annually in the United States [40]. The peak age of incidence is 50 to 60 years of age with a male to female ratio of 2 to 1 [40]. Tumors are usually solitary. In approximately 5 percent of patients tumors are multiple. Patients usually present late in the course of the disease when tumors are large and in an advanced stage due to a lack of symptoms from small tumors. Renal-cell cancer is associated with a myriad of presenting features including paraneoplastic phenomena.

Staging of renal-cell cancer can be performed by either Robson's or TNM classification (Table 1). Robson's classification is frequently used and is described in this text. Both MRI and current-generation CT scanners are able to detect renal cancers that measure 1 cm in diameter. In a study comparing dynamic contrast-enhanced CT imaging and MRI, these techniques detected 54 and 58 of 61 renal tumors that were present in 53 patients, respectively [41]. CT imaging and MRI correctly staged 24 and 29 of 31 renal cancers that were resected [41].

Conventional MRI sequences have been useful in evaluating renal tumors to assess the presence of tumor thrombus or extension of tumor to adjacent organs [42]. Thrombus is well-shown on spin-echo images due to high contrast between tumor thrombus and signal-void blood on spin-echo sequences [43–47]. MRI using gadolinium-enhanced breath-hold SGE and fat-suppressed sequences is superior to CT imaging in differentiating cysts from solid tumors due to the higher sensitivity of MRI for gadolinium than that of CT imaging for iodine contrast [1,11,41].

The typical appearance of a renal-cell cancer is an irregular mass with ill-defined margins. Tumors are generally slightly hypointense on T1-weighted images and slightly hyperintense on T2-weighted images relative to renal cortex [42]. The minimal difference from renal cortex renders tumors poorly visualized on noncontrast images. Following gadolinium administration, heterogeneous enhancement is apparent on immediate postgadolinium images, and enhancement diminishes on more delayed postcontrast images. Tumors are frequently hypervascular and demonstrate intense enhancement on immediate postgadolinium capillary-phase images, usually in a heterogeneous fashion with more intense peripheral enhancement [1,11,41,48,49]. Homogeneous enhancement does occur, and is typical of small, low-grade cancers [41]. Homogeneously enhancing small tumors may be difficult to distinguish from renal cortex on immediate postgadolinium images. As a result, it is important that a renal MRI protocol include not only immediate postgadolinium capillary-phase images, but also more delayed interstitial-phase images (Fig. 9.28). Diminished

Table 9.1 Renal-Cell Cancer Staging Systems		
Robson Stage	Description	TNM Stage
I	Tumor contained within renal capsule	
	Small tumor (<2.5 cm)	T1
	Large tumor (>2.5 cm)	T2
II	Tumor spread to perinephric fat	T3a
III-A	Venous tumor thrombus	
	Renal vein tumor thrombus only	T3b
	Infradiaphragmatic caval thrombus	T3c
	Supradiaphragmatic caval thrombus	T4b
III-B	Regional lymph node metastasis	N1–N3
III-C	Venous tumor thrombus and regional lymph node metastasis	
IV-A	Direct invasion of adjacent organs outside Gerota's fascia	T4a
IV-B	Distant metastasis	M1a–M1d, N4

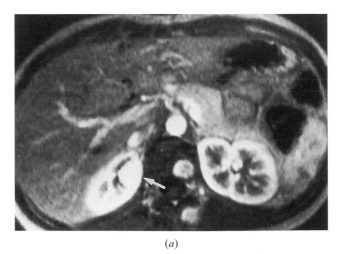

(a)

FIG. 9.28 Hypervascular renal-cell cancer. Immediate postgadolinium SGE (a) and gadolinium-enhanced T1-weighted fat-suppressed spin-echo (b) images demonstrate a small uniform-enhancing Stage I renal-cell cancer.

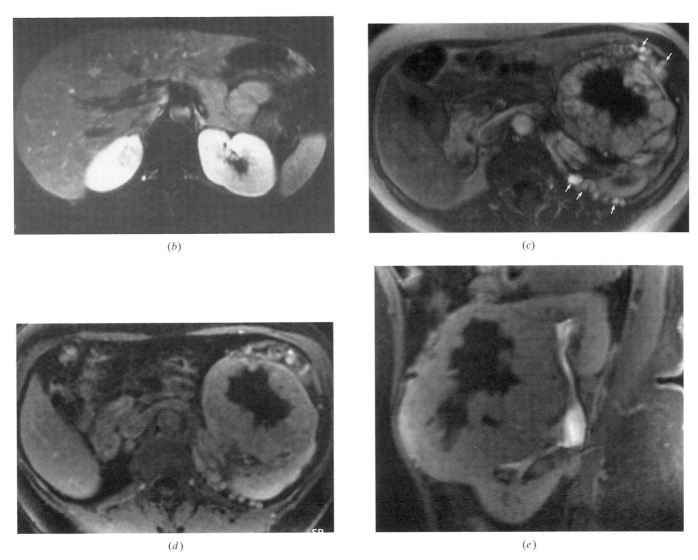

(b)

(c)

(d)

(e)

F IG . 9.28 (*Continued*)   A 2-cm renal cancer arises from the upper pole of the right kidney. The cancer enhances in a uniform intense fashion (*arrow, a*) on the immediate postgadolinium image, comparable in signal intensity to renal cortex. On the later interstitial-phase image the tumor is heterogeneous and lower in signal intensity than cortex. Immediate postgadolinium SGE (*c*), 90 second postgadolinium fat-suppressed SGE (*d*) and sagittal 5-minute postgadolinium SGE (*e*) images in a second patient demonstrates a 7 cm hypervascular renal-cell cancer arising from the left kidney. On the immediate postgadolinium image (*c*) viable tumor enhances intensely with lack of enhancement of the central portion of the tumor. Intense enhancement of multiple enlarged feeding vessels is present (*arrows, c*). On the 90 second postgadolinium image (*d*) the tumor has diminished in signal lower than renal cortex. The sagittal image (*e*) displays the location of the tumor in the midportion of the kidney.

enhancement on interstitial-phase images is observed for the great majority of tumors. Hypervascular cancers tend to wash out of contrast, whereas renal cortex remains high in signal intensity due to retention of contrast in renal tubules (see Fig. 9.28). Approximately 20 percent of renal cancers may be hypovascular. Hypovascular renal cancers enhance minimally on capillary-phase images and remain low in signal intensity relative to cortex on interstitial-phase images. These tumors may be sharply marginated and may resemble cysts on contrast-enhanced CT images. Diagnosis of a hypovascular renal cancer requires identification of small, short curvilinear

enhanced structures that are present on postgadolinium images but not apparent on precontrast images. Interstitial-phase images acquired with fat suppression are the most reliable at demonstrating these enhancing structures (Fig. 9.29).

Hemorrhage occurs occasionally in patients with normal renal function. This is different from tumors in patients with chronic renal failure, in which hemorrhage is relatively common (see later). Hemorrhage appears high in signal intensity on T1-weighted images (Fig. 9.30). Tumor size is not a reliable criterion for diagnosing renal cancer nor for distinguishing cancer from adenoma [32–

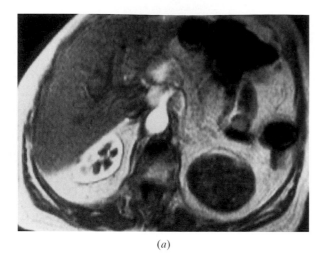

(a)

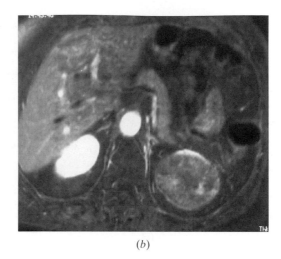

(b)

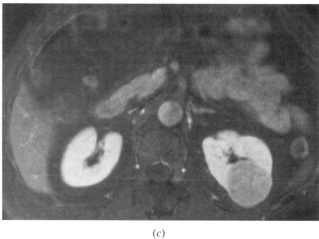

(c)

FIG. **9.29** Hypovascular Stage 2 renal-cell cancer. Immediate post-gadolinium SGE (*a*) and gadolinium-enhanced T1-weighted fat-suppressed spin-echo (*b*) images. The tumor shows diminished enhancement immediately following contrast (*a*). The interstitial-phase fat-suppressed image demonstrates small irregular enhancing structures within the mass (*b*), which distinguishes this lesion from a complicated cyst. T1-weighted fat-suppressed spin-echo image (*c*) in a second patient shows small irregular enhancing structures in a hypovascular renal cancer arising from the left kidney.

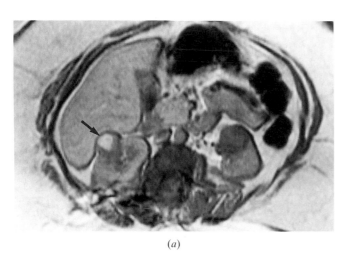

(a)

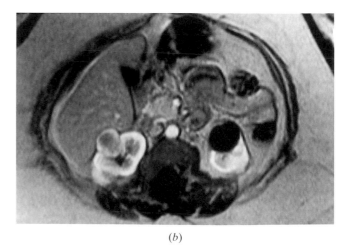

(b)

FIG. **9.30** Stage 2 renal-cell cancer with central hemorrhage. Precontrast SGE (*a*), immediate postgadolinium SGE (*b*) and gadolinium-enhanced T1-weighted fat-suppressed spin-echo (*c*) images.

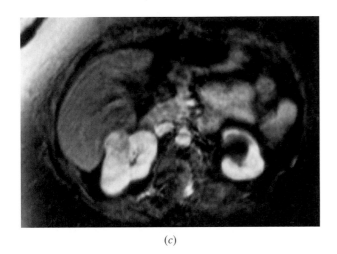

(c)

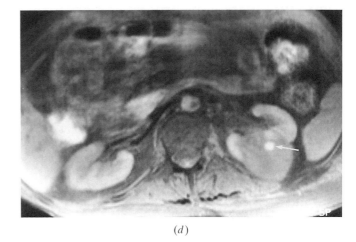

(d)

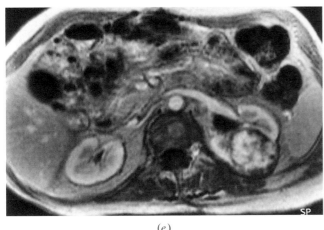

(e)

F IG . 9.30 (*Continued*) Hemorrhage is present in a 2.5-cm Stage 2 renal cancer arising from the right kidney, which appears as high-signal-intensity substance on the precontrast T1-weighted image (*arrow, a*). The tumor shows intense rim enhancement on the immediate postgadolinium image (*b*). Heterogeneous enhancement of the tumor is apparent on the interstitial-phase fat-suppressed image (*c*). Precontrast fat-suppressed SGE (*d*) and immediate postgadolinium SGE (*e*) images in a second patient demonstrate a 5-cm tumor arising in the left kidney. Foci of central high signal intensity on the postcontrast image (*arrow, d*) are consistent with hemorrhage. The tumor exhibits an unusual central radiating enhancement pattern on the immediate postgadolinium SGE image (*e*). This pattern of enhancement may be more typical of oncocytoma, but was present in this renal-cell cancer.

38]. Renal-cell cancers occasionally show no change in size in intervals of greater than 1 year [34,37]. Any solid renal tumor that is nonfatty should be considered a possible renal-cell cancer and should at the least be followed by serial imaging.

Stage 1 renal cancers are confined within the renal capsule (Fig. 9.31). Stage 2 cancers extend beyond the renal capsule (Fig. 9.32). Cancers that are completely intraparenchymal are Stage 1 cancers. Based on imaging features, distinction between Stage 1 and Stage 2 cancers cannot be reliably made for tumors that extend beyond the cortical margins. Large exophytic tumors may be Stage 1, and tumors with a small extrarenal component may be Stage 2. Surgical management is identical for disease stages 1 and 2, so differentiation by imaging is not essential. Renal-cell cancers stages 1 and 2 are associated with a high survival rate since the tumor is amenable to complete resection.

Stage 3a renal cancer is defined by tumor extension into the renal vein (Fig. 9.33). Tumor thrombus frequently extends into the inferior vena cava (IVC) and grows superiorly with the direction of blood flow toward and, in advanced cases, into the right atrium. MRI is superior to

CT imaging in determining the presence and superior extent of thrombus. Modern-generation CT imaging is not substantially inferior to MRI in detecting the presence of thrombus. However, the major advantages of MRI are demonstration of the superior extent of thrombus and

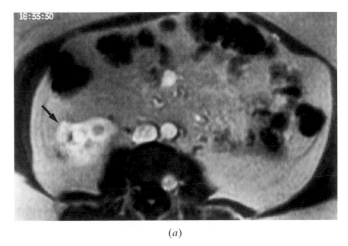

(a)

F IG . 9.31 Small renal cancer (Stage 1). One-second postgadolinium SGE (*a*) and 7-minute postgadolinium sagittal SGE (*b*) images.

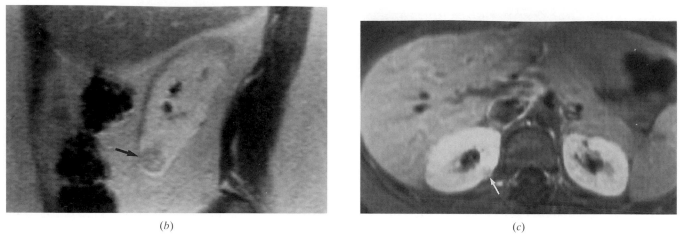

(b)   *(c)*

F I G . 9.31 (*Continued*)   A small renal cancer arises from the lower pole of the right kidney. The tumor demonstrates marked enhancement immediately after contrast administration (*arrow, a*) and diminished enhancement on the delayed postcontrast SGE image (*arrow, b*). Gadolinium-enhanced T1-weighted fat-suppressed spin-echo image (*c*) in a second patient demonstrates a heterogeneously enhanced 1-cm tumor (*arrow, c*) that is lower in signal intensity than adjacent cortex.

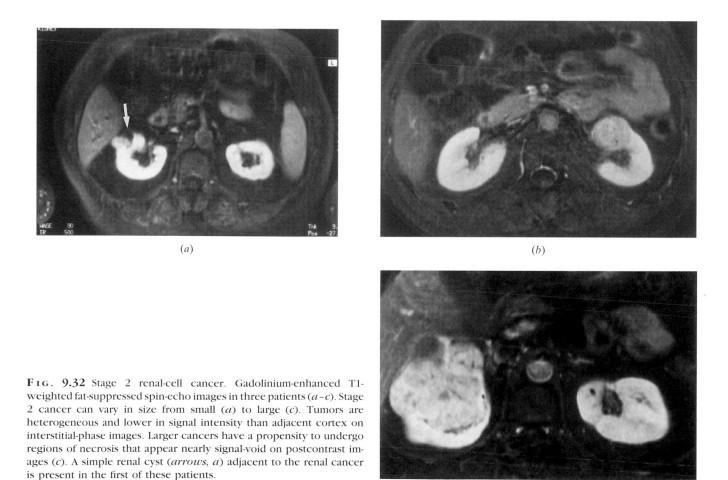

(a)   *(b)*

F I G . 9.32 Stage 2 renal-cell cancer. Gadolinium-enhanced T1-weighted fat-suppressed spin-echo images in three patients (*a – c*). Stage 2 cancer can vary in size from small (*a*) to large (*c*). Tumors are heterogeneous and lower in signal intensity than adjacent cortex on interstitial-phase images. Larger cancers have a propensity to undergo regions of necrosis that appear nearly signal-void on postcontrast images (*c*). A simple renal cyst (*arrows, a*) adjacent to the renal cancer is present in the first of these patients.

(c)

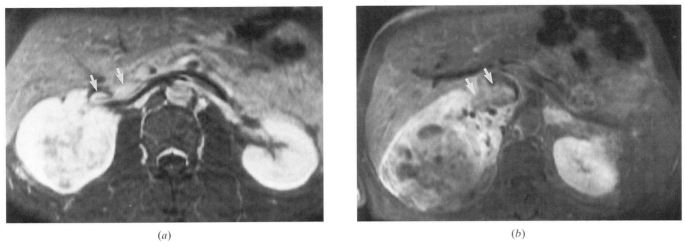

(a) (b)

F I G . 9.33 Stage 3a renal-cell cancer. Gadolinium-enhanced T1-weighted fat-suppressed spin-echo images in two patients (*a,b*). Enhancing tumor thrombus can be appreciated extending along the right renal vein into the IVC (*arrows a,b*). Enhancement of tumor thrombus is well-shown on fat-suppressed postgadolinium images acquired in the interstitial phase.

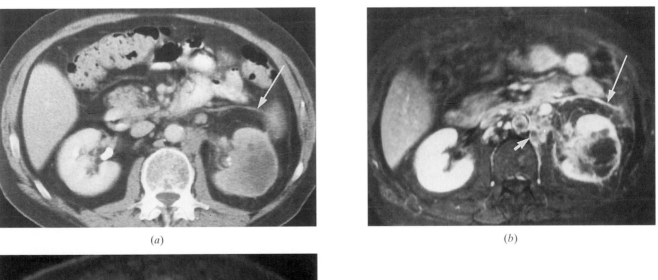

(a) (b)

(c)

F I G . 9.34 Stage 3b renal-cell cancer. Contrast-enhanced CT (*a*) and gadolinium-enhanced T1-weighted fat-suppressed spin-echo (*b*) images. A necrotic 6-cm tumor is present in the left kidney. Enlarged para-aortic nodes are identified on the CT scan. On the postcontrast T1-weighted fat-suppressed image the nodes enhance in a heterogeneous fashion with central low signal intensity (*short arrow, b*), with an appearance similar to that of the primary tumor. Note the thickening of Gerota's fascia (*long arrows, a,b*) shown on the CT and MR images. Gadolinium-enhanced T1-weighted fat-suppressed image of a Stage 3b cancer in a second patient demonstrates a heterogeneous necrotic primary renal cancer of the left kidney with central necrosis and para-aorta lymph nodes with a similar heterogeneous appearance (*arrow, c*).

determination whether thrombus is tumor or blood thrombus. Direct coronal or sagittal plane images are important for the demonstration of the superior extent of thrombus. This information is useful in that it assists in surgical planning for thrombus extraction. Thrombus extension above the hepatic veins requires a thoracoabdominal approach rather than an abdominal approach, which is used if thrombus extends below the hepatic veins. Gadolinium administration is generally useful for the evaluation of thrombus composition because tumor thrombus virtually always enhances with gadolinium. In comparison, in one CT imaging series, tumor thrombus was correctly detected in 18 of 19 patients on CT images of the patients, but only three of these thrombi demonstrated appreciable enhancement [50]. A gradient-echo technique that refocuses the signal of flowing blood (e.g., gradient recalled acquisition in steady state) has been proposed as another method for evaluating tumor thrombus [51]. On these images, tumor thrombus is intermediate in signal intensity (i.e., soft tissue signal intensity) whereas blood thrombus is low in signal intensity due to the presence of blood breakdown products. Because contrast enhancement should be routinely employed in evaluating kidneys and flow-sensitive gradient-echo is rapid to perform, it may be reasonable to use both methods to evaluate thrombus in order to increase confidence of characterization.

Stage 3b renal cancer is defined by presence of malignant nodes (Fig. 9.34). MRI is occasionally able to detect necrosis in lymph nodes, which appears as irregular low-signal-intensity centers that may not be identified on CT images. In the presence of a necrotic primary tumor, necrosis of lymph nodes may be specific for nodal involvement. The presence of enlarged lymph nodes does not necessarily indicate Stage 3b or 3c disease because adenopathy also may be benign. Studer et al. [52] reported that 58 percent of 163 patients with renal-cell cancer had enlarged hyperplastic lymph nodes. Stage 3c is tumor extension into the renal vein and nodal involvement (Fig. 9.35).

Stage 4 disease is extension to local (4a) or distant (4b) sites. Renal cancer metastasizes to lung, adrenal glands, mediastinum, axial skeleton, and liver (Fig. 9.36). The lung is the most common site of metastases. Lung metastases measuring 3 mm in diameter are detected on CT images. Reliable detection of metastases measuring

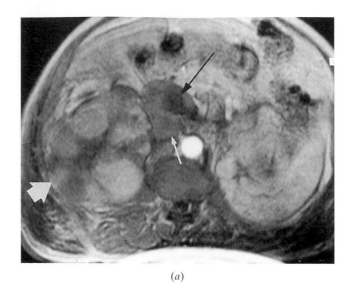

(a)

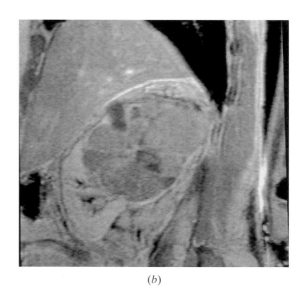

(b)

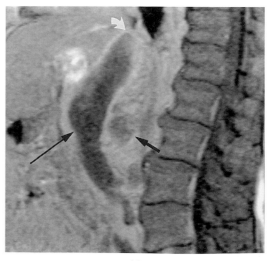

(c)

F I G . **9.35** Stage 3c renal-cell cancer. Forty-five-second transverse (a) and 90-second sagittal (b,c) postgadolinium SGE images. A 7-cm heterogeneously enhancing renal cancer is present in the right kidney (*arrow, a*). Thrombus is present in the IVC (*long arrow, a,c*). Retrocaval (*short arrows a,c*) and paracaval nodes are identified. The thrombus (*long arrow, c*) is noted to terminate approximately 1 cm below the level of the diaphragm on the sagittal projection (*curved arrow, c*).

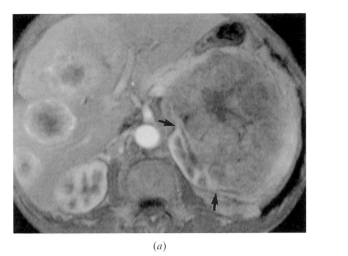

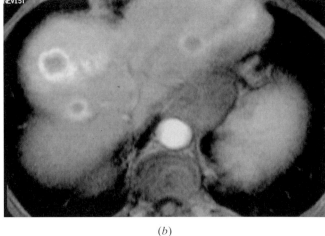

(a)

(b)

F I G . 9.36 Stage 4 renal cancer. Immediate postgadolinium SGE images (*a,b*) demonstrate a 12-cm renal cancer arising from the left kidney (*arrows, a*). Multiple hypervascular ring enhancing liver metastases are noted. Renal cancer metastases are frequently hypervascular.

5 mm in diameter may be made using a combination of T2-weighted images, gated T1-weighted spin-echo images, and 2- to 5-minute delayed postgadolinium breath-hold SGE images. Further sequence development is necessary for MRI to demonstrate 3-mm metastases reliably.

In rare instances renal-cell cancer is largely or completely cystic (Fig. 9.37). In particular, patients with multiple bilateral renal cancers have a propensity to develop cystic cancers, which may arise from intraparenchymal seeding of cysts or from de novo intramural growth (see

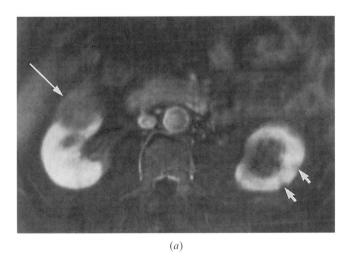

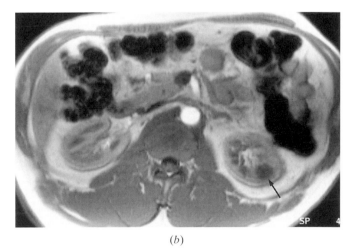

(a)

(b)

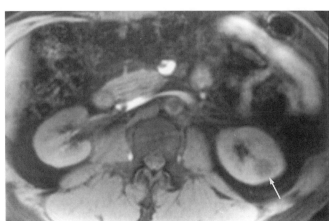

F I G . 9.37 Purely cystic renal-cell cancer. Gadolinium-enhanced T1-weighted fat-suppressed spin-echo image (*a*) in a patient with bilateral renal cancers. A 4-cm renal cancer is demonstrated in the right kidney (*long arrow, a*). Two 5-mm subcapsular low-signal-intensity lesions (*short arrows, a*) are present in the lower pole of the left kidney.

(c)

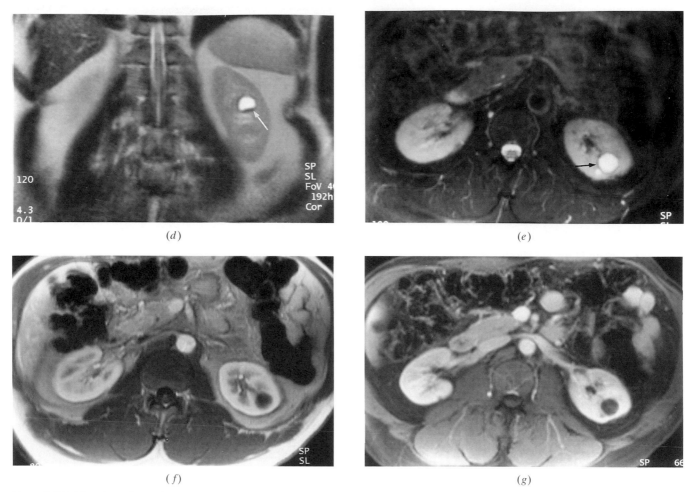

(d)   *(e)*

(f)   *(g)*

F IG . 9.37 (*Continued*)   At histopathological examination these lesions represented cysts with a thin lining of tumor cells found in part of their walls. SGE (*b*), fat-suppressed SGE (*c*), coronal HASTE (*d*), T2-weighted echo-train spin-echo (*e*), immediate postgadolinium SGE (*f*), and interstitial-phase gadolinium-enhanced fat-suppressed SGE (*g*) images. A well-defined cystic lesion with mural calcification was demonstrated on CT images (not shown). The lesion is well-circumscribed and low in signal intensity on T1-weighted images (*arrow, b,c*), high in signal intensity on T2-weighted images, and does not enhance following gadolinium administration (*f,g*). A low-signal-intensity mural rim on the T2-weighted images (*arrow, d,e*) corresponds to calcification as shown on the CT image. At surgery the lesion was considered to represent a cyst, but at histological examination a thin sheet of tumor cells was present in part of the cyst wall.

Fig. 9.37). Tumors can grow in a sheet-like fashion along the liver capsule and into the renal hilum (Fig. 9.38). Cysts in patients with multiple bilateral renal cancers have a high incidence of tumor seeding. Cystic cancers also are not uncommon in the setting of bilateral renal cancers (Fig. 9.39). Renal-cell cancer also may have a multicystic appearance resembling multilocular cystic nephroma (Fig. 9.40) and may cause substantial hemorrhage in the perinephric space (Fig. 9.41).

Renal Cancer in Chronic Renal Failure.   Patients with chronic renal failure have a substantial risk of developing renal-cell carcinoma, which has a reported incidence of approximately 7 percent [16]. Tumors in patients with chronic renal failure are much more commonly hypovascular than tumors in patients with normal renal function. The frequent occurrence of hypovascular cancers and the suboptimal enhancement of renal parenchyma in patients with chronic renal failure on iodine contrast-enhanced CT images renders chronic renal-failure patients difficult to evaluate with CT imaging examination. In comparison, MRI is able to demonstrate diminished heterogeneous enhancement of tumors and enhancement of background renal parenchyma, thereby improving detection of cancer in this patient group (Fig. 9.42). Cancers in patients with diminished renal function have a great propensity to undergo hemorrhage [53] (Fig. 9.43), which may be so extensive that the cancer can resemble a hemorrhagic cyst (Fig. 9.44). Therefore, caution must be exercised in interpreting hemorrhagic renal lesions as cysts in patients with chronic renal failure. Renal cancer also may arise in patients with other under-

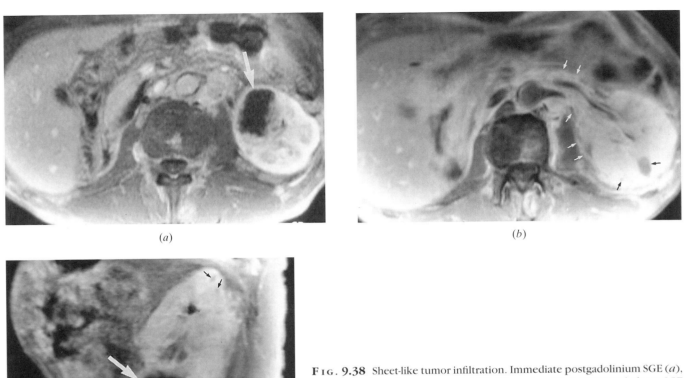

(a)

(b)

(c)

FIG. 9.38 Sheet-like tumor infiltration. Immediate postgadolinium SGE (*a*), interstitial-phase fat-suppressed SGE (*b*), and sagittal interstitial-phase SGE (*c*) images in a patient with prior right nephrectomy for renal cancer. A predominantly cystic renal cancer is present in the lower pole of the left kidney (*large arrow, a,c*). Extensive tumor infiltration in a sheet-like pattern is identified along the renal capsule and into the renal hilum (*small white arrows, b*). Numerous small cysts are also present (*small black arrows, b,c*), which are seeded with tumor.

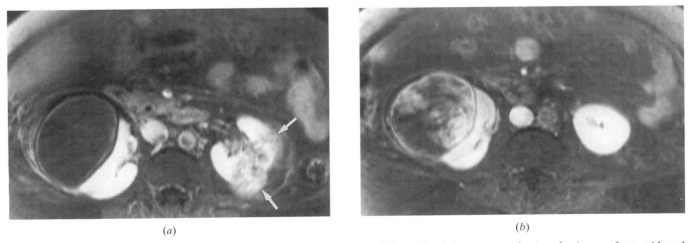

(a)

(b)

FIG. 9.39 Bilateral renal-cell cancer. Interstial-phase gadolinium-enhanced T1-weighted fat-suppressed spin-echo images from midrenal (*a*) and lower renal (*b*) levels. A large cystic/solid renal cancer arises from the right kidney. Two smaller renal cancers (*arrows, a*) are identified at the level of the renal hilum in the left kidney.

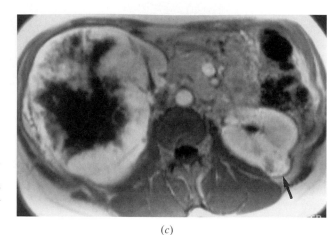

(c)

FIG. 9.39 (*Continued*)   Immediate postgadolinium SGE image (*c*) in a second patient demonstrates bilateral hypervascular renal-cell cancers. The large right renal cancer demonstrates a necrotic center, whereas the 2 cm left renal cancer (*arrow, c*) demonstrates intense heterogeneous enhancement.

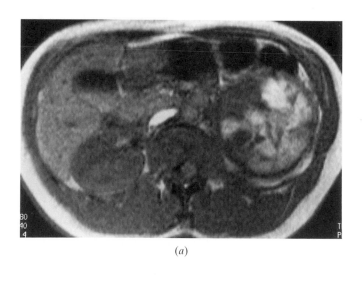

(a)

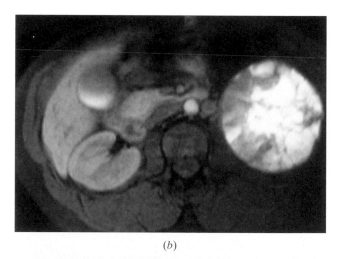

(b)

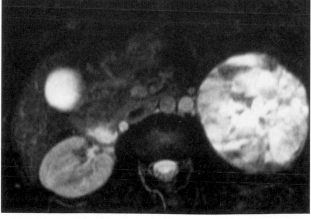

(c)

FIG. 9.40 Multicystic hemorrhagic renal-cell cancer. SGE (*a*), T1-weighted fat-suppressed spin-echo (*b*) and T2-weighted fat-suppressed spin-echo (*c*) images. T1- and T2-weighted images demonstrate an 8-cm tumor arising from the left kidney that contains regions of mixed low and high signal intensity compatible with blood products of varying ages. Small nodular masses of intermediate signal intensity are consistent with solid tumor.

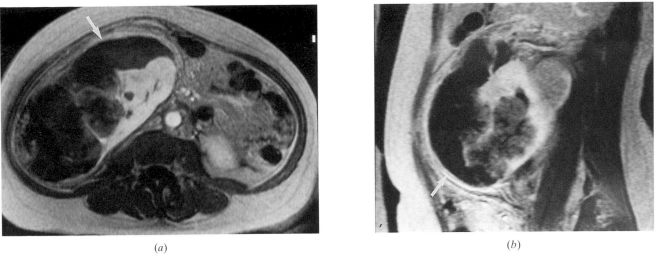

(a)   (b)

FIG. 9.41 Renal-cell cancer with perirenal hemorrhage. Ninety-second transverse (a) and 120-second sagittal (b) postgadolinium SGE images. An 8-cm irregular cystic/solid renal cancer arises from the mid and lower aspect of the right kidney. A large perirenal collection of blood surrounds the kidney (arrows a,b). The blood appears low in signal intensity on postcontrast images due to rescaling of abdominal tissue signal intensities.

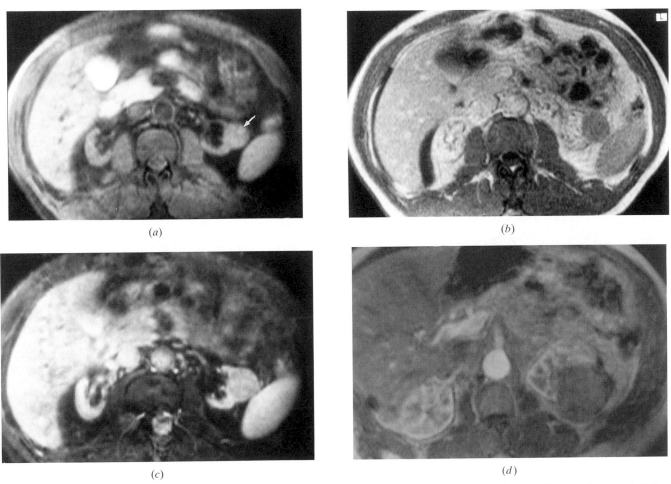

(a)   (b)

(c)   (d)

FIG. 9.42 Hypovascular renal-cell cancer in chronic renal failure. T1-weighted fat-suppressed spin-echo (a), 90-second postgadolinium SGE (b), and interstitial-phase gadolinium-enhanced T1-weighted fat-suppressed spin-echo (c) images. The kidneys are chronically failed and appear atrophic with no corticomedullary differentiation on the precontrast image. A 2.5-cm renal cancer arises from the lateral aspect of the left kidney and contains a punctate high-signal-intensity focus consistent with hemorrhage (arrow, a). The tumor enhances minimally on the 90-second postgadolinium SGE image (b). Small irregular enhancing structures are apparent on the gadolinium-enhanced T1-weighted fat-suppressed image (c), which represents enhancing stroma in a hypovascular renal cancer. Immediate postgadolinium SGE image (d) in a second patient in chronic renal failure with a hypovascular 5.5-cm renal cancer in the left kidney.

413

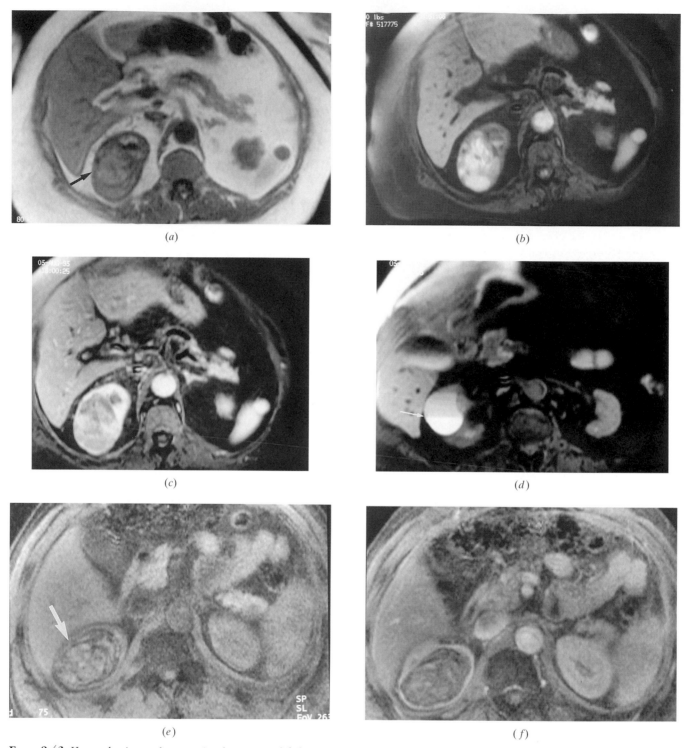

(a)

(b)

(c)

(d)

(e)

(f)

FIG. 9.43 Hemorrhagic renal cancer in chronic renal failure. SGE (a), T1-weighted fat-suppressed spin-echo (b), and interstitial-phase gadolinium-enhanced T1-weighted fat-suppressed spin-echo (c) images. A 5-cm renal cancer is present in the right kidney (arrow, a) that is heterogeneously high in signal intensity on precontrast T1-weighted images (a,b), consistent with hemorrhage, and shows heterogeneous high-signal-intensity stroma on the postgadolinium image (c). T1-weighted fat-suppressed spin-echo image (d) at a level immediately inferior to the renal cancer shows a hemorrhagic renal cyst with a fluid level (arrow, d). Fat-suppressed SGE (e) and 90-second postgadolinium SGE (f) images in a second patient demonstrate a 5-cm tumor that is heterogeneously high in signal intensity on the precontrast fat-suppressed image (arrow, e) and is heterogeneously diminished in signal intensity on the postgadolinium image (f).

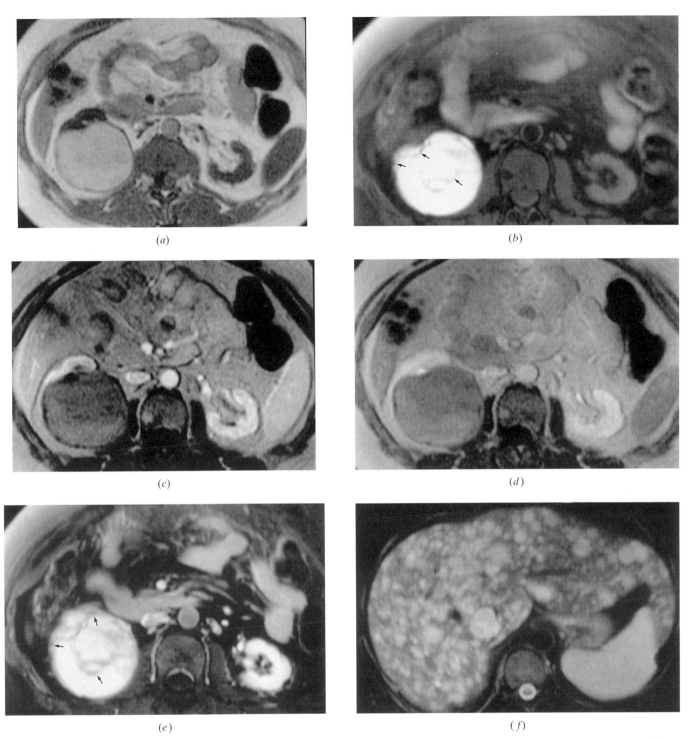

F IG . 9.44 Hemorrhagic cystic renal-cell cancer in chronic renal failure. SGE (*a*), T1-weighted fat-suppressed spin-echo (*b*), immediate postgadolinium SGE (*c*), and interstitial-phase gadolinium-enhanced T1-weighted fat-suppressed spin-echo (*e*) images. A largely cystic hemorrhagic renal mass is noted arising from the lower pole of the right kidney. Small mural-based nodular densities and reticular markings are apparent on precontrast and postcontrast images, which are best shown on the fat-suppressed images (*arrows, b,e*). Multiple surgical biopsies did not reveal renal cancer. T2-weighted fat-suppressed spin-echo (*f*), immediate postgadolinium SGE (*g,b*) and interstitial-phase gadolinium-enhanced T1-weighted fat-suppressed spin-echo (*i*) images obtained 2½ years later. Numerous liver metastases are apparent which are small and high in signal intensity on T2-weighted images (*f*) and enhance in a uniform intense fashion on immediate postgadolinium SGE images (*g,b*).

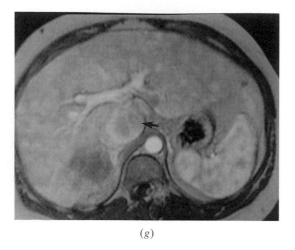

(g)

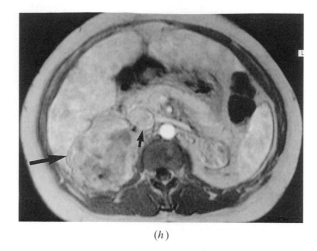

(h)

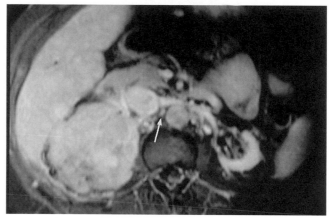

(i)

FIG. 9.44 (*Continued*) An 8-cm hypervascular renal cancer has developed from the cystic cancer (*large arrows, h*), and tumor thrombus expands the IVC (*small arrow, g,h*). Gadolinium-enhanced T1-weighted fat-suppressed spin-echo image shows the heterogeneous cancer, tumor thrombus, and small lymph nodes (*arrow, i*).

lying renal diseases such as polycystic kidney disease (Fig. 9.45).

MRI is slightly superior to dynamic contrast-enhanced CT imaging for the detection, characterization, and staging of renal cancer [1,11,41]. There is, however, little difference between dual-phase spiral CT imaging and MRI in the routine investigation of renal masses. There are definite indications for the use of MRI, which include (1) allergy to iodine contrast; (2) indeterminate, particularly calcified renal masses; and (3) renal failure [53–56]. The greater enhancement of renal parenchyma in patients with renal failure, the smaller volume of contrast, and lesser renal toxicity justify the routine use of contrast-enhanced MRI in these patients [53–56]. If necessary, gadolinium also may be hemodialyzed [57]. There may be no indication to perform noncontrast CT imaging alone in the investigation of renal masses.

Early detection of renal cancer is critical to improving patient survival [33,58,59]. Due to the ability of MRI to detect renal tumors smaller than 1 cm in diameter, the role of MRI in detecting and characterizing renal masses may become increasingly important in patients with bilateral renal tumors or in patients scheduled for renal-spar-

ing surgery because both CT imaging and ultrasound miss at least 50 percent of tumors smaller than 1 cm [60]. This may have a greater impact in the future, because renal-sparing surgery is becoming a more prevalent practice [61–64].

Wilms Tumor

Wilms tumor is a rare solid tumor of the kidney found in children with a peak occurrence at 2 years of age and 75 percent occurring before the age of 5. Wilms has a triphasic histology composed of blastema, epithelial, and stromal elements. Focal hemorrhage and necrosis are not uncommon. The lesions are usually solitary but may be multiple in 5 to 10 percent of cases. Wilms tumors present as large masses that calcify in only 5 percent of cases, in contrast to neuroblastomas, which calcify in 50 percent of cases. Unilateral Wilms tumor is associated with a 41 percent incidence of nephrogenic rests, whereas multifocal Wilms has a 99 percent incidence of nephrogenic rests [65]. Associated congenital abnormalities include aniridia and hemihypertrophy as well as Beckwith-Wiedeman and Drash syndromes.

Current staging of Wilms involves a 5-stage system

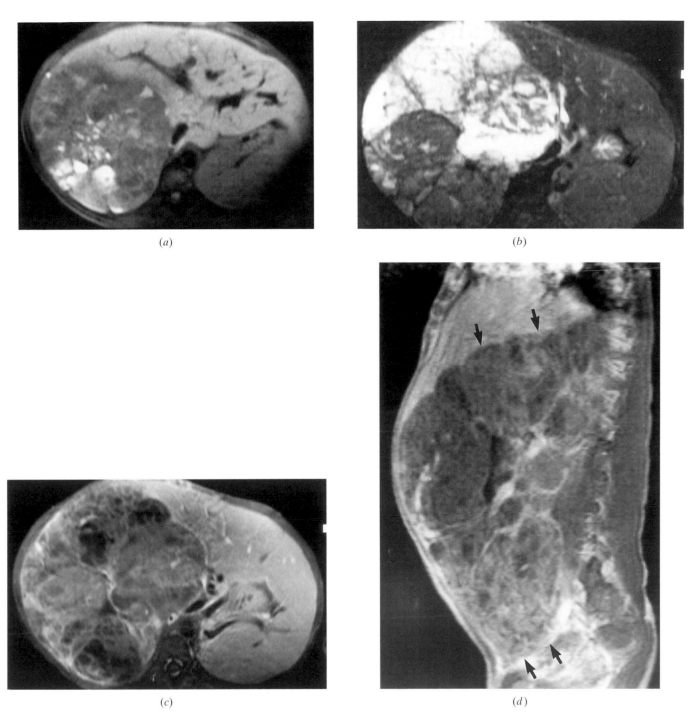

(a)

(b)

(c)

(d)

FIG. 9.45 Renal cell cancer in autosomal dominant polycystic kidney disease. T1-weighted fat-suppressed spin-echo (a), T2-weighted fat-suppressed spin-echo (b), interstitial-phase gadolinium-enhanced T1-weighted fat-suppressed spin-echo (c) and sagittal interstitial-phase gadolinium-enhanced SGE (d) images. A large multilocular renal mass is present involving the entire right kidney. Cystic spaces vary in signal on T1-weighted (a) and T2-weighted (b) images, consistent with blood products of differing age. Enhancement of septations and more solid tissue is present on postgadolinium images (c,d). The superior-inferior extent of the massive tumor is shown on the sagittal-plane image (arrows, d). Tumor infiltration of the entire kidney was present at histopathology. The left kidney had been removed with the same histological findings.

in which Stage 1 is a tumor confined to the kidney and completely excised; Stage 2 is a tumor extended beyond the kidney and completely excised; Stage 3 is a residual tumor after surgery confined to the abdomen; Stage 4 is hematogeneous metastases; and Stage 5 is bilateral renal involvement [66]. Metastases occur to the lungs, liver, and lymph nodes. Wilms tumor, in rare instances, may be highly cystic. Tumors arise from the kidney with an appearance at times indistinguishable from that of renal-cell cancer. Age constitutes a criterion for predicting the diagnosis. The most common renal malignancy in the pediatric patient is Wilms tumor. A transition occurs in the midteens after which renal-cell cancer is the most common renal tumor. Features suggestive of Wilms tumor are large renal tumors that cross the midline. Central necrosis and tumor thrombus are less common in large

Wilms tumors compared to renal-cell cancer, but this does not provide useful differentiating information. Wilms tumors commonly contain central hemorrhage.

Wilms tumors are slightly hypointense on T1-weighted images and slightly hyperintense on T2-weighted images [65]. Large cancers are frequently heterogeneous with regions of high signal intensity on T1-weighted images due to the presence of hemorrhage (Fig. 9.46). Tumors enhance heterogeneously on postgadolinium images, but tend to be less intensely enhanced and less heterogeneous than renal-cell cancer on early postcontrast images. Nephrogenic rests are typically smaller than 2 cm and enhance minimally on postgadolinium images [65]. As with renal cancer, tumor thrombus in Wilms tumor is well-shown on MR images (Fig. 9.47) and is better defined than on CT images [67].

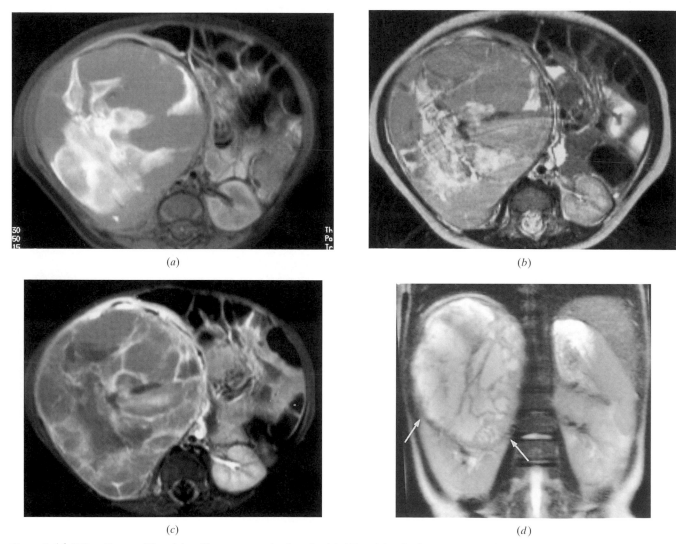

(a)   (b)

(c)   (d)

F I G . 9.46 Wilms Tumor. T1-weighted fat-suppressed spin-echo (*a*), T2-weighted echo-train spin-echo (*b*), and interstitial-phase gadolinium-enhanced T1-weighted fat-suppressed spin-echo (*c*) images. A large mass arises from the right kidney, and demonstrates central linear regions of high signal intensity on T1- and T2-weighted images consistent with blood. No substantial central necrosis is identified on the postcontrast images despite the large size of the tumor.

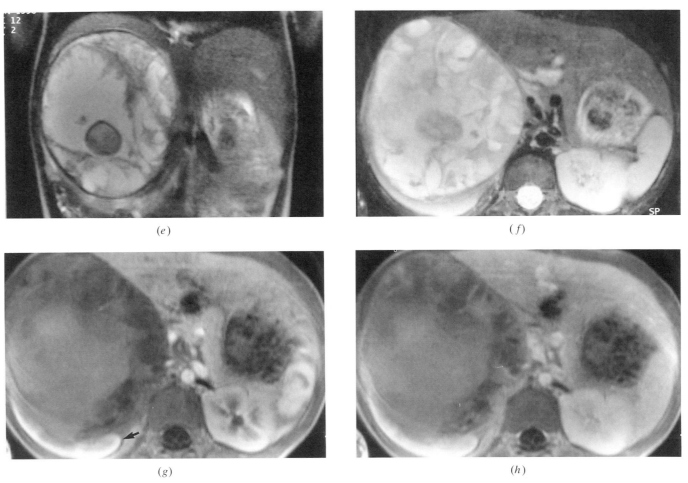

(e)

(f)

(g)

(h)

Fig. 9.46 (*Continued*) Coronal HASTE (*d,e*), T2-weighted fat-suppressed spin-echo (*f*), immediate (*g*), and 90-second (*h*) postgadolinium SGE images in a second patient. A large heterogeneous Wilms tumor arises from the upper pole of the right kidney (*arrows, d*). A rim of posterior normal renal cortex is apparent (*arrow, g*).

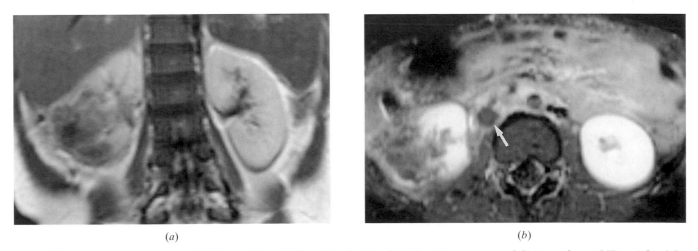

(a)

(b)

Fig. 9.47 Wilms tumor. Coronal gadolinium-enhanced T1-weighted spin-echo (*a*) and transverse gadolinium-enhanced T1-weighted fat-suppressed spin-echo (*b*) images. A heterogeneously enhancing tumor is present arising from the mid and lower pole of the right kidney (*a,b*). Thrombus is noted in the IVC (*arrow, b*), which represents blood thrombus at this tomographic section inferior to the renal vein.

Lymphoma

Lymphomatous involvement of the kidneys generally occurs in the context of widespread disease. However, isolated focal involvement of the kidney does occur [68–70]. Non-Hodgkin's lymphoma more commonly involves the kidneys than does Hodgkin's, and is most commonly the B-cell type [68]. Three basic patterns of involvement occur, which are (1) direct invasion from adjacent disease, most commonly large retroperitoneal masses (Fig. 9.48); (2) focal masses that may be solitary or multiple (Fig. 9.49 and 9.50); and (3) diffuse infiltration (Fig. 9.51) [68–70]. Lymphoma commonly extends along the subcapsular surface of the kidney, particularly in the setting of invasion from adjacent disease. Renal parenchyma lacks lymphoid tissue, so primary renal lymphoma usually arises from lymphatic tissue in the renal sinus.

Lymphoma is generally slightly hypointense relative to renal cortex on T1-weighted images and heterogeneous and slightly hypointense to isointense on T2-weighted images. Gadolinium enhancement of most lymphomas is mildly heterogeneous and minimal on early postcontrast images and remains minimal on late postcontrast images [70].

Lymphoma tends to infiltrate the renal medulla. Retroperitoneal lymphoma that invades the kidney usually extends through the renal sinus into the renal medulla (see Fig. 9.48). Diffuse infiltration of the kidney predominantly affects the medulla with relative sparing of the renal cortex (see Fig. 9.51) [67]. Focal masses arise in the renal medulla or cortex (see Fig. 9.49) [70,71]. Cortex-based masses tend to enhance more intensely than other forms of renal involvement [70,71], which may reflect the

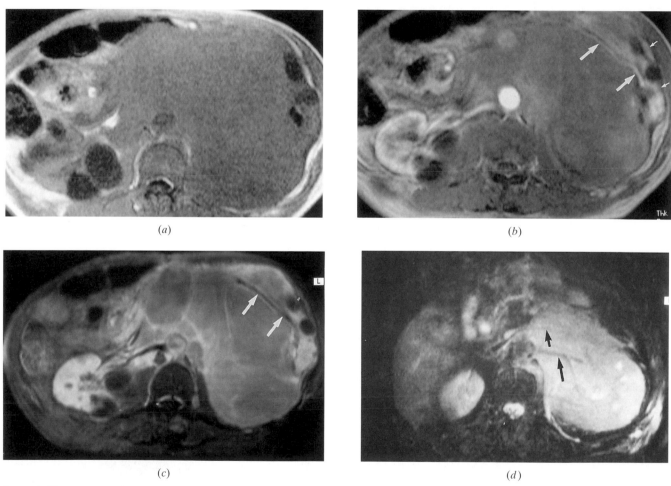

(a)

(b)

(c)

(d)

FIG. 9.48 Renal lymphoma, large retroperitoneal mass invading kidney. SGE (*a*), immediate postgadolinium SGE (*b*), and gadolinium-enhanced T1-weighted fat-suppressed spin-echo (*c*) images. A large retroperitoneal mass is present that is homogeneous and soft tissue signal intensity on the SGE image (*a*), and enhances minimally on capillary-phase (*b*) and interstitial-phase (*c*) images. On postcontrast images lymphoma is moderately heterogeneous with no evidence of necrosis. A thin rim of spared renal cortex is evident (*small arrows, b*), and the kidney is displaced anterolaterally. Tumor invades through the renal pelvis into the renal medulla. The renal artery is patent (*arrows, b,c*) but encased by lymphoma. Patency is shown by the presence of high-signal-intensity gadolinium in the artery on the immediate postgadolinium SGE image (*b*) and by flow-void on the spin-echo image (*c*). In a second patient, a similar appearance of lymphoma is shown on T2-weighted fat-suppressed spin-echo (*d*), immediate (*e*), and 90-second (*f*) postgadolinium SGE, and gadolinium-enhanced T1-weighted fat-suppressed spin-echo (*g*) images.

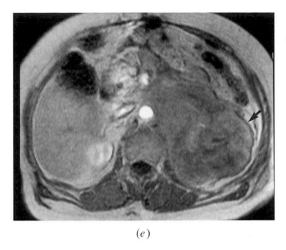

(e)

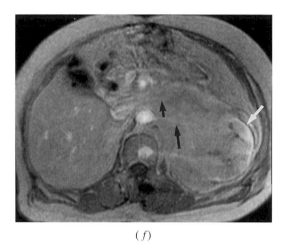

(f)

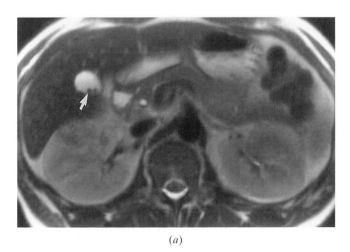

(g)

FIG. 9.48 (*Continued*) Lymphoma is mildly hyperintense on the T2-weighted image (*d*), and heterogeneous and mildly enhanced on capillary-phase (*e*) and interstitial-phase (*f,g*) gadolinium-enhanced images. The renal artery (*arrow d,f,g*) and renal vein (*small arrow d,f,g*) are encased by tumor but patent. Patency is demonstrated by the presence of high signal intensity on the SGE image (*f*) and signal-void on the spin-echo images (*d,g*). The involved kidney demonstrates diminished cortical enhancement (*arrow, e*) relative to the normal contralateral right kidney on the capillary-phase image (*e*). Lymphoma has extensively invaded the medulla, but relative sparing of cortex is observed (*white arrow f,g*).

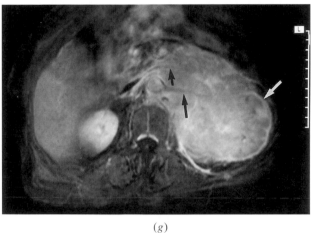

(a)

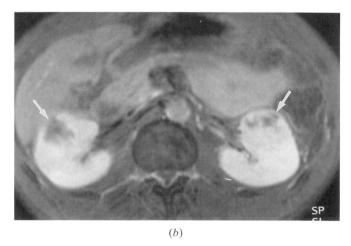

(b)

FIG. 9.49 Lymphoma, multifocal renal involvement. T2-weighted breathing-independent HASTE (*a*) and gadolinium-enhanced T1-weighted fat-suppressed spin-echo (*b*) images. Lymphoma masses are mildly hypo- to isointense on T2-weighted images (*a*) and heterogeneous with low-signal-intensity centers (*arrows, b*) on interstitial-phase gadolinium-enhanced images. Incidental note is made of gallstones, which are well-shown on the breathing-independent T2-weighted image (*arrow, a*).

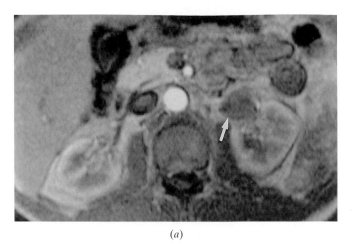

(a)

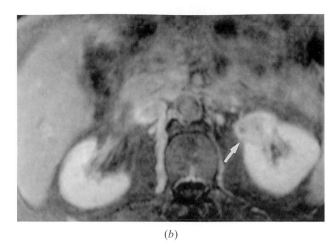

(b)

FIG. **9.50** Lymphoma, solitary mass. Immediate postgadolinium SGE (*a*) and gadolinium-enhanced T1-weighted fat-suppressed spin-echo (*b*) images. A solitary lymphoma mass is present in the left kidney (*arrow a,b*) that is minimally enhanced on the capillary-phase image (*a*) and heterogeneous and moderately enhanced on the interstitial phase image (*b*). (Reproduced with permission from Semelka RC, Kelekis NL, Burdeny DA, Mitchell DG, Brown JJ, Siegelman ES: Renal lymphoma: Demonstration by MR imaging. AJR Am J Roentgenol 166:823–827, 1996)

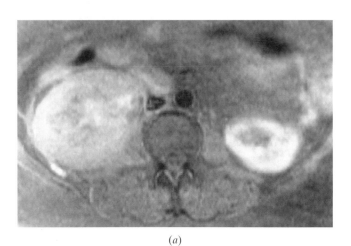

(a)

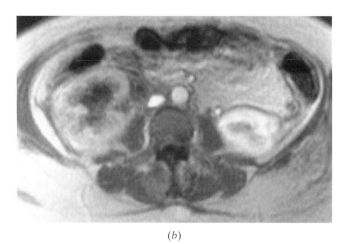

(b)

FIG. **9.51** Lymphoma, diffuse infiltration. T1-weighted fat-suppressed spin-echo (*a*), immediate postgadolinium SGE (*b*), and gadolinium-enhanced T1-weighted fat-suppressed spin-echo (*c*) images. The right kidney is enlarged in a generalized fashion (*a–c*). Corticomedullary differentiation is not well-shown on the precontrast T1-weighted image (*a*). On the immediate postgadolinium image (*b*) diminished enhancement of the renal cortex is present. However the cortex has a normal thickness and uniformity. On the later interstitial phase image increased enhancement is present of the outer medulla, and multiple low-signal-intensity foci (*arrow, c*) are present in the inner medulla, which likely represent focal aggregates of lymphoma. (Reproduced with permission from Semelka RC, Kelekis NL, Burdeny DA, Mitchell DG, Brown JJ, Siegelman ES: Renal lymphoma: Demonstration by MR imaging. AJR Am J Roentgenol 166:823–827, 1996)

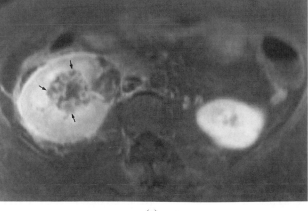

(c)

greater blood supply of the cortex. As most forms of lymphoma involve the medulla, these tumors can be distinguished from renal cancer because renal cancers originate in the renal cortex. Other distinguishing features include (1) the degree of vascularity (lymphoma shows mild diffuse heterogeneous enhancement, whereas renal cancer shows intense early heterogeneous enhancement), (2) the presence of necrosis (necrosis is uncommon in lymphoma, even in large masses, whereas central necrosis is very common in large renal cancers), (3) the presence of tumor thrombus (lymphoma rarely results in tumor thrombus, whereas tumor thrombus is common in large renal cancers), (4) the center of the tumor (in lymphoma the center is most often outside the contour of the kidney, whereas in renal cancer it is in the renal cortex), (5) the renal artery encasement with diminished capillary-phase enhancement of the entire kidney (diffusely infiltrative lymphoma commonly encases the renal artery and results in generalized diminished renal enhancement (70), which is a rare finding in renal cancer), and (6) direct extension and involvement of the psoas muscle (common in lymphoma and rare in renal cancer). Solitary focal renal cortical involvement of lymphoma, however, may resemble renal cancer. Focal masses usually arise in the setting of recurrent disease, so the history of lymphoma is known, and diagnosis can be established based on clinical history.

Chloromas (Leukemic Focal Infiltrates)

Chloromas, focal aggregates of leukemic cells in tissues, may appear as focal masses arising in kidney or the perirenal space. Chloromas are frequently hypovascular

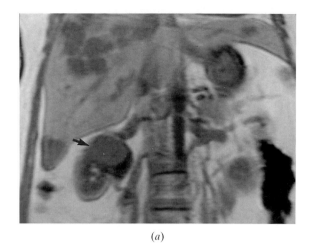

(a)

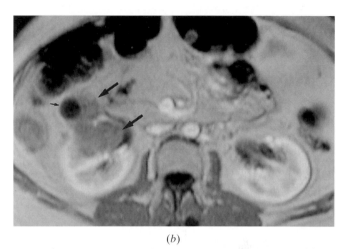

(b)

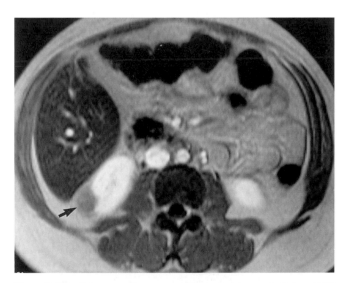

FIG. 9.52 Chloroma. Transverse 90-second postgadolinium SGE image in a patient with acute myelogenous leukemia. A homogeneous minimally enhanced 2-cm chloroma (arrow) arises from the upper pole of the right kidney. The liver is low in signal intensity secondary to transfusional hemosiderosis.

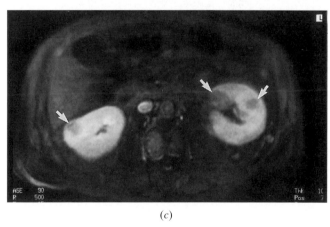

(c)

FIG. 9.53 Renal metastases. Coronal SGE (a) and immediate postgadolinium transverse SGE (b) images. On the precontrast image (a), a homogeneous intermediate signal-intensity mass is noted in the right kidney (arrow, a). In addition, multiple leiomyosarcoma liver metastases are present. On the immediate postcontrast image the renal metastasis (arrow, b) is noted to involve cortex and medulla (arrow, b) and extend into the perirenal space. The mass contains a small cystic component (small arrow, b). Gadolinium-enhanced T1-weighted fat-suppressed image (c) in a second patient who has renal metastases from lung cancer and demonstrates multiple low-signal-intensity metastatic lesions in both kidneys (arrows, c).

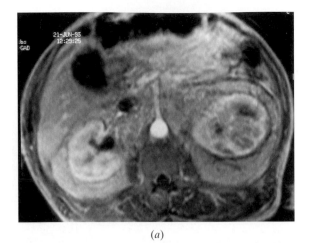

(a)

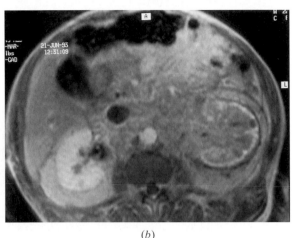

(b)

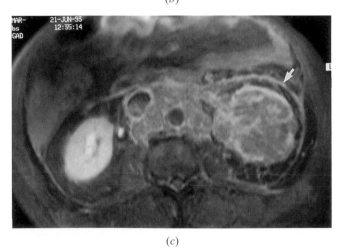

(c)

FIG. 9.54 Renal metastases, undifferentiated adenocarcinoma. Immediate (a) and 90-second (b) postgadolinium SGE and gadolinium-enhanced T1-weighted fat-suppressed spin-echo (c) images. Massive retroperitoneal adenopathy with extension through the renal hilum and invasion of the renal medulla is present (a-c). Extensive infiltration of the medulla with relative sparing of the cortex is well-shown on interstitial-phase images (b,c). The appearance of renal involvement resembles lymphoma. Thickening of Gerota's fascia (arrow, c) and retroperitoneal adenopathy are best shown on the gadolinium-enhanced fat-suppressed image. This reflects good conspicuity of enhanced malignant tissue in a background of suppressed fat.

and are low in signal intensity on precontrast T1- and T2-weighted images and on postgadolinium images (Fig. 9.52).

Metastases

Metastases to the kidney are a late manifestation of advanced disease. Lung and breast cancer are the two most common primaries, but metastases may occur in the setting of many malignant diseases. Metastases usually appear as multiple bilateral renal masses, but solitary masses may occur (Fig. 9.53). Anaplastic adenocarcinomas may diffusely infiltrate the kidneys with a similar appearance to that of lymphoma (Fig. 9.54).

DIFFUSE RENAL PARENCHYMAL DISEASE

Diffuse renal parenchymal diseases are common medical conditions. A variety of disease processes may result in parenchymal disease, and they may be classified into the following broad categories: glomerular disease; acute and chronic tubulointerstitial disease; diabetic nephropathy and nephrosclerosis, collectively referred to as microvascular disease; and ischemic nephropathy caused by disease of the main renal arteries; obstructive nephropathy; and infectious renal disease [72].

MRI has played a limited role in the evaluation of diffuse renal parenchymal disease. The intrinsic high soft-tissue contrast resolution of breath-hold SGE and fat-suppressed images, and the clear definition of the renal cortex on immediate postgadolinium images does provide useful information for the evaluation of morphological changes associated with these entities [72]. The renal cortex is most distinctly shown on immediate postgadolinium SGE images, and alterations of thickness, regularity, and temporal enhancement of the cortex provides information that correlates with underlying pathophysiology [72]. A recent study of 121 patients with renal disease [72] described MRI findings for diffuse parenchymal diseases. The presence of corticomedullary differentiation (CMD) demonstrated a strong inverse relationship with serum creatinine (sCr) ($r = -.568$, $p < .001$). The mean cortex thickness for normal kidney and kidneys with glomerular disease was 8.4 and 7.8 mm, respectively, which were significantly thicker ($p < .01$) than renal cortex in patients with microvascular disease (5.2 mm), tubulointerstitial disease secondary to antineoplastic chemotherapy (5.6 mm), ischemic nephropathy (5.5 mm), and obstructive nephropathy (4.3 mm). Irregularity of the renal cortex was common in microvascular disease (60.9%), infectious renal disease (62.5%), obstructive nephropathy (55.6%), and nonchemotherapy tubulointerstitial disease (53.8%), compared to chemotherapy-induced tubulointerstitial disease (5.9%), glomerular disease (3.8%), and normal kidneys (0%). Diffuse high signal intensity of the entire medulla on delayed postcontrast images was observed in 20.7 percent of patients with diffuse renal disease and in none of the patients with normal kidneys. Combining this information with other imaging findings, such as dilation of the renal collecting system in obstructive nephropathy or atherosclerotic disease of the aorta in ischemic nephropathy and microvascular disease, allows prediction of the probable underlying type of diffuse renal parenchymal disease. Dynamic changes of temporal enhancement of the cortex and medulla in normal kidneys, obstructive nephropathy, and post extracorporeal shock wave lithotripsy for renal calculous disease has been described [5,13,54]. Temporal changes in other causes of diffuse renal parenchymal disease remains to be established.

Diminished Renal Function

Loss of corticomedullary differentiation on T1-weighted images in patients with elevated sCr has been described [73]. This is a nonspecific finding observed in virtually all renal diseases that result in diminished renal function [73]. Demonstration of corticomedullary differentiation is best made on precontrast T1-weighted fat-suppressed images [73]. Fat-suppressed SGE imaging may be superior to fat-suppressed spin-echo imaging because breath-holding results in greater image sharpness. In one study that described the relationship of corticomedullary differentiation to the level of sCr using precontrast T1-weighted fat-suppressed spin-echo and immediate postgadolinium SGE imaging, all patients with sCr greater than 3.0 mg/dL showed loss of corticomedullary differentiation on precontrast images (Fig. 9.55) [73]. In patients with sCr 1.5

to 2.9 mg/dL, the loss of corticomedullary differentiation occurred in approximately half of the patients. The loss of corticomedullary differentiation on immediate post-gadolinium SGE images was not observed until sCr exceeded 8.5 mg/dL. Changes in fluid content between cortex and medulla likely account for the changes on precontrast images. This reflects some combination of increased fluid in cortex and decreased fluid in the medulla. Corticomedullary differentiation on immediate postgadolinium images reflects autoregulatory blood flow distribution in the kidney that may be lost in advanced renal disease. This may reflect irreversible renal parenchymal damage [73].

Not all patients with elevated sCr will show loss of CMD. Loss of corticomedullary differentiation on precontrast images presumably develops over some period of time. Patients with acute renal failure who are imaged within 1 week of onset may show preservation of corticomedullary differentiation [72].

Glomerular Disease

The clinical manifestations of glomerular disease are varied and range from asymptomatic urinary abnormalities to acute nephritis, nephrotic syndrome, and chronic renal failure. In patients with nephrotic syndrome, the majority have membranous nephropathy, and MRI findings are generally minimal (Fig. 9.56) [72]. Diffuse high signal intensity of the medulla on delayed postgadolinium images may be observed. In chronic disease, cortical thinning is smooth, and medullary atrophy may be substantial (Fig. 9.57). Nephrotic syndrome may also be associated with renal-vein thrombosis. Renal-vein thrombus may be well-shown using a number of MRI techniques [41,51,72,74]. SGE images acquired 45 to 120 seconds

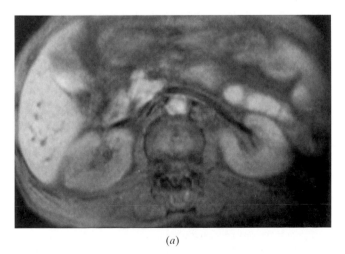

(a)

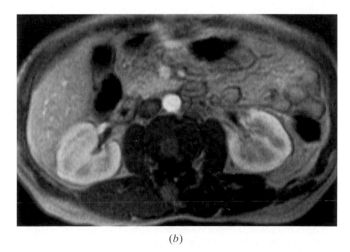

(b)

FIG. 9.55 Elevated serum creatinine (3 mg/dL) with loss of CMD. T1-weighted fat-suppressed spin-echo (a) and immediate postgadolinium SGE (b) images. Loss of corticomedullary differentiation on the precontrast image (a) is noted with preservation of corticomedullary differentiation on the immediate postgadolinium SGE (b) image. Loss of corticomedullary differentiation on precontrast T1-weighted images is a nonspecific finding of diminished renal function.

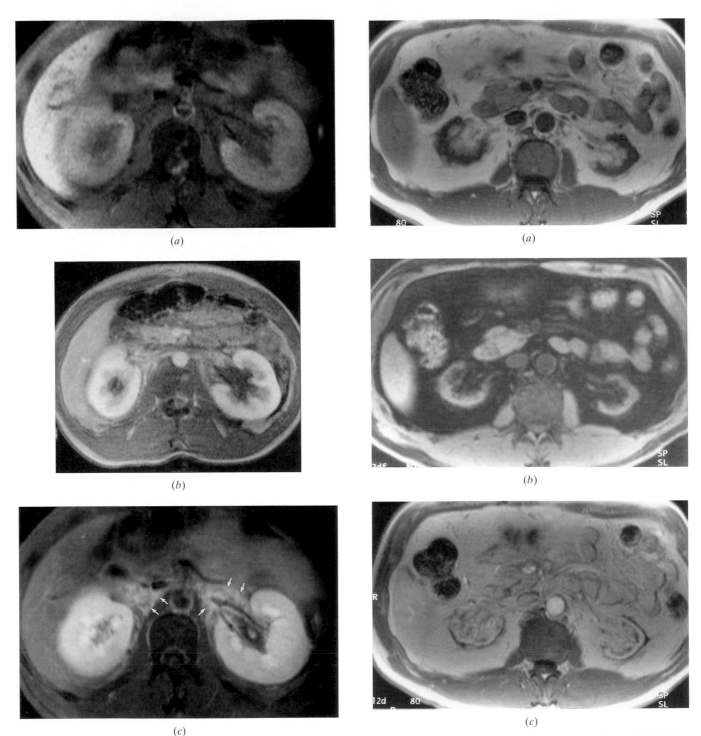

(a)

(b)

(c)

(a)

(b)

(c)

FIG. 9.56 Recent onset membranous nephropathy. T1-weighted fat-suppressed spin-echo (a), immediate postgadolinium SGE (b), and gadolinium-enhanced T1-weighted fat-suppressed spin-echo (c) images. Corticomedullary differentiation is diminished on the precontrast image (a). Renal cortex is uniform and of normal thickness on the immediate postgadolinium image (b). Diffuse increased enhancement of the medulla is noted on the interstitial-phase image (c). Enhancing plate-like retroperitoneal tissue is present that extends into the left renal hilum (arrow, b). This represents acute benign retroperitoneal fibrosis.

FIG. 9.57 Chronic membranous glomerulonephritis. SGE (a), fat-suppressed SGE (b), and immediate postgadolinium SGE (c) images. No corticomedullary differentiation is appreciated on precontrast images (a,b). The immediate postgadolinium image (c) demonstrates uniform cortical thinning and disproportionate atrophy of the renal medulla. Fat in the renal sinus has increased in volume to supplant the atrophic medulla.

after gadolinium serve as an effective technique for demonstrating renal-vein thrombus (Fig. 9.58). Detection of thrombus is important because it is treatable with thrombolytic agents, and successful treatment may result in improvement of the condition.

Tubulointerstitial Disease

A variety of underlying etiologies may result in tubulointerstitial disease of which drug-related causes are among the most common. Tubulointerstitial disease secondary to analgesic drug overuse results in irregular cortical thinning (Fig. 9.59) [72]. The irregularity presumably reflects the intermittent nature of the insult because drug intake is intermittent. Tubulointerstitial disease from antineo-

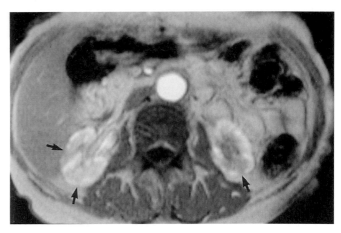

F I G . **9.59** Tubulointerstitial disease secondary to analgesic abuse. Immediate postgadolinium SGE image demonstrates irregular cortical thinning ranging in thickness from 1 to 4 mm. Regions of extreme cortical thinning are apparent (*arrows*). (Reproduced with permission from Kettritz U, Semelka RC, Brown ED, Sharp TJ, Lawing WL, Colindres RE: MR findings in diffuse renal parenchymal disease. J Magn Reson Imaging 6:136–144, 1996)

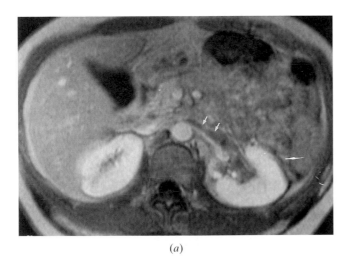

(*a*)

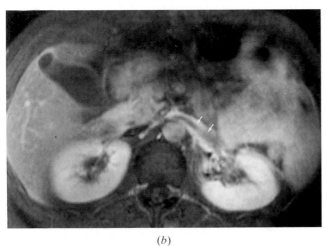

(*b*)

F I G . **9.58** Renal-vein thrombosis with nephrotic syndrome. Ninety-second gadolinium-enhanced SGE (*a*) and gadolinium-enhanced T1-weighted fat-suppressed spin-echo (*b*) images. Low-signal bland thrombus is identified in the left renal vein (*arrows a,b*). Flow in the vein surrounding the thrombus is identified as high signal intensity on these images. Greater conspicuity of gadolinium in the patent periphery of the vein is apparent on the fat-suppressed image due to suppression of the competing signal intensity of fat (*b*).

plastic chemotherapy results in more uniform cortical thinning (Fig. 9.60) [72]. This presumably reflects the fact that the cortical insult is more constant due to the regular rate of chemotherapy drug administration.

Acute Tubular Necrosis

Acute tubular necrosis results from metabolic or toxic etiologies in the majority of cases. Within 1 week of onset of this condition corticomedullary differentiation may be preserved despite substantial elevation of sCr (Fig. 9.61). This likely reflects the fact that the loss of corticomedullary differentiation may take more than 1 week to develop.

Tubular Blockage

A number of etiological agents may result in tubular blockage. Renal failure may result from blockage of a substantial portion of the renal tubules by various substances. The classical example of diffuse tubular blockage is by Bence-Jones proteinuria in multiple myeloma (Fig. 9.62).

Iron Deposition

Iron deposition occurs in the renal cortex in the setting of intravascular hemolysis with hemoglobin accumulation in renal glomeruli. Sickle-cell disease is the most common entity to result in this condition [75,76]. The usual appearance is low signal intensity of the renal cortex due to the T2*-shortening effects of iron. This is best appreciated on gradient-echo or T2-weighted images (Fig. 9.63). On immediate postgadolinium images the T1-shortening effects usually exceed the T2-shortening

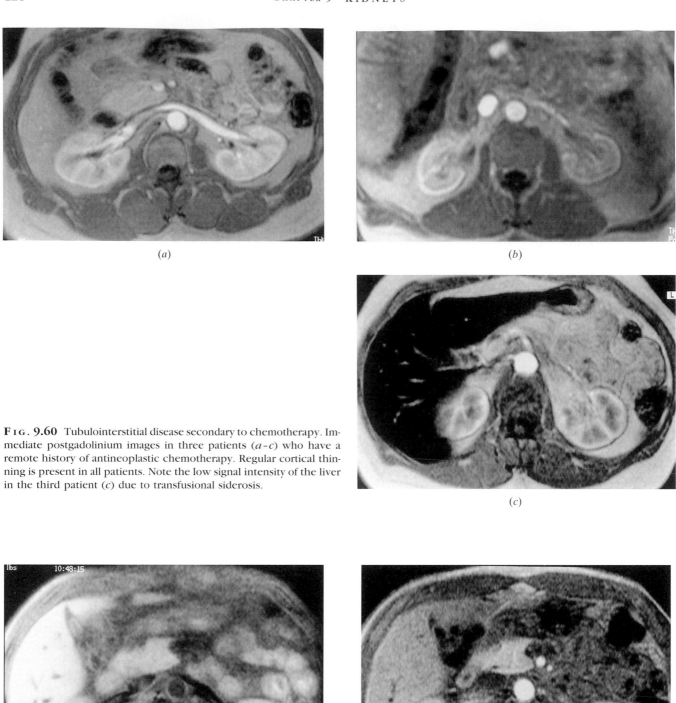

(a)

(b)

FIG. 9.60 Tubulointerstitial disease secondary to chemotherapy. Immediate postgadolinium images in three patients (*a-c*) who have a remote history of antineoplastic chemotherapy. Regular cortical thinning is present in all patients. Note the low signal intensity of the liver in the third patient (*c*) due to transfusional siderosis.

(c)

(a)

(b)

FIG. 9.61 Acute tubular necrosis. T1-weighted fat-suppressed spin-echo (*a*) and immediate postgadolinium SGE (*b*) images. Corticomedullary differentiation is demonstrated on both precontrast (*a*) and immediate postcontrast (*b*) images in a patient with acute tubular necrosis and serum creatinine of 6.3 mg/dL. Acute tubular necrosis developed within 1 week prior to MRI examination, and presumably the acute nature of the injury accounts for the presence of corticomedullary differentiation on the precontrast image.

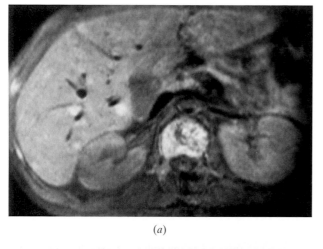

(a)

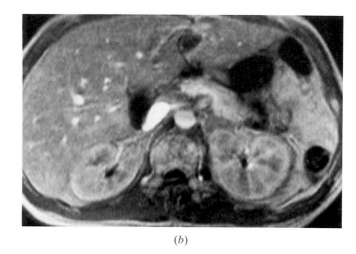

(b)

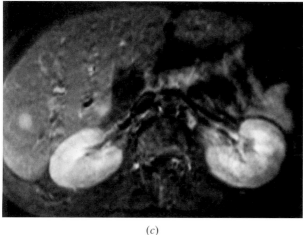

(c)

FIG. 9.62 Tubular blockage from Bence-Jones proteinuria. Precontrast T1-weighted fat-suppressed spin-echo (*a*), immediate postgadolinium SGE (*b*), and gadolinium-enhanced T1-weighted fat-suppressed spin-echo (*c*) images. This patient with multiple myeloma has high-signal-intensity lesions in the bone marrow and liver and absent corticomedullary differentiation on precontrast T1-weighted fat-suppressed spin-echo images (*a*). On immediate postgadolinium images (*b*), corticomedullary differentiation is present, but cortical enhancement is not intense. On interstitial-phase T1-weighted fat-suppressed spin-echo images (*c*) diffuse high signal intensity is present in the renal medulla suggesting the presence of tubular leakage of gadolinium.

effects of the iron in the renal cortex, resulting in high-signal-intensity-enhanced renal cortex. On interstitial-phase images, passage of contrast into the tubules and enhancement of the medulla results in signal reversal, with the cortex becoming lower in signal intensity than the medulla (Fig. 9.64). Less commonly, dilute concentration iron in the glomeruli may result in a high-signal-intensity renal cortex (Fig. 9.65). The spleen in sickle-cell disease is also affected with iron deposition, and splenic infarcts are observed.

Paroxysmal nocturnal hemoglobinuria results in iron deposition in the renal cortex [77]. Iron deposition in the liver and spleen are variable and related to blood transfusions or portal hypertension [77].

Parenchymal Changes From Obstruction

Acute and chronic obstruction are well-shown on MR images. In acute obstruction kidney size is enlarged, and contrast persists in the renal parenchyma for a prolonged

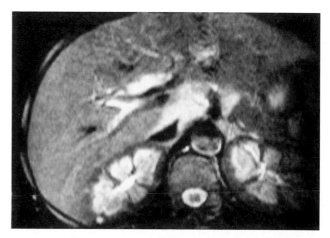

FIG. 9.63 Sickle cell disease. T2-weighted fat-suppressed spin-echo image demonstrates low signal intensity of renal cortex secondary to accumulation of free hemoglobin. High-signal-intensity celiac and porta hepatic nodes are also present.

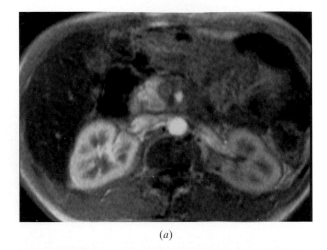

(*a*)

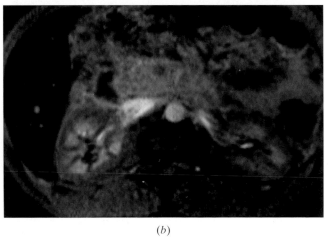

(*b*)

FIG. 9.64 Sickle-cell disease. Immediate (*a*) and 2-minute (*b*) postgadolinium SGE images. On the immediate postgadolinium image (*a*), the renal cortex is high in signal intensity, which reflects that the T1-shortening effect of gadolinium exceeds the T2-shortening effects of iron. At 2 minutes after injection (*b*), the T2-shortening of iron in the cortex exceeds the T1-shortening of gadolinium, causing diminished signal intensity of the cortex. The relative washout of gadolinium from the cortex coupled with the transit of gadolinium into the medulla results in this signal reversal of cortex and medulla. Signal intensity changes in renal parenchyma on postgadolinium images in patients with sickle-cell disease reflect the changing balance of T2-shortening effects of iron and T1-shortening effects of gadolinium.

period of time resulting in a prolonged nephrogram phase (Fig. 9.66). The appearance of gadolinium in the collecting system is usually dilute due to a combination of the excretion of dilute urine, which occurs in the setting of acute severe obstruction, and the dilutional effect of gadolinium within a large volume of urine in a dilated collecting system. Corticomedullary differentiation is diminished on immediate postgadolinium images [5]. In chronic obstruction, the kidney initially is enlarged and, over time, gradually decreases in size with diminished renal perfusion (Fig. 9.67) [5]. Renal cortical thinning

develops and in pure renal obstruction is usually uniform. Irregular cortical thinning, however, is not unusual. The regularity of cortical thinning presumably reflects the tissue pressure experienced in different portions of the kidney. Irregular thinning may be related to variations in calyceal dilatation and pressure. The presence of associated reflux in some conditions also contributes to irregular cortical thinning (Fig. 9.68). The collecting system generally remains dilated when the kidney atrophies, which permits distinction of chronic obstruction from chronic ischemia.

Reflux Nephropathy and Chronic Pyelonephritis
Reflux nephropathy represents renal parenchymal changes secondary to urine reflux into the renal collecting system. Changes of reflux nephropathy are more common in the polar regions due to the presence of compound papillae. Renal scarring is a frequent sequela of reflux nephropathy and occurs superficial to dilated calyces (Fig. 9.69). The renal cortex is thin and usually very irregular [72]. Chronic pyelonephritis is characterized by the combination of extensive calyceal dilatation and irregularity with overlying cortical scarring.

Renal Arterial Disease
Disease of the renal arterial system may be thrombotic/arterial wall or embolic in nature. Thrombosis/arterial-wall disease may be further subdivided into large-vessel, medium-vessel, and small-vessel disease.

Ischemic nephropathy results from atherosclerotic disease of the main renal artery. Concomitant changes of atherosclerotic disease of the abdominal aorta are virtually always present. MRI studies can be tailored to demonstrate both the anatomic change of renal artery disease and the functional consequences of renal artery perfusion

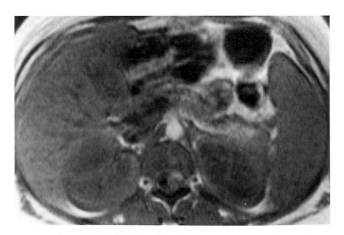

FIG. 9.65 Sickle-cell disease. SGE image demonstrates preservation of corticomedullary differentiation in a patient with sickle-cell disease due to the presence of dilute iron in the renal cortex that results in a T1-shortening paramagnetic effect.

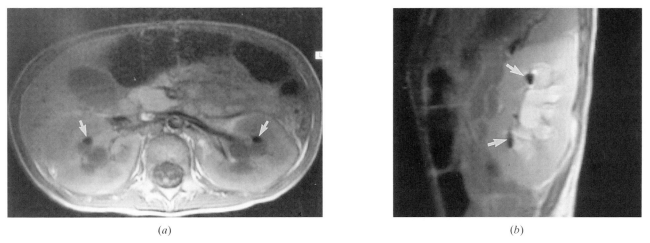

(a)   (b)

FIG. 9.66 Acute obstruction. T1-weighted spin-echo (a) and sagittal-plane gadolinium-enhanced T1-weighted spin-echo (b) images. The kidneys are enlarged in a globular fashion. Corticomedullary differentiation is preserved reflecting the acuteness of the obstruction (a). Gadolinium excreted into the collecting system is dilute and high in signal intensity (b). Signal-void foci located in the nondependent portions of the renal collecting system demonstrate blooming artifact (arrows a,b) that represent air introduced by Foley catheterization.

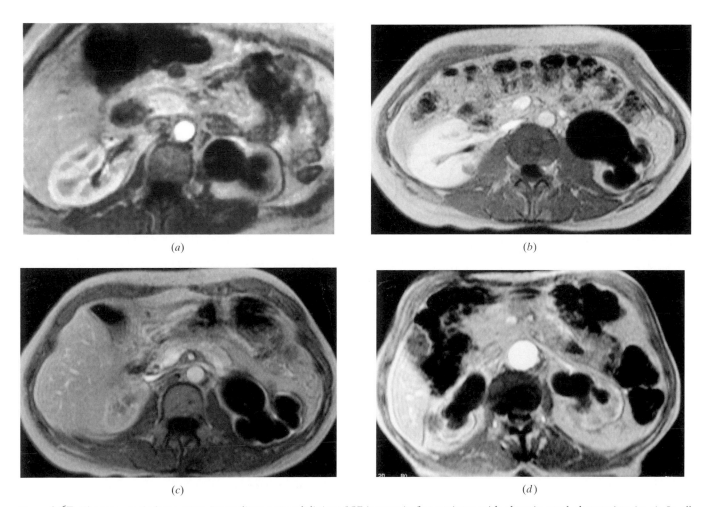

(a)   (b)

(c)   (d)

FIG. 9.67 Chronic renal obstruction. Immediate postgadolinium SGE images in five patients with chronic renal obstruction (a–e). In all cases of unilateral obstruction (a–c) the degree of cortical enhancement is less than that of the contralateral normal kidney.

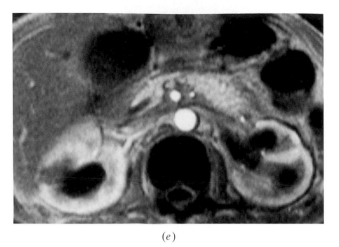

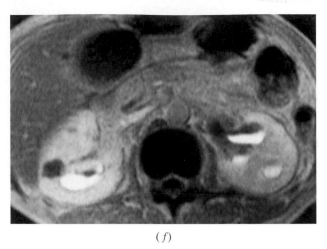

(e)   (f)

FIG. 9.67 (*Continued*) Substantial pelvicalyceal dilatation is present in all cases. Corticomedullary differentiation is diminished, and the cortex is thinned and relatively smooth. These factors reflect the duration and severity of obstruction. Excreted urine is dilute in the setting of chronic obstruction because kidneys lose concentrating ability. Excretion of dilute gadolinium is shown on a 4-minute postgadolinium SGE image (*f*) obtained from the same MRI study shown in image (*e*).

and contrast excretion. Anatomical changes of renal artery disease are shown on MR angiographic sequences. The most reproducible techniques for demonstrating changes of main artery disease include gadolinium-enhanced SGE and gadolinium-enhanced 3D fast imaging with steady state precession (FISP) [2,3]. It is critical that, in addition to the three-dimensional (3D) reconstructed images, the source images be examined to determine normal arteries (Fig. 9.70), number of arteries, and the

presence of stenosis (Fig. 9.71).The renal arteries are more clearly demonstrated if fat suppression is added to SGE sequences to remove the competing high signal intensity of fat and render small enhanced vessels more conspicuous. Imaging with 3D sequence acquisition achieves section thickness of 2 mm, which markedly improves detection of stenosis. Kidneys with ischemic nephropathy typically are small and smooth and show minimal early enhancement on immediate postgadolin-

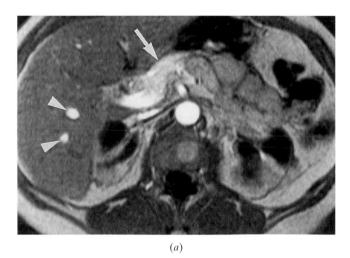

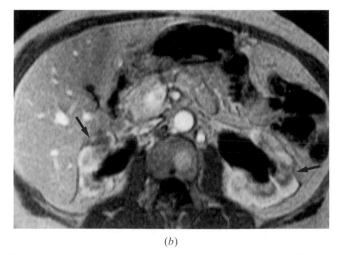

(a)   (b)

FIG. 9.68 Complicated chronic renal obstruction. Immediate (*a*) and 45-second (*b*) postgadolinium SGE images. Dilatation of both renal collecting systems has resulted from multiple urological procedures, including creation of an ileal conduit for obstruction of the distal ureters. Minimal cortical enhancement is shown on the immediate postgadolinium image. Image acquisition has been timed in the capillary phase of enhancement as evidenced by high signal intensity of the body of the pancreas (*arrow, a*) and contrast in portal veins (*arrowheads, a*). Cortical enhancement has developed in a delayed fashion and is apparent at 45 seconds. The combination of obstruction associated with reflux has resulted in variation in calyceal dilatation and tissue pressure experienced by the different regions of the kidneys. The result is severe irregularity of the renal cortex (*arrow, b*). (Reproduced with permission from Kettritz U, Semelka RC, Brown ED, Sharp TJ, Lawing WL, Colindres RE: MR findings in diffuse renal parenchymal disease. J Magn Reson Imaging 1:136–144, 1996)

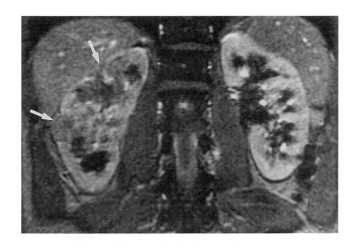

F i g. 9.69 Reflux nephropathy. Coronal 2.5-minute postgadolinium gradient-echo image. Reflux nephropathy of the right kidney is shown by irregular thinning of the renal cortex overlying renal calyces. Damage in this patient is most severe in the upper and mid renal regions (*arrows*).

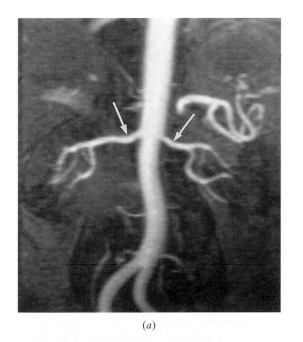

(*a*)

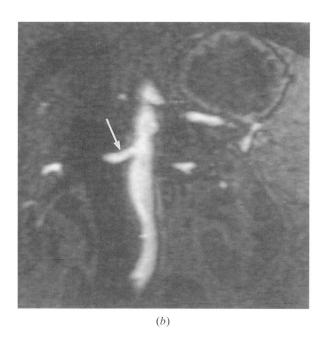

(*b*)

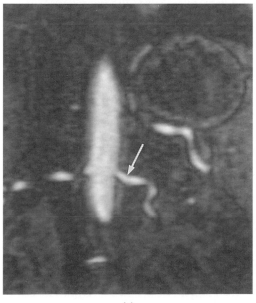

(*c*)

F i g. 9.70 MR angiogram using coronal 3D FISP. Coronal maximum-intensity projection (MIP) reconstructed image (*a*) and individual 2-mm-thin 3D FISP source image of the right (*b*) and left (*c*) renal artery origin. The MIP reconstructed image displays a normal aorta and renal arteries (*arrows, a*). Areas of stenosis, however, can be masked in reconstructed images. The individual source images of the right (*arrow, b*) and left (*arrow, c*) renal artery are normal.

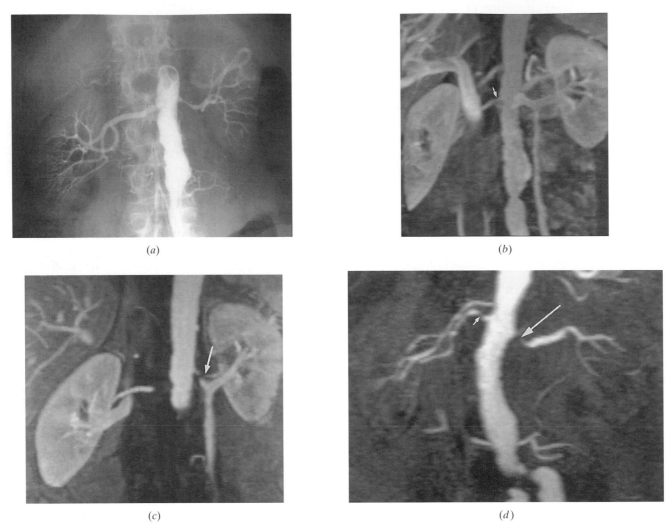

(a)   (b)

(c)   (d)

Fig. 9.71 Renal artery stenosis. Angiogram (*a*) and tailored 3D MIP projections, using an interactively selected volume of interest of a gadolinium-enhanced 3D FISP sequence (*b,c*). Mild stenosis of the right and severe stenosis of the left renal arteries are shown on the angiogram. MIP projection tailored for the right renal artery demonstrate minimal stenosis (*arrow, b*). MIP projection tailored for the left renal artery demonstrates severe stenosis (*arrow, c*). Coronal 3D MIP gadolinium-enhanced 3D FISP (*d*) in a second patient demonstrates two right renal arteries with moderate stenosis of the lower artery (*short arrow, d*) and moderately severe stenosis of a solitary left renal artery (*long arrow, d*). Breath-hold gadolinium-enhanced MR angiography is efficient at depicting the main as well as accessory renal arteries, which is important for preoperative planning (e.g., surgical repair of atherosclerotic aneurysms of the abdominal aorta).

ium images with delayed development and persistence of corticomedullary differentiation (Fig. 9.72) [72,78]. The renal cortex is thin and frequently smooth, which reflects the global nature of the ischemic injury.

Aortic dissection also may result in changes of diminished renal arterial blood flow to the kidney fed by the false lumen [78]. This may occur either by occlusion/thrombosis of the renal artery by the intimal flap or false channel, or by decreased arterial flow through the renal artery fed by the false lumen. Capillary-phase gadolinium-enhanced SGE imaging is effective at demonstrating differences in enhancement between the kidneys, where

one is fed by the true lumen and the other (usually the left) is fed by the false lumen (Fig. 9.73) [79].

Renal artery injury sustained by trauma or surgery may result in changes of ischemic nephropathy (Fig. 9.74). This may result in an acute or chronic ischemic process depending on the extent of injury. Associated perirenal hemorrhage is usually present. Fibromuscular dysplasia is a disease that affects the main renal arteries. Gadolinium-enhanced 3D FISP and 3D fat-suppressed SGE may be the most accurate MRI methods for demonstrating this entity. Carefully controlled comparisons with conventional angiography, however, are lacking.

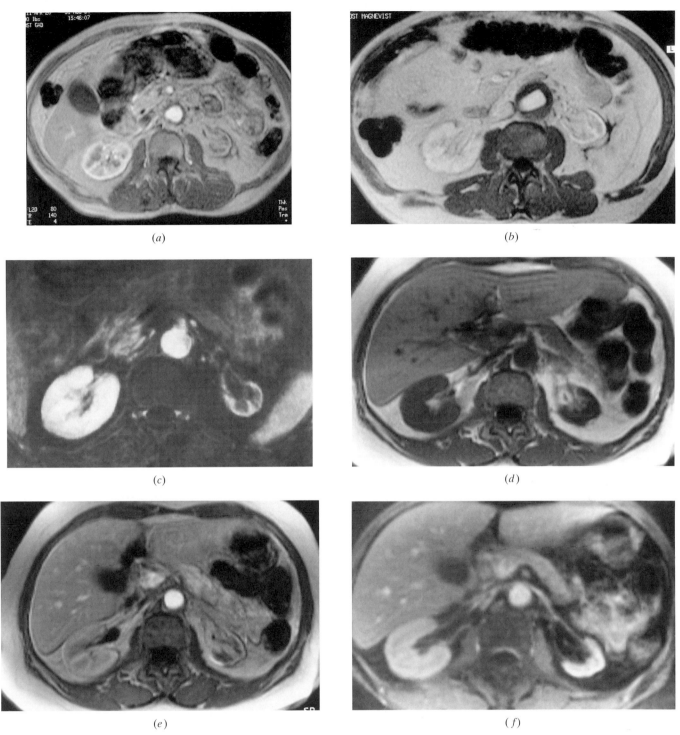

F IG. 9.72 Ischemic nephropathy. Immediate postgadolinium SGE (*a*), 2-minute postgadolinium SGE (*b*), and interstitial-phase gadolinium-enhanced T1-weighted fat-suppressed spin-echo (*c*) images in three different patients. In all three patients atherosclerotic disease of the aorta is present, and the involved left kidney is small, smooth and has uniform cortical thinning. The diseased kidneys enhance in a diminished fashion compared to the normal right kidneys on immediate postgadolinium images (*a*). Corticomedullary differentiation develops later and persists in a more prolonged fashion on interstitial-phase images (*b,c*). The renal collecting systems are normal in caliber, which is an important observation to exclude obstructive nephropathy. Precontrast SGE (*d*), 45-second postgadolinium SGE (*e*), and 90-second postgadolinium SGE (*f*) in a fourth patient. No corticomedullary differentiation is present on the precontrast image (*d*), reflecting diminished renal function. Enhancement of a thin uniform renal cortex is present on the 45-second postgadolinium image (*e*). Minor atherosclerotic changes of the abdominal aorta are also present, appearing as a thickened low-signal-intensity wall. Note that cortical enhancement of the ischemic kidney is more intense than the normal side at 45 seconds. More pronounced cortical enhancement is also present at 90 seconds (*f*).

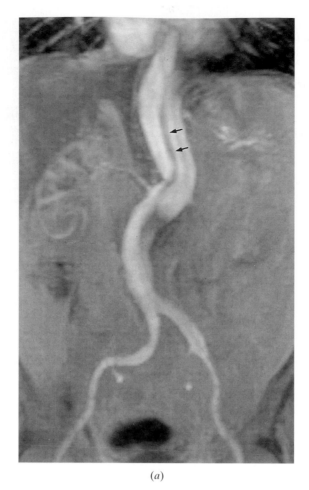

(a)

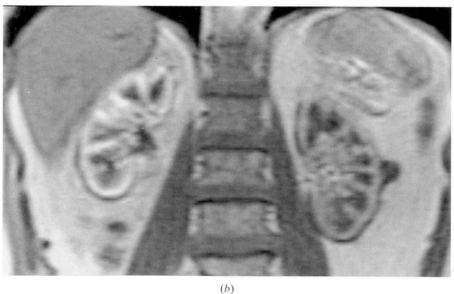

(b)

FIG. 9.73 Aortic dissection with differential renal perfusion. Coronal MIP reconstructed projection of coronal immediate postgadolinium 2D SGE images (a) and coronal 2D immediate postgadolinium source SGE image (b). Aortic dissection (*small arrows, a*) is shown on the MIP reconstructed gadolinium-enhanced SGE image (a). On an individual coronal acquired SGE image (b), lesser enhancement of the left renal cortex is present, reflecting diminished perfusion of the kidney caused by its blood supply by the false lumen, which has slower flow.

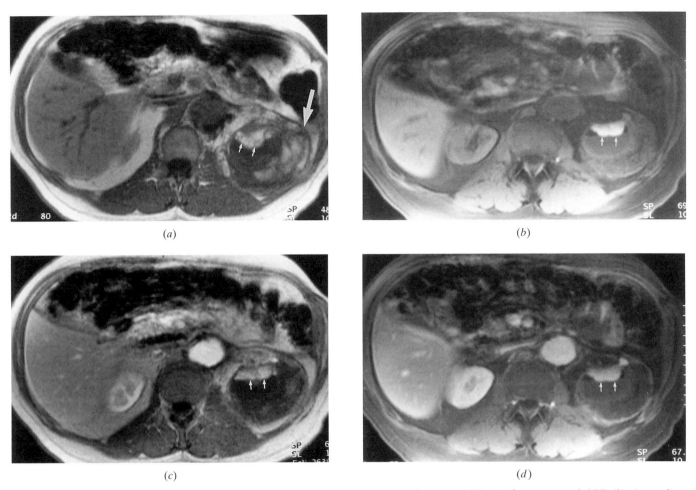

(a)

(b)

(c)

(d)

F IG . 9.74 Renal-artery injury secondary to abdominal aortic aneurysm surgical repair. SGE (*a*), fat-suppressed SGE (*b*), immediate postgadolinium SGE (*c*), and 90-second postgadolinium fat-suppressed SGE (*d*) images. Abdominal aortic surgery was performed 1 year earlier in which the left renal artery was injured. The left kidney is atrophic and high in signal intensity on T1-weighted images (*small arrows, a,b*), reflecting intraparenchymal hemorrhage. Associated subcapsular fluid collection and high-signal-intensity perirenal fluid (*large arrow, a*) are present. The kidney remains unchanged in signal intensity on postcontrast images (*small arrows, c,d*).

Medium-vessel disease is often observed in combination with large- or small-vessel disease. Atherosclerotic disease, for example, results in disease of all three types of vessels (Fig. 9.75). Various immunologic vasculitis such as Wegener's granulomatosis or polyarteritis involve medium and small vessels.

Small-vessel disease is a very common cause of renal vascular disease. Nephrosclerosis caused by hypertension and diabetic angiopathy are the most frequently observed disease entities, but a variety of vasculitis also results in this pattern of renal vascular disease. Changes of small-vessel disease are best shown on immediate postgadolinium SGE images as irregular areas of focal cortical thinning or focal perfusion defects [72]. As diabetes and hypertension tend to be chronic and progressive

in nature, cortical irregularity is due to irreversible scarring. On serial postgadolinium MR images areas of cortical thinning appear as fixed irregularities that are unchanged from capillary-phase to interstitial-phase images (Fig. 9.76). Vasculitis may be secondary to a number of etiologies, the most common of which are drugs or collagen vascular diseases. Onset of vascular changes is typically more acute than with diabetes or hypertension. Early in the course of vasculitis, MR images may demonstrate multiple transient perfusional defects that are observed on immediate postgadolinium images and that resolve on more delayed images (Fig. 9.77). Acute cortical necrosis may result from rapid-onset diffuse small-vessel disease (Fig. 9.78).

Renal emboli are a relatively common occurrence in

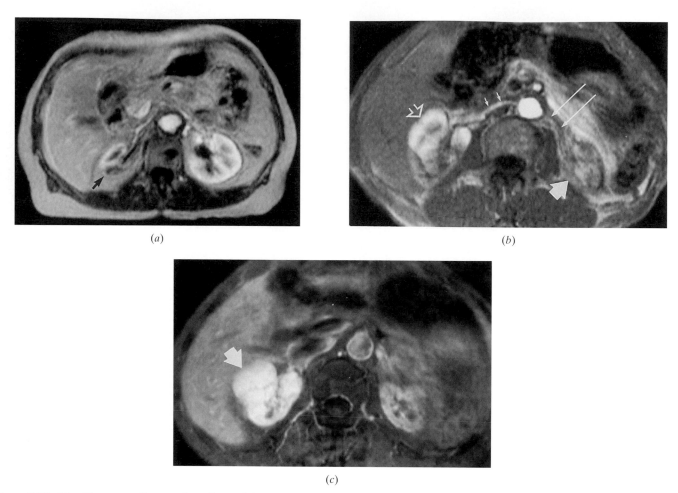

(a)

(b)

(c)

Fig. 9.75 Mixed large-, medium-, and small-vessel disease. Immediate postgadolinium SGE image (*a*) demonstrates unilateral renovascular disease The right kidney is noted to be globally small in size with a thin renal cortex. Cortical thinning is greater in the posterior aspect of the kidney (*arrow, a*) associated with greater decrease in enhancement. Immediate postgadolinium SGE (*b*) and gadolinium-enhanced T1-weighted fat-suppressed SGE (*c*) images in a second patient demonstrate bilateral renovascular disease. Global severe diminished enhancement of the left kidney and asymmetric renovascular disease of the right kidney are apparent. The posterior portion of the right kidney has severe disease as shown by severe cortical thinning and diminished enhancement (*b*). The main right renal artery is normal in caliber for most of its length, reflecting the presence of predominant medium- and small-vessel disease. The main left renal artery is small in caliber (*long arrows, b*) and, combined with global diminished enhancement of the left kidney (*large arrow, b*), reflects the severity of the main renal-artery disease. Hypertrophy of the anterior cortex of the right kidney has developed (*hollow arrow, b*) in compensation for the renovascular disease of the posterior aspect of the kidney. Uniform cortical thickness with presence of corticomedullary differentiation of the anterior portion of the right kidney on the immediate postgadolinium image shows that the enlargement is due to hypertrophy and not tumor. Later interstitial-phase gadolinium-enhanced T1-weighted fat-suppressed spin-echo image (*c*) in this patient demonstrates relatively uniform enhancement of this region of renal hypertrophy (*large arrow, c*), which mimics the appearance of a tumor. Atherosclerotic disease of the aorta is apparent in both patients.

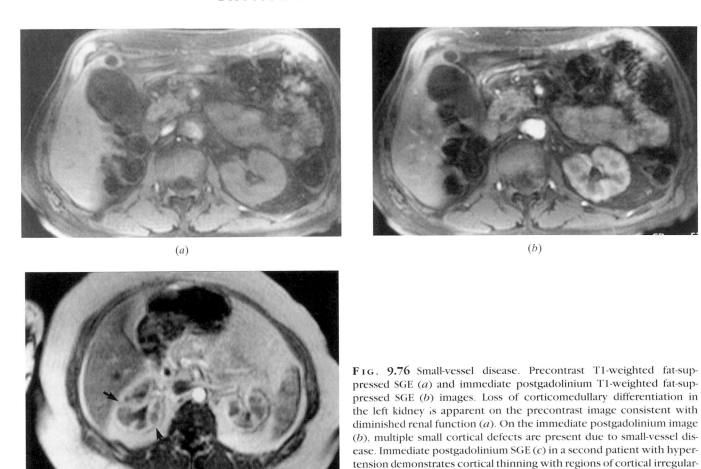

(a)

(b)

(c)

FIG. 9.76 Small-vessel disease. Precontrast T1-weighted fat-suppressed SGE (*a*) and immediate postgadolinium T1-weighted fat-suppressed SGE (*b*) images. Loss of corticomedullary differentiation in the left kidney is apparent on the precontrast image consistent with diminished renal function (*a*). On the immediate postgadolinium image (*b*), multiple small cortical defects are present due to small-vessel disease. Immediate postgadolinium SGE (*c*) in a second patient with hypertension demonstrates cortical thinning with regions of cortical irregularity (*arrows, c*).

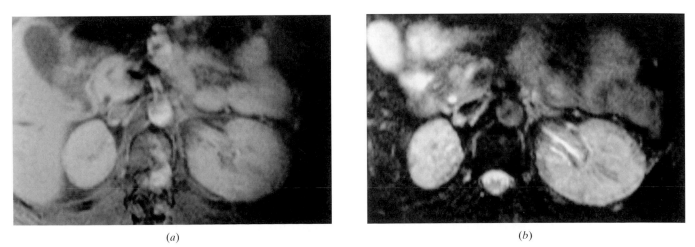

(a)

(b)

FIG. 9.77 Small vessel disease due to thrombotic microangiopathy. T1-weighted fat-suppressed spin-echo (*a*), T2-weighted fat-suppressed spin-echo (*b*), immediate (*c*), and 90 second (*d*) postgadolinium SGE images. No corticomedullary differentiation is apparent on the precontrast T1-weighted fat-suppressed spin-echo image (*a*). On the T2-weighted image (*b*), numerous 5-mm cortical defects are present.

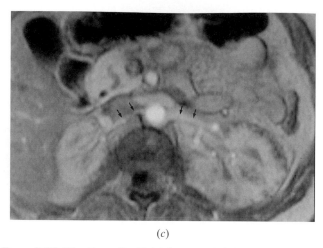

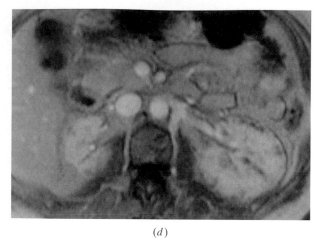

(c)

(d)

FIG. 9.77 (*Continued*) Multiple cortical defects are clearly shown on the immediate postgadolinium image (*c*). In addition, the main renal arteries are noted to be normal (*arrows, c*). On the more delayed image (*d*) some defects have resolved. However, many defects persist consistent with necrosis. Histology revealed thrombotic microangiopathy with acute tubular necrosis and cortical necrosis.

patients who have a source of emboli because the kidneys receive approximately 20 percent of the cardiac output. The most common cause of renal emboli is embolism of mural thrombi in patients with atrial arrythmias or prior myocardial infarction [80]. Renal infarction from embolic events tends to occur between calyces and demonstrates well-defined wedge-shaped defects in the renal outline. A thin enhancing peripheral rim is present due to enhancement of renal capsular vessels (Fig. 9.79) [78].

Renal Scarring
Renal scarring results from irreversible damage to renal parenchyma with regional loss of cortex. Scarring arises from a great variety of renal insults, which include vascu-

lar and collecting system disease. Scarring defects are well-shown on postgadolinium images, with immediate postgadolinium images clearly defining the extent of cortex loss (Fig. 9.80).

End-Stage Kidney
End-stage kidney appears as an atrophic diminutive kidney reflecting severe hypovascularity secondary to the loss of renal arterial supply. A variety of diffuse renal parenchymal diseases will result in end-stage kidneys. Kidneys may be markedly atrophied on MR images and demonstrate the enhancement pattern of scar tissue: negligible capillary-phase enhancement with slight enhancement on later postcontrast images (Fig. 9.81).

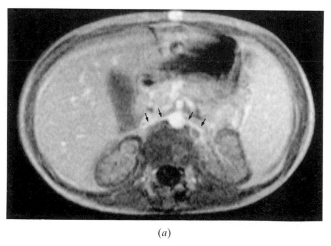

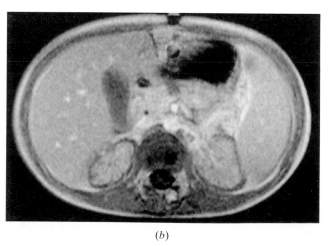

(a)

(b)

FIG. 9.78 Acute cortical necrosis secondary to small-vessel disease from mixed connective tissue disease. Immediate (*a*) and 45-second (*b*) postgadolinium SGE images demonstrate low-signal-intensity renal cortex due to lack of contrast enhancement. This appearance reflects acute cortical necrosis. Normal-appearing main renal arteries are present (*arrows, a*). (Reproduced with permission from Kettritz U, Semelka RC, Brown ED, Sharp TJ, Lawing WL, Colindres RE: MR findings in diffuse renal parenchymal disease. J Magn Reson Imaging 1:136–144, 1996)

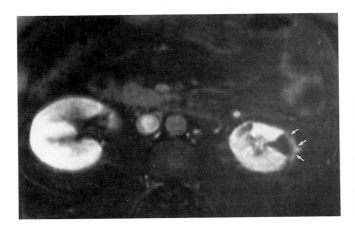

FIG. 9.79 Renal emboli. Interstitial-phase gadolinium-enhanced T1-weighted fat-suppressed spin-echo image demonstrates a nearly signal-void wedge-shaped defect in the inferior pole of the left kidney. Linear enhancement peripheral to the wedge-shaped defect (*arrows*) is due to enhancement of capsular based vessels. This is a classic feature of renal emboli. (Reproduced with permission from Semelka RC, Shoenut JP, Greenberg HM. The Kidney. In: Semelka RC, Shoenut JP, eds. MRI of the abdomen with CT correlation. Raven Press, 1993. New York, NY. p. 91–118)

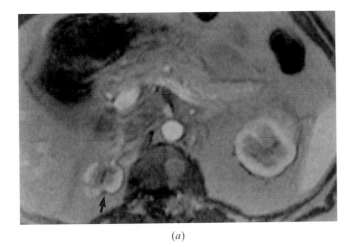

(a)

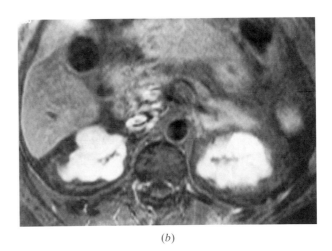

(b)

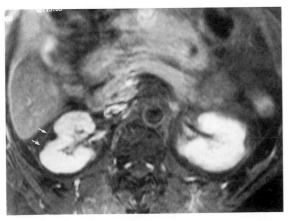

(c)

FIG. 9.80 Renal scarring. Immediate postgadolinium SGE image (*a*) demonstrates a well-defined cortical defect in the upper pole of a small right kidney (*arrow, a*). In a second patient, wedge-shaped defects are noted in both kidneys, but are more extensive in the right kidney on gadolinium-enhanced T1-weighted fat-suppressed spin-echo images (*b,c*). Many of the scars are located between calyces showing that they are not related to reflux. Enhancement of capsular based vessels is also noted (*arrows, c*).

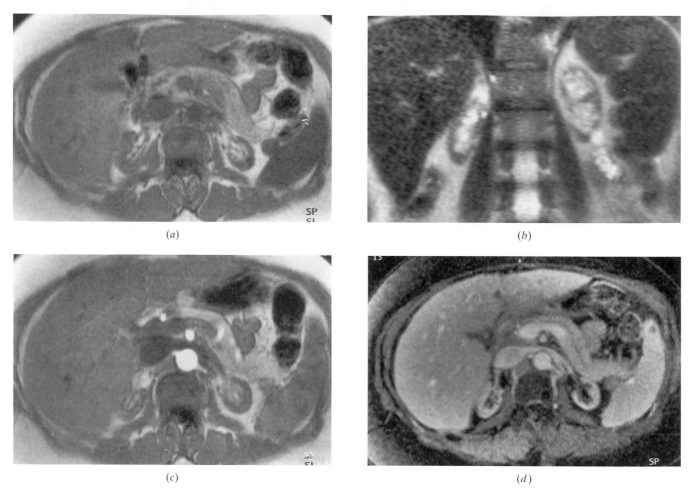

(a)   (b)

(c)   (d)

FIG. 9.81 End-stage kidney secondary to sustained hypertension. SGE (a), coronal HASTE (b), immediate postgadolinium SGE (c), and 2-minute postgadolinium fat-suppressed SGE (d) images. Bilateral diminished atrophic kidneys are apparent on precontrast images (a,b). Negligible enhancement is appreciated on the immediate postgadolinium SGE image (c). On more delayed images (d), renal parenchymal enhancement has increased.

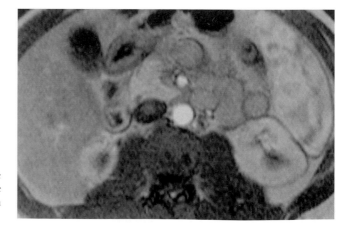

FIG. 9.82 Hypoplastic kidney. Immediate postgadolinium SGE image demonstrates symmetric enhancement of both renal cortices. Note that the renal cortex of the hypoplastic right kidney is uniform in thickness and commensurate in thickness to the size of the kidney.

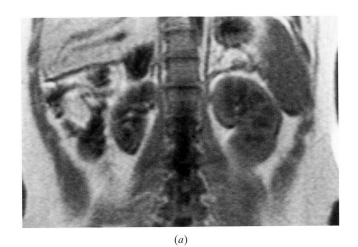

(a)

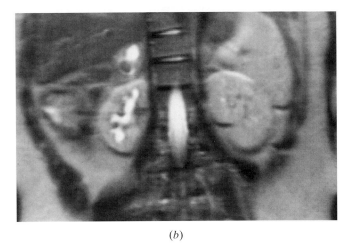

(b)

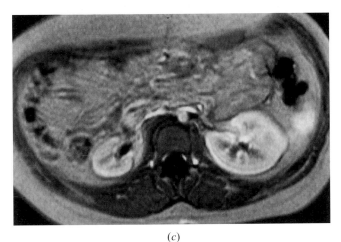

(c)

F IG . 9.83 Small kidney secondary to ureter reimplantation in infancy. Coronal SGE (*a*), coronal breath-hold echo-train spin-echo (*b*), and immediate postgadolinium SGE (*c*) images. The right kidney is small, smooth in contour, and has uniform cortical thickness (*a*-*c*). Corticomedullary differentiation is preserved on precontrast T1-weighted images. Mild caliectasis with dilatation of the intrarenal collecting system is demonstrated on the T2-weighted image (*b*), reflecting the underlying disease of the collecting system. On the immediate postgadolinium SGE image (*c*), the renal cortex is thin but uniform in thickness, and enhancement is symmetric with the normal left kidney.

Hypoplastic Kidney

The true hypoplastic kidney is a kidney that is congenitally small, with fewer papillae than a normal kidney. Hypoplastic kidneys have a normal collecting system and normal cortical enhancement (Fig. 9.82). The renal artery, however, is diminutive suggesting that in utero vascular compromise may be the underlying cause. Renal injury sustained in childhood such as surgery, radiation, or reflux may result in a small smooth kidney similar in appearance to a true hypoplastic kidney (Fig. 9.83).

Hyperplastic (Hypertrophic) Kidney

Renal hyperplasia that results in renal enlargement occurs in the setting of long-standing compromise or absence of the contralateral kidney. Hyperplasia is most pronounced if the original stimulus for renal enlargement occurs in childhood. Generalized, globular renal enlargement with increased thickness of renal cortex is observed on immediate postgadolinium SGE images (Fig. 9.84).

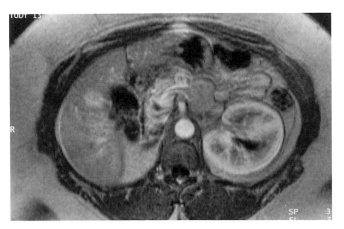

F IG . 9.84 Renal hypertrophy. Immediate postgadolinium SGE image demonstrates generalized enlargement of the left kidney with uniform thickness of renal cortex. This adult patient had undergone right nephrectomy in childhood.

INFECTION

Acute Infection

Acute pyelonephritis usually results in enlargement of the infected kidney [81]. The infection is most commonly caused by a gram-negative bacilli as an ascending infection from the lower urinary tract. Perinephric fluid may be observed, which is best shown on postgadolinium images (Fig. 9.85). Proteinaceous material in the renal tubules may result in high signal intensity on T1-weighted fat-suppressed images (see Fig. 9.85).

Abscess

Renal abscess usually occurs as a complication of an ascending urinary tract infection, but hematogenous infections also occur [82]. Hematogenous infection may be seen in tuberculosis secondary to other sites of infection, or in the setting of intravenous drug use. On MR images, renal abscesses appear as irregular mass lesions with a

signal-void center (Fig. 9.86) [83]. Perinephric stranding is frequently prominent [83]. Perinephric linear densities are more prominent in renal abscesses than in necrotic renal cancers because these reflect inflammatory tissue. It may not, however, always be possible to distinguish abscesses from cancer based on imaging findings, and follow-up studies may be needed to ensure resolution following treatment [84]. Patients with multifocal or diffuse renal abscesses frequently have elevated serum creatinine (see Fig. 9.86). Ultrasound and noncontrast CT imaging perform poorly at detecting renal abscesses; therefore, in patients with renal dysfunction, MRI is the procedure of choice [83].

Xanthogranulomatous Pyelonephritis

Xanthogranulomatous pyelonephritis (XGPN) is an unusual chronic infection that develops in the presence of chronic obstruction [85]. Sixty percent of cases are associated with proteus infection, which usually involves

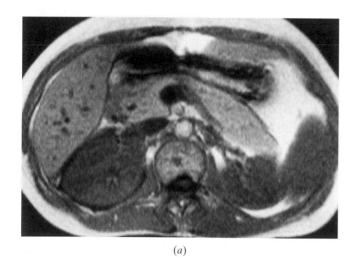

(a)

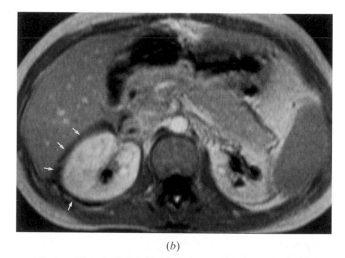

(b)

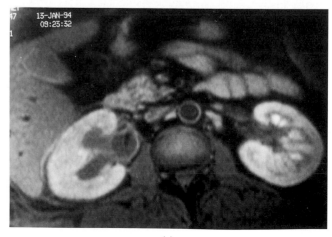

(c)

FIG. 9.85 Acute pyelonephritis. SGE (a) and 2-minute postgadolinium SGE (b) images. The right kidney is swollen, and perinephric fluid (arrows, b) is present. No focal parenchymal abnormalities are identified. Precontrast T1-weighted fat-suppressed spin-echo image (c) in a second patient demonstrates striated cone-shaped regions of high signal intensity in the medulla of the left kidney consistent with proteinaceous material in acute pyelonephritis. Hydronephrosis of the right kidney is identified.

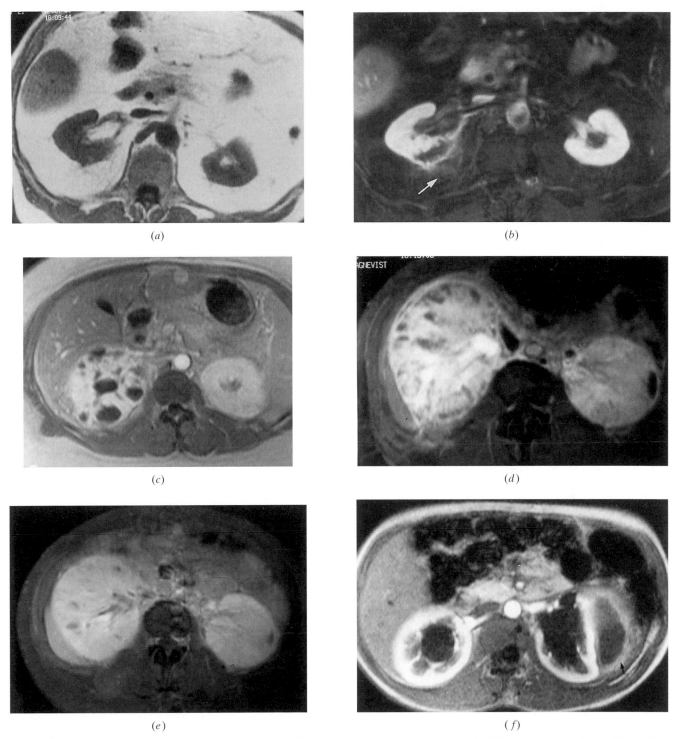

(a)   (b)

(c)   (d)

(e)   (f)

FIG. 9.86 Renal abscess. SGE (*a*) and gadolinium-enhanced T1-weighted fat-suppressed spin-echo (*b*) images in a patient with a solitary abscess in the posterior aspect of the right kidney. Perirenal stranding is noted on the precontrast image, but the abscess is not well-seen. On the gadolinium-enhanced fat-suppressed spin-echo image a signal-void intraparenchymal renal abscess is noted. The inner aspect of the abscess wall is irregular. Prominent perirenal stranding (*arrow, b*) is an important imaging feature of renal abscess. Ninety-second postgadolinium SGE image (*c*) in a second patient demonstrates multiple signal-void abscesses in the right kidney. Bilateral renal abscesses with substantial renal enlargement is demonstrated on a gadolinium-enhanced T1-weighted fat-suppressed spin-echo image (*d*) in a third patient with HIV infection and elevated serum creatinine. Ultrasound and noncontrast CT imaging demonstrated renal enlargement with no definition of abscesses. In the same patient, a repeat MRI study was performed after a 15-day course of antibiotics. The gadolinium-enhanced T1-weighted fat-suppressed spin-echo image (*e*) demonstrates decrease in renal size with decrease in size and number of abscesses.

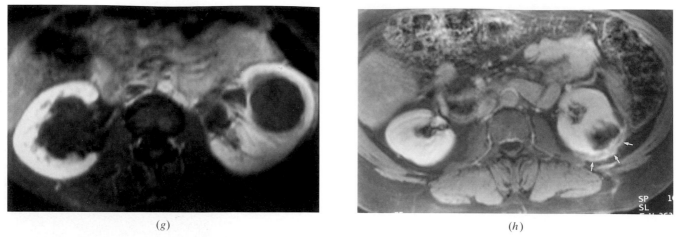

(g)   (h)

F I G . 9.86 (*Continued*) Immediate postgadolinium SGE (*f*) and gadolinium-enhanced T1-weighted fat-suppressed spin-echo (*g*) images in a fourth patient demonstrate a renal abscess with a prominent extrarenal component (*arrow, f*). Multiple parapelvic cysts are present in both kidneys. Three-minute postgadolinium fat-suppressed SGE image (*h*) in a fifth patient who is a diabetic. A left renal abscess is present that appears as a low-signal-intensity cystic lesion with an irregular wall. Prominent thickening and increased enhancement of adjacent fascia (*small arrows, h*) is present.

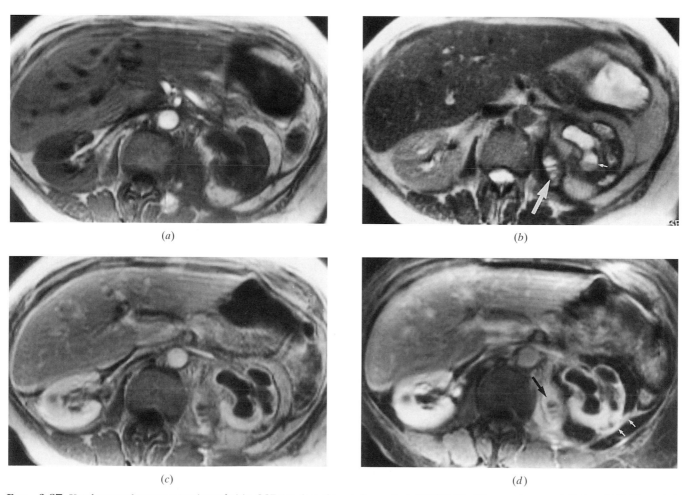

(a)   (b)

(c)   (d)

F I G . 9.87 Xanthogranulomatous pyelonephritis. SGE (*a*), breathing-independent HASTE (*b*), 90-second postgadolinium SGE (*c*), and 4-minute postgadolinium fat-suppressed SGE (*d*) images. The left renal collecting system is noted to be dilated (*a*–*d*). A large extrarenal component of the infection is noted in the psoas muscle (*arrow b,d*). Layering of low-signal-intensity material (*small arrows, b*) is noted in calyces on the T2-weighted image (*b*). No excretion of gadolinium by the involved kidney is apparent on the 4-minute postgadolinium image. Inflammatory changes in Gerota's fascia and lateral conal fascia (*small arrows, d*) and psoas abscess are most clearly defined on the gadolinium-enhanced fat-suppressed image (*d*). The combination of dilatation of the collecting system, lack of contrast excretion, and prominent extrarenal inflammatory changes are features observed for xanthogranulomatous pyelonephritis.

the kidney globally, although focal XGPN has been described [85].

On MR images, the kidney usually is enlarged. After gadolinium administration, minimal enhancement is present on capillary-phase images with progressively intense enhancement on interstitial-phase images (Fig. 9.87). This enhancement pattern reflects poor renal perfusion (minimal early enhancement) with substantial capillary leakage due to inflammatory change (increased delayed enhancement). Perinephric inflammatory changes are prominent. The renal collecting system almost invariably is dilated, and signal-void calculi may be identified. No evidence of gadolinium excretion in the collecting system is present.

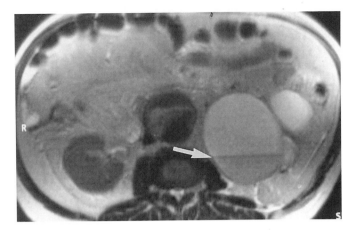

FIG. 9.89 Pyonephrosis. Breathing-independent HASTE image. Severe dilatation of the collecting system of the left kidney is present. Layering of low-signal-intensity debris (*arrow*) in the dependent portion of the renal pelvis is a common appearance in infection.

Candidiasis

Renal candidiasis occurs in the context of hepatosplenic candidiasis. These lesions are typically small (5 mm) and well-defined. Lesions are best shown on gadolinium-enhanced interstitial-phase fat-suppressed images (Fig. 9.88) [86].

Fungus balls also may develop in the collecting system. Diabetes predisposes to this condition.

Pyonephrosis

Pyonephrosis develops when a dilated, obstructed renal collecting system becomes infected. MRI features consistent with pyonephrosis include debris layering in the obstructed renal pelvis and enhancement of the wall of the renal pelvis on gadolinium-enhanced images (Fig. 9.89).

HEMORRHAGE

Renal/perirenal hemorrhage occurs in the context of bleeding disorders, trauma, and neoplasms. Large perinephric hematomas occur not infrequently in patients who have undergone renal lithotripsy on renal biopsy. MRI is more sensitive than CT imaging to the presence of hemorrhage in fluid collections. Parenchymal or subcapsular hemorrhage appears as high- or mixed high-signal-intensity fluid on both T1- and T2-weighted images (Fig. 9.90) [13]. Perirenal hemorrhage frequently has an unusual multilayered appearance due to blood layering along bridging renal septae.

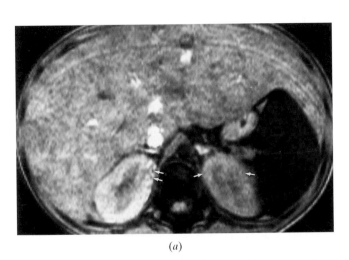

(*a*)

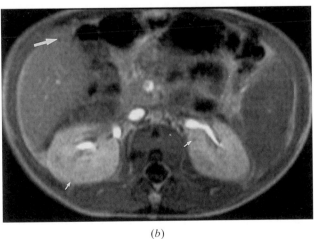

(*b*)

FIG. 9.88 Renal candidiasis. Immediate (*a*) and 90-second (*b*) postgadolinium SGE images in two patients with renal candidiasis. Multiple low-signal-intensity lesions less than 5 mm in size are present in the kidneys in both patients (*small arrows, a,b*). Extensive hepatic involvement is apparent in the first patient (*a*), whereas fewer liver lesions are apparent in the second patient (*arrow, b*).

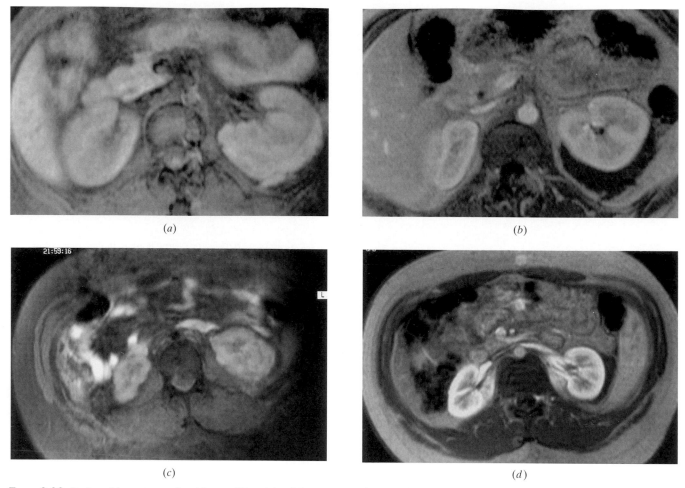

(a)

(b)

(c)

(d)

FIG. 9.90 Perirenal hematoma after biopsy. T1-weighted fat-suppressed spin-echo (a) and immediate postgadolinium SGE (b) images in one patient, and the same sequences, respectively (c,d), in a second patient. On the precontrast fat-suppressed spin-echo images (a,c) high-signal-intensity fluid is present in the perirenal space of the left kidney consistent with subacute blood. On the immediate postgadolinium SGE images (b,d) the fluid appears low in signal intensity due to rescaling of the tissue signal intensities after gadolinium administration.

■ DISEASE OF THE RENAL COLLECTING SYSTEM

MASS LESIONS

Primary Tumors

Transitional-Cell Cancer

The majority of primary tumors of the urothelium are malignant. Transitional-cell cancer (TCC) is the most common malignancy of the urothelium accounting for more than 90 percent of tumors [87]. Squamous-cell cancer accounts for 8 percent and adenocarcinoma for less than 1 percent [87]. TCC represents 8 percent of all renal tumors, rarely occurring in patients younger than 30 years of age. Males are more commonly affected in a 3 to 1 ratio with females. Risk factors include analgesics, tobacco, caffeine, chronic infection, and urolithiasis. Staging of transitional-cell cancer is as follows: Stage 1, limited to

uroepithelial mucosa and lamina propria; Stage 2, invasion to, but not beyond, pelvic/ureteral muscularis; Stage 3, invasion beyond muscularis into adventitial fat or renal parenchyma; and Stage 4, distant metastasis.

Tumors usually appear as eccentric filling defects in the renal pelvis (Fig. 9.91) [87,88]. On occasion they may cause concentric wall thickening (87,88). Tumors usually spread superficially (Fig. 9.92), but in rare instances may be large focal masses. TCC has a propensity to invade renal parenchyma, but invasion may be difficult to detect. Invasion of or along the IVC may occur and is well-depicted on MR images (Fig. 9.93) [88,89]. Although these tumors are hypovascular, they may be moderately high in signal intensity on gadolinium-enhanced interstitial-phase T1-weighted fat-suppressed images, presumably due to diminished clearance of contrast from the interstitial space [88]. Tumors tend to invade locally with spread to adjacent lymph nodes. There is a great propensity for the tumor to be multifocal; 30 to 50 percent of cases are

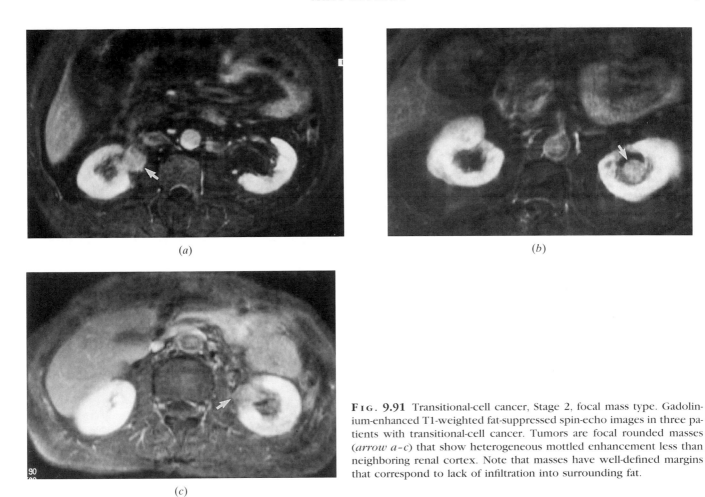

(a)

(b)

(c)

FIG. 9.91 Transitional-cell cancer, Stage 2, focal mass type. Gadolinium-enhanced T1-weighted fat-suppressed spin-echo images in three patients with transitional-cell cancer. Tumors are focal rounded masses (*arrow a–c*) that show heterogeneous mottled enhancement less than neighboring renal cortex. Note that masses have well-defined margins that correspond to lack of infiltration into surrounding fat.

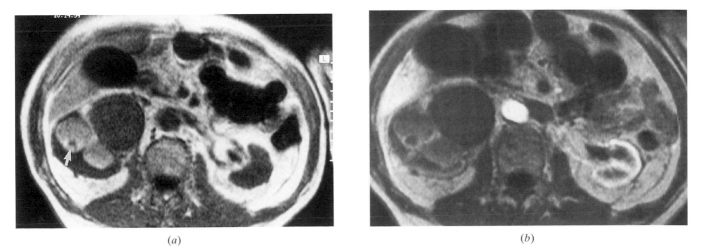

(a)

(b)

FIG. 9.92 Transitional-cell cancer, Stage 3, superficially spreading pattern. SGE (*a*), immediate postgadolinium SGE (*b*), and gadolinium-enhanced T1-weighted fat-suppressed spin-echo (*c*) images. Severe dilatation of the right renal collecting system is present (*a–c*). Blood is identified as high-signal-intensity substance in dilated calyces on the precontrast image (*a*), and a small low-signal-intensity blood clot is also apparent (*arrow, a*). The renal pelvis is filled with a large signal-void blood clot. Diminished cortical enhancement is present on the immediate postgadolinium image (*b*).

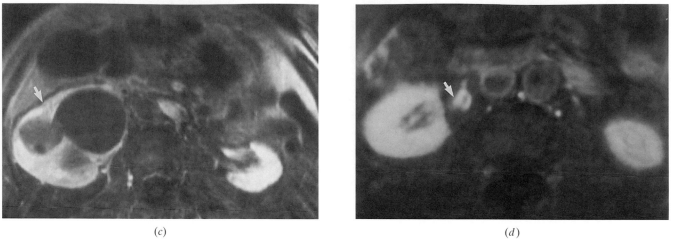

(c)   (d)

FIG. 9.92 (*Continued*) Thickening of the proximal aspect of the renal pelvis urothelium is noted with invasion of the renal cortex (*arrow, c*), which is best appreciated on the gadolinium-enhanced T1-weighted fat-suppressed spin-echo image (*c*). Gadolinium-enhanced T1-weighted fat-suppressed spin-echo image (*d*) in a second patient shows increased thickness and intense enhancement of the proximal ureter. Ill-defined external margin of the tumor (*arrow, d*) on the lateral aspect of the ureter wall is consistent with tumor extension into the periureteral fat.

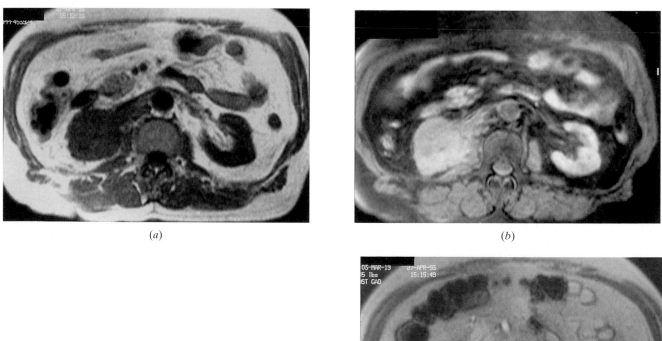

(a)   (b)

FIG. 9.93 Transitional-cell carcinoma, Stage 4. SGE (*a*), T1-weighted fat-suppressed spin-echo (*b*), immediate postgadolinium SGE (*c*), and coronal gadolinium-enhanced images. T1-weighted fat-suppressed spin-echo images from posterior (*d*) and anterior (*e*) sections. Low-signal-intensity tumor is seen involving kidney and extending posterior to the IVC on the precontrast images (*a,b*). On the immediate postgadolinium image (*c*), the tumor is noted to involve predominantly the medulla with relative sparing of the renal cortex.

(c)

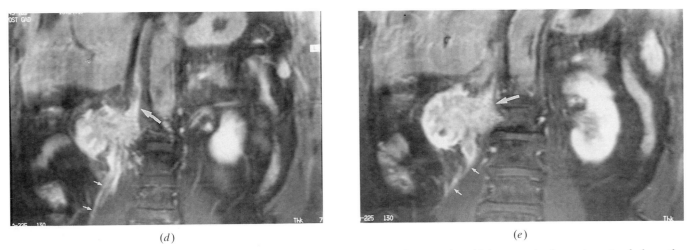

(d)   (e)

FIG. 9.93 (*Continued*)   The extent of tumor is best displayed on the coronal images in which tumor is shown to extend along the psoas muscle and ureter inferiorly (*small arrows, d,e*) and along the vertebral bodies and IVC superiorly (*arrows, d,e*).

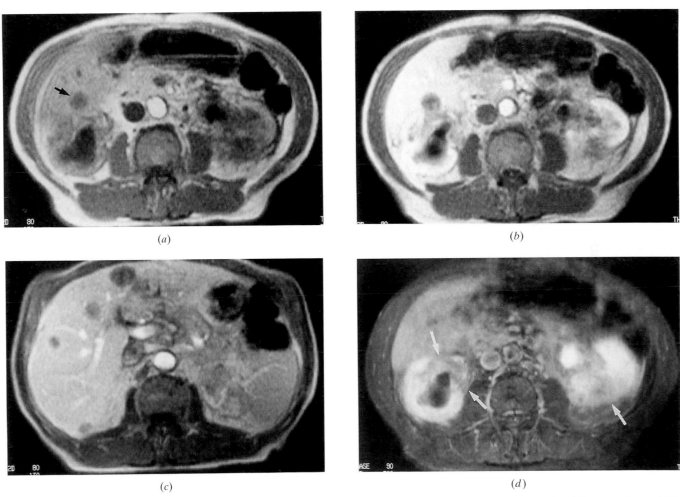

(a)   (b)

(c)   (d)

FIG. 9.94 Transitional-cell cancer, Stage 4. SGE (*a*), immediate (*b*), and 90-second (*c*) postgadolinium SGE and gadolinium-enhanced T1-weighted fat-suppressed spin-echo (*d*) images. Bilateral infiltrative tumors are present arising from the collection system of both kidneys (*a,b,d*). The transitional-cell tumors are low in signal intensity on precontrast T1-weighted images (*a*) enhance minimally on immediate postgadolinium images (*b*) and show heterogeneous enhancement less than renal parenchyma on later images (*arrow, d*). Liver metastases are also present (*c*). Liver metastases from transitional-cell cancer are generally hypovascular and are low in signal intensity on precontrast T1-weighted images (*arrow, a*), show faint rim enhancement on immediate postgadolinium images (*b*), and often remain well-defined and hypointense on later postcontrast images (*c*). Liver metastases frequently are poorly seen on T2-weighted images (not shown) due to their hypovascularity.

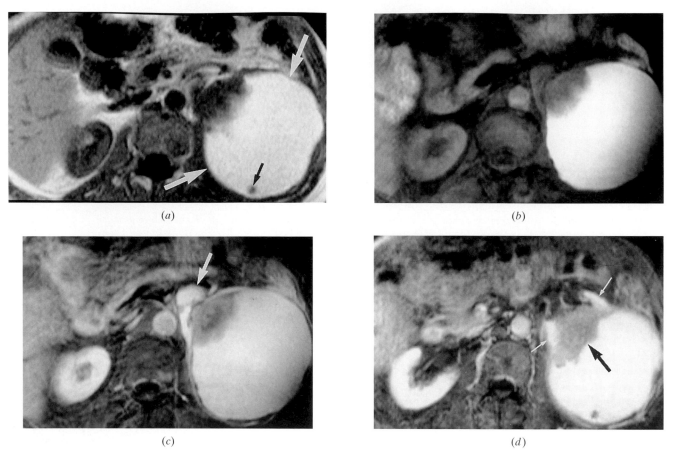

(a)

(b)

(c)

(d)

FIG. 9.95 Transitional-cell carcinoma, poorly differentiated. SGE (*a*), T1-weighted fat-suppressed spin-echo (*b*), and gadolinium-enhanced T1-weighted fat-suppressed spin-echo (*c,d*) images. An irregular tumor arises from the midportion of the kidney and is associated with a large hemorrhagic fluid collection (*large arrows, a*). A small tumor nodule is present in the cystic hemorrhagic component (*small arrow, a*). On the gadolinium-enhanced image, renal parenchyma is well-defined as uniformly enhancing tissue (*arrow, c*). The tumor mass extends from the renal pelvis through the renal parenchyma into the cystic space. Anterior and posterior cortices (*arrows, d*) are splayed by the irregular tumor mass (*black arrow, d*).

multifocal, and 15 to 25 percent are bilateral. Evaluation of the entire urothelium with retrograde pyelography is essential to establish the full extent of disease. The role of MR urography is not established at present. Liver metastases from TCC tend to be hypovascular (Fig. 9.94). In rare instances TCC may have poorly differentiated histology and act as a locally aggressive malignancy (Fig. 9.95).

Squamous-Cell Carcinoma

A predisposing cause for squamous-cell malignancy is usually present. Calculi are present in 50 to 60 percent of cases, and chronic infection, leukoplakia, and chronic drug overuse (e.g., phenacetin) are also associated with this malignancy [87]. Squamous cell carcinoma cannot be distinguished from transitional-cell cancer based on imaging findings (Fig. 9.96). Early tumors tend to spread superficially [87]. As tumors enlarge they may develop irregular margins, which is somewhat uncommon for transitional-cell carcinoma.

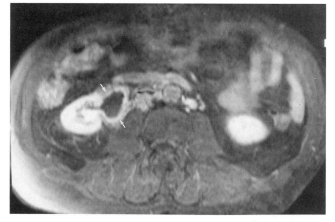

FIG. 9.96 Squamous-cell cancer. Gadolinium-enhanced T1-weighted fat-suppressed spin-echo image demonstrates dilatation of the right renal pelvis with irregularly thickened and intensely enhancing urothelium, which represents squamous-cell cancer (*arrows*). Surrounding peripelvic fat contains ill-defined enhancing tissue consistent with tumor extension.

Secondary Tumors

Lymphoma

Lymphoma is the most common secondary tumor to invade the urothelium. Direct coronal imaging with MRI allows visualization of the extent of disease [90].

Metastases from Other Primary Tumors

Breast, gastrointestinal tract, prostate, cervix, and kidney are the malignancies that most frequently metastasize to the ureters [87]. Metastases to the ureter are nevertheless rare. Small enhancing nodules of tumor may be appreciated on gadolinium-enhanced fat-suppressed images.

Filling Defects in the Collecting System

Calculi are the most common filling defects in the renal collecting system. Calcium oxalate stones are the most common form of renal calculi in North America, accounting for approximately 65 percent of cases [91]. Regardless of calcium composition, renal calculi are signal-void on MR images (Fig. 9.97). To maximize conspicuity of signal-

void calculi, they are best displayed on sequences in which urine is high in signal intensity. Echo-train spin-echo sequences such as the HASTE technique generate MR urographic images that can be reconstructed to resemble conventional intravenous urography [4,92]. MR urography may be effective at demonstrating ureteric calculi due to the high contrast between high-signal-intensity urine in dilated ureter and obstructing low-signal-intensity calculus (Fig. 9.98). Because HASTE images have less than 1 second temporal resolution, MRI may be a very time-efficient and cost-effective method of evaluating obstructing calculi. Calculi are well-shown using these sequences because urine is high and calculi are low in signal intensity. After gadolinium administration, detection of calculi is feasible when gadolinium is sufficiently dilute to render urine high in signal intensity. This is best accomplished by ensuring that the patient is well-hydrated and by delay of image acquisition 10 to 30 minutes following injection [5]. Signal-void calculi may be detected as small as 1 to 2 mm in diameter in a background of high-signal-intensity urine. Obstruction by calculi causes alteration in renal parenchymal en-

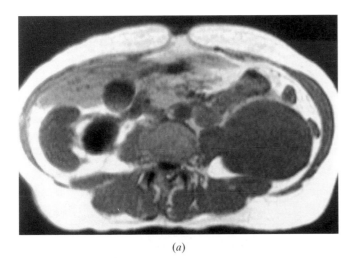

(a)

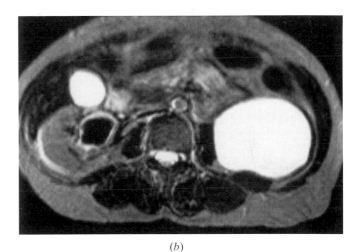

(b)

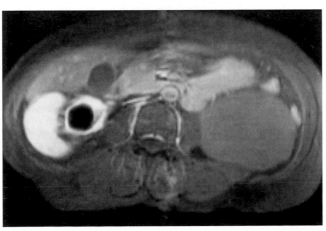

(c)

FIG. 9.97 Renal calculi. SGE (a), T2-weighted spin-echo (b), 10-minute postgadolinium T1-weighted fat-suppressed spin-echo (c) images. The renal calculus in the right renal pelvis is signal-void on all sequences (a–c). Conspicuity of the calculus is greatest on the T2-weighted image and the dilute gadolinium (high-signal-intensity)-enhanced image. Urine is high in signal intensity on these sequences and contrasts well with the signal-void calculus.

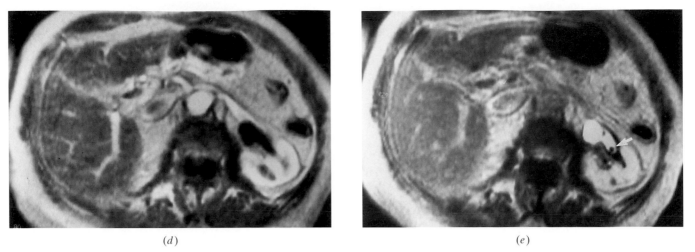

(d)   (e)

FIG. 9.97 (*Continued*)   Immediate (*d*) and 10-minute (*e*) postgadolinium images in a second patient demonstrate a signal-void small calculus, which is not apparent in gadolinium-free signal-void urine (*d*), but is well-shown on late postgadolinium image (*arrow, e*) due to the high signal intensity of dilute gadolinium-containing urine.

hancement and in the transit of contrast material within the kidney, which is well-shown on MR images (see section on Renal Function later).

Other filling defects such as blood clots or fungus balls are also well-depicted on MR images as low-signal-intensity mass lesions in high-signal-intensity urine on T2-weighted sequences, and as nonenhancing mass le-

sions seated in the high-signal-intensity contrast-filled collecting system on delayed postgadolinium SGE images. Foci of air in the collecting system may be distinguished from solid lesions by the presence of susceptibility artifact and by the observation that air foci locate in nondependent positions and solid lesions tend to layer in dependent positions (Fig. 9.99).

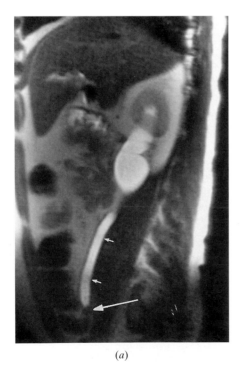

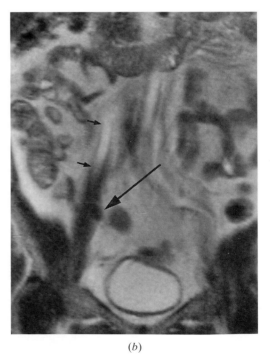

(a)   (b)

FIG. 9.98   Ureteric calculi. Sagittal (*a*), and coronal (*b*) HASTE images. The proximal two-thirds of the ureter are dilated and urine-filled, resulting in high signal intensity on the HASTE image (*small arrows, a,b*). A low-signal-intensity calculus is demonstrated obstructing the ureter (*long arrow, a,b*), which forms a convex meniscus sign within the urine-filled ureter.

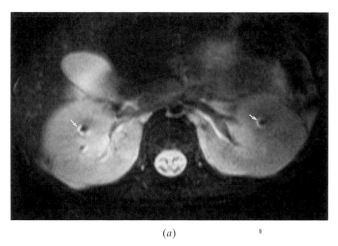

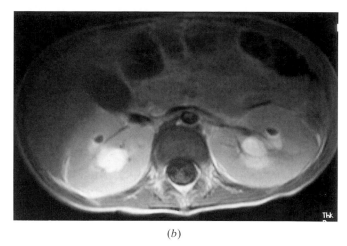

(a) *(b)*

FIG. 9.99 Air in the collecting system. T2-weighted fat-suppressed spin-echo (*a*) and gadolinium-enhanced T1-SE (*b*) images. Foci present in the nondependent portions of the renal collecting system that are signal-void on T2-weighted (*a*) and gadolinium-enhanced T1-weighted (*b*) images. These foci possess bright external rings on the T2-weighted images from air-fluid magnetic susceptibility artifact (*arrows, a*).

Dilation of the Collecting System

Dilation of the renal collecting system may arise as a variant of normal (Fig. 9.100), congenital anomaly, obstruction, reflux-related or post obstruction. Relatively little has been described on the MRI appearance of many of these entities. Recent implementations of MR urography may increase the role of MRI in the investigation of renal collecting system dilatation (Fig. 9.101). The combination of MR urography, tissue imaging sequences to evaluate renal cortex, and dynamic serial postcontrast imaging to assess renal function provides comprehensive information on the morphological and functional status of kidneys with dilated collecting systems (Fig. 9.102). As

with intravenous urography and CT imaging, gadolinium-enhanced SGE images can demonstrate delayed excretion of contrast (Fig. 9.103).

Calyceal Diverticulum

Calyceal diverticula may be shown on MR images using a combination of MR urography and delayed postgadolinium images. The MR urogram demonstrates the fluid-filled structure (Fig. 9.104), but the communication with the collecting system is confirmed by demonstration of high-signal-intensity fluid in the diverticulum on delayed images due to the presence of dilute gadolinium. Calyceal diverticula frequently contain calculi, which can be well-

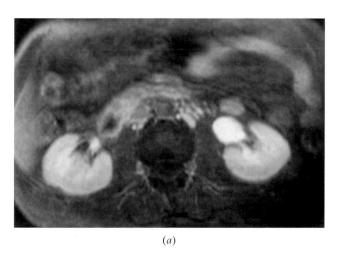

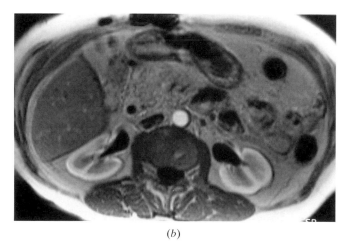

(a) *(b)*

FIG. 9.100 Extrarenal pelvis. Gadolinium-enhanced T1-weighted fat-suppressed spin-echo. Dilute, high-signal-intensity gadolinium is present in a prominent extrarenal pelvis in the left kidney. The calyces are normal and small in size, reflecting the absence of obstruction. This establishes the diagnosis of extrarenal pelvis. Immediate postgadolinium SGE image (*b*) in a second patient demonstrates bilateral extrarenal pelves. Calyces are normal in size, and cortical enhancement is symmetric and normal.

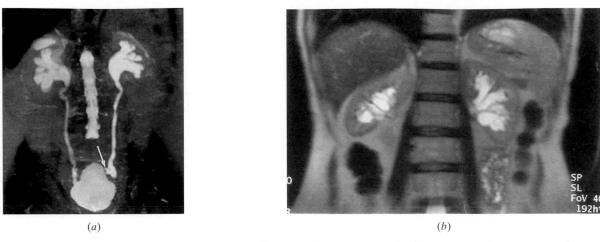

(a)   (b)

FIG. 9.101 MR urogram. Coronal MIP reconstructed MR urogram from 20 multisection coronal echo-train spin-echo sections (a) demonstrates bilateral severe dilatation of the renal collecting systems secondary to bladder outlet obstruction from prostate cancer. Superior deviation of the left ureter (arrow) results from superior extension of cancer. Coronal HASTE image (b) demonstrates moderate calicectasis bilaterally from chronic ureteropelvic junction obstruction.

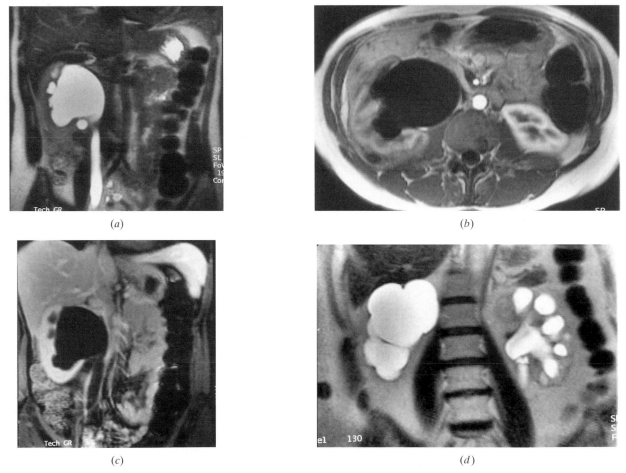

(a)   (b)

(c)   (d)

FIG. 9.102 Comprehensive evaluation of renal obstruction. Coronal HASTE (a), immediate postgadolinium SGE (b), and coronal 3-minute postgadolinium fat-suppressed SGE (c) images in a patient with distal ureteral obstruction secondary to gynecological malignancy. The coronal HASTE image (a) demonstrates the severe dilatation of the renal collecting system and ureter. The immediate postgadolinium SGE image (b) demonstrates diminished cortical enhancement of the obstructed right kidney compared to the left. The thickness of the renal cortex is well-preserved. The coronal gadolinium enhanced SGE image (c) demonstrates signal void urine in the ureter and renal pelvis and enhanced renal cortex. Coronal HASTE (d,e) and coronal 2-minute postgadolinium fat-suppressed SGE image (f) in a second patient with bilateral distal ureteral obstruction. Massive hydronephrosis is present of the right renal collecting system and severe dilatation is present of the left one (d,e).

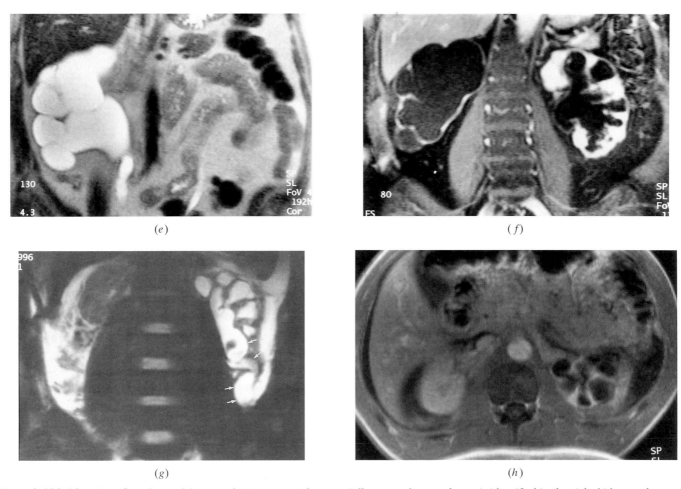

(e)

(f)

(g)

(h)

F IG . 9.102 (*Continued*) After gadolinium administration (*f*), essentially no renal parenchyma is identified in the right kidney, whereas moderately severe thinning is present in the left kidney. Coronal HASTE (*g*) and 90-second postgadolinium SGE (*h*) images in a third patient with long-standing ureterovesical obstruction secondary to childhood ureteric reimplantation. Coronal HASTE (*g*) shows severe hydronephrosis and tortuosity of the ureter (*small arrows, g*) of the left kidney. The transverse gadolinium enhanced image demonstrates extreme thinning of the renal parenchyma in the left kidney, which is effectively nonfunctioning. A normal-appearing right kidney is seen. Intraperitoneal high signal intensity on the T2-weighted image and low signal intensity on the postgadolinium T1-weighted image represents ascites.

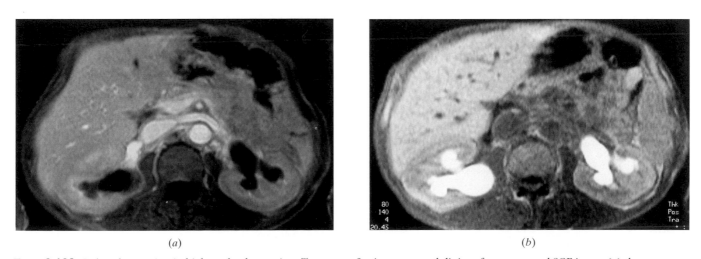

(a)

(b)

F IG . 9.103 Delayed excretion in high-grade obstruction. Transverse 2-minute postgadolinium fat-suppressed SGE image (*a*) demonstrates severe dilatation of the renal collecting system secondary to bladder cancer. SGE image (*b*) obtained 24 hours later demonstrates delayed excretion of gadolinium.

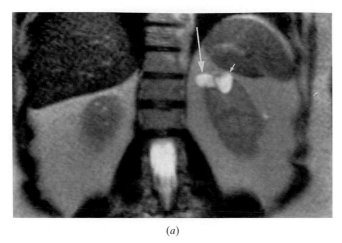

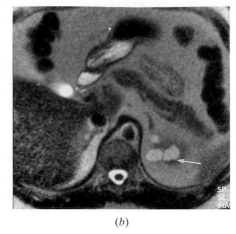

(a)   (b)

FIG. 9.104 Calyceal diverticulum. Coronal (a) and transverse (b) HASTE images. The coronal image demonstrates a calyceal diverticulum (*small arrow, a*) adjacent to a renal cyst (*long arrow, a*). The calyceal diverticulum extends to the surface of the kidney and contains low-signal-intensity milk of calcium, which is commonly observed in these lesions. Minute low-signal-intensity calculi are apparent in the dependent portion of the diverticulum (*arrow, b*) on the transverse image (b). Atrophy of the overlying renal cortex is apparent.

shown using sequences that result in high-signal-intensity urine. The diverticula not uncommonly extend to the cortical surface.

JUXTARENAL PROCESSES

Tumor, hemorrhage, abscess, and urine leaks all may occur in a juxtarenal location. Urine extravasation most commonly occurs either as a result of trauma or secondary to calyceal rupture due to elevated intracollecting system pressure. Although acute obstruction on the basis of renal calculi is the most common cause of calyceal rupture, this also may be seen in other causes of obstruction (Fig. 9.105).

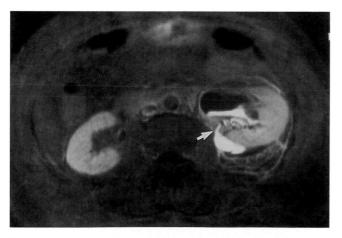

FIG. 9.105 Pyelosinus rupture. Gadolinium-enhanced T1-weighted fat-suppressed spin-echo image demonstrates leakage of dilute high-signal-intensity gadolinium (*arrow*) from a dilated, obstructed left renal collecting system.

TRAUMA

Renal trauma is a common occurrence in abdominal injury. Tomographic imaging is the most accurate method for assessing the severity of injury, which is generally classified as mild (contusion), moderate (laceration into the collection system), or severe (disruption of renal pedicle or complete crush). Precontrast T1-weighted images are sensitive to the presence of blood. Dynamic gadolinium-enhanced images demonstrate renal vessels as high in signal intensity and are useful for assessing their integrity. Degree of renal injury is well-shown on postgadolinium images by the demonstration of lacerations, hemorrhage, or areas of diminished enhancement (Fig. 9.106).

RENAL FUNCTION

Gadolinium-enhanced dynamic serial imaging of the kidneys demonstrates distinct phases of contrast enhancement based on the location of the bulk of the contrast agent. The phases of enhancement can be separated into (1) capillary, (2) early tubular, (3) ductal, and (4) excretory [5]. Evaluation of the concentrating ability of the kidneys may be made by the observation of signal-intensity changes in renal tissue based on the presence of gadolinium of varying concentrations (Fig. 9.107). When dilute, gadolinium renders tissues high in signal intensity, and when concentrated, gadolinium renders tissues signal-void. The assessment of these phases of enhancement has been shown to distinguish normal kidneys and those with dilated nonobstructed collecting systems from acute and chronic obstruction. Patients must be mildly dehydrated in order to provide the physiologic condition for

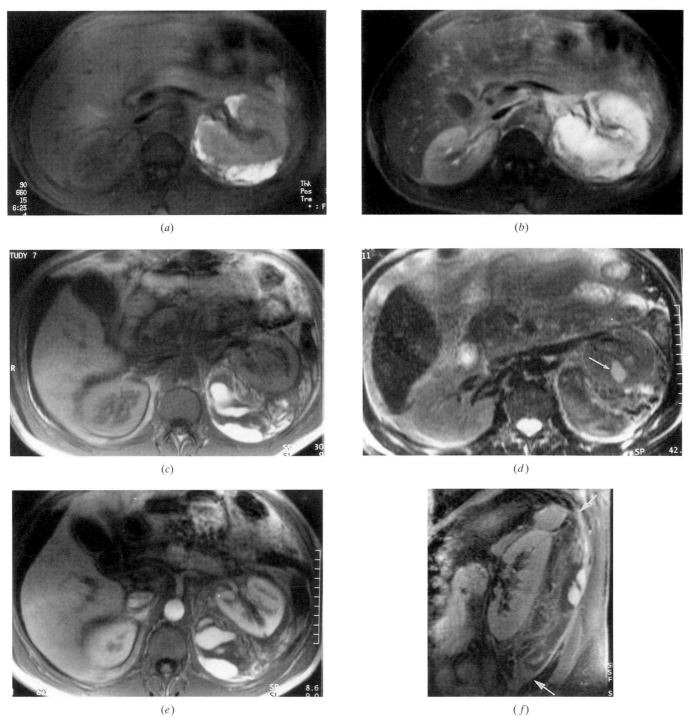

F IG . 9.106 Renal trauma. T1-weighted fat-suppressed spin-echo (*a*) and interstitial-phase gadolinium-enhanced T1-weighted fat-suppressed spin-echo (*b*) images. High-signal-intensity perirenal hematoma is present surrounding an enlarged left kidney on the precontrast image. The interstitial-phase gadolinium-enhanced image demonstrates greater enhancement of the left kidney, compared to the normal right kidney. This excludes renal-artery compromise but implies increased intrarenal tissue pressure, capillary leakage, and/or renal vein compromise. SGE (*c*), HASTE (*d*), immediate postgadolinium SGE (*e*), and sagittal 90-second postgadolinium SGE (*f*) images in a second patient who sustained abdominal trauma. High-signal-intensity hemorrhage is noted in the perirenal and posterior pararenal space in the left kidney with a multilayered appearance (*c*). Mixed high signal intensity is apparent on the T2-weighted image (*d*), which is consistent with blood products of varying age. In addition a tubular-shaped focus of high signal intensity is present, a finding consistent with an intraparenchymal laceration (*arrow, d*). The kidney enhances normally immediately after contrast administration excluding a major renal arterial injury. The sagittal image (*f*) demonstrates the full renal length and the volume of posterior pararenal blood (*arrows, f*).

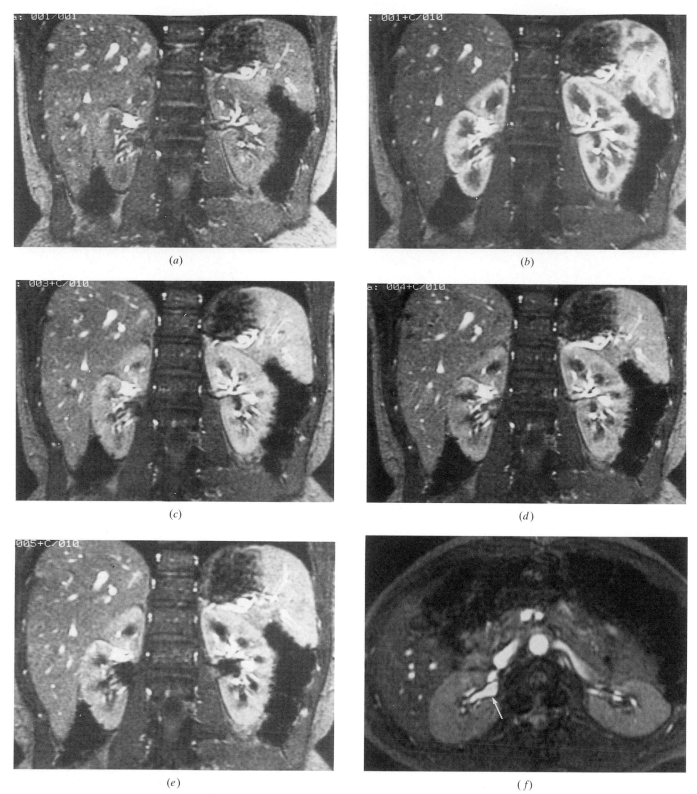

(a)

(b)

(c)

(d)

(e)

(f)

FIG. 9.107 Normal renal function. Precontrast image (*a*). Minimal corticomedullary differentiation is present. Cortical enhancement (capillary)-phase image (*b*). Cortex signal intensity is increased by 17 percent. Corticomedullary differentiation is distinct because of differential blood flow and increased delivery of gadolinium to the renal cortex. Early tubular-phase (*c*) image. Signal intensity of medulla is transiently increased, whereas there is little change in cortical signal intensity. Ductal-phase image (*d*). Signal intensity of medulla is decreased (6% from vascular phase) due to the concentration of gadolinium in distal convoluted tubules and collecting ducts. There is minimal decrease in cortical signal intensity (2%). Decreased signal intensity is apparent in the inner medulla and therefore mainly represents concentrated gadolinium in collecting ducts. Excretory-phase image (*e*). Urine containing concentrated gadolinium appears in renal collecting systems as signal-void fluid. Excretory-phase image (*f*) obtained 15 minutes after injection. No corticomedullary differentiation is present. Urine contains dilute (high-signal-intensity) gadolinium (*arrows, f*) because of rapid clearance of gadolinium from the body. (Reprinted with permission from Semelka RC, Hricak H, Tomei E, Floth A, Stoller M: Obstructive nephropathy: Evaluation with dynamic Gd-DTPA enhanced MR imaging. Radiology 175:797–803, 1990)

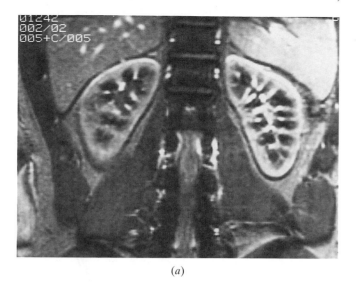

(a)

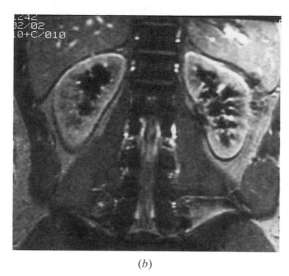

(b)

FIG. 9.108 Dilated nonobstructed kidney. Gradient-echo images of subject with a dilated nonobstructed right kidney. Ductal-phase image (a). Low signal intensity of the medulla appears simultaneously in the dilated nonobstructed right kidney and in the normal left kidney. Excretory-phase image (b). Excretion of concentrated urine is bilaterally symmetric. Susceptibility-induced image distortion of the renal collecting systems is due to the high concentration of gadolinium. (Reprinted with permission from Semelka RC, Hricak H, Tomei E, Floth A, Stoller M: Obstructive nephropathy: Evaluation with dynamic Gd-DTPA enhanced MR imaging. Radiology 175:797–803, 1990)

renal concentration. This can be achieved by a 5-hour fast. Dilated, nonobstructed kidneys have a temporal pattern of signal-intensity changes similar to that of normal kidneys because renal transit is not abnormal (Fig. 9.108). Acutely obstructed kidneys are enlarged and have increased renal transit time. This corresponds to an appearance of a prolonged increasing signal-intensity nephrogram and delayed appearance of contrast in the renal ducts and collecting system (Fig. 9.109). Chronic obstruction has diminished cortical enhancement and increased transit time (Fig. 9.110).

Functional changes of cortical and medullary en-

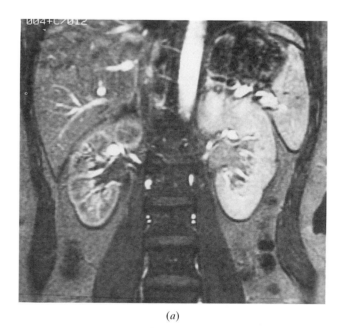

(a)

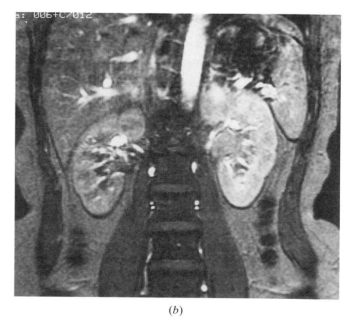

(b)

FIG. 9.109 Acute obstruction. Gradient-echo images of subject with an acutely obstructed left kidney and normal right kidney. Cortical enhancement (capillary)-phase image (a). The acutely obstructed left kidney is larger and swollen compared with the right kidney. Obstruction to venous drainage results in an abnormal pattern of contrast enhancement of the obstructed kidney. The parenchymal signal intensity is greater, and corticomedullary differentiation is diminished. Ductal-phase image (b). Tubular concentration is apparent on the normal right kidney but not on the obstructed left kidney. Cortical enhancement is persistent on the obstructed side, analogous to the persistent nephrogram on intravenous urogram (IVU) examination. Excretory-phase image (c).

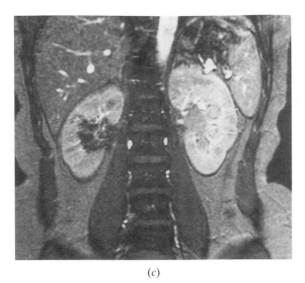

(c)

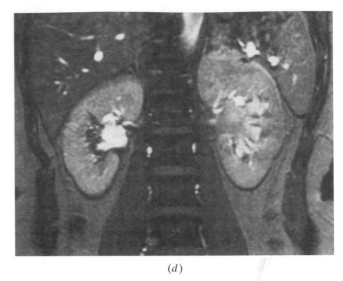

(d)

FIG. 9.109 (*Continued*)   The delayed image obtained at 3.5 minutes shows dilute (high-signal-intensity) urine in dilated calyces (*arrows, c*) of the left kidney. Concentrated (low-signal-intensity) urine is excreted from the right kidney. Excretory-phase image (*d*) obtained 15 minutes after injection. Dilute urine is excreted by the normal right kidney. Further excretion into the dilated left renal collecting system can be appreciated. (Reprinted with permission from Semelka RC, Hricak H, Tomei E, Floth A, Stoller M: Obstructive nephropathy: Evaluation with dynamic Gd-DTPA enhanced MR imaging. Radiology 175:797–803, 1990)

hancement also may be observed in the context of renal ischemia [93].

RENAL TRANSPLANTS

Loss of renal corticomedullary differentiation on T1-weighted images is an observation found in renal allo-

grafts undergoing rejection [94–96]. In a study comparing the accuracy of MRI, quantitative scintigraphy, and sonography for the detection of renal transplant rejection, the sensitivities for these modalities was 97, 80, and 70 percent, respectively [95]. Loss of corticomedullary differentiation, however, is nonspecific and observed also in cyclosporine toxicity and other infiltrative or diffuse renal parenchymal diseases [72,97]. Normal functioning trans-

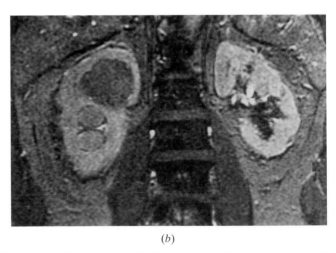

(a)   (b)

FIG. 9.110   Chronic obstruction. Gradient-echo images of a subject with a chronically obstructed right kidney and a dilated nonobstructed left kidney. Cortical enhancement (capillary)-phase image (*a*). Normal cortical enhancement is appreciated in the left kidney, which demonstrates corticomedullary distinction. Cortical enhancement is lower in the chronically obstructed right kidney with no definition of CMD. Low-signal-intensity gadolinium-free urine is present in both collecting systems (*arrows, a*). Excretory-phase image (*b*). Concentrated urine is excreted by the dilated nonobstructed left kidney. There is no apparent excretion by the chronically obstructed right kidney, no development of cortico-medullary differentiation, and no significant changes in parenchymal signal intensity from the cortical enhancement phase. (Reprinted with permission from Semelka RC, Hricak H, Tomei E, Floth A, Stoller M: Obstructive nephropathy: Evaluation with dynamic Gd-DTPA enhanced MR imaging. Radiology 175:797–803, 1990)

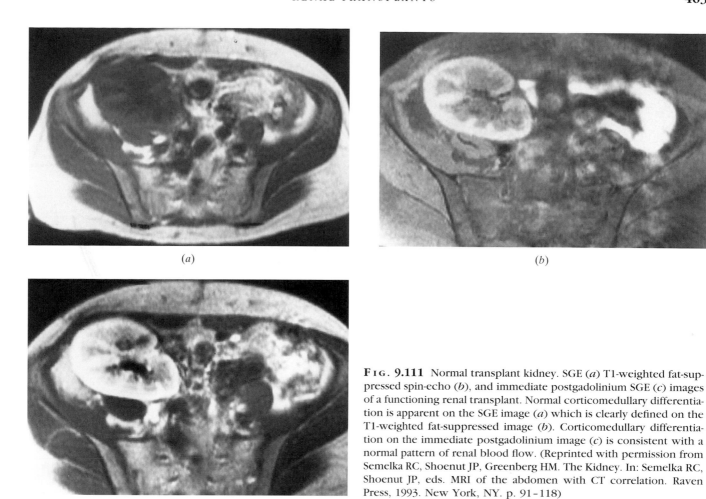

(a)

(b)

(c)

FIG. 9.111 Normal transplant kidney. SGE (a) T1-weighted fat-suppressed spin-echo (b), and immediate postgadolinium SGE (c) images of a functioning renal transplant. Normal corticomedullary differentiation is apparent on the SGE image (a) which is clearly defined on the T1-weighted fat-suppressed image (b). Corticomedullary differentiation on the immediate postgadolinium image (c) is consistent with a normal pattern of renal blood flow. (Reprinted with permission from Semelka RC, Shoenut JP, Greenberg HM. The Kidney. In: Semelka RC, Shoenut JP, eds. MRI of the abdomen with CT correlation. Raven Press, 1993. New York, NY. p. 91–118)

(a)

(b)

FIG. 9.112 Chronic rejection of renal transplant. SGE (a), T1-weighted fat-suppressed spin-echo (b), and immediate postgadolinium SGE (c) images in a renal transplant undergoing chronic rejection. Loss of corticomedullary differentiation is apparent on precontrast T1-weighted images (a,b). The presence of corticomedullary differentiation on the capillary-phase image shows persistence of a normal pattern of renal blood flow, which is consistent with preservation of some renal function. Fat-suppressed SGE (d) and immediate postgadolinium SGE (e) images in a second patient with chronic rejection.

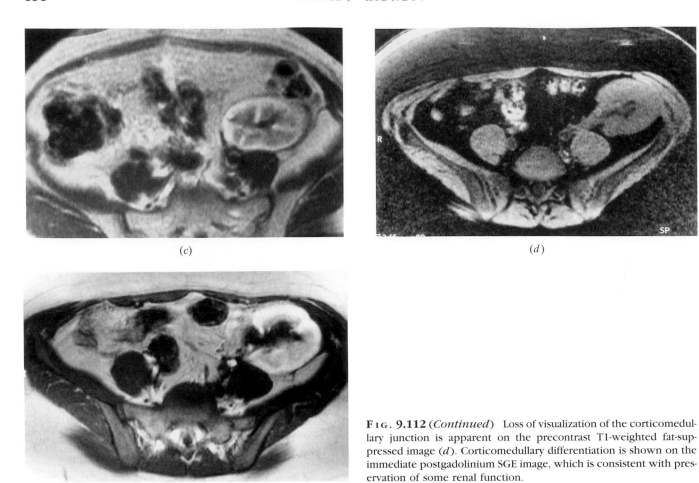

(c)

(d)

(e)

FIG. 9.112 (*Continued*)   Loss of visualization of the corticomedullary junction is apparent on the precontrast T1-weighted fat-suppressed image (*d*). Corticomedullary differentiation is shown on the immediate postgadolinium SGE image, which is consistent with preservation of some renal function.

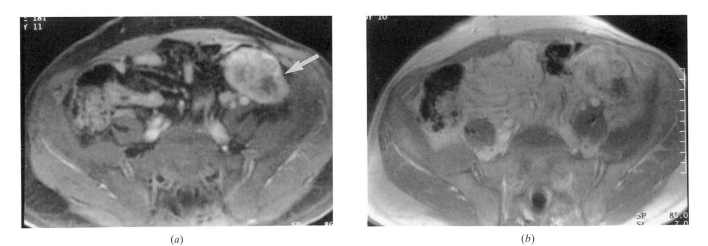

(a)

(b)

FIG. 9.113 Severe chronic rejection. Transverse 45-second postgadolinium fat-suppressed SGE (*a*) and 90-second postgadolinium SGE (*b*) images. The transplanted kidney has an irregular contour (*arrow, a*). Irregularly margined central areas of diminished enhancement are present on 45- and 90-second images. By 90 seconds, enhancement of renal medulla should equilibrate with the cortex, and therefore this central diminished enhancement does not reflect normal medulla.

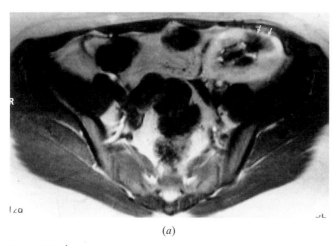

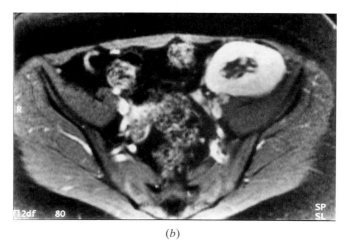

(a)   (b)

F IG. 9.114 Acute focal pyelonephritis in a renal transplant. Immediate postgadolinium SGE (*a*) and 90-second postgadolinium T1-weighted fat-suppressed SGE (*b*) images demonstrate a focal region anteriorly in the transplant kidney that shows a striated nephrogram appearance on the capillary-phase image (*arrow, a*), which resolves on the interstitial-phase image (*b*). This appearance is consistent with acute focal pyelonephritis without abscess formation.

plants have good corticomedullary differentiation on precontrast T1-weighted fat-suppressed images and immediate postgadolinium-enhanced images (Fig. 9.111). Chronic rejection results in loss of corticomedullary differentiation on T1-weighted fat-suppressed images (Fig. 9.112). The degree of loss of corticomedullary differentiation on dynamic contrast-enhanced images may correlate with the severity of rejection. Long-standing severe rejection may result in morphological alterations of the kidney (Fig. 9.113). Serial enhancement changes of cortex and medulla on dynamic gadolinium-enhanced studies may

indicate the severity of rejection and may permit differentiation between rejection, cyclosporine toxicity, and acute tubular necrosis. Definitive studies, however, are lacking at present. Assessment of surgical complications such as urinoma formation and renal vascular patency or stenosis are well-evaluated with MRI [98,99]. Infection or abscess formation in the transplant are also well-shown (Fig. 9.114). The gadolinium-enhanced 3D FISP technique is an accurate reproducible technique for evaluating renal artery complications [2,3]. Normal transplant arteries and veins are clearly identified (Fig. 9.115). Steno-

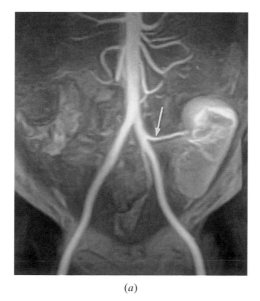

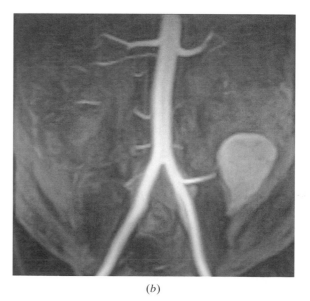

(a)   (b)

F IG. 9.115 Normal renal artery of a renal transplant. Coronal 3D maximum-intensity projection (MIP) reconstruction (*a*) and individual source section (*b*) of a 2-mm thin section bolus gadolinium 3D FISP acquisition. A normal caliber renal artery (*arrow, a*) is well-shown on the 3D MIP reconstructed image (*a*). Review of the individual source image confirms that no subtle stenotic lesions are apparent (*b*).

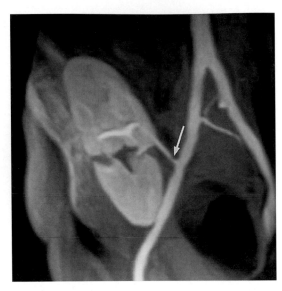

F IG. 9.116 Renal artery stenosis in a transplant kidney. Renal MR angiography (MRA) using bolus gadolinium enhanced 3D FISP demonstrates stenosis of the renal artery (*arrow*) approximately 2 cm distal to the anastomosis with the internal iliac artery.

sis or thrombosis of artery or vein are similarly demonstrated in a reproducible fashion with this technique (Fig. 9.116).

FUTURE DIRECTIONS

Anatomic display of kidneys is accurate using current imaging techniques and phased-array multicoil imaging. Although gadolinium-enhanced 3D FISP is the most reproducible MR angiography (MRA) technique, advances in noncontrast MRA continue to develop [100–102]. It remains to be determined whether noncontrast MRA may be sufficiently accurate to assess renal transplant donors. Further understanding of renal function and functional and morphological disturbance caused by various renal diseases are currently under investigation [103–109]. Fast imaging techniques such as turboFLASH and echoplanar imaging [105,106,110], new contrast agents [104], or a combination of both [105,106] are being employed to examine renal function. Flow quantification may provide useful information on renal perfusion [107,108]. Pharmacological stresses also may develop into a clinical routine for evaluating renal vascular disease [109].

CONCLUSIONS

MRI performs well at detecting and characterizing renal masses and staging renal cancer. Because CT imaging is also an effective modality and greater clinical experience

has been established with this modality, the current role of MRI is to study patients who are not ideal candidates for CT imaging or to solve problems. Indications for MRI include (1) evaluation of tumor thrombus; (2) characterization of complicated renal lesions, particularly calcified cysts; (3) allergy to iodinated contrast; (4) elevated sCr (in order not to worsen renal failure and because of adequate contrast enhancement of diseased renal parenchyma); and (5) evaluation of chronically impaired kidneys for renal cancer. In diffuse renal parenchymal disease MRI is able to provide useful information that can help to determine underlying etiology. Current high-quality MRA using gadolinium-enhanced 3D FISP and 3D fat-suppressed SGE allows adequate evaluation of many patients with renal-artery disease. MR urography evaluates dilatation of the renal collection system in a rapid, noninvasive fashion. The combination of tissue-imaging sequences, MRA and MR urography, renders MRI a modality that can comprehensively evaluate the full spectrum of renal diseases.

REFERENCES

1. Semelka RC, Shoenut JP, Kroeker MA, MacMahon RG, Greenberg HM: Renal lesions: Controlled comparison between CT and 1.5 T MR imaging with nonenhanced- and gadolinium-enhanced fat-suppressed spin-echo and breath-hold FLASH techniques. Radiology 182:425–430, 1992.

2. Prince MR, Narasimham DL, Stanley JC, Chenevert TL, Williams DM, Marx MV, Cho KJ: Breath-hold gadolinium-enhanced MR angiography of the abdominal aorta and its major branches. Radiology 197:785–792, 1995.

3. Snidow JJ, Johnson MS, Harris VJ, Margosian PM, Aisen AM, Lalka SG, Cikrit DF, Trerotola SO: Three-dimensional gadolinium-enhanced MR angiography for aortoiliac inflow assessment plus renal artery screening in a single breath-hold. Radiology 198:725–732, 1996.

4. Rothpearl A, Frager D, Subramanian A, Bashist B, Baer J, Kay C, Cooke K, Raia C: MR urography: Technique and application. Radiology 194:125–130, 1995.

5. Semelka RC, Hricak H, Tomei E, Floth A, Stoller M: Obstructive nephropathy: Evaluation with dynamic Gd-DTPA-enhanced MR imaging. Radiology 175:797–803, 1990.

6. Choyke PL, Frank JA, Girton ME, et al: Dynamic Gd-DTPA-enhanced MR imaging of the kidney: Experimental results. Radiology 170:713–720, 1989.

7. Kikinis R, von Schulthess GK, Jager P, et al: Normal and hydronephrotic kidney: Evaluation of renal function with contrast-enhanced MR imaging. Radiology 165:837–842, 1987.

8. Ros PR, Gauger J, Stoupis C, Burton SS, Mao J, Wilcox C, Rosenber EB, Briggs RW: Diagnosis of renal artery stenosis: Feasibility of combining MR angiography, MR renography, and gadopentetate-based measurements of glomerular filtration rate. AJR Am J Roentgenol 165:1447–1457, 1995.

9. Barnhart JL, Kuhnert N, Douglas BA, et al: Biodistribution of Gd-CL and Gd-DTPA and their influence on proton magnetic relaxation in rat tissues. Magn Reson Imaging 5:221–231, 1987.

10. Dalton D, Neiman H, Grayhack JT: The natural history of simple renal cysts: A preliminary study. J Urol 135:905–908, 1986.

11. Semelka RC, Hricak H, Stevens SK, Fingold R, Tomei E, Carroll PR:

Combined gadolinium-enhanced and fat saturation MR imaging of renal masses. Radiology 178:803–809, 1991.

12. Gabow PA: Autosomal dominant polycystic kidney disease. Review article. N Engl J Med 329:332–342, 1993.

13. Huch Boni RA, Debatin JF, Krestin GP: Contrast-enhanced MR imaging of the kidneys and adrenal glands. Contrast Agents for Body MR Imaging. MRI Clinics of North Amer 1064–1089, 1996.

14. Cho C, Friedland GW, Swenson RS: Acquired renal cystic disease and renal neoplasms in hemodialysis patients. Urol Radiol 6:153–157, 1984.

15. Ishikawa I: Uremic acquired cystic disease of kidney. Urology 26:101–107, 1985.

16. Levine E, Grantham JJ, Slucher SL, Greathouse JL, Krohn BP: CT of acquired cystic kidney disease and renal tumors in long term dialysis patients. AJR Am J Roentgenol 142:125–131, 1984.

17. Mitnick JS, Bosniak MA, Mitton S, Raghavendra BN, Subramanyan BR, Genieser NB: Cystic renal disease in tuberous sclerosis. Radiology 147:85–87, 1983.

18. Van Ball JG, Smits NJ, Keeman JN, et al: The evolution of renal angiomylipomas in patients with tuberous sclerosis. J Urol 152:35–38, 1994.

19. Lemaitre L, Robert Y, Dubrulle F, Claudon M, Duhamel A, Danjou P, Mazeman E: Renal angiomyolipoma: Growth followed up with CT and/or US. Radiology 197:598–602, 1995.

20. Choyke PL, Glenn GM, Wlather MM, Patronas NJ, Linehan WM, Zbar B: von Hippel-Lindau disease: Genetic, clinical, and imaging features. Radiology 194:629–642, 1995.

21. Agrons GA, Wagner BJ, Davidson AJ, Suarez ES: Multilocular cystic renal tumor in children: Radiologic-pathologic correlation. Radiographics 15:653–669, 1995.

22. Kettritz U, Semelka RC, Siegelman ES, Shoenut JP, Mithell DG: Multilocular cystic nephroma: MR imaging appearance with current techniques, including gadolinium enhancement. J Magn Reson Imaging 1:145–148, 1996.

23. Dikengil A, Benson M, Sanders L, Newhouse JH: MRI of multilocular cystic nephroma. Urol Radiol 10:95–99, 1988.

24. Bellin MF, Richard F, Attias S, et al: Renal angiomyolipoma: Comparison of MRI and CT results for diagnosis. Eur Radiol 2:465–472, 1992.

25. Steiner MS, Goldman SM, Fishman EK, Marshall FF: The natural history of renal angiomyolipoma. J Urol 150:1782–1786, 1993.

26. Wills, JS: Management of small renal neoplasms and angiomyolipoma: A growing problem. Radiology 197:583–586, 1995.

27. Burdeny DA, Semelka RC, Kelekis NL, Reinhold C, Ascher SM: Small (<1.5 cm) angiomyolipomas of the kidney: Characterization by combined use of in-phase and fat attenuated MR techniques. Magn Reson Imag (in press).

28. Osterling JE, Fishman EK, Goldman SM, Marshall FF: The management of renal angiomyolipoma. J Urol 135:1121–1124, 1986.

29. Strotzer M, Lehner KB, Becker K: Detection of fat in a renal cell carcinoma mimicking angiomyolipoma. Radiology 188:427–428, 1993.

30. Quinn MJ, Hartman DS, Friedman AC, et al: Renal oncocytoma: New observations. Radiology 153:49–53, 1984.

31. Press GA, McClennan BL, Melson GL, Weyman PJ, Mauro MA, Lee JKT: Papillary renal cell carcinoma: CT and sonographic evaluation. AJR Am J Roentgenol 143:1005–1010, 1984.

32. Davidson AJ, Hayews WS, Hartman DS, McCarthy WF, Davis CJ: Renal oncocytoma and carcinoma: Failure of differentiation with CT. Radiology 186:693–696, 1993.

33. Bosniak MA: The small (≤3.0 cm) renal parenchymal tumor: Detection, diagnosis, and controversies. Radiology 179:307–317, 1991.

34. Birnbaum BA, Bosniak MA, Megibow AJ, Lubat E, Gordon RB: Observations on the growth of renal neoplasms. Radiology 176:695–701, 1990.

35. Levine E, Huntrakoon M, Wetzel LH: Small renal neoplasms: Clinical, pathologic, and imaging features. AJR Am J Roentgenol 153:69–73, 1989.

36. Curry, NS: Small renal masses (lesions smaller than 3 cm): Imaging evaluation and managment. AJR Am J Roentgenol 164:355–362, 1995.

37. Bosniak MA, Birnbaum BA, Krinsky GA, Waisman J: Small renal parenchymal neoplasms: Further observations on growth. Radiology 197:589–597, 1995.

38. Bosniak MA, Rofsky NM: Problems in the detection and characterization of small renal masses. Radiology 198:638–641, 1996.

39. Ball DS, Friedman AC, Hartman DS, Radecki PD, Caroline DF: Scar sign of renal oncocytoma: Magnetic resonance imaging appearance and lack of specificity. Urol Radiol 8:46–48, 1986.

40. Boring CC, Squires TS, Tony T: Cancer statistics, 1991. CA Cancer J Clin 41:19, 1991.

41. Semelka RC, Shoenut JP, Magro CM, Kroeker MA, MacMahon R, Greenberg HM: Renal cancer staging: Comparison of contrast-enhanced CT and gadolinium-enhanced fat-suppressed spin-echo and gradient-echo MR imaging. J Magn Reson Imaging 3:597–602, 1993.

42. Hricak H, Thoeni RF, Carroll PR, Demas BE, Marotti M, Tanagho EA: Detection and staging of renal neoplasms: A reassessment of MR imaging. Radiology 166:643–649, 1988.

43. Hricak H, Amparo E, Fisher MR, Crooks L, Higgins CB: Abdominal venous system: Assessment using MR. Radiology 156:415–422, 1985.

44. Hricak H, Demas BE, Williams RD, et al: Magnetic resonance imaging in the diagnosis of renal and perirenal neoplasms. Radiology 154:709–715, 1985.

45. Patel SK, Stack CM, Turner DA: Magnetic resonance imaging in staging of renal cell carcinoma. Radiographics 156:415–422, 1987.

46. Pritchett TR, Raval JK, Benson RC, et al: Preoperative magnetic resonance imaging of vena caval tumor thrombi: Experience with five cases. J Urol 138:1220–1222, 1987.

47. Fein AB, Lee JKT, Balfe DM, et al: Diagnosis and staging of renal cell carcinoma: A comparison of MR imaging and CT. AJR Am J Roentgenol 148:749–753, 1987.

48. Eilenberg SS, Lee JKT, Brown JJ, Mirowitz SA, Tartar VM: Renal masses: Evaluation with gradient-echo Gd-DTPA-enhanced dynamic MR imaging. Radiology 176:333–338, 1990.

49. Rominger MB, Kenney PJ, Morgan DE, Bernreuter WK, Listinsky JJ: Gadolinium-enhanced MR imaging of renal masses. Radiographics 12:1097–1116, 1992.

50. Zeman RK, Cronan JJ, Rosenfield AT, Lynch JH, Jaffe MH, Clark LR: Renal cell carcinoma: Dynamic thin-section CT assessment of vascular invasion and tumor vascularity. Radiology 167:393–396, 1988.

51. Roubidoux MA, Dunnick NR, Sostman HD, Leder RA: Renal carcinoma: Detection of venous extension with gradient echo MR imaging. Radiology 182:269–272, 1992.

52. Studer UE, Scherz S, Scheidegger J, et al: Enlargement of regional lymph nodes in renal cell carcinoma is often not due to metastases. J Urol 144:243–245, 1990.

53. John G, Semelka RC, Burdeny DA, Kelekis NL, Kettritz U, Freeman JA: Renal cell cancer: Incidence of hemorrhage on MR images in patients with renal insufficiency. J Magn Reson Imag 7:157–160, 1997.

54. Terens WL, Gluck R, Golimbu M, Rofsky NM: Use of gadolinium-DTPA-enhanced MRI to characterize renal masses in patient with renal insufficiency. Urology 40:152–154, 1992.

55. Rofsky NM, Weinreb JC, Bosniak MA, Libes RB, Birnbaum BA: Renal lesion characterization with gadolinium-enhanced MR imaging: Efficacy and safety in patients with renal insufficiency. Radiology 180:85–89, 1991.

56. Haustein J, Niendorf HP, Krestin G, et al: Renal tolerance of gadolinium-DTPA/dimeglumine in patients with chronic renal failure. Invest Radiol 27:153–156, 1992.

57. Choyke PL, Girton ME, Vaughn EM, Frank JA, Austin HA. Clearance of gadolinium chelates by hemodialysis: An in vitro study. J Magn Reson Imaging 4:470–472, 1995.

58. Thompson IM, Peek M: Improvement in survival of patients with renal cell carcinoma: The role of the serendipitous detected tumor. J Urol 140:487–490, 1988.

59. Smith SJ, Bosniak MA, Megibow AJ, Hulnick DH, Horii SC, Raghavendra BN: Renal cell carcinoma: Earlier detection and increased detection. Radiology 170:699–703, 1989.

60. Jamis-Dow CA, Choyke PL, Jennings SB, Linehan WM, Thakore KN, Walther MM: Small (≤3 cm) renal masses: Detection with CT versus US and pathologic correlation. Radiology 198:785–788, 1996.

61. Butler BP, Novick AC, Miller DP, et al: Management of small unilateral renal cell carcinomas: Radical versus nephron-sparing surgery. Urology 45:34–41, 1995.

62. Novick AC: Partial nephrectomy for renal cell carcinoma (editorial). Urology 46:149–152, 1995.

63. Nissenkorn I, Bernheim J: Multicentricity in renal cell carcinoma. J Urol 153:620–622, 1995.

64. Pronet J, Tessler A, Brown J, Golimbu M, Bosniak M, Morales P: Partial nephrectomy for renal cell carcinoma: Indications, results and implications. J Urol 145:472–476, 1991.

65. Gylys-Morin V, Hoffer FA, Kozakewich H, Shamberger RC: Wilms tumor and nephroblastomatosis: Imaging characteristics at gadolinium-enhanced MR imaging. Radiology 188:517–521, 1993.

66. Cohen MD: Review. Staging of Wilms' tumour. Clin Radiol 14:77–81, 1993.

67. Weese DL, Applebaum H, Taber P: Mapping intravascular extension of Wilms' tumor with magnetic resonance imaging. J Pediatr Surg 1:64–67, 1991.

68. Richards MA, Mootoosamy I, Reznek RH, Webb JA, Lister TA: Renal involvement in patients with non-Hodgkin's lymphoma: Clinical and pathological features in 23 cases. Hematol Oncol 8:105–110, 1990.

69. Heiken JP, McClennan BL, Gold RP: Renal lymphoma. Semin Ultrasound CT MR 7:58–66, 1986.

70. Semelka RC, Kelekis NL, Burdeny DA, Mitchell DG, Brown JJ, Siegelman ES: Renal lymphoma: Demonstration by MR imaging. AJR Am J Roentgenol 166:823–827, 1996.

71. Hauser M, Krestin GP, Hagspiel KD: Bilateral solid multifocal intrarenal and perirenal lesions: Differentiation with ultrasonography, computed tomography and magnetic resonance imaging. Clin Radiol 50:288–294, 1995.

72. Kettritz U, Semelka RC, Brown ED, Sharp TJ, Lawing WL, Colindres RE: MR findings in diffuse renal parenchymal disease. J Magn Reson Imaging 6:136–144, 1996.

73. Semelka RC, Corrigan K, Ascher SM, Brown JJ, Colindres RE: Renal corticomedullary differentiation: Observation in patient with differing serum creatinine levels. Radiology 190:149–152, 1994.

74. Tempany CMC, Morton RA, Marshall FF: MRI of the renal veins: Assessment of nonneoplastic venous thrombosis. J Comput Assist Tomogr 16(6):929–934, 1992.

75. Lande IM, Glazer GM, Sarnaik S, Aisen A, Rucknagel D, Martel W: Sickle-cell nephropathy: MR imaging. Radiology 158:379–383, 1986.

76. Siegelman ES, Outwater E, Hanau CA, Ballas SK, Steiner RM, Rao VM, Mitchell DG: Abdominal iron distribution in sickle cell disease: MR finding in transfusion and nontransfusion dependent patients. J Comput Assist Tomogr 18(1):63–67, 1994.

77. Roubidouz MA: MR of the kidneys, liver, and spleen in paroxysmal nocturnal hemoglobinuria. Abdom Imaging 19:168–173, 1994.

78. Saunders HS, Dyer RB, Shifrin RY, Scharling ES, Bechtold RE, Zagoria RJ: The CT nephrogram: Implications for evaluation of urinary tract disease. Radiographics 15:1069–1085, 1995.

79. Kelekis NL, Semelka RC, Molina P, Warshauer DM: Abdominal

aorta: Evaluation with immediate post gadolinium spoiled gradient echo. J Magn Reson Imaging (submitted).

80. Lessman RK, Johnson SF, Coburn JW, et al: Renal artery embolism: Clinical features and long-term follow-up of 17 cases. Ann Intern Med 89:477–481, 1978.

81. Goldman SM, Fishman EK: Upper urinary tract infection: The current role of CT, ultrasound, and MRI. Semin Ultrasound CT MR 4:335–360, 1991.

82. Fowler JE Jr, Perkins T: Presentation, diagnosis and treatment of renal abscesses: 1972–1988. J Urol 151:847–851, 1994.

83. Brown ED, Semelka RC: Renal abscesses: Appearance on gadolinium-enhanced magnetic resonance images. Abdom Imaging 21:172–176, 1996.

84. Bova JG, Potter JL, Arevalos E, Hopens T, Goldstein HM, Radwin HM: Renal and perirenal infection: The role of computerized tomography. J Urol 133:375–378, 1985.

85. Mulopulos GP, Patel SK, Pessis D: MR imaging of xanthogranulomatous pyelonephritis. J. Comput Assist Tomogr 10:154–156, 1986.

86. Semelka RC, Shoenut JP, Greenberg HM, Bow EJ: Detection of acute and treated lesions of hepatosplenic candidiasis: Comparison of dynamic contrast-enhanced CT and MR imaging. J Magn Reson Imaging 2:414–420, 1992.

87. Winalski CS, Lipman JC, Tumeh SS: Ureteral neoplasms. Radiographics 10:271–283, 1990.

88. Weeks SM, Brown ED, Brown JJ, Adamis MK, Eisenberg LB, Semelka RC: Transitional cell carcinoma of the upper urinary tract staging by MRI. Abdom Imaging 20:365–367, 1995.

89. Leo ME, Petrou SP, Barrett DM: Transitional cell carcinoma of the kidney with vena caval involvement: Report of 3 cases and a review of the literature. J Urol 148:398–400, 1992.

90. Lebowitz JA, Rofsky NM, Weinreb JC, Friedmann P: Ureteral lymphoma: MRI demonstration. Abdom Imaging 20:173–175, 1995

91. Coe FL, Parks JH, Asplin JR: The pathogenesis and treatment of kidney stones. N Engl J Med 327:1141–1152, 1992.

92. Regan F, Bohlman ME, Khazan R, Rodriguez R, Schultze-Haakh H. MR urography using HASTE imaging in the assessment of ureteric obstruction. Am J Roentgen 167:1115–1120, 1996.

93. Laissy J-P, Faraggi M, Lebtahi R, et al: Functional evaluation of normal and ischemic kidney by means of gadolinium-DOTA enhanced TurboFLASH MR imaging: A preliminary comparison with 99mTc-MAG3 dynamic scintigraphy. Magn Reson Imaging 12:413–419, 1994.

94. McCreath GT, McMillan N, Patterson J, et al: Magnetic resonance imaging of renal transplants: Initial experience. Br J Radiol 61:113–118, 1988.

95. Hricak H, Terrier F, Marotti M, et al: Post-transplant renal rejection: Comparison of quantitative scintigraphy, ultrasonography and magnetic resonance imaging. Radiology 162:685–688, 1987.

96. Hanna S, Helenon O, Legendre C, et al: MR imaging of renal transplant rejection. Acta Radiol 32:42–46, 1991.

97. Liou JTS, Lee JKT, Heiken JP, Totty WG, Molina PL, Flye WM: Renal transplants: Can acute rejection and acute tubular necrosis be differentiated with MR imaging. Radiology 179:61–65, 1991.

98. Brichaux J-C, Grenier N, Douws C, Degreze P, Palussiere J, Trillaud H, Morel D, Potaux L: Time-of-flight MR angiography of kidney transplants. Eur Radiol 5:406–413, 1995.

99. Gedroyc WMW, Negus R, Al-Kutoubi A, Palmer A, Taube D, Hulme B: Magnetic resonance angiography of renal transplants. Lancet 339:789–791, 1992.

100. Edelman RR, Siewert B, Adamis M, Gaa J, Laub G, Wielopolski P: Signal targeting with alternating radiofrequency (STAR) sequences. Magn Reson Med 31:233–238, 1994.

101. Li D, Haacke EM, Muyler JP III, Berr S, Brookeman JR, Hutton MC: Three-dimensional time-of-flight MR angiography using selective

inversion recovery RAGE with fat saturation and ECG-triggering: Application to renal arteries. Magn Reson Med 31:414–422, 1994.

102. Yucel EK, Kaufman JA, Prince M, Bazari H, Fang LST, Waltman AC: Time-of-flight renal MR angiography: Utility in patients with renal insufficiency. Magn Reson Imaging 11:925–930, 1993.

103. Kim SH, Byun H, Park JH, Han JK, Lee JS: Renal parenchymal abnormalities associated with renal vein thrombosis: Correlation between MR imaging and pathologic findings in rabbits. AJR Am J Roentgenol 162:1361–1365, 1994.

104. Vexler VS, Bethezene Y, Clement O, Muhler A, Rosenau W, Moseley ME, Brasch RC: Detection of zonal renal ischemia with contrast-enhanced MR imaging with a macromolecular blood pool contrast agent. J Magn Reson Imaging 2:311–319, 1992.

105. Trillaud H, Grenier N, Degreze P, Louail C, Chambon C, Francoi J: First-pass evaluation of renal perfusion with TurboFLASH MR imaging and 'superparamagnetic iron oxide particles. J Magn Reson Imaging 3:83–91, 1993.

106. Wolf GL, Hoop B, Cannillo JA, Rogowska JA, Halpern EF: Measurement of renal transit of gadopentetate dimeglumine with echoplanar MR imaging. J Magn Reson Imaging 4:365–372, 1994.

107. Wolf RL, King BF, Torres VE, Wilson DM, Ehman RL: Measurement of normal renal arterial blood flow: Cine phase-contrast MR imaging vs. clearance of p-Aminohippurate. AJR Am J Roentgenol 161:995–1002, 1993.

108. Debatin JF, Ting RH, Wegmuller H, et al: Renal artery blood flow: Quantification with phase-contrast MR imaging with and without breath holding. Radiology 190:371–378, 1994.

109. Trillaud H, Roques F, Degreze P, Combe C, Grenier N: Gd-DOTA tubular transit asymmetry induced by angiotensin-converting enzyme inhibitor in experimental renovascular hypertension. J Magn Reson Imaging 1:149–155, 1996.

110. Müller MR, Prasad PV, Bimmler D, Kaiser A, Edelman RR: Functional imaging of the kidney by means of measurement of the apparent diffusion coefficient. Radiology 193:711–715, 1994.

RETROPERITONEUM AND BODY WALL

N. L. KELEKIS, M.D. AND R. C. SEMELKA, M.D.

■ THE RETROPERITONEUM

NORMAL ANATOMY

The retroperitoneum is limited anteriorly by the parietal peritoneum and posteriorly by the transversalis fascia, extending from the level of the diaphragm to the level of the pelvic inlet. It is divided into the perirenal, anterior, and posterior pararenal spaces. Recent work suggests that additional dissectable planes exist between the retroperitoneal spaces: the retromesenteric plane formed by retromesenteric fusion planes anteriorly and the anterior renal fascia (Gerota's) posteriorly, and the retrorenal plane formed by retromesenteric fusion planes and the posterior renal fascia (Zückerkandl's fascia). These potential spaces may form the pathway by which rapidly accumulating fluid collections in the retroperitoneal space may extend to the pelvis [1].

The kidneys, adrenals, and pancreas are discussed in individual chapters.

MRI TECHNIQUE

The retroperitoneum can be reliably assessed by MRI. An imaging protocol should be designed to (1) maximize the signal-intensity differences between suspected pathology and background tissues, (2) directly image the full extent of disease processes, and (3) define their boundaries with adjacent organs. The combination of breath-hold and breathing-independent sequences acquired in at least two different planes is able to achieve these goals without substantially prolonging the examination time. In the investigation of abnormal retroperitoneal tissue (enlarged lymph nodes, retroperitoneal fibrosis, tumors), the imaging protocol should include precontrast SGE, fat-suppressed T2-weighted images and postgadolinium fat-suppressed SGE images. In the investigation of retroperitoneal hemorrhage, precontrast fat-suppressed SGE images should be obtained because this technique has the greatest sensitivity for subacute hemorrhage. Image acquisition in two orthogonal planes permits direct evaluation of the extent of retroperitoneal disease.

MR angiographic techniques, particularly breath-hold three-dimensional (3D) gradient-echo sequences, play an important role in imaging the aorta and its branches. The combined use of 3D gradient-echo MR angiography (MRA) and tissue-imaging sequences provides information on vessel lumen, vessel wall, and surrounding organs. Imaging directly in the coronal plane provides an overview of the entire abdominal aorta.

Oral contrast also may be used in selected cases to provide better delineation of bowel and to facilitate distinction of bowel from retroperitoneal tissue. Orally administered water provides adequate bowel opacification as a positive contrast medium for short-duration T2-weighted echo-train spin-echo (e.g., half Fourier single-shot turbo spin-echo [HASTE]) sequences, and as a negative contrast medium for breath-hold T1-weighted (e.g., SGE) sequences.

The selection of sequences may vary according to the clinical history, the other organs that are examined, and the capabilities of the equipment.

MASS LESIONS

Benign Masses

Retroperitoneal Fibrosis

Retroperitoneal fibrosis is most frequently an idiopathic disease [2]. Benign retroperitoneal fibrosis also may arise secondary to certain drugs (classically methysergide), inflammatory aortic aneurysm, retroperitoneal hemorrhage, infection, surgery, or radiation therapy [3]. Idiopathic retroperitoneal fibrosis is considered part of a more extensive systemic fibrotic disorder related to mediastinal fibrosis, sclerosing cholangitis, Riedel's thyroiditis, orbital and sinus pseudotumors [4,5], and pulmonary hyalinizing granulomas [6].

The most important differential diagnosis is between idiopathic benign and malignant retroperitoneal fibrosis, particularly because malignant neoplasms may coexist with benign retroperitoneal fibrosis [7]. Retroperitoneal fibrosis most commonly appears as oval-shaped tissue that encases the aorta. The extent of disease may vary from a focal region of fibrosis to dense infiltration of the retroperitoneum encasing the aorta, inferior vena cava (IVC) and ureters. The disease in its acute stage may present as a focal unilateral mass in the region of the common iliac vessels. Over time fibrosis extends superiorly in the retroperitoneum along the major vessels. In rare instances, thrombosis of the iliac veins [8] and portal vein [9] may be encountered. In the majority of cases the fibrous tissue is located around the abdominal aorta below the level of the renal vessels. A feature distinguishing retroperitoneal fibrosis from retroperitoneal malignant adenopathy and lymphomas is that the fibrous tissue envelopes the aorta, IVC, and ureters, but does not displace the aorta substantially anteriorly.

Early reports suggested that MRI may be able to distinguish benign from malignant retroperitoneal fibrosis [3,10]. Acute benign retroperitoneal fibrosis may, however, resemble malignant retroperitoneal fibrosis because both may enhance substantially with contrast and may be high in signal intensity on T2-weighted sequences (Fig. 10.1) [11–13]. This enhancement pattern is due to the extensive capillary network of acute benign granulation tissue similar to that in the postoperative spine [14]. Even-

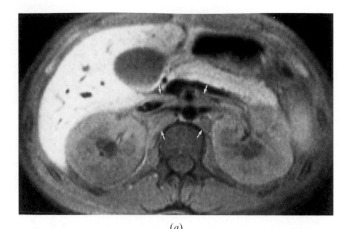

(*a*)

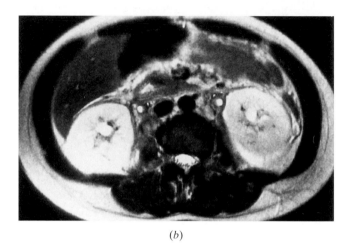

(*b*)

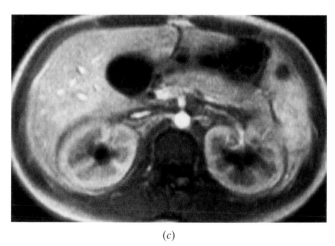

(*c*)

FIG. 10.1 Acute benign retroperitoneal fibrosis. T1-weighted fat-suppressed spin-echo (*a*), T2 spin-echo (T2-SE) (*b*), immediate postgadolinium SGE (*c*), and delayed postgadolinium T1-weighted fat-suppressed spin-echo (*d*) images. The aorta, IVC, renal arteries, and ureters are encased by soft tissue (*arrows, a*), which is low in signal intensity on T1-weighted (*a*) and heterogeneously high in signal intensity on T2-weighted (*b*) images, and has ill-defined margins. There is bilateral hydronephrosis and ureteral dilatation (*b*) caused by ureteral obstruction at a lower level. The fibrous tissue demonstrates heterogeneous enhancement on the immediate postgadolinium SGE image (*c*), which progresses on the more delayed T1-weighted fat-suppressed spin-echo image (*d*).

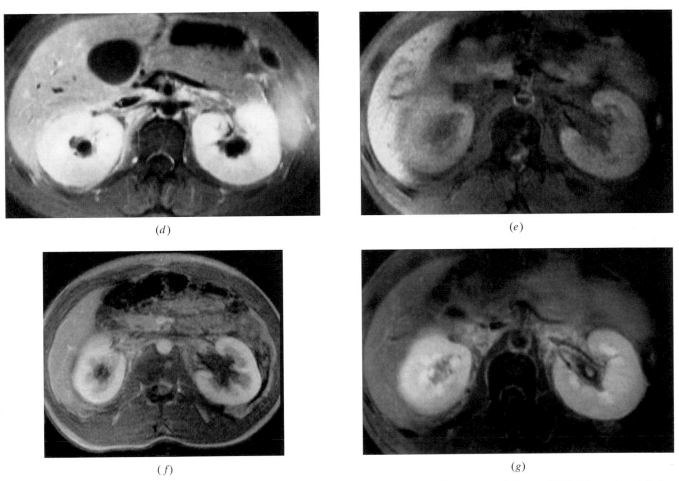

(d)

(e)

(f)

(g)

F IG. 10.1 (*Continued*) Precontrast T1-weighted fat-suppressed spin-echo (*e*), immediate postgadolinium SGE (*f*), and gadolinium-enhanced T1-weighted fat-suppressed spin-echo (*g*) images in a second patient with biopsy-proven membranous glomerulonephritis and benign retroperitoneal fibrosis. Ill-defined soft tissue is present in the retroperitoneum. The fibrous tissue is low on the precontrast T1-weighted image (*e*), demonstrates moderate heterogeneous enhancement on the immediate postgadolinium image (*f*), and is more conspicuous on the gadolinium-enhanced T1-weighted fat-suppressed spin-echo image (*g*) due to the removal of the competing high signal intensity of the fat. Corticomedullary differentiation is absent in both kidneys on the precontrast T1-weighted fat-suppressed spin-echo image (*e*) due to elevated serum creatinine level. Corticomedullary differentiation, however, is present on the immediate postgadolinium SGE image (*f*) reflecting some preservation of renal function. Increased medullary enhancement is shown in both kidneys on the gadolinium-enhanced T1-weighted fat-suppressed spin-echo image (*g*) reflecting tubulointerstitial damage.

tually, the granulation tissue alters to a more collagenous fibrotic form after approximately 1 year of development. During the course of maturation, signal intensity on T2-weighted images decreases, enhancement on immediate postgadolinium SGE images decreases, and the pattern of enhancement appears as a delayed, progressive increase in signal intensity (see Fig. 10.1). Granulation tissue on T2-weighted images generally shows decrease in signal intensity after approximately 1 year. Interstitial-phase gadolinium-enhanced fat-suppressed SGE images may show enhancement of acute fibrous tissue for approximately 1.5 year from onset. Mature chronic benign retroperitoneal fibrosis is low in signal intensity on T2-weighted images and demonstrates negligible contrast enhancement (Fig. 10.2), facilitating differentiation from malignancy. Imaging findings that may favor benign fi-

brosis include a well-marginated mass with smooth borders and a decrease in size and/or progressive smoothing of the borders on follow-up examinations.

Retroperitoneal Tumors

Benign retroperitoneal tumors are rare [15,16]. Therefore, any retroperitoneal tumor should initially be considered malignant. Retroperitoneal neurilemoma may have a characteristic high signal intensity on T2-weighted images [17]. Retroperitoneal plexiform neurofibromas are usually bilateral [18], slightly higher in signal intensity than muscles on T1-weighted images, and high in signal intensity on T2-weighted images [19–21] (Fig. 10.3). Other rare neoplasms include paragangliomas, hemangiomas/lymphangiomas, and lipomas [15]. Paragangliomas of Zückerkandl's organ may be hormone-secreting.

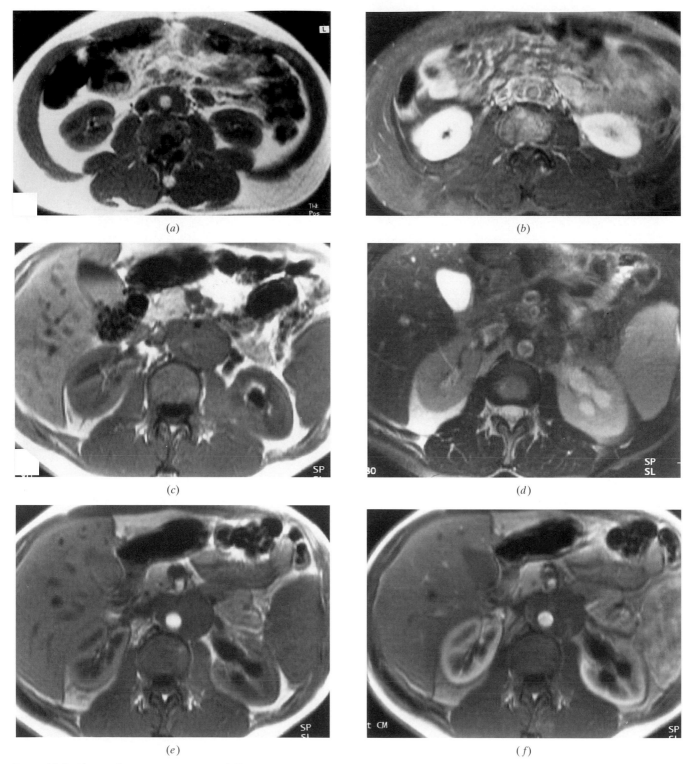

FIG. 10.2 Chronic benign retroperitoneal fibrosis. SGE (*a*) and gadolinium-enhanced fat-suppressed spin-echo (*b*) images. Low-signal-intensity oval-shaped tissue surrounds the aorta. The fibrous tissue has well-defined margins and shows minimal enhancement on the gadolinium-enhanced T1-weighted fat-suppressed spin-echo image (*b*), findings that are typical of mature fibrous tissue. SGE (*c*), T2-weighted echo-train spin-echo (*d*), arterial-phase (*e*) and capillary-phase (*f*) postgadolinium SGE, and 90-second postgadolinium fat-suppressed SGE (*g*) images in a second patient. The fibrotic tissue is oval-shaped with well-defined margins and encases the aorta. Note that, despite its size, the tissue does not substantially displace the aorta anteriorly. The fibrotic tissue is low in signal intensity on the T1-weighted image (*c*), is heterogeneously low with focal areas of high signal intensity on the T2-weighted image (*d*), demonstrates minimal enhancement on the arterial-phase (*e*) and capillary-phase (*f*) postgadolinium SGE images, and enhances moderately on the more delayed fat-suppressed SGE (*g*) image.

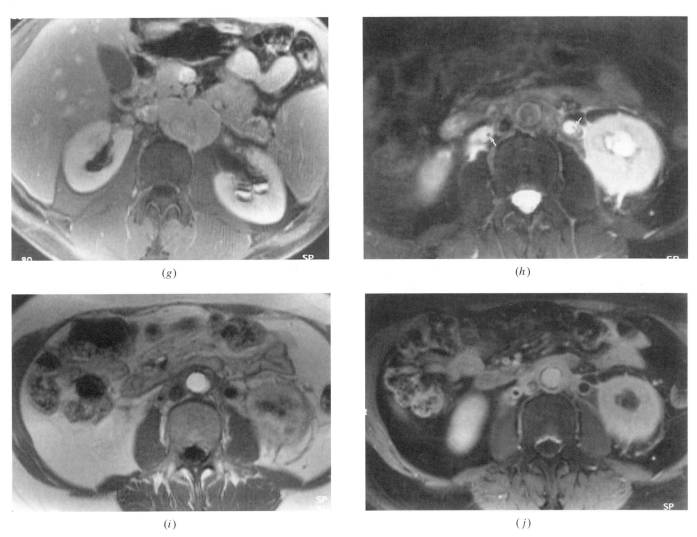

(g)   *(h)*

(i)   *(j)*

F ɪ ɢ . 10.2 (*Continued*) Delayed enhancement is characteristic of relatively mature fibrous tissue. Greater enhancement of the fibrotic tissue in the second patient reflects a more active stage in the transition between acute and chronic fibrosis than in the first patient. The pyelocalyceal system of the left kidney is dilated due to concomitant ureteral obstruction. T2-weighted echo-train spin-echo (*h*), immediate postgadolinium SGE (*i*), and interstitial-phase gadolinium-enhanced fat-suppressed SGE (*j*) images in a third patient. Again noted is relatively well-marginated oval tissue encasing the aorta, IVC, and both ureters. The fibrous tissue is heterogeneously low in signal intensity on the T2-weighted image (*h*) and demonstrates minimal enhancement on the immediate postgadolinium SGE image (*i*), progressing to moderate enhancement on the interstitial-phase gadoliniumenhanced fat-suppressed SGE image (*j*), indicating some degree of disease activity. Bilateral ureteral obstruction with hydronephrosis is present and signal-void ureteral stents (*arrows, h*) are demonstrated in both ureters on the T2-weighted image (*h*). The majority of the fibrous tissue is located anterior to the aorta and IVC, which are not displaced substantially anteriorly.

Imaging follow-up after surgery is advisable because 30 percent of the tumors are malignant and show late manifestation of remote disease [22]. Inflammatory pseudotumor is a rare benign mass lesion which is minimally low in signal intensity on T1-weighted images, heterogeneous and moderately high in signal intensity on T2-weighted images, and demonstrates moderately intense diffuse heterogeneous enhancement on immediate postgadolinium SGE images (Fig. 10.3). This appearance may mimic that of malignant tumors.

Lymphadenopathy

Benign lymphadenopathy may occur secondary to inflammatory or infectious disease. Sequences suited for detection of lymph nodes include precontrast SGE, fat-suppressed T2-weighted spin-echo or echo-train spin-echo, and gadolinium-enhanced fat-suppressed SGE techniques. In each of these techniques the signal difference between lymph nodes and background tissue is substantial. The enlarged lymph nodes appear low in signal on precontrast SGE and high in signal on fat-sup-

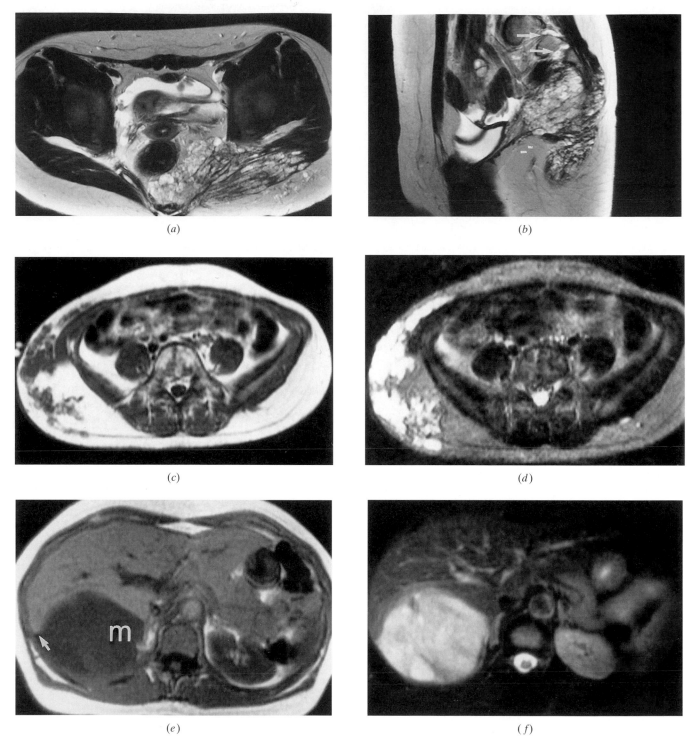

(a)

(b)

(c)

(d)

(e)

(f)

FIG. 10.3 Benign retroperitoneal tumors. Transverse (*a*) and sagittal (*b*) 512-resolution T2-weighted echo-train spin-echo images in a patient with plexiform neurofibroma of the pelvis and neurofibromatosis Type 1. The plexiform neurofibroma appears as a large heterogeneous mass that occupies the majority of the left posterior pelvis and infiltrates the left gluteus maximus and pyriformis muscles. Extension into the sacral neural foramina is present (*arrows, b*). T1-weighted spin-echo (*c*) and T2-weighted spin-echo (*d*) images in a second patient demonstrate an extensive plexiform neurofibroma in the right subcutaneous tissues that is low in signal intensity on the T1-weighted image (*c*) and high in signal intensity on the T2-weighted image (*d*). The tumors are high in signal intensity on the T2-weighted images in both patients, which is characteristic for tumors of neural origin. SGE (*e*), T2-weighted fat-suppressed echo-train spin-echo (*f*), and immediate post gadolinium SGE (*g*), images in a patient with inflammatory pseudotumor arising from the renal capsule. A large mass (mass = m, e) is noted posterior to the liver. The mass is well-marginated, heterogeneous and low in signal intensity on the T1-weighted image (*e*), moderately high in signal on the T2-weighted image (*f*) and demonstrates intense diffuse heterogeneous enhancement on the immediate post gadolinium SGE image (*g*). These findings mimic the appearance of a malignant neoplasm.

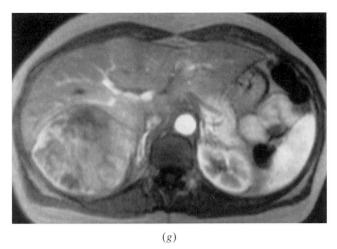

(g)

FIG. 10.3 (*Continued*) The posterior liver margin at the interface with the mass forms an obtuse angle consistent with an extrahepatic origin of the mass. The right kidney (not demonstrated) was displaced but not invaded by the mass. Inflammatory pseudotumor may have an aggressive appearance that mimics the appearance of a malignant tumor.

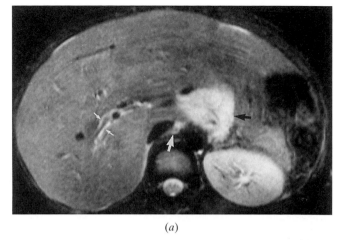

(a)

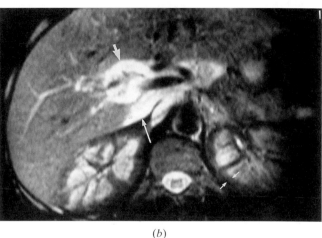

(b)

FIG. 10.4 Para-aortal adenopathy. T2-weighted fat-suppressed spin-echo image (*a*) in a patient with sclerosing cholangitis demonstrates para-aortic (*black arrow*) and aortocaval (*white arrow*) lymphadenopathy. Enlarged lymph nodes are readily distinguished in a dark background. Periportal high signal intensity is also noted (*small arrows*). T2-weighted fat-suppressed image in a second patient (*b*) shows inflammatory portal (*arrow, b*) and portocaval (*thin arrow, b*) nodes as high-signal-intensity structures. Note also that the cortex of the kidneys (*small arrows, b*) in this patient with sickle-cell anemia is low in signal intensity secondary to iron deposition.

pressed T2-weighted and gadolinium-enhanced images. Fat-suppressed T2-weighted images are very sensitive in the detection of lymph nodes, and exceed computed tomography (CT) imaging particularly in pediatric patients or patients with minimal retroperitoneal fat (Fig. 10.4). *Mycobacterium avium intracellulare* infection is common in immunocompromised patients and may feature enlarged lymph nodes and evidence of liver involvement (Fig. 10.5). Massive retroperitoneal adenopathy mimicking lymphoma may be an uncommon manifestation of sarcoidosis. Lymph nodes enhance with gadolinium and may have a speckled appearance on T2-weighted images [23–25]. Substantial benign adenopathy resembling malignant disease may also be found in Castleman's disease (Fig. 10.6), also known as giant lymph node hyperplasia. The lymph nodes have a heterogeneous appearance on the MR images with increased vascularity of the adjacent fat [26]. Retroperitoneal adenopathy is commonly observed in Kawasaki's disease, and involved lymph nodes are hemorrhagic, demonstrating characteristic high signal intensity on T1-weighted images (Fig. 10.7).

Miscellaneous

Masses of extramedullary hematopoiesis are more commonly found in patients with hereditary hemolytic anemias, particularly thalassemia major, but may be encountered in chronic leukemias, polycythemia vera, and diseases with extensive bone marrow infiltration [27]. Common locations in the retroperitoneum are the retrocrural and presacral spaces, and occasionally, they may have an aggressive appearance with bone destruction [27]. The masses are intermediate in signal intensity on T1-weighted images, intermediate to moderately high in signal intensity on T2-weighted images, enhancing moderately after gadolinium administration (Fig. 10.8).

Retroperitoneal hematomas may occur in patients with coagulation disorders or hemophilia, and after renal biopsy (Fig. 10.9).

Malignant Masses

Retroperitoneal Fibrosis

Malignant retroperitoneal fibrosis is most commonly associated with cervical, bowel, breast, prostate, lung, and kidney cancers [3,28]. The tumor consists of malignant

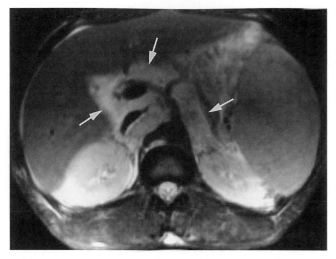

FIG. 10.5 Retroperitoneal lymphadenopathy from *Mycobacterium avium intracellulare* in a 13-year-old female patient. T2-weighted fat suppressed echo-train spin-echo image shows extensive para-aortic, aortocaval, paracaval, portocaval, and celiac lymphadenopathy (*arrows*). Retroperitoneal lymph nodes are conspicuous on T2-weighted fat-suppressed images as high-signal-intensity masses, and this permits detection of very small lymph nodes, particularly in thin or pediatric patients, who have little retroperitoneal fat.

cell infiltration of the retroperitoneum with associated desmoplastic reaction and encases the aorta, IVC, and ureters. The contour of the mass is not lobular, distinguishing malignant retroperitoneal fibrosis from adenopathy, and may be infiltrative and irregular (Fig. 10.10), a finding that favors malignant rather than benign retroperitoneal fibrosis. Ureteral obstruction with bilateral hydronephrosis is common. Malignant retroperitoneal fibrosis is usually moderately high in signal intensity on T2-weighted images, exhibiting increased enhancement with gadolinium [3,10,11]. Malignant retroperitoneal fibrosis will usually demonstrate enhancement on the immediate postgadolinium images. MRI can distinguish chronic benign from malignant retroperitoneal fibrosis, but distinction from acute benign retroperitoneal fibrosis is not always possible. Findings favoring malignancy include a more irregular contour and increase in size and irregularity on follow-up examinations. In indeterminate cases that have somewhat well-defined borders, high signal intensity on T2-weighted images, and increased enhancement on the immediate postgadolinium SGE images are findings that should be evaluated with caution. Biopsies from multiple sites should be obtained because benign retroperitoneal fibrosis may coexist with malig-

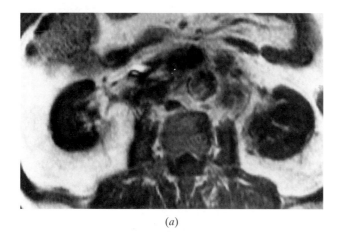

(a)

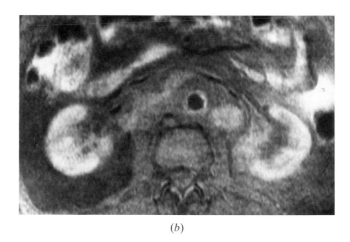

(b)

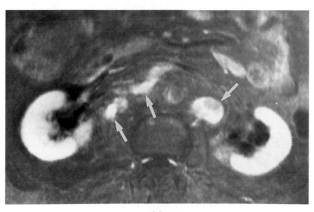

(c)

FIG. 10.6 Castleman's disease. SGE (*a*), T1 fat-suppressed spin-echo (*b*) and gadolinium-enhanced T1-weighted fat-suppressed spin-echo (*c*) images. Enlarged retroperitoneal lymph nodes are present. The lymph nodes are low in signal intensity on the SGE image (*a*) and intermediate to moderate in signal intensity on the T1-weighted fat-suppressed spin-echo image (*b*), with several of them demonstrating substantial enhancement (*arrows, c*) on the gadolinium-enhanced image (*c*). (Reproduced with permission from Semelka RC, Shoenut JP, Kroeker MA: The retroperitoneum and the abdominal wall. In Semelka RC, Shoenut JP (eds.). MRI of the Abdomen with CT Correlation. New York: Raven Press, pp. 13–41, 1993)

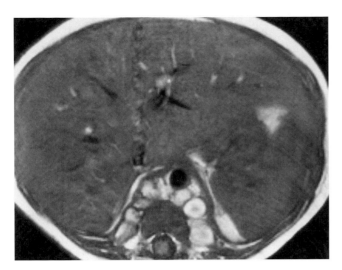

FIG. 10.7 Hemorrhagic lymph nodes in Kawasaki's disease. T1-SE image shows multiple retrocrural lymph nodes that are high in signal intensity due to the presence of subacute blood. (Reproduced with permission from Semelka RC, Shoenut JP, Kroeker MA: The retroperitoneum and the abdominal wall. In Semelka RC, Shoenut JP (eds.). MRI of the Abdomen with CT Correlation. New York: Raven Press, pp. 13–41, 1993)

nant neoplasms that are known to induce malignant retroperitoneal fibrosis [7].

Lymphoma

Lymphoma is the most common retroperitoneal malignancy, and both Hodgkin's and non-Hodgkin's lymphomas may involve the retroperitoneum [29–33]. Non-Hodgkin's lymphoma more commonly involves a variety of nodal groups (in particular, mesenteric nodes are involved in more than 50 percent of the cases) and extra-

nodal sites [30]. Intra-abdominal Hodgkin's lymphoma tends to be limited to the spleen and retroperitoneum [29].

MRI performs well in the demonstration of enlarged lymph nodes (Figs. 10.11, 10.12, and 10.13) [33–35] and outperforms CT imaging in the upper abdominal para-aortic region and in patients who are thin [33]. Short tau inversion recovery (STIR), T2-weighted fat-suppressed spin-echo or echo-train spin-echo technique results in excellent conspicuity of moderately high-signal-intensity nodes in a suppressed background. The fat-suppressed HASTE sequence may be used with good results as an alternative in uncooperative or pediatric patients. Persistent tissue after therapy also may be better characterized by MRI as recurrent disease or fibrosis [31,32,36]. After approximately 1 year, fibrotic tissue is low in signal intensity on T2-weighted images, unlike recurrent disease, which is high or mixed high in signal intensity on T2-weighted images. Chronic fibrotic tissue will enhance minimally with gadolinium compared with the enhancement of persistent or recurrent disease, which is moderate or marked and often heterogeneous. In rare instances, lymphoma may appear as a large solitary retroperitoneal mass (Fig. 10.12), that mimics the appearance of a primary malignant retroperitoneal tumor.

Retroperitoneal Lymphadenopathy

Carcinomas associated with retroperitoneal lymphadenopathy include kidney, colon, pancreas, lung, breast, testes, and melanoma [34,37,38]. Enlarged lymph nodes are usually moderate in signal intensity on T2-weighted images and higher than that of adjacent psoas muscle (Fig. 10.14). T2-weighted fat-suppressed spin-echo or echo-train spin-echo images are particularly effective at demonstrating nodes in patients who are thin. The addi-

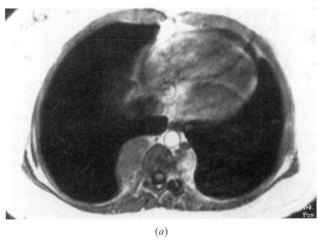

(a)

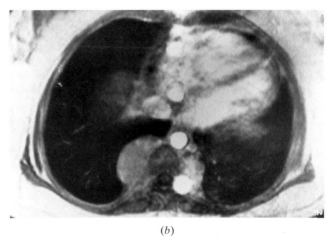

(b)

FIG. 10.8 Extramedullary hematopoiesis in thalassemia major. SGE (a) and immediate postgadolinium SGE (b) images. Soft tissue paravertebral masses in the lower thorax and abdomen are demonstrated. The hematopoietic masses are low in signal intensity on the SGE image (a) and demonstrate moderate enhancement on the immediate postgadolinium SGE image (b). (Reproduced with permission from Semelka RC, Shoenut JP, Kroeker MA: The retroperitoneum and the abdominal wall. In Semelka RC, Shoenut JP (eds.). MRI of the Abdomen with CT Correlation. New York: Raven Press, pp. 13–41, 1993.)

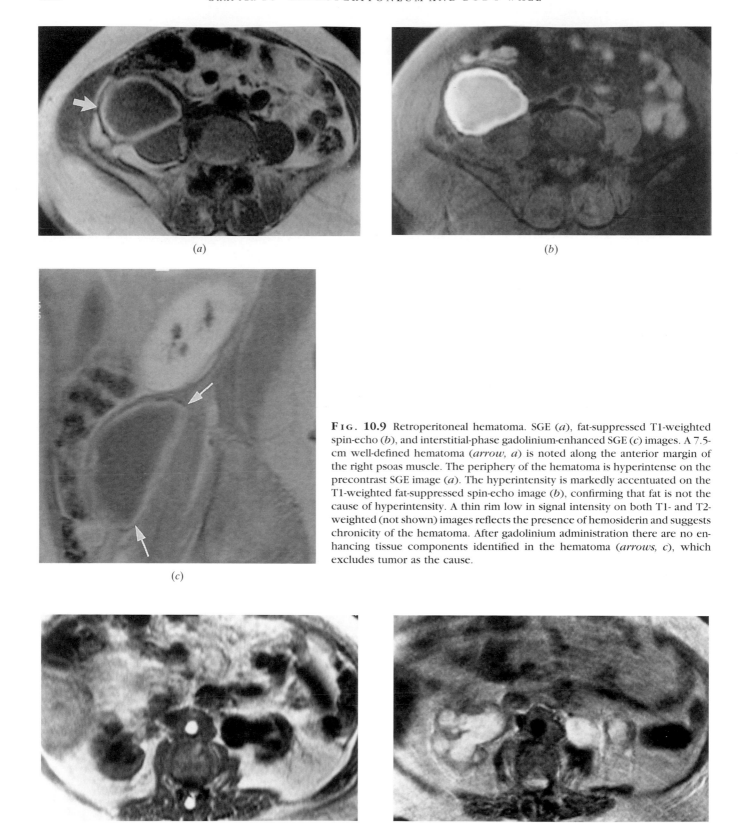

FIG. 10.9 Retroperitoneal hematoma. SGE (*a*), fat-suppressed T1-weighted spin-echo (*b*), and interstitial-phase gadolinium-enhanced SGE (*c*) images. A 7.5-cm well-defined hematoma (*arrow, a*) is noted along the anterior margin of the right psoas muscle. The periphery of the hematoma is hyperintense on the precontrast SGE image (*a*). The hyperintensity is markedly accentuated on the T1-weighted fat-suppressed spin-echo image (*b*), confirming that fat is not the cause of hyperintensity. A thin rim low in signal intensity on both T1- and T2-weighted (not shown) images reflects the presence of hemosiderin and suggests chronicity of the hematoma. After gadolinium administration there are no enhancing tissue components identified in the hematoma (*arrows, c*), which excludes tumor as the cause.

FIG. 10.10 Malignant retroperitoneal fibrosis from cervical cancer. SGE (*a*), T2-weighted echo-train spin-echo (*b*), and immediate postgadolinium SGE (*c*) images. The aorta is encased by abnormal soft tissue, which has slightly ill-defined margins. The soft tissue is low in signal intensity on the SGE image (*a*), heterogeneous and moderate in signal intensity on the T2-weighted echo-train spin-echo image (*b*), and demonstrates diffuse heterogeneous enhancement after gadolinium administration (*c*).

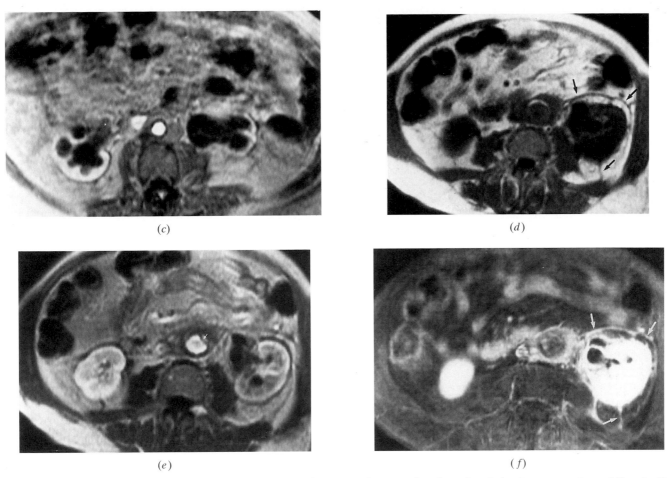

(c)

(d)

(e)

(f)

FIG. 10.10 (*Continued*) This appearance is compatible with active malignant rather than chronic benign retroperitoneal fibrosis. Note bilateral hydronephrosis resulting from ureteral obstruction at a lower level. SGE (*d*), immediate postgadolinium SGE (*e*), and postgadolinium T1-weighted fat-suppressed spin-echo (*f*) images in a second patient with malignant retroperitoneal fibrosis. An oval-shaped mass is encasing the aorta. The mass is low in signal intensity on the SGE image (*d*) and demonstrates moderate heterogeneous enhancement on the immediate postgadolinium image (*e*) that progresses on the postgadolinium T1-weighted fat-suppressed spin-echo (*f*) image. The mass has aggressive infiltrating (*arrows, f*) margins. The left perirenal fascia and perirenal septae are thickened (*arrows, d*) and demonstrate enhancement (*arrows, f*) on the gadolinium-enhanced T1-weighted fat-suppressed spin-echo (*f*) image. Incidentally noted is a dissection involving the abdominal aorta with good demonstration of the intimal flap (*small arrow, e*).

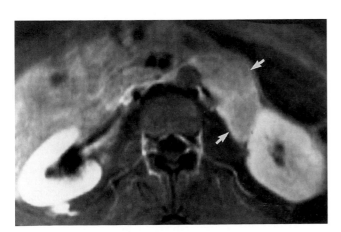

FIG. 10.11 Retroperitoneal lymphadenopathy from Hodgkin's lymphoma. Gadolinium-enhanced T1-weighted fat-suppressed spin-echo image shows a 4-cm moderately enhancing lymphomatous nodal mass (*arrows*) in a left periaortic location at the level of the left renal hilum. (Reproduced with permission from Semelka RC, Shoenut JP, Kroeker MA: The retroperitoneum and the abdominal wall. In Semelka RC, Shoenut JP (eds.). MRI of the Abdomen with CT Correlation. New York: Raven Press, pp. 13–41, 1993.)

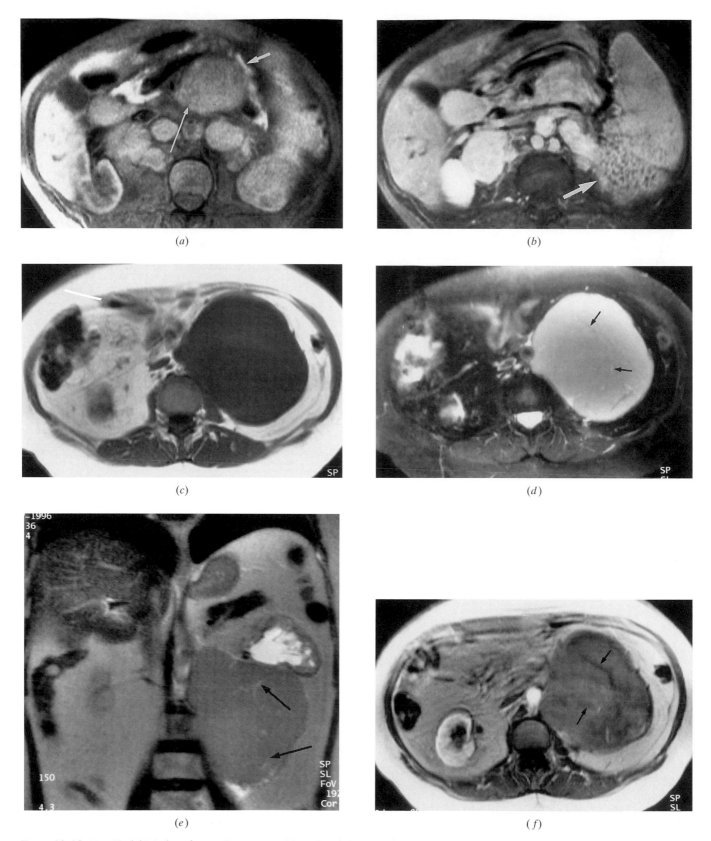

FIG. 10.12 Non-Hodgkin's lymphoma. Precontrast (*a*) and gadolinium-enhanced (*b*) T1-weighted fat-suppressed spin-echo images in a patient with retroperitoneal lymphadenopathy from non-Hodgkin's lymphoma. Extensive retroperitoneal and mesenteric lymphadenopathy is noted. The precontrast T1-weighted fat-suppressed spin-echo image (*a*) permits distinction of the normal high-signal-intensity pancreas (*short white arrow, a*) from the retropancreatic nodal mass (*long white arrow, a*) and documents the extrapancreatic location of the mass.

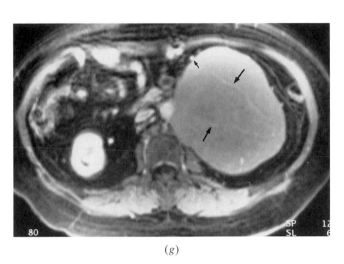

(g)

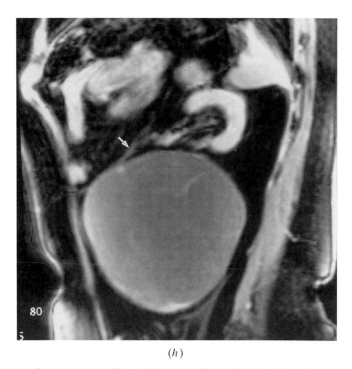

(h)

FIG. 10.12 (*Continued*) The nodal masses show moderate to intense enhancement on the gadolinium-enhanced image (*b*), whereas abnormal enhancement of the spleen (*arrow, b*) reflects lymphomatous infiltration. SGE (*c*), T2-weighted fat-suppressed echo-train spin-echo (*d*), coronal HASTE (*e*), immediate postgadolinium SGE (*f*), axial (*g*) and sagittal (*h*) interstitial phase gadolinium-enhanced fat-suppressed SGE images in a patient with lymphoma presenting as a solitary retroperitoneal mass. A large well-defined retroperitoneal mass is present. The mass is mildly heterogeneous and low in signal intensity on the T1-weighted image (*c*) and moderately high signal intensity on the T2-weighted image (*d*). Thin septations (*arrows, d,e*) are present in the mass. The coronal HASTE image demonstrates superior displacement and hydronephrosis of the left kidney secondary to ureteral compression caused by the mass. The lymphoma mass demonstrates mild to moderate diffuse heterogeneous enhancement on the immediate postgadolinium SGE (*f*), which becomes more homogeneous over time on the interstitial-phase fat-suppressed SGE image (*g*). Note that the internal septations (*arrows, f,g*) show minimal enhancement on the immediate postgadolinium SGE image (*f*) and show progressive enhancement on the more delayed fat-suppressed SGE images (*g,h*) consistent with fibrous tissue. The anteriorly displaced ureter is identified at the anterior margin of the mass on the interstitial phase fat-suppressed SGE image (*small arrow, g*). Note that the sagittal image clearly demonstrates the fat plane between the kidney and the mass, and depicts a segment of the anterosuperiorly displaced ureter (*small arrow, h*). A solitary mass lesion with no evidence of other sites of nodal or organ disease is a rare appearance for lymphoma. (Reproduced with permission from Semelka RC, Shoenut JP, Kroeker MA: The retroperitoneum and the abdominal wall. In Semelka RC, Shoenut JP (eds.). MRI of the Abdomen with CT Correlation. New York: Raven Press, pp. 13–41, 1993.)

tion of fat suppression is important, particularly when echo-train spin-echo sequences are used, because fat is high in signal intensity on these images (Fig. 10.15). Adenopathy, whether benign or malignant, will enhance on postgadolinium SGE images. A feature favoring malignancy is the depiction of necrotic lymph nodes in a patient in whom the primary tumor is also necrotic. The MRI and CT imaging criteria for pathologic lymph nodes to the present rely on their diameter being greater than 1.5 cm. Benign reactive lymph nodes may exceed 2 cm in diameter in the vicinity of malignant neoplasms, whereas gastrointestinal and cancers may involve lymph nodes without causing nodal enlargement. Tissue-specific contrast agents may increase the diagnostic accuracy of MRI in characterizing retroperitoneal lymphadenopathy. MR lymphography using iron oxide particles is currently under investigation. This technique has been shown to distinguish contrast-enhanced, low-signal-intensity benign lymph nodes from nonenhanced, intermediate, heterogeneous-signal-intensity malignant nodes on T2 weighted images in animal models [39]; initial clinical trials are promising [40].

Testicular Cancer
Testicular cancer may arise in an undescended testis located in the retroperitoneum [41], in the mediastinum or the retroperitoneum without evidence of primary testicular tumor [15], or in the testicles, metastasizing along the lymphatic pathway of testicular arteries and veins into para-aortic and paracaval nodes at the level of the renal hila. It is the most common solid cancer in men between the ages of 15 and 34 years, and in 95 percent of the

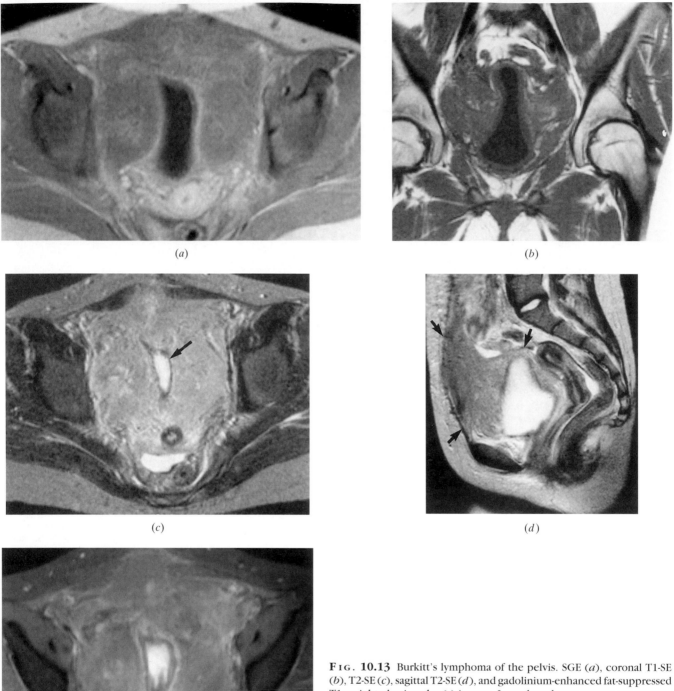

(a)

(b)

(c)

(d)

(e)

FIG. 10.13 Burkitt's lymphoma of the pelvis. SGE (*a*), coronal T1-SE (*b*), T2-SE (*c*), sagittal T2-SE (*d*), and gadolinium-enhanced fat-suppressed T1-weighted spin-echo (*e*) images. Large lymphoma masses are present in the pelvis and cause compression of the urinary bladder (*arrow, c*), which has an hourglass configuration better seen on the coronal T1-SE image (*b*). The sagittal T2-SE image depicts the large lymphomatous mass (*arrows, d*) that extends over the top of the bladder in the uterovesicular space. The masses are heterogeneous on both T1- and T2-weighted images and show minimal enhancement after gadolinium administration (*e*).

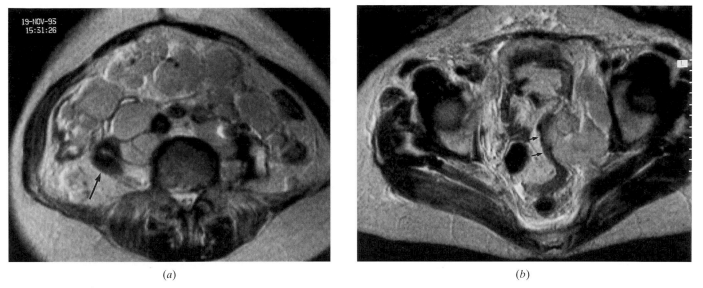

(a)   (b)

Fig. 10.14 Retroperitoneal adenopathy. T2-weighted spin-echo images from cranial (*a*) and more caudal (*b*) level. Enlarged retroperitoneal lymph nodes are demonstrated as rounded, well-defined masses of moderate signal intensity on both images. Note lateral displacement of the right psoas muscle (*arrow, a*) by enlarged paracaval lymph nodes and medial displacement of the sigmoid colon (*arrows, b*) by enlarged left obturator lymph nodes.

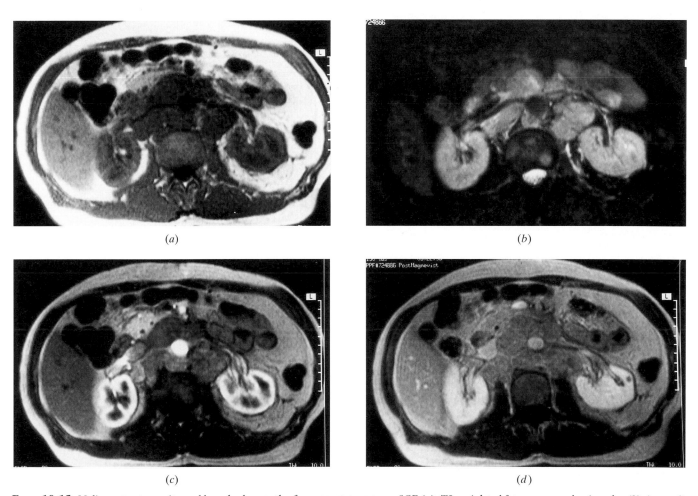

(a)   (b)

(c)   (d)

Fig. 10.15 Malignant retroperitoneal lymphadenopathy from prostate cancer. SGE (*a*), T2-weighted fat-suppressed spin-echo (*b*), immediate (*c*), and 90-second (*d*) postgadolinium SGE images. Multiple enlarged lymph nodes are present in the retroperitoneum displacing the aorta and the IVC anteriorly. The lymph nodes are low in signal intensity on the SGE image (*a*) and high in signal intensity on the T2-weighted fat-suppressed spin-echo image (*b*). Fat suppression removes the competing high signal intensity of fat and renders the lymph nodes particularly conspicuous on the T2-weighted image. The lymph nodes enhance minimally on the immediate postgadolinium SGE image (*c*) and show progressive enhancement on the 90-second postgadolinium SGE image (*d*).

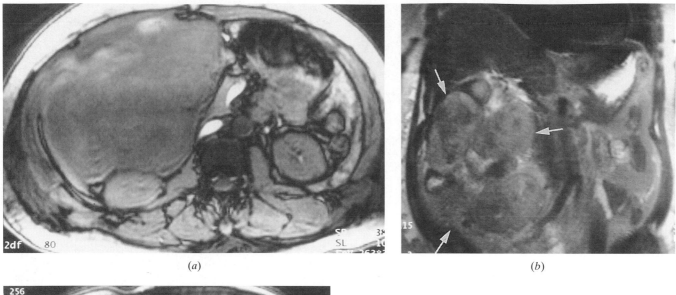

(a)   (b)

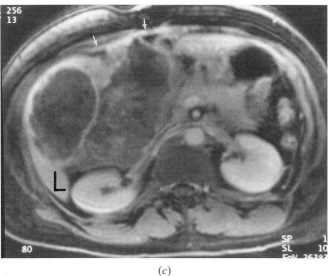

(c)

FIG. 10.16 Retroperitoneal carcinoma. Out-of-phase SGE (a), coronal HASTE (b), and interstitial-phase gadolinium-enhanced fat-suppressed SGE (c) images. A large, lobulated, heterogeneous mass is present, located in the right abdomen. The mass is heterogenous on both T1- (a) and T2-weighted (arrows, b) images, displacing the aorta and IVC medially, and the right kidney posteriorly. Areas of high signal intensity on the T2-weighted image (b) represent necrotic areas. The mass demonstrates peripheral and patchy heterogeneous enhancement on the interstitial-phase gadolinium-enhanced fat-suppressed SGE image (c). Invasion of the right lobe of the liver ("l",c) is clearly demonstrated. The mass abuts the anterior abdominal wall, and enhancement of the anterior peritoneum (small arrows, c) is evident secondary to recent laparotomy attempt, aborted due to the large size of the mass.

cases it is of germ cell origin, either seminomatous (40%) or nonseminomatous (embryonal cell tumors, teratocarcinomas, teratomas, choriocarcinomas, and mixed histology tumors). The remaining 5 percent are of stromal origin (Sertoli, Leydig, or mesenchymal-cell carcinomas). MRI and CT imaging have comparable ability to detect lymphadenopathy associated with testicular cancer [42]. MRI is useful in detecting undescended testes, which may be the site of origin of testicular neoplasms. T2-weighted fat-suppressed images may show the undescended testis as a moderate- to high-signal-intensity structure along the anatomic course of the spermatic vessels. In tumors arising in undescended testes MRI may perform better than CT imaging in lesion characterization [41].

Primary Retroperitoneal Tumors

The majority of primary retroperitoneal tumors (70 to 90%) are malignant [15,16,43,44]. The most common his-

tological type is liposarcoma, followed by leiomyosarcoma and malignant fibrous histiocytoma [15,16,43,44]. A male predominance exists for liposarcomas and malignant fibrous histiocytomas, whereas leiomyosarcomas are more common in women [15,16]. The tumors are typically large (Fig. 10.16), which is due to their silent clinical course. Presenting symptoms include abdominal mass, pain, weight loss, and nausea and vomiting [16]. In a review of leiomyosarcomas of the retroperitoneum and IVC, leiomyosarcomas with no major vascular involvement have been classified as Pattern 1 and comprise 62 percent of the total cases [16]. On MR images, tumors are generally mixed low and intermediate in signal intensity on T1-weighted images, and mixed medium and high in signal intensity on T2-weighted images [16,44]. Tumors enhance in a heterogeneous fashion, and leiomyosarcomas, in particular, are hypervascular and demonstrate intense enhancement (Fig. 10.17). Areas of

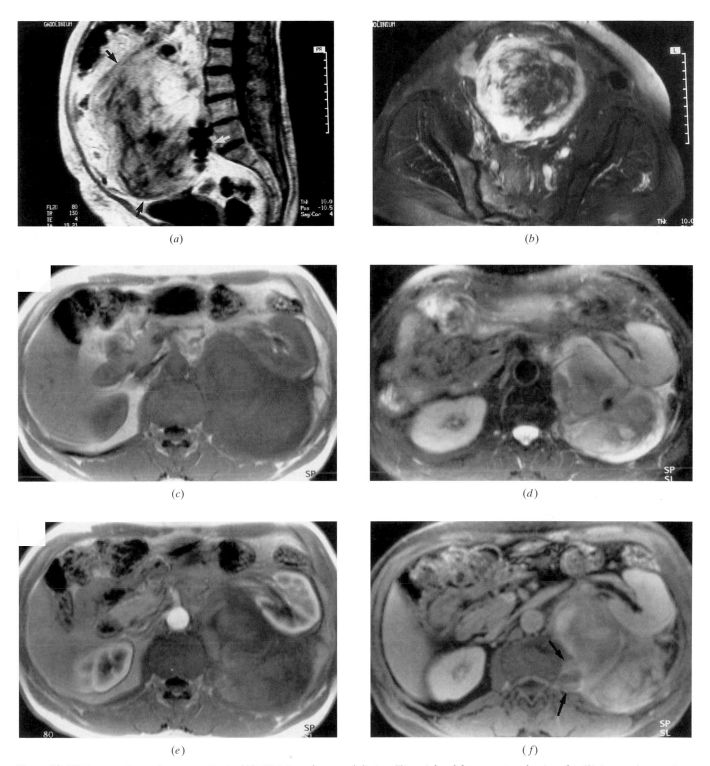

F IG. 10.17 Retroperitoneal sarcoma. Sagittal T1-SE (*a*), and postgadolinium T1-weighted fat-suppressed spin-echo (*b*) images in a patient with recurrent retroperitoneal leiomyosarcoma. A large, markedly heterogeneous mass (*arrows, a*) arises in the retroperitoneum immediately anterior to the lumbar spine and extends inferiorly to the pelvis. The mass is hypervascular and demonstrates intense heterogeneous enhancement after gadolinium administration. Magnetic susceptibility artifacts are present caused by surgical clips (*white arrow, a*). SGE (*c*), T2-weighted fat-suppressed echo-train spin-echo (*d*), immediate postgadolinium SGE (*e*), transverse (*f*) and sagittal (*g*) interstitial-phase gadolinium-enhanced fat-suppressed SGE images in a patient with pleomorphic rhabdomyosarcoma. A large, left-sided retroperitoneal rhabdomyosarcoma mass is present. The mass displaces the left kidney anterolaterally, consistent with the retroperitoneal origin of the mass. The mass is heterogeneous and low in signal intensity on the precontrast SGE image (*c*), and heterogeneous and mixed high signal intensity on the T2-weighted image (*d*). The mass demonstrates moderate and heterogeneous enhancement on the immediate postgadolinium SGE image (*e*) with progressive enhancement on the interstitial-phase fat-suppressed SGE images (*f,g*).

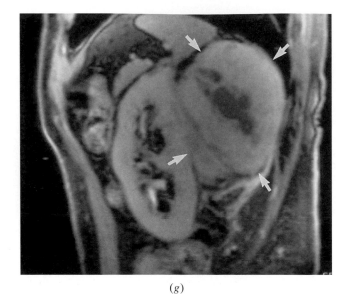

(g)

FIG. 10.17 (*Continued*) Invasion of the left psoas muscle (*arrows, f*) is better seen on the interstitial-phase fat-suppressed SGE image (*f*) as an enhancing area with irregular margins within the muscle. The sagittal image demonstrates the longitudinal extent of the mass (*arrows, g*) and anterior displacement of the kidney. Central necrosis is present which appears as a central area of lack of enhancement within the mass.

necrosis may be present, which is common in leiomyosarcomas [15,16], and are demonstrated as areas that are low signal intensity on T1-weighted images, high signal intensity on T2-weighted images, and lack enhancement on postgadolinium images (see Fig. 10.17). Hemorrhage occasionally occurs in the liquefied necrotic areas and may be demonstrated as high in signal intensity on T1-weighted images and as a low signal-intensity dependent layer on T2-weighted images [16]. The various histological types share common MRI appearances, and differentiation may not be possible. In rare cases liposarcomas may be sufficiently well-differentiated (lipogenic liposarcoma) to contain mature fat, which is high in signal intensity on T1- and T2-weighted echo-train spin-echo images, intermediate in signal intensity on T2-weighted spin-echo images, and suppresses on fat-suppressed images. In these cases, soft tissue strands are present within the fatty mass, and tumor nodules may enhance after gadolinium administration. These tumors are better assessed by MRI, which provides direct imaging of the craniocaudal and transverse extent of the tumor.

Neuroblastoma-Ganglioneuroblastoma

These tumors are discussed in Chapter 8 on the Adrenal Glands. Extra-adrenal involvement increases with age [45]. MRI with the use of phased-array multicoil, T2-weighted fat-suppressed echo-train spin-echo, and gadolinium-enhanced T1-weighted fat-suppressed images provides excellent morphological detail and tumor/background contrast. MRI is superior to CT imaging because CT imaging may not detect small tumor masses or involved lymph nodes in this mainly pediatric population due to small patient size and lack of retroperitoneal fat. The HASTE sequence should be part of the imaging protocol because it provides sharp motion and breathing-artifact-free images in pediatric patients who may move during the acquisition and in problematic areas such as the subdiaphragmatic paraspinal retroperitoneum. Added advantages of MRI include the lack of ionizing radiation and direct imaging in the coronal and sagittal plane, which provides direct evaluation of the craniocaudal extent and facilitates detection of tumor extension into the neural foramina, a common feature of these neoplasms.

AORTA

The aorta and its branches are well-evaluated by MRI due to the variety of techniques available. Techniques employed are termed black blood (flowing blood appears as signal-void) or bright blood (flowing blood appears bright).

Conventional T1- and T2-weighted spin-echo images will demonstrate the aortic lumen as a signal-void area (dark-blood technique) because the excited blood leaves the slice in the time interval between excitation pulse and echo sampling. Despite the use of presaturation pulses and a long echo time, slow blood flow may appear bright on T1-weighted spin-echo images, causing confusion with thrombus.

Bright-blood techniques include sequences that refocus blood signal intensity with gradient pulses or gadolinium-enhanced gradient-echo sequences. Sequences that refocus blood signal include cine gradient-echo, time-of-flight MR angiography and phase-contrast MR angiography. Time-of-flight MRA techniques [46–52] rely on the inflow of unsaturated spins into the examined slice (2D) or volume (3D). Although these techniques perform well in the central nervous system, they do not achieve reproducible image quality in the abdomen due to respiratory and peristaltic motion and larger volume of examined tissues and vessels. As the majority of these techniques are nonbreath-hold they have limited reproducibility in patients who are uncooperative, a circumstance that may be observed in patients with substantial disease. Furthermore, slow or turbulent flow in aortic aneurysms and poststenotic turbulent flow (e.g., in aortic occlusive disease or renal artery stenosis) cause dephasing that leads to signal loss and impaired vessel visualization [49,52–54]. Phase-contrast techniques may be used when flow velocity and direction information is required (Fig. 10.18). They require cardiac triggering and are time consuming.

For the assessment of aortic pathology, early (up to

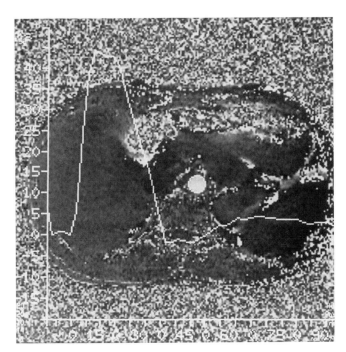

Fig. 10.18 Phase map of the normal aorta. The abdominal aorta (*encircled*) appears high in signal intensity on this phase map in the systolic phase of antegrade blood flow. A blood velocity tracing obtained throughout the cardiac cycle is superimposed on the phase image, demonstrating the normal velocity profile of blood in the abdominal aorta. (Reproduced with permission from Semelka RC, Shoenut JP, Kroeker MA: The retroperitoneum and the abdominal wall. In Semelka RC, Shoenut JP (eds.). MRI of the Abdomen with CT Correlation. New York: Raven Press, pp. 13–41, 1993.)

2 minutes after injection) postgadolinium images obtained for investigation of diseases of solid abdominal organs provide a fast and reproducible technique incorporated into the routine abdominal MRI protocol. Immediate postgadolinium SGE images also generate information on capillary blood flow, which may provide important insight into the impact of anatomical vessel abnormalities on organ perfusion. When angiographic sequences are not available, an anteroposterior projection of a maximum-intensity projection (MIP) reconstruction using immediate postgadolinium coronal SGE sections (6 to 8 mm thick) results in angiographic-like images.

The disadvantages of time-of-flight techniques include signal loss in low-flow and turbulent-flow states and saturation of in-plane flow. To overcome these disadvantages of time-of-flight techniques, gadolinium enhancement has been employed in conjunction with 2D or 3D fast gradient-echo acquisitions yielding reproducible, good results [53–59]. A 3D gadolinium-enhanced gradient-echo MRA does not rely on time-of-flight effects, but rather on the T1-shortening provided by gadolinium. Advantages compared to 2D techniques include a high sig-

nal-to-noise ratio permitting nearly isotropic resolution (typically 2-mm effective slice thickness), acquisition of the central-phase encoding steps at the same time point for all the slices, and avoidance of slice misregistration [54]. Recent advances in MRI, including the use of phased-array coils that increase the signal-to-noise ratio and faster rising gradient times, have led to the implementation of fast 3D gradient-echo acquisitions in a breath-hold [60]. We currently use a breath-hold 3D fast imaging in the steady state precession (FISP) sequence with a repetition time of 5 msec and an echo time of 2.3 msec. Two complete datasets are acquired in sequential breath-holds with a short interval between acquisitions to allow for patient respiration. The sequence is initiated shortly after the administration of 40 mL of gadolinium, either as a bolus injection or an infusion. Timing of the injection depends on the vessels studied and the length of the breath-hold, in an effort to maximize intravascular gadolinium concentration during the acquisition of the central phase-encoding steps [56]. A tight bolus technique is useful when examining renal arteries because the venous return from the kidneys is rapid and overlap from renal veins is more difficult to control with infusion techniques. A slower infusion technique may be used when smaller and/or distal vessels are imaged, as in combined examinations of aortoiliac and lower extremity vessels. An important advantage of our protocol is that two datasets are obtained, providing both arterial-phase and venous-phase datasets. The second dataset serves also as a backup in patients with low cardiac output in the event that the first dataset is acquired too early.

The data acquired can be postprocessed either by multiplanar reconstructions or by 3D reconstruction using an MIP algorithm. The small size of the individual slices permits reconstructions and 3D MIP projections at any level without image degradation. MIP images provide a quick overview and are useful in tracking vessels that have a tortuous course in and out of the section plane. They are also useful for identifying smaller vessels (e.g., accessory renal arteries) (Fig. 10.19). The diagnosis, however, is usually based on the individual source sections, and evaluation should not rely solely on the MIP images. The source images are superior to MIP reconstructions in the depiction of vessel wall, presence of mural thrombus, renal artery ostia, small vessels running in plane, and intimal flap in aortic dissections [47].

A useful adjunct, particularly in uncooperative patients, is a HASTE sequence combined with a set of preparatory inversion pulses (black-blood technique): A non-slice selective 180-degree inversion pulse is applied, which is followed by a slice selective 180-degree inversion pulse prior to the start of the echo-train sequence. The first pulse inverts the longitudinal magnetization of the whole body, whereas the second pulse selectively restores the longitudinal magnetization of the examined

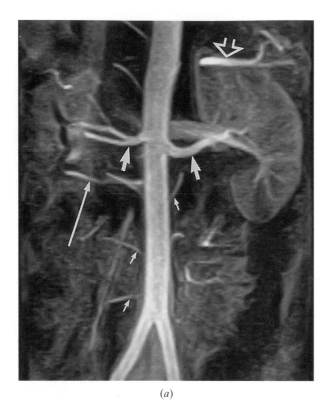

(a)

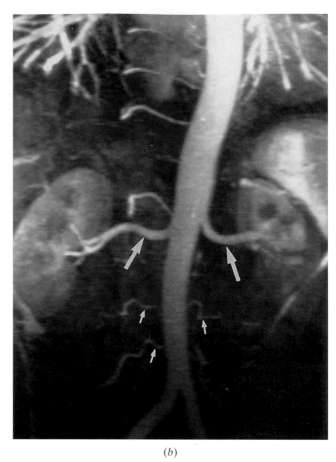

(b)

FIG. 10.19 Normal abdominal aorta and iliac vessels. Anteroposterior projection (*a*) from a 3D MIP reconstruction of a set of immediate postgadolinium coronal breath-hold 3D FISP sections with effective slice thickness of 2 mm. The abdominal aorta, left and right renal arteries (*arrows, a*) and a right accessory lower pole renal artery (*long arrow, a*), common iliac arteries, and lumbar arteries (*small arrows, a*) are well-visualized with good lumen enhancement and smooth contours. The celiac axis and superior mesenteric artery are not visualized because they course outside the narrow (4-cm) coronal slab. A segment of the splenic artery is identified reentering the acquired slab in its posterior course toward the hilum of the spleen (*hollow arrow, a*). Anteroposterior projection (*b*) from a 3D MIP reconstruction of a set of immediate postgadolinium coronal breath-hold 3D FISP sections with effective slice thickness of 2 mm in a second patient. The normal aorta, renal arteries (*arrows, b*) and lumbar arteries (*small arrows, b*) are well demonstrated.

slice. The time delay of the first inversion pulse is selected so that the central-phase encoding steps are acquired when blood reaches the null point, resulting in no signal from blood [61].

For clinical examinations, it may be of value to obtain a bright-blood and a black-blood technique for studying the aorta [48,62]. An attractive feature of MRI is its ability to image the aorta along its longitudinal length, which has particular advantage in studying the length of a disease process such as aneurysm [48,59,62].

Aortic Aneurysm

Abdominal aortic aneurysm (AAA) is a common disease entity in North America. The incidence is 21.1 per 100,000, and men are five times more likely than women to be affected by AAA. The median age at diagnosis is 69 years for men and 78 years for women [63]. Important

diagnostic information for patient management includes diameter of the aneurysm, its longitudinal length, and its relationship to renal, common iliac, and femoral arteries. Spontaneous rupture is a frequent complication of aneurysms 6 cm or more in diameter, but it is relatively uncommon for AAAs smaller than 5 cm [64,65]. MR images with black-blood and white-blood techniques are successful at demonstrating aneurysms [32,48,59,62,66–69]. Gadolinium-enhanced 3D gradient-echo MR angiography (e.g., 3D FISP) demonstrates the full extent of the aneurysm and its relationship to the renal arteries, celiac axis, and superior mesenteric artery (SMA) (Fig. 10.20). In patients with atherosclerotic disease, renal-artery stenosis may coexist and is well-depicted on gadolinium-enhanced 3D FISP images. Stenosis of the SMA also can be assessed reliably, and this is of importance in patients with suprarenal aortic aneurysms because postoperative

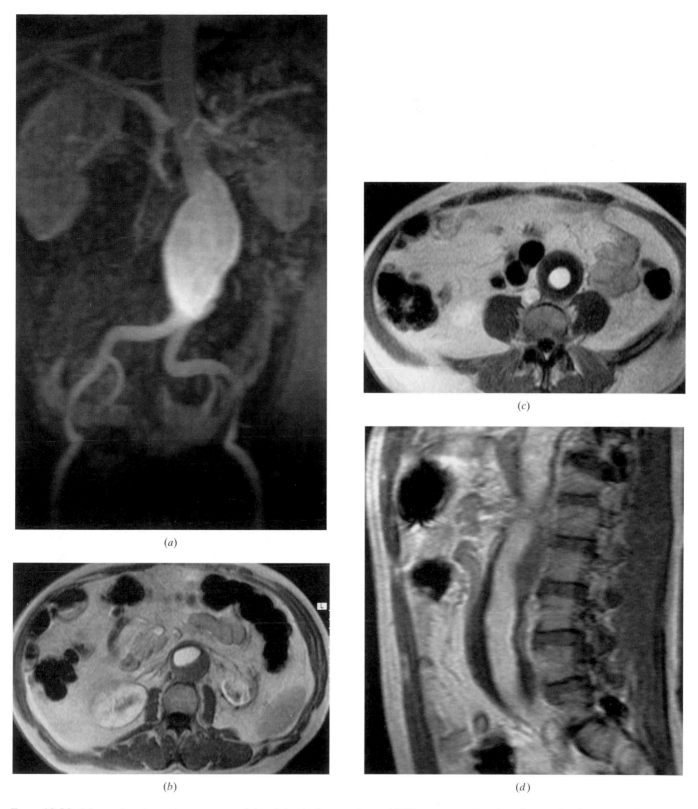

F ɪ ɢ . 10.20 Atherosclerotic aortic aneurysm of the abdominal aorta. Coronal MIP reconstruction (*a*) of a set of gadolinium enhanced 2-mm thin section coronal 3D FISP sections in a patient with an infrarenal aortic aneurysm. The MIP images demonstrate a large fusiform infrarenal aortic aneurysm. The aneurysm is shown not to extend into the common iliac arteries. Transverse 45-second postgadolinium SGE (*b*), interstitial-phase gadolinium-enhanced SGE (*c*), and sagittal interstitial-phase SGE (*d*) images in a second patient. An abdominal aortic aneurysm containing high-signal-intensity gadolinium in the lumen and low-signal-intensity wall thrombus is evident on the 45-second postgadolinium SGE image (*b*).

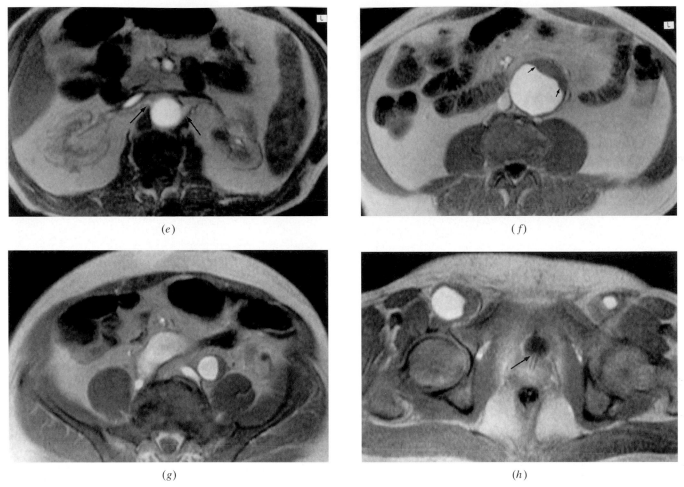

(e)

(f)

(g)

(h)

FIG. 10.20 (*Continued*) The left kidney is small and demonstrates delayed enhancement of a uniform thin cortex, findings consistent with left renal artery stenosis. Note that the signal intensity of the cortex and medulla of the right kidney has equilibrated at this tubular phase of enhancement. Good delineation of the patent lumen and mural thrombus is provided by gadolinium enhancement on early postgadolinium SGE images (*c,d*), while imaging in the sagittal plane demonstrates the longitudinal extent of disease. Immediate postgadolinium (*e*), transverse (*f,g,h*) and sagittal (*i*) interstitial-phase gadolinium-enhanced SGE images in a third patient, and coronal immediate postgadolinium SGE (*j*) and coronal 3D MIP reconstruction (*k*) of a set of coronal immediate postgadolinium SGE images obtained in a follow-up study on the same patient. The abdominal aorta is normal in diameter at the level of the origins (*arrows, e*) of the renal arteries. At lower tomographic levels (*f–h*) enlargement of the aortic lumen with sharp demarcation of the high-signal-intensity patent lumen and low-signal-intensity wall thrombus (*small arrows, f*) is noted. Involvement of the infrarenal aorta (*f*), common iliac arteries (*g*) and common femoral arteries (*h*) is demonstrated. A Foley catheter is also noted in place (*arrow, h*). The sagittal interstitial-phase image provides direct visualization of the site of maximal anteroposterior diameter (*arrow, i*) with depiction of low-signal-intensity thrombus (*small arrows, i*) in the anterior abdominal wall. The origin of the superior mesenteric artery (*thin arrow, i*) is also demonstrated. The origin of the aneurysm is shown to be inferior to the origins of the renal arteries (*small arrows, j,k*) on both the coronal immediate postgadolinium SGE image (*j*) and the coronal projection from the 3D MIP reconstruction (*k*). The projection from the 3D MIP reconstruction (*k*) demonstrates an overview of the aneurysm and its peripheral extent in an angiographic fashion. Enhancement of the IVC is also present, which causes overlap (*arrow, k*) of enhancing veins and arteries at the level of the common iliac vessels. This approach can be used to generate angiographic images. It is limited to a single projection plane because section thickness is too large to permit image rotation. T1-weighted fat-suppressed spin-echo image (*l*) in a fourth patient with aortic aneurysm demonstrates an aortic aneurysm with atherosclerotic plaque in its right posterior aortic wall with a high-signal-intensity focus (*arrow, l*) representing a blood clot.

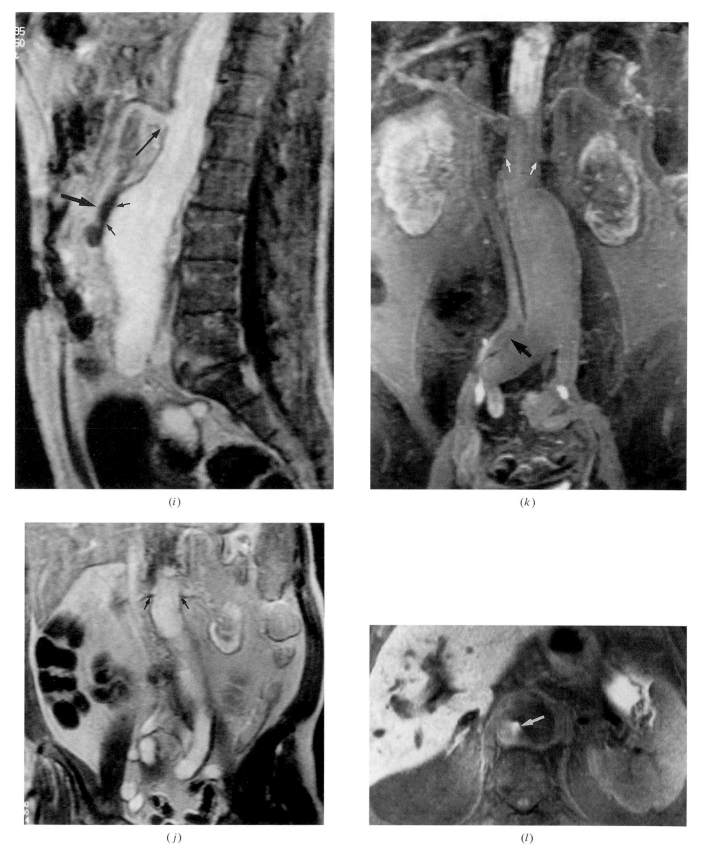

(i)

(k)

(j)

(l)

FIG. 10.20 (Continued)

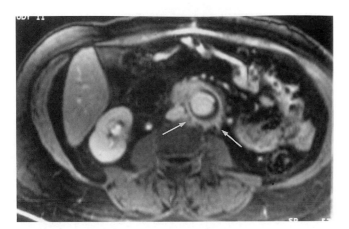

FIG. 10.21 Inflammatory aortitis. Interstitial-phase gadolinium-enhanced fat-suppressed SGE image. An aortic aneurysm is present with diffusely thickened wall and enhancing ill-defined tissue that projects (*arrows*) into the retroperitoneal fat surrounding the aneurysm. Enhancement of the lumen and nearly signal-void wall thrombus are also shown.

bowel ischemia may complicate the aneurysmal repair [70]. Assessment of the aortic wall, mural thrombus, and abdominal viscera is accomplished on the postgadolinium SGE or fat-suppressed SGE images following the 3D acquisition (see Fig. 10.20).

Inflammatory aortitis, also termed inflammatory aortic aneurysm, is an uncommon entity in which an inflammatory reaction develops around an aortic aneurysm [13,71]. Etiological factors proposed by some investigators include an immune response to ceroid produced in atheromatous plaque [25], whereas other investigators have found evidence of vasculitis involving the aortic wall in patients with inflammatory aortic aneurysms and have postulated that the combination of retroperitoneal fibrosis, vasculitis, and aortic aneurysm may represent a distinct pathological entity [71]. Gadolinium-enhanced fat-suppressed SGE images demonstrate infiltrative enhancing tissue surrounding an aortic aneurysm (Fig. 10.21).

Aortic Dissection

Aortic dissection usually originates in the thoracic aorta. MRI has been shown to be accurate in the detection of aortic dissection [65,72,73]. The noninvasive nature of the technique and the lack of nephrotoxicity are important features of MRI. Because patients may frequently have diminished renal function, the lack of nephrotoxicity is an advantage over angiography and CT imaging. Strengths of MRI include the ability to demonstrate the intimal flap [72] and entry site [54], to examine the whole length of the aorta, and occasionally to demonstrate so-called "aortic cobwebs," which are fibroelastic bands formed during the dissection process that project from the false lumen wall [74]. The detection of these bands

facilitates the distinction of the false from the true lumen because they are located in the false lumen. On spin-echo images, flow in the true lumen is usually signal-void, whereas flow in the false lumen can be signal-void or high in signal intensity depending upon the velocity of blood flow (Fig. 10.22). Slow flow in the false lumen of a dissection may be difficult to differentiate from thrombosis on spin-echo images.

The role of conventional spin-echo imaging is limited because gadolinium-enhanced SGE (2D or 3D), gadolinium-enhanced 3D gradient-echo (e.g., 3D FISP), and gad-

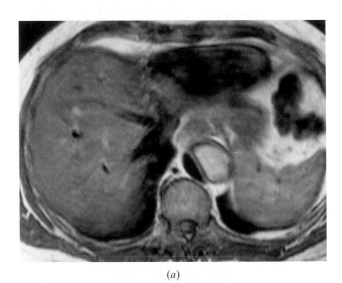

(a)

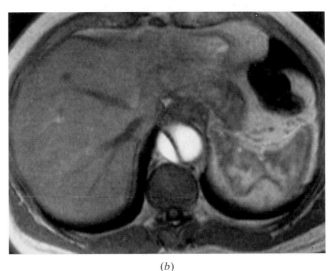

(b)

FIG. 10.22 Aortic dissection with perfusion differential between the kidneys. T1-weighted spin-echo (*a*), immediate (*b,c*) and 90-second (*d*) postgadolinium SGE images. The T1-weighted spin-echo image (*a*) shows enlargement of the abdominal aorta, which contains an intimal flap and has a true and a false lumen. High signal intensity is noted in the false lumen due to slow flow. Note that the true lumen has a biconvex configuration due to the higher blood pressure. The immediate postgadolinium SGE image (*b*) acquired at the same tomographic level shows enhancement of both lumens with sharp demarcation of the intimal flap.

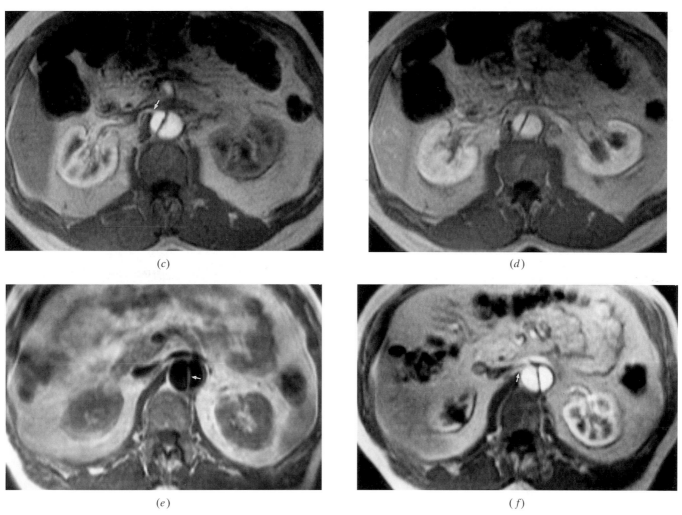

(c)

(d)

(e)

(f)

FIG. 10.22 (*Continued*) The false lumen enhances substantially less than the true lumen on the immediate postgadolinium SGE image (*c*) at a lower tomographic level due to diminished contrast delivery secondary to slow flow in the false lumen. The right renal artery (*arrow, c*) is demonstrated originating from the true lumen. Intense cortical enhancement of the right kidney and minimal cortical enhancement of the left kidney is evident, reflecting the origin of the left renal artery from the false lumen. Note that on the 90-second postgadolinium SGE image (*d*) both lumen and kidneys enhance to the same extent. T1-weighted spin-echo (*e*) and immediate postgadolinium SGE (*f*) images in a second patient with aortic dissection. The T1-weighted spin-echo image shows an aortic aneurysm with an intimal flap (*arrow, e*). Both lumen are signal-void on this image reflecting higher blood velocity in the false lumen than observed in the first patient. The right lumen has a biconvex configuration consistent with the true lumen. High flow in both lumen is also reflected as equal enhancement on the immediate postgadolinium SGE image. The origin of the right renal artery (*arrow, f*) from the true lumen is well-shown. Immediate postgadolinium SGE images in patients with aortic dissection provide hemodynamic information that is helpful in determining true and false lumens and abdominal organ arterial perfusion.

olinium-enhanced fat-suppressed SGE (2D or 3D) imaging are all fast, accurate, and reproducible techniques for the demonstration of dissection. Gadolinium-enhanced SGE and 3D gradient-echo techniques reliably differentiate slow flow, which is high in signal intensity on these images, from thrombus, which is low to intermediate in signal intensity (Fig. 10.22). Breath-hold gadolinium-enhanced 3D FISP images provide sharp detail and demonstrate the full extent of dissection, the entry site, the location of the intimal flap, and the relation of the visceral vessels to the true and false lumen (Fig. 10.23). The entry site, intimal flap, and origins of the vessels are better shown on the individual sections than on the 3D MIP reconstructions. The acquisition of two datasets provides dynamic flow information with delayed enhancement of the false lumen (see Fig. 10.23), which is apparent in cases with slow flow. Immediate postgadolinium SGE images also provide this information. Postgadolinium SGE and fat-suppressed SGE images delineate the intimal flap, demonstrate the origins of the aortic branches, and may show extension of the dissection into the splanchnic vessels (Fig. 10.24). This extension is evaluated better on transverse than on sagittal or coronal plane images.

In rare instances the only finding may be wall thick-

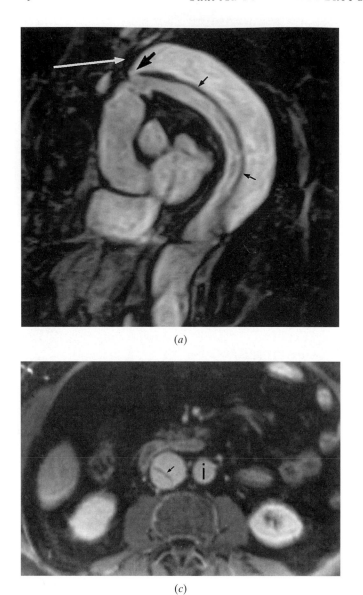

(a)

(c)

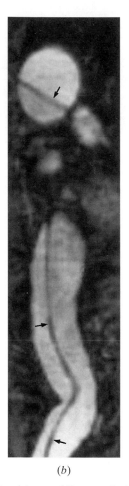

(b)

FIG. 10.23 Aortic dissection. Gadolinium-enhanced 2-mm thin section 3D FISP (a) obtained in an oblique sagittal plane through the center of the lumen of the aortic arch, coronal multiplanar reconstruction (b) from the set of gadolinium enhanced 2-mm thin oblique sagittal 3D FISP sections and transverse interstitial-phase gadolinium-enhanced fat-suppressed SGE (c) images in a patient with type B aortic dissection. The oblique sagittal gadolinium-enhanced 3D FISP image (a) demonstrates an aortic dissection originating in the thoracic aorta. The intimal flap (small arrows, a–c) is readily demonstrated as a low signal intensity curvilinear structure. The entry site (arrow, a) identified immediately distal to the origin of the left subclavian artery (long arrow, a). The multiplanar reconstruction (b) outlines the course of the dissection and demonstrates the intimal flap (small arrows, b) from the thoracic to the abdominal aorta. The intimal flap is well seen on the interstitial phase gadolinium enhanced fat suppressed SGE image (c) at the level of the abdominal aorta. Incidental note is made of a left-sided IVC ("i",c).

ening with or without high-signal-intensity areas on T1-weighted images [75,76]. The high-signal-intensity areas on T1-weighted images reflect the presence of intramural hematoma. This pattern may be missed on angiography and has been postulated to represent the early stage of dissection with hemorrhage from the vasa vasorum that leads to aortic wall weakening and subsequent intimal rupture [75,76]. In one report the transition from this

appearance to classic dissection with intimal flap and blood flow in the false lumen was documented on follow-up studies in two patients [76].

Penetrating Aortic Ulcers and Intramural Dissecting Hematoma

Penetrating aortic ulcers result from ulcerated atherosclerotic plaques that penetrate the internal elastic lamina

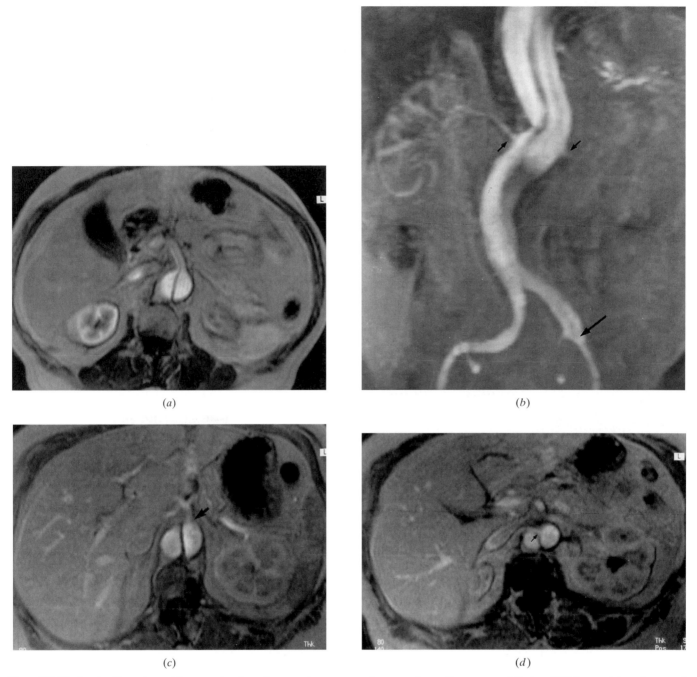

F I G. 10.24 Aortic dissection with extension into the superior mesenteric artery. Immediate postgadolinium SGE image (*a*) and coronal projection (*b*) from 3D MIP reconstruction of a set of coronal immediate postgadolinium SGE images obtained in a follow-up study. The immediate postgadolinium SGE image (*a*) at the level of the origin of the superior mesenteric artery shows high-signal-intensity, gadolinium-containing true (*right*) and false (*left*) lumens and extension of the intimal flap into the superior mesenteric artery. The coronal projection from the 3D MIP reconstruction shows the abdominal aorta and iliac arteries, with the intimal flap extending into the external iliac artery (*arrow, b*). The ostia of the renal arteries are clearly depicted (*small arrows, b*), whereas the left renal artery and kidney are not visualized due to decreased enhancement from slow blood flow in the false lumen. Immediate postgadolinium SGE images (*c,d*) at different tomographic levels in a second patient. The high-signal-intensity gadolinium-containing aorta is clearly shown on both images. The intimal flap is well-shown as are the origins of the celiac axis (*arrow, c*) and right renal artery (*small arrow, d*) from the true lumen.

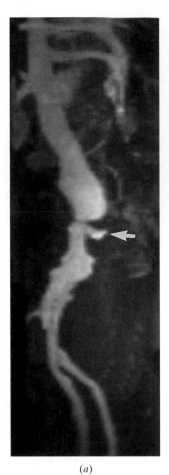

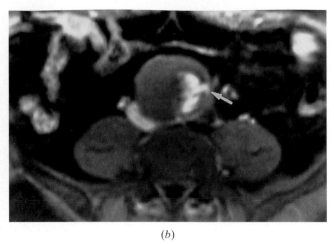

(b)

FIG. 10.25 Penetrating aortic ulcer. Lateral MIP projection of a set of gadolinium-enhanced 2-mm thin section coronal 3D FISP sections (*a*), and transverse interstitial-phase gadolinium-enhanced fat-suppressed SGE (*b*) images. An atherosclerotic aneurysm of the infrarenal abdominal aorta is present. An ulceration of the atherosclerotic plaque (*arrow, a,b*) is demonstrated on the lateral MIP projection. On the interstitial-phase gadolinium-enhanced fat-suppressed SGE image (*b*) the diameter of the aortic aneurysm and the presence of mural thrombus are well evaluated. The depth of the ulceration in relation to the outer aortic wall is appreciated. Interstitial-phase gadolinium-enhanced fat-suppressed SGE images provide information on the aortic wall and the surrounding tissues that are not available on MR angiographic images.

(a)

and may lead to hematoma formation within the media of the aortic wall, false aneurysm, and finally transmural rupture of the aorta. They are more commonly located in the descending thoracic or upper abdominal aorta (Fig. 10.25) [77]. In cases of intramural dissecting hematoma the intimal flap is not often seen and is irregular and thick. The intramural hematoma rarely fills with contrast and is usually seen to extend both cephalad and caudal to the entry site, which is at the penetrating atherosclerotic ulcer. Extensive atherosclerotic changes are usually present in the aorta [77]. It is important to differentiate this entity from aortic dissection because management may be different. MRI can demonstrate the intramural hematoma, atherosclerotic ulcer, and false aneurysm [77,78], and is superior to angiography in depicting the extent of intramural thrombus. MRI is also superior to CT imaging in differentiating acute hematoma from atherosclerotic plaque and chronic thrombus [78]. Intramural hematoma is high in signal intensity on both T1- and T2-weighted images and can be differentiated from chronic mural thrombus which is low in signal intensity [78]. The combination of gadolinium-enhanced 3D FISP images to define the aortic lumen and gadolinium-enhanced fat-suppressed SGE images to demonstrate the wall thickness

in deep aortic ulcers may be the most effective means for evaluating this entity (see Fig. 10.25).

Aortoiliac Atherosclerotic Disease—Thrombosis

Gadolinium-enhanced SGE or fat-suppressed SGE images may demonstrate gross atherosclerotic changes of the aorta and iliac arteries. Gadolinium-enhanced 3D FISP images can reliably assess atherosclerotic changes and stenoses of the aorta (Figs. 10.26 and 10.27) and iliac arteries and are able to demonstrate the lumen of the stenotic segment and the immediate poststenotic area (see Fig. 10.27) because they do not suffer from dephasing phenomena compared with time-of-flight techniques.

Occlusion of the abdominal aorta and its branches may occur in advanced thrombotic disease or dissection. Gadolinium-enhanced SGE images permit clear distinction between high-signal-intensity patent lumen and low-signal-intensity thrombosed lumen (Fig. 10.28). Coronal or sagittal images are useful to confirm the level of occlusion (Figs. 10.28 and 10.29).

Postoperative Aortic Graft Evaluation

Postoperative complications of abdominal aortic graft surgery include occlusion, hemorrhage with false aneu-

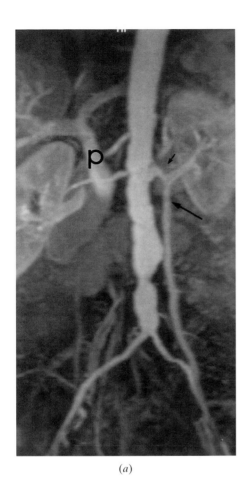

(a)

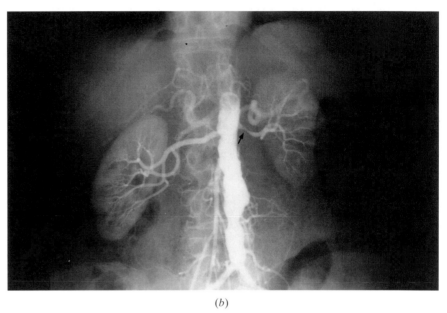

(b)

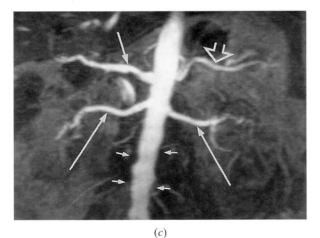

(c)

FIG. 10.26 Atherosclerotic disease of the abdominal aorta. Coronal 3D MIP reconstruction (a) of a set of immediate postgadolinium 3D FISP sections with effective slice thickness of 2 mm and anteroposterior conventional arteriography image (b). Diffuse atherosclerotic disease of the abdominal aorta with irregularity of the contour and focal stenotic and dilated segments is demonstrated on the 3D MIP image (a). Close correlation of the MRI findings with the intra-arterial catheter angiographic image (b) is present. The image acquisition timing in this case was slightly delayed, and the 3D FISP images were acquired during the capillary rather than the arterial phase of enhancement, as evidenced by the presence of enhanced portal vein (p,a) and right renal vein. Enhancement of the left renal vein partially masks a stenosis (small arrow, a,b) of the left renal artery. Targeted 3D MIP reconstructions of the left renal artery revealed this stenosis. Note early retrograde filling of the left ovarian vein (arrow, a). Coronal 3D MIP reconstruction (c) of a set of immediate postgadolinium 3D FISP sections with effective slice thickness of 2 mm in a second patient shows irregular contour of the aorta (small arrows, c) due to diffuse atherosclerotic changes. Note normal renal arteries (long arrows, c) bilaterally. The common hepatic artery (short arrow, c) and splenic artery (hollow arrow, c) are also demonstrated.

rysm formation, infection, and aortoenteric fistula formation. Complications are well-shown on MR images [62]. Fluid is frequently present surrounding the graft within 3 months following surgery (Fig. 10.30). Fluid surrounding the graft beyond 3 months or an increasing volume of perigraft fluid after 3 months is suggestive of infection on T1- and T2-weighted images [62,79,80]. Gadolinium-enhanced fat-suppressed imaging may also be an ideal technique for evaluating inflammatory en-

hancement in aortic graft infections (Fig. 10.31). Gadolinium-enhanced fat-suppressed SGE images are preferable to gadolinium-enhanced T1-weighted fat-suppressed spin-echo images because patency of the graft lumen can also be assessed reliably with the SGE sequence. Patent lumen is high in signal intensity, and intraluminal thrombus is low to intermediate in signal intensity. Inflammatory tissue shows substantial enhancement, and fluid collections/abscesses will be low in signal intensity.

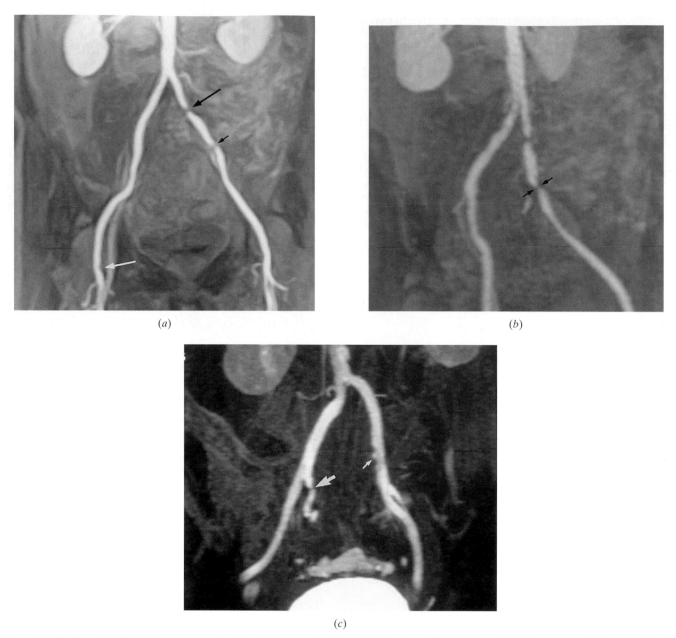

(a)

(b)

(c)

FIG. 10.27 Stenosis of the left common and external iliac arteries. Coronal (*a*) and magnified oblique (*b*) (right anterior oblique equivalent) 3D MIP reconstructions from a set of immediate postgadolinium 3D FISP images with effective slice thickness of 2 mm. High-grade stenoses are demonstrated at the left common iliac (*black arrow, a*) and left external iliac (*small black arrow, a*) arteries. Irregularity of the vessel contour from diffuse atherosclerotic disease and a more prominent eccentric plaque at the right common femoral artery (*white arrow, a*) are also noted. On the magnified image (*b*) vessel lumen distal to the high-grade stenoses and the lumen of the stenotic segment (*small arrows, b*) are well-visualized, reflecting negligible signal loss from dephasing. This is due to the very short echo time of the sequence combined with the T1-shortening from the gadolinium enhancement. The internal iliac arteries are not adequately visualized due to their location outside the obtained 3D slab. Coronal 3D MIP reconstruction (*c*) from a set of immediate postgadolinium coronal breath-hold 3D FISP images with effective slice thickness of 2 mm in a second patient with diabetes mellitus and recent onset of impotence. A high-grade stenosis (*arrow, c*) of the right internal iliac artery is demonstrated 1 cm from its origin. The lumen immediately distal to the stenotic area is well-visualized due to minimized dephasing despite turbulent flow. An ulcerated atherosclerotic plaque (*small arrow, c*) in the left common iliac artery is also present. The peripheral segments of the internal iliac arteries are not visualized due to their course outside the acquired 3D slab.

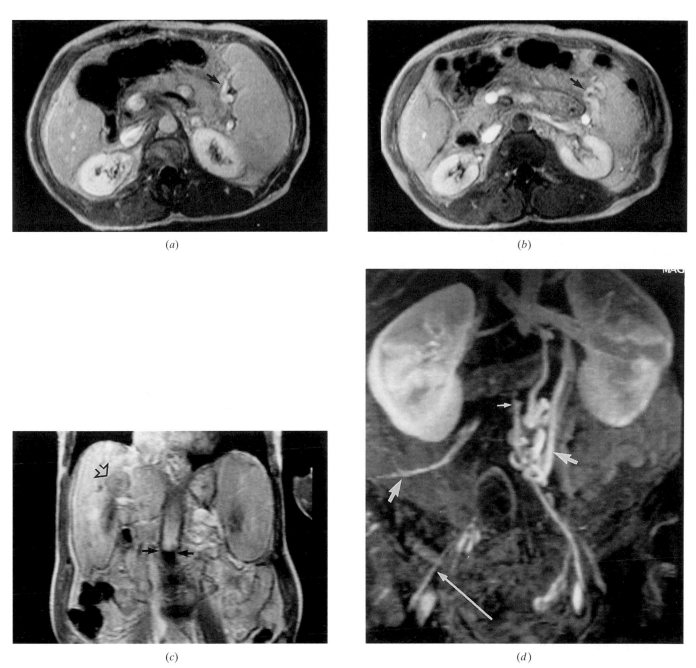

FIG. 10.28 Thrombotic occlusion of the infrarenal aorta. Transverse (*a,b*) and coronal (*c*) interstitial-phase gadolinium-enhanced SGE images. The lumen of the abdominal aorta demonstrates normal enhancement at the level of celiac axis origin (*a*). On the SGE image at a lower tomographic level (*b*), lack of enhancement of the aortic lumen reflects thrombotic occlusion. The abrupt transition (*arrows, c*) of enhancing patent to low-signal-intensity thrombosed lumen is demonstrated on the coronal image. This patient was assessed for multifocal hepatocellular carcinoma, and a tumor nodule (*hollow arrow, c*) is demonstrated in the right lobe of the liver. Splenomegaly with varices (*arrows, a,b*) is also present in this patient due to portal hypertension secondary to alcoholic cirrhosis. Coronal MIP reconstruction (*d*) of a set of gadolinium-enhanced 2-mm thin section coronal 3D FISP sections, coronal interstitial-phase gadolinium-enhanced fat-suppressed SGE (*e*), and sagittal multiplanar reconstruction (*f*) from the set of gadolinium-enhanced 2-mm thin section coronal 3D FISP sections in a second patient with infrarenal aortic occlusion. Complete occlusion of the infrarenal aorta 1 cm below the level of the renal arteries is demonstrated on the coronal MIP image (*d*). The lumen of the aorta (*small arrow, d*) is reconstituted distally, through numerous retroperitoneal collateral vessels (*arrows, d*). The left common iliac artery is patent, while the right common iliac artery is occluded at its origin with reconstitution at the level of the distal external iliac artery (*long arrow, d*).

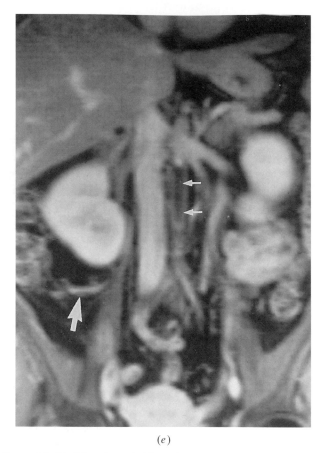

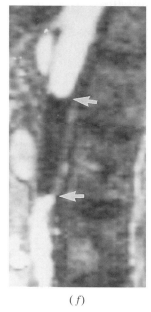

(e)   *(f)*

FIG. **10.28** (*Continued*) Thrombus (*small arrows*, *e*) in the infrarenal aorta and a large retroperitoneal collateral (*arrow*, *e*) are demonstrated on the interstitial-phase gadolinium-enhanced fat-suppressed SGE image (*e*). The sagittal 2-mm thin reconstruction (*f*) through the center of the aortic lumen clearly demonstrates the superior and inferior margins (*arrows*, *f*) of the near signal void thrombus against the homogeneous high-signal-intensity gadolinium-enhanced patent lumen. The acquisition of a volume of data with thin sections permits excellent resolution for multiplanar reconstructions.

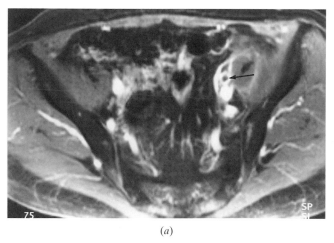

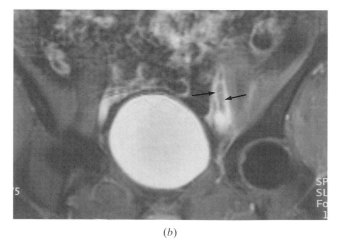

(a)   *(b)*

FIG. **10.29** External iliac artery thrombosis. Transverse (*a*) and coronal (*b*) interstitial-phase gadolinium-enhanced fat-suppressed SGE images. The left external iliac artery is identified medially to the psoas muscle on the transverse image (*a*), and contains low-signal-intensity thrombus (*arrow*, *a*). The presence of intraluminal thrombus (*arrows*, *b*) is confirmed on the coronal image. Post-gadolinium SGE images, acquired within 2 minutes after gadolinium injection and performed as part of routine abdominal and pelvic MR imaging protocols, provide a reproducible technique for the assessment of the patency of large and medium-sized arteries and veins.

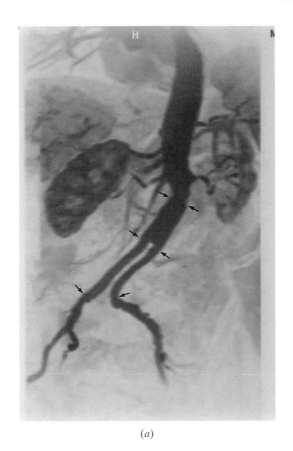

(a)

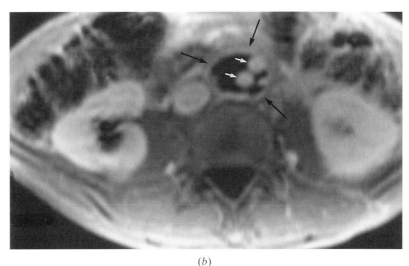

(b)

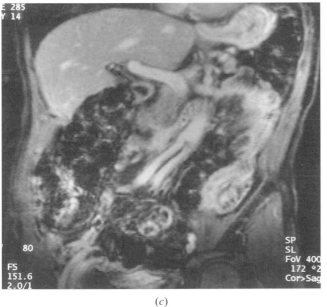

(c)

F IG. 10.30 Aortobifemoral graft in a patient with Marfan's syndrome 1 month after surgery. A 3D MIP reconstruction (*a*) from a set of coronal 2-mm-thin immediate postgadolinium 3D FISP images, and transverse (*b*) coronal (*c*) interstitial-phase gadolinium-enhanced fat-suppressed SGE images. The MIP image (*a*) demonstrates an abdominal aortic aneurysm with a maximal diameter of 4.5 cm at the level of the upper pole of the left kidney. More distally within the abdominal aorta, an aortoiliac graft is identified (*small arrows, a*). Irregularity of the arterial contour is noted distal to the graft due to atherosclerotic disease. The transverse 1 minute postgadolinium fat-suppressed SGE image shows the patent lumens of the limbs of the graft (*small arrows, b*) surrounded by low-signal-intensity postoperative fluid contained within the wall (*arrows, b*) of the native aorta. The patency of the graft is also shown on the coronal interstitial-phase gadolinium-enhanced fat-suppressed SGE image (*c*).

INFERIOR VENA CAVA

As with the aorta, the IVC may be evaluated with bright-blood and black-blood techniques [81,82]. The IVC may be evaluated for the presence of thrombus, differentiation of blood from tumor thrombus, and in rare instances, for the evaluation of primary tumors. In the vast majority of cases an abdominal protocol employing precontrast SGE and postgadolinium SGE and/or fat-suppressed SGE images provides sufficient evaluation of the IVC for patient management. At least one sequence should be performed in the sagittal or coronal plane such as gadolinium-enhanced SGE or, preferably, fat-suppressed SGE images because it permits direct visualization of the longitudinal

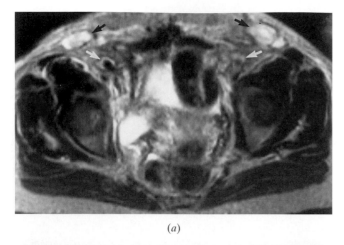

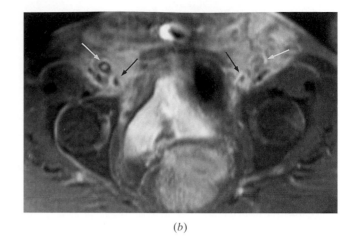

(a)

(b)

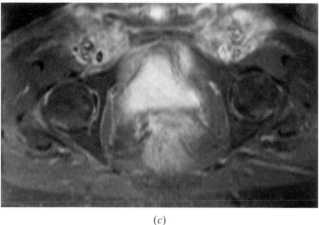

(c)

FIG. 10.31 Infected aortobifemoral graft. T2-weighted spin-echo (*a*) and gadolinium-enhanced T1-weighted fat-suppressed spin-echo (*b,c*) images. High-signal-intensity fluid (*white arrows, a*) is demonstrated on the T2-weighted image (*a*) surrounding the wall of the infected grafts. The subcutaneous fat in the groins and anterior abdominal wall is heterogeneously high in signal intensity reflecting the presence of inflammation, and bilateral enlarged inguinal lymph nodes (*black arrows, a*) are noted. Intense enhancement of the surrounding soft tissue and the walls of the grafts (*black arrows, b*) as well as the walls of the common femoral veins (*white arrows, b*) is demonstrated on gadolinium-enhanced T1-weighted fat-suppressed spin-echo images, reflecting severe inflammatory changes.

extent of the IVC, which is ideal in examining for the extent of blood or tumor thrombus. Breath-hold time-of-flight techniques are less effective at demonstrating slow flow than gadolinium-enhanced SGE techniques. Gadolinium-enhanced MRA of the IVC is not usually performed because preferential venous enhancement requires suppression of the arterial signal by presaturation pulses, which are not effective at overcoming the extreme T1-shortening caused by gadolinium. Alternatively when 3D venography-like images are required to answer complicated clinical problems, immediate postgadolinium breath-hold 3D gradient-echo techniques (e.g., breath-hold coronal 3D FISP acquisition) may be performed during the simultaneous injection of gadolinium in peripheral veins of both legs. This technique provides thin-slice (2-mm) resolution, but is seldom needed in routine clinical practice.

Congenital Abnormalities

Congenital abnormalities of the inferior vena cava and related veins are common [81–85]. The most common venous anomalies are those of the left renal vein. Retroaortic left renal vein is the most common (Fig. 10.32)

[83–85], with other anomalies such as circumaortic left renal vein (Fig. 10.33) being less common. A combination of a black-blood technique (e.g., T1-weighted spin-echo or SGE with inferior presaturation pulses) and a bright-blood technique (dynamic gadolinium-enhanced SGE,

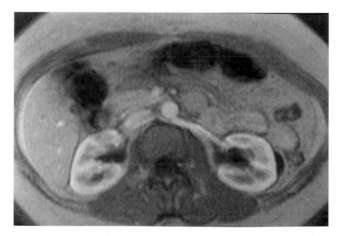

FIG. 10.32 Retroaortic left renal vein. The immediate postgadolinium SGE image demonstrates a retroaortic left renal vein entering the IVC.

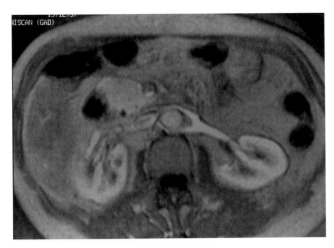

F I G. 10.33 Circumaortic left renal vein. Immediate postgadolinium SGE image clearly defines both limbs of the circumaortic left renal vein with their entry into the IVC.

or preferably fat-suppressed SGE imaging) are useful in order to determine that rounded or tubular retroperitoneal structures are vascular in nature [86]. Left-sided vena cava (Fig. 10.34), duplicated vena cava (Fig. 10.35), and IVC interruption with azygous/hemiazygous continuation are not uncommon anomalies, which are well-shown by MRI. Gadolinium enhancement is useful because in noncontrast images duplicated IVC, thrombophlebitis of the left-sided IVC, and existing retroperitoneal collateral vessels may mimic retroperitoneal lymphadenopathy [87].

Venous Thrombosis

MRI performs well in evaluating IVC thrombosis [88,89] and distinguishing tumor from blood thrombus. Gadolinium-enhanced SGE or fat-suppressed SGE images are

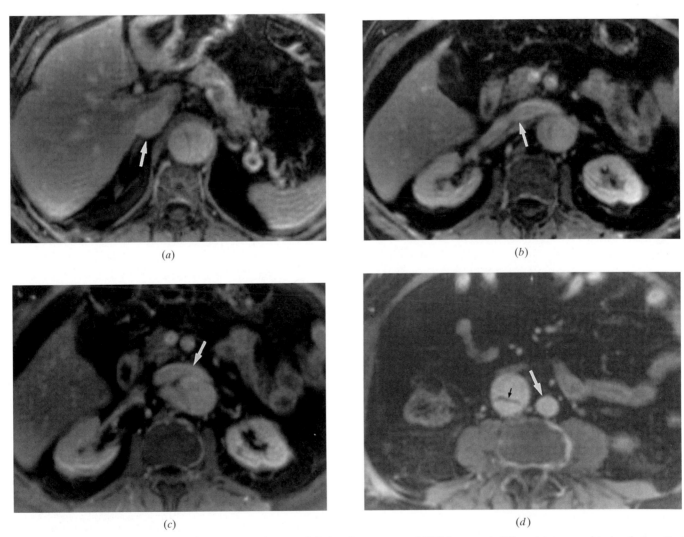

(a)

(b)

(c)

(d)

F I G. 10.34 Left sided IVC. Pictured are 90-second postgadolinium fat-suppressed SGE images at different tomographic levels (a–d). A right-sided suprarenal IVC is demonstrated on the most cranial image (arrow, a). At the level of the renal veins the IVC (arrow, b) crosses over the aorta to the left and the infrarenal IVC (arrow, c,d) is left-sided (c). An aortic dissection is also present with the intimal flap (small arrow, d) shown in the contrast enhanced aortic lumen.

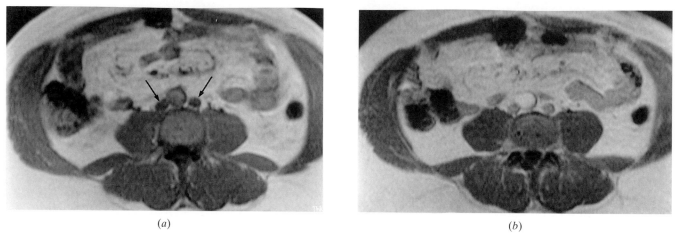

(a)   (b)

FIG. 10.35 Duplicated IVC. SGE (*a*) and immediate postgadolinium SGE (*b*) images. A duplicated IVC (*arrows, a*) is present. The venae cavae are low in signal intensity on the precontrast image (*a*), whereas a mild degree of high signal intensity is present in the aorta due to inflow of unsaturated blood in a craniocaudal direction. On the immediate postgadolinium SGE image (*b*), the venae cavae enhance, but to a lesser degree than the abdominal aorta because in this early phase of enhancement the majority of the contrast is in the arterial and capillary circulation. Combining morphological and directional flow information on the precontrast images with dynamic temporal flow information on serial postgadolinium SGE images permits evaluation of congenital vascular variations and malformations.

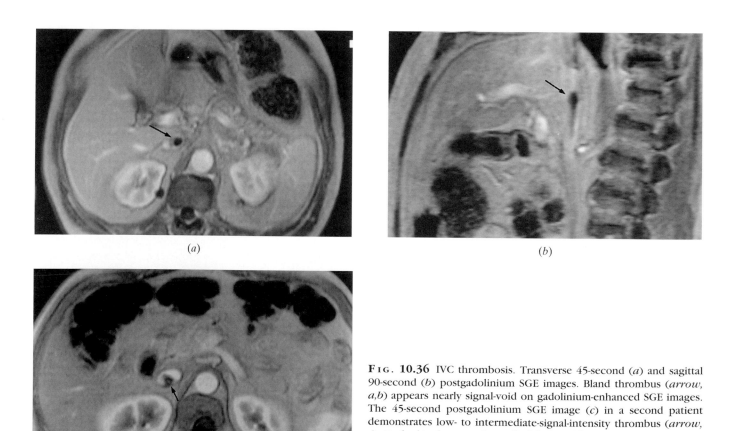

(a)   (b)

(c)

FIG. 10.36 IVC thrombosis. Transverse 45-second (*a*) and sagittal 90-second (*b*) postgadolinium SGE images. Bland thrombus (*arrow, a,b*) appears nearly signal-void on gadolinium-enhanced SGE images. The 45-second postgadolinium SGE image (*c*) in a second patient demonstrates low- to intermediate-signal-intensity thrombus (*arrow, c*) attached to the posterior wall of the IVC. The combination of intense enhancement of the IVC on gadolinium-enhanced SGE images with multiplanar imaging renders MRI an excellent noninvasive modality for the assessment of venous thrombosis.

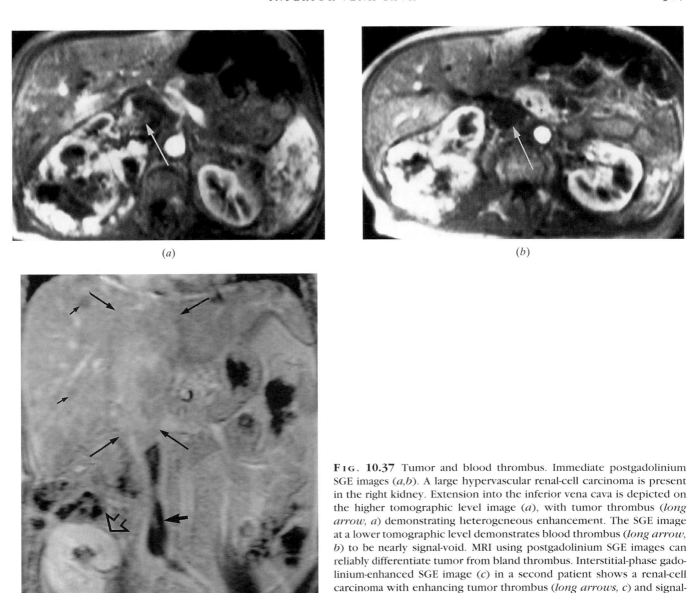

(a)

(b)

(c)

Fig. 10.37 Tumor and blood thrombus. Immediate postgadolinium SGE images (*a,b*). A large hypervascular renal-cell carcinoma is present in the right kidney. Extension into the inferior vena cava is depicted on the higher tomographic level image (*a*), with tumor thrombus (*long arrow, a*) demonstrating heterogeneous enhancement. The SGE image at a lower tomographic level demonstrates blood thrombus (*long arrow, b*) to be nearly signal-void. MRI using postgadolinium SGE images can reliably differentiate tumor from bland thrombus. Interstitial-phase gadolinium-enhanced SGE image (*c*) in a second patient shows a renal-cell carcinoma with enhancing tumor thrombus (*long arrows, c*) and signal-void blood thrombus (*arrow, c*) extending distally to the left common iliac vein. Multiple hepatic metastases (*small arrow, c*) and a renal transplant (*hollow arrow, c*) curved arrow are also noted.

useful for these determinations. Tumor thrombus enhances, whereas blood thrombus does not enhance with contrast (Figs. 10.36 and 10.37) [90]. Signal-intensity measurements of thrombus before and after gadolinium administration may be necessary because blood thrombus, which is subacute or responding to anticoagulant therapy, may be high in signal intensity on precontrast images. Lack of increase in signal intensity on postcontrast images would confirm the blood nature of the thrombus. Flow-sensitive gradient-echo techniques with a lower flip angle (30 to 45°) may distinguish tumor from blood thrombus. Tumor thrombus is intermediate (soft tissue) in signal intensity on these sequences, whereas blood thrombus is generally very low in signal intensity [91].

Blood thrombus frequently exists at the tail of tumor thrombus (see Fig. 10.37), and the two components can be distinguished readily on postgadolinium SGE and fat-suppressed SGE images. The combination of gadolinium-enhanced and flow-sensitive techniques to assess thrombus is useful, and evaluation of the degree of expansion of the IVC is also contributory because pronounced expansion rules against blood thrombus. MRI, because of its direct multiplanar capability and serial dynamic postcontrast imaging, is superior to CT imaging in determining the presence and extent of tumor thrombus. MRI outperforms CT imaging in detecting the extension of tumor thrombus supradiaphragmatically into the right atrium. This is an important evaluation in the preopera-

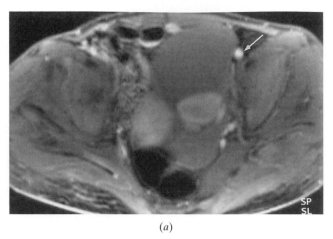

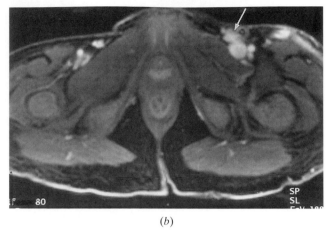

(a)   (b)

FIG. 10.38 Chronic venous thrombosis. Interstitial-phase gadolinium-enhanced fat-suppressed SGE images at superior (a) and more inferior (b) tomographic levels. At the level of the midpelvis, only the left external iliac artery (arrow, a) is identified, while the chronically thrombosed left external iliac vein appears as linear nonenhancing tissue immediately posterior to the artery. A collateral enhancing vessel (arrow, b) is noted reconstituting the left common femoral vein at a lower tomographic level (b). SGE images obtained from 45 seconds to 2 minutes after gadolinium administration provide reproducible uniform intense enhancement of normal veins, rendering this technique sensitive to the presence of thrombus even in medium and small diameter vessels. Imaging within 40 seconds permits evaluation of arteries, often without the presence of contrast in veins.

tive setting because supradiaphragmatic thrombus requires combined thoracoabdominal surgery, whereas tumor thrombus whose superior extension is below the hepatic veins may require just an abdominal approach.

In cases of chronic venous thrombosis the affected vessel may not be identified if the thrombus is organized but the vein is not recanalized. In these cases careful evaluation may reveal the absence of thrombosed vessel enhancement with the presence of collateral vessel network (Fig. 10.38). IVC filters can be recognized by the symmetrical arrangement of their elements and the magnetic susceptibility artifact on SGE images (Fig. 10.39).

In a fashion similar to that of IVC evaluation, MRI is

effective at demonstrating renal and gonadal veins as well as retroperitoneal collaterals in cases of venous thrombosis [82]. Compression of the left renal vein between the aorta and superior mesenteric artery may result in the "nutcracker syndrome," and when a pressure gradient is present it may occasionally lead to development of varicocele, ovarian vein or pelviureteral varices, hematuria, and flank pain [92]. Thrombosed, enlarged retroperitoneal collateral veins may mimic lymphadenopathy on imaging studies [87]. In these cases careful following of the course of the structures on transverse images may indicate the vascular nature of the masses [87]. Direct coronal or sagittal imaging is also helpful because these planes demonstrate the tubular shape of these vessels. Gadolinium-enhanced fat-suppressed SGE images provide a definitive answer because they demonstrate lack of enhancement in thrombosed vessels compared to moderate enhancement of lymph nodes. Gonadal veins may be enlarged in cases of varicoceles in men and varices of the ovarian venous plexus in women (Fig. 10.40). Early retrograde filling of a large and/or tortuous gonadal vein may be demonstrated on immediate post-gadolinium SGE or arterial-phase bolus-enhanced 3D FISP images (see Fig. 10.26). Markedly enlarged ovarian veins are commonly encountered during pregnancy due to compression by the pregnant uterus and increased venous flow (Fig. 10.41). Thrombosis of the ovarian veins may complicate puerperal infection and is readily detected on gadolinium-enhanced fat-suppressed SGE images.

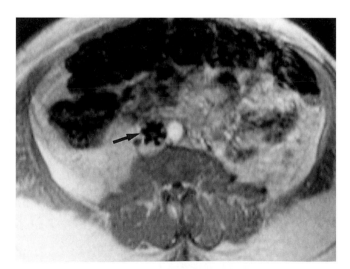

FIG. 10.39 IVC filter. A 45-second postgadolinium SGE image demonstrates a Gianturco IVC filter (arrow) in the inferior vena cava. The filter is readily recognized by the magnetic susceptibility effect and the symmetric configuration of its pedicles.

Primary Malignant Tumors

Primary malignant tumors of the IVC are rare. The most common histological type is leiomyosarcoma, followed

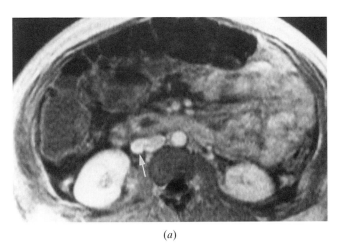
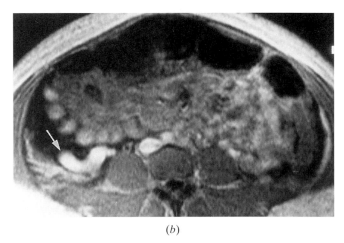

(a)   (b)

FIG. 10.40 Dilated gonadal vein. Pictured are 90-second postgadolinium SGE images at superior (a) and more inferior (b) tomographic levels. A dilated right gonadal vein is demonstrated at its drainage into the IVC (arrow, a). At the lower tomographic level, the enhancing vessel (arrow, b) follows a serpiginous course. Low-signal-intensity ascites with centrally displaced bowel loops is also identified.

by angiosarcoma [16]. In a review of leiomyosarcomas of the retroperitoneum and inferior vena cava, leiomyosarcomas involving the IVC have been classified as Pattern 2 when completely intraluminal and Pattern 3 in cases of combined extraluminal and intraluminal components, which comprise 5 and 33 percent, respectively, of the total cases [16]. These tumors are frequently large at presentation (Fig. 10.42), but tend to present earlier than their completely extraluminal counterparts because of symptoms related to obstruction of the IVC. Signal intensity of these tumors is moderately low on T1-weighted images and mixed moderate to high on T2-weighted images. Areas of intermixed tumor and blood thrombus may have bright signal intensity on the T1-weighted images, a finding accentuated on fat-suppressed images (see Fig. 10.42). These tumors, which are usually hyper-

vascular, demonstrate intense heterogeneous enhancement on gadolinium-enhanced images [93]. Bright-blood MRI techniques are useful for demonstrating IVC patency and extent of tumor [93], and may provide individual sections for MR angiographic MIP reconstructions. On occasion it may be difficult to distinguish neoplasms with completely intraluminal growth from tumor thrombus. Expansion of the IVC and enhancement on postgadolinium SGE images are features favoring neoplasm and tumor thrombus. In rare cases of hypovascular neoplasms (e.g., malignant fibrous histiocytoma) IVC expansion and demonstration of arterial feeders on immediate postgadolinium SGE images may help to distinguish the neoplasm from blood thrombus (Fig. 10.43) [94]. In rare instances, leiomyosarcomas originating in the renal veins may extend intraluminally into the IVC, and they are demon-

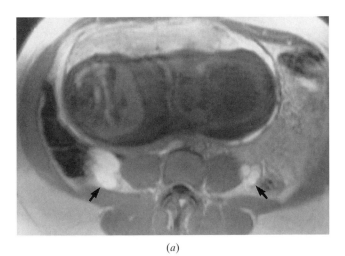
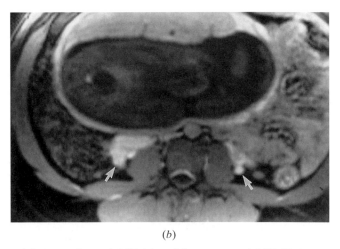

(a)   (b)

FIG. 10.41 Dilated ovarian veins during pregnancy. Interstitial-phase gadolinium-enhanced SGE (a) and fat-suppressed SGE (b) images in a pregnant woman. The inferior vena cava is compressed by the pregnant uterus and the ovarian veins (arrows, a,b) are enlarged, more prominent on the right. The patient was scanned for evaluation of persistent right flank pain, and her pain was attributed to the venous engorgement.

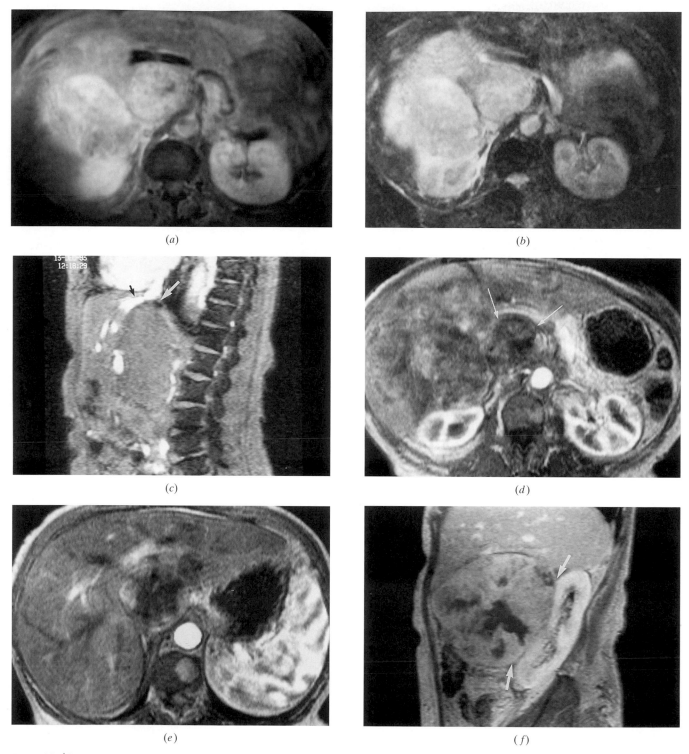

FIG. 10.42 Leiomyosarcoma of the IVC. T1-weighted fat-suppressed spin-echo (*a*), T2-weighted fat-suppressed spin-echo (*b*), sagittal gradient-refocused (time-of-flight) SGE (*c*), immediate (*d,e*) postgadolinium SGE, and sagittal 90-second postgadolinium SGE (*f*) images. A large tumor is present with a large IVC component and a large retroperitoneal component. The tumor is heterogeneous on both T1- (*a*) and T2-weighted (*b*) images. The hyperintense areas on the T1-weighted fat-suppressed image (*a*) reflect the presence of subacute blood products admixed in the tumor thrombus. The superior extent of the tumor within the IVC (*arrow, c*) is immediately below the diaphragm. The IVC and the anteriorly displaced left hepatic vein (*small arrow, c*) immediately above the tumor are patent as shown by the presence of high signal intensity on the flow-sensitive SGE image (*c*). On the immediate postgadolinium SGE images (*d,e*) the mass (*long arrows, d*) enhances in a diffuse heterogeneous fashion. The sagittal 90-second postgadolinium SGE image (*f*) demonstrates the mass (*arrows, f*) invading and compressing the kidney posteriorly. An intense enhancing tumor containing central nonenhancing areas of necrosis is a common appearance for leiomyosarcomas.

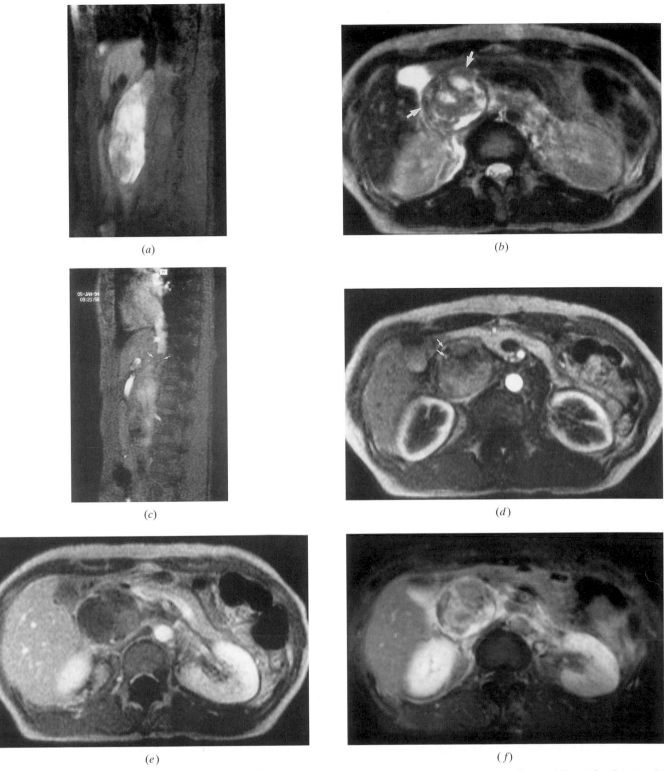

(a)

(b)

(c)

(d)

(e)

(f)

FIG. 10.43 Primary malignant fibrous histiocytoma of the IVC. Sagittal T1-weighted fat-suppressed spin-echo (*a*), T2-weighted spin-echo (*b*), sagittal gradient-refocused (time-of-flight) SGE (*c*), immediate (*d*) and 90-second (*e*) postgadolinium SGE, and transverse gadolinium-enhanced T1-weighted fat-suppressed spin-echo (*f*) images. The tumor (*arrows, b*) is heterogeneous in signal intensity on the T1- (*a*) and T2-weighted (*b*) images and contains areas of high signal intensity on the T1-weighted fat-suppressed spin-echo (*a*) image, reflecting the presence of subacute methemoglobin in the thrombus. The neoplasm expands the IVC, but is contained within the vessel lumen, which is consistent with its primary origin from the vessel wall. The superior extent of the neoplasm (*small arrows, c*) is clearly depicted at the level of the intrahepatic IVC, the patent portion of which is high in signal on the flow-sensitive gradient-refocused SGE image (*c*). Arterioles (*small arrows, d*) are demonstrated as tubular enhancing structures on the immediate postgadolinium SGE image (*d*). The neoplasm enhances minimally in a heterogeneous fashion on the immediate (*d*) and 90-second (*e*) postgadolinium SGE images, reflecting its hypovascular nature. Progressive enhancement is noted on the more delayed T1-weighted fat-suppressed spin-echo image (*f*), which is consistent with delayed enhancement of fibrotic tumor components. The superior extension of tumor thrombus in the IVC is important for surgical planning because the demonstration of supradiaphragmatic extension requires a combined abdominothoracic surgical approach. Sagittal images are superior to transverse sections for demonstrating the craniocaudal extent and defining the superior border of tumor thrombus in the IVC.

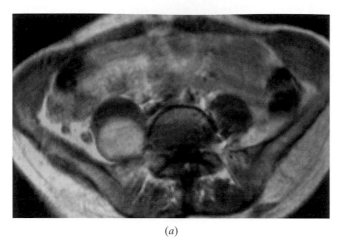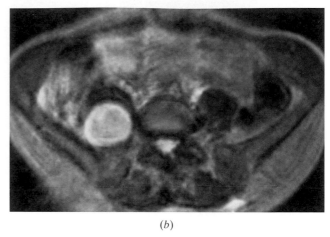

(a)   *(b)*

FIG. 10.44 Neurogenic psoas tumor. T1-weighted spin-echo (*a*) and T2-weighted spin-echo (*b*) images. A well-defined rounded tumor is noted in the right psoas muscle. The tumor is moderate in signal intensity on the T1-weighted image and high in signal intensity on the T2-weighted image. High signal intensity on T2-weighted images is a common feature of tumors of neural origin.

strated as tumors in the medial portion of the kidney with tumor thrombus in the renal vein and IVC [95].

PSOAS MUSCLE

Diseases affecting the psoas muscle more commonly originate from adjacent structures and involve the muscle by direct tissue spread. These include malignant and infectious processes of the spine, kidney, bowel, pancreas, and retroperitoneal lymph nodes [96,97]. Atrophy of the iliopsoas from neuromuscular disease can occur. Spontaneous hemorrhage may also occur in the iliopsoas muscle and is most frequently observed in patients on anticoagulant therapy or in hemophiliacs. Primary tumors

of the muscle are rare, but the psoas can be the site of metastatic deposits.

The psoas muscle is well-evaluated by MRI. The normal muscle is low in signal intensity on T2-weighted images, and because most disease processes are high in signal intensity on T2-weighted images (Fig. 10.44), they can be detected readily [96,97]. Imaging in the coronal or sagittal planes provides direct evaluation of the full craniocaudal extent of the muscle. Lymph nodes are well-evaluated on precontrast sagittal SGE images in a background of retroperitoneal fat, but they are isointense with psoas muscle. Lymph nodes are readily distinguished from psoas muscle on T2 weighted images because muscle is low in signal intensity compared to the moderate signal intensity of lymph nodes [96,97]. Metastatic disease

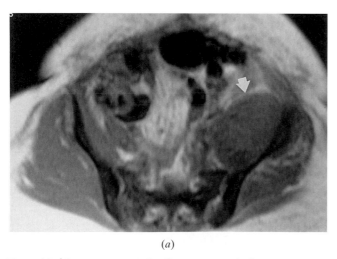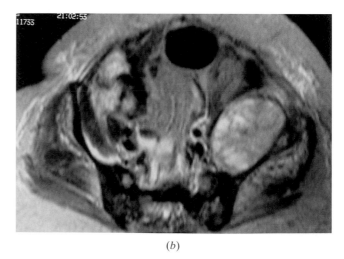

(a)   *(b)*

FIG. 10.45 Metastasis to the iliopsoas muscle from carcinoma of the breast. SGE (*a*) and T2-weighted spin-echo (*b*) images. A large heterogeneous mass (*arrow, a*) is present in the left iliopsoas muscle. The metastasis is low in signal intensity on the SGE image (*a*) and high in signal intensity on the T2-weighted spin-echo image (*b*).

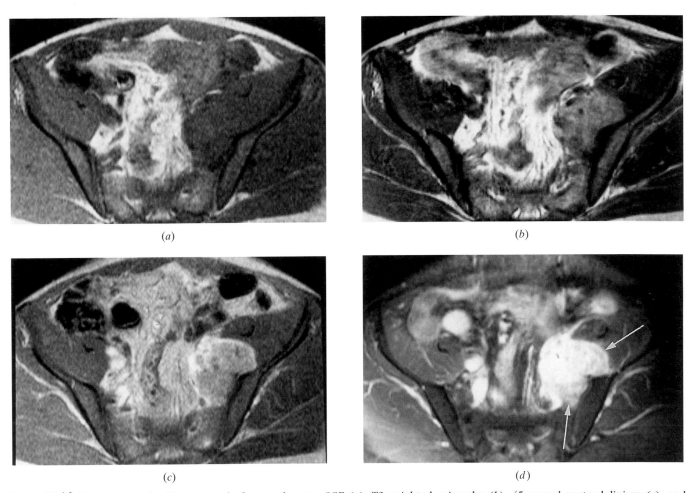

(a)   (b)

(c)   (d)

F I G . 10.46 Metastasis to the iliacus muscle from melanoma. SGE (*a*), T2-weighted spin-echo (*b*), 45-second postgadolinium (*c*), and gadolinium-enhanced T1-weighted fat-suppressed spin-echo (*d*) images. A mass is identified in the posterior portion of the left iliacus muscle. The mass is isointense to muscle on the SGE image (*a*), heterogeneously high in signal intensity on the T2-weighted image (*b*), and enhances in a heterogeneous fashion after gadolinium administration (*c,d*). The degree of enhancement and delineation of its borders are best appreciated on the postgadolinium T1-weighted fat-suppressed spin-echo image (*arrows, d*).

to the iliopsoas muscle is moderate to high in signal intensity on T2 weighted images and shows substantial enhancement on gadolinium-enhanced fat-suppressed SGE images (see Figs. 10.45 and 10.46). Infection is well-shown on MR images as high-signal-intensity areas on T2-weighted images and intense enhancement on gadolinium-enhanced SGE images (Fig. 10.47). Destruction of adjacent vertebral body is common with associated extension into the disc space. Disc space involvement is more typical of infection than of malignancy. On postgadolinium images, abscesses are shown as expansile lesions with signal-void centers, intense peripheral enhancement, and enhancement of the periabscess tissues (see Fig. 10.47).

Hemorrhage is well-shown on MR images due to the high signal intensity of subacute blood on T1-weighted images [98–100]. The use of fat suppression permits the detection of even small amounts of blood, and imaging in different planes provides direct evaluation of the dimensions and extent of the hematoma (Fig. 10.48).

■ THE BODY WALL

Neoplasms

Benign Tumors

Cysts and desmoid tumors are two common benign body wall tumors [101]. Desmoids may be encountered in the setting of Gardner's syndrome and are relatively avascular, locally aggressive masses with a propensity for recurrence, occurring more commonly in middle-aged women [102]. They arise most commonly from the aponeurosis

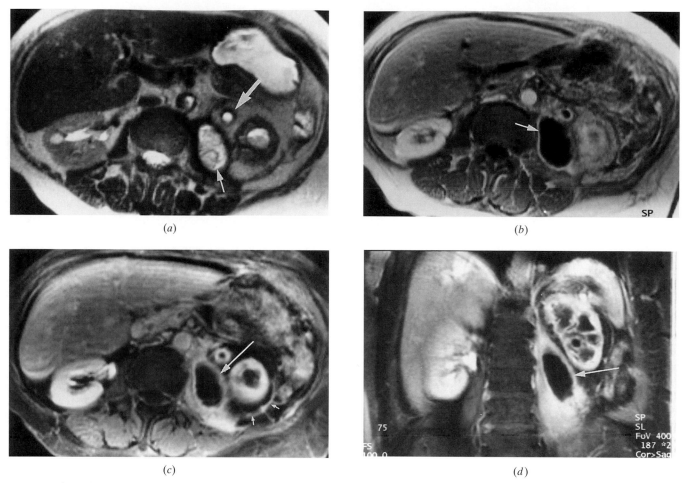

(a) *(b)*

(c) *(d)*

F IG. 10.47 Psoas abscess in a patient with xanthogranulomatous pyelonephritis. HASTE (*a*), 45-second postgadolinium SGE (*b*), and axial (*c*) and coronal (*d*) interstitial-phase gadolinium-enhanced fat-suppressed SGE images. A complex fluid collection is present in an enlarged left psoas muscle. The fluid is heterogeneously high in signal intensity on the T2-weighted image (*arrow, a*) and contains low-signal-intensity necrotic debris. The left ureter (*large arrow, a*) is dilated and has a thick wall. The abscess wall (*arrow, b*) and the ureteral wall demonstrate enhancement on the 45-second postgadolinium SGE image (*b*), which progresses on the interstitial-phase images (*c,d*) to intense enhancement of the abscess-containing psoas muscle (*long arrows, c,d*) and the ureteral wall. Ill-defined borders with linear enhancing strands reflect the extension of the inflammation into the pararenal and perirenal fat. Enhancement of the thickened left perirenal fascia (*small arrows, c*) is also noted. The contents of the abscess are signal-void on the postgadolinium images (*b–d*). Imaging in the coronal plane (*d*) provides direct evaluation of the craniocaudal extent of the abscess. The right psoas muscle is uninvolved and remains low in signal intensity on the postgadolinium images. The collecting system of the left kidney is dilated and low in signal intensity on the interstitial-phase gadolinium-enhanced fat-suppressed SGE images (*c,d*) due to absent gadolinium excretion in a kidney with xanthogranulomatous pyelonephritis.

of the rectus abdominis muscle, and may on occasion be very large mimicking intra-abdominal masses [102]. They are readily detected on T1-weighted images as low-signal-intensity masses in a background of high-signal-intensity fat (Fig. 10.49). In mature desmoids, areas of abundant fibrosis result in low signal intensity on T2-weighted images [102].

The body wall also may be involved in cases of endometriosis occurring almost exclusively along scars from previous surgery. Endometriomas are generally shown better on fat-suppressed SGE images as high-signal-intensity foci.

Malignant Tumors

Direct tumor spread, hematogenous metastases (Fig. 10.50), sarcomas (Figs. 10.51 and 10.52), and lymphomas can involve the body wall. Tumors are medium-signal-intensity masses that are well-defined in the background of high-signal-intensity subcutaneous fat on SGE images, and that on gadolinium-enhanced fat-suppressed images are moderate to high in signal intensity in a background of low-signal-intensity fat. Imaging in the sagittal plane permits direct visualization of the extent of the tumor and its relationship to the abdominal wall muscles.

Tumors arising in or involving the skeletal structures

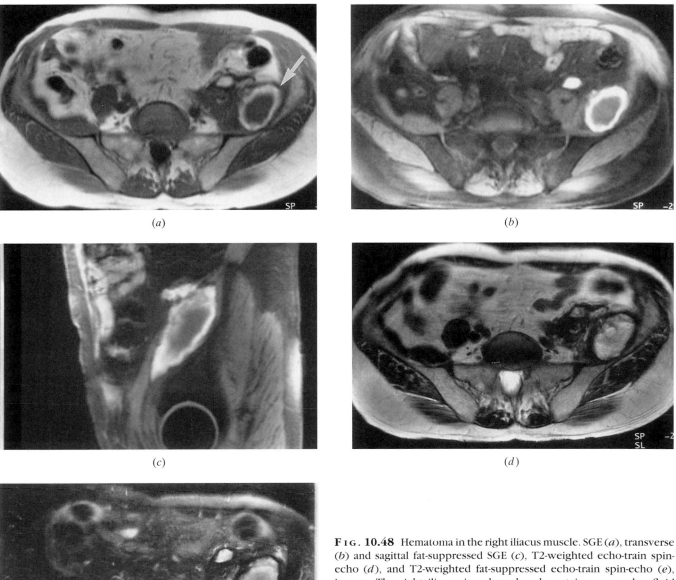

(a)

(b)

(c)

(d)

(e)

FIG. 10.48 Hematoma in the right iliacus muscle. SGE (*a*), transverse (*b*) and sagittal fat-suppressed SGE (*c*), T2-weighted echo-train spin-echo (*d*), and T2-weighted fat-suppressed echo-train spin-echo (*e*), images. The right iliacus is enlarged and contains a complex fluid collection which is low in signal intensity centrally with a high-signal-intensity peripheral rim (*arrow, a*) on the T1-weighted images (*a–c*) and heterogeneously high in signal intensity on the T2-weighted images (*d,e*). The hyperintensity of the peripheral rim is accentuated with the use of fat suppression on the T1-weighted images (*b,c*). The sagittal fat-suppressed SGE image (*c*) demonstrates the craniocaudal extent of the hematoma. The mixed signal intensity of the hematoma reflects blood products in different stages of degradation.

of the abdomen and pelvis are well-shown on a combination of T1-weighted images, T2-weighted fat-suppressed spin-echo, and gadolinium-enhanced fat-suppressed SGE images (Figs. 10.53 and 10.54).

Miscellaneous

Hernias, hematomas, infection, arteriovenous malformations, and varices (Fig. 10.55) may involve the abdominal wall. (Hernias are discussed in Chapter 7 on the Peritoneal Cavity.) Hematomas and vascular abnormalities are well-shown on MR images, and malignant or vascular lesions are well-shown on SGE and gadolinium-enhanced fat-suppressed SGE images. Vascular structures are shown as low-signal-intensity structures on SGE images and enhance after gadolinium administration. The enhancement is rendered more conspicuous with the

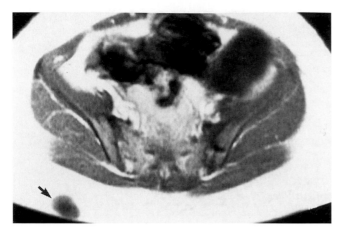

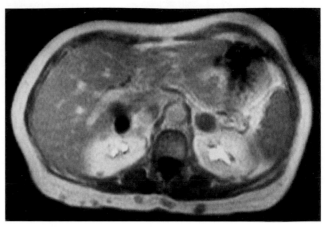

FIG. 10.49 Desmoid. SGE image in a patient with Gardner's syndrome demonstrates a subcutaneous desmoid (*arrow*) in the right gluteal region. Fibrous tumors are low in signal intensity on T1-weighted images and are readily detected against a background of high-signal-intensity fat.

FIG. 10.50 Subcutaneous metastases. Delayed postgadolinium SGE image demonstrates multiple subcutaneous metastases from breast cancer.

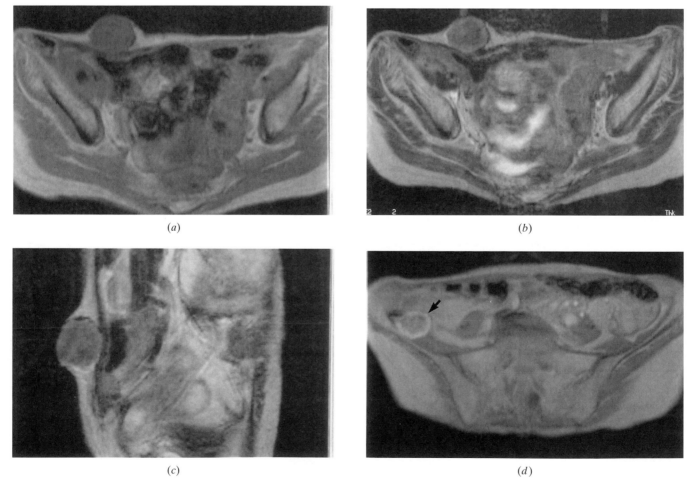

(a)

(b)

(c)

(d)

FIG. 10.51 Malignant fibrous histiocytoma of the right anterior abdominal wall. SGE (*a*), transverse (*b*) and sagittal (*c*) T2-weighted echo-train spin-echo, 90-second postgadolinium SGE images at superior (*d*) and inferior (*e*) tomographic levels, and gadolinium-enhanced T1-weighted fat-suppressed spin-echo (*f*) images. The tumor is readily identified as a low-signal-intensity well-defined mass against the high-signal-intensity background of subcutaneous fat on the T1-weighted image (*a*), and is heterogeneously low to intermediate in signal intensity on the T2-weighted images (*b,c*).

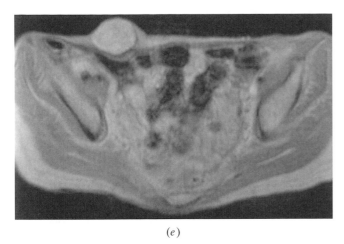

(e)

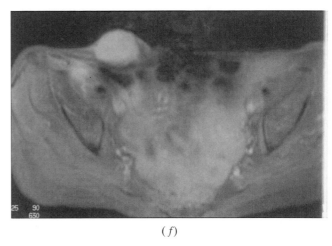

(f)

F IG . 10.51 (*Continued*) The tumor abuts and displaces the right rectus abdominis muscle, which is well-shown on the sagittal T2-weighted image (*c*). The tumor enhances in a mildly heterogeneous fashion on the 45-second postgadolinium SGE image (*e*). A metastatic tumor nodule (*arrow, d*) with predominantly peripheral heterogeneous enhancement is also present at a higher tomographic level (*d*) in the right iliacus muscle. Enhancement of the tumor is more uniform on the more delayed gadolinium-enhanced T1-weighted fat-suppressed spin-echo image (*f*), reflecting delayed enhancement of the fibrotic components of the tumor. The use of fat suppression increases the conspicuity of the abnormally enhancing tumor.

addition of fat suppression on postcontrast images. Involvement of the abdominal wall in cases of hemangiomas/lymphangiomas is not infrequent and may be part of a larger mass, usually of congenital origin. MRI demonstrates multiple ovoid and tubular structures infiltrating subcutaneous tissue and abdominal wall muscles (Fig. 10.56). The hemangiomatous component is comprised of smaller vascular spaces that may enhance after gadolinium administration, whereas the lymphangiomatous components, which are generally cystic, greater in size, and high in signal intensity on T1-weighted images, demonstrate dependent low-signal-intensity layers on T2-weighted images (see Fig. 10.56). MRI using multiplanar imaging demonstrates the extent of the abnormality and degree of infiltration of muscles and abdominal structures. Heavily T2-weighted echo-train spin-echo images have been used to scan patients with generalized lymphangiomatosis, because the fluid-filled cystic spaces are high in signal intensity on these images. Differentiation from hemangiomatous malformations or the hemangiomatous component of mixed malformations may also be possible with this technique because the vascular hemangiomatous spaces will be low in signal intensity on these images [103].

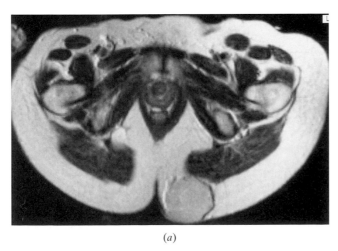

(a)

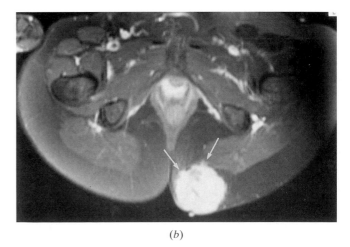

(b)

F IG . 10.52 Well-differentiated subcutaneous fibrosarcoma. T2-weighted spin-echo (*a*), and gadolinium-enhanced T1-weighted fat-suppressed spin-echo (*b*) images. The tumor is located in the subcutaneous tissue of the right buttock, is moderate in signal intensity on the T2-weighted image (*a*), and shows intense enhancement on the gadolinium-enhanced T1-weighted fat-suppressed image (*b*). The anterior margin of the mass appears irregular (*arrows, b*) and abuts the gluteus maximus muscle. Note the presence of chemical-shift artifact on the lateral edges of the mass on the T2-weighted image (*a*).

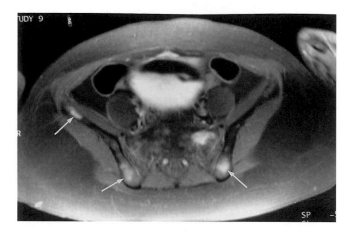

FIG. 10.53 Leukemic bone infiltrates. Gadolinium-enhanced T1-weighted fat-suppressed spin-echo image in a patient with leukemia shows focal enhancing leukemic lesions (*arrows*) in the bone marrow of the iliac bones bilaterally. Normal fat-containing marrow is low in signal intensity rendering enhancing tumors conspicuous.

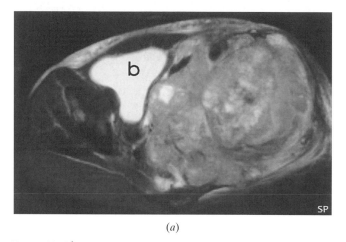

(*a*)

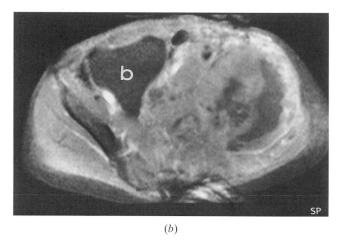

(*b*)

FIG. 10.54 Extensive Ewing's sarcoma of the pelvis. T2-weighted fat-suppressed echo-train spin-echo (*a*) and gadolinium-enhanced fat-suppressed SGE (*b*) images. An extensive heterogeneous mass originating from the left iliac bone is demonstrated. The mass invades all the muscles of the left pelvis and displaces the bladder (*"b"*,*a*,*b*) to the right. The tumor is heterogeneous with mixed high-signal-intensity areas on the T2-weighted image (*a*) and demonstrates heterogeneous enhancement after gadolinium administration (*b*).

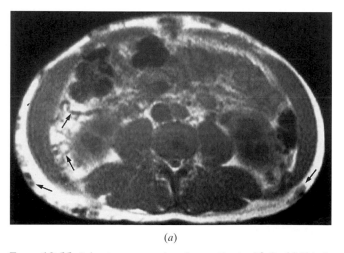

(*a*)

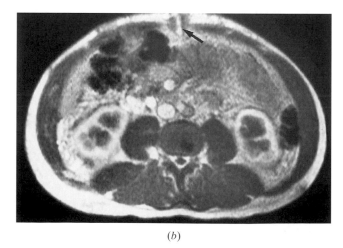

(*b*)

FIG. 10.55 Subcutaneous varices in a patient with Budd-Chiari syndrome and extensive varices. SGE (*a*) and immediate postgadolinium SGE (*b*) images. The precontrast image (*a*) demonstrates numerous signal-void serpiginous subcutaneous and perirenal collateral vessels (*small arrows, a*). The varices are not well-demonstrated on the immediate postgadolinium SGE image (*b*) because they become isointense with surrounding fat. A large recanalized umbilical vein, however, is demonstrated clearly (*arrow, b*) on the postcontrast image due to the presence of surrounding low-signal-intensity fibrous tissue.

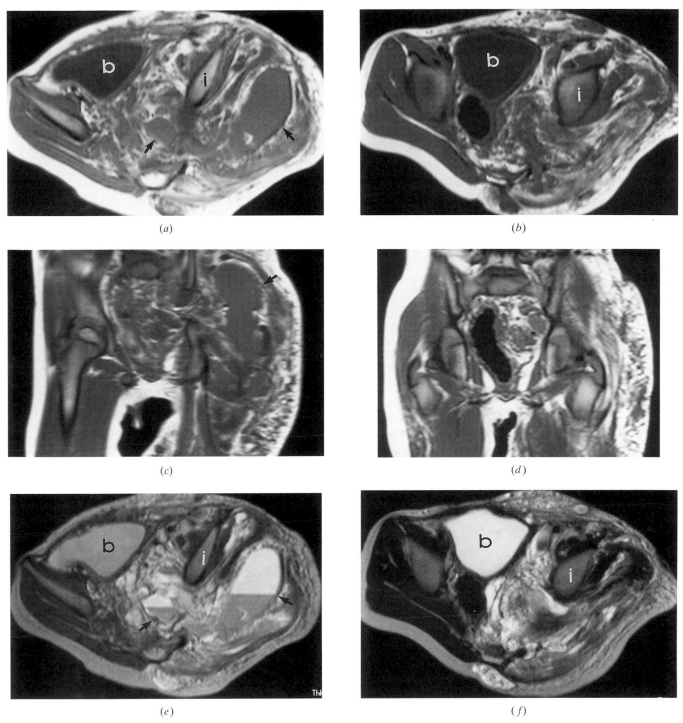

FIG. 10.56 Lymphangioma-hemangioma of the pelvis. Transverse (*a,b*) and coronal (*c,d*) T1-weighted spin-echo, and transverse (*e,f*) and sagittal (*g*) T2-weighted spin-echo images. An extensive heterogeneous mass is present in the left and central pelvis. The mass infiltrates the subcutaneous tissue of the entire left hemipelvis, the gluteus maximus, intermedius and minor muscles, and extends into the true pelvis causing extensive deformity and displacing the bladder ("*b*",*a,b,e–g*) and left iliac bone ("*i*",*a,b,e,f*) anteriorly to the right. The mass consists of numerous tubular and ovoid cystic structures, representing malformed blood and lymph vessels. The cystic spaces are low in signal intensity on the T1-weighted images and high in signal intensity on the T2-weighted images, reflecting their fluid content. Larger fluid-filled cystic spaces (*arrows, a,c,e*) have fluid-fluid levels on the T2-weighted image (*e*) with the dependent lower-signal-intensity level representing fluid of higher protein concentration. The presence of large fluid-filled cystic spaces is characteristic of lymphangiomatous rather than hemangiomatous malformations.

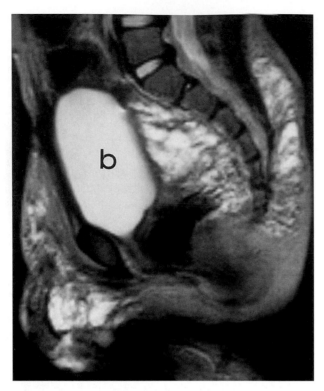

F I G. 10.56 (*Continued*) The coronal images (*c,d*) demonstrate the extent of the pelvic deformity and extension of the vascular malformation to the muscles and subcutaneous tissues of the left thigh, which are enlarged compared to the contralateral side.

Cellulitis can be differentiated from abscess on MR images by the demonstration of a signal-void center in an abscess. The extent of inflammatory or infectious disease is well-defined on gadolinium-enhanced fat-suppressed SGE images by the demonstration of high-signal-enhancing tissue.

CONCLUSION

MRI is effective at defining the full range of disease processes affecting the retroperitoneum and body wall. Recent advances in MRA, specifically development of the dynamic gadolinium enhanced gradient echo technique, have resulted in an increasing role for MRI in the evaluation of aorto-iliac disease.

REFERENCES

1. Molmenti EP, Balfe DM, Kanterman RY, Bennet HF: Anatomy of the retroperitoneum: Observations of the distribution of pathologic fluid collections. Radiology 200:95–103, 1996.
2. Lepor H, Walsh PC: Idiopathic retroperitoneal fibrosis. J Urol 122:1–6, 1979.
3. Arrive L, Hricak H, Tavares NJ, Miller TR: Malignant versus nonmalignant retroperitoneal fibrosis: Differentiation with MR imaging. Radiology 172:139–143, 1989.
4. Comings DE, Skubi KB, Van Eyes J, Motulsky AG: Familial multifocal fibrosclerosis. Findings suggesting that retroperitoneal fibrosis, mediastinal fibrosis, sclerosing cholangitis, Riedel's thyroiditis, and pseudotumor of the orbit may be different manifestations of a single disease. Ann Intern Med 66:884–892, 1967.
5. Van Hoe L, Oyen R, Gryspeerdt S, Baert AL, Bobbaers H, Baert L: Case report: Pseudotumoral pelvic retroperitoneal fibrosis associated with orbital fibrosis. Br J Radiol 68:421–423, 1995.
6. Dent RG, Godden DJ, Stovin PG, Stark JE: Pulmonary hyalinising granuloma in association with retroperitoneal fibrosis. Thorax 38:955–956, 1983.
7. Connolly J, Eisner D, Goldman S, Stutzman R, Steiner M: Benign retroperitoneal fibrosis and renal cell carcinoma. J Urol 149:1535–1537, 1993.
8. Rhee RY, Gloviczki P, Luthra HS, Stanson AW, Bower TC, Cherry KJ, Jr: Iliocaval complications of retroperitoneal fibrosis. Am J Surg 168:179–183, 1994.
9. Gatanaga H, Ohnishi S, Miura H, Kita H, Matsuhashi N, Kodama T, Minami M, Okudaira T, Imawari M, Yazaki YRC: Retroperitoneal fibrosis leading to extrahepatic portal vein obstruction. Intern Med 33:346–350, 1994.
10. Hricak H, Higgins CB, Williams RD: Nuclear magnetic resonance imaging in retroperitoneal fibrosis. AJR Am J Roentgenol 141:35–38, 1983.
11. Mulligan SA, Holley HC, Koehler RE, Koslin DB, Rubin E, Berland LL, Kenney PJ: CT and MR imaging in the evaluation of retroperitoneal fibrosis. J Comput Assist Tomogr 13:277–281, 1989.
12. Rubenstein WA, Gray G, Auh YH, Honig CL, Thorbjarnason B, Williams JJ, Haimes AB, Zirinsky K, Kazam E: CT of fibrous tissues and tumors with sonographic correlation. AJR Am J Roentgenol 147:1067–1074, 1986.
13. Cullenward MJ, Scanlan KA, Pozniak MA, Acher CA: Inflammatory aortic aneurysm (periaortic fibrosis): Radiologic imaging. Radiology 159:75–82, 1986.
14. Ross JS, Delamarter R, Hueftle MG, Masaryk TJ, Aikawa M, Carter J, VanDyke C, Modic MT: Gadolinium-DTPA-enhanced MR imaging of the postoperative lumbar spine: Time course and mechanism of enhancement. AJR Am J Roentgenol 152:825–834, 1989.
15. Lane RH, Stephens DH, Reiman HM: Primary retroperitoneal neoplasms: CT findings in 90 cases with clinical and pathologic correlation. AJR Am J Roentgenol 152:83–89, 1989.
16. Hartman DS, Hayes WS, Choyke PL, Tibbetts GP: From the archives of the AFIP. Leiomyosarcoma of the retroperitoneum and inferior vena cava: Radiologic-pathologic correlation. Radiographics 12:1203–1220, 1992.
17. Kim SH, Choi BI, Han MC, Kim YI: Retroperitoneal neurilemoma: CT and MR findings. AJR Am J Roentgenol 159:1023–1026, 1992.
18. Bass JC, Korobkin M, Francis IR, Ellis JH, Cohan RH: Retroperitoneal plexiform neurofibromas: CT findings. AJR Am J Roentgenol 163:617–620, 1994.
19. Ros PR, Eshaghi N: Plexiform neurofibroma of the pelvis: CT and MRI findings. Magn Reson Imaging 9:463–465, 1991.
20. Bequet D, Labauge P, Larroque P, Renard JL, Goasguen J: [Peripheral neurofibromatosis and involvement of lumbosacral nerves. Value of imaging]. Rev Neurol (Paris) 146:757–761, 1990.
21. Burk DL, Jr., Brunberg JA, Kanal E, Latchaw RE, Wolf GL: Spinal and paraspinal neurofibromatosis: Surface coil MR imaging at 1.5 T1. Radiology 162:797–801, 1987.
22. Pagliano G, Michel P, la Fay T, Duverger V: [Paraganglioma of the organ of Zuckerkandl]. Chirurgie 120:128–133, 1994.
23. Kessler A, Mitchell DG, Israel HL, Goldberg BB: Hepatic and splenic sarcoidosis: Ultrasound and MR imaging. Abdom Imaging 18:159–163, 1993.

24. Warshauer DM, Semelka RC, Ascher SM: Nodular sarcoidosis of the liver and spleen: Appearance on MR images. J Magn Reson Imaging 4:553–557, 1994.

25. Mitchinson MJ: Retroperitoneal fibrosis revisited. Arch Pathol Lab Med 110:784–786, 1986.

26. Johnson WK, Ros PR, Powers C, Stoupis C, Segel KH: Castleman disease mimicking an aggressive retroperitoneal neoplasm. Abdom Imaging 19:342–344, 1994.

27. Vlahos L, Trakadas S, Gouliamos A, Plataniotis G, Papavasiliou C: Retrocrural masses of extramedullary hemopoiesis in beta-thalassemia. Magn Reson Imaging 11:1227–1229, 1993.

28. Koep L, Zuidema GD: The clinical significance of retroperitoneal fibrosis. Surgery 81:250–257, 1977.

29. Blackledge G, Best JJ, Crowther D, Isherwood I: Computed tomography (CT) in the staging of patients with Hodgkin's Disease: A report on 136 patients. Clin Radiol 31:143–147, 1980.

30. Neumann CH, Robert NJ, Canellos G, Rosenthal D: Computed tomography of the abdomen and pelvis in non-Hodgkin lymphoma. J Comput Assist Tomogr 7:846–850, 1983.

31. Rahmouni A, Tempany C, Jones R, Mann R, Yang A, Zerhouni E: Lymphoma: Monitoring tumor size and signal intensity with MR imaging. Radiology 188:445–451, 1993.

32. Amparo EG, Hoddick WK, Hricak H, Sollitto R, Justich E, Filly RA, Higgins CB: Comparison of magnetic resonance imaging and ultrasonography in the evaluation of abdominal aortic aneurysms. Radiology 154:451–456, 1985.

33. Hanna SL, Fletcher BD, Boulden TF, Hudson MM, Greenwald CA, Kun LE: MR imaging of infradiaphragmatic lymphadenopathy in children and adolescents with Hodgkin disease: Comparison with lymphography and CT. J Magn Reson Imaging 3:461–470, 1993.

34. Lee JK, Heiken JP, Ling D, Glazer HS, Balfe DM, Levitt RG, Dixon WT, Murphy WA, Jr: Magnetic resonance imaging of abdominal and pelvic lymphadenopathy. Radiology 153:181–188, 1984.

35. Dooms GC, Hricak H, Crooks LE, Higgins CB: Magnetic resonance imaging of the lymph nodes: Comparison with CT. Radiology 153:719–728, 1984.

36. Glazer HS, Lee JK, Levitt RG, Heiken JP, Ling D, Totty WG, Balfe DM, Emani B, Wasserman TH, Murphy WA: Radiation fibrosis: Differentiation from recurrent tumor by MR imaging. Radiology 156:721–726, 1985.

37. Hricak H, Demas BE, Williams RD, McNamara MT, Hedgcock MW, Amparo EG, Tanagho EA: Magnetic resonance imaging in the diagnosis and staging of renal and perirenal neoplasms. Radiology 154:709–715, 1985.

38. Fein AB, Lee JK, Balfe DM, Heiken JP, Ling D, Glazer HS, McClennan BL: Diagnosis and staging of renal cell carcinoma: A comparison of MR imaging and CT. AJR Am J Roentgenol 148:749–753, 1987.

39. Guimaraes R, Clement O, Bittoun J, Carnot F, Frija G: MR lymphography with superparamagnetic iron nanoparticles in rats: Pathologic basis for contrast enhancement. AJR Am J Roentgenol 162:201–207, 1994.

40. Anzai Y, Blackwell KE, Hirschowitz SL, Rogers JW, Sato Y, Yuh WT, Runge VM, Morris MR, McLachlan SJ, Lufkin RB: Initial clinical experience with dextran-coated superparamagnetic iron oxide for detection of lymph node metastases in patients with head and neck cancer [see comments]. Radiology 192:709–715, 1994.

41. Williams WM, Kosovsky PA, Rafal RB, Markisz JA: Retroperitoneal germ cell neoplasm: MR and CT. Magn Reson Imaging 10:325–331, 1992.

42. Ellis JH, Bies JR, Kopecky KK, Klatte EC, Rowland RG, Donohue JP: Comparison of NMR and CT imaging in the evaluation of metastatic retroperitoneal lymphadenopathy from testicular carcinoma. J Comput Assist Tomogr 8:709–719, 1984.

43. Cohan RH, Baker ME, Cooper C, Moore JO, Saeed M, Dunnick NR: Computed tomography of primary retroperitoneal malignancies. J Comput Assist Tomogr 12:804–810, 1988.

44. Bretan PN, Jr., Williams RD, Hricak H: Preoperative assessment of retroperitoneal pathology by magnetic resonance imaging. Primary leiomyosarcoma of inferior vena cava. Urology 28:251–255, 1986.

45. Feinstein RS, Gatewood OM, Fishman EK, Goldman SM, Siegelman SS: Computed tomography of adult neuroblastoma. J Comput Assist Tomogr 8:720–726, 1984.

46. Swan JS, Grist TM, Weber DM, Sproat IA, Wojtowycz MM: MR angiography of the pelvis with variable velocity encoding and a phased-array coil. Radiology 190:363–369, 1994.

47. Arlart IP, Guhl L, Edelman RR: Magnetic resonance angiography of the abdominal aorta. Cardiovasc Intervent Radiol 15:43–50, 1992.

48. Sallevelt PE, Barentsz JO, Ruijs SJ, Heijstraten FM, Buskens FG, Strijk SP: Role of MR imaging in the preoperative evaluation of atherosclerotic abdominal aortic aneurysms. Radiographics 14:87–98; 1994.

49. Kim D, Edelman RR, Kent KC, Porter DH, Skillman JJ: Abdominal aorta and renal artery stenosis: Evaluation with MR angiography. Radiology 174:727–731, 1990.

50. Mulligan SA, Doyle M, Matsuda T, Koslin DB, Kenney PJ, Barton RE, Pohost GM: Aortoiliac disease: Two-dimensional inflow MR angiography with lipid suppression. J Magn Reson Imaging 3:829–834, 1993.

51. Ecklund K, Hartnell GG, Hughes LA, Stokes KR, Finn JP: MR angiography as the sole method in evaluating abdominal aortic aneurysms: Correlation with conventional techniques and surgery [see comments]. Radiology 192:345–350, 1994.

52. Durham JR, Hackworth CA, Tober JC, Bova JG, Bennett WF, Schmalbrock P, Van Aman ME, Horowitz JD, Wright JG, Smead WL: Magnetic resonance angiography in the preoperative evaluation of abdominal aortic aneurysms. Am J Surg 166:173–177, 1993.

53. Kaufman JA, Geller SC, Petersen MJ, Cambria RP, Prince MR, Waltman AC: MR imaging (including MR angiography) of abdominal aortic aneurysms: Comparison with conventional angiography. AJR Am J Roentgenol 163:203–210, 1994.

54. Prince MR, Narasimham DL, Jacoby WT, Williams DM, Cho KJ, Marx MV, Deeb GM: Three-dimensional gadolinium enhanced MR angiography of the thoracic aorta. AJR Am J Roentgenol 166:1387–1397, 1996.

55. Douek PC, Revel D, Chazel S, Falise B, Villard J, Amiel M: Fast MR angiography of the aortoiliac arteries and arteries of the lower extremity: Value of bolus-enhanced, whole-volume subtraction technique. AJR Am J Roentgenol 165:431–437, 1995.

56. Prince MR, Yucel EK, Kaufman JA, Harrison DC, Geller SC: Dynamic gadolinium-enhanced three-dimensional abdominal MR arteriography. J Magn Reson Imaging 3:877–881, 1993.

57. Snidow JJ, Aisen AM, Harris VJ, Trerotola SO, Johnson MS, Sawchuk AP, Dalsing MC: Iliac artery MR angiography: Comparison of three-dimensional gadolinium-enhanced and two-dimensional time-of-flight techniques. Radiology 196:371–378, 1995.

58. Sivananthan UM, Ridgway JP, Bann K, Verma SP, Cullingworth J, Ward J, Rees MR: Fast magnetic resonance angiography using turbo-FLASH sequences in advanced aortoiliac disease. Br J Radiol 66:1103–1110, 1993.

59. Prince MR: Gadolinium-enhanced MR aortography. Radiology 191:155–164, 1994.

60. Leung DA, McKinnon GC, Davis CP, Pfammatter T, Krestin GP, Debatin JF: Breath-hold, contrast-enhanced, three-dimensional MR angiography. Radiology 200:562–571, 1996.

61. Sinha S, Atkinson D, Mather R, Lucas-Quesada A: Improved depiction of vascular lumen: Fast black blood imaging of the carotids with HASTE. Proceedings of the ISMRM fourth scientific meeting and exhibition 2:1265, 1996.

62. Auffermann W, Olofsson P, Stoney R, Higgins CB: MR imaging of complications of aortic surgery. J Comput Assist Tomogr 11:982–989, 1987.

63. Bickerstaff LK, Hollier LH, Van Peenen HJ, Melton LJd, Pairolero PC, Cherry KJ: Abdominal aortic aneurysms: The changing natural history. J Vasc Surg 1:6–12, 1984.

64. Szilagyi DE, Elliott JP, Smith RF: Clinical fate of the patient with asymptomatic abdominal aortic aneurysm and unfit for surgical treatment. Arch Surg 104:600–606, 1972.

65. Dinsmore RE, Wedeen VJ, Miller SW, Rosen BR, Fifer M, Vlahakes GJ, Edelman RR, Brady TJ: MRI of dissection of the aorta: Recognition of the intimal tear and differential flow velocities. AJR Am J Roentgenol 146:1286–1288, 1986.

66. Herfkens RJ, Higgins CB, Hricak H, Lipton MJ, Crooks LE, Sheldon PE, Kaufman L: Nuclear magnetic resonance imaging of atherosclerotic disease. Radiology 148:161–166, 1983.

67. Lee JK, Ling D, Heiken JP, Glazer HS, Sicard GA, Totty WG, Levitt RG, Murphy WA: Magnetic resonance imaging of abdominal aortic aneurysms. AJR Am J Roentgenol 143:1197–1202, 1984.

68. Flak B, Li DK, Ho BY, Knickerbocker WJ, Fache S, Mayo J, Chung W: Magnetic resonance imaging of aneurysms of the abdominal aorta. AJR Am J Roentgenol 144:991–996, 1985.

69. Evancho AM, Osbakken M, Weidner W: Comparison of NMR imaging and aortography for preoperative evaluation of abdominal aortic aneurysm. Magn Reson Med 2:41–55, 1985.

70. LaRoy LL, Cormier PJ, Matalon TA, Patel SK, Turner DA, Silver B: Imaging of abdominal aortic aneurysms. AJR Am J Roentgenol 152:785–792, 1989.

71. Lindell OI, Sariola HV, Lehtonen TA: The occurrence of vasculitis in perianeurysmal fibrosis. J Urol 138:727–729, 1987.

72. Amparo EG, Higgins CB, Hricak H, Sollitto R: Aortic dissection: Magnetic resonance imaging. Radiology 155:399–406, 1985.

73. Geisinger MA, Risius B, JA OD, Zelch MG, Moodie DS, Graor RA, George CR: Thoracic aortic dissections: Magnetic resonance imaging. Radiology 155:407–412, 1985.

74. Williams DM, Joshi A, Dake MD, Deeb GM, Miller DC, Abrams GD: Aortic cobwebs: An anatomic marker identifying the false lumen in aortic dissection—imaging and pathologic correlation [see comments]. Radiology 190:167–174, 1994.

75. Yamada T, Tada S, Harada J: Aortic dissection without intimal rupture: Diagnosis with MR imaging and CT. Radiology 168:347–352, 1988.

76. Wolff KA, Herold CJ, Tempany CM, Parravano JG, Zerhouni EA: Aortic dissection: Atypical patterns seen at MR imaging. Radiology 181:489–495, 1991.

77. Welch TJ, Stanson AW, Sheedy PFd, Johnson CM, McKusick MA: Radiologic evaluation of penetrating aortic atherosclerotic ulcer. Radiographics 10:675–685, 1990.

78. Yucel EK, Steinberg FL, Egglin TK, Geller SC, Waltman AC, Athanasoulis CA: Penetrating aortic ulcers: Diagnosis with MR imaging. Radiology 177:779–781, 1990.

79. Justich E, Amparo EG, Hricak H, Higgins CB: Infected aortoiliofemoral grafts: Magnetic resonance imaging. Radiology 154:133–136, 1985.

80. Auffermann W, Olofsson PA, Rabahie GN, Tavares NJ, Stoney RJ, Higgins CB: Incorporation versus infection of retroperitoneal aortic grafts: MR imaging features. Radiology 172:359–362, 1989.

81. Hricak H, Amparo E, Fisher MR, Crooks L, Higgins CB: Abdominal venous system: Assessment using MR. Radiology 156:415–422, 1985.

82. Colletti PM, Oide CT, Terk MR, Boswell WD, Jr: Magnetic resonance of the inferior vena cava. Magn Reson Imaging 10:177–185, 1992.

83. Cory DA, Ellis JH, Bies JR, Olson EW: Retroaortic left renal vein demonstrated by nuclear magnetic resonance imaging. J Comput Assist Tomogr 8:339–340, 1984.

84. Schultz CL, Morrison S, Bryan PJ: Azygos continuation of the inferior vena cava: Demonstration by NMR imaging. J Comput Assist Tomogr 8:774–776, 1984.

85. Fisher MR, Hricak H, Higgins CB: Magnetic resonance imaging of developmental venous anomalies. AJR Am J Roentgenol 145:705–709, 1985.

86. Semelka RC, Shoenut JP, Kroeker MA: The retroperitoneum and the abdominal wall. In Semelka RC, Shoenut JP (eds.). MRI of the Abdomen with CT Correlation. New York: Raven Press, pp. 13–41, 1993.

87. Silverman SG, Hillstrom MM, Doyle CJ, Tempany CM, Sica GT: Thrombophlebitic retroperitoneal collateral veins mimicking lymphadenopathy: MR and CT appearance. Abdom Imaging 20:474–476, 1995.

88. Erdman WA, Weinreb JC, Cohen JM, Buja LM, Chaney C, Peshock RM: Venous thrombosis: Clinical and experimental MR imaging. Radiology 161:233–238, 1986.

89. Higgins CB, Goldberg H, Hricak H, Crooks LE, Kaufman L, Brasch R: Nuclear magnetic resonance imaging of vasculature of abdominal viscera: Normal and pathologic features. AJR Am J Roentgenol 140:1217–1225, 1983.

90. Semelka RC, Shoenut JP, Magro CM, Kroeker MA, MacMahon R, Greenberg HM: Renal cancer staging: Comparison of contrast-enhanced CT and gadolinium-enhanced fat-suppressed spin-echo and gradient-echo MR imaging. J Magn Reson Imaging 3:597–602, 1993.

91. Roubidoux MA, Dunnick NR, Sostman HD, Leder RA: Renal carcinoma: Detection of venous extension with gradient-echo MR imaging. Radiology 182:269–272, 1992.

92. Wendel RG, Crawford ED, Hehman KN: The "nutcracker" phenomenon: An unusual cause for renal varicosities with hematuria. J Urol 123:761–763, 1980.

93. Cyran KM, Kenney PJ: Leiomyosarcoma of abdominal veins: Value of MRI with gadolinium DTPA. Abdom Imaging 19:335–338, 1994.

94. Kelekis NL, Semelka RC, Hill ML, Meyers DC, Molina PL: Malignant fibrous histiocytoma of the inferior vena cava: Appearances on contrast-enhanced spiral CT and MRI. Abdom Imaging 21:461–463, 1996.

95. Lipton M, Sprayregen S, Kutcher R, Frost A: Venous invasion in renal vein leiomyosarcoma: Case report and review of the literature. Abdom Imaging 20:64–67, 1995.

96. Lee JK, Glazer HS: Psoas muscle disorders: MR imaging. Radiology 160:683–687, 1986.

97. Weinreb JC, Cohen JM, Maravilla KR: Iliopsoas muscles: MR study of normal anatomy and disease. Radiology 156:435–440, 1985.

98. Hahn PF, Saini S, Stark DD, Papanicolaou N, Ferrucci JT, Jr: Intraabdominal hematoma: The concentric-ring sign in MR imaging. AJR Am J Roentgenol 148:115–119, 1987.

99. Rubin JI, Gomori JM, Grossman RI, Gefter WB, Kressel HY: High-field MR imaging of extracranial hematomas. AJR Am J Roentgenol 148:813–817, 1987.

100. Unger EC, Glazer HS, Lee JK, Ling D: MRI of extracranial hematomas: Preliminary observations. AJR Am J Roentgenol 146:403–407, 1986.

101. Brasfield RD, Das Gupta TK: Desmoid tumors of the anterior abdominal wall. Surgery 65:241–246, 1969.

102. Ichikawa T, Koyama A, Fujimoto H, Honma M, Saiga T, Matsubara N, Ozeki Y, Uchiyama G, Ohtomo K: Abdominal wall desmoid mimicking intra-abdominal mass: MR features. Magn Reson Imaging 12:541–544, 1994.

103. Stover B, Laubenberger J, Hennig J, Niemeyer C, Ruckauer K, Brandis M, Langer M: Value of RARE-MRI sequences in the diagnosis of lymphangiomatosis in children. Magn Reson Imaging 13:481–488, 1995.

BLADDER

E. D. BROWN, M.D. AND R. C. SEMELKA, M.D.

NORMAL ANATOMY

The bladder consists of three layers: an outer adventitial layer of connective tissue, a nonstriated muscle layer (the detrusor muscle), and an inner layer of mucous membrane. The ureteric orifices are placed at the angles of the trigone and are usually slit-like. The internal urethral orifice is at the apex of the trigone, the lowest part of the bladder.

On MR images, the thickness of the normal bladder wall ranges from 2.9 to 8.8 mm, with a mean of 5.4 mm. The normal wall appears as an intermediate-signal-intensity band on T1-weighted images. On T2-weighted images, the bladder wall has previously been reported as a low-signal-intensity band, which represents the entire muscular layer. More recently, this band has been divided into two bands of low signal intensity (inner) and intermediate signal intensity (outer) corresponding to the compact inner and looser outer smooth muscle layers [1].

MRI TECHNIQUES

A variety of MRI techniques have been employed to study the bladder. Techniques that are particularly useful include T2-weighted spin-echo or echo-train spin-echo, pre- and postintravenous gadolinium, T1-weighted fat-suppressed spin-echo, and dynamic immediate postgadolinium gradient-echo sequences. T1-weighted images are effective at demonstrating morphology, but are not as effective as the aforementioned techniques at demonstrating depth of tumor invasion. As in other organ systems, it is useful to combine imaging techniques that demonstrate different tissue contrasts. In the bladder it is useful to combine sequences that demonstrate high-signal-intensity urine (i.e., T2-weighted imaging and delayed postgadolinium imaging) with techniques which demonstrate low-signal-intensity urine (i.e., T1-weighted spin-echo imaging with or without fat suppression and immediate postgadolinium dynamic gradient-echo imaging). The acquisition of sequences that show different contrast between urine and bladder wall is important to effectively evaluate abnormalities in the bladder wall and lumen. Another important feature of MRI is the multiplanar imaging capability that permits image acquisition in different planes to minimize partial volume effects when evaluating depth of penetration of bladder cancer (i.e., sagittal imaging for anterior and posterior wall and dome lesions, and coronal imaging for lateral wall and dome lesions).

The critical artifacts in MRI of the bladder include motion, degree of bladder distention, and chemical shift. Involuntary motion artifacts include motion from respiration, intestinal peristalsis, and bladder motion. Respiratory movements can be reduced by the use of a tight abdominal band. Moderate bladder distention is important. If the bladder is not distended, the detrusor muscle is thickened, mimicking thickening from disease states and making it difficult to recognize small tumors. If the bladder is too distended, the patient becomes uncomfortable, and flat tumors can be missed secondary to overstretching of the muscle layer. Chemical-shift artifact occurs at the water-fat interface and appears as a dark band along the lateral wall on one side and a bright band along the lateral wall on the opposite side [2]. This appearance can mimic or mask an invasive bladder cancer. To correct for this, chemically selective fat suppression can be performed, or the frequency-encoding gradient can be rotated to select the direction that least interferes with examination of bladder wall adjacent to tumor [2].

The use of surface coils can significantly improve the image quality of the pelvic structures. Double surface coils have been shown to improve pelvic MR imaging [3–5]. Even greater image improvements occur with the use of a phased-array multicoil.

Currently, T1-weighted images performed as breath-hold spoiled gradient-echo (SGE) sequences have shown good spatial and temporal resolution. Recent implementation of breath-hold T2-weighted echo-train spin-echo sequences have been effective in examining the pelvis. One version of this, the half Fourier single-shot turbo spin-echo (HASTE) technique has the additional advantage of being breathing independent.

DISEASE ENTITIES

FOCAL DISEASE

Benign Masses

Leiomyoma

Leiomyoma is the most common of the rare benign bladder tumors, affecting women 30 to 55 years of age. The lesion most commonly arises at the trigone, but may be found on the lateral and posterior walls. Lesions may be intravesicular (60%), extravesicular (30%), or intramural (10%). Intramural and extravesicular tumors do not cause symptoms, but intravesicle lesions may present with hematuria or dysuria. Bladder neck tumors causing bladder outlet obstruction have been reported. Intravenous urography usually shows a fixed filling defect. Ultrasound and CT imaging are accurate in detection but not in the characterization of these lesions.

The lesion is intermediate in signal intensity on T1-weighted images and well-shown against a background of low-signal-intensity urine. On T2-weighted images, the high-signal-intensity of the lesion contrasts well with intermediate low-signal-intensity muscle in the bladder wall, and intramural extent can be assessed. Degenerating leiomyomas can have various appearances, including medium to high signal intensity on T1-weighted images, and heterogeneous mixed signal intensity on T2-weighted images. These appearances are thought to be

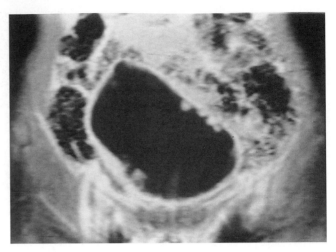

FIG. 11.1 Multiple papillary tumors. Coronal gadolinium-enhanced T1-weighted fat-suppressed spin-echo image. The enhancing papillomas are well-demonstrated in contrast to the low signal intensity of non-gadolinium containing urine.

secondary to hemorrhage, calcification, or cystic transformation [6].

Papilloma

Transitional-cell papilloma accounts for 2 to 3 percent of all primary bladder tumors and is histologically benign but may recur or become malignant. The lesion is an epithelial tumor without nuclear abnormalities covered with urothelium-like cell layers less than seven cells thick [7].

Bladder papillomas are most clearly shown on immediate postgadolinium MR images as small enhancing masses arising from lesser enhancing wall. Dynamic postgadolinium enhanced MR images (15 to 45 seconds) may be most useful to demonstrate the superficial nature of these lesions (Fig. 11.1).

Calcifications

Bladder calculi may be the result of foreign body nidus, stasis, or migration of upper tract calculi, or they may be idiopathic. Foreign bodies include catheters, nonabsorbable sutures, hair, or bone fragments. Stasis may result from bladder outlet obstruction, diverticula, cystocele, or postoperative states. Bladder calculi are well-shown on T2-weighted images or late postgadolinium T1-weighted images. These sequences show good contrast between high-signal-intensity urine and signal-void calculi (Fig. 11.2) [8].

Bilharziosis is caused by the organism *Schistosoma haematobium* in the majority of cases. Patients present with frequency, urgency, dysuria, flank pain, and hematuria. The characteristic calcifications are linear and continuous along the bladder wall. These bladder wall calcifications are signal-void on all MRI sequences [9].

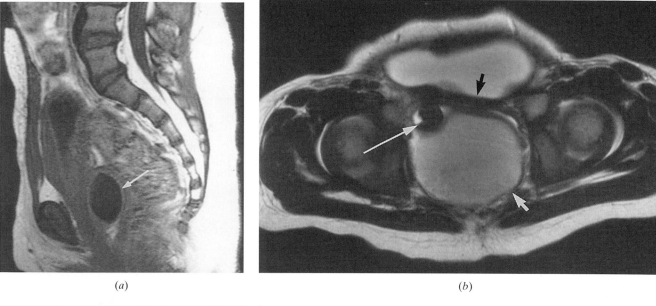

(a)

(b)

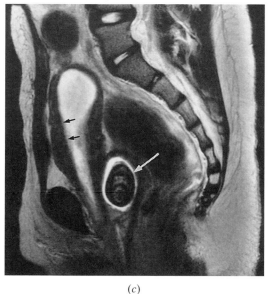

(c)

Fig. 11.2 Bladder calculus in a patient with a surgically repaired persistent cloaca. Sagittal T1-weighted spin-echo (*a*), T2-weighted fat-suppressed echo-train spin-echo (*b*), and sagittal 512 resolution T2-weighted echo-train spin-echo (*c*) images. A nearly signal-void oval structure (*long white arrows, a–c*) on the T1- and T2-weighted images represents a calculus in a bladder diverticulum. The bladder wall is thickened (*black arrows, b,c*), and the reconstructed rectum is dilated (*short white arrow, b*).

Neurofibromatosis

Neurofibromatosis, the most common phakomatosis, is characterized by cafe-au-lait spots, optic gliomas, Lisch nodules, distinctive bone lesions, and neurofibromas. Genitourinary tract neurofibromas are rare. Obstructive hydronephrosis, a common complication, is presumably due to neurofibromas involving the trigone. Pelvic side-wall tumors appear nodular and may extend into the obturator foramina.

Neurofibromas demonstrate distinct MRI features that allow better characterization of the extent of the tumor within the bladder, pelvic sidewalls, and surrounding soft tissues than does CT imaging. The MRI appearance for Type 1 neurofibromatosis (von Recklinghausen disease) is a T1-weighted signal intensity slightly greater than that of skeletal muscle and a markedly increased signal intensity relative to the surrounding tissues on the T2-weighted images. Most demonstrate enhancement with gadolinium administration [10].

Ganglioneuromas have a similar appearance; they are isointense on T1-weighted images, hyperintense on T2-weighted images, and enhance substantially with gadolinium (Fig. 11.3).

Granulomatous Disease

In the setting of genitourinary tuberculosis, bladder involvement is common. Patients present with dysuria and frequency. The earliest manifestations are mucosal edema and ulcerations, primarily surrounding the ureteral orifices, which can produce obstruction. Tuberculo-

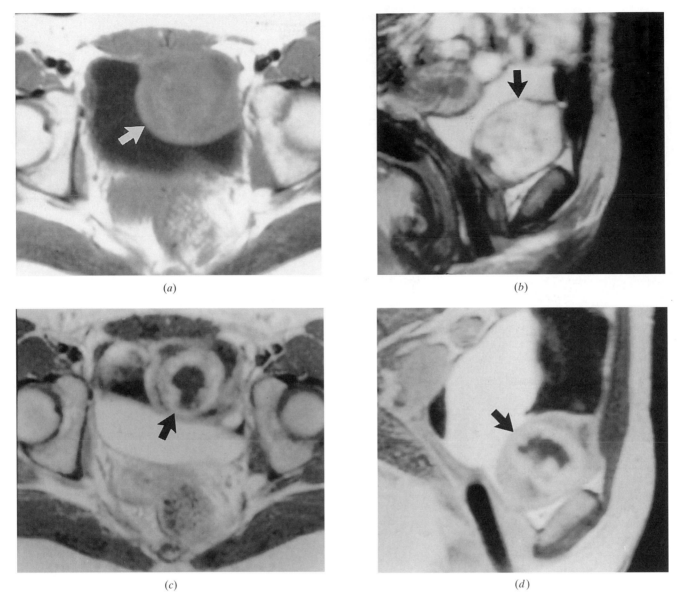

(a)

(b)

(c)

(d)

FIG. 11.3 Ganglioneuroma. T1-weighted spin-echo (*a*), sagittal T2-weighted spin-echo (*b*), transverse (*c*) and sagittal (*d*) gadolinium-enhanced T1-weighted spin-echo images. A 4-cm ganglioneuroma arises from the anteroinferior bladder wall. The tumor is intermediate in signal intensity on the T1-weighted image (*arrow, a*), moderately hyperintense on the T2-weighted image (*arrow, b*), and showing substantial enhancement on interstitial-phase gadolinium-enhanced images (*arrow, c,d*) with central necrosis. (Courtesy of Hedvig Hricak, M.D., Ph.D.).

mas in the bladder wall can be large and simulate mass lesions [11]. Focal granulomatous reactions appear as intravesical lesions with high signal intensity on T2-weighted images [8]. Epithelioid granulomatous lesions, which can occur in patients undergoing immunotherapy for the treatment of malignant bladder lesions, may appear similar to malignant tumors on MRI. Although MRI accurately shows these lesions to be confined to the vesical wall, their presence can lead to false-positive findings [8].

Pheochromocytoma

Pheochromocytomas can occur anywhere along the sympathetic nervous system from the neck to the sacrum. Ten to 15 percent occur in an extraadrenal location. One percent are located in the bladder and have a predilection for the trigone. Episodes of paroxysmal hypertension may be associated with micturition. Seven percent of bladder pheochromocytomas are malignant [7].

Bladder pheochromocytoma occurs most commonly in the trigone or near the ureteral orifices. It is found

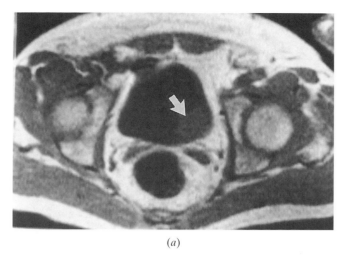

(a)

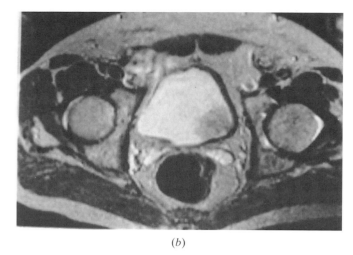

(b)

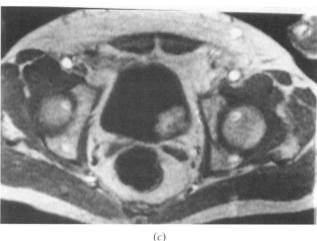

(c)

Fig. 11.4 Transitional-cell cancer, superficial invasion. A superficial T1 transitional-cell cancer is identified on SGE (a), T2 echo-train spin-echo (b), and immediate postgadolinium SGE (c) images. The tumor is intermediate in signal intensity on the T1-weighted image (arrow, a) and moderately high in signal intensity on the T2-weighted image (b). Tumor enhancement is appreciated on the postgadolinium image (c), and lack of wall invasion is shown. Intact low-signal-intensity muscular wall deep to the tumor is appreciated on the T2-weighted (b) and immediate postgadolinium SGE (c) images.

less frequently in the dome and lateral walls of the bladder. Characteristic MRI features help to distinguish this tumor from other tumors, including carcinoma [12–13]. Typically, these tumors show markedly increased, homogeneous signal intensity on T2-weighted spin-echo sequences.[14–16] T1-weighted images demonstrate hypointense or isointense signal intensity [6].

Pelvic Lipomatosis

Pelvic lipomatosis predominantly affects black males between the ages of 25 and 55 years. Some patients present with frequency, dysuria, perineal pain, or suprapubic discomfort. Although the process is benign, the effects may be damaging, including renal failure and rectal compression [17].

The diagnosis of pelvic lipomatosis can be supported with the use of MRI. It characteristically appears as an extensive amount of fat, which appears high in signal intensity on T1-weighted images surrounding the bladder [18].

Malignant Masses

Primary Epithelial Neoplasm

Classification of bladder tumors is based on three criteria: cell type (urothelial, squamous, or glandular), pattern of growth (papillary, nonpapillary, noninfiltrating, or infiltrating), and grading (degree of cellular differentiation). The nonpapillary urothelial tumors include invasive transitional-cell carcinoma, squamous-cell carcinoma, adenocarcinoma, and spindle-cell carcinoma.

Transitional-cell carcinoma is the most common primary bladder malignancy and accounts for 85 percent of all bladder malignancies. Nonpapillary or sessile urothelial tumors are typically more invasive and higher grade than exophytic types. Most patients history of papillary tumors, which abnormalities adjacent to papillar sion of the lymphatics and inf are common finding prognosis [7].

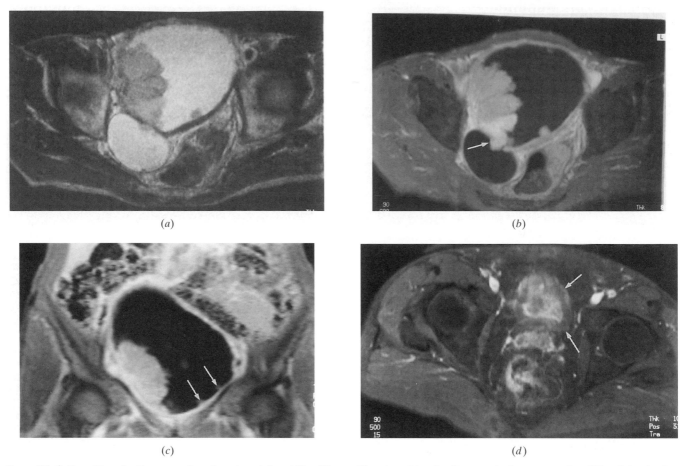

(a) (b)

(c) (d)

FIG. 11.5 Transitional-cell cancer, deep invasion. A frond-like, T3a papillary transitional-cell cancer is demonstrated on T2-weighted echo-train spin-echo (a), gadolinium-enhanced T1-weighted fat-suppressed spin-echo (b), and coronal interstitial-phase gadolinium-enhanced SGE (c) images. A large tumor arises from the right lateral wall of the bladder. Note that the lesion extends into a diverticulum (arrow, b). On the T2-weighted echo-train spin-echo image, the low-signal-intensity muscular wall is not infiltrated by tumor. Multiple small papillomas are also identified (arrows, c). Diffuse relative symmetric thickening of the bladder wall from transitional-cell cancer (arrows, d) is demonstrated on postgadolinium T1-weighted fat-suppressed (d) image in a second patient. Heterogeneous moderate enhancement is present.

The staging of bladder neoplasms is as follows:

T0   No evidence of primary tumor.
Ta   Noninvasive papillary carcinoma.
Tis   Carcinoma in situ: "flat tumor."
T1   Tumor invades subepithelial connective tissue.
T2   Tumor invades superficial muscle.
T3   Tumor invades deep muscle or perivesical fat.
T3a   Tumor invades deep muscle (outer half).
T3b   Tumor invades perivesical fat.
T4   Tumor invades any of the following: prostate, uterus, vagina, pelvic wall, or abdominal wall.
T4a   Tumor invades the prostate, uterus, or vagina.
T4b   Tumor invades the pelvic or abdominal wall [19].

Both T1 and T2-weighted images are useful in staging bladder cancers [20–27]. The use of T1-weighted se-

quences is recommended to determine invasion of the perivesical fat and surrounding organs (except the prostate) and involvement of lymph nodes and bone marrow. T2-weighted images are recommended for assessment of the extent of tumor invasion into the muscle layer of the bladder wall and prostate [2,20–24,27,28].

The use of intravenous gadolinium contrast agents has improved the imaging of bladder carcinomas. Gadolinium quickly distributes in the extracellular space without passing through intact cell membranes [28] and typically provides substantial enhancement of urinary bladder carcinomas [29–37]. Bladder carcinomas tend to enhance more than the surrounding bladder wall early after injection of contrast. Tumors are well-seen approximately 5 to 15 seconds after arterial enhancement [36]. This early phase of enhancement also demonstrates good conspicuity of bladder tumor against gadolinium-free urine in the bladder. Delayed postcontrast T1-weighted

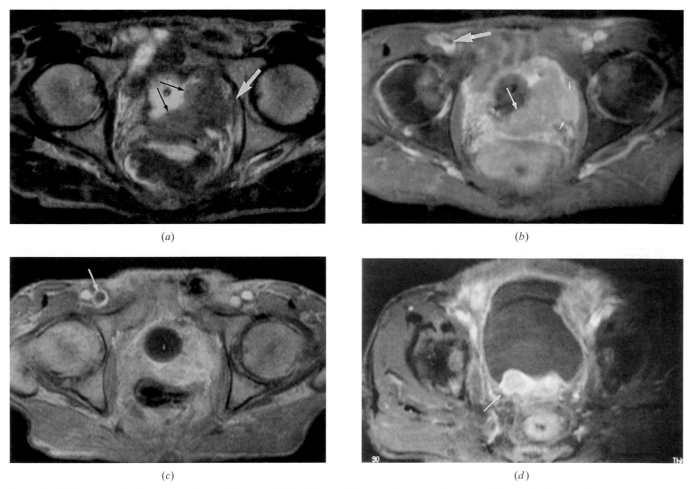

FIG. 11.6 Transitional-cell cancer, advanced disease. T4bN1M0 transitional-cell cancer shown on T2-weighted spin-echo (*a*), postgadolinium T1-weighted fat-suppressed spin-echo (*b*), and postgadolinium SGE (*c*) images. A large cancer arises from the left and posterior aspect of the bladder (*black arrows, a*). Invasion of the obturator internus muscle is shown (*large arrow, a*). The tumor enhances heterogeneously after gadolinium administration (*large white arrow, b*). Tumor extension into the obturator internus (*small arrows, b*) is relatively high in signal intensity compared to muscle. Thrombus in the right common iliac vein is identified (*large arrow, b* and *arrow, c*). A Foley catheter is present in the bladder (*large arrow, c*). Deeply invasive transitional-cell cancer on gadolinium-enhanced T1-weighted fat-suppressed (*d*) image in a second patient. The tumor invades the posterior wall of the bladder. Deep invasion is evidenced by irregular enhancing tissue (*arrow, d*).

images show high signal intensity of urine, and the intraluminal portion of a bladder tumor is usually well-delineated, although small tumors may be obscured.

MRI may be able to differentiate between superficial (Stage T1) (Fig. 11.4) and deep invasion of the muscle layer of the bladder wall (Stage T3a) (Fig. 11.5). Immediate postgadolinium SGE images acquired in an oblique projection to demonstrate tumor-bladder wall interface in profile may be the most effective approach. This distinction is not possible with clinical staging, CT imaging, or intravesical sonography.

Accuracy of MRI in the staging of bladder carcinoma has been reported to range from 69 to 89 percent. Staging of small tumors, particularly, is improved with the use of immediate postgadolinium imaging [30,33,34,36,37]. MRI offers several advantages over CT imaging, including

higher contrast resolution and multiplanar imaging, which permits better imaging of the bladder dome, trigone, perivesical fat, prostate, and seminal vesicles. The higher contrast resolution is most useful in the differentiation between muscular invasion (Stage T3a) and invasion into the perivesical fat (Stage T3b) [20–24,26,31]. Bladder tumors at the base or dome are better staged with MRI. For deeply infiltrative tumors (stages T3b, T4a, and T4b), MRI is generally considered to be the most accurate method of staging (Fig. 11.6). The most common cause of staging error in MRI and CT imaging studies is overstaging, and prior cystoscopic biopsy is likely a common cause of this overstaging [38]. For this reason, it is recommended that MRI studies be performed at least 3 weeks after bladder biopsy.

Acquisition of MR images in oblique planes to demonstrate the tumor-bladder wall interface in profile has been effective for assessing depth of bladder wall invasion, with overall staging accuracy of 78 percent for gadolinium-enhanced T1-weighted images and 60 percent for T2-weighted images. Improved staging accuracy with oblique imaging was noted after gadolinium administration, especially in the differentiation of superficial tumors and tumors with superficial muscle invasion [31].

MRI is useful in the distinction between late fibrosis and recurrence of carcinoma. One year after transurethral resection, following resolution of the acute edema, residual scar can be distinguished from recurrence of tumor using T2-weighted images [27–39]. Fibrosis is low in signal intensity, whereas tumor recurrence is heterogeneous and moderate in signal intensity. Prior to resolution of the edema, distinction between granulation tissue and recurrence is problematic [27,30,33,34,36,37].

In the staging of lymph node metastases, MRI and CT imaging appear to be comparable. Accuracy is 83 to 97 percent for CT imaging and 73 to 98 percent for MRI. At present, distinction between enlarged hyperplastic nodes and malignant nodes cannot be made, which can result in overstaging of tumors. (Fig. 11.7) MRI, however, is superior to CT imaging in the diagnosis of bone marrow metastases [36,40].

MRI and clinical staging have complementary roles, and staging of urinary bladder tumors is best achieved with the use of both approaches. Because of the limitations in differentiating acute edema from tumor tissue, MRI is most helpful if performed prior to the clinical staging [41].

Squamous-cell carcinoma is rare in Western countries, but is the most frequent form of bladder neoplasm (55%) in patients with schistosomiasis and is often associated with squamous metaplasia. Histologically, these tumors form squamous pearls and are graded based on the varying degrees of cellular differentiation and histological appearance [7]. Tumors are intermediate in signal intensity on T1-weighted images and enhance with gadolinium (Fig. 11.8). Their appearance is usually not distinguishable from that of transitional-cell carcinoma.

Adenocarcinoma of the bladder is rare and is the most common tumor to arise at the vesicourachal remnant of the bladder dome (Fig. 11.9). The tumor may however arise in any location. It is also found in patients with exstrophy of the bladder. Adenocarcinoma most commonly arises secondarily as extension from adjacent organs (see later discussion). As with squamous-cell carcinoma, the prognosis is poor.

Spindle-cell carcinoma, also known as carcinosarcoma, contains spindle and giant cells. The epithelial component is most often transitional-cell carcinoma. These tumors are bulky and invariably deeply invade the bladder wall. Prognosis is poor [7].

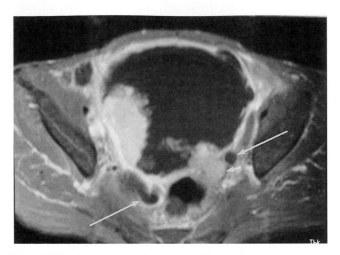

F IG . 11.7 Transitional-cell cancer and hyperplastic lymph node. Multiple varying-sized papillary cancers are present on the gadolinium-enhanced T1-weighted fat-suppressed spin-echo image. Substantial enhancement of the mucosa with gadolinium is identified. A 1.2 cm lymph node (*arrow*) is shown, which was considered consistent with nodal disease. At histopathology the enlarged nodes were benign and hyperplastic. Note also the dilated ureters (*long arrows*).

Metastatic Neoplasms

Direct invasion of the bladder may occur secondary to prostate, rectosigmoid, and uterine adenocarcinomas, and adenocarcinomas of stomach and breast may metastasize to the bladder [7]. The most common metastases to the bladder from distant sites are melanoma and gastric carcinoma. However, more commonly, metastases to the bladder arise from direct extension of pelvic neoplasms. The diagnostic accuracy of MRI in the detection of bladder mucosal invasion by pelvic tumors was reported to be 81 percent in one series [42]. The types of tumors studied in this series were cervical, colon, urethral, vaginal, vulvar, and lymphoid tissue. False negative findings may arise from microscopic foci of invasion, whereas false positive findings may stem from muscularis invasion without mucosal invasion. In this series, it was noted that postradiation changes and bullous edema are distinguishable from tumor [42].

Multiplanar imaging with precontrast T1- and T2-weighted images as well as postcontrast T1-weighted images is effective at defining tumor extension to the bladder (Fig. 11.10). Sagittal-plane imaging is particularly effective for rectal and gynecological malignancies, and fat suppression combined with gadolinium enhancement is useful. Cervical carcinoma Stage 4a has a particular propensity to invade bladder mucosa. This invasion is well-shown with the use of sagittal-plane imaging and gadolinium-enhanced T1-weighted images, which provide accurate diagnosis [43,44].

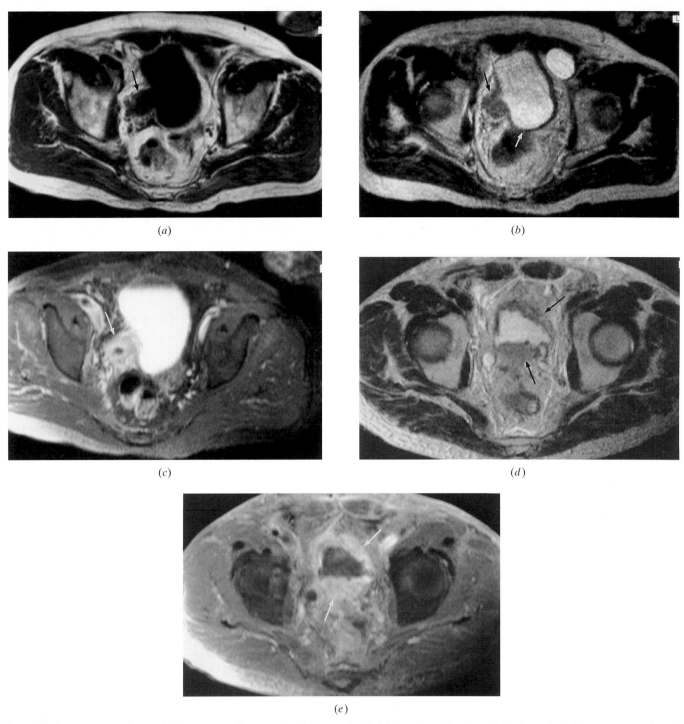

(a)

(b)

(c)

(d)

(e)

FIG. 11.8 Squamous-cell cancer. Squamous-cell cancer involving the distal right ureter and adjacent bladder wall is shown on T1-weighted spin-echo (a), T2-weighted spin-echo (b), and postgadolinium T1-weighted fat-suppressed spin-echo (c) images. On the T1-weighted spin-echo image (a), the tumor is low to intermediate in signal intensity (*arrow, a*). The tumor is minimally hyperintense on the T2-spin-echo image (*black arrow, b*). A transition is identified between intermediate signal intensity of the involved bladder wall and low signal intensity of the normal wall (*white arrow, b*). On the gadolinium-enhanced image (c) the tumor shows moderate, heterogeneous enhancement (*arrow, c*). The fat planes around the tumor are ill-defined with high-signal-intensity reticular strands on the gadolinium-enhanced fat-suppressed image, which is consistent with perivesicular fat infiltration. T2-weighted spin-echo (d) and postgadolinium T1-weighted fat-suppressed spin-echo (e) images in a second patient with squamous-cell cancer of the bladder. The tumor is irregular in contour, and heterogeneously and minimally hyperintense on the T2-weighted spin-echo image (*arrows, d*). Heterogeneous enhancement is apparent following gadolinium administration (*arrows, e*).

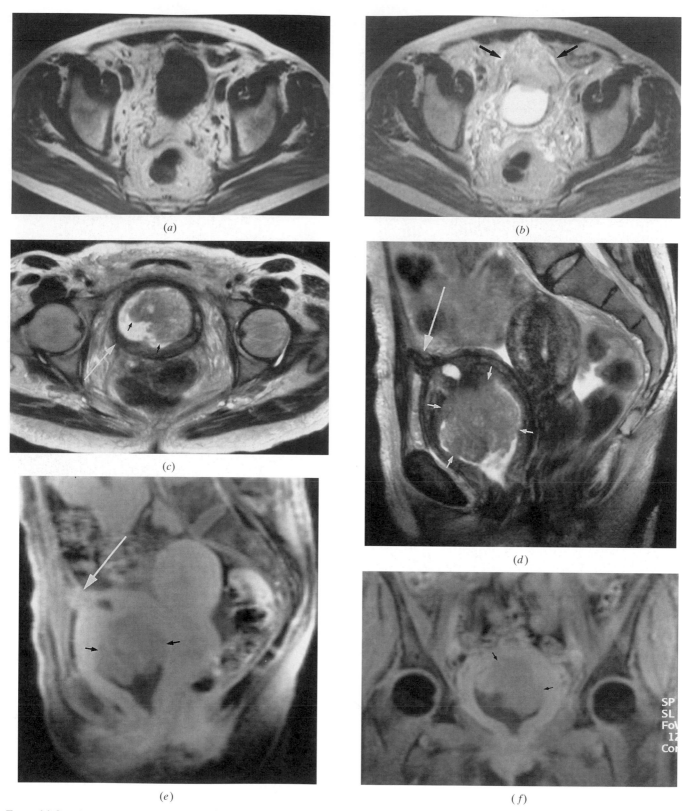

(a)

(b)

(c)

(d)

(e)

(f)

FIG. 11.9 Adenocarcinoma. T1-weighted spin-echo (*a*) and T2-weighted spin-echo (*b*) images. This patient has a patent urachus. The tumor is low in signal intensity on the T1-weighted image (*a*) and heterogeneous and moderately high in signal intensity (*arrows, b*) on the T2-weigthed image (*b*). The tumor extends anteriorly along the urachus. T2-weighted echo-train spin-echo (*c*), sagittal T2-weighted echo-train spin-echo (*d*), sagittal (*e*), and coronal (*f*) interstitial-phase gadolinium-enhanced fat-suppressed SGE images in a second patient. A large pedunculated adenocarcinoma (*short arrows, c–f*) arises from the dome of the bladder. Origin of the tumor is well shown on sagittal (*d,e*) and coronal (*f*) images. Diffuse bladder well thickening is noted (*long arrow, c*). Heterogeneous signal of the bladder wall on the T2-weighted image reflects deep bladder wall invasion. The bladder wall is more homogeneous on the post gadolinium image because it was acquired late following contrast administration. Definition of tumor invasion of the wall is not feasible on these late post contrast images due to equilibration of contrast between wall and tumor. A urachal remnant is apparent on sagittal plane images (*long arrow, d,e*).

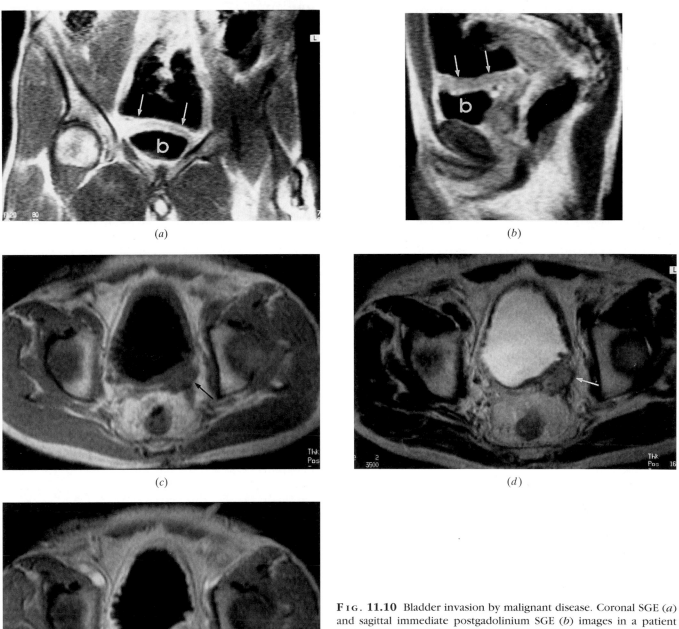

FIG. 11.10 Bladder invasion by malignant disease. Coronal SGE (*a*) and sagittal immediate postgadolinium SGE (*b*) images in a patient with rectal cancer. Tumor is identified arising from the rectum and extending along the superior bladder (*b*) wall (*arrows, a,b*). SGE (*c*), T2-weighted echo-train spin-echo (*d*), and postgadolinium SGE (*e*) images in a patient with recurrent prostate cancer invading the bladder. Tumor is intermediate in signal intensity on T1- (*arrow, c*) and T2-weighted (*arrow, d*) images, and enhances minimally with gadolinium (*arrow, e*).

DIFFUSE CHANGES

Hypertrophy

Muscular hypertrophy of the bladder wall results from bladder outlet obstruction. Underlying causes include benign prostatic enlargement (the most common cause in males), prostatic cancer, large pelvic tumors, bladder neck obstruction (functional or anatomic), and hydrocolpos.

Bladder wall hypertrophy appears as an increased thickness of the bladder wall, which is low in signal intensity on T2-weighted images and does not enhance substantially with gadolinium. Signal-intensity features are similar to those of normal bladder wall (Fig. 11.11).

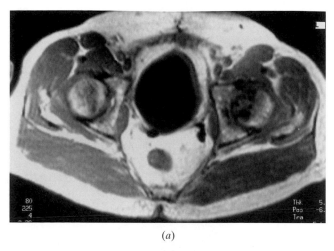

(a)

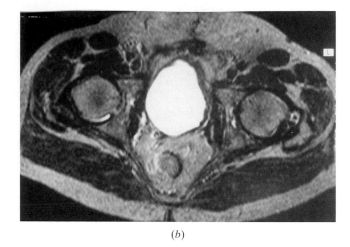

(b)

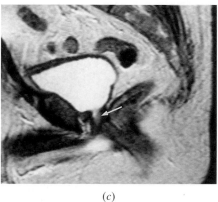

(c)

FIG. 11.11 Bladder wall hypertrophy secondary to chronic outlet obstruction by prostate enlargement. SGE (*a*), transverse (*b*), and sagittal (*c*) T2-weighted echo-train spin-echo images. The bladder wall is asymmetrically thickened, with low signal intensity on T1- and T2-weighted images. Note the transurethral prostatectomy defect in the bladder base on the sagittal image (*arrow, c*).

Radiation Changes

As a sequela of pelvic radiation, bullous edema may arise in the bladder and may persist for months or years. Over time, patients may develop radiation cystitis with fibrosis and a contracted bladder.

Radiation changes in the bladder increase with increasing radiation dose. Radiation-induced disease is common when the dose exceeds 4,500 cGy. In one study, the incidence of bladder changes increased from 8 to 51 percent as the dose surpassed 4,500 cGy [45]. In patients with moderate or severe symptoms, radiation changes are detectable on MRI. However, abnormalities on MRI may be present in the absence of symptoms. Postradiation changes of the bladder have MRI appearances that correlate with the severity of histological features. The mildest form of radiation change results in a high signal intensity of the bladder mucosa with preservation of the bladder wall thickness on T2-weighted images. The high signal intensity typically is seen at the trigone, but may spread to involve the entire mucosa and could be the result of mucosal edema. With more severe injury, the wall increases in thickness (greater than 5 mm when fully distended), and the signal characteristics are one of two patterns. Either the wall has a uniformly high signal inten-

sity or a low signal intensity in the inner layer with high signal intensity at the periphery. With extreme radiation change, formation of fistula or sinus tracts are seen in addition to the thickening and abnormal signal intensity. On gadolinium-enhanced studies, the bladder wall shows increased enhancement, sometimes without other morphological changes on noncontrast images. This enhancement may occur up to 2.5 years after irradiation [46]. Other findings are commonly present (Fig. 11.12).

Edema

Edema of the bladder wall as a result of acute bladder disease can be distinguished from bladder wall hypertrophy by its longer T2, which renders it high in signal intensity on T2-weighted images [47].

Hemorrhagic Cystitis

Hemorrhagic cystitis is a severe form of cystitis characterized by hematuria. It may be secondary to radiation of the pelvis or infectious agents including *Escherichia coli* and viruses.

Hemorrhagic cystitis demonstrates a complex appearance on MR images based on the T1 and T2 characteristics of aging blood products. Active bleeding (oxyhe-

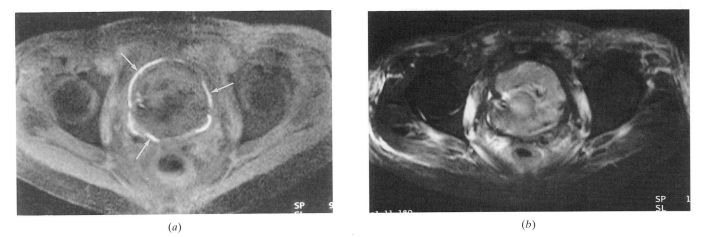

(a) (b)

FIG. 11.12 Radiation changes. Fat-suppressed SGE (a) and T2-weighted fat-suppressed spin-echo (b) images. High-signal-intensity obturator internus muscles and high-signal-intensity strands in the perirectal space, consistent with radiation-induced tissue damage, are present on the T2-weighted image (b). High signal intensity within the bladder wall on the fat-suppressed SGE image and low signal intensity on the T2-weighted fat-suppressed spin-echo images are consistent with intracellular methemoglobin due to the radiation-induced hemorrhagic cystitis. The fluid in the bladder is predominantly high in signal intensity on T1- and T2-weighted images, which is consistent with extracellular methemoglobin.

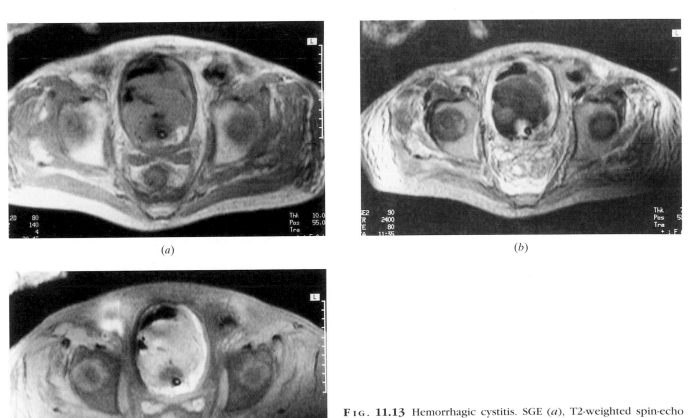

(a) (b)

(c)

FIG. 11.13 Hemorrhagic cystitis. SGE (a), T2-weighted spin-echo (b), and T1-weighted fat-suppressed spin-echo (c) images in a patient with hemorrhagic cystitis. The bladder contains fluid of varying signal intensities due to the presence of blood products of varying ages. Note that the signal intensity of the bladder wall has variations due to the presence of blood products of differing ages.

moglobin) has limited paramagnetic properties and behaves like simple fluid with a long T1 (low signal intensity on T1-weighted images) and a long T2 (high signal intensity on T2-weighted images). Acute blood (intracellular deoxyhemoglobin) has a long T1 (low signal intensity on T1-weighted images) and a short T2 (low signal intensity on T2-weighted images). Intracellular methemoglobin has a short T1 (high signal intensity on T1-weighted images) and a short T2 (low signal intensity on T2-weighted images). Extracellular methemoglobin has a short T1 (high signal intensity on T1-weighted images) and a long T2 (high signal intensity on T2-weighted images), and this appearance is most typical for subacute hemorrhage. Intracellular hemosiderin in an old hematoma has a medium T1 (intermediate signal intensity on T1-weighted images) and a short T2 (low signal intensity on T2-weighted images) [48]. Thus, the appearance of hemorrhagic cystitis demonstrates not only a thickened bladder wall, but also the complex signal characteristics of hemorrhage (Fig. 11.13).

INFLAMMATION

Cystitis
Inflammation of the bladder wall may be the result of infection, foreign bodies within the bladder, peritonitis, drug toxicity, or other causes. The appearance is a thickened bladder wall that may be focal or diffuse. On T2-weighted images four layers can be appreciated within the inflamed bladder wall. An innermost low signal intensity and an inner high-signal-intensity band represent the thickened epithelium and lamina propria, respectively. An outer low-signal-intensity band and outermost intermediate-signal-intensity bands represent the inner compact muscle layer and outer loose muscle layer, respectively [1]. Increased enhancement after gadolinium administration is observed. The extent of enhancement reflects the severity of the inflammatory process (Fig. 11.14).

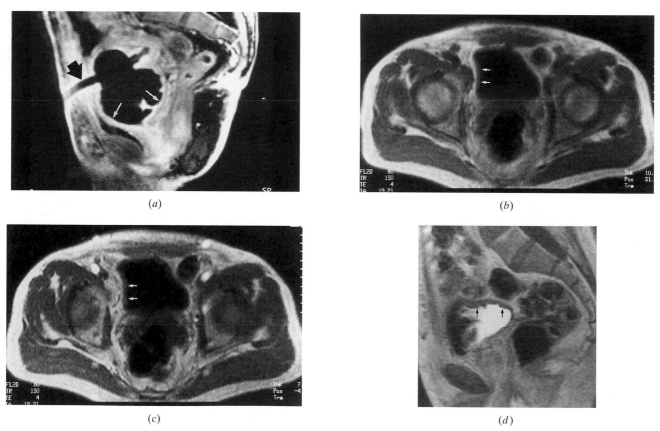

(a)

(b)

(c)

(d)

FIG. 11.14 Inflammation. Sagittal immediate postgadolinium SGE image (*a*) in a patient with a suprapubic catheter (*black arrow, a*). Substantial enhancement of the bladder wall is demonstrated (*small arrows, a*). Mild inflammatory cystitis on SGE (*b*), immediate postgadolinium SGE (*c*), and sagittal 5-minute postgadolinium SGE (*d*) images in a second patient. The bladder wall is irregularly thickened (*arrows, b*) with minimal enhancement on the postgadolinium images (*arrows, c,d*). Marked inflammation secondary to infection on 90-second postgadolinium SGE (*e*) and gadolinium-enhanced T1-weighted fat-suppressed spin-echo (*f*) images in a third patient. Diffuse bladder wall thickening is present (*arrows, f*) and a large gadolinium-containing diverticulum (*arrows, e*) is identified arising from the right aspect of the bladder.

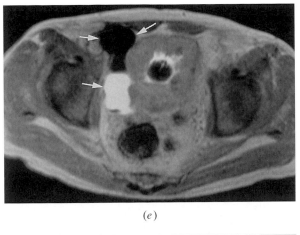

(e)

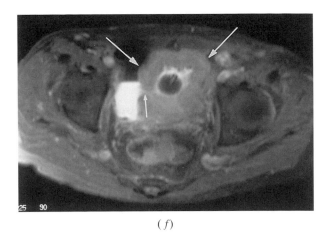

(f)

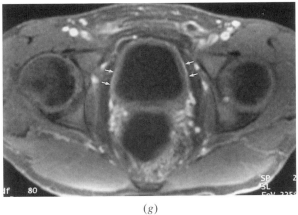

(g)

FIG. 11.14 (*Continued*) A small high-signal-intensity tract represents the communication between the bladder and the diverticulum (*short arrow, f*). Chemical peritonitis demonstrated on a 90-second postgadolinium fat-suppressed SGE image (*g*) in a patient who had undergone intraperitoneal chemotherapy. Increased enhancement of the serosal surface of the bladder (*small arrows, g*) is present as a result of chemical peritonitis.

Cystitis Cystica

Cystitis cystica is a cystic lesion that appears in the lamina propria. The lesion may be an incidental finding at biopsy, but is more common in the clinical setting of chronic cystitis. Grossly, the appearance may be that of large cysts, resembling cobblestones (Fig. 11.15) [49].

Fistulas

Pelvic fistulas may result from obstetrical procedures, surgery, trauma, radiation, infection, inflammatory bowel disease, or pelvic malignancies. Typically, patients present with urinary or fecal incontinence, pneumaturia, fecaluria, or vaginal discharge. Patients can be evaluated

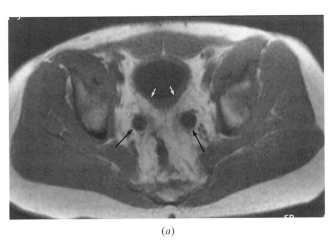

(a)

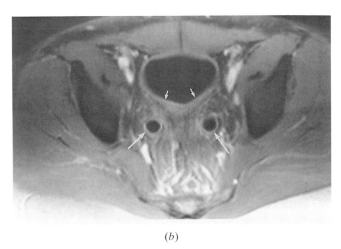

(b)

FIG. 11.15 Cystitis cystica. SGE (*a*) and 90-second postgadolinium fat-suppressed SGE (*b*) images. Note that the bladder wall is uniformly thickened (*short arrows*), and the distal ureters are thick-walled and substantially dilated (*long arrows*).

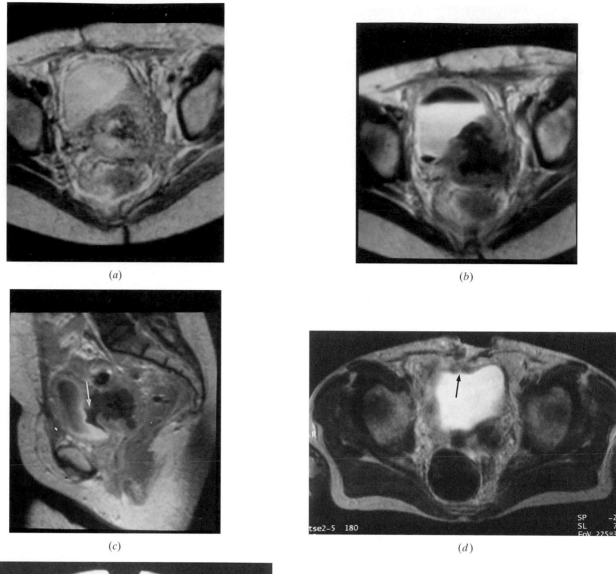

(a)

(b)

(c)

(d)

(e)

F IG. 11.16 Bladder fistula. Cervicovesical fistula formation following radiation for cervical cancer shown on T2-weighted spin-echo (*a*), transverse (*b*), and sagittal (*c*) gadolinium-enhanced T1-weighted spin-echo images. The fistula tract is best shown on the sagittal postgadolinium image (*arrow, c*). (Courtesy of Hedvig Hricak, M.D., Ph.D.). Vesicocutaneous fistula shown on T2-weighted echo-train spin-echo (*d*) and gadolinium-enhanced T1-weighted fat-suppressed spin-echo (*e*) images. The bladder wall shows focal, irregular thickening. An overlying skin defect is noted. A thin fistula tract is apparent and is high in signal intensity on the T2-weighted echo-train spin-echo image (*arrow, d*) and low in signal intensity on the postgadolinium T1-weighted fat-suppressed spin-echo image (*arrow, e*). There is substantial enhancement on the postgadolinium images of the soft tissues surrounding the fistula and of the skin, which is consistent with inflammatory changes.

with cystoscopy, vaginoscopy, colonoscopy, fistulography, gastrointestinal contrast radiographic studies, sonography, scintigraphy, computed tomography, or magnetic resonance.

The sagittal plane is particularly effective at demon-

strating vesicocervical fistulas because it displays these fistulas in profile. They typically insert low in the bladder, a region less well evaluated on transverse images due to volume averaging of the pelvic floor musculature. Gadolinium-enhanced T1-weighted images best demonstrate

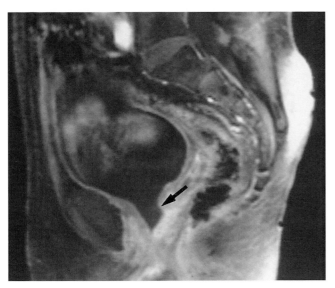

F I G. 11.17 Transurethral prostatectomy defect. Sagittal gadolinium-enhanced fat-suppressed SGE image showing the characteristic widening of the prostatic urethra (*arrow*).

Surface Coils

The use of specialized surface coils improves the signal-to-noise ratio in imaging of the abdomen. Endorectal coils specifically improve imaging in the pelvis. Use of an endorectal coil combined with an external anterior coil may increase the signal-to-noise ratio for larger spatial coverage.

Contrast Agents

Lymph-node-specific contrast agents have been investigated that may permit differentiation of lymph-node malignant involvement versus hyperplastic enlargement. Thus, the staging of bladder carcinomas may be improved [53].

bladder fistulas. On early postgadolinium images, the fistula wall has a high signal intensity, and the tract has a low signal intensity. Late postgadolinium images may show high-signal-intensity fluid within the fistula tract [50]. The addition of fat suppression increases the conspicuity of enhancing fistulous tract walls (Fig. 11.16).

CONCLUSION

MRI is an effective technique for evaluating the full range of bladder disease. Staging of transitional-cell carcinoma is the most common indication for bladder MRI investigation and is well-performed with a combination of breath-hold SGE, 512 resolution T2-weighted echo-train spin-echo, and immediate and delayed postgadolinium fat-suppressed SGE techniques, with image acquisition in multiple planes and the concurrent use of a phased-array multicoil.

POSTOPERATIVE CHANGES

Widening of the prostatic urethra occur following all forms of prostatectomies. Immediately following prostatectomy, the prostatic fossa is quite wide, but it rapidly involutes to a more normal configuration over several weeks. However, a residual prostatectomy defect typically is observed for years. The configuration of the widening after cryocaustic prostate surgery is bottle-shaped and different from that of transurethral resection (Fig. 11.17) [51].

FUTURE DIRECTIONS

MRI Sequences

Cine MRI has been evaluated for urodynamic studies, with 30 scans of the same slice acquired during micturition. Maximal and mean flow rate, total voiding time, residual volume, and pattern of bladder emptying can be studied as a function of time. Additionally, detrusor muscle activity, opening of the bladder neck, and external sphincter are displayed in the dynamic mode [52].

REFERENCES

1. Narumi Y, Kadota T, Inoue E, et al: Bladder wall morphology: In vitro MR imaging-histopathologic correlation. Radiology 187:151–155, 1993.
2. Lee JKT, Rholl KS: MRI of the bladder and prostate (review). AJR Am J Roentgenol 147:732–736, 1986.
3. Barentsz JO, Lemmens JAM, Ruijs SHJ, et al: Carcinoma of the urinary bladder: MR imaging using a double surface coil. AJR Am J Roentgenol 151:107–112, 1988.
4. Reiman TH, Heiken JP, Totty WG, Lee JKT: Clinical MR imaging with a Helmholtz-type surface coil. Radiology 169:564–566, 1988.
5. Requardt H, Sauter R, Weber H: Helmholtzspulen in der Kernspintomographie. Electromed 55:61–72, 1987.
6. Menahem MM, Slywotzky C. Urinary bladder leiomyoma: Magnetic resonance imaging findings. Urol Radiol 14:197–199, 1992.
7. Hahn D. Neoplasms of the urinary bladder. In Pollack HM (ed.). Clinical Urography, volume 2. Philadelphia: WB Saunders pp. 1355–1377, 1990.
8. Arrive L, Malbec L, Buy JN, Guinet C, Vadrot D: Male pelvis In Vanel D, McNamara MT (eds.). MRI of the Body. New York: Springer-Verlag, pp. 242–255, 1989.
9. Bryan PJ, Butler HE, Nelson AD, Lipuma JP, Kopiwoda SY, et al: Magnetic resonance imaging of the prostate. AJR Am J Roentgenol 146:543–548, 1986.
10. Shonnard KM, Jelinek JS, Benedikt RA, Kransdorf MJ: CT and MR of neurofibromatosis of the bladder. J Comput Assist Tomgr 16:433–438, 1992.

11. Elkin M. Urogenital tuberculosis. In Pollack HM (ed.). Clinical Urography volume 1. Philadelphia: WB Saunders pp. 1020–1046, 1990.

12. Warshawsky R, Bow SN, Waldbaum RS, Cintron J: Bladder pheochromocytoma with MR correlation. J Comput Assist Tomogr 13:714–716, 1989.

13. Heyman J, Cheung Y, Ghali V, Leiter E: Bladder pheochromocytoma: Evaluation with magnetic resonance imaging. J Urol 141:1424–1426, 1989.

14. Fink JIJ, Reinig JW, Dwyer AJ, et al: MR imaging of pheochromocytoma. J Comput Assist Tomogr 9:454–458, 1985.

15. Falke ThM, LeStrake L, Shaff MI, et al: MR imaging of the adrenals: Correlated with computed tomography. J Comput Assist Tomogr 10:242–253, 1986.

16. Quint LE, Glazer GM, Francis IR, Shapiro B, Chenevert TL: Pheochromocytoma and paraganglioma: Comparison of MR imaging with CT and I-131 MIB6 scintigraphy. Radiology 165:89–93, 1987.

17. Saxton HM. Pelvic lipomatosis. In Pollack HM, (ed.). Clinical Urography, volume 3. Philadelphia: WB Saunders pp. 2458–2461, 1990.

18. Schnall MD, Connick T, Hayes CE, Lenkinski RE, Kressel HY: MR imaging of the pelvis with an endorectal-external multicoil array. J Magn Reson Imaging 2:229–232, 1992.

19. Beahrs OH, Henson DE, Hetter RVP, eds: Manual for Staging of Cancer, (4th ed.). Philadelphia: LIppincott 1992.

20. Fisher MR, Hricak H, Tanagho EA: Urinary bladder MR imaging. Part II. Neoplasm. Radiology 157:471–477, 1985.

21. Amendola MA, Glaser GM, Grossman HB, et al: Staging of bladder carcinoma: MRI-CT-surgical correlation. AJR Am J Roentgenol 146:1179–1183, 1986.

22. Bryan PJ, Butler HE, LiPuma JP, et al: CT and MR imaging in staging bladder neoplasms. J Comput Assist Tomogr 11:96–101, 1987.

23. Rholl KS, Lee JKT, Heiken JP, et al: Primary bladder carcinoma: Evaluation with MR imaging. Radiology 163:117–123, 1987.

24. Buy JN, Moss AA, Guinet C, et al: MR staging of bladder carcinoma: Correlation with pathologic findings. Radiology 169:695–700, 1988.

25. Koebel G, Schmeidl U, Griebel J, et al: MR imaging of urinary bladder neoplasms. J Comput Assist Tomogr 12:98–103, 1988.

26. Husband JE, Oliff JF, Williams MP, Heron CW, Cherryman GR: Bladder cancer: Staging with CT and MR imaging. Radiology 173:435–440, 1989.

27. Barentsz JO, Debruyne FMJ, Ruijs SHJ: Magnetic Resonance Imaging of carcinoma of the Urinary Bladder. Boston: Kluwer, 1990.

28. Persad R, Kabala J, Gillatt D, Penry B, Gingell JC, Smith JB. Magnetic resonance imaging in the staging of bladder cancer. Br J Urol 71:566–573, 1993.

29. Strich G, Hagan P, Gerber KH, et al: Tissue distribution and magnetic resonance spin lattice relaxation effects of gadolinium-DTPA. Radiology 154:723–726, 1985.

30. Tachibana M, Baba S, Daguchi N, et al: Efficacy of gadolinium-diethylene-triaminepentaacetic acid-enhanced magnetic resonance imaging for differentiation between superficial and muscle-invasive tumor of the bladder: A comparative study with computerized tomography and transurethral ultrasonography. J Urol 145:1169–1173, 1991.

31. Narumi Y, Kadota T, Inoue E, et al. Bladder tumors: Staging with gadolinium-enhanced oblique MR imaging. Radiology 187:145–150, 1993.

32. Neuerburg JM, Bohndorf K, Sohn M, et al: Urinary bladder neoplasms: Evaluation with contrast-enhanced MR imaging. Radiology 172:739–743, 1989.

33. Neuerburg JM, Bohndorf K, Sohn M, Teufl F, Gunther RW: Staging of urinary bladder neoplasms with MR imaging: Is Gd-DTPA helpful? J Comput Assist Tomogr 15:780–786, 1991.

34. Sohn M, Neuerburg JM, Teufl F, Bohndorf K: Gadolinium-enhanced magnetic resonance imaging in the staging of urinary bladder neoplasms. Urol Int 45:142–147, 1990.

35. Barentsz JO, van Erning LJThO, Ruijs JHJ, Bors WG, Jager G, Oosterhof G: Dynamic turbo-FLASH subtraction MR imaging: Perfusion of pelvic tumors (abstr). Radiology 185:340, 1992.

36. Nicolas V, Spielmann R, Maas R, et al: The diagnostic value of MR tomography following gadolinium-DTPA compared to computed-tomography in bladder tumors. Fortschr Rontgenstr 154:357–363, 1991.

37. Sparenberg A, Hamm B, Hammerer P, Samberger V, Wolf KJ: The diagnosis of bladder carcinomas by NMR tomography: Any improvement with Gd-DTPA? Fortschr Rontgenstr 155:117–122, 1991.

38. Kim B, Semelka RC, Ascher SM, Chalpin D, Carroll P, Hricak H: Bladder tumor staging: Comparison of contrast enhanced CT, T1- and T2- weighted MR imaging, dynamic gadolinium-enhanced imaging, and late gadolinium-enhanced imaging. Radiology 193:239–245, 1994.

39. Ebner F, Kressel HY, Mintz MC, et al: Tumor recurrence versus fibrosis in the female pelvis: Differentiation with MR imaging at 1.5T. Radiology 166:333–340, 1988.

40. Algra PR, Bloem JL, Tissing H, Falke ThM, Arndt J-W, Verboom LJ: Detection of vertebral metastases: Comparison between MR imaging and bone scintigraphy. Radiographics 11:219–232, 1991.

41. Barentsz JO, Ruijs SHJ, Strijk SP: The role of MR imaging in carcinoma of the urinary bladder. AJR Am J Roentgenol 160:937–947, 1993.

42. Popovich MJ, Hricak H, Sugimura Kazuro, Stern JL: The role of MR imaging in determining surgical eligibility for pelvic exenteration. AJR Am J Roentgenol 160:525–531, 1993.

43. Hricak H, Hamm B, Semelka R, Cann CE, Nauert T, Secaf E, Stern JL, Wolf K-J: Carcinoma of the uterus: Use of gadopentetate dimeglumine in MR imaging. Radiology 181:95–106, 1991.

44. Janus CL, Mendelson DS, Moore S, Gendal EL, Dottino P, Brodman M: Staging of cervical carcinoma: Accuracy of magnetic resonance imaging and computed tomography. Clin Imaging 13:114–116, 1989.

45. Sugimura K, Carrington, BM, Quivey JM, et al: Postirradiation changes in the pelvis: Assessment with MR imaging. Radiology 175:805–813, 1990.

46. Hricak H: Magnetic resonance imaging evaluation of the irradiated female pelvis. Semin Roentgenol 29:70–80, 1994.

47. Rifkin MD, Piccoli CW: Male pelvis and bladder. In Stark DD, Bradley WG (eds.). Magnetic Resonance Imaging, volume 2. Baltimore: Mosby pp. 2044–2057, 1992.

48. Bradley, WG Jr: Hemorrhage and brain iron. In Stark DD, Bradley WG Jr (eds.): Magnetic Resonance Imaging, volume 1. Baltimore: Mosby pp. 721–728, 1992.

49. Hahn D. Neoplasms of the urinary bladder. In Pollack HM (ed.). Clinical Urography, volume 2. Philadelphia: WB Saunders 1353–1354, 1990.

50. Semelka RC, Hricak H, Kim B, Forstner R, Bis KG, Ascher SM, Reinhold C. Pelvic fistulas: Appearances on MR images. Abdom Imaging 22:91–95, 1997.

51. Mindell HJ, Quiogue T, Lebowitz RL: Postoperative uroradiological appearances. In Pollack HM, (ed.). Clinical Urography, volume 3. Philadelphia: WB Saunders 2510–2531, 1990.

52. Gupta RK, Kapoor R, Poptani H, Rastogi H, Gujral RB. Cine MR voiding cystourethrogram in adult normal males. Magn Reson Imaging 10:881–885, 1992.

53. Guimaraes R, Clemont O, Bittoun J, Carnot F, Frija G: MR lymphadenopathy with superparamagnetic iron manoparticles in rats: Pathologic basis for contrast enhancement. AJR Am J Roentgenol 162:201–207, 1994.

chapter 12

MALE PELVIS

T. C. NOONE, M.D., R. A. HUCH BÖNI, M.D., AND R. C. SEMELKA, M.D.

MRI TECHNIQUE

MRI is an effective modality for the diagnosis, staging, and, follow-up of a variety of diseases of the male pelvis. Our standard male pelvis imaging protocol includes 512-resolution transverse and sagittal T2-weighted echo-train spin-echo, postgadolinium transverse and sagittal fat-suppressed SGE sequences. The routine use of a phased-array multicoil results in reproducible high image quality. Endorectal coil imaging generates higher spatial resolution imaging, but the impact on patient management is presently not clear. Recent reports have emphasized the value of the high spatial resolution achieved with endo-rectal coil imaging [1–3]. Supplemental T1-weighted imaging through the abdomen and pelvis should be performed to assess for lymphadenopathy.

■ PROSTATE AND POSTERIOR URETHRA

NORMAL ANATOMY

The prostate is divided anatomically into central, transitional, and peripheral zones. The *peripheral zone* comprises the greatest percentage of the gland and is most extensive within the prostatic apex, where it forms the majority of the gland, and in the midgland where it is posterior and posterolateral in location. The *central zone* is periurethral in location and is situated superiorly within the base of the gland. It surrounds the verumontanum. The *transitional zone* surrounds the central zone and also is located predominately within the base of the prostate. The transitional zone increases in size with patient age.

The prostate appears homogeneous and intermediate in signal intensity on T1-weighted images, and zonal anatomy is not demonstrable. The zonal anatomy of the prostate is well-demonstrated on T2-weighted images (Fig. 12.1). Signal intensity on T2-weighted images is directly related to the proportion of glandular elements and inversely related to the density of stromal or muscular elements. Thus, there is increased signal intensity in the peripheral zone, where there is abundant glandular material, and decreased signal intensity in the central zone, where more striated muscle and stroma are present. The signal intensity of the transitional zone, where there is also a large volume of stroma, is similar to that of the central zone. Differentiation between the two cannot be made by imaging appearances, but is based primarily on anatomic location.

The anterolateral prostate is cloaked by the anterior fibromuscular band, which is low in signal intensity on both T1- and T2-weighted images. It serves as a landmark dividing the prostate from the tissues of the preprostatic space. The prostate capsule also consists of fibromuscular

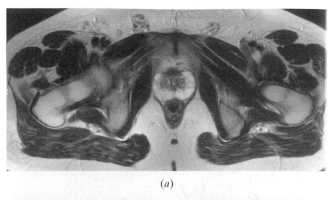

(a)

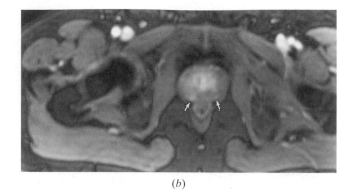

(b)

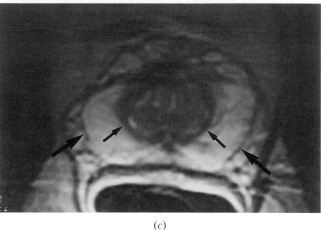

(c)

FIG. 12.1 Normal prostate midgland level. Transverse 512-resolution T2-weighted echo-train spin-echo (*a*) and immediate postgadolinium fat-suppressed SGE (*b*) images. The peripheral zone is high in signal intensity on T2-weighted images and surrounds the lower-signal-intensity transitional and central zones (*a*). Note the vascular enhancement delineating the neurovascular bundles (*arrows, b*) on the postgadolinium image (*b*). T2-weighted endorectal coil image (*c*) in a second patient with a normal prostate. The zonal anatomy of the prostate is well-demonstrated on T2-weighted images. The normal central zone and transitional zones are low in signal intensity (*short arrows, c*), and the normal peripheral zone is high in signal intensity (*long arrows, c*).

tissue and is low in signal intensity on T2-weighted images. The verumontanum, a central ovoid high-signal-intensity structure, is located in the periurethral region at the midgland level. The neurovascular bundles are located posterolaterally at 5 and 7 o'clock within the rectoprostatic angles.

The prostatic and membranous portions of the urethra form the posterior urethra. The distal prostatic ure-

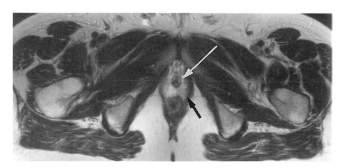

FIG. 12.2 Normal prostate level of apex. Transverse 512-resolution T2-weighted echo-train spin-echo image. At the level of the prostatic apex the gland is comprised predominantly of the peripheral zone, which is high in signal intensity on T2-weighted images (*black arrow*). The muscular wall of the urethra, which is low in signal intensity on T2-weighted images, is clearly depicted (*white arrow*).

thra is demonstrated as a low-signal-intensity rounded structure within the high-signal-intensity peripheral zone at the apex of the prostate (Fig. 12.2). The membranous urethra extends from the prostatic apex to the bulb of the penis. The muscular wall of the membranous urethra forms the external sphincter, and embedded within its adventitia are the paired Cowper's glands.

DISEASE ENTITIES

Congenital Abnormalities

Prostatic agenesis and hypoplasia are very rare anomalies that are often associated with other anomalies of the genitourinary tract. Cysts are the most commonly encountered congenital anomalies of the prostate. Congenital prostatic cysts are generally high in signal intensity on T2-weighted images and of variable signal intensity on T1-weighted images, depending on the presence of infection or hemorrhage. Characterized by their location in relation to the prostate, which may be midline, paramedian, or lateral, they occur between the prostatic urethra or bladder anteriorly, and the rectum posteriorly.

Midline cysts include utricular and Müllerian duct cysts. Utricular cysts arise from dilatation of the prostatic utricle, originating from the verumontanum. Frequently

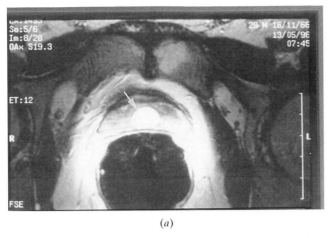

(a)

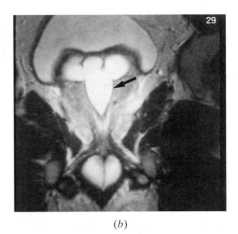

(b)

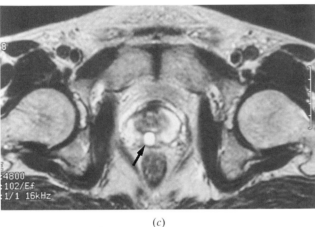

(c)

FIG. 12.3 Utricular cyst in an infertile 29-year-old male. Transverse (a) and coronal (b) T2-weighted spin-echo endorectal coil images. A rounded, central structure, which is high in signal intensity on the T2-weighted images represents a utricular cyst (*white arrow, a; black arrow, b*). Transverse T2-weighted spin-echo image (c) in a second patient. A utricular cyst located in the region of the verumontanum is high in signal intensity on this T2-weighted image (*black arrow, c*).

associated with other genital anomalies, they are usually teardrop-shaped and communicate with the posterior urethra (Fig. 12.3) [4,5].

In contrast, müllerian duct cysts do not communicate with the posterior urethra, but are connected to the verumontanum by a stalk. Generally retrovesical in location

(Fig. 12.4), they are remnants of the müllerian duct system and are rarely associated with renal agenesis. Patients may present with urinary retention, infection, and stone formation. There are associated increased incidences of both squamous-cell carcinoma and adenocarcinomas [4–6].

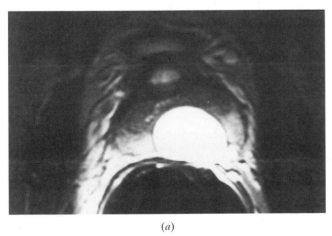

(a)

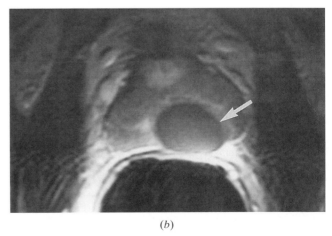

(b)

FIG. 12.4 Müllerian cyst. Transverse T2-weighted spin-echo (a) and immediate postgadolinium fat-suppressed T1 SGE (b) endorectal coil images. A large, ovoid müllerian cyst is seen in the dorsal aspect of the prostate near the midline, which is high in signal intensity on the T2-weighted image (a) and intermediate in signal intensity on the postgadolinium image (*white arrow, b*).

Cysts arising from the vas deferens or ejaculatory ducts are paramedian in location. Ejaculatory duct cysts may be either congenital or postinflammatory and generally result from obstruction along the expected course of the ductal system. Cysts of the vas deferens, although extremely rare, most frequently involve the ampulla. When large, either of these paramedian cystic structures may appear identical to utricular or müllerian duct cysts. Aspirated cyst fluid contains spermatozoa, permitting differentiation from müllerian duct cysts [4,5,7,8]. Cysts are high in signal intensity on high-resolution T2-weighted images and appear as signal-void on postgadolinium images.

MASS LESIONS

Benign Masses

Proliferation of glandular, or, less commonly, interstitial elements of the transitional zone leads to benign prostatic hyperplasia (BPH), a disease entity observed in approximately 50 percent of the male population older than 45

years of age [9]. When changes are focal, they may result in the formation of nodules or adenomyomata.

Glandular hyperplasia frequently results in enlargement of the central aspect of the prostate. BPH is low in signal intensity on T1-weighted images. On T2-weighted images BPH may be homogeneous or heterogeneous in appearance, ranging from medium to high in signal intensity [10–12]. Compression of the adjacent peripheral zone results in a low-signal-intensity band referred to as the surgical pseudocapsule [12,13]. Adenomatous changes may result in focal, nodular enlargement of the gland. Signal characteristics may be variable on T2-weighted images [10,14]. BPH commonly occurs in conjunction with prostate cancer because both are disease processes that increase in incidence with patient age (Fig. 12.5).

Distinction between interstitial hyperplasia and glandular hyperplasia has been described on MR images [11,15]. Hyperplastic changes that predominately involve the interstitium result in heterogeneous low signal intensity of the enlarged gland on T2-weighted images [11]. Focal alterations in signal intensity may result from infarction or cystic changes within nodules of glandular

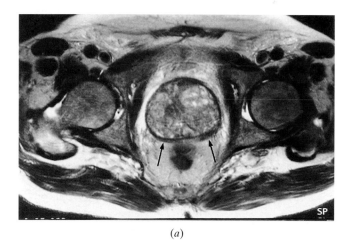

(*a*)

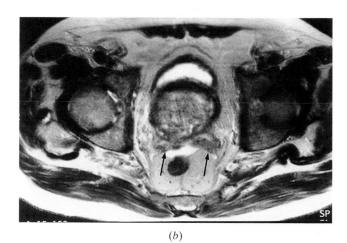

(*b*)

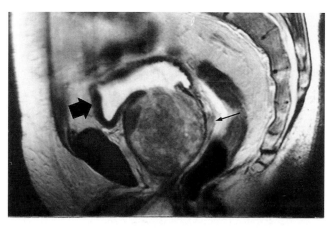

(*c*)

FIG. 12.5 Prostate cancer with seminal vesicle extension in the setting of massive BPH. Transverse (*a,b*) and sagittal (*c*) 512-resolution T2-weighted echo-train spin-echo images. The transitional zone, which is greatly enlarged, is heterogeneous and moderately high in signal intensity. The peripheral zone of the prostate (*thin arrows, a*) is thin and diffusely low in signal intensity secondary to tumor involvement (*a*). The seminal vesicles (*thin arrows, b,c*) also are low in signal intensity secondary to invasion by tumor (*b,c*). The bladder (*large arrow, c*) is elevated by the enlarged prostate and thick walled from resultant outlet obstruction.

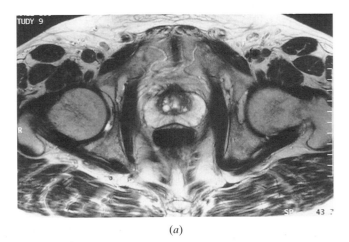

(a)

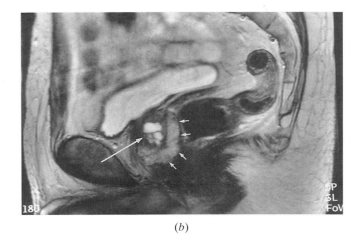

(b)

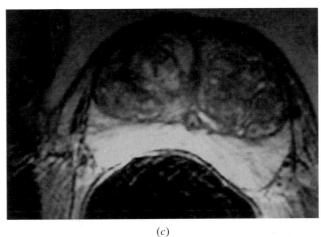

(c)

Fig. 12.6 Benign prostatic hyperplasia. Transverse (*a*) and sagittal (*b*) 512-resolution T2-weighted echo-train spin-echo image. High signal intensity foci are present representing cystic elements of interstitial BPH (*long arrow, b*). Normal signal intensity is seen within the surrounding peripheral zone (*short arrows, b*). Transverse T2-weighted echo-train spin-echo endorectal coil image (*c*) in a second patient. Diffuse heterogeneous low signal intensity within an enlarged central gland is consistent with the predominately glandular subtype of BPH.

BPH [5,15–17]. Areas of infarction may demonstrate low signal intensity on T2-weighted images [17]. Cystic ectasia, corresponding to dilatation of glandular elements, results in high signal intensity on T2-weighted images (Fig. 12.6) [11,15]. BPH may occasionally infiltrate the peripheral zone, making its distinction from carcinoma problematic [15].

Progressive enlargement of the central portion of the prostate with resultant protrusion into the bladder leads to partial bladder outlet obstruction [11]. After the surgical removal of periurethral tissue by transurethral, transvesical, or retropubic approaches, the adjacent prostatic urethra dilates to the level of the verumontanum. Residual hyperplastic tissue may be low to medium in signal intensity on T2-weighted images (Fig. 12.7) [8]. Radical prostatectomy may result in periurethral scarring, which also is low in signal intensity on T2-weighted images (Fig. 12.8). Fibrosis in the bed of the prostate and seminal vesicles following total prostatectomy is low in signal intensity on T2-weighted images and may mimic the appearance of a small low-signal-intensity prostate and seminal vesicles.

Malignant Masses

Rare Tumors

Squamous-cell cancer, transitional-cell cancer, and sarcoma are uncommon malignancies that involve the prostate and account for less than 5 percent of malignant tumors. In the pediatric population, prostate rhabdomyosarcoma is the most common tumor to arise from the bladder region (Fig. 12.9) [8].

Prostate Adenocarcinoma

Approximately 95 percent of malignant prostate lesions are adenocarcinomas. Prostatic carcinoma is frequently latent. It may occur in as many as 80 percent of men 80 years of age or older and in as many as 50 percent of men 50 years of age or older [15]. Its behavior depends on histological grade/stage and tumor volume [19,20]. Thus, tremendous controversy regarding diagnostic and treatment options remains.

Approximately 70 percent of prostate cancers arise from the peripheral zone, and the remainder arise in the transitional and central zones. Detection of prostate

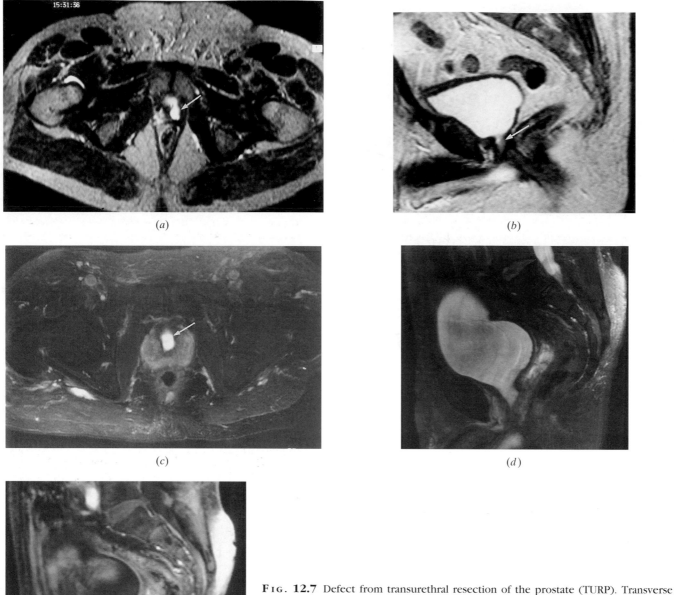

FIG. 12.7 Defect from transurethral resection of the prostate (TURP). Transverse (*a*) and sagittal (*b*) T2-weighted echo-train spin-echo images. The TURP defect is seen within the base of the prostate. The posterior urethra (*arrow, a,b*) is dilated following the surgical removal of periurethral tissue. Transverse 512-resolution T2-weighted fat-suppressed echo-train spin-echo (*c*), sagittal 512-resolution T2-weighted fat-suppressed echo-train spin-echo (*d*), and sagittal postgadolinium T1-weighted fat-suppressed SGE (*e*) images in a second patient. Dilatation of the prostatic urethra (*arrow, c*) is observed following TURP.

carcinoma with MRI is limited primarily to tumors involving the peripheral zone. These tumors are generally isointense relative to surrounding peripheral zone tissue on T1-weighted images. The majority of prostate cancers are hypointense on T2-weighted images (Fig. 12.10). In rare instances, tumors may be isointense or hyperintense [21–23]. These tumors frequently contain numerous mucinous elements [23,24]. When isolated to the transition zone, adenocarcinomas may appear heterogeneous,

isointense, or hypointense relative to surrounding tissue [16]. Thus, these lesions may be difficult to differentiate from BPH. Tumors in the peripheral zone demonstrate increased enhancement on immediate postgadolinium fat-suppressed SGE images (Fig. 12.11).

Tumors spread first to penetrate the prostatic capsule (Fig. 12.12). After capsular penetration, tumor extends to the neurovascular bundles and seminal vesicles (Fig. 12.13). Bladder invasion occurs commonly in advanced-

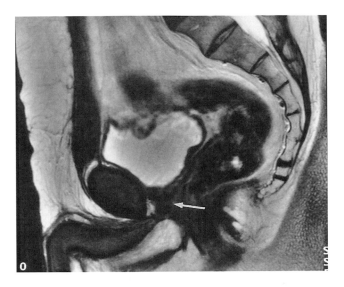

FIG. 12.8 Post-prostatectomy pelvis. Sagittal 512-resolution T2-weighted echo-train spin-echo image. Low-signal-intensity tissue surrounds the posterior urethra within the prostatic bed (*white arrow*) of this patient after prostatectomy. This appearance results from fibrosis and scarring at the operative site.

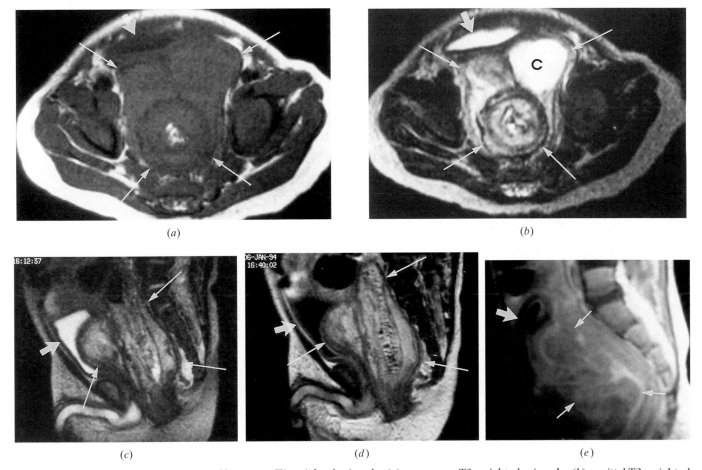

(*a*) (*b*)

(*c*) (*d*) (*e*)

FIG. 12.9 Prostatic rhabdomyosarcoma. Transverse T1-weighted spin-echo (*a*), transverse T2-weighted spin-echo (*b*), sagittal T2-weighted spin-echo (*c*) and sagittal postgadolinium T1-weighted spin-echo (*d*) images. A complex, predominantly solid mass (*long arrows, a–c*) compresses and displaces the bladder anteriorly (*arrow, a–d*). An area of cystic ("*c*",*b*) change within the left aspect of the tumor is shown on the T2-weighted image (*b*). Sagittal immediate postgadolinium SGE image (*e*) in a second patient with prostatic rhabdomyosarcoma. A predominantly solid complex mass (*thin arrows, e*) impresses upon the bladder posteriorly and displaces it anteriorly. There is bladder wall thickening from outlet obstruction (*large arrow, e*).

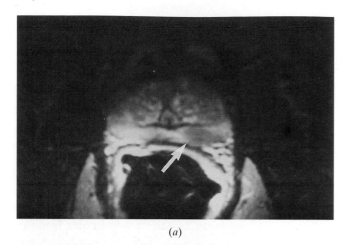

(a)

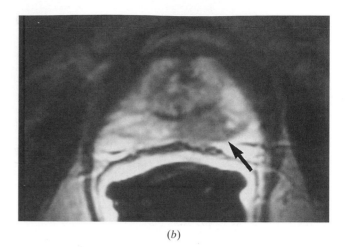

(b)

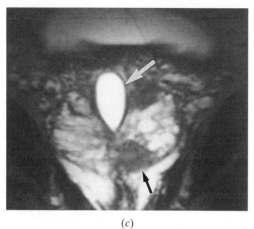

(c)

FIG. 12.10 Prostate adenocarcinoma Stage T2. Transverse T2-weighted echo-train spin-echo endorectal image (*a*). A focus of low signal intensity is seen within the peripheral zone in this patient with Stage T2 adenocarcinoma of the prostate (*arrow*). Endorectal transverse T2-weighted echo-train spin-echo image (*b*) in a second patient with prostate carcinoma. A hypointense tumor is seen within the peripheral zone of the prostate at the level of the apex (*arrow, b*). Endorectal coronal T2-weighted echo-train spin-echo (*c*) in a third patient with prostate carcinoma. A low-signal-intensity focus within the apex of the prostate represents primary adenocarcinoma (*black arrow, c*). Note the incidental, midline utricular cyst, which is high in signal intensity on the T2-weighted image (*white arrow, c*).

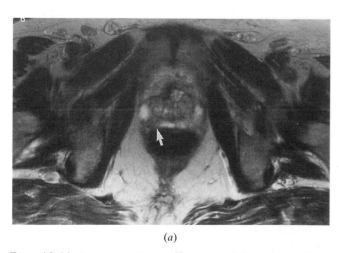

(a)

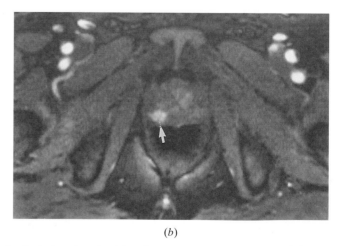

(b)

FIG. 12.11 Prostate carcinoma. Transverse 512-resolution T2-weighted echo-train spin-echo (*a*) and transverse immediate postgadolinium fat-suppressed SGE (*b*) images. High-resolution T2-weighted image (*a*) reveals a well-defined carcinoma within the peripheral zone of the right lobe of the prostate (*arrow, a*). Smaller tumor volume is present within the left lobe (*a*). Immediate postgadolinium image demonstrates enhancement of the tumor focus within the right lobe (*arrow, b*). More ill-defined enhancement is seen within the left lobe (*b*).

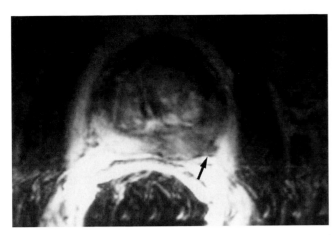

FIG. 12.12 Prostate carcinoma with capsular penetration. T2-weighted echo-train spin-echo endorectal image demonstrates low-signal-intensity tumor within the peripheral zone of the prostate that extends posterolaterally (*arrow*), indicating capsular penetration.

tumor staging is essential for appropriate clinical decision making.

Detection of extracapsular extension precludes radical prostatectomy in the younger patient. A variety of signs have been used to predict Stage C disease by MRI. These include focal contour abnormalities within the prostatic capsule, tumor volume, apical location, broad margins with the prostate capsule, and infiltration of the periprostatic fat [10,24,26,27]. Seminal vesicle invasion is demonstrated by low signal intensity on T2-weighted images (Fig. 12.13). Increased staging accuracy can be achieved with the use of T2-weighted endorectal coil MRI and prostate specific antigen values [28–30].

Identifying invasion of the neurovascular bundles can have important clinical implications because preservation of one or both bundles during radical prostatectomy results in a significantly decreased incidence of postoperative impotency. Identification of direct tumor extension posterolaterally into the neurovascular bun-

stage prostate cancer and may be extensive (Fig. 12.14). The most common sites of metastasis are the bone marrow and lymph nodes. Infiltration of the pelvic lymphatics, particularly the obturator, external and internal iliac chains, precedes distant metastases to the bones and retroperitoneum. Bone marrow in the iliac bones is frequently marbled in signal intensity on T1- and T2-weighted images rendering detection of bone metastases at times problematic. On gadolinium-enhanced fat-suppressed images metastases appear as relatively well-defined focal mass lesions or diffusely enhancing extensive bony infiltration in a low-signal-intensity background of fatty or fibrotic marrow (Fig. 12.15).

Table 12.1 outlines the American Joint Committee on Cancer's TNM staging classification of prostate carcinoma [20]. The American Urological Association staging system, developed by Whitmore and Jewett, assigns alphabetical stages (A through D) to disease extent that corresponds roughly to the primary tumor staging (T1 through T4) of the TNM system [25], which is outlined briefly in Table 12.2. Histologic grading may be by degree of anaplasia, DNA ploidy (diploid, tetraploid, or anaploid), or by Gleason Score, which sums the scores of the two most predominant glandular patterns of the tumor to predict aggressivity.

Currently accepted therapies for Stages A, B, and C disease include radical prostatectomy and radiation therapy, including both external beam irradiation and radioisotope implants. Radical prostatectomy is generally reserved for patients with either Stage A or Stage B disease. Stage D disease is treated palliatively with either hormonal or radiation therapies. Clinical assessment and treatment decisions are based on imaging stage, pathological grade, and prostate specific antigen levels, as well as the patient's age and general state of health. Accurate

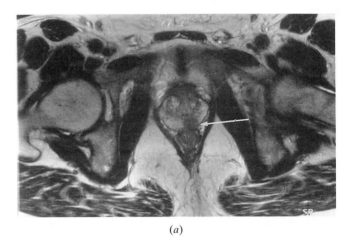

(a)

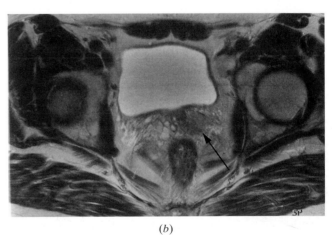

(b)

FIG. 12.13 Prostate cancer with seminal vesicle invasion. Transverse (*a,b*) and sagittal (*c*) 512-resolution T2-weighted echo-train spin-echo images. A 1-cm tumor (*white arrow, a*) within the left aspect of the prostate at the midgland level is low in signal intensity on the T2-weighted image (*a*).

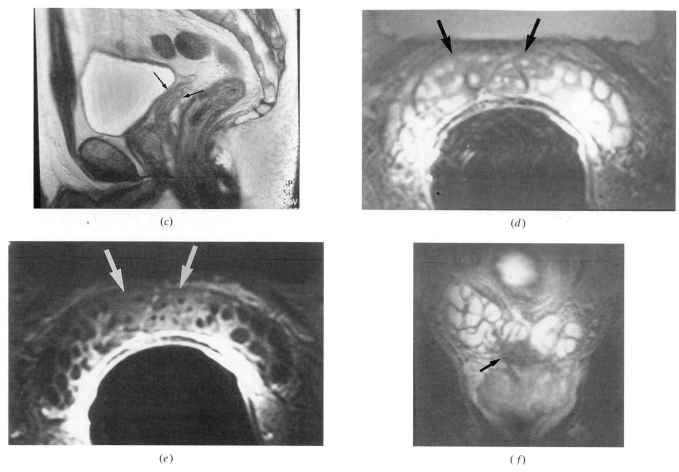

(c)

(d)

(e)

(f)

F IG . 12.13 (*Continued*) The left seminal vesicle (*black arrow, b*) is diffusely low in signal intensity secondary to diffuse tumor involvement. Note the normal high-signal-intensity cluster-of-grapes appearance of the right seminal vesicle (*b*). Loss of normal architecture and diffuse low signal intensity of the left seminal vesicle (*black arrows, c*) is confirmed on the sagittal image (*c*). Transverse T2-weighted echo-train spin-echo endorectal coil (*d*) and postgadolinium T1-weighted fat-suppressed SGE endorectal coil (*e*) images. There is ill-defined low-signal-intensity tissue (*arrows, d*) within the medial aspects of the seminal vesicles on the T2-weighted image (*d*) corresponding to tumor invasion. Loss of the normal architecture of the seminal vesicles, medially (*arrows, e*), indicates tumor invasion on the postgadolinium T1-weighted image (*e*). Coronal T2-weighted echo-train spin-echo endorectal coil image (*f*) in a third patient with seminal vesicle invasion. There is low signal intensity within the inferomedial aspects of the seminal vesicles (*arrow, f*) secondary to tumor invasion.

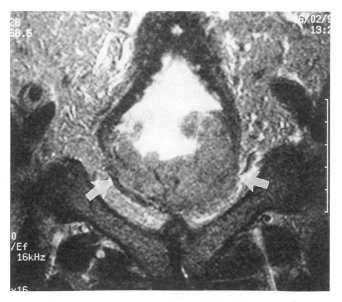

F IG . 12.14 Anaplastic prostate carcinoma. Coronal T2-weighted echo-train spin-echo endorectal coil image. Lobular low-signal-intensity tissue invading the urinary bladder (*arrows*) represents invasive prostate carcinoma in this patient with a normal prostate specific antigen level.

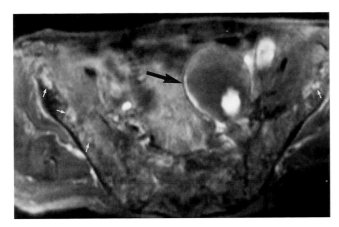

F IG. 12.15 Osseous metastases secondary to prostate carcinoma. Transverse 90-second postgadolinium fat-suppressed SGE image. Metastatic lesions are focal, well-defined enhancing lesions in a background of low-signal-intensity fatty marrow on gadolinium-enhanced fat-suppressed images. Gadolinium-enhanced fat-suppressed technique enables accurate differentiation of enhancing metastatic foci (*white arrows*) from the frequently marbled appearance of normal bone marrow in the older patient. High-signal-intensity intraluminal flow surrounded by low-signal-intensity mural thrombus is seen in an incidental left internal iliac artery aneurysm (*black arrow*).

dles, decreased signal intensity obliterating the rectoprostatic angle, and focal contour abnormalities within the posterolateral aspect of the gland on transverse T2-weighted images have been shown to be valuable in the prediction of neurovascular invasion [31].

Table 12.1 American Joint Committee on Cancer Staging of Prostate

Carcinoma	
Primary Tumor	
T0	No evidence of primary tumor
T1	Clinical inapparent, not visible by imaging
T2	Tumor confined to the prostate (may involve capsule)
T3	Tumor extends beyond capsule (may involve seminal vesicles)
T4	Invasion of adjacent structures other than seminal vesicles (bladder, rectum, levator m.)
Regional Lymph Nodes	
N0	No regional lymph node metastasis
N1	Metastasis in a single node, 2 cm or smaller
N2	Metastasis in a single node between 2 and 5 cm in size, or in multiple nodes each 5 cm or smaller
N3	Metastasis in a single node larger than 5 cm
Distant Metastasis	
M0	No distant metastasis
M1	Distant metastasis (regional nodes, bone, other sites)

Table 12.2 American Urological Association Staging of Prostate Carcinoma

A	Clinical inapparent
B	Tumor confined to the prostate
C	Tumor extends beyond capsule (may involve seminal vesicles)
D	Metastatic disease to pelvic or distant nodes, bones, soft tissues, or organs

Hormonal and radiation therapies may result in low signal intensity within the prostate. Postbiopsy changes also may mask prostate cancer. High signal intensity in the peripheral zone or seminal vesicles on T1- and T2-weighted images reflects postbiopsy hemorrhage, which can thereby conceal underlying tumor. Cryosurgery may result in necrosis and loss of zonal anatomy [26,32]. Because either recent biopsy or cryosurgery may hinder differentiation from residual carcinoma, MRI should generally be delayed at least 3 weeks following intervention [26].

DIFFUSE DISEASE

Prostatic Calcifications

Prostatic calcifications may be either primary or secondary in origin. Primary prostatic calcifications form within the ductal and acinar components of the gland. Acquired calcifications include those arising within the prostatic urethra or secondary to other etiologies, including infection, obstruction, necrosis, and radiation therapy [33].

Calcification appears as a signal-void focus on both T1- and T2-weighted images. Primary prostatic calcifications classically have a curvilinear configuration. Secondary dystrophic calculi are generally larger and more irregular in appearance [8,13,33].

Several age-related changes within the prostate are well-recognized. The peripheral zone enlarges approximately 67 percent, and the central gland, which includes both the central and transitional zones, enlarges approximately 175 percent between the second and eighth decades [34]. Although the zonal anatomy becomes more clearly defined, the periprostatic venous plexus and anterior fibromuscular stroma are less easily distinguished in the older patient [34,35].

INFLAMMATION AND INFECTION

Inflammatory processes of the prostate may be classified as either bacterial or nonbacterial in origin. Gram-negative organisms are responsible for 90 to 95 percent of infectious prostatitis cases. Approximately 80 percent of these result from infection with *Escherichia coli*, whereas

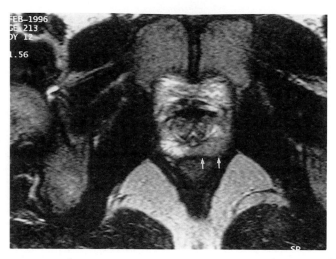

FEB–1996
GE 213
DY 12
1.56

FIG. 12.16 Chronic prostatitis. Transverse 512-resolution T2-weighted echo-train spin-echo image at the midgland level reveals low signal intensity within the peripheral zone of the prostate (*arrows*). This entity may mimic the appearance of carcinoma.

10 to 15 percent are the consequences of klebsiella, serratia, proteus, pseudomonas and enterobacter infections. The remaining cases result from infection by gram-positive organisms, including enterococcus, streptococcus, and staphylococcus [36].

MRI of acute prostatitis frequently reveals an enlarged gland with abnormal signal intensity within the peripheral zone. Low signal intensity on T1-weighted images and higher signal intensity on T2-weighted images are often observed. Areas of inflammation demonstrate diffusely increased signal intensity following the intravenous administration of gadolinium. Infiltration of the adjacent periprostatic fat and involvement of the seminal vesicles are frequent associated findings [8]. Chronic prostatitis results in lesser inflammatory changes. Focal low signal intensity within the peripheral zone may result from chronic granulomatous prostatitis, simulating the MRI appearance of prostate carcinoma (Fig. 12.16) [37].

Abscesses can result in ill-defined, focal enlargement of the prostate that is appreciable on T1- and T2-weighted images. Abscesses are often very high in signal intensity on T2-weighted images. There are frequently associated inflammatory changes in the periprostatic fat [13]. Enhancement of the abscess wall and inflammatory tissue surrounding a signal-void center is demonstrated on gadolinium-enhanced T1-weighted fat-suppressed images.

TRAUMA

Posterior urethral trauma may occur in association with crush injuries or extensive pelvic fracturing. There may be complete disruption of the prostatomembranous urethra with resultant erectile dysfunction and stricture forma-

tion. Demonstration of superior prostatic displacement on imaging studies is useful because it may alter the surgical approach [38].

Disruption of the posterior urethra is identified by urethral discontinuity and a low-signal-intensity band on T2-weighted images. Stricture-associated fibrosis is shown on T1- and T2-weighted images as low-signal-intensity tissue. Sagittal T2-weighted images clearly depict displacement and elevation of the prostatic apex above the pubic symphysis, which may necessitate a suprapubic approach or pubectomy [8,38,39].

■ PENIS AND ANTERIOR URETHRA

NORMAL ANATOMY

The anterior urethra is separated into bulbous and penile portions by the suspensory ligament of the penis. It is surrounded by the *corpus spongiosum*, which in turn is enveloped by a thin layer of the *tunica albuginea*. These structures comprise the ventral compartment of the penis. The dorsal compartment contains the paired *corpora cavernosa*. The two compartments are separated by *Buck's fascia*, which encases both the thin layer of *tunica albuginea* surrounding the ventral compartment and a thicker layer surrounding the dorsal compartment [39].

The posterior portion of the corpus spongiosum expands to form the *bulb* of the penis, which is attached to the urogenital diaphragm. Immediately inferior and lateral to the bulb lies the *bulbospongiosus muscle*. The posterior aspects of the corpora cavernosa form the *crura*, which are attached to the *ischiopubic ramus* and are contiguous with the *ischiocavernosus muscles*, inferomedially [40].

MRI studies should be performed with a circular surface coil or a phased-array multicoil to achieve a good signal-to-noise ratio and spatial resolution. On T1-weighted images both the corpora spongiosa and cavernosa demonstrate homogeneous, medium signal intensity. The corpus spongiosum demonstrates a homogeneous high signal intensity on T2-weighted images, whereas, the corpora cavernosa may demonstrate homogeneous or heterogeneous increases in signal intensity, depending on perfusion distribution (Fig. 12.17). The bulb of the penis is a useful landmark due to its high signal intensity on T2-weighted images.

The urethra and cavernous arteries are identified as low-signal-intensity tubular structures within the centers of the corpus spongiosum and corpora cavernosa, respectively. The fascial layers demonstrate low signal intensity on both T1- and T2 weighted images. Gadolinium

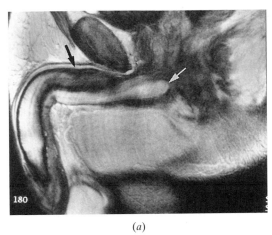

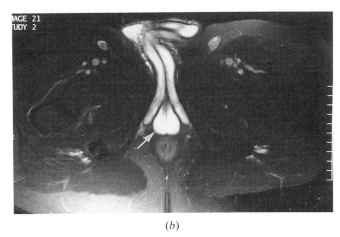

(a)   (b)

F I G . 12.17 Normal penis. Sagittal 512-resolution T2-weighted echo-train spin-echo image (*a*). The corpus cavernosum is high in signal intensity on the T2-weighted image (*black arrow, a*). The high signal intensity of the bulb of the penis is seen posteriorly (*white arrow, a*). A 512-resolution T2-weighted fat-suppressed echo-train spin-echo image (*b*) in a second patient. The bulb of the penis is well-defined as a high-signal-intensity structure (*white arrow, b*).

administration results in an increased signal intensity of both the corpus spongiosum and corpora cavernosa, enabling improved differentiation from the surrounding muscle and fascial layers (Fig. 12.18). Greater delineation of anterior urethral and penile anatomy is achieved with the application of fat saturation techniques.

DISEASE ENTITIES

Congenital Abnormalities

Epispadias is a rare anomaly characterized by absence of the dorsal covering of the distal urethra and ectopic placement of the proximal urethral aperture, which may be located anywhere along the length of the penis. This entity is almost always associated with bladder exstrophy and accompanying pubic diastasis.

MRI reveals separation of the corpora cavernosa and inversion of their normal relationship with the corpus spongiosum at the level of the pubic symphysis. Hence, the urethra assumes a more cephalad position. The detailed anatomic display provided by MRI enables careful surgical planning.

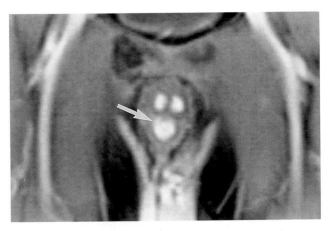

F I G . 12.18 Normal progression of enhancement of the penis. Coronal immediate postgadolinium SGE image. Enhancement of the corpus spongiosum (*arrow*) and corpora cavernosa commences proximally and centrally, as seen on this immediate postgadolinium image. There is subsequent progression of enhancement outward and distally within the erectile bodies.

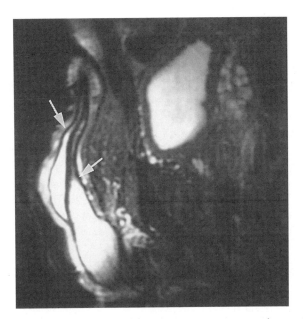

F I G . 12.19 Partial aplasia of the corpora cavernosa and spongiosum. Sagittal T2-weighted echo-train spin-echo image. The distal aspects of the corpora cavernosa and spongiosa are atrophic and demonstrate a dramatic change in caliber (*arrows*) in this patient presenting with distal erectile dysfunction. The patient had other concomitant urogenital anomalies.

Hypospadias denotes a proximal, ventral location of the meatus. Perineal hypospadias is frequently associated with a ventral fibrous band, resulting in a chordee deformity. There may be foreshortening of the urethra with either epispadias or hypospadias [41].

In rare instances, partial aplasia of the corpora cavernosa may lead to erectile dysfunction. Patients frequently have other associated anomalies within the genitourinary tract. Irregularity of length and caliber are well-shown on T2-weighted images (Fig. 12.19). Diphallus is another rare anomaly resulting in partial or complete duplication of the erectile bodies and urethra. Frequently, there is associated shortening of the perineum or asymmetric development of the corpora cavernosa and ischiocavernosus muscles. Again, the detailed anatomic information provided by MRI permits accurate surgical planning. The MRI signal characteristics of the supernumerary corpora are identical to those of normally configured corpora [39,40].

MASS LESIONS

Benign Masses

Penile Prostheses
MRI may be helpful in the postoperative evaluation of penile prostheses. These are identified as tubular structures within the central corpora cavernosa. Solid silicone prostheses appear signal-void on all imaging sequences. Inflatable prostheses, however, follow the signal charac-

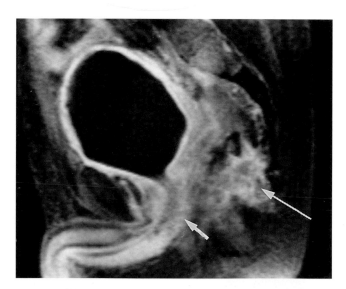

F IG . 12.20 Invasion of prostate and membranous urethra by recurrent rectal carcinoma. Sagittal 90-second postgadolinium fat-suppressed SGE image. Heterogeneously enhancing recurrent rectal carcinoma is seen in the presacral space (*long arrow*). There is invasion of the prostate and membranous urethra (*short arrow*). Note the increased enhancement of the bladder wall secondary to radiation changes.

teristics of the fluid they contain. Progressive decreased signal intensity on T2-weighted images within the corpora cavernosa may reflect the development of fibrosis. Other complications detected by MRI include infection and hematoma formation [39,40].

Malignant Masses

Carcinomas of the urethra and penis are extremely rare, accounting for less than 1 percent of genitourinary cancers in males. Histologic examination reveals squamous-cell carcinoma in more than 95 percent of cases of penile carcinoma. Approximately 78 percent of urethral carcinomas demonstrate this histology, whereas transitional-cell carcinomas constitute approximately 15 percent of tumors. Adenocarcinomas account for 6 percent of cases, and undifferentiated carcinomas the remainder [40,42]. Metastatic penile lesions may result from contiguous spread of prostatic, testicular, bladder, and osseous neoplasms, as well as from disseminated leukemia and lymphoma [39,40].

Primary neoplasms of the urethra and penis demonstrate isointense to low signal intensity relative to the surrounding corpus spongiosum on both T1- and T2-weighted images. Metastatic lesions are also of low or intermediate signal intensity on T1-weighted images, but they may appear hypointense, isointense, or hyperintense relative to the corpus spongiosum on T2-weighted images. Heterogeneous enhancement paralleling the appearance of the remainder of the malignant process is apparent (Fig. 12.20). Regardless of the organ of origin, MRI aids in the delineation of the extent of tumor dissemination, enabling detection of invasion into the corpora cavernosa or tunica albuginea.

DIFFUSE DISEASE

MRI may be employed to evaluate normal and abnormal flow phenomena within the corpora spongiosum and cavernosa. Alteration in the normal vascular flow progression, which extends from the central cavernosal arteries outward and distally, may provide evidence for erectile dysfunction. Vascular disorders may result from impairment of the arterial supply, intracorporeal sinusoids, or venous drainage networks [43].

Amyloid may also affect the anterior urethra. Although the majority of cases represent amyloid secondary to other disease states, very rarely primary amyloid of the urethra occurs, which is identified by immunohistochemical stains. The disease may result in stricture formation and calcified plaques within the anterior urethra [44]. Focal low signal intensity on T2-weighted images may reflect amyloid deposition.

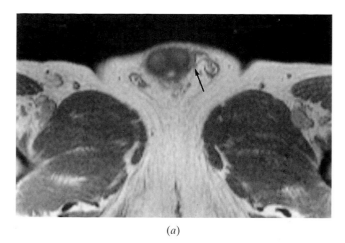
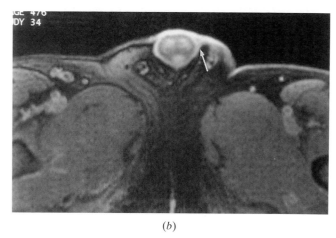

(a)   (b)

F ɪ ɢ . 12.21 Fibrosis of Buck's fascia. Transverse T1-weighted SGE (*a*) and 90-second postgadolinium fat-suppressed SGE (*b*) images. There is increased thickness of the left aspect of Buck's fascia (*black arrow, a*). Note the low-signal-intensity linear markings in the adjacent fat (*a*). The thickened fascia enhances diffusely after gadolinium administration (*white arrow, b*). These changes are compatible with early Peyronie's disease.

INFLAMMATION

Peyronie's disease (induratio penis plastica) is caused by focal inflammation of the tunica albuginea and corpora cavernosa. Resultant fibrosis and plaque formation lead to painful, deviated erections. Various etiologies including trauma, diabetes, gout, and hormonal dysfunction have been implicated in the development of the disease. It is most commonly observed in patients between the ages of 30 and 60 years, although occasional cases have been reported in men younger than 20 [45,46].

On T2-weighted images heterogeneity of the corpora cavernosa may be demonstrated. In addition, low-signal-intensity plaques may be visualized within the corpora cavernosa and tunica albuginea on T1- and T2-weighted images [39,45]. Plaque detection is improved by the administration of gadolinium, with increased enhancement apparent in areas of active inflammation [45].

In rare instances fibrosis may affect Buck's fascia. This entity may be observed in cases of early Peyronie's disease. Alternatively, it may represent extension of fibrosis resulting from other causes including trauma, sustained priapism, and collagen vascular disease (Fig. 12.21).

INFECTION

Urethritis may be secondary to infection with *Neisseria gonococcus, Chlamydia trachomatis, Condylomata acuminatum* or *Mycobacterium tuberculosis*. The periurethral glands of Littre may become distended with bacteria and leukocytes. Spread to adjacent periurethral tissues may lead to abscess formation. Aggressive infections also may result in perineal or scrotal sinus formation [47]. MRI may prove helpful in the detection of these associated complications.

TRAUMA

Penile trauma usually results from direct, blunt injury. The most common finding is a tear in the tunica albuginea. An adjacent hematoma is frequently visualized. There also may be fracture or avulsion of the corpora cavernosa from their ischial attachments.

MRI demonstrates discontinuity of the normal low-signal-intensity ring of the tunica albuginea on T2-weighted images following a tear. Discontinuity between the corpus cavernosum and ischium also results in focal low signal intensity on T2-weighted images. Signal characteristics of associated hematomas reflect the acuity of the traumatic event [38–40]. MRI has been shown to alter surgical planning in as many as 26 percent of cases [38].

■ SEMINAL VESICLES

NORMAL ANATOMY

The seminal vesicles are paired accessory glands located superior to the prostate gland. Each is comprised of a single tube coiled upon itself. It is surrounded by a dense fibromuscular sheet and narrows medially, forming an excretory duct that joins with the vas deferens to form the ejaculatory duct.

Both the width and fluid content of the seminal vesicles increase after puberty, peaking within the fifth and

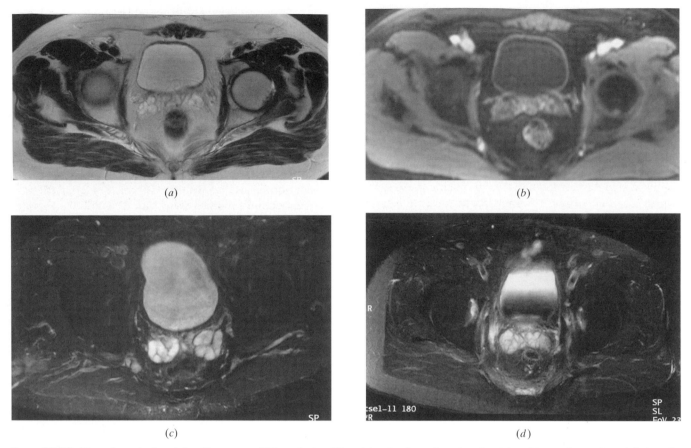

(a)   (b)

(c)   (d)

FIG. 12.22 Normal seminal vesicles. Transverse 512-resolution T2-weighted echo-train spin-echo (a) and immediate postgadolinium fat-suppressed SGE (b) images. High signal intensity is seen within the normal fluid-filled seminal vesicles on the T2-weighted image (a). Fat suppression increases conspicuity of the convoluted walls of the seminal vesicles, which enhance relative to the fluid that they contain (b). Transverse 512-resolution T2-weighted fat-suppressed echo-train spin-echo (c) in a second patient. Normal, fluid-filled seminal vesicles exhibit high signal intensity on T2-weighted images. The low signal intensity of the walls of the tubules gives the glands a cluster-of-grapes appearance. They are clearly demarcated after the application of fat suppression. Transverse 512-resolution T2-weighted fat-suppressed echo-train spin-echo image (d) in a third patient. The seminal vesicles are high in signal intensity on this high-resolution T2-weighted image. Image acquisition after gadolinium administration accounts for the low signal intensity within the dependent portion of the urinary bladder.

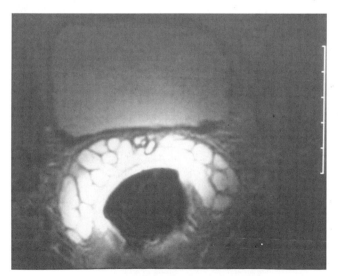

FIG. 12.23 Normal seminal vesicles in the presence of adenocarcinoma of the prostate. Transverse T2-weighted fat-suppressed echo-train spin-echo endorectal coil image. Normal, high signal intensity is present within the seminal vesicles in this patient with Stage T2 adenocarcinoma of the prostate.

sixth decades. On T1-weighted images the seminal vesicles demonstrate homogeneous signal intensity similar to that of muscle tissue. On T2-weighted images the signal intensity varies with the composition of fluid content. In normal men younger than 60 years of age fluid is abundant, and the seminal vesicles appear as high-signal-intensity "cluster of grapes" structures (Fig. 12.22). After the administration of intravenous gadolinium, the convoluted walls of the vesicles enhance. The walls can be more clearly defined with concomitant application of fat saturation techniques. The surrounding walls appear higher in signal intensity than the fluid using these techniques (see Fig. 12.22). The high contrast resolution for the appearance of normally uninvolved seminal vesicles is an important feature in the staging of prostate cancer by MRI (Fig. 12.23).

Beyond 60 years of age fluid content decreases, and the seminal vesicles may appear progressively lower in signal intensity. In the normal process of aging, low signal intensity is symmetric bilaterally and associated with a decrease in size.

DISEASE ENTITIES

Congenital Abnormalities

Congenital abnormalities of the seminal vesicles including ectopia, hypoplasia, and agenesis are frequently associated with other anomalies of the genitourinary tract. Detection of congenital seminal vesicle abnormalities therefore warrants evaluation of the remainder of the genitourinary tract. Congenital seminal vesicle cysts are the most commonly encountered abnormalities. Approximately 80 percent of cases are associated with ipsilateral renal dysgenesis and approximately 8 percent with collecting system duplication. Seminal vesicle cysts are frequently asymptomatic, but may become large enough to cause dysuria, perineal pain, increased frequency, or bladder outlet obstruction [48,49]. Seminal vesicle cysts are easily differentiated from müllerian or utricular cysts on MRI because of their typical lack of connection to the prostate. They are of variable signal intensity on T1-weighted-images and high in signal intensity on T2-weighted images. Variable signal intensity on T1-weighted images reflects the presence of hemorrhage or highly proteinaceous material.

MASS LESIONS

Benign Masses

Vesicular tumors are rare, and among benign mass lesions leiomyomas are the most common histological type. They generally appear well-circumscribed and are of interme-

diate signal intensity on T1-weighted images and high signal intensity on T2-weighted images. In rare cases, lipomas, fibromas, cystadenomas and angiomas may occur in the seminal vesicles.

Malignant Masses

Most malignant disease of the seminal vesicles results from local extension of prostatic, urinary bladder, or rectal carcinomas. Invasion by prostate carcinoma results in loss of normal architecture and decreased signal intensity on T2-weighted images (see Figs. 12.5 and 12.13). Primary malignancies are rare and usually adenocarcinomas. Leiomyosarcomas and fibrosarcomas also have been reported.

DIFFUSE DISEASE

Calcifications within the seminal vesicles are most commonly associated with diabetes mellitus. Less often, calcifications may arise secondary to infectious etiologies, which include tuberculosis and schistosomiasis [49]. Calcifications are low in signal intensity on both T1- and T2-weighted images. Abnormally low signal intensity on T2-weighted images also may be seen following prostatic biopsy [50]. This finding, if confused with tumor invasion, may prevent radical prostatectomy in eligible patients. Senile amyloidosis of the seminal vesicles is a common finding at autopsy. Appearing as low signal intensity on T2-weighted images, it also can mimic malignancy (Fig. 12.24) [24,51].

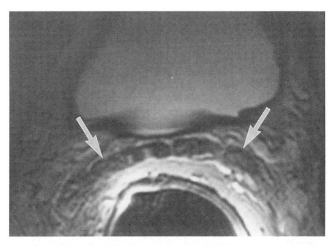

FIG. 12.24 Amyloidosis of the seminal vesicles. Transverse T2-weighted echo-train spin-echo endorectal coil image. There is bilateral decreased signal intensity of the seminal vesicles secondary to amyloid deposition (*arrows*).

INFECTION

Infection of the seminal vesicles is diagnosed primarily on the basis of clinical presentation. Patients usually have associated prostatitis or epididymitis. Rare, isolated infection of the seminal vesicles classically results in hemospermia. Signal characteristics on MR images therefore reflect the presence or absence of blood products. The acutely inflamed gland also may appear enlarged and of lower signal intensity than the contralateral side. Chronic infection may result in fibrosis with concomitant loss of fluid content and a resultant decrease in signal intensity on T1- and T2-weighted images. Abscess formation may manifest as an ill-defined focus of decreased signal intensity on T1-weighted images.

■ TESTES, EPIDIDYMIS, AND SCROTUM

NORMAL ANATOMY

The testes lie within the *scrotum*, a sac comprised of internal cremasteric and external fascial layers, dartos muscle, and skin. They are encased by the *tunica albuginea*, a fibrous capsule that invaginates into the testis posteriorly to form the *mediastinum testis*. The *processus vaginalis* represents an extension of peritoneum, projecting between the tunica albuginea and dartos layers. The posterior testis and mediastinum testis are not undermined by the tunica vaginalis, resulting in the bare area through which vascular structures and tubules pass. Approximately 400 to 600 *seminiferous tubules* are coiled within each testis. These converge to form the *rete testis* and, ultimately, the *efferent ductules*. The efferent ductules form the epididymal head posterior to the testis. They then unify into a single coiled duct representing the epididymal body. The narrowed tail of the epididymis ultimately leads into the vas deferens.

MRI TECHNIQUE

MRI studies should be performed with a phased-array surface coil or a circular surface coil overlying the testes, which should be elevated above a folded towel placed between the thighs. The testes are clearly demarcated on both T1- and T2-weighted images by the low signal intensity of the surrounding tunica albuginea. The testes are homogeneous and isointense to muscle on T1-weighted images and higher in signal intensity on T2-weighted images. The mediastinum testis can be identified as a low-signal-intensity band within the posterior testis on T2-weighted images. Low-signal-intensity fi-

brous projections emanating from the mediastinum testis represent septulae, which divide the testis into lobules. The gubernaculum may be recognized on T2-weighted images as a low-signal-intensity curvilinear rim along the inferoposterior aspect of the testis. The signal intensity of the epididymis is slightly heterogeneous and hypo- to isointense to the testis on T1-weighted images. The epididymis is more clearly differentiated from the testis on T2-weighted images because it is lower in signal intensity than the adjacent testis. Gadolinium administration results in hyperintensity of the epididymis relative to the testis [52].

DISEASE ENTITIES

Congenital Abnormalities

Congenital abnormalities of the testes include unilateral or bilateral hypoplasia and agenesis, as well as duplication and cryptorchidism. Congenitally duplicated testes may be classified by their location within the scrotum, inguinal canal, or retroperitoneum. Supernumerary scrotal testes are usually associated with duplication of the vas deferens and epididymis. There may be an associated ipsilateral inguinal hernia. Inguinal testes have duplicated draining systems in the majority of cases and also may have associated inguinal hernias. Retroperitoneal testes, frequently occurring near the deep inguinal ring, are always associated with ipsilateral inguinal hernias. They may or may not demonstrate separate draining structures. Polyorchia is associated with an increased incidence of testicular malignancy [53].

Cryptorchidism
MRI may be employed to localize a clinically suspected undescended testis. The testes normally descend into the scrotum during the 8th month of gestation, accounting for the increased incidence of cryptorchidism in premature births. Approximately 80 percent of undescended testes are located distal to the external inguinal ring [54]. A significant number of cryptorchid testes will descend spontaneously during an infant's first year of life. Fibrosis and impaired spermatogonia have been observed in undescended testes not surgically corrected by 2 years of age. Hence, as a result of subsequent increased incidences of both infertility and carcinoma, it is recommended that orchiopexy be performed between the first and second years of life [55,56].

Undescended testes demonstrate low signal intensity on T1-weighted images and intermediate to high signal intensity on T2-weighted images. Low signal intensity on T2-weighted images may be observed in more fibrotic or atrophic testes [12,56]. Identification of the undescended testis may be aided by identifying the mediastinum testis as a low-signal-intensity structure on T2-weighted images and recognizing that undescended testes often have a

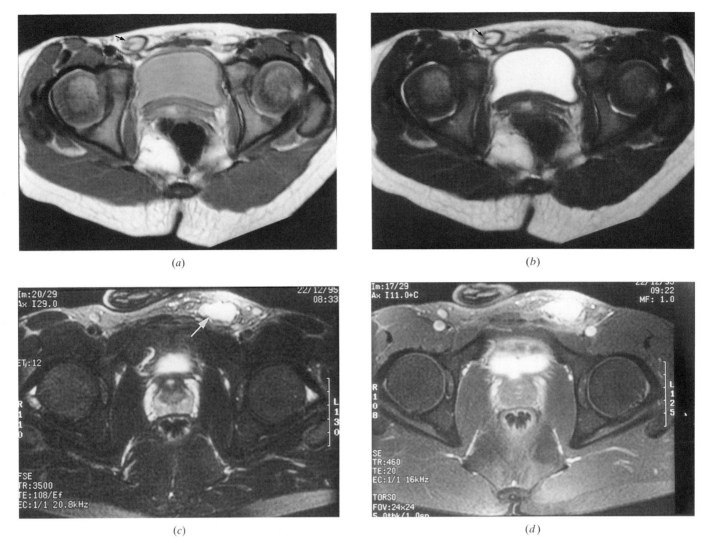

(a)   *(b)*

(c)   *(d)*

FIG. 12.25 Cryptorchidism. Transverse T1-weighted spin-echo (*a*) and T2-weighted echo-train spin-echo (*b*) images. The undescended testis within the right inguinal canal is intermediate to high in signal intensity on both T1- and T2-weighted images. The mediastinum testis is shown as a low-signal-intensity transverse band (*arrow, a,b*). Transverse T2-weighted fat-suppressed echo-train spin-echo (*c*) and transverse T1-weighted postgadolinium fat-suppressed SGE (*d*) images in a second patient. The undescended testis in the left inguinal canal (*arrow, c*) is high in signal intensity on both T2-weighted and postgadolinium T1-weighted images. Note the greater transverse than antero-posterior dimension of the ovoid testis, aiding differentiation from inguinal adenopathy.

larger transverse than antero-posterior (AP) diameter (Fig. 12.25). In comparison, lymph nodes usually have a larger AP than transverse diameter. The low-signal-intensity remnant of the gubernaculum testis on coronal T2-weighted images also serves as a helpful landmark because the testis frequently lies along its medial border [56].

MASS LESIONS

Benign Masses

Testicular Prostheses

Testicular prostheses usually contain silicone. The older, fluid-filled silicone prostheses demonstrate low signal intensity on both T1- and T2-weighted images. Newer prostheses are composed of solid elastomers and demonstrate signal characteristics similar to those of native testes: They are of intermediate signal intensity on T1-weighted images and of high signal intensity on T2-weighted images. They are generally recognized by the presence of chemical-shift artifact and the absence of spermatic cord or other scrotal structures [57].

Cystic Lesions

Intratesticular cysts may be solitary or multiple and may occur in up to 10 percent of the male population. They are characterized by distinct margins and most commonly demonstrate simple fluid signal characteristics [12].

Seminiferous tubular ectasia in the region of the rete

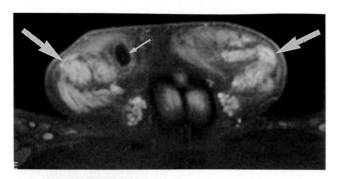

FIG. 12.26 Spermatocele and bilateral varicoceles. Transverse gadolinium-enhanced T1-weighted fat-suppressed spin-echo image demonstrates a nonenhancing ovoid structure within the right epididymal head consistent with a spermatocele (*small arrow*). There are also bilateral, enhancing varicoceles (*large arrows*).

testis may produce ovoid lesions in continuity with the edge of the testis. These cystic lesions, which contain spermatozoa, are bilateral in approximately 71 percent of cases and associated with an ipsilateral spermatocele in approximately 92 percent of cases. Centered at the mediastinum testis, they are contiguous with the adjacent spermatocele along the bare area of the testis. Seminiferous tubular ectasia is lower in signal intensity than the normal surrounding testis on T1-weighted images and nearly isointense to the surrounding testis on T2-weighted images. It has been postulated that pure intratesticular cysts originate from progressive seminiferous tubular ectasia [58]. Occasionally, cysts also may be localized to the tunica albuginea [52].

Epididymal cysts can occur along the length of the epididymis. They contain simple fluid and are low in signal intensity on T1-weighted images and high in signal intensity on T2-weighted images [12]. Spermatoceles, small cystic structures that occur most commonly in the epididymal head, may be either solitary or multiloculated. They demonstrate variable signal intensity, depending on the presence of spermatozoa, fat, lymphocytes, and cellular debris (Fig. 12.26) [12,59].

Benign Neoplasms

Only 5 percent of testicular neoplasms are benign. Of these, 90 percent are nongerm-cell tumors. They may arise from Leydig cells, Sertoli cells, or connective tissue stroma [59].

The most common extratesticular neoplasm is the adenomatoid tumor. It most commonly arises in the epididymis, but may be located in the spermatic cord or tunica. Adenomatoid tumor may be round and well-defined (Fig. 12.27) or occasionally, plaque-like and less well-defined [60,61]. Lipomas also may arise within the spermatic cord. They demonstrate high signal intensity on T1-weighted images and follow the signal intensity of other adipose tissues on T2-weighted images [62]. As

with other fatty lesions, loss of signal intensity on fat-suppressed images is a diagnostic finding.

The paratesticular tissues also may harbor benign, fibroproliferative tumors classified as fibrous pseudotumors. They are the second most common extratesticular neoplasm after adenomatoid tumors. They may originate from the tunica albuginea or vaginalis, spermatic cord, or epididymis [63], and their etiology is uncertain [64,65].

Patients most commonly present with painless masses. Slightly less than half of fibrous pseudotumors are associated with hydroceles or hematoceles [63]. These masses are frequently lobulated, demonstrating frond-like projections, but they also may be characterized by circumferential thickening of the tunica albuginea. They are low in signal intensity on both T1- and T2-weighted images and enhance negligibly with gadolinium [62,63].

Other Benign Scrotal Lesions

Fluid may accumulate between the parietal and visceral layers of the tunica vaginalis, producing hydroceles, pyoceles, or hematoceles. Hydroceles may occur in association with infection, tumor, or trauma. They demonstrate signal characteristics typical of simple fluid, and are low in signal intensity on T1-weighted images, high in signal intensity on T2-weighted images, and nearly signal-void on postgadolinium images (Fig. 12.28). Pyoceles may appear complicated with heterogeneous low signal intensity on T1-weighted images and heterogeneous high signal intensity on T2-weighted images. Hematoceles may exhibit varied signal characteristics, depending on the chronicity of the blood products they contain.

Varicoceles may occur as the result of thrombosis or extrinsic compression of the testicular venous system by organomegaly or retroperitoneal masses. They are more commonly left-sided as a result of testicular vein drainage into the left renal vein, which is lengthier and more prone to compression than the right testicular vein. MRI reveals multiple serpiginous structures in the region of the pampiniform plexus, epididymal head, and spermatic cord. Signal intensity is dependent on flow velocity. Varicoceles often appear intermediate in signal intensity on T1-weighted images and higher in signal intensity on T2-weighted images [12,59,62]. On early postgadolinium gradient-echo images varicoceles are well-shown as high-signal-intensity tubular structures (Fig. 12.29). Varicoceles often exist with hydroceles (Fig. 12.29).

Scrotal hernias are most frequently diagnosed by clinical inspection. MRI evaluation may prove helpful in equivocal cases, particularly when there is marked associated pain or when physical examination is limited.

The MRI appearance of the hernia may vary with its contents. A complex mass is frequently visualized within an enlarged inguinal canal. Mesenteric fat, loops of bowel, and intraluminal air may be visualized within the scrotal sac. Imaging with a half Fourier single-shot turbo

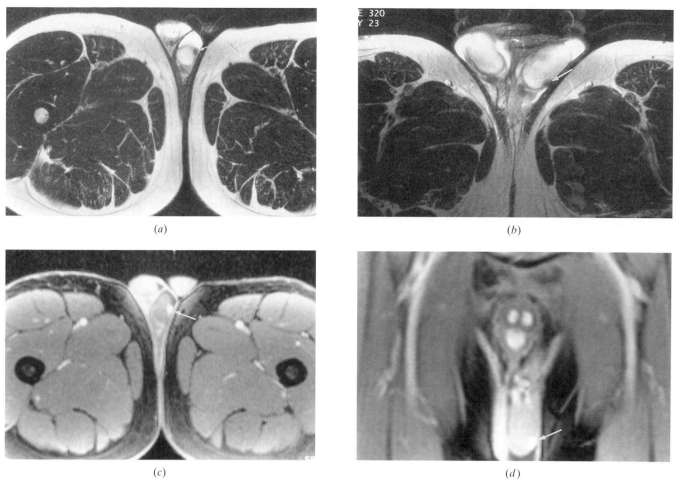

(a)   (b)

(c)   (d)

F IG. 12.27 Adenomatoid neoplasm. Transverse phased-array body coil 512-resolution T2-weighted echo-train spin-echo (*a*), transverse circular surface coil 512-resolution T2-weighted echo-train spin-echo (*b*), transverse phased-array body coil T1-weighted immediate postgadolinium fat-suppressed SGE (*c*), and coronal phased-array coil T1-weighted immediate postgadolinium fat-suppressed SGE images (*d*). The tumor is hypointense to the normal surrounding testis on T2-weighted imaging (*arrow, a,b*). After the administration of gadolinium, there is immediate increased enhancement of the tumor relative to the surrounding testis (*arrow, c,d*). Note that the higher signal-to-noise ratio of the circular surface coil permits higher spatial resolution imaging (*b*) compared to the phased-array body coil (*a*). This is useful for imaging superficial structures such as the testicles.

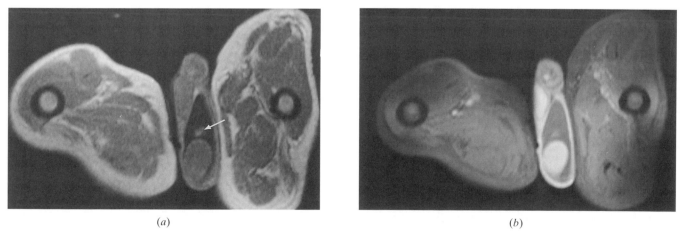

(a)   (b)

F IG. 12.28 Hydrocele. Transverse T1-weighted SGE (*a*) and transverse 1-minute postgadolinium T1-weighted fat-suppressed SGE (*b*) images. A left-sided hydrocele is low in signal intensity on the T1-weighted image (*a*). A focus of high signal intensity within the fluid represents the spermatic cord (*arrow, a*). There is uniform enhancement of the testes on the postgadolinium image (*b*).

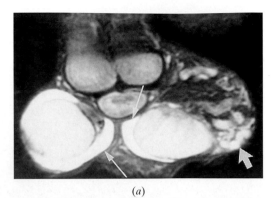

(a)

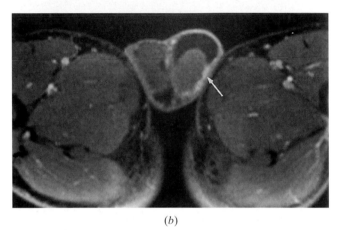

(b)

FIG. 12.29 Varicocele with bilateral hydroceles. Coronal T2-weighted echo-train spin-echo image (*a*) demonstrates high-signal-intensity, serpiginous structures within the left scrotal sac representing a varicocele (*thick arrow, a*). There are also bilateral hydroceles (*thin arrows, a*). Transverse 90-second postgadolinium fat-suppressed SGE image (*b*) in a second patient with a varicocele and bilateral hydroceles. High-signal-intensity tubular structures represent a varicocele (*arrow, b*).

spin-echo (HASTE) and immediate postgadolinium fat-suppressed spoiled gradient-echo (SGE) sequence may provide helpful information regarding entrapped bowel viability.

Malignant Masses

Although testicular carcinomas comprise less than 1 percent of tumors in the male population, a significant number of these occur in males under the age of 40 years, and approximately 95 percent are malignant [66,67]. Early detection and treatment are crucial, particularly for seminomas, which are chemotherapy and radiotherapy sensitive.

Testicular carcinomas may be divided into germ-cell and nongerm-cell subtypes. Approximately 95 percent of malignant neoplasms are of germ-cell origin [68]. These include seminomas (approximately 40%) and nonseminomatous tumors. Nonseminomatous tumors may be subclassified into embryonal carcinomas (~30%), terato-

carcinomas (~25%), teratoma (10%), and choriocarcinomas (1%). Another 30 percent of the cases are of mixed histology [69]. The remainder are comprised of Sertoli, Leydig, or mesenchymal-cell carcinomas. There may also be involvement by leukemia, lymphoma, or in rare instances, metastatic disease from lung, melanoma, genitourinary, or gastrointestinal malignancies [59,68]. Lymphatic drainage of the testes follows the gonadal vessels to the retroperitoneum. In the presence of epididymis or spermatic cord invasion, lymphatic drainage also extends to the pelvic nodes. Tumors are staged according to TNM criteria as outlined in Table 12.3 [70].

MRI of testicular neoplasms may reveal relative enlargement of the involved testis. Tumors are low in signal intensity on T2-weighted images, and there is degradation of normal testicular morphology. Lack of visualization of the normal septulae has been found to be a sensitive indicator of malignant infiltration [62].

Seminomas are isointense to normal tissue on T1-weighted images and hypointense to normal tissue on T2-weighted images. They most commonly demonstrate homogeneous low signal intensity on T2-weighted images (Fig. 12.30) [54,62]. They may exhibit lobulation or, occasionally, central necrosis [62,67]. Tumors enhance to a lesser degree than normal testicular tissue. Thus, gadolinium administration may increase lesion conspicuity and aid detection of extension into the surrounding tunica albuginea [52,62].

Nonseminomatous tumors appear more heterogeneous on T2-weighted images, and have more ill-defined margins (Fig. 12.31). Areas of increased and decreased

Table 12.3 American Joint Committee on Cancer Staging of Testicular Carcinoma

Carcinoma	
Primary Tumor	
T0	No evidence of primary tumor
T1	Tumor limited to testis, including rete testis
T2	Tumor extends beyond tunica albuginea or into epididymis
T3	Tumor invades spermatic cord
T4	Tumor invades scrotum
Lymph Nodes	
N0	No lymph node metastasis
N1	Metastasis to a single lymph node 2 cm or smaller
N2	Metastasis to a single lymph node between 2 and 5 cm in size, or to multiple nodes each 5 cm or smaller
N3	Metastasis to a single lymph node larger than 5 cm
Distant Metastases	
M0	No distant metastases
M1	Distant metastases

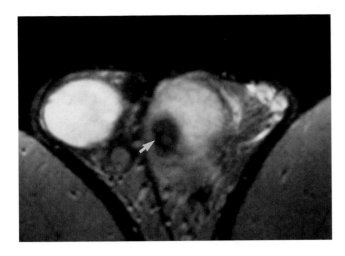

F IG . 12.30 Testicular seminoma. T2-weighted fat-suppressed echo-train spin-echo image using a surface coil demonstrates a well-defined, homogeneously low-signal-intensity, one cm semionoma (*arrow*) arising in the left testicle. (Courtesy of Evan S. Siegelman, M.D.)

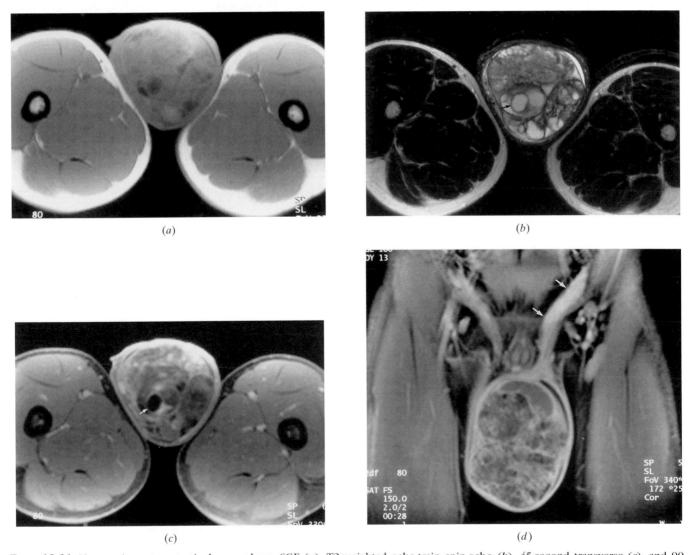

(*a*)

(*b*)

(*c*)

(*d*)

F IG . 12.31 Non-seminomatous testicular neoplasm. SGE (*a*), T2-weighted echo-train spin-echo (*b*), 45-second transverse (*c*), and 90-second coronal (*d*) gadolinium-enhanced fat-suppressed SGE images. The left testicle is greatly enlarged, measuring 5 cm in diameter. Tumor replaces the testicle and is mildly heterogeneous on the T1-weighted image (*a*) and considerably heterogeneous on the T2-weighted image (*b*). The tumor contains multiple cystic spaces that are well-defined, high signal intensity foci (*arrow, b*) on the T2-weighted image, and show lack of enhancement on the postgadolinium images (*arrow, c*). The coronal image demonstrates the vertical size of the tumor and enlargement of testicular vessels in the left inguinal canal (*arrows, d*).

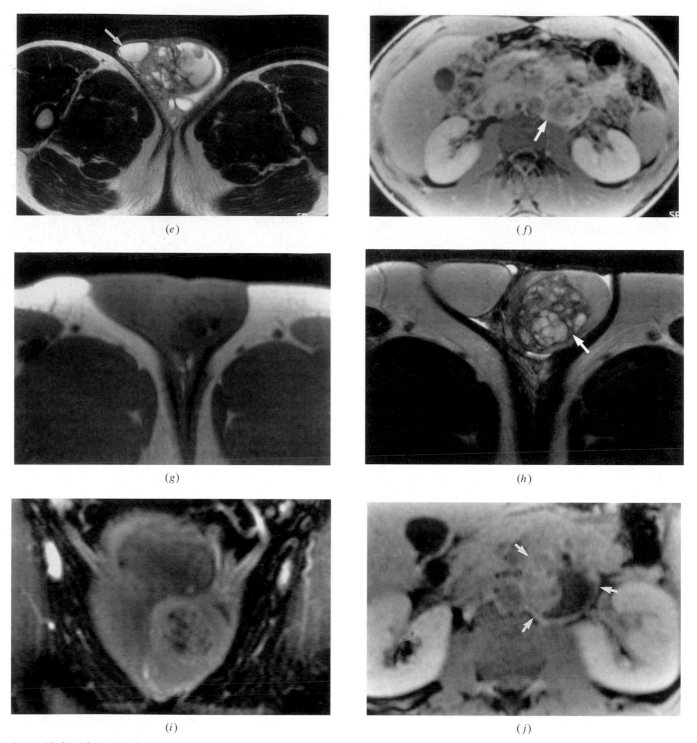

FIG. 12.31 (*Continued*) T2-weighted echo-train spin-echo image (*e*) from a more superior tomographic section through the scrotum demonstrates a normal high signal intensity right testicle (*arrow, e*). On a 3 minute postgadolinium fat-suppressed SGE image (*f*) a 3 cm left para-aortic lymph node (*arrow, f*) is present at the level of the left renal hilum that demonstrates a similar heterogeneous appearance to the primary tumor. SGE (*g*), T2-weighted echo-train spin-echo (*h*), and coronal interstitial phase gadolinium enhanced fat-suppressed SGE (*i*) images in a second patient. A 2.5 cm tumor is present in the left testicle (*arrow, h*). The appearance is similar to the prior case. Note in particular the well-defined high signal intensity foci within the mass on the T2-weighted image (*h*). Heterogeneous appearance of the involved left para-aortic lymph nodes on the interstitial phase gadolinium-enhanced fat-suppressed SGE (*arrows, j*) is also comparable.

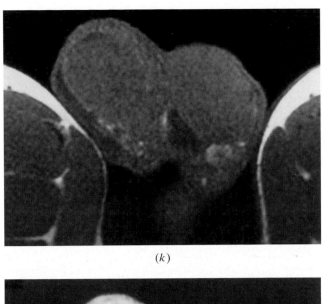

(k)

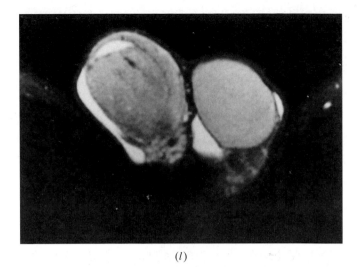

(l)

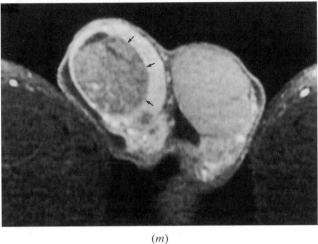

(m)

FIG. 12.31 (*Continued*) T1-weighted spin-echo (*k*), T2-weighted echo-train spin-echo (*l*), and gadolinium-enhanced T1-weighted spin-echo (*m*) images in a third patient. The tumor in this patient is mixed embryonal carcinoma/seminoma. The tumor has a relatively homogeneous and mildly low signal intensity on the T2-weighted image (*l*). Tumor enhancement is slightly heterogeneous on postgadolinium images (*m*) and has a relatively sharp margination (*arrows, m*) from background testicle.

signal intensity on T1- and T2-weighted images correspond to foci of hemorrhage and necrosis, respectively, on histologic specimens [54,67]. These features are most marked within tumors demonstrating mixed histologies [62,67].

TESTICULAR TORSION

Acute testicular torsion arises when the bare area is not sufficiently broad to anchor the testis and its supporting structures in place, resulting in a "bell clapper" deformity. It results in irreversible ischemia in less than 30 percent of cases if diagnosis and surgical correction occur within 12 hours of the event. The salvage rate decreases rapidly thereafter with minimal surgical success following 24 hours of ischemia [71]. Ultrasound and nuclear medicine examinations enable timely diagnosis in the acute setting. However, bilateral orchiopexy is still indicated in the subacute period, when findings may be equivocal with either of these modalities. In the setting of subacute torsion, MRI may provide assistance in differentiating this entity from epididymo-orchitis.

Common findings on MRI in the subacute setting include an enlarged spermatic cord with diminished flow, diffusely decreased signal intensity of the testis, decreased testicular size, and mild to moderate thickening of the tunica albuginea and epididymis [71]. There also may be increased-signal-intensity foci on T1-weighted images, reflecting hemorrhage, visualization of the pedicular attachment of the testicle in a bell-clapper deformity, or an associated hematocele. The identification of a whirling pattern within the spermatic cord and an associated low-signal-intensity knot at the point of maximal torsion on T2-weighted images provides specific evidence for the diagnosis [62,71]. Initial studies with P-31 MR spectroscopy in an animal model have revealed additional promise for the evaluation of testicular torsion in the acute setting [72].

INFECTION

The vast majority of acute epididymitis cases are isolated, but up to 20 percent may be associated with orchitis [59]. Therapy is conservative and limited to antibiotics unless there is concomitant infarction from extensive edema or abscess formation necessitating surgery [71]. With the exception of mumps orchitis, isolated acute infection of the testes is rare [36]. When pyogenic abscesses occur, they are frequently accompanied by pyoceles [59,71].

On MRI, epididymal inflammation is most commonly manifested by generalized enlargement of the organ [52,62]. The involved epididymis may be hyperintense on T1-weighted images and of variable signal intensity relative to the contralateral side on T2-weighted images [52,59,62]. There is heterogeneous enhancement after gadolinium administration [52].

Testicular inflammation also is commonly manifested by generalized enlargement (Fig. 12.32) [12,52,71]. There is frequently decreased signal intensity of the involved testis on T2-weighted images [52,59,62]. The testicular septulae remain well-defined but thickened, a finding that is in contrast to the loss of normal architecture frequently observed with invasive neoplastic disease [62]. Intense enhancement of the involved testis is seen after gadolinium administration [52]. Abscesses are accompanied by pyoceles in the majority of patients [71]. Heterogeneous high signal intensity on T2-weighted images is observed both in these extratesticular fluid collections and in the infected fluid intercalating between the testicular septulae (Fig. 12.33) [62].

Acute inflammation often results in enlargement and edema of the spermatic cord [52,71]. However, in contrast to the avascularity of the cord observed in cases of torsion, there is increased vascularity of the cord in the setting of infection. On gadolinium-enhanced images, there is marked enhancement of the inflamed structure and surrounding tissues [52]. These findings serve as helpful differentiating factors in equivocal cases. Identi-

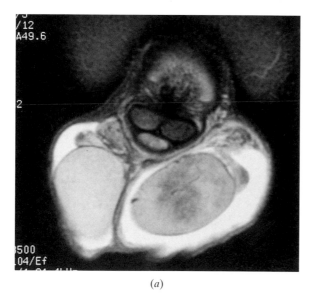

(a)

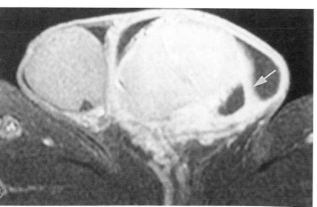

(c)

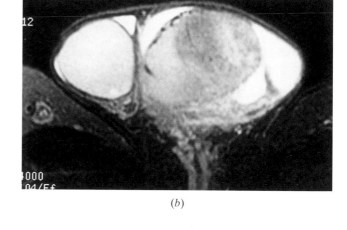

(b)

FIG. 12.32 Mumps orchitis. Coronal T2-weighted fat-suppressed echo-train spin-echo (*a*), transverse T2-weighted fat-suppressed echo-train spin-echo (*b*), and T1-weighted postgadolinium fat-suppressed spin-echo (*c*) images. There is enlargement of the left testis relative to the contralateral side (*b,c*). The affected testis is heterogeneous and low in signal intensity on the T2-weighted images (*a,b*) and enhances slightly more than the unaffected testis on the postgadolinium image (*c*). Note the enhancing, thickened septations within the scrotal sac (*arrow, c*). There are accompanying hydroceles, bilaterally.

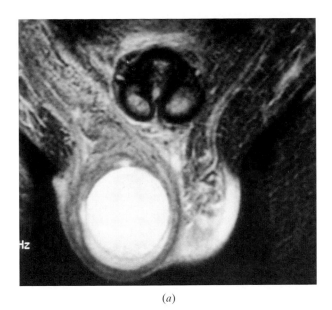
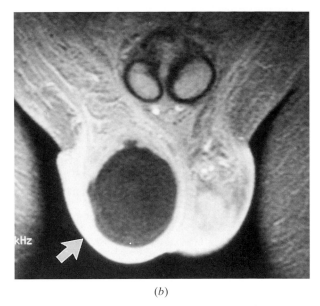

(a)   (b)

F I G . 12.33 Testicular abscess. Coronal T2-weighted echo-train spin-echo (*a*) and gadolinium-enhanced T1-weighted spin-echo (*b*) images. A complex fluid collection within the right testis is heterogeneously high in signal intensity on the T2-weighted image (*a*) and heterogeneously low in signal intensity on the postgadolinium T1-weighted image, which is consistent with an abscess. There is extensive enhancement of the surrounding scrotal tissues secondary to adjacent inflammatory changes (*arrow, b*).

fication of the bare area of the testis also virtually excludes the possibility of a bell-clapper deformity, and thus of torsion as well [71].

TRAUMA

MRI may provide information important for clinical management following testicular trauma. Hemorrhage is well-demonstrated on T1- and T2-weighted images. Intratesticular hematomas may appear high in signal intensity on T1-weighted images and variable in signal intensity on T2-weighted images [52,62]. They may also result in alternating bands of increased and decreased signal intensity on T1-weighted images [62]. Blood intersecting between the layers of the tunica vaginalis may result in hematoceles, which also follow the signal intensity of blood products.

Contusion in the absence of focal hemorrhage may also be detected by MRI. There is a resultant decrease in signal intensity of the involved testis on T2-weighted images, as well as a relative decrease in gadolinium enhancement [52].

Careful inspection of the tunica albuginea is necessary to evaluate for the possibility of acute testicular rupture. This may be manifested by discontinuity in the normal low signal intensity of the tunica albuginea on T2-weighted images. Detection of testicular rupture often necessitates surgical intervention [62].

FUTURE DIRECTIONS

The high signal-to-noise ratio, spatial resolution, and lack of difficulty with localization achievable with endorectal coils for prostate disease and surface coils for testicular disease have resulted in clinical applicability of spectroscopy for distinguishing prostate cancer from fibrosis and testicular cancer from other disease entities [72–74].

CONCLUSIONS

MRI is an effective modality for detecting the full range of disease entities involving the male pelvis due to high intrinsic soft tissue contrast resolution, high spatial resolution, and multiplanar imaging. The greatest role for MRI has been in the staging of prostate cancer. The variety of diagnostic options and uncertainty in patient outcome following therapeutic intervention has limited the widespread use of MRI in this setting. Although MRI is excellent at evaluating testicular disease, the lower cost and acceptable accuracy of other imaging approaches has relegated MRI to a problem-solving modality.

REFERENCES

1. Mirowitz SA, Heiken JP, Brown JJ: Evaluation of fat saturation technique for T2-weighted endorectal coil MRI of the prostate. Magn Reson Imaging 12:743–747, 1994.

2. Nunes LW, Scheibler MS, Rauschning W, Schnall MD, Tomaszewski JE, Pollack H, Kressel H: The normal prostate and periprostatic structures: Correlation between MR images made with an endorectal coil and cadaveric microtome sections. AJR Am J Roentgenol 164:923–927, 1995.

3. Hricak H, White S, Vigneron D, et al: Carcinoma of the prostate gland: MR imaging with pelvic phased-array coils versus integrated endorectal-pelvic phased-array coils. Radiology 193:703–709, 1994.

4. McDermott VG, Meakem III TJ, Stolpen AH, Schnall MD: Prostatic and periprostatic cysts: Findings on MR imaging. AJR Am J Roentgenol 164:123–127, 1995.

5. Nghiem HT, Kellman GM, Sandberg SA, Craig BM: Cystic lesions of the prostate. Radiographics 10:635–650, 1990.

6. Thurnher S, Hricak H, Tanagho EA: Müllerian duct cyst: Diagnosis with MR imaging. Radiology 168:25–28, 1988.

7. Gevenois PA, Van Sinoy ML, Sintzoff Jr SA, Stallenberg B, Salmon I, Regemorter GV, Struyven J: Cysts of the prostate and seminal vesicles: MR findings in 11 cases. AJR Am J Roentgenol 155:1021–1024, 1990.

8. Hricak H: The prostate gland. In Hricak H, Carrington BM (eds.). MRI of the Pelvis. Norwalk: Appleton & Lange, pp. 249–312, 1991.

9. Keetch DW, Andriole GL: Medical therapy for benign prostatic hyperplasia. AJR Am J Roentgenol 164:11–15, 1995.

10. Kahn T, Burrig K, Schmitz-Drager B, Lewin JS, Furst G, Modder U: Prostatic carcinoma and benign prostatic hyperplasia: MR imaging with histopathologic correlation. Radiology 173:847–851, 1989.

11. Schiebler ML, Tomaszewski JE, Bezzi M, Pollack HM, Kressel HY, Cohen EK, Altman HG: Prostatic carcinoma and benign prostatic hyperplasia: Correlation of high resolution MR and histopathologic findings. Radiology 172:131–137, 1989.

12. Fritzsche PJ, Wilbur MJ: The male pelvis. Semin Ultrasound CT MR 10:11–28, 1989.

13. Chang Y, Hricak H: Magnetic resonance imaging of the prostate gland. Semin Ultrasound CT MR 9:343–351, 1988.

14. Way WG, Brown JJ, Lee JKT, Gutierrez E, Andriole GL: MR imaging of benign prostatic hypertrophy using a Helmholtz-type surface coil. Magn Reson Imaging 10:341–349, 1992.

15. Lovett K, Rifkin MD, McCue PA, Choi H: MR imaging characteristics of noncancerous lesions of the prostate. J Magn Reson Imaging 2:35–39, 1992.

16. Sommer FG, Nghiem HV, Herfkens R, McNeal J: Gadolinium-enhanced MRI of the abnormal prostate. Magn Reson Imaging 11:941–948, 1993.

17. Phillips M, Kressel H, Spritzer C, et al: Prostatic disorders: MR imaging at 1.5 T. Radiology 164:386–392, 1987.

18. Hricak H, Thoeni R: Neoplasms of the prostate gland. In Pollack H (ed.). Clinical Urography. Philadelphia: WB Saunders. pp. 1382–1383, 1990.

19. Hricak H: Imaging prostatic carcinoma. Radiology 169:569–571, 1988.

20. American Joint Committee on Cancer: Prostate. In Manual for Staging Cancer (4th ed.). Philadelphia: Lippincott, pp. 181–183, 1992.

21. Schnall M, Imai Y, Tomaszewski J, Pollack H, Lenkinski R, Kressel H: Prostate cancer: Local staging with endorectal surface coil MR imaging. Radiology 178:797–802, 1991.

22. Carter H, Brem R, Tempany C, Yang A, Epstein J, Walsh P, Zerhouni E: Nonpalpable prostate cancer: Detection with MR imaging. Radiology 178:523–525, 1991.

23. Outwater E, Schiebler M, Tomaszewski J, Schnall M, Kressell H: Mucinous carcinomas involving the prostate: Atypical findings at MRI. J Magn Reson Imaging 2:597–600, 1992.

24. Schiebler M, Schnall M, Pollack H, Lenkinski R, Tomaszewski J, Wein A, Whittington R: Current role of MR imaging in the staging of adenocarcinoma of the prostate. Radiology 189:339–352, 1993.

25. Steinfeld A: Questions regarding the treatment of localized prostate cancer. Radiology 184:593–598, 1992.

26. Quinn S, Franzini D, Demlow T, Rosencrantz D, Kim J, Hanna R, Szumowski J: MR imaging of prostate cancer with an endorectal surface coil technique: Correlation with whole mount-specimens. Radiology 190:323–327, 1994.

27. Harris R, Schned A, Heaney J: Staging of prostate cancer with endorectal MR imaging: Lessons from a learning curve. Radiographics 15:813–829, 1995.

28. Huch Boni R, Boner J, Debatin J, Trinkler F, Knonagel H, Von Hochstetter A, Helfenstein U, Krestin G: Optimization of prostate carcinoma staging: Comparison of imaging and clinical methods. Clin Radiol 50:593–600, 1995.

29. Huch Boni R, Boner J, Lutolf U, Trinkler F, Pestalozzi D, Krestin G: Contrast-enhanced endorectal coil MRI in local staging of prostate carcinoma. J Comput Assit Tomogr 19(2):232–237, 1995.

30. Huch Boni R, Meyenberger C, Pok Lundquist J, Trinkler F, Lutolf U, Krestin G: Value of endorectal coil versus body coil MRI for diagnosis of recurrent pelvic malignancies. Abdom Imaging 21:345–352, 1996.

31. Tempany C, Rahmouni A, Epstein J, Walsh P, Zerhouni E: Invasion of the neurovascular bundle by prostate cancer: Evaluation with MR imaging. Radiology 181:107–112, 1991.

32. Kalbhen CL, Hricak H, Shinohara K, et al: Prostate carcinoma: MR imaging findings after cryosurgery. Radiology 198:807–811, 1996.

33. McCollum RW, Banner MP: Calculous disease of the urinary tract. In Pollack H (ed.). Clinical Urography. Philadelphia: WB Saunders, pp. 1908–1912, 1990.

34. Allen KS, Kressel HY, Arger PH, Pollack HM: Age-related changes of the prostate. AJR Am J Roentgenol 152:77–81, 1989.

35. Hricak H, Dooms GC, Jeffrey RB, et al: Prostatic carcinoma: Staging by clinical assessment, CT, and MR imaging. Radiology 162:331–336, 1987.

36. Rifkin M: Inflammation of the lower genitourinary tract: The prostate, seminal vesicles and scrotum. In Pollack H (ed.). Clinical Urography. Philadelphia: WB Saunders, pp. 940–960, 1990.

37. Gevenois PA, Stallenberg B, Sintzoff SA, Salmon I, Van Regemorter G, Struyven J: Granulomatous prostatitis: A pitfall in MR imaging of prostatic carcinoma. Eur Radiol 2:365–367, 1992.

38. Narumi Y, Hricak H, Armenakas NA, Dixon CM, McAninch JW: MR imaging of traumatic posterior urethral injury. Radiology 188:439–443, 1993.

39. Hricak H, Marotti M, Gilbert TJ, Lue TF, Wetzel LH, McAninch JW, Tanagho EA: Normal penile anatomy and abnormal penile conditions: Evaluation with MR imaging. Radiology 169:683–690, 1988.

40. Hricak H: The penis and male urethra. In Hricak H, Carrington BM (eds.). MRI of the Pelvis. Norwalk: Appleton & Lange, pp. 383–416, 1991.

41. Amis ES, Newhouse JH: Essentials of uroradiology. Boston: Little, Brown, & Company p. 69, 1991.

42. McCollum RW: Urethral neoplasms. In Pollack HM (ed.). Clinical Urography. Philadelphia: WB Saunders, pp. 1406–1409, 1990.

43. Kaneko K, De Mouy EH, Lee BE: Sequential contrast-enhanced MR imaging of the penis. Radiology 191:75–77, 1994.

44. Noone T, Clark R: Primary, isolated urethral amyloidosis. Abdom Imag In press.

45. Helweg G, Judmaier W, Buchberger W, Wicke K, Oberhauser H, Knapp R, Ennemoser O, Zur Nedden D: Peyronie's disease: MR findings in 28 patients. AJR Am J Roentgenol 158:1261–1264, 1992.

46. Schneider HJ, Rufendorff EW, Rohrborn C: Pathogenesis, diagnosis, and therapy of induratio penis plastica. Int Urol Nephrol 17:235–244, 1985.

47. Di Santis D: Urethral inflammation. In Pollack H (ed.). Clinical Urography. Philadelphia: WB Saunders, pp. 925–939, 1990.

48. King BF, Hattery RR, Lieber MM, Berquist TH, Williamson Jr B, Hartman GW: Congenital cystic disease of the seminal vesicle. Radiology 178:207–211, 1991.

49. King BF, Hattery RR, Lieber MM, Williamson Jr B, Hartman GW, Berquist TH: Seminal vesicle imaging. Radiographics 9:653–676, 1989.

50. Mirowitz S: Seminal vesicles: Biopsy-related hemorrhage simulating tumor invasion at MR imaging. Radiology 185:373–376, 1992.

51. Ramchandani P, Schnall MD, LiVolsi VA, Tomaszewski JE, Pollack HM: Senile amyloidosis of the seminal vesicles mimicking metastatic spread of prostatic carcinoma on MR images. AJR Am J Roentgenol 161:99–100, 1993.

52. Muller-Leisse C, Bohndorf K, Stargardt A, et al: Gadolinium-enhanced T1-weighted imaging of scrotal disorders: Is there an indication for MR imaging? J Magn Reson Imaging 4:389–395, 1994.

53. Hancock RA, Hodgins TE: Polyorchidism. Urology 24:303–307, 1984.

54. Johnson JO, Mattrey RF, Philipson J: Differentiation of seminomatous from nonseminomatous testicular tumors with MR imaging. AJR Am J Roentgenol 154:539–543, 1990.

55. Giwercman A, Grindsted J, Hansen B, et al: Testicular cancer risk in boys with maldescended testis: A cohort study. J Urol 138:1214–1216, 1987.

56. Kier R, McCarthy S, Rosenfield AT, Rosenfield NS, Rapoport S, Weiss RM: Nonpalpable testes in young boys: Evaluation with MR imaging. Radiology 169:429–433, 1988.

57. Semelka R, Anderson M, Hricak H: Prosthetic testicle: Appearance at MR imaging. Radiology 173:561–562, 1989.

58. Tartar VM, Trambert MA, Balsara ZN, Mattrey RF: Tubular ectasia of the testicle. AJR Am J Roentgenol 160:539–542, 1993.

59. Hricak H: The testis. In Hricak H, Carrington BM (eds.). MRI of the Pelvis. Norwalk: Appleton & Lange, pp. 343–382, 1991.

60. Faysal MH, Strefling A, Kosek JC: Epididymal neoplasms: A case report and review. J Urol 129:843–844, 1983.

61. Pavone-Macaluso M, Smith PH, Bagshaw MA: Testicular cancer and other tumors of the genitourinary tract. New York: Plenum Press, 1985.

62. Cramer BM, Schiegel E, Thuroff J: MR imaging in the differential diagnosis of scrotal and testicular disease. Radiographics 11:9–21, 1991.

63. Grebenc ML, Gorman JD, Sumida FK: Fibrous pseudotumor of the tunica vaginalis testis: Imaging appearance. Abdom Imaging 20:379–380, 1995.

64. Sajjad SM, Azizi MR, Llamas L: Fibrous pseudotumor of the testicular tunic. Urology 19:86–88, 1982.

65. Parveen T, Fleischmann, J, Petrelli M: Benign fibrous tumor of the tunica vaginalis testis. Arch Pathol Lab Med 116:277–280, 1992.

66. Parker SL, Tong T, Bolden S, Wingo PA: Cancer statistics, 1996. CA Cancer J Clin 65:5–27, 1996.

67. Reinges MHT, Kaiser WA, Miersch WD, Vogel J, Reiser M: Dynamic MRI of benign and malignant testicular lesions: Preliminary observations. Eur Radiol 5:615–622, 1995.

68. Richie JP: Detection and treatment of testicular cancer. CA Cancer J Clin 43:151–175, 1993.

69. Mostofi FK: Proceedings: Testicular tumors: Epidemiologic, etiologic, and pathologic features. Cancer 32:1186–1201, 1973.

70. American Joint Committee on Cancer: Testis. In Manual for Staging Cancer (4th ed.). Philadelphia: Lippincott, pp. 187–189, 1992.

71. Trambert MA, Mattrey RF, Levine D, Berthoty DP: Subacute scrotal pain: Evaluation of torsion versus epididymitis with MR imaging. Radiology 175:53–56, 1990.

72. Tzika AA, Vigneron DB, Hricak H, Moseley ME, James TL, Kogan BA: P-31 MR spectroscopy in assessing testicular torsion: Rat model. Radiology 172:753–757, 1989.

73. Chew W, Hricak H: P-31 MRS of human testicular function and viability. Invest Radiol 24:997–1000, 1989.

74. Cornel E, Smits G, Oosterhof G, Karthaus H, Deburyne F, Schalken J, Heerschap A: Characterization of human prostate cancer, benign prostatic hyperplasia and normal prostate by in vitro ^{1}H and ^{31}P magnetic resonance spectroscopy. Urology 150:2019–2024, 1993.

CHAPTER 13

FEMALE URETHRA AND VAGINA

L. B. EISENBERG, M.D. AND S. M. ASCHER, M.D.

■ FEMALE URETHRA

Evaluation and diagnosis of pathology involving the female urethra has been challenging and difficult due to the poor specificity of clinical symptoms and the lack of a suitable imaging modality. MRI has proven to be the most sensitive modality for detection and staging of benign and malignant urethral pathology.

MRI TECHNIQUE

Routine imaging for urethral pathology should include transverse, high-resolution, small field-of-view T1-weighted images before and after intravenous contrast administration, particularly in cases of suspected tumor. The addition of fat suppression may increase conspicuity of disease. Orthogonal transverse and sagittal T2-weighted images are also routinely obtained [1].

Normal Anatomy

The female urethra originates at the trigone of the bladder and terminates anterior to the opening of the vagina. It is a thin-walled muscular channel and measures approximately 4 cm in length. On transverse T2- and enhanced T1-weighted images the female urethra demonstrates a

"target" appearance with a low-signal-intensity outer ring, a high-signal-intensity middle ring, and a low-signal-intensity central dot (Fig. 13.1) [1]. The dark outer ring likely corresponds to both the outer striated and inner longitudinal and circular smooth muscle layers [1,2,3]. The middle high-signal-intensity ring is thought to represent the vascular submucosal layer [1], whereas the dark central dot is believed to represent the mucosal layer. This target appearance is seen more commonly in the middle urethra than in the proximal or distal urethra. The low-signal-intensity outer layer thins toward the distal urethra.

On enhanced T1-weighted images, the most common pattern seen is marked enhancement in the middle submucosal layer with little to no enhancement of the remaining urethra [1,4].

CONGENITAL LESIONS

Congenital anomalies include abnormalities of number, morphology, or both.

Duplication
Urethral duplication may occur alone or in concert with duplication of the bladder. Associated genital abnormalities also have been described. Surface coil imaging and postcontrast T1-weighted fat-suppressed SGE techniques

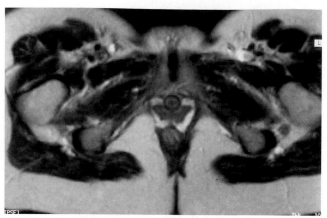

FIG. 13.1 Normal urethra. T2-weighted echo-train spin-echo image. Note the central low-signal-intensity mucosal layer, higher-signal-intensity surrounding submucosal layer, and low-signal-intensity outer ring representing the muscular layer.

may be useful in the evaluation of suspected urethral duplication.

Diverticula

Urethral diverticula may be congenital or acquired and is discussed fully in the Inflammatory Conditions section.

MASS LESIONS

Benign Masses

Urethral papillomas are benign lesions in the spectrum of venereal condylomas, which occur just inside or on the outside of the external meatus [3]. The MRI appearance of these lesions has not yet been described. These lesions, however, are usually visible clinically, and imaging is not necessary.

Malignant Masses Lesions

Carcinomas of the urethra are uncommon lesions that occur in middle-aged or older women. These lesions tend to originate in the external meatus or surrounding tissues. Most urethral carcinomas are of squamous-cell origin, but transitional-cell carcinomas and adenocarcinomas also occur [3]. In rare instances, metastases from renal-cell carcinoma and melanoma may be seen. Patients often present with advanced disease owing to nonspecific symptomatology combined with difficulty in detecting lesions clinically. A TNM staging approach is used for urethral carcinomas (Table 13.1). Urethral carcinoma spreads contiguously to adjacent tissues and then lymphatically to distant sites. Nodal involvement relates to the initial location of the tumor. Anterior urethral lesions usually involve the inguinal nodes with subsequent

Table 13.1 TNM Staging for Female Urethral Carcinoma

Primary Tumor	
Tx	Primary tumor cannot be assessed
T0	No evidence of primary tumor
Tis	Carcinoma in situ
T1	Tumor invades subepithelial connective tissue
T2	Tumor invades periurethral muscle
T3	Tumor invades the bladder neck or anterior vaginal wall
T4	Tumor invades other adjacent organs
Regional Lymph Nodes	
Nx	Regional lymph nodes cannot be assessed
N0	No regional lymph node metastasis
N1	Metastasis in one lymph node is 2 cm or smaller
N2	Metastasis in one node in between 2 and 5 cm in size
N3	Metastasis in one node is larger than 5 cm
Metastases	
Mx	Distant metastases cannot be assessed
M1	No distant metastases
M2	Distant metastases

spread to pelvic nodal groups. Posterior urethral lesions, in contrast, tend to involve pelvic nodes initially [1,5].

The combination of transverse T2- and T1-weighted images before and after contrast administration provides complementary information (Fig. 13.2). T2-weighted images are useful for depicting tumor invasion of the muscular wall of the vagina and pelvic floor. Postgadolinium T2-weighted sequences provide a novel approach for assessing bladder base involvement, especially in the coronal and sagittal planes. The low signal intensity of concentrated gadolinium on T2-weighted images contrasts with the high signal intensity of tumor involvement of the bladder. T1-weighted images, on the other hand, demonstrate extension into periurethral fat [4]. Although proven to be a sensitive modality for this entity, MRI is limited by difficulty in differentiating tumor from secondary inflammatory change, which can lead to overestimation of disease extent [1,4].

INFLAMMATORY CONDITIONS

Diverticula

Urethral diverticula are saccular outpouchings from the urethra, which are thought to originate from dilated periurethral glands [6]. They are often asymptomatic but can become infected, form stones, or less often, cause dyspareunia, dribbling, or a palpable mass [6]. These lesions often are difficult to diagnose because of the nonspecific

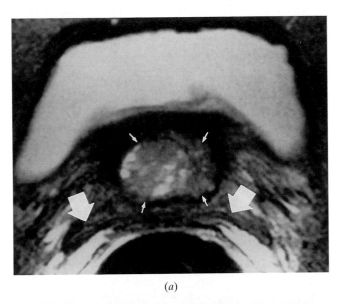

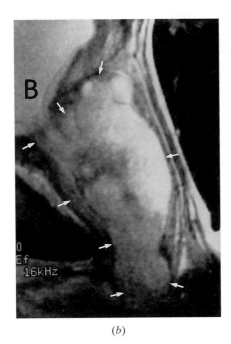

(a)

(b)

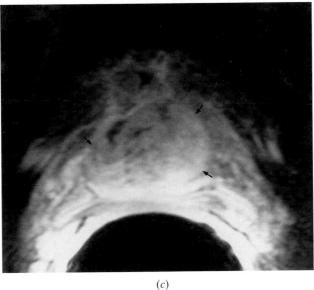

(c)

FIG. 13.2 Urethral carcinoma. Transverse (*a*) and sagittal (*b*) T2-weighted fat-suppressed echo-train spin-echo and transverse interstitial-phase gadolinium-enhanced T1-weighted fat-suppressed spin-echo (*c*) images obtained using an endorectal coil. A bulky urethral carcinoma is present, that is hetergeneous in signal intensity on T2-weighted image (*arrows, a*). The full extent of the tumor is clearly shown from the external meatus to the base of the bladder (''*B*'',*b*) on the sagittal phase image (*arrows, b*). Moderately heterogeneous enhancement of the tumor is shown on the postgadolinium image (*arrows, c*). The vagina (*large arrows, a*) is noted to be separate from the tumor. (Courtesy of Evan S. Siegelman, M.D.)

symptoms. Traditional evaluation for urethral diverticula has been done with voiding cystourethrography, double-balloon urethrography, and/or urethroscopy [1]. These modalities are not always successful. Ultrasound has been advocated by some as an economical way to evaluate this condition, but ultrasound may not be able to distinguish a diverticulum from vaginal cysts and Gartner's duct cysts, nor can it localize the ostium of the diverticulum [7,8].

MRI is an excellent imaging modality for evaluating symptomatic urethral diverticulum. Its accuracy and sensitivity exceeds both urethrography and urethroscopy, and MRI has the added advantage of visualizing the sur-

rounding anatomy [8]. MRI findings include an enlarged urethra with a focal area of low signal intensity on T1-weighted images and high signal intensity on T2-weighted images corresponding to the diverticulum. Multiplanar T2-weighted images are useful for the accurate localization of diverticula (Fig. 13.3). Gadolinium-enhanced T1-weighted fat-suppressed images have proven useful in demonstrating the cystic nature of diverticula. Contrast-enhanced images may also detect the presence of granulation tissue or carcinoma [8]. Carcinomas arising within diverticula are very rare and most often adenocarcinomas, reflecting the ductal origin of the diverticula [8,9].

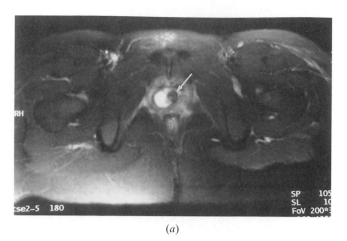

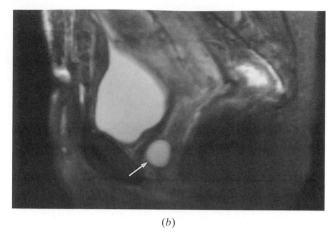

(a)   (b)

FIG. 13.3 Urethral diverticulum. Axial (*a*) and sagittal (*b*) T2-weighted fat-suppressed echo-train spin-echo images. The axial image (*a*) shows the high-signal-intensity diverticulum surrounding the lower-signal-intensity urethra (*arrow*), which is displaced laterally. The sagittal image (*b*) demonstrates the high-signal-intensity diverticulum (*arrow*), which projects posteriorly and causes mass effect on the adjacent vagina.

Caruncle

Urethral caruncles are benign, painful, small inflammatory masses that typically occur in older women and arise on or near the external meatus. The MRI appearance of this lesion has not been described.

Strictures

Urethral strictures in females are exceedingly rare. MRI has been helpful in the evaluation of stricture disease in men, but the role in women has not been described.

Collagen Injection

Collagen injection into the periurethral tissues may be performed as a means of controlling stress incontinence. Periurethral collagen is well-shown on T2-weighted images and appears high in signal intensity (Fig. 13.4) [10].

■ THE VAGINA

The high contrast resolution, large field of view, and multiplanar capability renders MRI superior to CT imaging and ultrasound for evaluation of many benign and malignant conditions of the vagina. In addition, the lack of invasiveness and added extraluminal anatomic detail makes MRI preferable to vaginography for evaluation of congenital anomalies.

MRI TECHNIQUE

As in the evaluation of the pelvis in general, T2-weighted images are critical because they differentiate the layers of the vaginal wall to the best advantage. T1-weighted images are complementary, particularly combining fat suppression with contrast administration. The transverse plane is ideal for evaluation of pathology with respect to the vaginal wall, and sagittal plane imaging demonstrates the relationship with bladder and rectum. Coronal images can demonstrate levator ani muscle involvement. Thin (≤5 mm) sections are preferable [4]. Patients should be asked to remove tampons before imaging to avoid obscuring detail (Fig. 13.5).

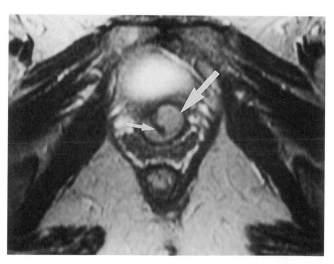

FIG. 13.4 Periurethral collagen injection. Transverse T2-weighted spin-echo image demonstrates high-signal-intensity collagen (*large arrow*) surrounding the low-signal-intensity urethra (*small arrow*).

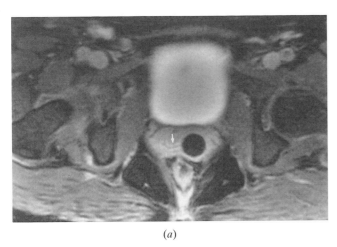

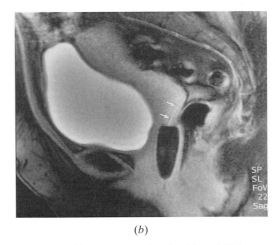

(a) (b)

F IG . 13.5 Tampon. Axial (*a*) and sagittal (*b*) postgadolinium fat-suppressed SGE image. Tampons are signal-void on MR images. They distort the vaginal anatomy and interfere with visualization of surrounding tissue. Enhancing vaginal mucosa is apparent (*arrows, a,b*).

NORMAL ANATOMY

The vagina is a muscular tube lying between the bladder and rectum. The upper one-third is derived from müllerian duct fusion, whereas the lower two-thirds originate from the urogenital sinus [11]. T2-weighted images of the vagina demonstrate high signal intensity centrally due to the presence of intraluminal fluid and mucus, and the wall of the vagina is largely low in signal intensity reflecting the muscular layers of the wall. The surrounding high-signal-intensity pelvic fat provides excellent contrast with the vagina (Fig. 13.6) [2,12]. The thickness of the central high-signal-intensity area has been shown to cor-

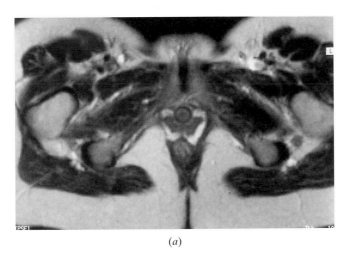

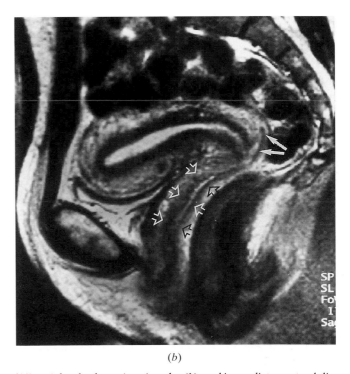

(a) (b)

F IG . 13.6 Normal vagina. Transverse T2 echo-train spin-echo (*a*), sagittal T2-weighted echo-train spin-echo (*b*), and immediate postgadolinium fat-suppressed SGE (*c*) images. On the T2-weighted images the low-signal-intensity muscular wall and the central higher-signal-intensity mucosal layer of the vagina are apparent. The transverse T2-weighted image (*a*) shows vagina clearly demarcated by surrounding fat. The relationship of the urethra and rectum to the vagina is well-seen. The sagittal T2-weighted image (*b*) shows vagina (*open arrows*) as well as the posterior vaginal fornix (*closed arrows*).

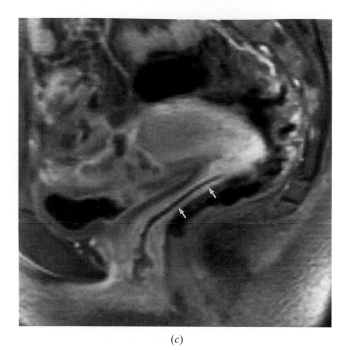

(c)

FIG. 13.6 (*Continued*)   Relationship with uterus and cervix is well-seen. On the immediate postgadolinium fat-suppressed image (*c*), intense enhancement of vaginal mucosa (*arrows, c*) is present.

relate with estrogen levels and becomes more prominent during the late proliferative and early secretory phases. A thick mucus-containing region is also seen in infants less than 1 month old [12]. Pregnant patients often have medium to high signal intensity of the mucus layer, vaginal wall, and surrounding tissues. In contrast, premenarchal females and postmenopausal females have a low-signal-intensity wall and a very thin high-signal-intensity mucus layer. The anterior, posterior, and lateral fornices of the vagina surround the cervix and are best seen on sagittal and transverse images. For descriptive purposes, it is useful to divide the vagina into thirds. The upper third is considered to be at the level of the lateral fornices, the middle third at the level of the base of the bladder, and the lower third at the level of the urethra [4,12]. After gadolinium administration, the vaginal wall enhances, and occasionally, a low-signal-intensity line is present centrally, which may represent the lumen or inner epithelial layer [4,13].

CONGENITAL LESIONS

Congenital and developmental anomalies of the vagina can be divided into four categories: absence and partial absence, duplication and partial duplication, abnormalities of gonadal differentiation, and ambiguous genitalia.

MRI provides a noninvasive method of determining the presence of the uterus, cervix, vagina, gonads, and penile bulb and thus is ideally suited for evaluation of these abnormalities [12,14–16].

Vaginal agenesis and partial agenesis are rare conditions that are classified under the larger category of Müllerian duct anomalies. The incidence of all Müllerian duct anomalies in women has been reported to be 1 to 15 percent [17]. One in 4,000 to 5,000 women are estimated to have vaginal agenesis [14,18]. These patients typically have normal ovaries and external genitalia, but can have associated abnormalities of the uterus, cervix, upper urinary tract, and skeleton. If no functioning endometrium is present, these patients will often present with primary amenorrhea. If functioning endometrium is present, however, patients present after menarche with pain and mass effect from hematometra [14,18].

The surgical management of these patients is determined by the presence of functioning endometrium and a cervix. Complete vaginal agenesis with no functioning endometrium and only a small uterine bulb is treated with vaginoplasty. If the uterine bulb contains functioning endometrium, vaginoplasty along with open surgery to remove the uterine remnant are required to prevent endometriosis. When complete agenesis is accompanied by a uterus with endometrium but no cervix, hysterectomy and vaginoplasty are required. If patients have a partial vaginal agenesis with a normal uterus and cervix, creation of an external vaginal opening alone is required, and pregnancy is possible [18].

Mayer-Rokitansky-Küster-Hauser syndrome is the name given to the müllerian duct anomaly with vaginal and uterine agenesis, normal tubes and ovaries, and variable urinary tract anomalies (Fig. 13.7). Uterine and/or vaginal rudiments may be present, and documentation of their presence is also important for planning of the surgical approach [15]. Vaginal agenesis, partial agenesis, and cloacal abnormalities (Fig. 13.8) are best imaged using MRI. Five-mm thick T2-weighted transverse image accurately demonstrate agenesis, and in cases of partial agenesis, combined transverse and sagittal images delineate vaginal length, which is important in surgical planning [4,12,14,15]. MRI also shows the presence or absence of the uterus, cervix, and kidneys. Exquisite sensitivity in evaluating blood makes MRI ideal for identifying functioning endometrium.

Duplication and partial duplication of the vagina are typically seen in association with the didelphys anomaly of the uterus. This anomaly is well-seen on transverse T2-weighted images. (A more complete discussion of uterine anomalies is present in Chapter 14 on the Uterus and Cervix.)

Abnormalities of gonadal differentiation include true hermaphroditism and gonadal dysgenesis. True hermaphrodites have both ovarian and testicular tissues,

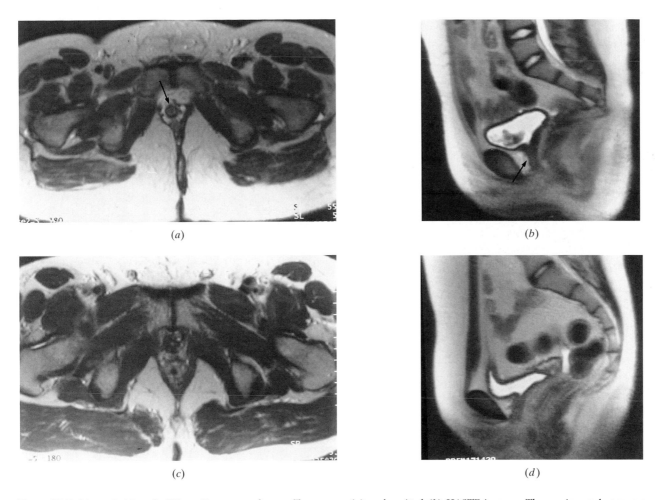

(a)

(b)

(c)

(d)

F IG. 13.7 Mayer-Rokitansky-Küster-Hauser syndrome. Transverse (*a*) and sagittal (*b*) HASTE images. The vagina and uterus are absent, and the urethra (*arrow, a,b*) is more posteriorly positioned than normal. Partial absence of the sacrum with abnormal elevation of the pelvic floor is present. Transverse 512-resolution echo-train spin-echo (*c*) and sagittal HASTE (*d*) images in a second patient demonstrate similar findings of absent vagina and uterus with posterior positioned urethra.

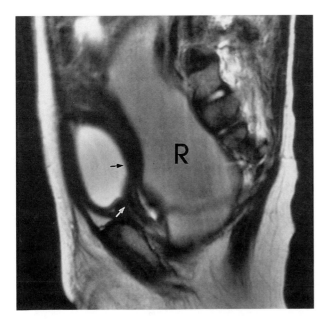

F IG. 13.8 Vaginal agenesis in patient with surgically repaired persistent cloaca. Sagittal HASTE image. No vagina is seen. The urethra (*white arrow*) is elongated and superiorly positioned. The bladder has a thickened wall (*black arrow*). The reconstructed rectum (*R*) is dilated.

which can exist together as an ovotestis or in separate discrete gonads [4,19,20]. Although the internal genitalia is variable, most patients have a uterus. Ovatestes and testes are often intra-abdominal or cryptorchid, whereas ovaries are typically intra-abominal [19]. Most (80%) have XX karyotype, with the remaining 20 percent evenly divided between XY and mosaic karyotypes [19,20]. Development of the internal ducts usually corresponds with the gonad on that side [4]. Sex assignment of true hermaphrodites is usually made by the external genitalia, which are variable in appearance. MRI evaluation can be helpful in demonstrating the internal anatomy. Presence of the vagina or prostate are well-established with transverse imaging, and sagittal views display the uterus, penile bulb, and prostate well [4,12,19,21]. The gonads in these patients are at increased risk of neoplasms.

The term pure gonadal dysgenesis refers to the presence of bilateral streak gonads, which are fibrous in nature and contain no germ cells [4,19]. The basic underlying defect is typically an abnormal second sex chromosome. The majority of these patients are of the XO phenotype known as Turner's syndrome. These patients have infantile external genitalia, a uterus and vagina, as well as bilateral streak ovaries [4,19]. They often have other abnormalities such as a webbed neck and short stature. Other karyotypes occur with gonadal dysgenesis and include mixed gonadal dysgenesis in which the patients have a mosaic karyotype (XO/XY, XO/XYY). These patients have one testis and one streak gonad [19]. A 46 XY combination also exists with abnormal testicular development. This entity differs from testicular feminization in that female internal ducts are usually present as well as external female genitalia. The feminization may be incomplete if the testes are able to produce some testosterone or müllerian regression factor [19]. In patients with gonadal dysgenesis, Y chromosome-containing gonads are at increased risk for malignant transformation and should be removed. Although karyotype analysis is the most critical in the evaluation of these patients, MRI can be helpful in demonstrating the degree of differentiation of internal organs as well as identifying streak gonads that are of low signal intensity on T2-weighted images [4].

Patients with normal genotype but ambiguous genitalia are classified as pseudohermaphrodites. Male pseudohermaphrodites have testes but possess ambiguous internal and/or external genitalia [19]. The most common etiology is testicular feminization, which is an X-linked recessive disorder in which there is an absence of cytoplasmic testosterone receptors. These patients are phenotypically female but have a blind-ended vagina with no uterus or fallopian tubes because the testes make normal müllerian regression factor (Fig. 13.9) [4,19,20]. T2-weighted MR imaging is helpful in preoperative location of the testes, which are removed because of increased

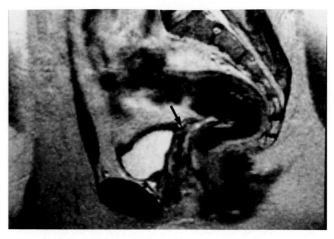

FIG. 13.9 Testicular feminization. Sagittal T2-weighted echo-train spin-echo image. Note absence of the uterus and the blind-ended vagina (*arrow*).

risk of malignancy [19]. Other forms of male pseudohermaphroditism include incomplete testicular feminization with partially masculinized genitalia, inability of tissues to convert testosterone to dihydrotestosterone, congenital errors of testosterone synthesis, and inability of the testes to respond to hypothalamic gonadotropins [19].

Female pseudohermaphrodites have normal 46 XX karyotypes and normal ovaries but have virilized external genitalia because of androgen exposure in utero [12,19]. The most common etiology is 21-hydroxylase deficiency, which is one form of congenital adrenal hyperplasia [4,19]. This deficiency leads to an excess of androgenic sex steroids, which leads in turn to ambiguous genitalia if exposure occurs before the 12th week of gestation and to clitoromegaly if exposure occurs later [19]. Development of male internal genitalia does not occur because this requires local androgen exposure rather than systemic exposure [19]. Other more rare causes of female pseudohermaphroditism include androgen-producing ovarian or adrenal tumors or maternal ingestion of androgen-containing drugs during the first trimester. With surgical and/or hormonal treatment, these females can have normal fertility and near normal female phenotype. MRI is important in identifying uterus, ovaries, vagina, and penile bulb if it is present.

MASS LESIONS

Benign Masses

Bartholin's Cysts

Bartholin's glands are mucus-secreting glands that open into the posterolateral aspect of the vaginal vestibule [11]. Trauma or chronic inflammation in this region is thought to lead to retention of secretion in these glands and cyst formation. Unless these cysts become infected, they usually do not incite symptoms [4]. They are seen on MR images as small fluid-filled structures in the lower third of the vagina. These cysts are high in signal intensity on T2-weighted images and medium to high in signal intensity on T1-weighted images, depending on the protein content of the fluid (Fig. 13.10).

Gartner's Duct Cysts

Gartner's duct cysts are formed from mesonephric duct and tubule remnants and represent the most common benign vulvovaginal lesion in children [11]. These lesions have signal characteristics typical for cysts that are low in signal intensity on T1-weighted images and high in signal intensity on T2-weighted images.

Malignant Masses

Primary Vaginal Malignancies

Up to 95 percent of primary vaginal malignancies are of squamous-cell histology, and they are usually well-differentiated [3,22]. This entity affects older patients with a peak age incidence of 60 to 70 years. Patients are often symptomatic but can present with increased vaginal discharge or spotting [3]. Either TNM or FIGO classification schemes can be used for staging (Table 13.2). These lesions typically arise from the upper posterior vagina and then spread through the wall to invade adjacent pelvic structures. Lesions in the upper third of the vagina spread to the iliac nodes, whereas tumors in the lower two-thirds initially involve the inguinal nodes [3].

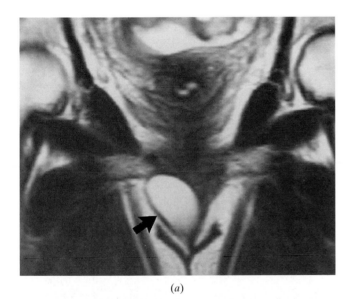

(a)

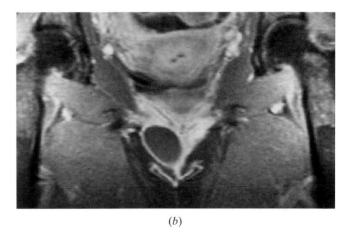

(b)

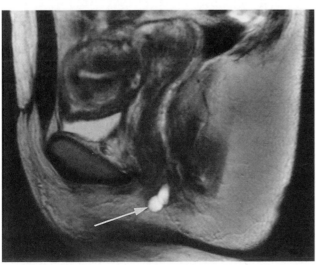

(c)

F IG. 13.10 Bartholin duct cyst. Coronal T2-weighted echo-train spin-echo (*a*) and coronal gadolinium-enhanced fat-suppressed SGE (*b*) images. The cyst is high in signal intensity on the T2-weighted image (*arrow, a*) and demonstrates an enhancing cyst wall with low-signal-intensity cyst contents on the postgadolinium image (*b*). Sagittal 512-resolution T2-weighted echo-train spin-echo image (*c*) in a second patient demonstrates two (*arrow, c*) Bartholin duct cysts.

Table 13.2 TNM Staging for Vaginal Carcinoma		
Primary Tumor		
Tx	Primary tumor cannot be assessed	
T0	No evidence of primary tumor	
Tis	Carcinoma in situ	
T1	Tumor confined to the vagina	
T2	Tumor invades paravaginal tissues but does not extend to the pelvic	
T3	Tumor extends to the pelvic wall	
T4	Tumor invades mucosa of bladder or rectum and/or extends beyond	
Regional Lymph Nodes		
Nx	Regional lymph nodes cannot be assessed	
N0	No regional lymph node metastasis	
	Upper two-thirds of vagina	
N1	Regional lymph node metastasis	
	Lower third of vagina	
N2	Regional lymph node metastasis	
	Bilateral inguinal lymph node metastasis	
Metastases		
M1	Distant metastases	

Clear-cell adenocarcinomas are primary vaginal malignancies that occur in less than 0.14 percent of women who have suffered in utero diethylstilbestrol (DES) exposure [23]. Most of these patients were born between 1951 and 1953. These tumors most often arise from the anterior aspect of the upper third of the vagina. There is an 80 percent 5-year survival rate for women with this entity [11].

Sarcoma botryoides or embryonal rhabdomyosarcoma is an uncommon tumor that originates from mesenchymal tissue of the lamina propria in children typically under 5 years of age [3,11]. These patients usually present with vaginal bleeding or with a polypoid mass protruding from the vagina [3,4]. These tumors then spread locally and can obstruct the ureters or penetrate into the peritoneal cavity [3].

The contrast resolution of MRI has made it the modality of choice in the evaluation of vaginal tumors. It can be used to assess the extent of disease at initial presentation, and it can be used to detect tumor recurrence. Differentiation of inflammatory changes from primary or metastatic lesions may be problematic, but one group of investigators has shown MRI to be 92 percent accurate in demonstrating metastatic disease and 82 percent accurate in depicting recurrence [24]. Vaginal tumors are of intermediate signal intensity on T1-weighted images and may be occult when small. However, these lesions are well-seen on T2-weighted images and demonstrate moderately high signal intensity [4,25]. Vaginal neoplasms show variable enhancement after gadolinium administration (Figs. 13.11 and 13.12) [4,25].

Detection of tumor recurrence after hysterectomy may be an important role for MRI. The vaginal cuff can have a very irregular appearance due to postoperative fibrosis and granulation tissue. Tumor is generally irregular in contour and usually high in signal intensity on T2-weighted images, whereas fibrosis and granulation tissue are low in signal intensity on T2-weighted images [4,24,26–29]. Recurrent tumor frequently enhances in a heterogeneous intense fashion on gadolinium-enhanced fat-suppressed images (Figs. 13.12). Inflammatory changes within 9 months to 1 year following radiation

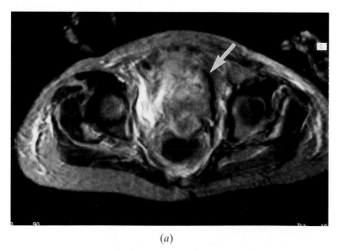

(a)

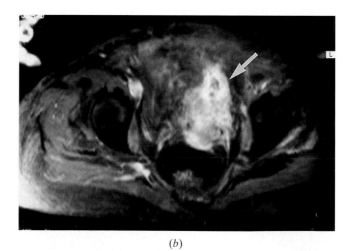

(b)

FIG. 13.11 Vaginal carcinoma with bladder and rectum invasion. Transverse T2-weighted spin-echo (*a*) and transverse gadolinium-enhanced T1-weighted fat-suppressed spin-echo (*b*) images. A large heterogeneous vaginal cancer is identified on the T2-weighted image (*arrow, a*). Postradiation changes in the pelvis are also heterogeneous in signal intensity and the margins of the tumor are not well-defined. The tumor enhances heterogeneously and intensely after gadolinium administration (*arrow, b*), and invasion of the anterior rectum and the bladder are clearly shown.

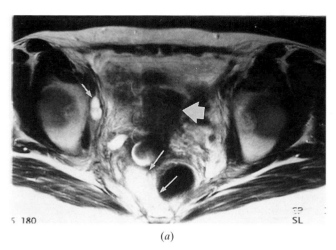
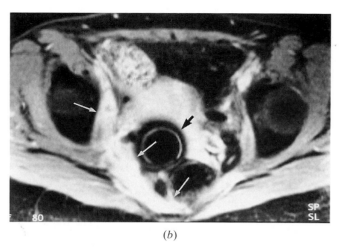

(a)   *(b)*

F I G . **13.12** Recurrent vaginal carcinoma. Transverse 512-resolution T2-weighted echo-train spin-echo (*a*) and gadolinium-enhanced fat-suppressed SGE (*b*) images. On the T2-weighted image (*a*) high-signal-intensity recurrent vaginal carcinoma is seen extending from the presacral space along the right lateral pelvic wall (*small arrows, a*). Low-signal-intensity uterus is demonstrated (*large arrow*). The tumor is very conspicuous on the enhanced image (*b*) and appears as enhancing soft tissue (*white arrows, b*) extending along the right pelvic side wall. Susceptibility artifact (*black arrow, b*) is from surgical clips.

therapy result in increased signal intensity on T2-weighted images and may mimic tumor recurrence [28]. Close follow-up with MRI may be useful in selected cases.

Other rare primary vaginal malignancies include leiomyosarcomas in adults, endodermal sinus tumors in infants as well as lymphoma and melanoma [30,31]. Leiomyosarcoma and endodermal sinus tumors are highly malignant with poor prognosis. Melanoma may be high in signal intensity on T1-weighted images, which reflects the paramagnetic properties of melanin [30].

Vaginal Metastases

Vaginal metastases are more common than primary vaginal neoplasms. Local spread from cervical and endome-

trial carcinoma occurs most frequently, although other sources including colon, melanoma, bladder, and kidney have been reported (Figs. 13.13 and 13.14) [3,4,32,33].

Sagittal- and transverse-plane images are useful for the demonstration of tumor extension to the vagina. Both T2-weighted ETSE images and gadolinium-enhanced T1-weighted fat-suppressed images define tumor involvement.

Radiation Changes

The appearance of radiation changes of the vagina varies depending on the time interval between therapy and imaging. Acute radiation changes in less than 1 year reflect histological changes of interstitial edema and capil-

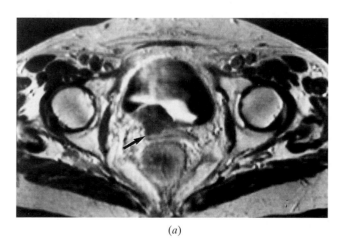
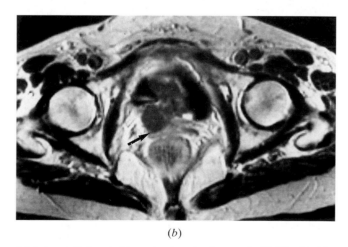

(a)   *(b)*

F I G . **13.13** Bladder carcinoma with vaginal invasion. Transverse T1-weighted gadolinium-enhanced spin-echo images (*a,b*). The bladder cancer (*arrow, a,b*) arises from the posterior wall and invades the anterior wall of the vagina. The tumor enhances modestly with gadolinium.

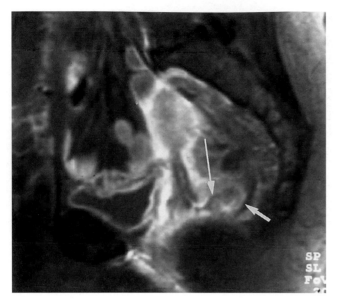

FIG. 13.14 Rectal carcinoma with spread to posterior vaginal fornix. Sagittal immediate postgadolinium fat-suppressed SGE image. Lobulated intermediate-signal-intensity mass (*arrow*) extends to involve the posterior vaginal fornix (*long arrow*), which appears expanded.

lary leakage. The vaginal wall shows generalized thickening and is high in signal intensity on T2-weighted and gadolinium-enhanced T1-weighted images. Enhancement is best appreciated if the T1-weighted images are fat suppressed (Fig. 13.15). Chronic changes after more than 1 year result in fibrosis, diminished interstitial fluid,

and diminished vascularity. The vaginal wall may become atrophic, has low signal intensity on T2-weighted images, and demonstrates diminished enhancement after gadolinium administration.

Fistulas

Fistulas to the vagina occur most commonly in the setting of gynecological malignancy after radiation therapy, hysterectomy, inflammatory bowel disease, or a combination of these. Imaging in the sagittal and transverse planes with T2-weighted and postgadolinium T1-weighted images is important to maximize detection (Fig. 13.16). The addition of fat suppression to the T1-weighted images increases the conspicuity of the enhancing sinus tract walls.

Vulvar Carcinoma

Vulvar carcinomas are uncommon lesions that occur in older patients and are typically of squamous cell origin. Most of the patients have vulvar pruritus, although pain, bleeding, and palpable mass are often typical symptoms. A TNM system is used for staging (Table 3). Modern treatment is somewhat conservative and includes topical 5-fluorouracil, laser ablation, and wide local excision. MRI is evolving as a sensitive modality for the evaluation of recurrent vulvar carcinoma (Fig. 13.17) [34].

Other more rare malignancies involving the vulva include: Bartholin gland carcinoma, Paget's disease, melanoma, basal-cell carcinoma, and sarcoma [34].

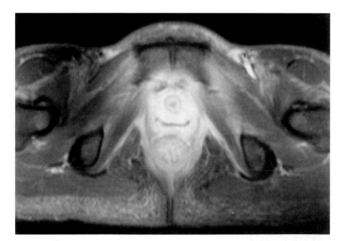

FIG. 13.15 Radiation changes following treatment for vaginal carcinoma. Transverse gadolinium-enhanced T1-weighted fat-suppressed spin-echo image. Enhancing tissue is seen involving the urethra, vagina, and anal canal. Diffuse thickening of the vaginal wall is appreciated. Enhancement from acute radiation changes cannot be easily distinguished from tumor, but symmetric changes favor benign disease.

Table 13.3 TNM Staging for Carcinoma of the Vulva

Primary Tumor

T1	Tumor 2 cm or smaller confined to the vulva
T2	Tumor larger than 2 cm confined to the vulva
T3	Tumor of any size with adjacent spread to the urethra and/or perineum
T4	Tumor of any size infiltrating the bladder mucosa and/or the rectum

Regional Lymph Nodes

N0	No nodes palpable
N1	Nodes palpable in either groin, not enlarged, mobile
N2	Nodes palpable in either one or both groins, enlarged, firm, and mobile
N3	Fixed or ulcerated nodes

Metastases

M0	No clinical metastases
M1	Palpable deep pelvic lymph nodes
M2	Other distant metastases

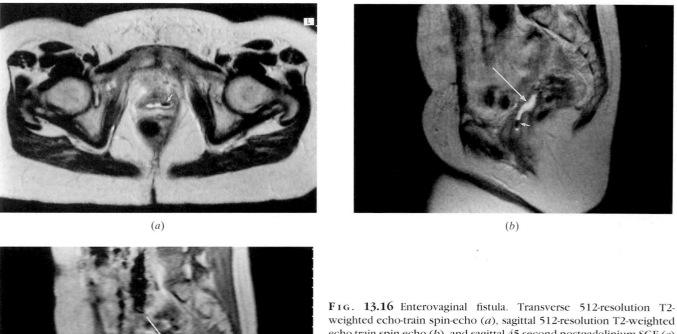

(a)

(b)

(c)

FIG. 13.16 Enterovaginal fistula. Transverse 512-resolution T2-weighted echo-train spin-echo (a), sagittal 512-resolution T2-weighted echo-train spin-echo (b), and sagittal 45-second postgadolinium SGE (c) images. This woman is status posthysterectomy for cervical cancer. A signal-void focus of air is present in the vagina on T2-weighted images (*small arrow, a,b*) consistent with a fistulous communication with bowel. The superior aspect of the vagina expands into an abscess cavity (*long arrow, b*), which is well-shown on sagittal plane images. The gadolinium-enhanced image shows increased enhancement and thickness of the vaginal wall, which is consistent with inflammatory changes (*short arrows, c*). A fistulous tract is apparent on this sagittal image (*long arrow, c*) in continuity with adjacent bowel.

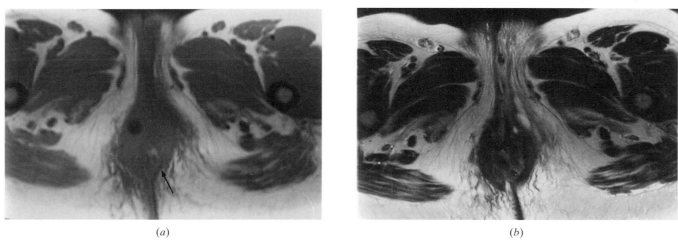

(a)

(b)

FIG. 13.17 Vulvar carcinoma. Transverse SGE (a), 512-resolution T2-weighted echo-train spin-echo (b), and 90-second postgadolinium fat-suppressed SGE (c) images. The T1-weighted image (a) shows an irregular low-signal-intensity mass arising from the vulva with posterior extension to involve the anus (*arrow*). On the T2-weighted image (b) the mass is intermediate in signal intensity.

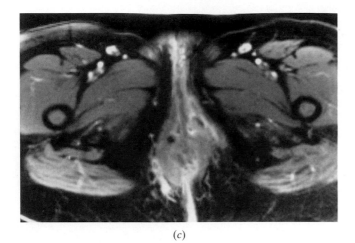

(c)

FIG. 13.17 (*Continued*) In part, this reflects the high signal intensity of fat on echo-train spin-echo sequences. Heterogeneous enhancement of tumor is seen on postgadolinium imaging (c).

REFERENCES

1. Hricak H, Secaf E, Buckley D, et al: Female urethra: MR imaging. Radiology 178:527–535, 1991.
2. Moore K: Clinically Orientated Anatomy (2nd ed.). Baltimore: Williams & Wilkins, pp. 365–373, 1985.
3. Cotran R, Kumar V, Robbins S: Pathologic Basis of Disease (4th ed.). Philadelphia: WB Saunders, pp. 1095–1097, 1133–1139, 1989.
4. Higgins C, Hricak H, Hilms C: Magnetic Resonance Imaging of the Body. New York: Raven Press, pp. 820–863, 977–980, 1992.
5. Benson RC Jr, Tunca JC, Buchler PA, Uehling DT: Primary carcinoma of the female urethra. Gynecol Oncol 14:313–318, 1982.
6. Davidson AJ, Hartman DS: Radiology of the Kidney and Urinary Tract. Philadelphia: WB Saunders, pp. 664–666, 1994.
7. Keefe B, Warshauer DM, Tucker MS, Mittelstaedt CA: Diverticula of the female urethra: Diagnosis by endovaginal and transperineal sonography. AJR Am J Roentgenol 156:1195–1197, 1991.
8. Kim B, Hricak H, Tanagho E: Diagnosis of urethral diverticula in women: Value of MR imaging. AJR Am J Roentgenol 161:809–815, 1993.
9. Thomas RB, Maguire B: Adenocarcinoma in a female urethral diverticulum. Aust N Z J Surg 61:869–871, 1991.
10. Carr LK, Herschorn S, Leonhardt C: Magnetic resonance imaging after intraurethral collagen injected for stress urinary incontinence. J Urol 155:1253–1255, 1996.
11. Moore KL. The devleoping human. Clinically oriented embryology. 2nd ed. Philadelphia, WB Saunders, pp. 220–258, 1977.
12. Hricak H, Chang YCF, Thurnher S: Vagina: Evaluation with MR imaging. Part I. Normal anatomy and congenital anomalies. Radiology 169:169–174, 1988.
13. Hricak H, Hamm B, Wolf KJ: Use of Gd-DTPA in MRI of the female pelvis. In Bydder G, Felix R, Bücheler E, et al., eds. Contrast media in MRI. Bussum, The Netherlands: Medicom, pp. 351–356, 1990.
14. Togashi K, Nishimujra K, Itoh K, et al: Vaginal agenesis: Classification by MR imaging. Radiology 162:675–677, 1987.
15. Fedele L, Dorta M, Brioschi D, Giudici MN, Candiani GB: Magnetic resonance imaging in Mayer-Rokitansky-Küster-Hauser syndrome. Obstet Gynecol 76(4):593–596, 1990.
16. Carrington BM, Hricak H, Nuruddin R, Secaf E, Laros RK, Hill EC: Müllerian duct anomalies: MR imaging evaluation. Radiology 176:715–720, 1990.
17. Sorenson SS: Estimated prevalence of müllerian anomalies. Acta Obstet Gynecol Scand 67:441–445, 1988.
18. Capraro VJ, Gallego MB: Vaginal agenesis. Am J Obstet Gynecol 124:98–107, 1976.
19. Gambino J, Caldwell B, Dietrich R, Walot I, Kangarloo H: Congenital disorders of sexual differentiation: MR findings. AJR Am J Roentgenol 158:363–367, 1992.
20. Saenger P: Abnormal sex differentiation. J Pediatr 104:1–16, 1984.
21. Secaf E, Hricak H, Gooding CA, et al: Role of MRI in the evaluation of ambiguous genitalia. Pediatr Radiol 24:231–235, 1994.
22. Pride GL, et al: Primary invasive squamous carcinoma of the vagina. Obstet Gynecol 53:218, 1979.
23. Herbst AL: Clear cell adenocarcinoma and the current status of DES-exposed females. Cancer 48:484, 1981.
24. Chang YCF, Hricak H, Thurnher S, Lacey C: Vagina: Evaluation with MR imaging. Part II. Neoplasms. Radiology 169:175–179, 1988.
25. Gilles R, Michel G, Chancellier MD, Vanel D, Masselot J: Case report: Clear cell adenocarcinoma of the vagina: MR features. Br J Radiol 66:168–170, 1993.
26. Ebner F, Kressel HY, Mintz MC, et al: Tumor recurrence versus fibrosis in the female pelvis: Differentiation with MR at 1.5T. Radiology 333–340, 1988.
27. Brown JJ, Gutierrez ED, Lee JKT: MR appearance of the normal and abnormal vagina after hysterectomy. AJR Am J Roentgenol 158:95–99, 1992.
28. Sugimura K, Carrington BM, Quivey JM, Hricak H: Post-irradiation changes in the pelvis: Assessment with MR imaging. Radiology 175:805–813, 1990.
29. Hricak H: Postoperative and postradiation changes in the pelvis. Magn Reson Q 6:276–297, 1990.
30. Moon WK, Kim SH, Han MC: MR findings of malignant melanoma of the vagina. Clin Radiol 48:326–328, 1993.
31. McNicholas MMJ, Fennely JJ, MacErlaine DP: Imaging of primary vaginal lymphoma. Clin Radiol 49:130–132, 1994.
32. Phillips GL, Prem KA, Adcock LL, et al: Vaginal recurrence of adenocarcinoma of the endometrium. Gynecol Oncol 13:323–328, 1982.
33. Chen NJ: Vaginal invasion by cervical carcinoma. Acta Med Okayama 38:305–313, 1984.
34. Jones HW, Wentz AC, Burnett LS: Novak's Textbook of Gynecology. Baltimore: Williams & Wilkins, pp. 599–613, 1988.

CHAPTER 14

UTERUS AND CERVIX

C. REINHOLD, M.D., B. P. GALLIX, M.D., AND S. M. ASCHER, M.D.

R ecent developments in magnetic resonance imaging (MRI), including the advent of fast pulse sequences and phased-array multicoil technology, has increased the role of MRI in evaluating pathology of the uterus [1]. Although ultrasound remains the procedure of choice for the initial evaluation of patients with suspected uterine disease, MRI is an important adjunct due to its excellent soft tissue differentiation [2,3]. Images of high diagnostic quality can be generated with endovaginal ultrasound, but the small field of view (FOV) makes it impossible to adequately evaluate large masses, tumor extension to the pelvic side wall, or the presence of lymphadenopathy. MRI is indicated in patients for whom the ultrasound examination is technically suboptimal or nondiagnostic. This is true, for example, in cases where the origin of a pelvic mass is uncertain and further tissue characterization is required. Patients with complex uterine congenital anomalies may benefit from MRI, particularly when endovaginal ultrasound is not feasible. In patients undergoing uterus-sparing surgery, MRI can be performed to accurately localize uterine leiomyomas for preoperative planning in selected cases. In addition, for patients receiving hormonal therapy in the treatment of leiomyomas or adenomyosis, MRI is ideal for monitoring the evolution of disease because standard and reproducible images can be obtained. MRI has been shown to be the modality of choice for tumor staging, particularly in the evaluation of patients with cervical carcinoma. Finally, MRI plays an important role as a problem-solving modality in evaluating the pregnant patient.

MRI TECHNIQUE

General Guidelines

Patient Preparation

No special patient preparation is required for MRI of the uterus. However, it is preferable that patients fast for a minimum of 6 hours to minimize bowel peristaltism. Immediately prior to the examination, patients should be asked to void. This minimizes phase ghost artifacts of the distended urinary bladder induced by patient motion. In addition, an overly distended bladder may result in uterine compression, which may alter the appearance of normal and pathological structures. Furthermore, the fundus of the uterus is displaced superiorly, frequently bringing it into close contact with the small bowel and, possibly, artifacts from intestinal peristaltism.

Although examinations are usually performed in the supine position, placing patients with claustrophobia in the prone position often obviates the need for administering a sedative. (A more complete discussion of MRI techniques for imaging the pregnant patient is presented in the subsection, MRI Technique, in the section on MRI and Pregnancy.)

Surface/Endoluminal Coils

A phased-array pelvic multicoil should be used routinely if available. Pelvic multicoils markedly increase the signal-to-noise ratio of the image and permit the use of a small FOV ranging from 20 to 26 cm, depending on the size of the patient [1]. Also, in conjunction with T2-weighted echo-train spin-echo sequences, higher matrix sizes of 512 in the frequency encode direction and 256 to 512 in the phase encode direction become feasible [4]. The combination of a small FOV and large matrix size results in high-resolution T2-weighted images of the uterus and cervix.

Although a larger field of view is usually prescribed for body coil imaging because of signal-to-noise considerations, the FOV should be maintained as small as possible, usually on the order of 28 to 32 cm, depending on the patient's size.

Little has been written to the present on the use of intravaginal coils, either alone or in combination with a pelvic multicoil. Excellent detail of the normal anatomy and vascularity of the cervix can be achieved with intravaginal coils [5]. However, when purchased commercially, intravaginal coils can add significant cost to the MRI examination. Further study is therefore needed to determine the exact role of intravaginal coils in evaluating uterine and cervical pathology [1].

Imaging Protocol

Pulse Sequences

We routinely perform a localizing sequence using a fast T2-weighted sequence such as an echo-train spin-echo sequence, (e.g., fast or turbo spin-echo) half Fourier single-shot turbo spin-echo (HASTE) sequence is an example. A localizing sequence can be acquired in less than 24 seconds, depending on the type of sequence used. We recommend using a fast T2-weighted sequence over a gradient-echo sequence because pelvic structures are better defined on T2-weighted sequences, allowing technologists to readily identify the uterus and other important landmarks.

T2- and T1-weighted sequences are standard techniques for evaluating the uterine corpus and cervix. The uterine and cervical zonal anatomy is best defined on T2-weighted sequences (see the later subsection, Uterine Corpus, in the section on Normal Anatomic Structures and Physiologic Variants). In the pelvis, T2-weighted echo-train spin-echo sequences have largely replaced conventional spin-echo sequences because of shortened acquisition times [6]. The imaging time with echo-train spin-echo sequences is inversely proportional to the number of 180-degree pulses applied, or the echo-train length. In the pelvis, where only a single-echo (T2-weighted) image is acquired, an echo-train length of 16 can potentially decrease the acquisition time by a factor of 16 if all other imaging parameters remain constant [7]. In the abdomen, where dual-echo (proton density and T2-weighted) images are routinely acquired, the echo-train length usually is maintained at 8. Longer echo-train lengths may further decrease imaging times, but at the

cost of image blurring in the phase encode direction, particularly when larger FOVs are used [8]. For the vast majority of uterine pathology, proton density-weighted images add little diagnostic information over that provided by T2-weighted images alone [4,9]. Therefore, since the acquisition of dual-echo images with a shorter echo-train length prolongs the imaging time, proton density-weighted images are not routinely obtained. The shorter acquisition time achievable with echo-train spin-echo sequences is partially offset by the use of higher matrix sizes, which would not be feasible with T2-weighted conventional spin-echo sequences, and longer repetition times (TR), which are needed to cover the desired anatomic region.

Echo-train spin-echo images with T2 contrast similar to that obtained with conventional spin-echo images can be achieved by using long repetition and long echo times. We routinely use a repetition time in the range of 3,000 to 5,000 msec and an effective echo time of 90 to 120 msec. Nevertheless, the contrast of certain tissues is altered with echo-train spin-echo imaging. For example, fat is of a higher signal intensity on echo-train spin-echo sequences due to altered J-coupling between neighboring protons in the hydrocarbon chains, whereas muscle shows lower signal intensity due to magnetization transfer effects [10,11].

T1-weighted sequences maximize the image contrast between muscle and fat. In addition, the presence of hemorrhage or fat within a lesion is best depicted on T1-weighted images. Because acquisition times are considerably shorter for T1-weighted images, conventional spin-echo sequences are usually performed. On MRI systems in which respiratory motion compensation techniques are not available, breath-hold T1-weighted spoiled gradient-echo (SGE) sequences can be obtained.

Gadolinium-enhanced studies are primarily reserved for evaluating the endometrium and for tumor staging. Staging of uterine neoplasms is performed using dynamic scanning—usually three sequential acquisitions beginning immediately after an intravenous bolus of gadolinium chelate. Dynamic scanning allows the tumor to be studied during the capillary and interstitial phases of enhancement. T1-weighted spin-echo or SGE techniques can be used for delayed imaging following gadolinium administration.

Imaging Planes

Three orthogonal planes (transverse, sagittal, and coronal), as well as off-axis imaging, can be performed with MRI. Each plane of a section has distinct advantages for imaging uterine and cervical pathology. Only general guidelines will be presented here, with more detail provided in the various sections dealing with uterine and cervical disease processes.

Transverse and sagittal planes are most commonly

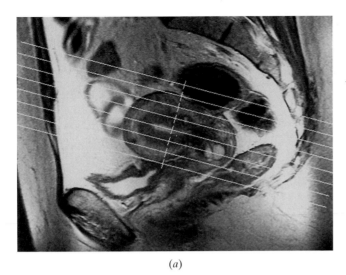

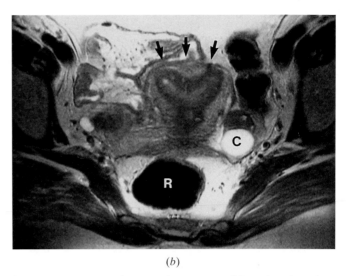

(a)   (b)

F IG. 14.1 Long-axis view of the uterus. T2-weighted echo-train spin-echo sequence. (*a*) On the sagittal section an oblique imaging plane parallel to the endometrium is prescribed graphically. (*b*) The resultant image shows the outward convexity of the fundal contour (*arrows*) in this patient with an arcuate uterus. *C*, ovarian cyst; *R*, rectum

used to image the uterus and cervix. Sagittal sections image the uterus in its long axis. In addition, the cervix, including the pars vaginalis and the posterior vaginal fornix are well-demonstrated on T2-weighted sequences. On sagittal images, the bladder, rectum, and anterior and posterior cul de sac are all visualized in a single plane of a section. Transverse sections demonstrate the uterus and cervix, as well as the parametrium. Transverse sections are most commonly used to detect the presence of lymphadenopathy. Coronal sections are supplementary and provide an additional view of the parametrium. In specific instances, off-axis imaging planes may be helpful. For example, an oblique transverse section parallel

to the endometrium results in a long-axis view and is ideal for imaging the fundal contour in congenital uterine anomalies (Fig. 14.1). A coronal oblique section obtained perpendicular to the endometrium, results in a short-axis view and allows accurate assessment of zonal anatomy, such as in the diagnosis of adenomyosis or in endometrial carcinoma staging (Fig. 14.2).

Artifacts

Motion Artifact Reduction
To minimize motion artifacts from intestinal peristaltism, patients should ideally be fasting before imaging for a

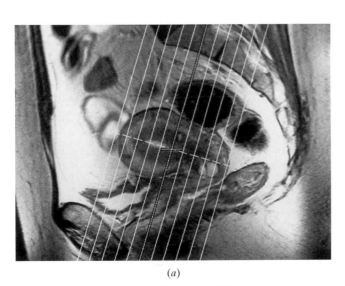

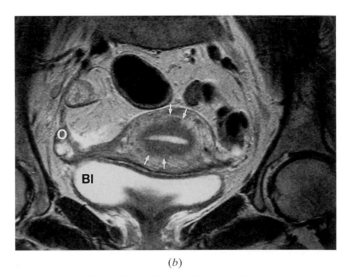

(a)   (b)

F IG. 14.2 Short-axis view of the uterus. T2-weighted echo-train spin-echo sequence. (*a*) On the sagittal section an oblique imaging plane perpendicular to the endometrium is prescribed graphically. (*b*) The zonal anatomy is well-depicted. Note the irregular thickening of the junctional zone (JZ) (*arrows*) consistent with adenomyosis. *Bl*, bladder; *O*, right ovary

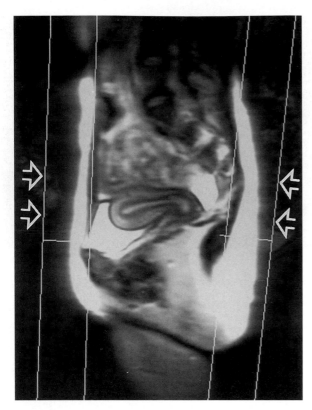

FIG. **14.3** In-field-of-view saturation bands. Sagittal T2-weighted echo-train spin-echo localizing sequence. In-field-of-view saturation bands (*open arrows*) are placed over the subcutaneous fat anteriorly and posteriorly to decrease the signal intensity of the fat adjacent to the multicoil.

minimum of 6 hours. In addition, an antispasmodic can be administered, provided no medical contraindications are present. Immediately prior to the examination, patients should be asked to void (see earlier subsection, Patient Preparation).

Respiratory motion artifacts are frequently accentuated with multicoil imaging for two reasons: (1) Superficial structures that generate artifact (e.g., subcutaneous fat, bladder, and bowel) are in close proximity to the coils and therefore have a relatively high signal intensity when compared to the uterus, for example, which is typically located farther from the coils. (2) The signal intensity of phase ghost artifacts generated by respiration is greater with a small voxel size [12]. The following steps can be taken to minimize respiratory motion with multicoil imaging. Motion of the coil itself should be restricted by binding the coil firmly to the patient's abdomen. In-field-of-view saturation bands are placed over the subcutaneous fat anteriorly and posteriorly to decrease the signal of the fat immediately adjacent to the coils (Fig. 14.3). For conventional spin-echo sequences, respiratory-ordered phase encoding can be used where it is available. This option is not compatible with fast

imaging sequences, but respiratory triggering (or gating) can be used in conjunction with echo-train spin-echo sequences on some MRI systems. The addition of respiratory triggering prolongs the image acquisition and allows only one set of images to be acquired at any given time. Therefore, although it is of considerable benefit in the upper abdomen, we do not routinely employ respiratory triggering for imaging the pelvis. However, for cases in which extensive respiratory artifact is present, the image quality can be significantly improved by the addition of respiratory gating. Breath hold echo-train spin-echo sequences are a useful alternative as breathing artifact is avoided, and image quality is often satisfactory because of the increase signal-to-noise of the phased array multicoil. In patients who are unable to cooperate, consideration should be given to using a single-shot sequence for T2-weighted imaging because it is relatively breathing independent. SGE sequences, where possible, are best performed during a breath-hold.

Metallic Artifacts

The usual contraindications to MRI also apply to examinations of the uterus. The presence of orthopedic devices, although not hazardous to the patient, can seriously impair image quality. Extensive signal loss is usually present at the site of a metallic device. In patients with a hip prosthesis, the signal loss may extend as far across as the midpelvis (Fig. 14.4). Most intrauterine contraceptive devices (IUD) do not cause sufficient signal loss to render the examination of the uterus nondiagnostic (Fig. 14.5) [13]. Surgical clips and certain types of surgical sutures also may result in areas of signal loss (Fig. 14.6) [14]. Magnetic susceptibility artifacts can be minimized by utilizing echo-train spin-echo sequences and are most accentuated with gradient-echo sequences [11]. HASTE images suffer the least artifact from metallic devices.

NORMAL ANATOMIC STRUCTURES AND PHYSIOLOGIC VARIANTS

Anatomic and Histologic Considerations

Uterine Corpus

The uterus is divided into three major segments: (1) the *fundus*, which consists of that portion of the uterus cephalad to the cornua; (2) the *body* or corpus; and (3) the *cervix*. In women of reproductive age the uterus measures 6 to 9 cm in length, of which the corpus measures 4 to 6 cm and the cervix 2.5 to 3.2 cm. The uterus measures approximately 4 cm in thickness and 6 cm in its maximal transverse dimension [15–19]. Histologically, the uterine corpus is divided into three tissue layers: (1) the *serosa*, which consists of the peritoneum; (2) the *myometrium*, which is largely made up of involuntary smooth muscle;

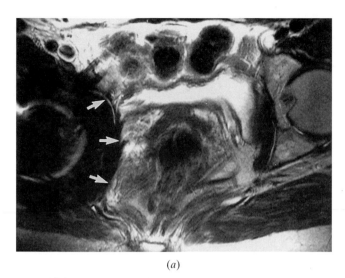

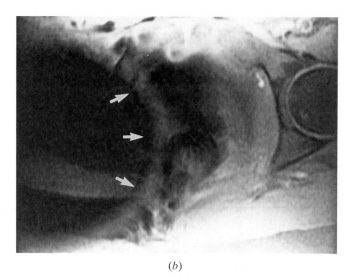

(a)   (b)

FIG. 14.4 Artifact related to hip prosthesis. Transverse (a) T2-weighted echo-train spin-echo sequence, (b) T1-weighted SGE sequence. The presence of a right hip prosthesis, although not a contraindication to MRI, results in signal loss radiating from the prosthesis (*arrows, a,b*). On the echo-train spin-echo sequence (a), the signal loss is limited to the immediate proximity of the prosthesis, whereas the artifact extends across the midpelvis on the SGE sequence (b).

and (3) the *endometrium*, composed of the *mucosal stratum functionalis* (responsive to hormonal stimuli) and the *stratum basale* (responsible for growth and regeneration of the endometrium) [20]. The inner third of the myometrium is composed of densely packed smooth muscle bundles with an orientation that is parallel to the stratum basale of the endometrium [21]. In contrast, the outer myometrium or myometrium proper consists of randomly oriented and loosely packed smooth muscle bundles. This difference in the orientation and density of smooth muscle bundles between the inner and outer myometrium is of interest because it may be one of the

factors contributing to the MRI appearance of the myometrium [22] (see later subsection, MRI Considerations).

Cervix

The cervix is separated from the corpus of the uterus by the *internal os*, which corresponds to a slight constriction visible externally and by the entrance of the uterine vessels. The cervical canal is lined by the *endocervix*, which is composed of columnar epithelium. Small folds in the mucous membrane called *plicae palmatae* are present [23]. Surrounding the endocervix is the *fibrous stroma*. The outermost layer of the cervix is composed of a mus-

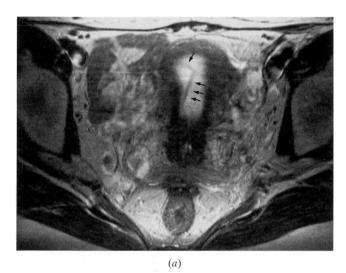

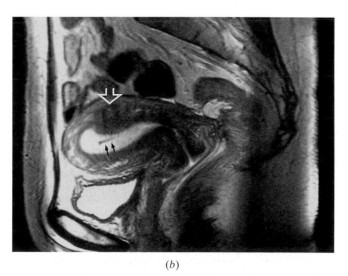

(a)   (b)

FIG. 14.5 Intrauterine device (IUD). (a) Transverse and (b) sagittal T2-weighted echo-train spin-echo images. A correctly positioned IUD (*arrows, a,b*) is shown as a low-signal-intensity linear structure within the endometrial cavity. Note that the IUD does not create any significant artifact. A contraction (*open arrow, b*) arising from the dorsal aspect of the uterus is also visualized.

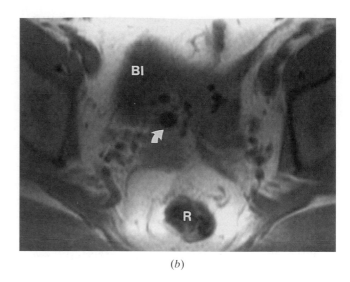

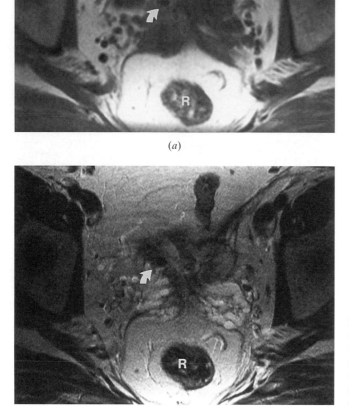

(a)

(b)

(c)

FIG. 14.6 Artifact related to surgical sutures. (*a*) T1-weighted spin-echo, *b*) T1-weighted SGE, and *c*) T2-weighted echo-train spin-echo images in a patient posthysterectomy. Several foci of low signal intensity consistent with surgical sutures are visible at the vaginal cuff (*curved arrows, a–c*). Note that the artifact is accentuated on the gradient-echo sequence (*b*) and minimized on the echo-train spin-echo sequence (*c*). *Bl*, bladder; *R*, rectum

cular coat that becomes increasingly thin in the lower portion of the cervix. The external os marks the opening between the cervix and vagina and is defined histologically by the *squamocolumnar junction*. The portion of the cervix protruding into the vagina is called the *pars* or *portio vaginalis* and is covered by stratified squamous epithelium [19].

Parametrium and Ligaments of the Uterus

It is important to be familiar with the ligaments of the uterus because they may serve as pathways for local spread of disease. The *parametrium* is located between the layers of the broad ligament adjacent to the lateral margins of the uterine corpus and cervix [19]. It is composed largely of loose connective and areolar tissue. The broad ligament consists of a double sheet of peritoneum that reflects off the ventral and dorsal surfaces of the

uterus and extends to the pelvic side wall. The lower border of the broad ligament is thickened, with a condensation of connective tissue and smooth muscle fibers forming the paired cardinal ligaments [19]. The paired uterosacral ligaments fuse anteromedially with the cardinal ligaments, as well as with the fascia surrounding the upper vagina and cervix, before coursing posteriorly to the sacrum. The paired round ligaments are muscular bands (5 to 6 mm in diameter) that arise from the lateral aspect of the uterine fundus, slightly below and anterior to the insertion of the fallopian tubes [19]. They pass through the inguinal canal to fuse with the subcutaneous tissue of the labia majora. The uterovesical ligaments extend from the cervix to the base of the urinary bladder [19]. The cardinal, uterosacral, and uterovesical ligaments are the main suspensory ligaments of the uterus. The main function of the round ligaments is to prevent retrodisplacement [19].

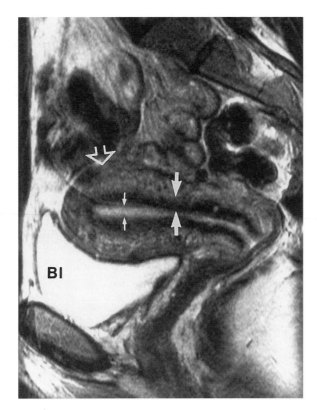

FIG. 14.7 Zonal anatomy of the uterine corpus. Sagittal T2-weighted echo-train spin-echo image. The central, high-signal-intensity stripe represents the endometrium (*small arrows*). The band of low signal intensity subjacent to the endometrial stripe represents the inner myometrium or junctional zone (JZ) (*arrows*). The outer layer of the myometrium (*open arrow*) is of intermediate signal intensity. *Bl*, bladder

MRI Considerations

Uterine Corpus

The uterus is optimally depicted with MRI using T2-weighted sagittal sequences. In women of reproductive age, three different zones can be identified within the uterine corpus on T2-weighted images [15,24,25]. A high-signal-intensity stripe representing the normal endometrium and secretions within the endometrial cavity is present centrally (Fig. 14.7). The width of the endometrial stripe varies with the menstrual cycle, being thinnest at the time of menstruation. The endometrium increases in width rapidly during the follicular or proliferative phase and continues to increase during the secretory phase, although at a slower rate [26]. The reported thickness of the endometrial stripe varies widely but averages from 3 to 6 mm in the follicular phase and 5–13 mm during the secretory phase (Fig. 14.8) [16,17,27,28]. Immediately subjacent to the endometrial stripe, a band of low signal intensity referred to as the junctional zone (JZ) is seen (see Fig. 14.7). Histologic studies have demonstrated that this zone corresponds to the innermost layer of the myo-

metrium [22,29]. The histological basis for the low signal intensity of the junction zone has not yet been established, but a number of factors likely contribute to this imaging appearance. Brown et al. [22] hypothesized that the compact smooth muscle bundles, as well as the orientation of the fibers within the junctional zone, may contribute to the low signal on T2-weighted images. McCarthy et al. [25] found that the water content of the junctional zone was significantly lower than that of the endometrium and outer myometrium. Scoutt et al. [30] found an increase in the percentage of nuclear area in the junctional zone in comparison with that of the outer myometrium. The outer layer of the myometrium is of intermedi-

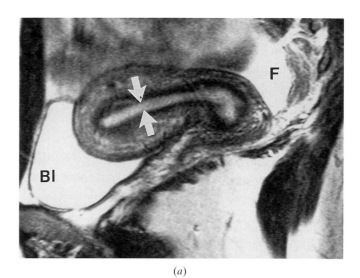

(a)

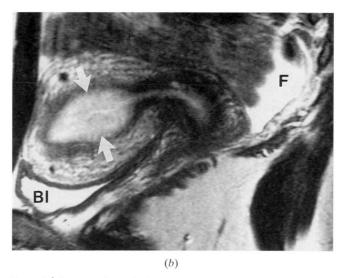

(b)

FIG. 14.8 Physiological changes during menstrual cycle. (*a,b*) Sagittal T2-weighted echo-train spin-echo images at different phases of the menstrual cycle. (*a*) During the follicular phase (day 6), the high-signal-intensity endometrial stripe is thin (*arrows*). (*b*) During the secretory phase (day 24), the endometrial stripe widens considerably (*arrows*), and the endometrial complex as well as the myometrium shows increased signal intensity. *Bl*, bladder; *F*, fluid

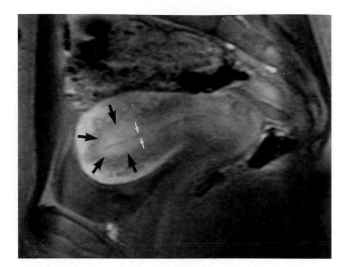

FIG. 14.9 Variable patterns of uterine enhancement. Early enhancement of the inner myometrium may be observed during the menstrual phase. Sagittal fat-suppressed SGE sequence obtained immediately after gadolinium administration. The endometrial stripe is thin and hypointense (*small arrows*). There is early enhancement of the JZ (*arrows*) relative to the outer myometrium.

ate signal intensity on T2-weighted images (see Fig. 14.7). During the menstrual cycle, the thickness of the myometrium increases slightly and is greatest during the secretory phase [26]. Considerable variation in the normal thickness of the junctional zone has been reported, with a mean thickness ranging from 2 to 8 mm [15,22,27,29,31]. In addition to an increase in thickness, the endometrium and myometrium both demonstrate a gradual increase in signal intensity from the follicular to the secretory phase (see Fig. 14.8) [16,17].

On T1-weighted images, the zonal anatomy of the uterine corpus is usually inapparent. The uterus is of intermediate and homogeneous signal intensity, aside from the midsecretory phase, during which the endometrium may exhibit slightly greater signal intensity than the adjacent myometrium [15,32].

Considerable variation in the pattern of uterine enhancement may be observed, depending on the hormonal status of the patient and the imaging delay after injection [33–35]. Although the endometrium shows little enhancement during the dynamic phase of gadolinium administration, it shows marked enhancement on the delayed T1-weighted images. Peak myometrial enhancement has been reported to occur 120 seconds after gadolinium administration [34]. During the menstrual phase, intense early enhancement of the junctional zone may be observed at dynamic imaging (Fig. 14.9) [34]. Enhancement of a thin subendometrial layer followed by enhancement of the myometrium has been reported in postmenopausal women and in women during the proliferative phase of their menstrual cycle [34]. During the secretory phase, enhancement of the entire myometrium, predominantly in the outer muscle layer, may be seen on early dynamic images (Fig. 14.10) [34]. Although this pattern of enhancement is most frequently encountered in women during the secretory phase of their cycle, it also may be seen during the menstrual phase and in postmenopausal women [34,35]. On postcontrast delayed images, the signal intensity of the uterine corpus may parallel that seen with T2-weighted sequences: endometrium—high signal intensity; junctional zone—low signal intensity; and outer myometrium—intermediate signal intensity. However, the difference in contrast between the various layers is considerably diminished compared

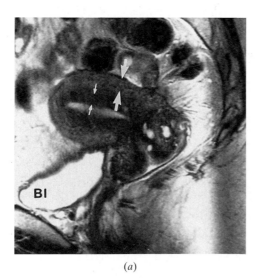

(a)

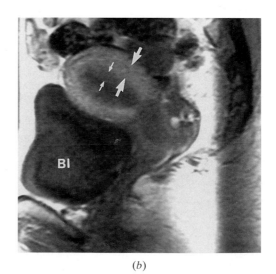

(b)

FIG. 14.10 Variable patterns of uterine enhancement. Early enhancement of the outer myometrium may be observed during the secretory phase. (*a*) Sagittal T2-weighted echo-train spin-echo sequence, (*b–d*) sagittal SGE sequences obtained serially after gadolinium administration.

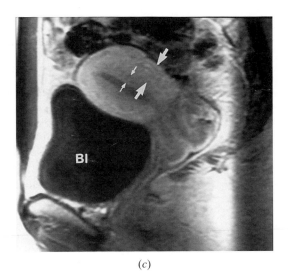

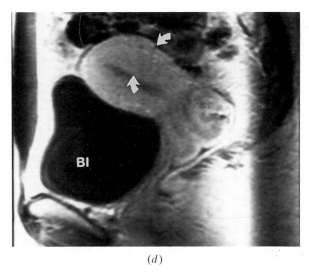

(c)

(d)

F IG. 14.10 (*Continued*) On the T2-weighted image (*a*), the inner (*small arrows, a*) and outer myometrium (*arrows, a*) are well-depicted. After contrast injection, there is early enhancement of the outer myometrium (*arrows b,c*) relative to the inner myometrium (*small arrows, b,c*). On the delayed sequence (*d*), the myometrium is homogeneously enhanced (*curved arrows, d*). *Bl,* bladder

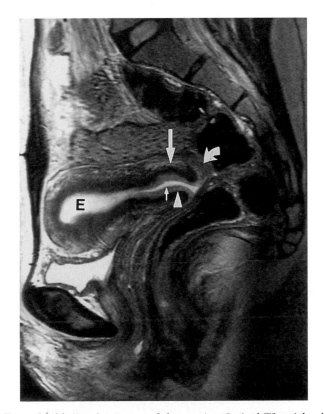

F IG. 14.11 Zonal anatomy of the cervix. Sagittal T2-weighted echo-train spin-echo sequence. The inner layer of high signal intensity represents mucous within the endocervical canal (*small arrow*). Immediately subjacent is a zone of intermediate signal intensity representing the cervical mucosa (*arrowhead*). The fibrous stroma is of low signal intensity (*arrow*). The outer muscular layer (*curved arrow*) is continuous with the outer myometrium of the uterine corpus. *E,* endometrium

to T2-weighted sequences, and frequently, the uterine zonal anatomy is completely obscured [36].

Cervix

Four distinct zones can be visualized in the cervix with high-resolution imaging on T2-weighted sequences (Fig. 14.11) [4,37]. Centrally, a hyperintense zone representing the mucous within the endocervical canal can be seen. Immediately subjacent is a zone of intermediate signal intensity representing the cervical mucosa. Mucosal folds termed *plica palmatae* are frequently identified in this layer (Fig. 14.12). The combined thickness of the endo-

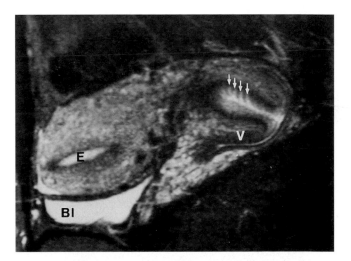

F IG. 14.12 Cervical plica palmatae. Sagittal T2-weighted echo-train spin-echo sequence. Cervical mucosal folds (*arrows*) are visible subjacent to the cervical fibrous stroma. *E,* endometrium; *Bl,* bladder; *V,* vaginal fornix

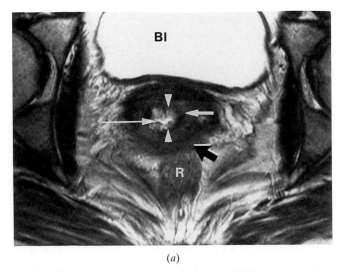

(a)

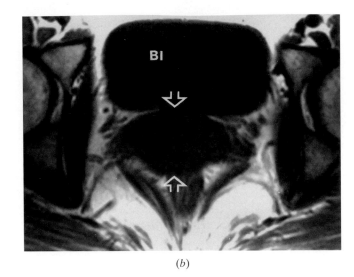

(b)

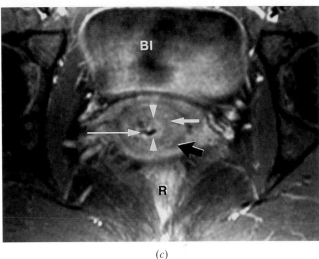

(c)

F IG. 14.13 Normal cervical enhancement. (*a*) T2-weighted echo-train spin-echo sequence, (*b*) T1-weighted spin-echo sequence, and (*c*) gadolinium-enhanced fat-suppressed SGE sequence. On the T2-weighted sequence (*a*), the mucus containing endocervical lumen (*long arrow*), mucosa (*arrowheads*), fibrous stroma (*arrow*), and outer muscular layer (*large arrow*) are well-demarcated. On the unenhanced T1-weighted sequence (*b*), the cervix (*open arrows*) is of low signal intensity and the zonal anatomy is not visualized. After contrast injection (*c*), the endocervical lumen (*long arrow*) does not enhance and remains low in signal intensity. The mucosa (*arrowheads*) enhances rapidly, whereas the fibrous stroma (*arrow*) enhances at a slower rate relative to the outer muscular layer (*large arrow*). Note the poor demarcation between the fibrous stroma and the outer muscular layer on the postcontrast image (*c*) relative to the T2-weighted image (*a*). *Bl*, bladder; *R*, rectum

cervical canal and mucosa on conventional T2-weighted spin-echo images ranges from 2 to 3 mm [37]. Surrounding the cervical mucosa is a hypointense zone corresponding to the fibrous stroma. The thickness of this zone varies from 3 to 8 mm [15,32,37]. An additional layer of intermediate signal intensity is usually seen at the periphery of the fibrous stroma. This layer is continuous with the outer myometrium of the uterine corpus and most probably represents smooth muscle (see Fig. 14.11). The MRI appearance of the cervical zonal anatomy does not appear to vary with the hormonal status of the patient.

On T1-weighted images the zonal anatomy of the cervix usually is not apparent (Fig. 14.13) [15,32]. However, the different layers may be identified with high-resolution, multicoil, or endocavitary imaging [5].

After gadolinium administration, the endocervical mucosa enhances rapidly, whereas the stroma shows more gradual enhancement. The fibrous stroma enhances at a slower rate relative to the outer zone of smooth muscle (see Fig. 14.13) [5].

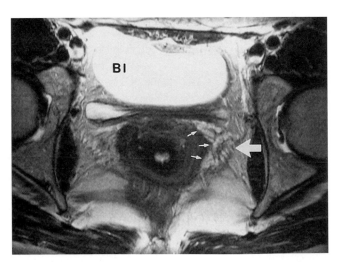

F IG. 14.14 Parametrium. T2-weighted echo-train spin-echo sequence. The hyperintense parametrium (*arrow*) is shown lateral to the cervix. Note the clear demarcation between the outer cervical muscular layer and the parametrium (*small arrows*). *Bl*, bladder

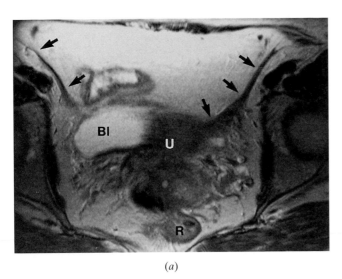

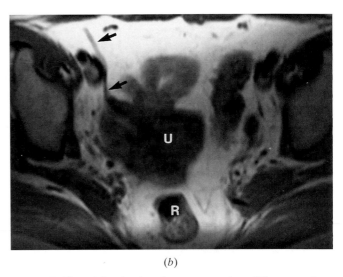

(a)   (b)

FIG. 14.15 Round ligament. (*a*) T2-weighted echo-train spin-echo sequence, (*b*) T1-weighted spin-echo sequence in a different patient. The round ligaments (*arrows, a,b*) are of low signal intensity on both T2- and T1-weighted sequences. *Bl*, bladder; *U*, uterus; *R*, rectum

Parametrium and Ligaments of the Uterus

The parametrium and cardinal ligaments contain multiple venous plexuses, and are therefore usually of intermediate signal intensity on T1-weighted sequences and iso- or hyperintense to fat on T2-weighted sequences [38,39]. On T2-weighted echo-train spin-echo sequences, the parametrium is frequently isointense to surrounding fat due to prolonged T2 values of fat with echo-train imaging (Fig. 14.14). On postcontrast images intense enhancement of the parametrium is noted. The round ligaments are hypointense on both T1- and T2-weighted sequences (Fig. 14.15). The uterosacral ligaments are hypointense on T1-weighted and of variable signal intensity on T2-weighted sequences.

Age-Related Physiologic Alterations

Premenarchal Uterus

In the premenarchal female the uterine corpus is small, and the cervix accounts for more than half of the total length of the uterus [16]. On T2-weighted sequences, the endometrium may be identified as a thin line. The junctional zone, although visible, appears indistinct. The overall signal intensity of the myometrium is lower than in women of reproductive age [16,32].

Postmenopausal Uterus

In postmenopausal women the uterus is small, with a 1 to 1 ratio of the corpus to the cervix. On T2-weighted sequences the endometrial stripe can be identified as a thin hyperintense structure (Fig. 14.16). A few small series using MRI have reported a maximal endometrial thickness of 3 mm in women not receiving exogenous hormones and a thickness of 4 to 6 mm in women receiving hormonal replacement therapy [16,32,40]. Several sono-

graphic studies of endometrial thickness in postmenopausal women have suggested an upper limit of 5 mm in patients who are not on hormone replacement and one of 8 mm for patients receiving hormonal therapy [41–43]. Although the upper limit of endometrial thick-

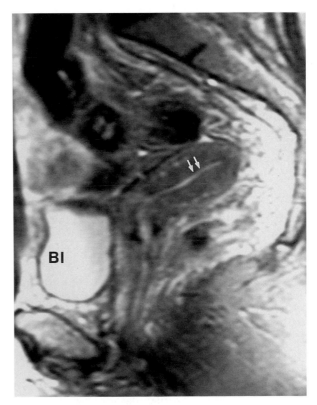

FIG. 14.16 Postmenopausal uterus. Sagittal T2-weighted spin-echo sequence. The uterus is small with a thin hyperintense endometrial stripe (*arrows*). Note that the myometrium is of low signal intensity and that the junctional zone is not visualized. *Bl*, bladder

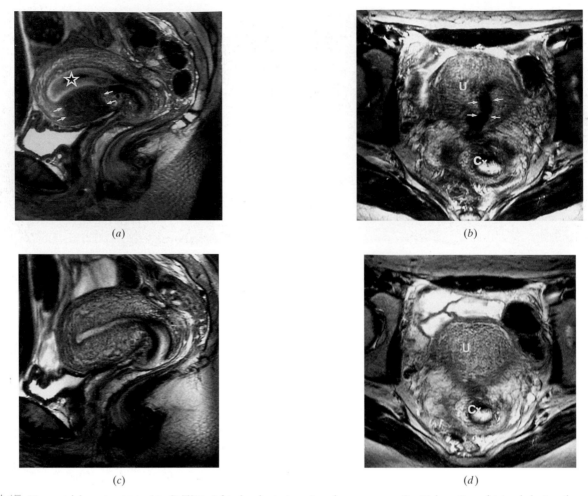

(a)

(b)

(c)

(d)

F I G . 14.17 Myometrial contraction. (*a–d*) T2-weighted echo-train spin-echo sequence. Sagittal section obtained during the menstrual phase shows a rectangular area of low signal intensity (*arrows, a*) in the ventral myometrium with distortion of the endometrial complex. However, no deformity of the outer uterine contour is present. Blood and sloughed endometrial lining are seen in the endometrial cavity (*asterisk, a*). Corresponding axial section shows the myometrial contraction to have a linear appearance (*arrows, b*). Repeat examination at a later date demonstrates a normal uterus (*c,d*). *Cx*, cervix; *U*, uterus

ness in postmenopausal women has not yet been firmly established with MRI, measurements of endometrial thickness on MR images are usually less than the corresponding measurements obtained with ultrasound [29]. The signal intensity of the myometrium on T2-weighted sequences is decreased and the junctional zone is not consistently visualized (see Fig. 14.16) [16].

Myometrial Contractions

Uterine contractions occurring during pregnancy have been well described on ultrasound and at times closely mimic the appearance of leiomyomas [44,45]. Although myometrial contractions are known to occur in the non-gravid uterus, their role in menstrual discharge and implantation is currently not well understood. On T2-weighted images, myometrial contractions appear as areas of low signal intensity within the myometrium that result in distortion of the endometrial complex but typically do not deform the outer uterine contour (Fig. 14.17) [46,47]. Myometrial contractions may closely resemble the appearance of focal adenomyosis or leiomyomas on MRI, depending on the shape and border definition of the resultant myometrial abnormality (Figs. 14.17 and 14.18). Contractions are differentiated from true myometrial pathology on sequential imaging acquisitions by their transient nature and changing appearance over time. Myometrial contractions usually resolve within 30 to 45 minutes of onset [44,45]. The cause of the low signal intensity on T2-weighted sequences observed with myometrial contractions is unknown but may relate to a regional decrease in vascularity [47].

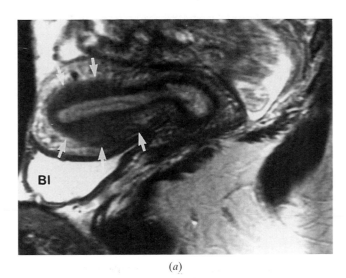

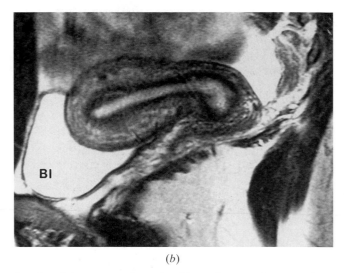

(a)   (b)

F IG . 14.18 Myometrial contraction. (*a,b*) Sagittal T2-weighted echo-train spin-echo sequence. Low-signal-intensity areas (*arrows, a*) are present in the ventral and dorsal myometrium representing contractions. The appearance mimics adenomyosis. Repeat examination 3 days later demonstrates a normal uterus (*b*). *Bl*, bladder

TREATMENT-INDUCED ALTERATIONS AND POSTSURGICAL CHANGE

Treatment-Induced Alterations

Oral Contraceptives

With prolonged use of oral contraceptives the uterine corpus may decrease in size [48]. The endometrial thickness averages 2 mm and does not vary during the course of the menstrual cycle (Fig. 14.19) [16,17]. Similarly, the junctional zone shows a decrease in maximal thickness compared to women who do not use oral contraceptives [17]. The signal intensity of the myometrium is increased, consistent with the known myometrial edema that occurs with oral contraceptive intake [48].

Exogenous Hormones

Changes induced by exogenous hormones will vary depending on the type of regimen used. The uterus of a postmenopausal woman on hormonal replacement therapy is similar in appearance to the premenopausal uterus. Exogenous hormones such as gonadotropin-releasing hormone (GnRH) used to treat leiomyomas, for example, will induce changes that parallel those of a postmenopausal uterus [16,49]. These changes will revert to normal once the treatment is stopped. Hormonal therapy for the treatment of endometrial hyperplasia induces changes similar to those seen with oral contraceptive use [50].

Radiation Therapy

Irradiation of the uterus in the premenopausal woman results in a decrease in the size of the uterus, thinning of the endometrium, decreased signal intensity of the myometrium, and loss of uterine zonal anatomy on T2-weighted sequences [51]. The MRI appearance resembles that of a nonirradiated postmenopausal uterus. These changes likely reflect a combination of direct radiation effects on the uterus and loss of hormonal stimulation from ovarian function suppression. The appearance of the uterus in postmenopausal women does not significantly change following radiation therapy [51].

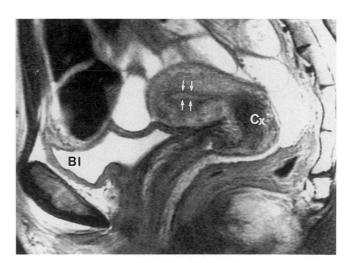

F IG . 14.19 Oral contraceptive changes. Sagittal T2-weighted echo-train spin-echo image obtained during the secretory phase (day 24) of the menstrual cycle. Note the thin endometrial stripe (*arrows*), the relative decreased thickness of the junctional zone (JZ), and the overall increased signal intensity of the myometrium, which is consistent with edema. *Bl*, bladder; *Cx*, cervical stroma

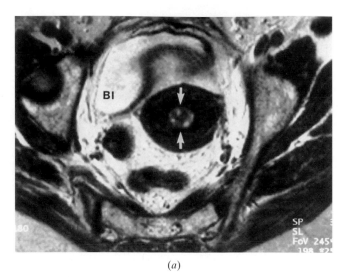

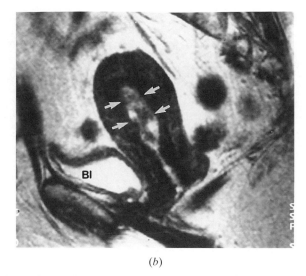

(a)   (b)

FIG. 14.20 Tamoxifen-induced changes. (*a*) Transverse and (*b*) sagittal T2-weighted echo-train spin-echo images show marked expansion and heterogeneity of the endometrial complex (*arrows, a,b*). A polyp with superficial carcinoma was found at histopathology. *Bl*, bladder

Tamoxifen

Tamoxifen is a nonsteroidal antiestrogen that binds to estrogen receptors and is used as an adjuvant therapy in women with breast carcinoma. In addition to its antiestrogen effects on breast cancer tissue, tamoxifen acts as a weak estrogen agonist on the postmenopausal uterus. A spectrum of endometrial abnormalities has been reported in patients receiving tamoxifen therapy, including proliferative changes, hyperplasia, polyps, and carcinoma [52–54]. Currently, no definitive screening guidelines for monitoring patients on tamoxifen therapy have been established, but a combination of endovaginal ultrasound and endometrial sampling is most frequently used [55].

There is a paucity of literature on the MRI appearance of uteri in women receiving tamoxifen therapy [56]. Consequently, the role of MRI in evaluating this group of patients is not yet known. However, in patients with technically inadequate or indeterminate endovaginal sonographic examinations, MRI may be helpful in determining which patients could benefit from further investigation. Ascher et al. [56] described two distinct MRI patterns in women receiving tamoxifen therapy and correlated these results with findings at histopathology. In patients with atrophy or proliferative changes at histopathology, the endometrium was homogeneously hyperintense on T2-weighted images. After contrast administration, there was enhancement of the endometrial-myometrial interface with a persistent signal void in the lumen. In patients with polyps the endometrium was of heterogeneous signal intensity on T2-weighted images (Figs. 14.20 and 14.21). On images obtained after gadolinium administration, a lattice-like pattern of enhancement was seen traversing the endometrial canal (Figs. 14.21 and 14.22).

Concomitant cystic atrophy was present in both groups at histopathology. The endometrial thickness was significantly greater in patients with polyps (mean, 1.8 cm) compared to that of patients with atrophic or proliferative changes (mean, 0.5 cm). Additional findings included subendometrial cysts, adenomyosis, leiomyomas, and a small amount of intraperitoneal fluid [56].

Diethylstilbesterol Exposure

Diethylstilbesterol (DES) is a synthetic estrogen agent frequently used until 1970 to treat pregnant women with vaginal bleeding in an attempt to prevent miscarriage. Women exposed to DES in utero have an almost 50 percent incidence of congenital uterine anomalies and are at risk for developing clear-cell carcinoma of the vagina [57]. (A more detailed discussion of the MRI findings associated with DES exposure is presented in the later subsection, Class VI: DES-Related, in the section on Congenital Uterine Anomalies.)

Postsurgical Change

Changes after Dilatation and Curettage

Dilatation and curettage (D&C) may precede MRI, such as in patients referred for endometrial carcinoma staging. Knowledge of the MRI findings after D&C is important so as not to mistake postinstrumentation changes for actual disease processes. Ascher at al. [58] found curvilinear areas of low signal intensity, most likely representing a clot in the endometrial cavity, within 2 days of D&C (Fig. 14.23). Significant widening of the endometrial stripe or disruption of the junctional zone was not observed after uncomplicated D&C.

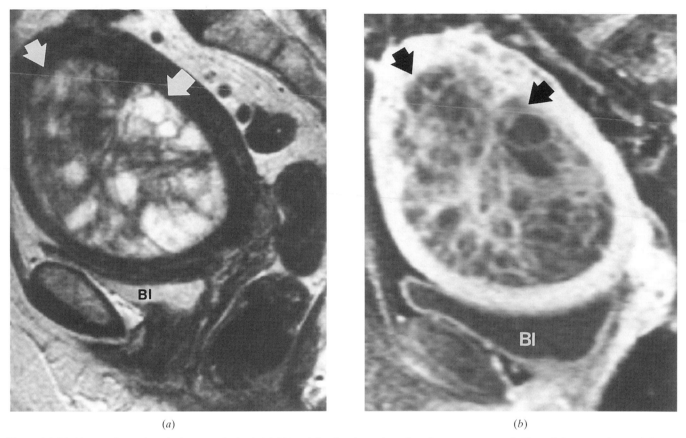

FIG. 14.21 Tamoxifen-induced changes. Sagittal (*a*) T2-weighted echo-train spin-echo sequence and (*b*) gadolinium-enhanced fat-suppressed SGE sequence. The endometrial complex is markedly enlarged (*arrows, a,b*) and shows heterogeneous signal intensity. A lattice-like pattern of enhancement is present. A benign polyp was found at histopathology. *Bl*, bladder

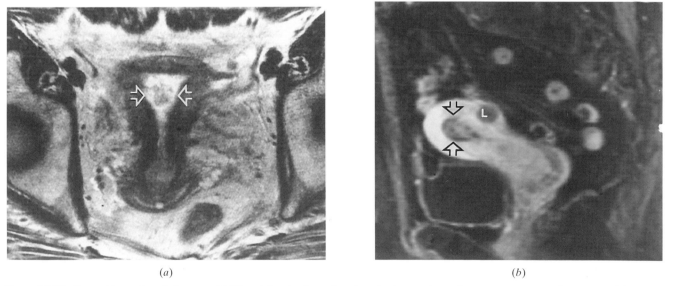

FIG. 14.22 Tamoxifen-induced changes. (*a*) T2-weighted echo-train spin-echo image shows heterogeneous signal intensity of the endometrial complex (*open arrows*). (*b*) Sagittal gadolinium-enhanced fat-suppressed SGE sequence shows a lattice-like pattern of enhancement traversing the endometrial canal, which is consistent with a polyp (*open arrows*). *L*, leiomyoma

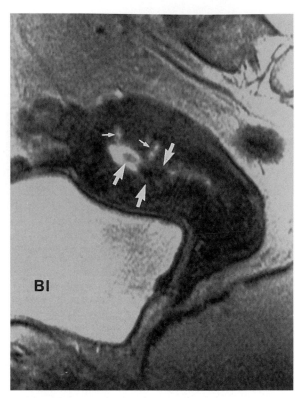

F IG . 14.23 Postdilatation and curettage (D&C) changes. Sagittal T2-weighted echo-train spin-echo sequence. Areas of low signal intensity (*arrows*) consistent with blood clot are seen within the endometrial cavity. No interruption of the inner myometrium is present. Bright foci visible in the dorsal myometrium (*small arrows*) represent areas of adenomyosis. *Bl*, bladder

Postmyomectomy

In women undergoing myomectomy, the surgical bed may be seen as an area of moderately high signal intensity on both T1- and T2-weighted sequences. These signal characteristics suggest the presence of a subacute hematoma within the myometrium at the myomectomy site (Fig. 14.24).

Postcesarean Section

(A description of the MRI findings in women who have undergone cesarean section is presented in the later subsection, Postcesarean section, in the section on MRI and Pregnancy.)

CONGENITAL UTERINE ANOMALIES

Müllerian Duct Anomalies

General Considerations

The incidence of uterine anomalies among women of reproductive age is estimated to range from 0.1 to 0.5 percent [59]. Although uterine anomalies may be entirely asymptomatic, their clinical significance lies in an increased incidence of impaired fertility, pregnancy wastage (recurrent miscarriage, premature labor, intrauterine growth retardation), and menstrual disorders [60,61].

The fallopian tubes, uterus, and upper two-thirds of the vagina are derived from paired müllerian ducts, which migrate caudally, then undergo fusion and subsequent canalization [62]. This process, which begins at approximately 10 weeks following conception, may be interrupted at any stage during development. Failure of the paired müllerian ducts to develop results in various degrees of uterine, cervical, and vaginal agenesis. Didelphys or bicornuate uteri result from absent or incomplete fusion of the uterine horns respectively. Finally, if fusion does occur but is followed by absent or incomplete resorption of the septum between müllerian duct components, a septate uterus will result. Due to the proximity

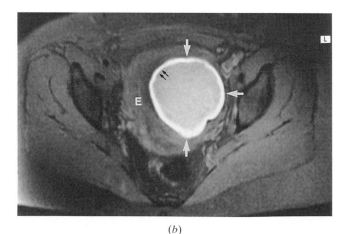

(a)   (b)

F IG . 14.24 Postmyomectomy hematoma. (*a*) T2-weighted echo-train spin-echo sequence, (*b*) fat-suppressed T1-weighted SGE sequence. A well delineated mass of moderately high signal intensity (*arrows, a,b*) consistent with a hematoma is present in the surgical bed. Note the peripheral rim of higher signal intensity (*small arrows, b*), which is typical of a subacute hematoma. *E*, endometrium of the müllerian and wolffian systems embryologically, müllerian duct anomalies are frequently associated with urinary anomalies, particularly renal agenesis or ectopia [60].

The treatment options for different uterine anomalies vary considerably, and accurate preoperative diagnosis is essential for appropriate patient management. The most widely used classification is that proposed by Buttram and Gibbons [63], which divides anomalies into classes with similar clinical features, prognoses, and treatment options (Table 14.1). It is important to emphasize that these anomalies represent a spectrum of disorders rather than discrete entities, and it may not be possible to group all malformations into one particular class.

Hysterosalpingography (HSG), laparoscopy, and laparotomy have been the standard techniques used to classify müllerian duct anomalies [60]. However, HSG has several limitations in classifying patients with uterine anomalies [64]. First, only horns that communicate with the main endometrial cavity are opacified at HSG. Second, the external contour of the uterus cannot be evaluated, thereby limiting accurate differentiation between bicornuate and septate uteri [63]. Transabdominal sonography has met with variable success in evaluating patients with müllerian duct anomalies [65–67]. More recently, endovaginal sonography and MRI have been shown to be highly accurate in diagnosing uterine malformations [64,68–71]. Endovaginal sonography can be used initially to classify patients with suspected uterine anomalies given the low cost and widespread availability of this technique. MRI should be reserved for (1) patients with a technically inadequate or indeterminate ultrasound examination; (2) patients in whom concomitant cervical or vaginal malformations, including septae, are suspected; and (3) patients with multiple and complex anomalies.

Class I: Müllerian Agenesis/Hypoplasia

Uterine agenesis or hypoplasia may occur as part of a congenital syndrome or as a result of chromosomal defects. In addition, uterine agenesis may be found in isolation in patients presenting with primary amenorrhea. Sagittal T2-weighted sequences are obtained for documenting the presence or absence of the uterus. In patients with uterine hypoplasia, the endometrial cavity is small, and the intercornual distance measures less than 2 cm [68]. When uterine hypoplasia is associated with hypogonadism, T2-weighted sequences demonstrate loss of the zonal anatomy and decreased signal intensity of the myometrium (Figs. 14.25 and 14.26) [68].

Class I-E is the most common type of Class I anomaly. Patients with Class I-E anomalies have frequently been categorized as belonging to the Mayor-Rokitanski-Küster-Hauser (MRKH) syndrome. In patients with MRKH syndrome, the presence of vaginal agenesis or hypoplasia with intact ovaries and fallopian tubes is accompanied

Table 14.1 Classification of Müllerian Anomalies[1]

Class I	Segmented agenesis or hypoplasia	
	A	Vaginal
	B	Cervical
	C	Fundal
	D	Tubal
	E	Combined anomalies
Class II	Unicornuate uterus	
	A1	Rudimentary horn with endometrium
		a. Communicating with main uterine cavity
		b. Not communicating with main uterine cavity
	A2	Rudimentary horn without endometrium
	B	No rudimentary horn
Class III	Uterus didelphys	
Class IV	Bicornuate uterus	
	A	Complete (division down to internal os)
	B	Partial
	C	Arcuate
Class V	Septate	
	A	Complete (down to internal or external os)
	B	Incomplete
Class VI	DES-related	

[1] After Buttram VC Jr, Gibbons WE: Müllerian anomalies: A proposed classification. (an analysis of 144 cases). Fertil Steril 32(1):40–46, 1979.

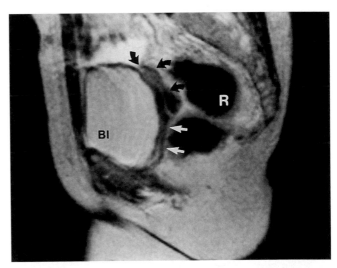

FIG. 14.25 Gonadal dysgenesis (Turner's syndrome). Sagittal T2-weighted spin-echo image through the midpelvis in a patient with Turner's syndrome. There is uterine hypoplasia (*curved arrows*) with a uterus to cervix ratio of 1 to 1. Vaginal hypoplasia (*arrows*) is also noted. Ovaries were not identified. *Bl*, bladder; *R*, rectum (Reprinted with permission from Reinhold C, Hricak H, Forstner R, et al: Primary amenorrhea: Evaluation with MR imaging. Radiology. In Press)

eventually closes, resulting in endometriosis (Fig. 14.28). Due to its excellent soft tissue differentiation, MRI can easily confirm the presence of an endometrial stripe by demonstrating the endometrial complex of high signal intensity on T2-weighted sequences. In addition, when using a combination of T1- and T2-weighted sequences, MRI is an excellent tool for documenting the presence of blood in the vagina or uterine cavity and the presence of retrograde endometriosis that may complicate Class I anomalies [78]. For patients who have not undergone

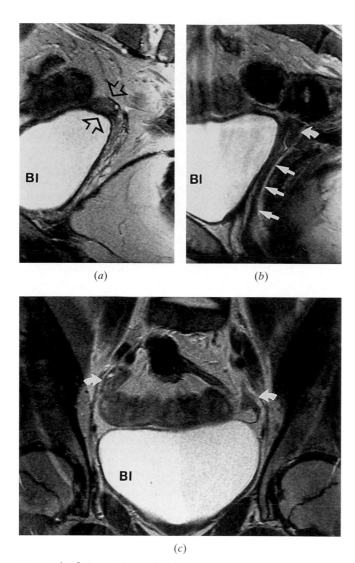

(a)   (b)

(c)

F IG . 14.26 Pure XY gonadal dysgenesis (Swyer syndrome). (*a,b*) Sagittal, and (*c*) coronal T2-weighted echo-train spin-echo sequence. The uterine corpus (*open arrows, a*) and cervix (*curved arrow, b*) are hypoplastic. Note the low signal intensity of the myometrium. The vagina (*arrows, b*) is present but hypoplastic. Bilateral streak gonads (*curved arrows, c*) are visualized. *Bl*, bladder

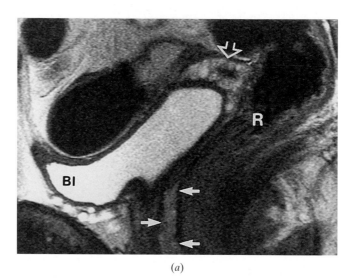

(a)

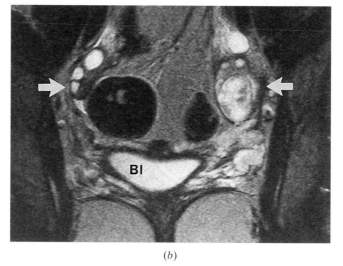

(b)

F IG . 14.27 Mayor-Rokitanski-Küster-Hauser (MRKH) syndrome. (*a*) Sagittal and (*b*) coronal T2-weighted echo-train spin-echo sequence in a 21-year-old patient presenting with primary amenorrhea. There is complete vaginal and uterine agenesis; only loose connective tissue and pelvic veins are present in the area of the expected vagina (*arrows, a*) and uterus (*open arrow, a*). Coronal section through the midpelvis shows both ovaries (*arrows, b*). A hemorrhagic cyst is present in the left ovary. *Bl*, bladder; *R*, rectum (Reprinted with permission from Reinhold C, Hricak H, Forstner R, et al: Primary amenorrhea: Evaluation with MR imaging. Radiology. In Press)

by variable anomalies of the uterus, urinary tract, and skeletal system (Fig. 14.27) [72–75]. The role of MRI is to provide a detailed map of the pelvic anatomy, including the presence and extent of any anomalies. Surgical management in patients with female anatomic anomalies is aimed at preventing endometriosis and preserving fertility [76,77]. Vaginal agenesis with a patent endometrial canal and a cervix can be treated by vaginoplasty to allow the egress of menstrual discharge. Isolated cervical or vaginal agenesis with a functioning endometrium but without a cervix requires hysterectomy because (1) a uterovaginal fistula or an artificial cervix cannot successfully sustain a pregnancy, and (2) the uterovaginal fistula

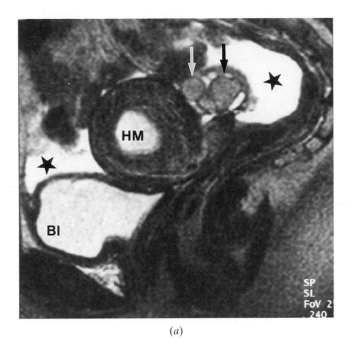

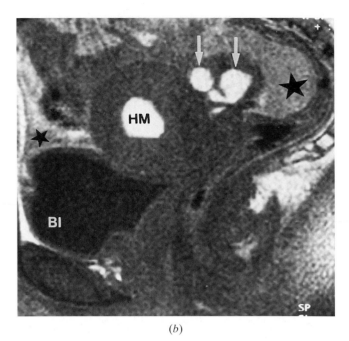

(a)   (b)

FIG. 14.28 Isolated cervical agenesis in a 21-year-old patient presenting with primary amenorrhea. (*a*) Sagittal T2-weighted echo-train spin-echo and (*b*) T1-weighted fat-suppressed spin-echo images show the presence of a hematometra (HM). There is complete cervical agenesis (*a,b*). The vagina was patent but atrophic. Small ovarian endometriomas (*arrows, a,b*) are present due to retrograde endometriosis. Note the associated hemoperitoneum both ventrally and dorsally (*asterisk, a,b*). *Bl*, bladder (Reprinted with permission from Reinhold C, Hricak H, Forstner R, et al: Primary amenorrhea: Evaluation with MR imaging. Radiology. In Press)

prior renal sonography, the renal fossa can be evaluated at the time of the pelvic MRI to exclude the presence of coexisting renal anomalies.

(A more detailed discussion of vaginal anomalies is presented in Chapter 13 on the Female Urethra and Vagina.)

Class II: Unicornuate Uterus

A unicornuate uterus is characterized on MRI by its elongated, curved, banana-shaped configuration. The unicornuate uterus demonstrates normal zonal anatomy on T2-weighted images, but the overall uterine volume is reduced [64]. In patients with unicornuate uteri that have an asociated rudimentary horn, three different subtypes are usually recognized: (1) rudimentary horn with communicating cavity (Class II-A-1a), (2) rudimentary horn with noncommunicating cavity (Class II-A-1b), and (3) noncavitary rudimentary horn (Class II-A-2). The differentiation of these subtypes is important because Class II-A-1a anomalies usually require no treatment, whereas Class II-A-1b and Class II-A-2 anomalies may benefit from removal of the rudimentary horn [79]. T2-weighted short- and long-axis views, as well as parasagittal sections, are used to image the rudimentary horn. The presence or absence of the hyperintense endometrial stripe, as well as its continuity with the main uterine cavity, can be accurately determined with MRI (Fig. 14.29) [68,79].

Class III: Uterus Didelphys

Uterus didelphys is diagnosed at MRI when two separate normal-sized uteri and cervices are seen [64,68]. Although a septate vagina may be seen with any of the müllerian duct anomalies, it is most commonly associated with uterus didelphys (Fig. 14.30) [60]. When transverse, the septum can obstruct the outflow of blood into the vagina and result in hematocolpometra. MRI demonstrates a distended vagina and uterine horn whose contents follow the signal characteristics of blood on T1- and T2-weighted images.

Class IV: Bicornuate Uterus

The following criteria are used to diagnose a bicornuate uterus with MRI: (1) divergent uterine horns with an intercornual distance exceeding 4 cm [68], and (2) a concavity of the fundal contour or external fundal cleft measuring more than 1 cm in depth (Fig. 14.31) [64]. In addition to standard MRI planes, long- and short-axis views of the uterus should be obtained (see Figs. 14.1 and 14.2). A T1-weighted, long-axis view obtained at the level of the endometrial stripe is best for evaluating the fundal contour. T2-weighted images are used to demonstrate the zonal anatomy and uterine septum. The septum of patients with a bicornuate uterus may terminate at the level of the internal os (uterus bicornuate unicollis) or extend down to the external os (uterus bicornuate bicollis). At times it may be difficult to differentiate a double

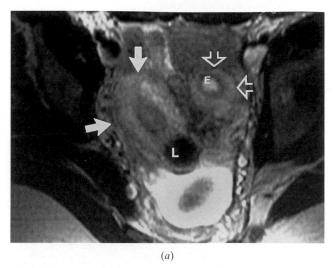 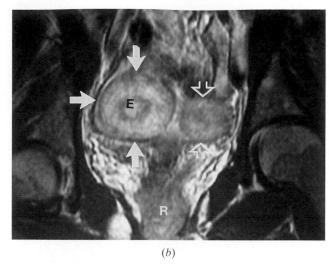

(a)   (b)

F IG . 14.29 Unicornuate uterus with rudimentary horn. (*a*) Transverse and (*b*) coronal oblique T2-weighted spin-echo sequence. The unicornuate uterus demonstrates normal zonal anatomy (*arrows, a,b*). The rudimentary horn (*open arrows, a,b*) is of small caliber and a hyperintense endometrial stripe is visualized (*a*). The continuity with the main uterine cavity was easily demonstrated on serial sections (not shown). Note the overall lower signal intensity of the myometrium of the rudimentary horn. *E*, endometrium; *L*, leiomyoma; *R*, rectum

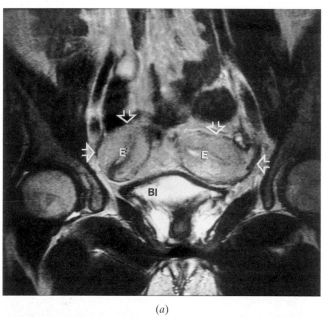 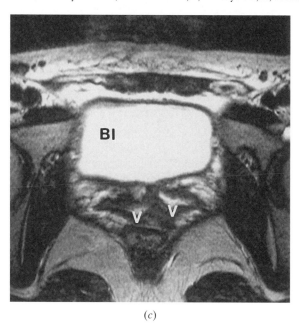

(a)   (c)

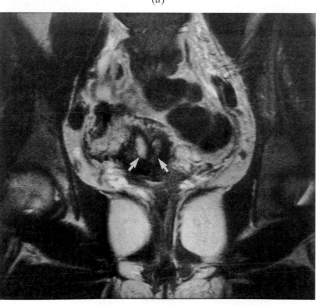

F IG . 14.30 Uterus didelphys. (*a,b*) Coronal oblique T2-weighted echo-train spin-echo images; (*c*) transverse T2-weighted echo-train spin-echo image in a different patient. Complete uterine duplication with two separate, normal-sized corpora (*open arrows, a*). On a more posterior section, a double cervix can be seen with two hyperintense endocervical canals (*arrows, b*). Two separate vaginas are present in another patient with uterus didelphys (*c*). (Figs. 14.30*a,b* courtesy of Dr. Shirley McCarthy, Yale University, New Haven, Connecticut) *Bl*, bladder; *V*, vagina; *E*, endometrium

(b)

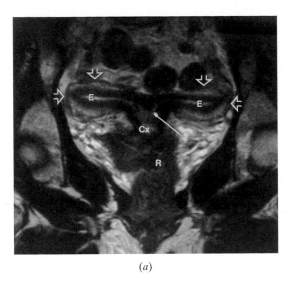

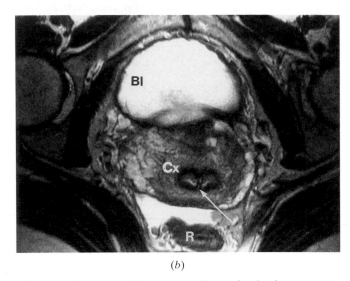

(a)   (b)

Fig. 14.31 Bicornuate uterus. (*a*) Coronal oblique T2-weighted echo-train spin-echo image; (*b*) transverse T2-weighted echo-train spin-echo image in a different patient. Widely divergent uterine horns (*open arrows, a*), with a large intercornual distance. The septum (*long thin arrow, a*) terminates at the level of the internal os (uterus bicornuate unicollis). When the septum (*long thin arrow, b*) extends to the external os, a uterus bicornuate bicollis results. (Fig. 14.31*a* courtesy of Dr. Shirley McCarthy, Yale University, New Haven, Connecticut) *Bl*, bladder; *E*, endometrium; *Cx*, cervix; *R*, rectum

cervix from a cervical septation at MRI. On T2-weighted sequences, the septum in a bicornuate uterus may consist of low-signal-intensity fibrous tissue in addition to intermediate-signal-intensity myometrium.

Although a bicornuate uterus infrequently requires surgery, a transabdominal approach is used to fuse the uterine horns in symptomatic patients.

Class V: Septate Uterus

The external contour of the uterine fundus is the main differentiating feature between a septate and bicornuate uterus (Figs. 14.32 and 14.33). Until recently, laparoscopy was the only reliable method of differentiating these enti-

ties. Several studies have demonstrated the accuracy of MRI in diagnosing septate and bicornuate uteri [64,68–70]. Septate uteri have a convex, flat, or minimally indented (≤1 cm) fundal contour, whereas bicornuate uteri have a large fundal cleft [64]. In addition, septate uteri maintain a normal intercornual distance (range, 2 to 4 cm) [68]. The signal intensity of the septum (muscular versus fibrous) cannot be used to differentiate septate from bicornuate uteri because fibrous tissue as well as

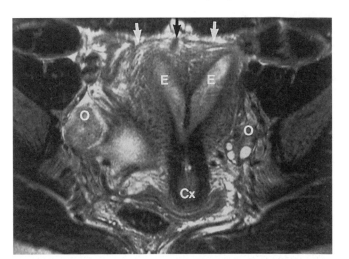

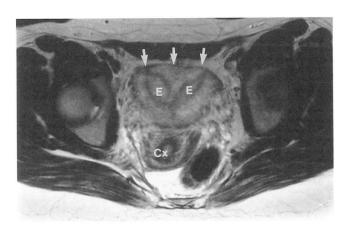

Fig. 14.32 Septate uterus. T2-weighted echo-train spin-echo image in a patient with a previous history of second trimester abortions. The fundal contour is convex (*arrows*), and the intercornual distance is less than 4 cm. A single cervix is present. *E*, endometrial cavity; *Cx*, cervix

Fig. 14.33 Septate uterus. T2-weighted echo-train spin-echo sequence, long-axis view. Two endometrial cavities and one cervix can be identified. The external fundal contour is convex (*arrows*). The superior portion of the septum consists of intermediate-signal-intensity myometrium; in its inferior aspect, fibrous tissue is present. Incidentally, a hemorrhagic cyst of intermediate signal is present in the right ovary. *E*, endometrial cavity; *Cx*, cervix; *O*, ovary

myometrium may be encountered in the septum of both anomalies (see Fig. 14.33) [64,68]. Accurate distinction between septate and bicornuate uteri is important for proper patient management. Septate uteri are associated with a higher rate of reproductive failure, with two-thirds of pregnancies terminating in abortion [60]. In contradistinction to bicornuate uteri, septate uteri are successfully treated with hysteroscopic excision of the septum and do not require abdominal surgery. The MRI protocol used for evaluating a septate uterus is the same as that described in the preceding section for a bicornuate uterus.

Class VI: DES-Related

Diethylstilbesterol (DES) is a synthetic estrogen agent used frequently until 1970 to treat pregnant women with vaginal bleeding. Women exposed to DES in utero have an almost 50% incidence of congenital uterine anomalies [57]. Hysterosalpingography (HSG) has been used most commonly to diagnose anomalies associated with DES exposure, including hypoplasia, T-shape, constrictions, polypoid defects, synechiae, and marginal irregularities of the uterine cavity [57,80]. No increased incidence of urinary tract anomalies has been reported in patients with DES exposure.

In a small series, van Gils et al. [81] reported that MRI correctly identified all anomalies diagnosed with HSG, aside from marginal irregularities of the uterine cavity. Long-axis views were best suited to demonstrate the anomalies of the endometrial cavity. At the site of uterine cavity constriction, localized thickening of the junctional zone was noted on T2-weighted images. The zonal anatomy of the uterus was preserved in all patients studied. In addition to hypoplasia of the uterine cavity (length <3.3 cm), the length of the cervix, including the endocervical canal, may be reduced. When associated with cervical incompetence, the endocervical canal usually measures shorter than 2.5 cm. The width of the internal os and the signal intensity of the cervical stroma, however, remain normal [81,82].

Congenital Disorders of Sexual Differentiation

Congenital disorders of sexual differentiation can be divided into genetic, gonadal, or phenotypic anomalies [83,84].

A multidisciplinary approach is usually required because hormonal studies, karyotyping, and anatomic information are all necessary for accurate diagnosis and treatment. The role of imaging includes (1) detailing the presence or absence of all pertinent pelvic anatomic structures, (2) identifying functioning uterine tissue in patients with a uterus in situ, (3) determining the length of the atretic segment in patients with vaginal agenesis, and (4) locating ectopic gonads for surgical removal because these are at increased risk for developing malig-

nancy (Figs. 14.34 and 14.35). The excellent soft tissue differentiation and multiplanar imaging capability of MRI make it a useful tool in the evaluation of patients with congenital disorders of sexual differentiation [78,85]. (A more detailed discussion of congenital disorders of sex-

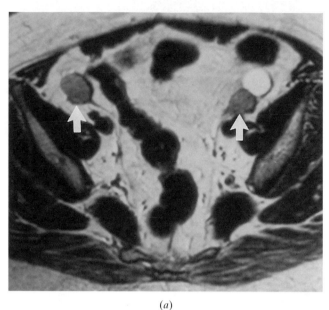

(a)

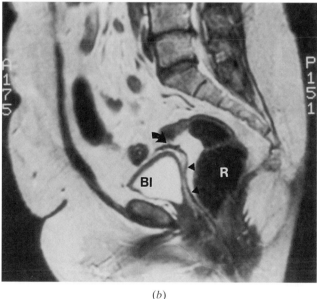

(b)

FIG. 14.34 Testicular feminization. A 39-year-old patient with a previous history of primary amenorrhea presented for evaluation of infertility. (*a*) Transverse and (*b*) sagittal T2-weighted spin-echo images. There are bilateral undescended testes (*arrows, a*). The small size and low signal intensity of the testes indicate atrophy. An inclusion cyst is present adjacent to the left testis. At histopathology, a focus of germinoma was found in the right testes. Sagittal image shows a hypoplastic vagina (*arrowheads, b*) and a small uterine remnant (*curved arrow, b*). *Bl*, bladder; *R*, rectum (Reprinted with permission from Reinhold C, Hricak H, Forstner R, et al: Primary amenorrhea: Evaluation with MR imaging. Radiology. In Press)

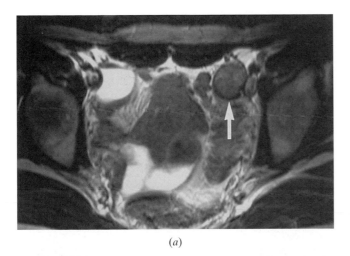

(a)

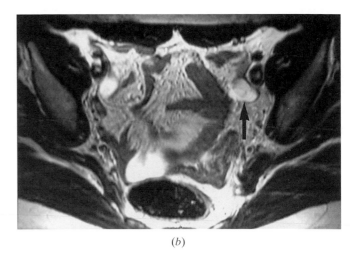

(b)

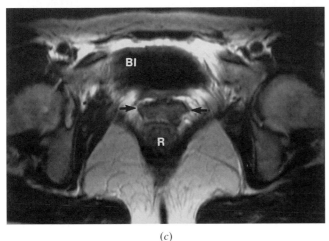

(c)

FIG. 14.35 True hermaphrodite (46,XY). A 39-year-old woman with a past medical history of primary amenorrhea, hysterectomy, and removal of a right ovotestis. (*a–c*) T2-weighted echo-train spin-echo sequence shows a testis (*arrow, a*) and adjacent epididymis (*arrow, b*) along the left external iliac chain. Because of gonadal enlargement and heterogeneous signal intensity, malignancy was suspected. However, at histopathology only hamartomatous smooth muscle hyperplasia was found. A caudal section shows a normal vagina (*arrows, c*) between the bladder base and rectum. *Bl*, bladder; *R*, rectum (Reprinted with permission from Reinhold C, Hricak H, Forstner R, et al: Primary amenorrhea: Evaluation with MR imaging. Radiology. In Press)

ual differentiation is presented in Chapter 13 on the Female Urethra and Vagina.)

BENIGN DISEASES OF THE UTERINE CORPUS

Endometrial Polyps and Hyperplasia

General Considerations

Endovaginal sonography (EVS) is currently the standard imaging modality for assessing the endometrium in symptomatic patients [41–43,86]. A major indication for endovaginal sonographic evaluation of the endometrium is abnormal postmenopausal bleeding. Sonographic studies of endometrial thickness in postmenopausal women have suggested an upper limit of 5 mm in patients who are not on hormone replacement and 8 mm for patients receiving hormonal therapy [41–43,86]. EVS is highly sensitive for detecting endometrial pathology when these cutoff values are used as guidelines to determine which patients would benefit from endometrial sampling. The presence of endometrial thickening on EVS is nonspecific

and may be due to endometrial hyperplasia, polyps, or carcinoma [86,87]. Endometrial sampling, however, is indicated in all cases of endometrial thickening in postmenopausal women because both endometrial hyperplasia and polyps may be seen in association with endometrial carcinoma [88]. Although submucosal leiomyomas are usually differentiated from endometrial pathology by their location and typical sonographic appearance, distinction may not always be possible. Improved differentiation between endometrial abnormalities and submucosal leiomyomas may be achieved with hysterosonography [89].

Nevertheless, EVS is a highly effective screening tool when the endometrium can be adequately visualized. In some patients, however, accurate measurements of endometrial thickness may not be possible due to a vertical orientation of the uterus, the presence of multiple leiomyomas, or extensive adenomyosis. Under these circumstances, MRI may be able to provide additional information on the appearance of the endometrium, particularly in patients for whom endometrial sampling would be difficult (e.g., patients with cervical stenosis). Currently MRI has no established role in screening for endometrial pathology, and the accuracy of MRI in evaluating this subgroup of patients is not known.

MRI Considerations

A combination of T2-weighted and contrast-enhanced T1-weighted sequences is used to evaluate benign endometrial pathology. Contrast-enhanced T1-weighted sequences considerably improve the detection rate of endometrial polyps. T2-weighted sagittal and transverse images are initially obtained through the pelvis. Short-axis views through the uterus may be helpful in selected cases. Dynamic and delayed T1-weighted contrast-enhanced sequences are obtained following the T2-weighted sequences.

To the present, the normal range of endometrial thickness in postmenopausal women with MRI has not been extensively studied. A few small series using MRI have reported a maximal endometrial thickness of 3 mm in women not receiving exogenous hormones and 4 to 6 mm in women receiving hormonal replacement therapy [16,32,40].

Endometrial hyperplasia usually presents as diffuse thickening of the endometrial stripe on T2-weighted images (Fig. 14.36). The signal intensity of the endometrial

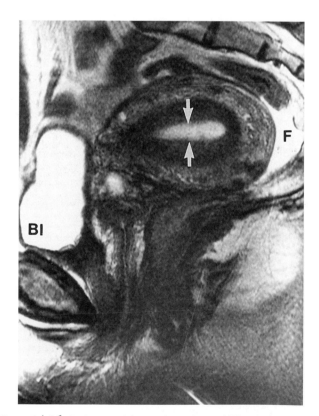

FIG. 14.36 Endometrial hyperplasia. Sagittal T2-weighted echo-train spin-echo image. The uterus is retroverted. The endometrial stripe is diffusely thickened (*arrows*) and of minimally decreased signal intensity. Endometrial hyperplasia was found at histopathology. *Bl*, bladder; *F*, fluid in cul de sac

stripe is isointense or slightly hypointense relative to normal endometrium [40]. These imaging characteristics, however, are nonspecific and are also seen with endometrial carcinoma.

On T2-weighted images, endometrial polyps most frequently present as masses of slightly lower signal intensity relative to normal endometrium (Fig. 14.37). At times, however, they may be entirely isointense and present as diffuse or focal thickening of the endometrial stripe [9]. Particularly when large, endometrial polyps may be markedly heterogeneous with areas of high and low signal intensity (Fig. 14.38). A linear area of low signal intensity corresponding to a stalk may be identified at the periphery of pedunculated polyps. After gadolinium administration, polyps show variable degrees of enhancement (see Figs. 14.37 and 14.38). Typically, polyps enhance less than the endometrium but similar to or greater than the adjacent myometrium. Although contrast-enhanced images improve detection of endometrial polyps, the pattern of contrast enhancement is nonspecific, and differentiation from early endometrial carcinoma is not possible [36].

Submucosal leiomyomas may be differentiated from endometrial polyps on T2-weighted images by confirming their myometrial origin. In addition, leiomyomas are typically of low signal intensity on T2-weighted images. However, leiomyomas may exhibit variable signal intensities, and overlap in signal characteristics between leiomyomas and endometrial polyps is frequently noted [40].

Leiomyomas

General Considerations

Leiomyoma, the most common type of uterine tumor, is estimated to be present in 20 percent of women over 35 years of age [90]. Leiomyomas are estrogen dependent, and therefore usually regress after the onset of menopause.

Leiomyomas are benign neoplasms of smooth-muscle cell origin. They are sharply demarcated from the surrounding myometrium by a pseudocapsule of light areolar tissue [90]. The smooth-muscle cells are arranged in a whorl-like interlacing pattern, giving leiomyomas their characteristic gross appearance. Cellular leiomyomas are a specific subtype composed of densely packed smooth-muscle tissue with little intervening collagen. Most leiomyomas undergo some degree of degeneration, which contributes to the variable appearance of these tumors on imaging [90,91]. Hyalin degeneration occurs to some extent in all leiomyomas except the very small. Leiomyomas may also undergo myxomatous, hyalin, cystic, fatty, or hemorrhagic (carneous) degeneration. In addition, leiomyomas frequently calcify, particularly in older women. Torsion, infection, and sarcomatous degeneration are rare complications.

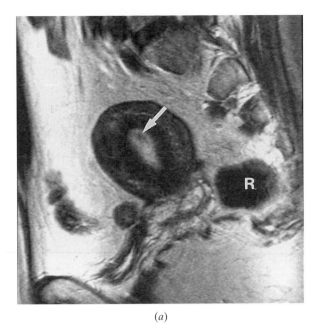

(a)

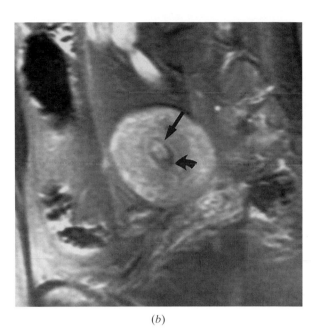

(b)

Fig. 14.37 Benign endometrial polyp. Sagittal (*a*) T2-weighted echo-train spin-echo sequence, and (*b*) immediate postgadolinium fat-suppressed SGE sequence. On the T2-weighted sequence (*a*), an area of decreased signal intensity (*arrow, a*) is seen within the endometrial stripe that may present a small polyp. The polyp (*arrow, b*) is better demonstrated after gadolinium administration and enhances to a greater degree than the normal endometrium (*curved arrow, b*). *R*, rectum

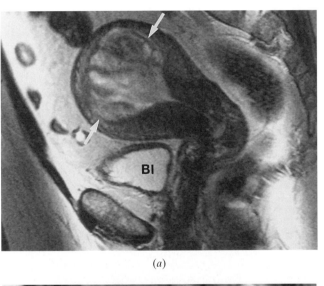

(a)

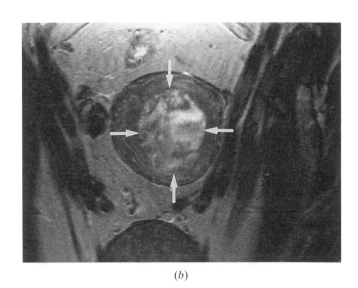

(b)

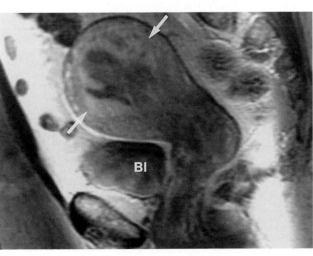

(c)

Fig. 14.38 Benign endometrial polyp. (*a*) Sagittal, (*b*) coronal oblique T2-weighted echo-train spin-echo sequences, and (*c*) sagittal gadolinium-enhanced T1-weighted spin-echo sequence. A large heterogeneous polyp distends the endometrial cavity (*arrows, a–c*). The polyp (*arrows, a,b*) is contained within the endometrial cavity and does not disrupt the inner myometrium. Variable enhancement of the polyp (*arrows, c*) is noted relative to the adjacent myometrium. *Bl*, bladder.

Leiomyomas are usually classified according to location: submucosal, intramural, subserosal, or cervical. Uncommonly, a leiomyoma may be situated in the broad ligament or be entirely detached from the uterus, parasitizing the blood supply from other vascular beds, usually the omentum [92]. Although leiomyomas may be entirely asymptomatic and present as incidental findings, they may be associated with a variety of symptoms, including menorrhagia, dysmenorrhea, pressure effects, infertility, second trimester abortions, and dystocia [90].

The role of imaging in evaluating patients with suspected leiomyomas is directed toward lesion detection, characterization, and localization. Ultrasound remains the initial imaging modality of choice for patients with suspected leiomyomas, and in the vast majority of routine clinical presentations no additional investigation is needed [93,94]. However, a number of limitations may be encountered with ultrasound when evaluating patients with suspected leiomyomas. Small leiomyomas (<2 cm) may not be consistently depicted with ultrasound, and although large leiomyomas are more likely to be symptomatic, small tumors also may produce symptoms, depending on their location [93]. The presence of multiple lesions and/or marked distortion of the uterus can adversely affect the ability of ultrasound to precisely locate leiomyomas [95,96]. In patients electing to undergo uterine-sparing surgery, accurate preoperative localization of leiomyomas is of paramount importance in planning myomectomy. Submucosal leiomyomas may be resected hysteroscopically, whereas laparoscopic or transabdominal myomectomy is required for intramural or subserosal leiomyomas. Similarly, visualization of the endometrium or ovaries may be obscured in patients with large or multiple leiomyomas [96]. Therefore, distinction

between a pedunculated leiomyoma and a solid ovarian mass may not always be possible [97]. Although leiomyomas are usually easily recognized at ultrasound as localized hypoechoic masses with or without attenuation, the appearance is nonspecific, and overlap with other disease entities (e.g., adenomyosis) may be present.

Under these circumstances, further evaluation with MRI is indicated. Several studies have demonstrated MRI to be superior to ultrasound for the detection and localization of uterine leiomyomas [95,97–99]. Furthermore, MRI is a useful adjunct for differentiating leiomyomas from other pathological conditions [97,100].

MRI Considerations

T2-weighted sequences provide optimal contrast between leiomyomas and the adjacent myometrium or endometrium [99]. In addition to standard sagittal and transverse views, coronal or oblique views may be indicated for accurate localization and for establishing the myometrial origin of a lesion [98]. T1-weighted sequences may be obtained if areas of degeneration are suspected. In addition, the presence of a fat plane on T1-weighted sequences may aid in differentiating a pedunculated leiomyoma from a solid ovarian mass. Contrast-enhanced T1-weighted images are not usually helpful in the detection or characterization of uterine leiomyomas. However, in cases where the myometrial origin of a mass has not been established with T2-weighted sequences, contrast-enhanced images with fat saturation may provide additional information by demonstrating the splaying of the myometrium around a portion of the lesion.

Leiomyomas typically appear as sharply marginated masses of low signal intensity relative to myometrium on T2-weighted sequences (Fig. 14.39). Lesions smaller than

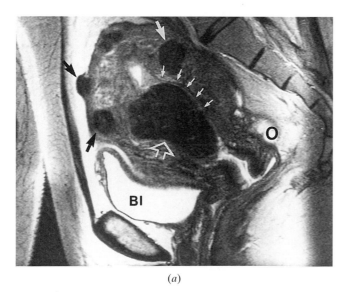

(a)

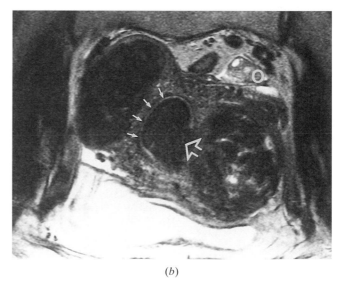

(b)

FIG. 14.39 Multiple uterine leiomyomas. (a) Sagittal and (b) coronal oblique T2-weighted echo-train spin-echo sequence. Multiple leiomyomas are shown as sharply marginated masses of low signal intensity (*arrows, a*). A submucosal leiomyoma (*open arrow, a,b*) displacing the endometrium (*small arrows, a,b*) is also seen. *Bl*, bladder; *O*, ovary

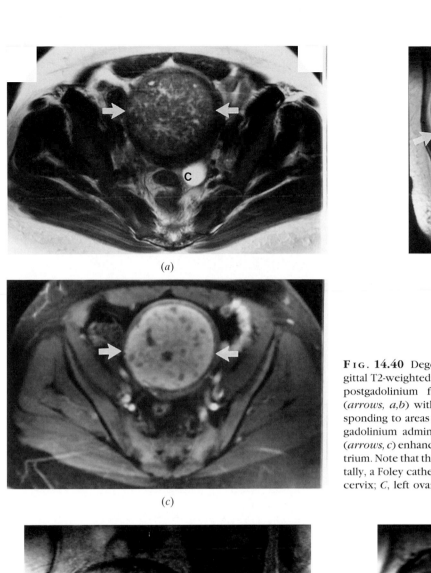

(a)

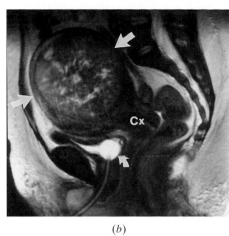

(b)

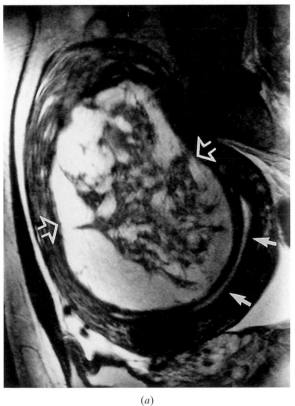

(c)

FIG. 14.40 Degenerated uterine leiomyoma. (*a*) Transverse, (*b*) sagittal T2-weighted echo-train spin-echo sequence, and (*c*) 120-second postgadolinium fat-suppressed SGE sequence. Large leiomyoma (*arrows, a,b*) with multiple foci of increased signal intensity corresponding to areas of degeneration is present within the uterus. After gadolinium administration, the solid component of the leiomyoma (*arrows, c*) enhances more than the surrounding rim of normal myometrium. Note that the foci of degenerated tissue do not enhance. Incidentally, a Foley catheter (*curved arrow, b*) is present in the bladder. *Cx*, cervix; *C*, left ovarian cyst

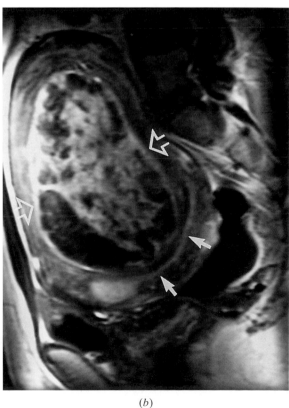

(a)   (b)

FIG. 14.41 Cystic uterine leiomyoma. Sagittal (*a*) T2-weighted echo-train spin-echo sequence, and (*b*) gadolinium-enhanced, fat-suppressed SGE sequence. A large intramural leiomyoma (*open arrows, a,b*) is seen displacing the endometrial cavity (*arrows, a,b*) inferiorly and posteriorly. Note the markedly heterogeneous appearance of this leiomyoma with extensive cystic degeneration.

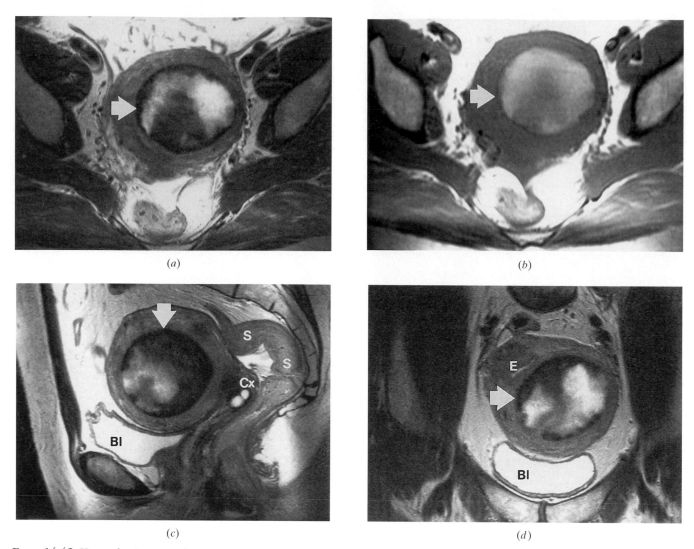

(a)   (b)

(c)   (d)

FIG. 14.42 Hemorrhagic uterine leiomyoma. (*a*) Transverse T2-weighted echo-train spin-echo sequence, (*b*) transverse T1-weighted spin-echo sequence, (*c*) sagittal and (*d*) coronal oblique T2-weighted echo-train spin-echo sequence. A large intramural leiomyoma (*arrow, a–d*) is shown with hemorrhagic degeneration resulting in increased signal intensity on both T2- and T1-weighted images. The endometrium (*E*) is easily identified separately from the leiomyoma on the coronal oblique image (*d*). *E*, endometrium; *Cx*, cervix with nabothian cysts; *Bl*, bladder; *S*, sigmoid

0.5 cm are frequently identified. A rim of high signal intensity representing a combination of dilated lymphatics, veins, or edema may at times be seen surrounding intramural or subserosal leiomyomas [101]. Care must be taken not to mistake this high-signal-intensity rim for a displaced endometrial stripe. Leiomyomas larger than 3 to 5 cm in diameter may demonstrate heterogeneous areas of increased signal intensity representing degeneration (Figs. 14.40 and 14.41) [99,102]. Accurate differentiation among the various types of degeneration is not possible with MRI, except for hemorrhagic degeneration, which typically demonstrates hyperintense areas on T1-weighted images (Fig. 14.42) [99]. Fatty degeneration in leiomyomas is rare, but may occur with advanced hyalin degeneration. However, when macroscopic areas of fat

are present within a leiomyoma, the diagnosis of a benign mixed müllerian tumor or lipoadenofibroma is probable (Fig. 14.43) [90,103]. Extensive peripheral cystic degeneration in large leiomyomas occasionally may be seen (Fig. 14.44). Cellular leiomyomas have been reported to be homogeneously hyperintense on T2-weighted sequences (Fig. 14.45) [102]. However, considerable overlap in the signal characteristics of cellular and degenerated leiomyomas is known to occur. Diagnosing cellular leiomyomas with MRI may be of interest because this subtype is reported to be more responsive to treatment with gonadotropin-releasing hormone (GnRH) analogues [102].

The appearance of leiomyomas following the administration of a gadolinium chelate is variable [9]. On dynamic and delayed contrast-enhanced images, the major-

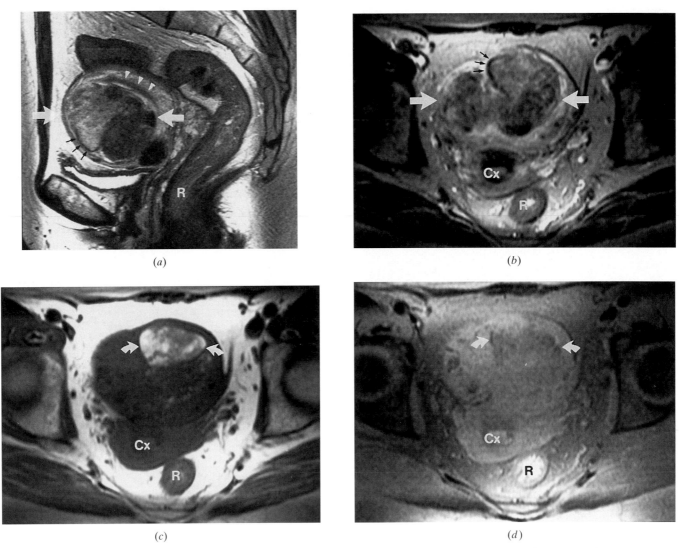

F IG. 14.43 Uterine lipoadenofibroma. (*a*) Sagittal T2-weighted echo-train spin-echo sequence, (*b*) T2-weighted spin-echo sequence, (*c*) T1-weighted spin-echo, and (*d*) fat-suppressed, T1-weighted spin-echo sequence. A heterogeneous mass (*arrows, a,b*) arising from the ventral myometrium displaces the endometrial stripe (*arrowheads, a*) superiorly. The presence of a chemical-shift artifact (*small arrows, a,b*) indicates fat within the lesion. The fatty component (*curved arrows, c,d*) of the tumor is clearly shown on the T1-weighted images with and without fat suppression. *Cx*, cervix; *R*, rectum

ity of leiomyomas enhance to a lesser degree than the surrounding myometrium and remain well-marginated (Fig. 14.46). However, intense early enhancement also may be seen and is reported to occur most frequently with the cellular subtype [102]. The enhancement pattern is heterogeneous in the majority of leiomyomas (see Figs. 14.40 and 14.46) [9].

Leiomyomas can be localized accurately with MRI as submucosal (Figs. 14.39 and 14.47), intramural (see Figs. 14.41 and 14.42), subserosal (Fig. 14.48), or cervical. In patients with prolapsed submucosal leiomyomas, accurate localization of the stalk may facilitate hysteroscopic resection (Fig. 14.49) [98].

MRI has proved useful in differentiating leiomyomas from other solid pelvic masses when sonographic find-

ings are indeterminate [97]. Establishing the myometrial origin of a mass by demonstrating splaying of the uterine serosa or myometrium usually allows a confident diagnosis of leiomyoma to be made (see Fig. 14.48). In addition, the presence of tumor-feeding vessels arising from the myometrium lends further support to the myometrial origin of a pelvic mass (see Fig. 14.44). Signal characteristics of a pelvic mass also can be used to suggest the diagnosis of a leiomyoma. If a mass is predominantly of low signal intensity relative to myometrium on T2-weighted images, the diagnosis of leiomyoma is probable. Although the signal characteristics of leiomyomas may be indistinguishable from those of fibrothecomas of the ovary, the consequence of a misdiagnosis is probably not significant because these tumors are rarely malignant [97,104,105].

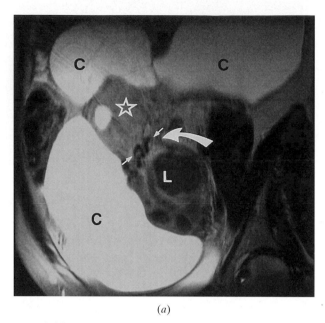

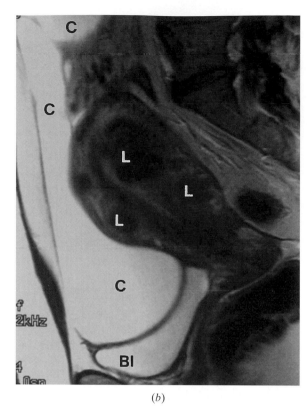

(a)   (b)

FIG. 14.44 Peripheral cystic degeneration in uterine leiomyoma. (*a*) Coronal and (*b*) sagittal T2-weighted echo-train spin-echo sequence. Large areas of peripheral cystic degeneration (*C*) can be seen in a subserosal leiomyoma (*asterisk, a*) originating off the right superior aspect (*curved arrow*) of the uterus. Tumor-feeding vessels (*arrows, a*) originating from the myometrium can be seen. Multiple intramural leiomyomas (*L*) of low signal intensity are also present within the uterus. *Bl*, bladder

However, if a mass adjacent to the uterus is of intermediate or increased signal intensity, the differential diagnosis includes a degenerated leiomyoma as well as benign or malignant extrauterine tumors. Under these circumstances, a specific diagnosis of leiomyoma should not be made unless the myometrial origin of a mass can be

unequivocally demonstrated [97]. Submucosal leiomyomas may be differentiated from endometrial polyps by confirming their myometrial origin and by their typical low signal intensity on T2-weighted images (Fig. 14.50). However, leiomyomas may exhibit variable signal intensities, and overlap in signal characteristics between leio-

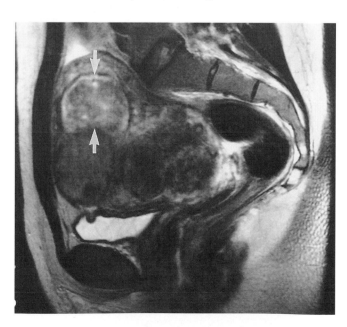

FIG. 14.45 Hyperintense uterine leiomyoma. Sagittal T2-weighted echo-train spin-echo sequence shows multiple uterine leiomyomas. Note the hyperintense signal of the most cranial lesion (*arrows*), which is consistent with a cellular leiomyoma.

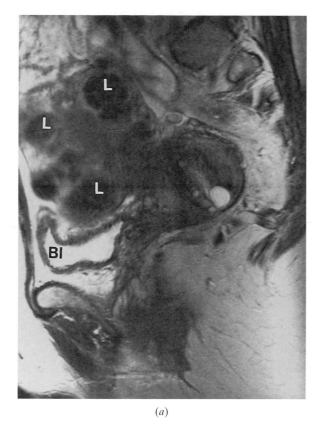

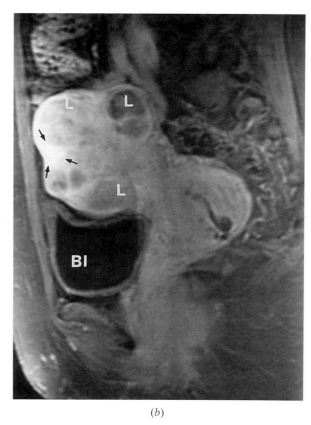

(a)   (b)

F I G . 14.46 Enhancement patterns in uterine leiomyomas. Sagittal (*a*) T2-weighted echo-train spin-echo sequence and (*b*) gadolinium-enhanced, fat-suppressed SGE sequence. Multiple hypointense masses consistent with leiomyomas (*L*) are present in the uterus. After gadolinium administration the enhancement of the leiomyomas (*L*) is variable. However, most enhance to a lesser degree than the surrounding myometrium (*small arrows, b*) and remain well-marginated. *Bl*, bladder

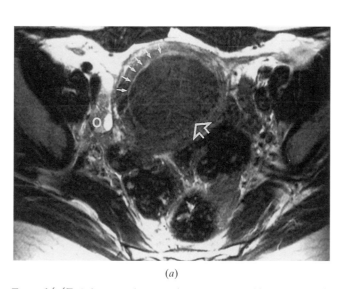

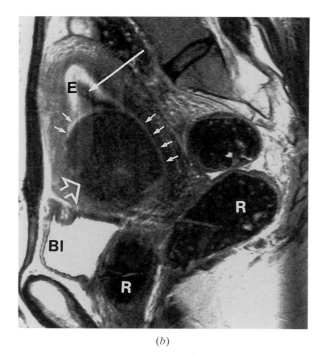

(a)   (b)

F I G . 14.47 Submucosal uterine leiomyoma. (*a*) Transverse and (*b*) sagittal T2-weighted echo-train spin-echo sequence. A sharply margin-ated mass (*open arrow, a,b*) with signal characteristics of a leiomyoma can be seen protruding into and splaying (*small arrows, a,b*) the endometrial cavity. Menstrual blood (*long arrow, b*) is present in the superior aspect of the endometrial cavity. *E*, endometrial cavity; *O*, ovary; *R*, rectum; *Bl*, bladder

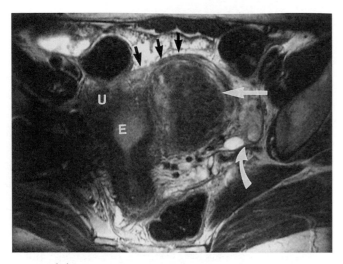

FIG. 14.48 Subserosal uterine leiomyoma. T2-weighted echo-train spin-echo sequence. A hypointense mass (*arrow*) is seen in the left adnexa. Splaying of the myometrium (*small arrows*) anterior to the lesion establishes the myometrial origin of the mass. Separate identification of a normal left ovary (*curved arrow*) excludes the presence of a solid ovarian mass. Both of these signs may be difficult to visualize with ultrasound in the presence of large or multiple leiomyomas. *E*, endometrium; *U*, uterus

myomas and endometrial polyps is frequently noted [40]. Leiomyomas must also be differentiated from adenomyosis on MRI. (For a discussion on the features distinguishing leiomyomas and adenomyosis see later subsection, Adenomyosis, MRI Considerations.) Myometrial contractions may mimic the appearance of leiomyomas on MRI. Contractions can be differentiated from true myometrial pathology on sequential imaging acquisitions by their transient nature and changing appearance over time (see also the earlier subsection, Myometrial Contractions, in the section on Normal Anatomic Structures and Physiologic Variants).

Malignant degeneration of a leiomyoma occurs rarely, but is suspected if a leiomyoma enlarges suddenly, especially following menopause, or if an indistinct border or irregular contour is noted. MRI signal characteristics are not reliable in differentiating leiomyomas from leimyosarcomas (Fig. 14.51).

Benign metastasizing leiomyoma is one of several unusual variants that includes intravenous leiomyomatosis, and leiomyomatosis peritonealis disseminata. In benign metastasizing leiomyoma, histologically appearing benign smooth-muscle tumors metastasize to dis-

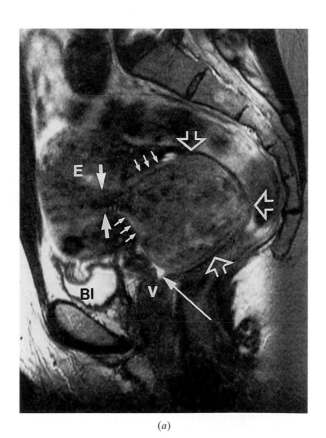

(a)

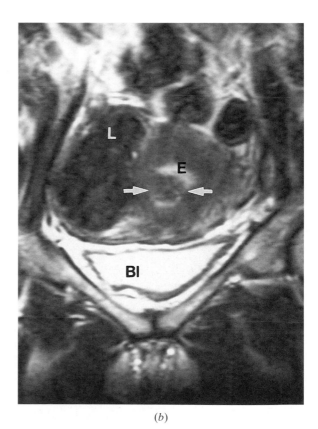

(b)

FIG. 14.49 Prolapsed submucosal leiomyoma. (*a*) Sagittal and (*b*) coronal oblique T2-weighted echo-train spin-echo sequence. A mass of intermediate signal intensity (*open arrows, a*) is seen protruding into the cervical canal (*small arrows, a*) and upper vagina, the latter being outlined by a small amount of fluid (*long arrow, a*). A stalk (*arrows, a,b*) attaches the mass to the ventral myometrium. In *b*, the stalk (*arrows*) is clearly visualized as it traverses the endometrial cavity. Note, in addition, the presence of a mural leiomyoma (*L*) in *b*. *E*, endometrium; *V*, vagina; *Bl*, bladder

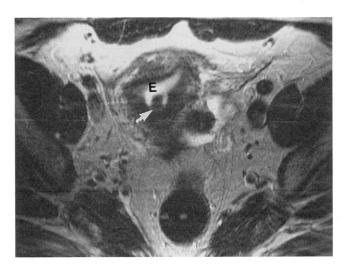

Fig. 14.50 Submucosal leiomyoma versus endometrial polyp. T2-weighted echo-train spin-echo sequence. A small mass (*arrow*) is seen protruding into the endometrial cavity. The marked decreased signal intensity favors the diagnosis of a submucosal leiomyoma. *E*, endometrium

tant organs, such as the lung (Fig. 14.52). Although histologically benign, this form of leiomyoma is generally believed to be a variant of low grade leiomyosarcoma [90].

Adenomyosis

General Considerations

Uterine adenomyosis is a common disease that results from the presence of heterotopic endometrial glands and stroma in the myometrium with adjacent myometrial hyperplasia. Cyclic hemorrhage is infrequently observed with adenomyosis because the ectopic endometrial tissue originates from the stratum basale and is typically unresponsive to hormonal stimuli. The associated myometrial hyperplasia interdigitates with the normal myometrium resulting in poorly marginated borders that are not encapsulated. Adenomyosis may be microscopic, focal, or diffuse. The term adenomyoma is reserved for the nodular form of adenomyosis [106]. The incidence of adenomyosis in unselected hysterectomy specimens ranges from 8.8 to 31 percent [107–110].

Although adenomyosis is most frequently diagnosed in multiparous, premenopausal women, it is not uncommon in postmenopausal women [111]. Although adenomyosis may be entirely asymptomatic, it frequently presents with symptoms of pelvic pain, hypermenorrhea, and uterine enlargement. These symptoms and signs, however, are nonspecific and can be seen in other common gynecological disorders such as dysfunctional uterine bleeding, leiomyomas, and endometriosis [106,112]. It is hardly surprising, therefore, that the clinical diagnosis of adenomyosis is fraught with error, and until recently the diagnosis of adenomyosis was rarely established prior to surgical exploration [107–109,113]. Establishing the correct diagnosis preoperatively is essential because uterine-conserving therapy is possible with leiomyomas, whereas hysterectomy is the definitive treatment for debilitating adenomyosis.

Studies published on the accuracy of sonography in diagnosing adenomyosis report a wide range of results. Early reports on transabdominal sonography concluded

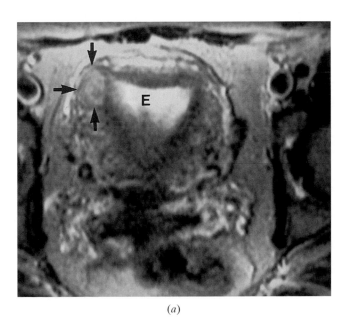

(*a*)

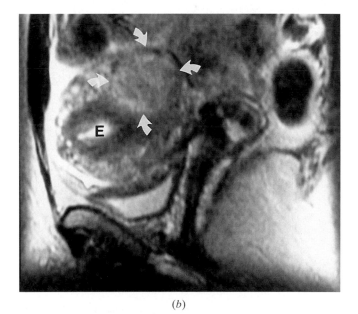

(*b*)

Fig. 14.51 Uterine leiomyoma and sarcoma. (*a*) Transverse and (*b*) sagittal T2-weighted spin-echo images. A small mass of intermediate signal intensity (*arrows, a*) is present adjacent to the right cornua. Although not diagnosed preoperatively, this mass was proven to be a uterine sarcoma at histopathology. Note the similar signal characteristics of the sarcoma (*arrows, a*) and leiomyoma (*curved arrows, b*) present in the same patient. *E*, endometrium

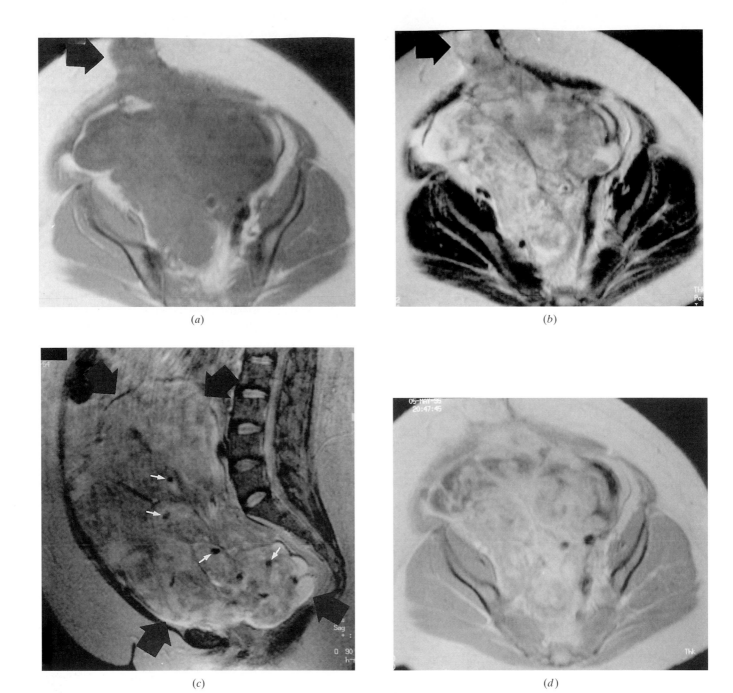

(a)

(b)

(c)

(d)

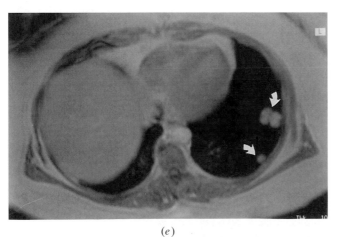

(e)

F IG. 14.52 Benign metastasizing leiomyoma (low grade leiomyosarcoma). SGE (*a*), transverse (*b*), and sagittal (*c*) T2-weighted echo-train spin-echo and one minute postgadolinium SGE (*d*) images. A massive uterine tumor is present involving the entire uterus. The tumor extends through the peritoneum at the level of the umbilicus into subcutaneous tissue (*arrows, a,b*). The tumor is moderately low in signal intensity, comparable to skeletal muscle on the T1-weighted image (*a*), and heterogeneous and moderately high in signal intensity on the T2-weighted images (*b,c*). The sagittal plane image clearly defines the longitudinal extent of tumor (*arrows, c*). Multiple signal void calcified foci are present in the mass (*small arrows, c*). Relatively intense diffuse heterogeneous enhancement is present on the early postgadolinium image (*d*). A 120-second postgadolinium SGE image (*e*) through the lung bases in this patient demonstrates several enhancing metastases in the left lung base (*curved arrows*).

that ultrasound is able neither to reliably diagnose adenomyosis nor to consistently differentiate it from leiomyomas [114,115]. However, the advent of endovaginal sonography (EVS) with its improved resolution has renewed interest in diagnosing this disease. Several series have reported the sensitivity of EVS for diagnosing adenomyosis as ranging from 53 to 89 percent with a specificity of 50 to 98 percent [31,111,116–119]. The wide range of reported accuracies reflects, in part, the high degree of operator-dependence. The findings of adenomyosis on EVS are subtle and can be diagnosed only if the exam is performed meticulously and in real time.

MRI offers several advantages over EVS in the diagnosis of adenomyosis. The presence of mural leiomyomas can limit the assessment of the adjacent myometrium with EVS. MRI is considerably less operator-dependent. MRI provides images that are standard and reproducible from one examination to another, whereas EVS may not be suitable for monitoring the evolution of adenomyosis because identical views from one examination to the next may be difficult to reproduce. Several studies have demonstrated MRI to be highly accurate in diagnosing adenomyosis, with a sensitivity and specificity ranging from 86 to 100 percent [9,31,100,118,120,121].

MR Imaging Considerations

T2-weighted sequences are used to diagnose adenomyosis because they provide optimal depiction of the uterine zonal anatomy. In addition to standard sagittal and transverse imaging planes, short-axis views of the uterine corpus may be indicated for accurate measurements of junctional zone thickness (see Fig. 14.2). On T1-weighted sequences, small hyperintense foci representing hemorrhage within the ectopic endometrial tissue may be seen in approximately 20 percent of patients

[9,31]. The addition of contrast-enhanced images does not improve the detection or characterization of adenomyosis [9].

Diagnostic criteria used for diagnosing adenomyosis on T2-weighted sequences include (1) a low-signal-intensity lesion adjacent to the endometrium presenting as focal or diffuse thickening of the junctional zone, or (2) the presence of a low-signal-intensity myometrial mass with ill-defined borders (adenomyoma). Cutoff values for junctional zone thickness used to differentiate patients with adenomyosis from those without have been variably reported as greater than 5 mm by some investigators and greater than or equal to 12 mm by others [31,100,118]. In practice, we have found that a maximal junctional zone thickness greater than or equal to 12 mm is highly predictive of the presence of adenomyosis, whereas a junctional zone thickness less than or equal to 8 mm usually excludes the disease (Fig. 14.53). In patients with a junctional zone thickness measuring between 8 and 12 mm, ancillary findings such as relative thickening of the junctional zone in a localized area, poor definition of borders, or the presence of high-signal foci on T2- or T1-weighted sequences can be used to diagnose adenomyosis (Fig. 14.54). High-signal-intensity foci within the lesion on T2-weighted sequences have been reported in 50 to 88 percent of cases and may represent islands of ectopic endometrium, cystically dilated endometrial glands, and/or hemorrhagic fluid (Figs. 14.55 and 14.56) [31,120,121]. In some patients, linear striations of increased signal intensity can be seen radiating out from the endometrium into the myometrium on T2-weighted sequences (Figs. 14.57 and 14.58). These striations likely represent direct invasion of the basal endometrium into the myometrium. On T1-weighted sequences, adenomyosis is isointense to the surrounding myometrium,

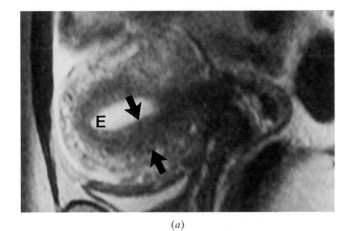
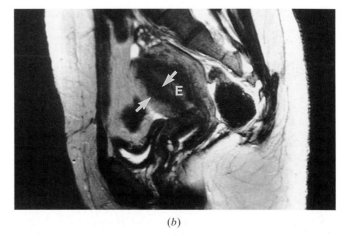

(a)   (b)

Fig. 14.53 Diffuse adenomyosis. Sagittal T2-weighted (a) spin-echo and (b) echo-train spin-echo sequences in two different patients. Diffuse thickening of the junctional zone (JZ) (≥ 12 mm) is present (arrows, a,b). The border of the JZ with the outer myometrium is poorly defined. E, endometrium (Fig. 14.53a Reprinted with permission from Reinhold C, McCarthy S, Bret PM et al: Diffuse adenomyosis: Comparison of endovaginal US and MR imaging with histopathologic correlation. Radiology 199:151–158, 1996)

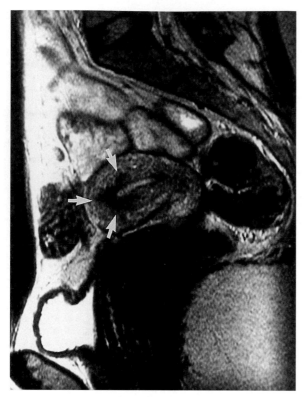

FIG. 14.54 Focal adenomyosis. Sagittal T2-weighted echo-train spin-echo sequence. Localized thickening of the junctional zone (JZ) (*arrows*) is present at the level of the uterine fundus. The border of the JZ with the outer myometrium is poorly defined.

except for the presence of bright foci, which have been shown to correspond to small areas of hemorrhage at histopathology (Fig. 14.58) [121].

Practically, the most important differential diagnosis of adenomyosis is leiomyoma. Differentiating the two conditions is essential because uterine-conserving ther-

apy is possible with leiomyomas, whereas hysterectomy is the definitive treatment for debilitating adenomyosis. Although MRI is shown to be highly accurate in differentiating adenomyosis from leiomyomas, the imaging characteristics may overlap, particularly in the case of adenomyomas (Fig. 14.59) [100,121]. Features that favor the diagnosis of adenomyosis include (1) a lesion with poorly defined borders, (2) a lesion that extends along endometrium and usually has an elliptical shape, (3) minimal mass effect on the endometrium relative to the size of the lesion (Fig. 14.60), and (4) linear striations radiating out from endometrium into the myometrium.

Myometrial contractions may closely resemble the appearance of focal adenomyosis on MRI. Contractions can be differentiated from true myometrial pathology on sequential imaging acquisitions by their transient nature and changing appearance over time (see also the earlier subsection, Myometrial Contractions, in the section on Normal Anatomic Structures and Physiologic Variants). In addition, the presence of muscular hypertrophy of the uterus may result in thickening of the junctional zone at MRI mimicking the appearance of diffuse adenomyosis (Fig. 14.61) [31].

BENIGN DISEASE OF THE CERVIX

Nabothian Cysts

General Considerations

Nabothian cysts result from mucous distention of endocervical glands or clefts, either as a result of an inflammatory process or due to squamous metaplasia [122]. Although nabothian cysts are common, they are rarely symptomatic and require no treatment. Occasionally, nabothian cysts reach 2 to 4 cm in diameter and, when multiple, result in marked enlargement of the cervix.

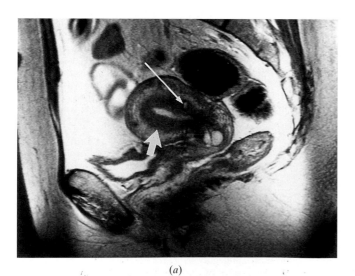

(a)

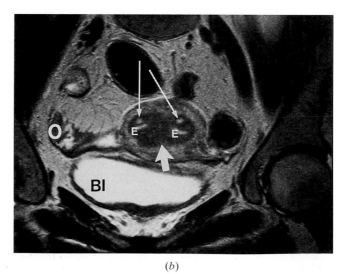

(b)

FIG. 14.55 Diffuse adenomyosis with high-signal-intensity foci. (*a*) Sagittal and (*b*) coronal oblique T2-weighted echo-train spin-echo sequence show an arcuate uterus. Mild diffuse thickening of the junctional zone (JZ) is present (*arrow, a,b*). Foci of high signal intensity are shown within the lesion (*long arrows*). *Bl*, bladder; *E*, endometrium; *O*, ovary

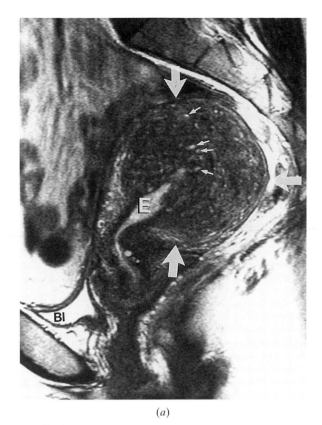
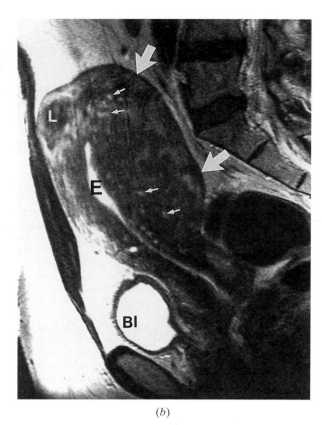

(a)

(b)

FIG. 14.56 Focal adenomyosis with high-signal-intensity foci. (*a,b*) Sagittal T2-weighted echo-train spin-echo images in two different patients. (*a*) Low-signal-intensity myometrial mass (*arrows, a*) is present in the fundus resulting in a globular appearance of the uterus. (*b*) In the second patient, there is marked thickening of the junctional zone (JZ) in the dorsal myometrium (*arrows, b*). Note numerous foci of high signal intensity within both lesions (*small arrows, a,b*). *Bl*, bladder; *E*, endometrium; *L*, leiomyoma

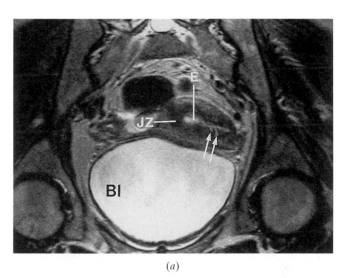
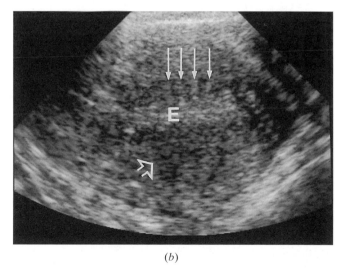

(a)

(b)

FIG. 14.57 Adenomyosis with linear striations. (*a*) Coronal oblique T2-weighted echo-train spin-echo image. Linear striations (*arrows, a*) of increased signal intensity are seen extending from the endometrium into the myometrium along the ventral aspect. The junctional zone (JZ) is unevenly thickened and has poorly defined borders. (*b*) Transverse oblique ultrasound image shows linear echogenic striations (*arrows, b*) radiating out from the endometrium ventrally. Note that the inner two-thirds of the myometrium is hypoechoic and heterogeneous (*open arrow, b*). This sonographic finding corresponds to the JZ thickening seen with MRI. *Bl*, bladder; *E*, endometrium

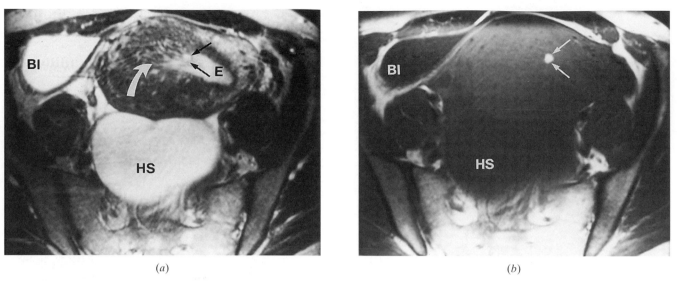

(a)   (b)

FIG. 14.58 Adenomyosis with linear striations. Transverse oblique (a) T2-weighted echo-train spin-echo and, (b) T1-weighted spin-echo sequences. Multiple linear striations of high signal intensity (curved arrow, a) are seen radiating out from the endometrium into the myometrium. In addition, a focus of high signal intensity (arrows, a,b) is shown on both the T2- and T1-weighted sequences. A large hydrosalpinx (HS) is present behind the uterus. E, endometrium; Bl, bladder

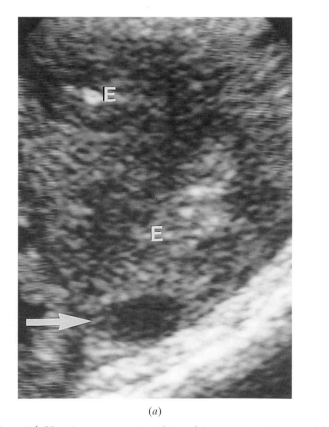

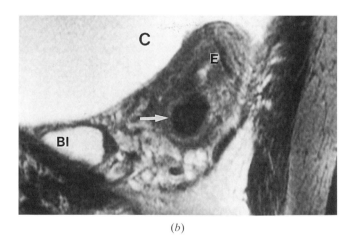

(a)   (b)

FIG. 14.59 Adenomyoma mimicking a leiomyoma. (a) Sagittal oblique endovaginal ultrasound image shows a septate uterus with a well-defined hypoechoic mass (arrow, a) that has the appearance of a leiomyoma. (b) Sagittal T2-weighted echo-train spin-echo image in the same patient demonstrates a well-defined hypointense mass (arrow, b) in the dorsal myometrium. This mass was falsely diagnosed as a leiomyoma preoperatively. (c) Corresponding histologic section through the uterus shows a nodular arrangement of ectopic endometrial tissue surrounded by hypertrophic smooth muscle fibers (arrows, c).

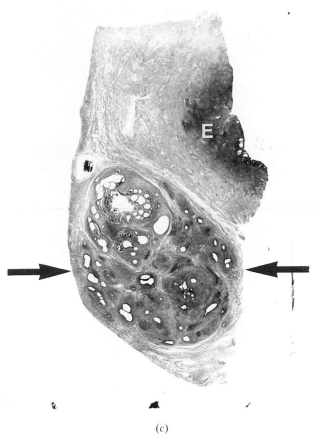

(c)

FIG. 14.59 (*Continued*) These findings are diagnostic of an adenomyoma. *E*, endometrium; *C*, large ovarian cyst (Fig. 14.59*a,c* Reprinted with permission from Reinhold C, Atri M, Mehio A, Zakarian R, Aldis AE, Bret PM: Diffuse uterine adenomyosis: Morphologic criteria and diagnostic accuracy of endovaginal sonography. Radiology 197:609–614, 1995)

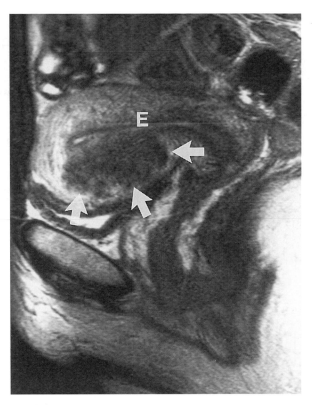

FIG. 14.60 Adenomyoma. Sagittal T2-weighted echo-train spin-echo sequence. Low-signal-intensity mass (*arrows*) with an elliptical shape in the ventral myometrium. Poorly defined borders and lack of significant mass effect differentiates the adenomyoma from a leiomyoma. *E*, endometrium

MRI Considerations

Nabothian cysts are well-depicted on T2-weighted sagittal and transverse images. Nabothian cysts demonstrate medium to high signal intensity on T1-weighted images and are hyperintense on T2-weighted images (Fig. 14.62). They show no enhancement after gadolinium chelate administration. Nabothian cysts are differentiated from most cervical neoplasms by their small size, well-defined margins, and very high signal intensity on T2-weighted images.

Adenoma malignum of the cervix has been reported to mimic nabothian cysts at MRI [123]. Adenoma malignum are rare tumors that represent approximately 3 percent of adenocarcinomas of the cervix and form nodular masses with mucin-rich cystic spaces. Therefore, if cystic lesions are observed in a patient with adenocarcinoma of the cervix at histopathology, adenoma malignum may be considered in the differential diagnosis. Furthermore, hemorrhagic foci associated with cervical

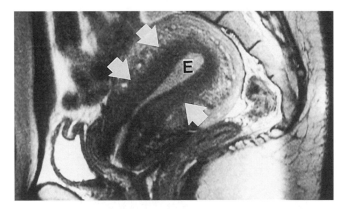

FIG. 14.61 Diffuse muscular hypertrophy. Sagittal T2-weighted echo-train spin-echo sequence. Diffuse thickening (*arrows*) of the junctional zone (JZ = 12 mm) is present in this patient with a retroverted uterus. At histopathologic examination diffuse muscular hypertrophy was found without evidence of adenomyosis. *E*, endometrium (Reprinted with permission from Reinhold C, McCarthy S, Bret PM et al: Diffuse adenomyosis: Comparison of endovaginal US and MR imaging with histopathologic correlation. Radiology 199:151–158, 1996)

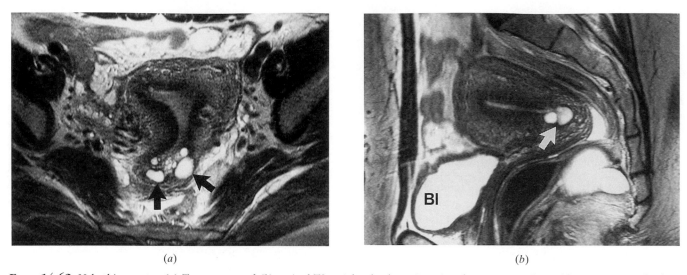

(a)   (b)

Fig. 14.62 Nabothian cysts. (*a*) Transverse and (*b*) sagittal T2-weighted echo-train spin-echo sequence. Several hyperintense nabothian cysts (*arrows*) are present in the cervix. *Bl*, bladder

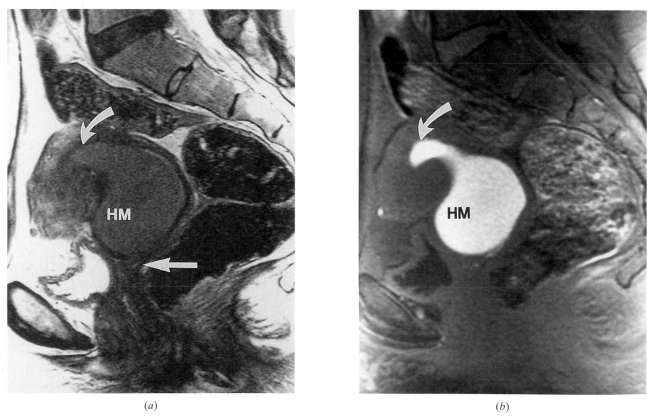

(a)   (b)

Fig. 14.63 Cervical stenosis. Sagittal (*a*) T2-weighted echo-train spin-echo, and (*b*) fat-suppressed T1-weighted spin-echo sequences. A fibrotic stenosis at the level of the external os (*arrow, a*) completely obstructs the endocervical canal. A hematometra (HM) markedly distends the endocervical canal and, to a lesser extent, the endometrial cavity (*curved arrow, a,b*).

endometriosis may mimic the MRI appearance of nabothian cysts.

Cervical Stenosis

General Considerations

Cervical stenosis may be congenital, inflammatory, neoplastic, or iatrogenic in origin [122]. Most cases of cervical stenosis involve the external os and are associated with extensive surgical manipulation (e.g., conization, electrocoagulation, cryotherapy) or are radiation-induced [122]. Senile atrophy also may result in cervical stenosis. The role of imaging is to exclude mechanical obstruction, most commonly due to the presence of endometrial or cervical carcinoma. When the obstruction of the cervix is complete, hematometra or pyometra may result.

MRI Considerations

T2- and T1-weighted sagittal images through the uterus are best to demonstrate the relationship of the distended uterine cavity to the cervical stenosis (Fig. 14.63). Unenhanced and contrast-enhanced sequences are necessary to differentiate tumor from debris or blood within the uterine cavity.

MRI can identify the presence and location of the cervical stenosis. In cases of complete obstruction, the uterine cavity is distended by material of variable signal intensity, depending on its composition (e.g., retained secretions, pus, blood, or tumor).

Cervical Incompetence

General Considerations

Cervical incompetence occurs in less than 1 percent of all pregnancies but may account for up to 16 percent of second- or third-trimester abortions [124]. The etiology of cervical incompetence is as follows: (1) congenital—including congenital uterine malformation, in-utero exposure to diethylstilbestrol (DES), and decreased collagen content, or (2) acquired—including obstetric or gynecologic trauma, multiple gestations, and hormonal disorders [124,125]. The MRI findings of the cervix in the nonpregnant woman with a history of cervical incompetence have been described and are addressed in the ensuing paragraph [82]. (A more complete discussion on cervical incompetence in the pregnant patient is provided later in the subsection, Cervical Incompetence, in the section on MRI and Pregnancy.)

MRI Considerations

One or more of the following findings at MRI can suggest the presence of cervical incompetence in the nonpregnant woman: (1) cervical length less than or equal to 3.0 cm (measured from the internal os to the external os), (2) internal cervical os greater than or equal to 4.3 mm (distance between inner margins of the fibrous stroma), (3) thinning or increased signal intensity of the cervical fibrous stroma, and (4) irregular asymmetric widening of the endocervical canal [82]. All measurements are obtained on T2-weighted sagittal images.

In patients with cervical incompetence related to DES exposure, the endocervical canal usually measures shorter than 2.5 cm. The width of the internal os and the signal intensity of the cervical stroma, however, remain normal. [81,82].

MALIGNANT DISEASE OF THE UTERINE CORPUS AND CERVIX

Endometrial Carcinoma

General Considerations

Carcinoma of the endometrium is the most common invasive malignancy of the female genital tract and the fourth most common cancer occurring in North American women. Endometrial carcinoma reaches a peak incidence between 55 and 65 years of age. Risk factors include obesity, diabetes mellitus, hypertension, polycystic ovary syndrome, nulliparity, unopposed estrogen replacement therapy, and adenomatous endometrial hyperplasia [126]. Most women present early during the course of their disease, with intermenstrual or postmenopausal bleeding as the presenting symptom in 75 to 90 percent of patients [127,128]. These patients are usually referred for dilatation and curettage (D&C) if a definite cause is not evident on clinical grounds, allowing for prompt diagnosis and treatment.

Adenocarcinomas account for 80 to 90 percent of all endometrial carcinomas and are composed of malignant glands that range from well-differentiated (Grade 1) to anaplastic carcinoma (Grade 3) [126]. Less common histologic subtypes include adenocarcinoma with squamous differentiation, adenosquamous carcinoma, papillary serous carcinoma, and clear-cell carcinoma. Papillary serous and clear-cell carcinomas carry a worse prognosis, with patterns of spread and clinical behavior similar to those of ovarian carcinoma [126]. Four pathways of spread have been described with endometrial carcinoma: (1) direct extension, (2) lymphatic metastases, (3) peritoneal metastases usually via transtubal spread, and (4) hematogenous metastases [126]. Para-aortic lymphadenopathy may occur without involvement of pelvic lymph nodes if the tumor spreads via lymphatics accompanying the ovarian vessels. Peritoneal metastases are rare with adenocarcinomas, but are frequently seen with papillary serous and clear-cell carcinomas. Hematogenous metastases occur in patients with disseminated disease and most frequently involve the lungs [126].

Table 14.2 **Revised FIGO Staging of Endometrial Carcinoma with Corresponding MRI Findings**

Revised FIGO Staging[1]

Stage 0		Carcinoma in situ
Stage I		Tumor confined to corpus
	IA	Tumor limited to endometrium
	IB	Invasion <50% of myometrium
	IC	Invasion >50% of myometrium
Stage II		Tumor invades cervix but does not extend beyond uterus
	IIA	Invasion of endocervix
	IIB	Cervical stromal invasion
Stage III		Tumor extends beyond uterus but not outside true pelvis
	IIIA	Invasion of serosa, adnexa, or positive peritoneal cytology
	IIIB	Invasion of vagina
	IIIC	Pelvic and/or para-aortic lymphadenopathy
Stage IV		Tumor extends outside of true pelvis or invades bladder or rectal mucosa
	IVA	Invasion of bladder or rectal mucosa
	IVB	Distant metastases (includes intra-abdominal or inguinal lymphadenopathy)

Corresponding MR Findings[2]

Stage 0		Normal or thickened endometrial stripe
Stage I	IA	Thickened endometrial stripe with diffuse or focal abnormal signal intensity. Endometrial stripe may be normal
		Intact junctional zone with smooth endometrial-myometrial interface[3]
	IB	Signal intensity of tumor extends into myometrium <50%
		Partial or full thickness disruption of junctional zone with irregular endometrial-myometrial interface
	IC	Signal intensity of tumor extends into myometrium >50%
		Full thickness disruption of junctional zone[3]
		Intact stripe of normal outer myometrium
Stage II	IIA	Internal os and endocervical canal are widened
		Low signal intensity of fibrous stroma remains intact
	IIB	Disruption of fibrous stroma
Stage III	IIIA	Disruption of continuity of outer myometrium
		Irregular uterine configuration
	IIIB	Segmental loss of hypointense vaginal wall
	IIIC	Regional lymph nodes larger than 1.0 cm in diameter
Stage IV	IVA	Tumor signal disrupts normal tissue planes with loss of low signal intensity of bladder or rectal wall
	IVB	Tumor masses in distant organs or anatomic sites

[1]All stages are further subdivided into three tumor grades (not shown).
[2]MRI findings seen on T2-weighted or contrast-enhanced T1-weighted images.
[3]For patients with adenomyosis, criteria may not apply.

The prognosis of patients with endometrial carcinoma is based largely on the surgical stage of the disease [129]. In response to this, the Fédération Internationale de Gynécologie et d'Obstétrique (FIGO) revised the staging of endometrial carcinoma in October 1988 (Table 14.2) [130]. Histologic grade of tumor, stage of disease, and depth of myometrial invasion are the most important prognostic factors [131]. These factors directly relate to regional lymph node involvement, tumor recurrence, and ultimately to 5-year survival. The depth of myometrial invasion is considered the factor most responsible for the extreme variation in the 5-year survival of patients with Stage I disease: from 40 to 60 percent in the most invasive cases to 90 to 100 percent in cases with little or no myometrial involvement [132–135]. Furthermore, the significant correlation between depth of myometrial invasion and presence of malignant lymphadenopathy has been well-documented [133,136]. Piver et al. [136] reported that the prevalence of para-aortic lymph node metastases varies from 3 percent among patients with tumor confined to the endometrium or superficial myometrium to 46 percent in patients with deep myometrial invasion. Approximately 75 percent of patients present with surgical Stage I tumors, which explains the overall favorable prognosis in patients with endometrial carcinoma. Five-year survival rates for the various surgical stages have been reported as follows: Stage I (85.3%), Stage II (70.2%), Stage III (49.2%), Stage IV (18.7%) [126].

Most patients with early-stage endometrial carcinoma are treated with hysterectomy. Adjuvant radiation therapy is frequently used to treat patients with endometrial carcinoma, but protocols vary among institutions regarding indications and optimal timing of treatments. Although the majority of patients are staged surgically, preoperative knowledge of advanced disease may have important therapeutic implications. Patients with Grade 3 endometrial carcinoma, papillary serous carcinoma, or clear-cell carcinoma frequently present with advanced disease, and thus may benefit from preoperative imaging [137,138]. In the presence of deep myometrial or cervical stromal invasion, preoperative intracavitary radiation therapy may be given at some centers. Extensive lymph node sampling at the time of hysterectomy may be planned with prior knowledge of the depth of myometrial invasion. In addition, preoperative staging may allow high-risk cases to be referred to specialized treatment centers.

A number of imaging modalities have been advocated in the pretreatment evaluation of endometrial carcinoma. On contrast-enhanced computed tomography (CT) imaging endometrial carcinoma may appear as a hypodense mass within the endometrial cavity [139]. Although CT imaging is useful in identifying extrauterine spread of disease, it cannot accurately predict the degree of myometrial invasion or the presence of cervical extension [140–142]. Several studies have investigated the use endovaginal sonography (EVS) in predicting the depth of myometrial invasion. Reported accuracies range from 68 to 99 percent, depending on the degree of rigor with which the FIGO staging system was applied and the type of patient population studied [143–147]. On EVS, the presence of an endometrial mass disrupting the subendometrial halo or extending asymmetrically into the myometrium has a high positive predictive value for the presence of myometrial invasion [143]. However, the degree of myometrial invasion may be overestimated in the setting of a large intraluminal tumor, adenomyosis, or lymphovascular space invasion [143,144,147]. Conversely, microscopic or minimal myometrial invasion cannot be excluded. In addition, EVS is not accurate in predicting cervical extension, parametrial invasion, or the presence of lymphadenopathy. In some patients, complete evaluation of the myometrium may not be possible with EVS due to a vertical orientation of the uterus or the presence of multiple leiomyomas.

The excellent contrast resolution and multiplanar capability of MRI renders it invaluable in staging patients with endometrial carcinoma [148,149]. Although a number of studies have demonstrated no significant difference in the accuracy of MRI and EVS in assessing myometrial invasion, more recently, contrast-enhanced MRI was found to be significantly superior [143–145]. MRI is indicated for patients in whom advanced disease is suspected on clinical grounds and for patients with histologic subtypes that signify a worse prognosis. In addition, MRI can be performed in cases where EVS is technically limited or indeterminate and in patients with coexisting myometrial pathology such as leiomyomas or adenomyosis. The decision to evaluate patients routinely with MRI or EVS will depend to a large extent on cost, availability of equipment, local expertise, and the potential impact on patient management.

MRI Considerations

T2-weighted sequences are used to identify and stage endometrial carcinoma because they provide optimal depiction of the uterine zonal anatomy. In addition to standard sagittal and transverse imaging planes, short-axis views of the uterine corpus are helpful for assessing myometrial invasion (see Fig. 14.2). Transverse T1-weighted sequences are used to detect the presence of lymphadenopathy. We routinely perform dynamic gadolinium-enhanced imaging, using fat-suppressed SGE sequences in the sagittal plane. Immediately after gadolinium administration, three sequential acquisitions are rapidly performed through the uterus. After dynamic scanning, delayed T1-weighted sequences are usually obtained. Gadolinium-enhanced T1-weighted sequences have been shown to improve the detection of endometrial carcinoma and to facilitate differentiation of tumor from debris when compared with T2-weighted spin-echo sequences [34,145,150,151]. In addition, improved as-

sessment of myometrial invasion has been reported. However, studies comparing gadolinium-enhanced T1-weighted sequences with T2-weighted echo-train spin-echo sequences using a dedicated pelvic multicoil have not been performed.

The MRI appearance of noninvasive endometrial carcinoma (Stage IA) is nonspecific. Therefore, MRI has no role as a screening modality. Histologic sampling is required to diagnose noninvasive endometrial carcinoma because accurate differentiation from other conditions, (e.g., endometrial polyps and adenomatous hyperplasia) is not possible [40]. Although the uterus may appear entirely normal, endometrial carcinoma most commonly presents as a widening of the endometrial stripe (more than 3 mm) in postmenopausal women [40,139,152]. The signal intensity of endometrial carcinoma on T2-weighted sequences is variable, ranging from iso- or slightly hypointense relative to normal endometrium to an intermediate signal intensity (isointense to myometrium) (Figs. 14.64 and 14.65). Alternatively, a heterogeneous mass with areas of high and low signal intensity may be noted distending the endometrial cavity [40,139,152]. On dynamic images obtained immediately after gadolinium ad-

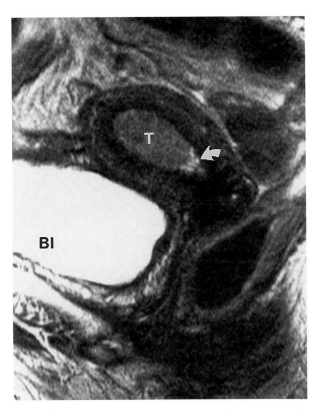

FIG. 14.64 Stage IA endometrial carcinoma, hypointense relative to endometrium. Sagittal T2-weighted echo-train spin-echo sequence. A tumor (*T*) of intermediate signal intensity is seen within the endometrial cavity. The tumor is confined to the endometrium and the junctional zone (JZ) remains intact. A small amount of fluid is present in the lower uterine segment (*curved arrow*). *Bl*, bladder.

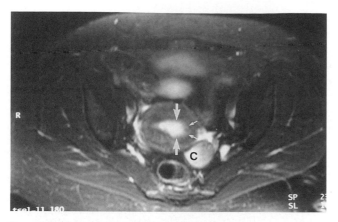

FIG. 14.65 Stage IB endometrial carcinoma, isointense relative to endometrium. T2-weighted, fat-suppressed echo-train spin-echo sequence. Asymmetric widening (*arrows*) of the endometrial stripe by a tumor isointense to normal endometrium is shown. The tumour invades the inner myometrium along the left lateral aspect (*small arrows*). *C*, left ovarian cyst

ministration, endometrial carcinoma typically enhances to a lesser extent than the adjacent myometrium. This difference in enhancement becomes less marked on the delayed images [33,34,151]. In patients with Stage IA disease (see Table 14.2), the junctional zone or endometrial-myometrial interface will remain intact (see Fig. 14.64). On dynamic images, a thin layer of subendometrial enhancement may be present in some patients and, when continuous, has been reported in a small series of patients to be highly accurate in excluding invasive disease [34]. The accuracy of MRI in differentiating noninvasive from invasive endometrial carcinoma has been reported to range from 69 to 88 percent [40,137,144,145,151,153].

In patients with myometrial invasion (Stages IB and IC), segmental or complete disruption of the junctional zone by an intermediate signal intensity mass can be seen on T2-weighted sequences (see Table 14.2; Fig. 14.66) [40,139,152]. Disruption of the junctional zone must be evaluated on two imaging planes. In the absence of a junctional zone, irregularity of the endometrial-myometrial interface is evidence of invasion (Fig. 14.67) [40]. Caution must be exercised when interpreting this finding

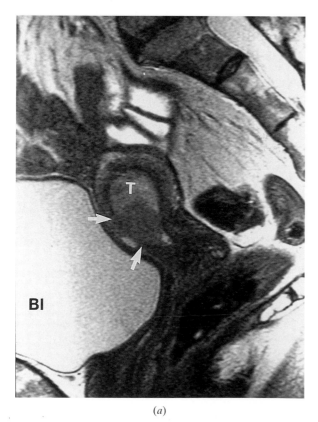

(*a*)

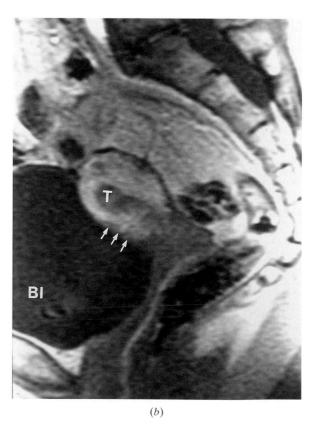

(*b*)

FIG. 14.66 Stage IB Endometrial carcinoma, disruption of junctional zone (JZ). Sagittal (*a*) T2-weighted echo train spin-echo and (*b*) 45-second postgadolinium fat-suppressed SGE sequences. A tumor (*T*) of mixed signal intensity that completely disrupts the JZ ventrally (*arrows, a*) is present within the endometrial cavity. Depth of myometrial invasion is difficult to determine on the T2-weighted sequence (*a*). After gadolinium administration, the outer myometrium (*small arrows, b*) is shown to be intact. At histopathology the diagnosis of a Stage IB endometrial carcinoma was confirmed. *Bl*, bladder

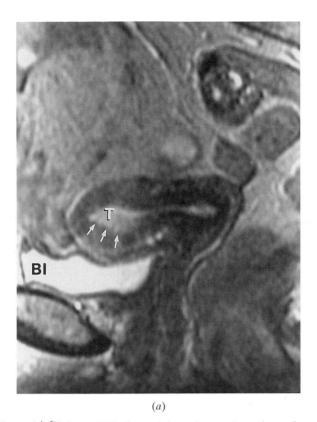

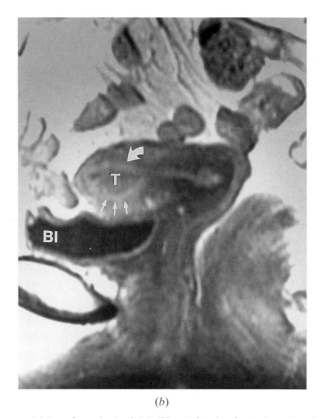

(a) (b)

F I G . 14.67 Stage IB Endometrial carcinoma, irregular endometrial-myometrial interface. Sagittal (*a*) T2-weighted echo-train spin-echo and (*b*) delayed postgadolinium T1-weighted spin-echo sequences. An endometrial tumor (*T*) of intermediate signal intensity is present. On the T2-weighted image (*a*), the ventral endometrial-myometrial interface (*small arrows, a*) is irregular, which is consistent with myometrial invasion. The delayed postgadolinium image (*b*), demonstrates the tumor (*T*) to be hypointense relative to the uninvolved dorsal endometrium (*curved arrow, b*), and iso- or slightly hypointense relative to myometrium. The band of increased signal ventrally (*small arrows, b*) represents compressed myometrium and must not be mistaken for subendometrial enhancement on dynamic images or for enhancing endometrium on delayed images. *Bl*, bladder

in patients with adenomyosis, where direct invasion of the basal endometrium into the myometrium may result in an irregular appearance of the endometrial-myometrial interface. The percentage of myometrial invasion is easily calculated, separating patients into Stage IB (<50% wall invasion) or Stage IC (>50% wall invasion) (Fig. 14.68). The accuracy of differentiating early disease (stages IA, IB) from deep myometrial invasion (Stage IC) has been reported to range from 71 to 100 percent [33,137, 142,143,145,150,153–155]. In these studies, an intact junctional zone was highly accurate in excluding the presence of deep myometrial invasion. Similarly, preservation of a thin layer of subendometrial enhancement on dynamic images is reported to have a high negative predictive value for excluding deep myometrial invasion [34]. However, MRI is considerably less accurate under the following circumstances: (1) when the myometrium is thinned by a large polypoid tumor or obstructed endometrial cavity, (2) in the presence of poor tumor-myometrial contrast on T2-weighted or gadolinium-enhanced sequences (Fig. 14.69), (3) when the junctional zone is

absent, and (4) in the presence of multiple or large leiomyomas [145,154,155].

Superficial extension of endometrial carcinoma to the cervical mucosa (Stage IIA) is demonstrated on T2-weighted images by widening of the internal os and endocervical canal (see Table 14.2). Invasion of the cervical fibrous stroma (Stage IIB) is diagnosed when the low-signal-intensity stroma is disrupted by the higher signal intensity of the tumor mass (Fig. 14.70). Only a limited number of patients with cervical invasion have thus far been studied with MRI, but MRI is reported to be sensitive in diagnosing Stage II disease and is indicated in patients with detached fragments of malignant tissue at endocervical curettage that are inclusive for cervical invasion [40,137,142]. A false diagnosis of cervical invasion may result when the endocervical canal is merely widened by a polypoid extension of the tumor, coexisting benign endocervical polyp, or debris. Although gadolinium enhancement is generally not helpful for evaluating cervical stromal invasion, it can be used to differentiate viable tumor from debris or blood clot within the endocervical

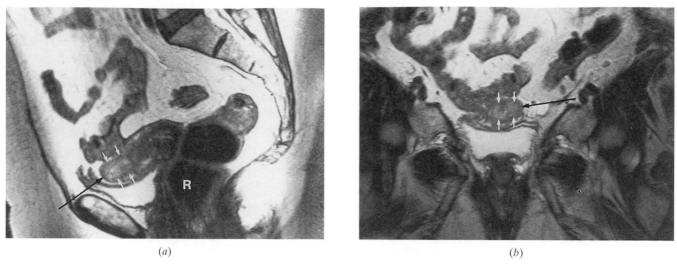

(a)   *(b)*

FIG. 14.68 Stage IC Endometrial carcinoma. (*a*) Sagittal and (*b*) coronal oblique T2-weighted echo-train spin-echo sequence. Sagittal section through the left lateral aspect of the uterus and coronal oblique section at the level of the fundus demonstrate an intermediate-signal-intensity endometrial mass (*arrows, a,b*). Note extension into the outer myometrium at the level of the left cornua (*long thin arrow, a,b*). *R*, rectum

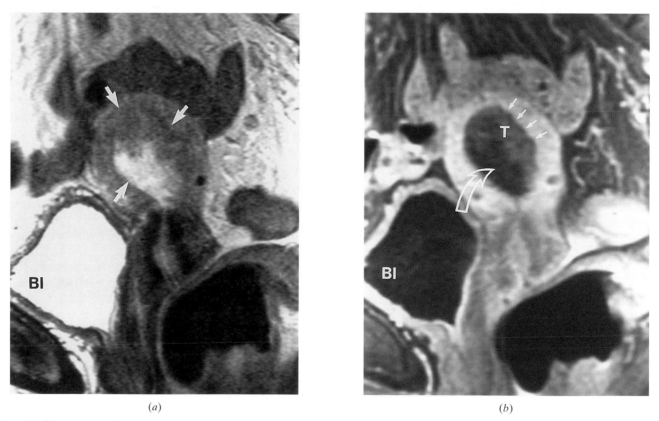

(a)   *(b)*

FIG. 14.69 Stage IB Endometrial carcinoma, poor tumor-myometrial contrast. Sagittal (*a*) T2-weighted echo-train spin-echo and (*b*) delayed postgadolinium T1-weighted fat-suppressed spin-echo sequences. A mass of mixed signal intensity is shown on the T2-weighted image (*arrows, a*). Depth of myometrial invasion cannot be accurately assessed on the T2-weighted image (*a*) due to poor tumor-myometrial contrast. After gadolinium administration (*b*), the ventral component of the mass does not enhance corresponding to fluid and debris within the endometrial cavity (*curved open arrow, b*). The tumor (*T*) remains hypointense relative to myometrium on the delayed postgadolinium image (*b*). Minimal irregularity at the dorsal endometrial-myometrial interface (*small arrows, b*) indicates superficial myometrial invasion. *Bl*, bladder

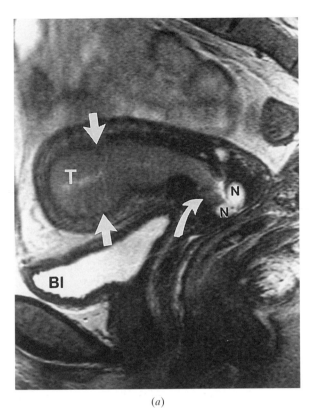

(a)

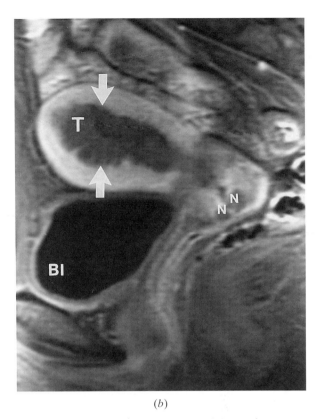

(b)

F IG. **14.70** Stage IIB Endometrial carcinoma. Sagittal (*a*) T2-weighted echo-train spin-echo and (*b*) 45-second postgadolinium fat-suppressed SGE sequences. (*a*) A large endometrial tumor (*T*) with inner myometrial invasion (*arrows, a,b*) is present. The tumor extends to the cervix and focally invades the cervical fibrous stroma (*curved arrow, a*). Note that the invasion of the fibrous stroma is not evident on the gadolinium-enhanced image (*b*) because of decreased contrast between the tumor and hypovascular fibrous stroma. *Bl*, bladder; *N*, nabothian cyst

canal [33,40]. Conversely, false negative results may occur in the setting of microscopic cervical invasion.

Experience in the evaluation of Stage III and Stage IV endometrial carcinoma with MRI is currently limited due to the preponderance of patients with Stage I and Stage II disease in most published series. In Stage III disease (see Table 14.2), transmyometrial extension of the tumor with interruption of the low-signal-intensity myometrium is noted on T2-weighted sequences [40]. When parametrial extension is present, the tumor mass can be seen to penetrate the serosal surface, disrupting the normal signal intensity of the parametrial fat [40]. The ovaries may be involved by contiguous spread or may present with discrete metastases (Fig. 14.71) [40,142]. Secondary involvement of the ovaries is suggested whenever a mass with indeterminate signal characteristics is noted within the ovary. Assessment of metastatic lymphadenopathy with MRI is based on the size of lymph nodes, with nodes larger than 1.0 cm short axis diameter considered pathologic [40,156]. Signal-intensity characteristics have not been useful in differentiating metastatic from hyperplastic lymphadenopathy. Lymphadenopathy in the up-

per abdomen may occur without involvement of pelvic lymph nodes if the tumor spreads via lymphatics accompanying the ovarian vessels (Figs. 14.72 and 14.73). Lymph nodes are well shown on T1-weighted images due to the good soft tissue contrast between low to moderate signal intensity nodes with the high signal intensity surrounding fat. Gadolinium-enhanced fat-suppressed SGE or T2-weighted fat suppressed echo-train spin-echo also are useful, showing moderately high signal intensity lymph nodes in the background of suppressed low signal intensity fat. In addition, flow phenomenon may be utilized to differentiate lymph nodes from adjacent vessels. The accuracy of MRI in evaluating bladder or rectal invasion (Stage IVA) has not been established. However, differentiation between contiguous spread and frank tumor invasion may be difficult. Pelvic manifestations of Stage IVB disease include ascites, peritoneal implants, and omental cakes [142]. Microscopic spread of disease, including peritoneal or omental implants smaller than 1 to 2 cm, are not consistently detected with MRI due to limitations in spatial resolution and the presence of motion artifact.

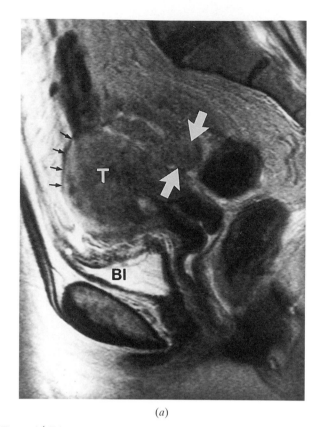
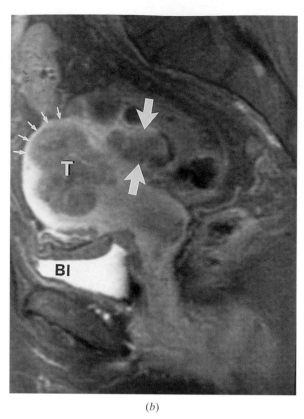

(a)   (b)

FIG. 14.71 Stage III endometrial carcinoma. Sagittal (*a*) T2-weighted echo-train spin-echo and (*b*) delayed postgadolinium T1-weighted fat-suppressed spin-echo sequences. A lobulated tumor (*T*) with deep myometrial invasion extending to the serosa (*small arrows, a,b*) is demonstrated. Left ovarian metastases (*arrows, a,b*) with the same signal intensity as the primary tumor are present dorsally. *Bl*, bladder

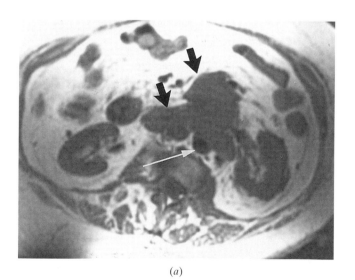
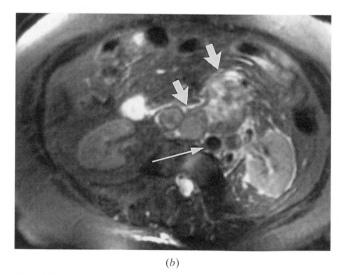

(a)   (b)

FIG. 14.72 Metastatic lymphadenopathy. (*a*) T1-weighted spin-echo and (*b*) T2-weighted fat-suppressed echo-train spin-echo sequences. Multiple confluent, enlarged lymph nodes (*arrows, a,b*) are seen anterior to the aorta (*long thin arrow, a,b*) at the level of the left renal hilum. The location of the lymphadenopathy suggests spread via lymphatics accompanying the left ovarian vessels.

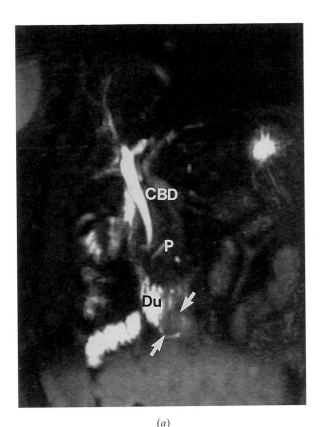

(a)

(b)

FIG. 14.73 Metastatic lymphadenopathy with invasion of duodenum. Patient with a previous hysterectomy for Stage I endometrial carcinoma presents with hematemesis. (*a*) Coronal reformation, heavily T2-weighted fat-suppressed echo-train spin-echo sequence, (*b*) postgadolinium T1-weighted fat-suppressed spin-echo sequence. A poorly defined mass (*arrows a,b*) is seen invading the duodenum (*curved arrow, b*). The mass is contiguous to, but does not invade, the aorta (*long arrow, b*). *CBD*, common bile duct; *P*, pancreatic duct; *Du*, second portion of duodenum

Uterine Sarcoma

General Considerations

Uterine sarcomas are rare, constituting only 2 to 3 percent of all uterine malignancies. Uterine sarcomas are generally classified into four histologic subtypes: malignant mixed mesodermal tumors (50%), leiomyosarcomas (35 to 40%), endometrial stromal sarcomas (8%), and adeno sarcomas (1 to 2%) [126]. With the exception of leiomyosarcomas, which are of smooth-muscle cell origin, all other sarcomas are believed to arise from undifferentiated endometrial stromal cells [126]. Malignant mixed mesodermal tumors contain malignant glands and heterotopic elements such as bone, striated muscle, cartilage, and fat, and have therefore been termed carcinosarcomas.

Leiomyosarcomas typically occur in the perimenopausal woman and most commonly present with abnormal vaginal bleeding. Although the majority of leiomyosarcomas arise de novo, 5 to 10 percent arise from sarcomatous degeneration of a preexisting leiomyoma [126]. Hysterectomy is usually required for histologic diagnosis because dilatation and curettage (D&C) is inaccurate unless the tumor is submucosal in location.

Malignant mixed mesodermal tumors and endometrial stromal sarcomas occur predominantly in postmenopausal women. Postmenopausal bleeding is the most common presenting symptom. A significant number of patients with malignant mixed mesodermal tumors have a history of prior pelvic irradiation [126]. Sarcomas of endometrial origin are usually accurately diagnosed by D&C. Malignant mixed mesodermal tumors are more aggressive than endometrial carcinomas, and approximately 70 percent of patients initially present with disease that has spread beyond the uterine corpus [157].

No specific staging system is designated for uterine sarcomas. Most authors stage uterine sarcomas using the revised FIGO system for endometrial carcinoma (see Table 14.2). Uterine sarcomas invade blood vessels, lymphatics, and contiguous pelvic structures once they have extended beyond the uterus. The lung is the most common site of distant metastases (see Fig. 14.52).

MRI Considerations

MRI techniques as well as criteria for staging uterine sarcomas are similar to those described in the earlier subsection, Endometrial Carcinoma. In addition, T1-weighted sequences with and without fat suppression are useful for confirming the presence of fat in malignant mixed mesodermal tumors.

Experience in the evaluation of uterine sarcomas with MRI is currently limited. Malignant degeneration of a leiomyoma occurs rarely but may be suspected if a leiomyoma enlarges suddenly, especially following menopause. MRI signal characteristics are not reliable in differentiating sarcomas from other benign or malignant

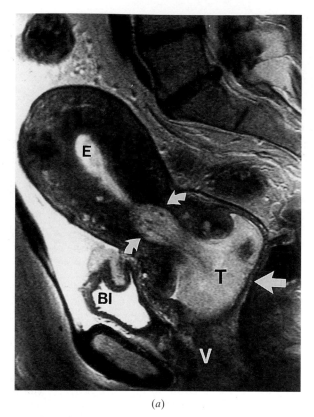
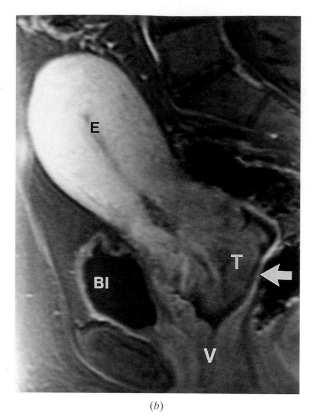

(a)   (b)

FIG. 14.74 Malignant mixed mesodermal tumor. Sagittal (*a*) T2-weighted echo-train spin-echo and (*b*) 45-second postgadolinium fat-suppressed SGE sequences. An exophytic tumor (*T*) is seen arising from the lower uterine segment (*curved arrows, a*). The tumor extends into the vagina but does not invade the vaginal wall (*arrow, a,b*). *Bl*, bladder; *E*, endometrium; *V*, vagina

uterine neoplasms, but the presence of a large, heterogeneous mass with indistinct borders or irregular contours should raise concern (Figs. 14.74, 14.75, and 14.76) [158,159].

Cervical Carcinoma

General Considerations

Invasive cervical carcinoma is the third most common malignancy of the female genital tract and the second most common cause of gynecologic malignancy death, following ovarian carcinoma. However, early detection with Papanicolaou (Pap) smears has led to a significant decrease in the mortality rate since the early 1950s [160]. The average age at diagnosis of patients with cervical carcinoma is 45 years. Risk factors include first intercourse at an early age, multiple sexual partners, low socioeconomic background, tobacco use, oral contraceptive use, immunocompromised host, and infection with human papilloma virus [160].

Cervical intraepithelial neoplasia (CIN) is considered a precursor lesion of cervical carcinoma. Patients with CIN or preclinical carcinoma are usually asymptomatic, and the diagnosis is most often based on cytological findings obtained during the course of a routine cervical Pap smear. Intermenstrual bleeding is the most common symptom of invasive cervical carcinoma.

Approximately 80 to 90 percent of all cervical carcinomas are squamous-cell carcinomas [160,161]. The remaining types consist of adenocarcinomas, adenosquamous carcinomas, and undifferentiated carcinomas. Adenocarcinomas and mucin-secreting tumors tend to have a worse prognosis. Other indicators of a poor prognosis include young age, lymphadenopathy, tumor diameter larger than 4 cm, depth of stromal invasion greater than 5 mm, and advanced stage at presentation [160,162]. Most cervical carcinomas arise from the squamocolumnar junction, which lies on the vaginal surface of the cervix (portio vaginalis) in women under 35 years of age, and most occur within the endocervical canal in older women. Cervical carcinomas arising from the portio vaginalis tend to grow in a polypoid fashion, whereas carcinomas arising from within the endocervical canal frequently result in a barrel-shaped cervix. Tumors located entirely within the cervical canal are difficult to evaluate clinically and have a higher incidence of parametrial invasion [163]. Cervical carcinoma spreads predominantly via direct extension and local spread. The external iliac lymph nodes

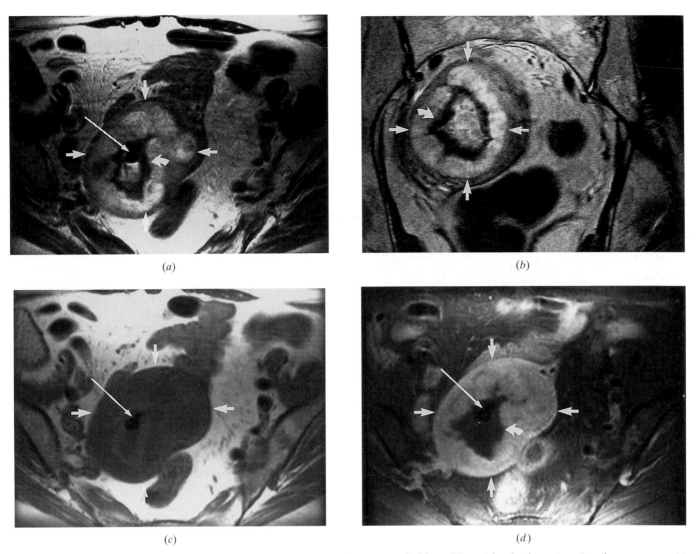

(a)

(b)

(c)

(d)

FIG. 14.75 Malignant mixed mesodermal tumor. (*a*) Transverse and (*b*) coronal oblique T2-weighted echo-train spin-echo sequence, (*c*) T1-weighted spin-echo sequence, and (*d*) postgadolinium T1-weighted fat-suppressed spin-echo sequence. A large, heterogeneous mass (*arrows, a–d*) with central necrosis (*curved arrow, a,b,d*) can be seen replacing the normal uterus. The mass demonstrates marked peripheral enhancement, whereas the necrotic center remains unenhanced (*curved arrow, d*). Air (*long thin arrow, a–d*) can be identified within the necrotic center.

are most frequently involved, followed by the obturator and the common iliac and internal iliac nodes [160]. Para-aortic lymph nodes are involved in approximately 45 percent of patients with tumor extension to the pelvic side wall or lower vagina. With tumor extension to the lower vagina, metastases may occur to inguinal lymph nodes. Hematogenous spread is rare and occurs only in the presence of advanced disease. The liver and lung are the most common sites of hematogenous metastases [160].

Cervical carcinoma is staged clinically according to the FIGO staging system (Table 14.3) [164]. Routine clinical staging is based on findings from chest radiography, intravenous pyelography, and bimanual pelvic examina-

tion performed under general anesthesia. In symptomatic patients or patients with advanced disease, barium enema, cystoscopy, and proctoscopy are performed [160]. Patients with carcinoma in situ (Stage 0) or microinvasive disease (Stage IA) are usually treated with simple hysterectomy, whereas patients with invasive carcinoma (Stage IB) or tumor extending to the upper vagina (Stage IIA) are generally treated with radical hysterectomy and pelvic lymph node dissection. In patients with tumors exceeding 3 to 5 cm in size, adjuvant radiation therapy followed by extrafascial hysterectomy has been shown to reduce pelvic recurrence [160]. Patients with more advanced disease (Stage IIB or beyond) are typically treated with radiation therapy. Five-year survival rates

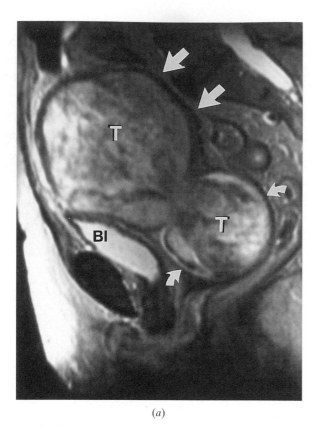

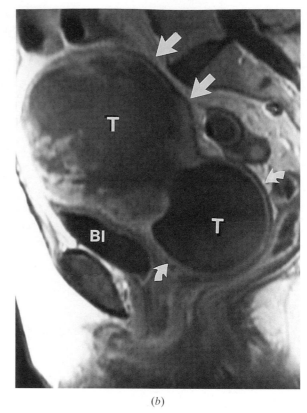

(a)   (b)

FIG. 14.76 Endometrial stromal sarcoma. Sagittal (*a*) T2-weighted echo-train spin-echo, and (*b*) postgadolinium T1-weighted spin-echo sequences. A large, heterogeneous, bilobed tumor (*T*) is seen originating within the uterus (*a,b*). The tumor invades the outer myometrium (*arrows, a,b*) but does not extend beyond the uterus. Caudally, the tumor prolapses into the cervix but does not invade the cervical wall (*curved arrows, a,b*). After gadolinium administration (*b*), the mass shows moderate peripheral enhancement. *Bl*, bladder

for the various clinical stages are estimated as follows: Stage I (79 to 92%), Stage II (67 to 75%), Stage III (38%), Stage IV (12%) [160].

Despite the well-known limitations of the FIGO staging system, clinical staging remains the standard of reference by which treatment protocols are instituted in patients with invasive cervical carcinoma, [163]. Staging errors ranging from 17 to 32 percent for Stage IB disease and from 39 to 64 percent for Stage II disease have been reported [165–167]. Furthermore, although the presence of lymphadenopathy, large tumor volume, and tumor extension to the uterine corpus may have important prognostic and therapeutic implications, these factors are not evaluated in the FIGO staging system [162,168].

Patients are usually referred for imaging studies only after the diagnosis of cervical carcinoma has been established. Therefore, the role of imaging is primarily to assess the regional and distant spread of disease. Numerous studies have investigated the role of cross-sectional imaging techniques in staging patients with carcinoma of the cervix. Transrectal ultrasound has been used by some investigators to stage cervical carcinoma and to assess tumor size [169,170]. Limitations of transrectal ultrasound include difficulty in evaluating the cephalad extent of

large tumors and inability to image pelvic lymph nodes [170]. CT imaging has been found useful for evaluating patients with advanced disease, with a reported accuracy ranging from 58 to 80 percent [171,172]. However, the relatively poor soft tissue contrast resolution of CT imaging precludes direct visualization of the tumor, thereby limiting accurate evaluation of tumor size and parametrial invasion [171,172]. Similarly, accurate diagnosis of tumor extension to the vagina or uterine corpus is not usually possible.

Recent studies suggest that MRI is an accurate and cost-effective means of staging patients with invasive cervical carcinoma [163,173,174]. MRI measurements of tumor size are reported to agree within 5 mm of measurements obtained at histopathology [175]. In addition, tumor size as measured on the MRI examination has been shown to correlate with the presence of parametrial and nodal disease [162,163]. MRI surpasses CT imaging and clinical staging in assessing the depth of stromal invasion, with reported accuracies ranging from 77 to 85 percent [176–178]. Similarly, MRI has been shown to be superior in assessing parametrial invasion, with accuracy rates ranging from 92 to 94 percent for MRI, 70 to 76 percent for CT imaging, and 78 percent for clinical staging

Table 14.3 FIGO Staging of Cervical Carcinoma with Corresponding MRI Findings

FIGO Staging[1]

Stage 0		Carcinoma in situ
Stage I		Tumor confined to cervix (extension to corpus should be disregarded)
	IA	Microinvasion
	IB	Clinically invasive. Invasive component >5mm in depth and >7mm in horizontal spread
Stage II		Tumor extends beyond cervix but not to pelvic side wall or lower third of vagina
	IIA	Vaginal invasion (no parametrial invasion)
	IIB	Parametrial invasion
Stage III		Tumor extends to lower third of vagina or pelvic side wall; ureter obstruction
	IIIA	Invasion of lower third of vagina (no pelvic side-wall extension)
	IIIB	Pelvic side wall extension or ureteral obstruction
Stage IV		Tumor extends outside true pelvis or invades bladder or rectal mucosa
	IVA	Invasion of bladder or rectal mucosa
	IVB	Distant metastases

Corresponding MRI findings[2]

Stage 0		No tumor mass present
Stage I	IA	No tumor mass or localized widening of the endocervical canal with a small tumor mass Fibrous stroma intact and symmetric
	IB	Partial or complete disruption of low-signal-intensity fibrous stroma Rim of intact cervical tissue surrounding tumor
Stage II	IIA	Segmental disruption of hypointense vaginal wall (upper two-thirds)
	IIB	Complete disruption of low signal intensity fibrous stroma with tumor signal extending into parametrium
Stage III	IIIA	Segmental disruption of hypointense vaginal wall (lower third)
	IIIB	Same findings as IIB with tumor signal, most frequently extending to involve obturator internus, piriformis, or levator ani muscles Dilated ureter
Stage IV	IVA	Tumor signal disrupts normal tissue planes with loss of low signal intensity of bladder or rectal wall
	IVB	Tumor masses in distant organs or anatomic sites

[1]The presence of metastatic lymph nodes is not included in the FIGO classificaiton.
[2]MRI findings seen on T2-weighted or contrast-enhanced T1-weighted images.

[177,179]. In addition, MRI is more accurate than CT imaging for selecting patients who will benefit from surgical intervention (94% versus 76%) [179]. MRI and CT imaging are comparable in diagnosing the presence of lymphadenopathy, with reported accuracies in the range of 77 to 90 percent [163,177,179,180]. Currently MRI may not be indicated in all patients with cervical carcinoma. Patients with tumors larger than 2 cm in size or with tumors located entirely within the endocervical canal have been shown to benefit most from undergoing MRI evaluation [163]. MRI is particularly useful in patients with concomitant pelvic masses and is currently the best imaging procedure for evaluating pregnant patients with cervical carcinoma. In addition, MRI may be useful in the assessment of patients with suspected recurrent disease.

MRI Considerations

T2-weighted sequences are used to identify and stage cervical carcinoma because they provide optimal contrast between the tumor and the residual cervix. Sagittal and transverse imaging planes are most commonly obtained to evaluate local tumor extension. Coronal sections may be performed in selected cases to provide additional views of the parametrium and lateral vaginal fornices. Transverse T1-weighted sequences are used to detect the presence of lymphadenopathy. The role for gadolinium-enhanced MRI in staging cervical carcinoma has not yet been established. However, in patients for whom the findings on T2-weighted images are indeterminate, gadolinium-enhanced sequences in the transverse or sagittal plane may be performed. We perform dynamic gadolinium-enhanced imaging, using fat-suppressed SGE sequences. Immediately after gadolinium administration, three sequential acquisitions are rapidly performed through the cervix. Following dynamic scanning, delayed T1-weighted sequences are usually obtained. In addition, in patients with tumors complicated by fistula formation to the bladder, gadolinium enhancement may facilitate visualization of the fistulous tract [181]. Little has been written to date on the use of intravaginal coils, either alone or in combination with a pelvic multicoil. Excellent detail of the normal anatomy and vascularity of the cervix can be achieved with intravaginal coils [5,182]. In addition, preliminary data has shown it to be an accurate technique in the evaluation of early cervical neoplasia [183–185]. However, when purchased commercially, intravaginal coils can add significant cost to the MRI examination. Further study is therefore needed to determine the exact role of intravaginal coils in evaluating uterine and cervical pathology [1].

Carcinomas in situ or microinvasive (Stage 1A) tumors are not routinely identified with MRI (see Table 14.3). However, MRI surpasses clinical examination in detecting tumors with stromal invasion covered by a normal-appearing surface epithelium [173,175,177]. In macroinvasive cervical carcinoma, the invasive component measures at least 5 mm in depth and 7 mm in horizontal spread. Macroinvasive cervical carcinoma (Stage IB) appears on T2-weighted images as an intermediate-signal-intensity mass that may deform the endocervical canal or disrupt the low-signal-intensity fibrous stroma (see

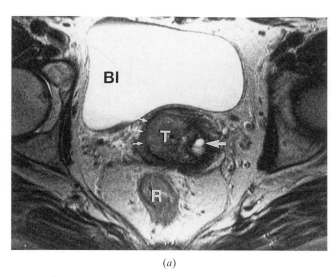

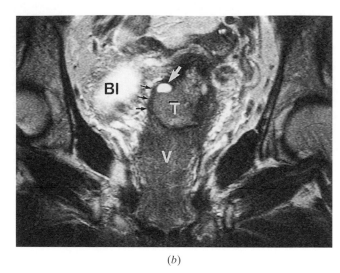

(a)   *(b)*

F IG . 14.77 Stage IB cervical carcinoma. (*a*) Transverse and (*b*) coronal T2-weighted echo-train spin-echo sequence. A tumor (*T*) of intermediate signal is shown within the cervix (*a,b*). Partial disruption of cervical stroma is noted, particularly along the right lateral aspect (*small arrows, a,b*). The parametrium is not invaded. Incidentally, nabothian cysts (*arrow, a,b*) are present within the cervix. *Bl*, bladder; *R*, rectum; *V*, vagina

Table 14.3) (Figs. 14.77 and 14.78) [173,175]. On T2-weighted images, the lateral margins of the cervix remain smooth. In addition, the normal signal intensity and symmetric configuration of the parametrium remain intact. On T1-weighted images, the mass is usually isointense relative to normal cervix and is therefore not visible unless associated contour abnormalities are present [38]. On dynamic images obtained 30 to 60 seconds after gado-

linium administration, cervical carcinoma demonstrates increased enhancement relative to the cervical stroma [33,186]. This difference in enhancement becomes less marked on delayed images resulting in decreased contrast between the tumor and surrounding stroma [150,178]. The MRI appearance of noninvasive cervical carcinoma is not specific, and its differentiation from cervical polyps or hyperintense submucosal leiomyomas

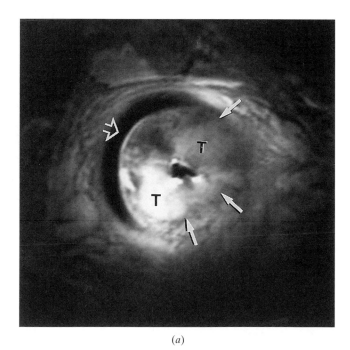

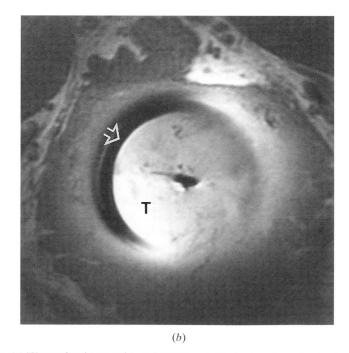

(a)   *(b)*

F IG . 14.78 Stage IB cervical carcinoma, endovaginal coil. Transverse (*a*) T2-weighted spin-echo and (*b*) T1-weighted spin-echo sequences using a solenoid geometry ring endovaginal coil (*open arrow, a,b*). A susceptibility artifact is present centrally within the cervix from a recent biopsy (*a,b*). An intermediate-signal-intensity tumor (*T*) is expanding the cervix (*a,b*), but an intact stripe of residual cervical stroma is seen around the periphery (*arrows, a*). (Courtesy of Dr. Naudita De Souza, MRI unit, Hammersmith Hospital, London, UK. Reprinted with permission from de Souza NM, Scoones D, Krausz T, Gilderale DJ, Soutter WP. High-resolution MR imaging of Stage I cervical neoplasia with a dedicated transvaginal coil: MR features and correlation of imaging and pathological findings. AJR 166:553–559, 1996) within the cervical canal, for example, may not be possible. In addition, MRI is unable to reliably discriminate postbiopsy changes from primary tumor [175]. The detection of macroscopic tumor on MRI is reported to have a 100 percent positive predictive value (PPV) for the presence of invasive disease (Stage IB or higher) [173]. Invasive cervical carcinoma may however on occasion appear subtle on MR examination [173,177,187]. When the criteria of partial or complete disruption of the low-signal-intensity fibrous stroma is used for detecting stromal invasion, the reported accuracy of MRI ranges from 76 to 85 percent [150,177,178,186]. However, when marked effacement (residual stroma less than 3 mm in width) or full thickness disruption of the cervical stroma occurs, microscopic parametrial extension may be present despite a smooth lateral cervical margin and a normal-appearing parametrium [174,188]. The role of gadolinium enhancement in evaluating Stage I cervical carcinoma has not yet been established. A number of studies have reported that gadolinium-enhanced delayed T1-weighted images are less accurate than T2-weighted images in assessing the depth of stromal invasion [150,178,186]. However, Yamashita et al. [186] reported in a small series of patients that dynamic gadolinium-enhanced images are more accurate than either T2-weighted or delayed enhanced T1-weighted images in evaluating stromal invasion.

A tumor is classified as Stage IIA when it invades the upper two-thirds of the vagina (see Table 14.3). On T2-weighted images, segmental disruption of the low-signal-intensity vaginal wall or the presence of a thickened hyperintense vagina indicate tumor invasion [173, 175,177]. Differentiation between a large polypoid tumor resulting in secondary effacement of the vaginal wall and frank vaginal invasion is frequently difficult. Of greater clinical significance is the presence or absence of parametrial invasion because patients with Stage IIB disease are not usually operative candidates. Parametrial extension is diagnosed with MRI when there is complete disruption of the cervical stroma associated with irregularity or stranding within the parametrial fat (Figs. 14.79 and 14.80) [173,175,177]. Studies have shown that a completely intact ring of low-signal-intensity cervical stroma is highly accurate in excluding parametrial invasion [173–175,177,178]. However, full thickness disruption of the fibrous cervical stroma by tumor, with or without abnormal signal intensity within the parametrium, has a PPV for parametrial invasion of only 39 to 86 percent [177,188]. The presence of peritumoral inflammatory tissue or exophytic Stage I tumors can lead to a false positive diagnosis of parametrial invasion. [178,179]. Furthermore, distinguishing tumor from normal parametrial tissue may at times be difficult due to the limited tissue contrast generated between the tumor and parametrium on T2-weighted sequences. Gadolinium-enhanced T1-weighted images have been shown to consistently over-

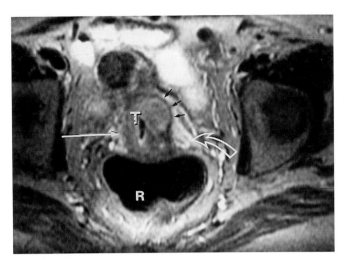

FIG. 14.79 Stage IIB cervical carcinoma. T2-weighted spin-echo sequence. The cervix is replaced by tumor (*T*) and there is right parametrial invasion (*long thin arrow*). Note complete disruption of the fibrous stroma along the right lateral aspect. On the left, a thin rim of intact cervical stroma is seen (*small arrows*). Note the hyperintense signal of the uninvolved left parametrium (*curved open arrow*) relative to the right. *R*, rectum

estimate parametrial invasion due to the lack of contrast between the tumor, enhancing parametrial vessels, and hyperintense parametrial fat [150,178,186]. The use of fat-suppressed imaging may improve the assessment of parametrial spread, but further investigation of the relative accuracy of this technique is needed (see Fig. 14.80) [186]. The overall accuracy of diagnosing parametrial invasion with MRI is reported to range from 80 to 92 percent [173,174,177,178,188].

Experience in the MRI evaluation of Stage III and Stage IV cervical carcinoma (see Table 14.3) is currently limited due the small number of cases with surgical correlation in most published series. In Stage IIIA disease, the tumor mass can be seen extending to the lower third of the vagina. Soft tissue stranding with or without an associated tumor mass extending to the pelvic side wall, or the presence of hydronephrosis identifies patients with Stage IIIB disease. Pelvic side-wall invasion is suggested when the normal low signal intensity of the levator ani, pyriformis, or obturator internus muscle is disrupted on T2-weighted images. Bladder or rectal involvement (Stage IVA) is suggested by focal disruption of the normal low-signal-intensity wall of these organs. In addition, nodular wall thickening or intraluminal masses may be present. In patients with tumors complicated by fistula formation to the bladder, the addition of gadolinium-enhanced sequences may facilitate visualization of the fistulous tract (Fig. 14.81) [181]. In a study of 23 patients (including 11 patients with cervical carcinoma) performed to evaluate the accuracy of MRI in the preoperative assessment of patients considered for pelvic exenteration, MRI had a 100 percent negative predictive value

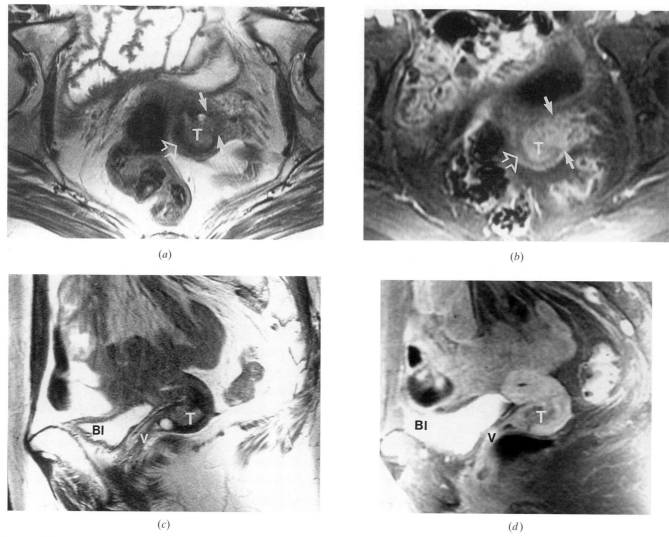

FIG. 14.80 Stage IIB cervical carcinoma. (*a*) T2-weighted echo-train spin-echo sequence, (*b*) 45-second postgadolinium fat-suppressed SGE sequence, (*c*) sagittal T2-weighted echo-train spin-echo sequence and (*d*) delayed postgadolinium T1-weighted fat-suppressed spin-echo sequence. A tumor (*T*) of intermediate signal intensity is present within the cervix (*a,c*). The tumor enhances more than the fibrous stroma on the early dynamic phase (*b*) and less on the delayed phase (*d*). Complete disruption (*arrows, a,b*) of the fibrous stroma (*open arrow, a,b*) with extension into the left parametrium is noted. Note that the extent of parametrial invasion may be overestimated on gadolinium enhanced images because of associated enhancement of parametrial vessels (*b*). The sagittal images (*c,d*) are useful for excluding vaginal invasion. *Bl*, bladder; *V*, vagina

for evaluating pelvic side-wall involvement [156]. In addition, the accuracy of assessing bladder and rectal invasion with MRI in this group of patients was 81 and 85 percent, respectively.

Although not evaluated by the FIGO staging system, the presence of lymph node metastases correlates significantly with adverse patient outcome. Moreover, lymphadenopathy precludes surgical cure and frequently necessitates the extension of radiation ports [156, 162,180]. Assessment of metastatic lymphadenopathy with MRI is based on the size of lymph nodes, with nodes larger than 1.0 cm in short axis diameter considered pathologic [156,180]. Signal intensity characteristics have not been useful in differentiating metastatic from hyper-

plastic lymphadenopathy. Similarly, the presence of microscopic disease in normal-sized lymph nodes cannot be detected. Lymph nodes are well shown on T1-weighted images, gadolinium-enhanced fat-suppressed SGE images and T2-weighted fat-suppressed echo-train spin-echo images. The accuracies of MRI and CT imaging in diagnosing lymph node metastases are essentially equivalent and reported to range from 76 to 93 percent [156,177,179,180,189].

Patients who have undergone radiation therapy present a diagnostic challenge because differentiation between radiation changes and residual or recurrent disease is frequently problematic. Early detection and accurate assessment of the regional extent of tumor recurrence

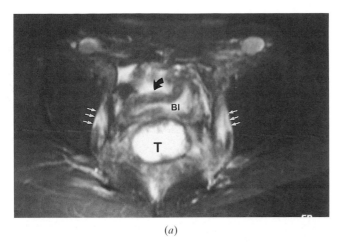

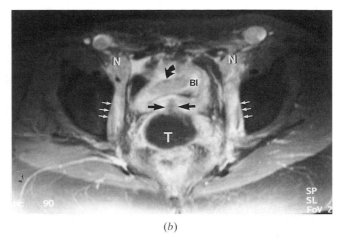

(a)   (b)

F I G . 14.81 Cervical carcinoma, postradiation necrosis. (*a*) T2-weighted echo-train spin-echo sequence, (*b*) interstitial-phase gadolinium enhanced fat-suppressed SGE sequence. A large necrotic tumor (*T*) is present in the cervix (*a,b*). Note marked thickening of the bladder wall (*curved arrow, a,b*) and increased signal intensity of the internal obturator muscles (*small arrows, a,b*) secondary to radiation therapy. A fistulous tract (*arrows, b*) to the bladder is shown to better advantage after gadolinium enhancement. Enlarged bilateral external iliac lymph nodes (*N*) are also present (*b*). *Bl*, bladder

are necessary for optimal treatment. Patients with locally recurrent disease may be candidates for pelvic exenteration if the disease does not extend to the pelvic side wall or outside the true pelvis [156]. However, patients with documented para-aortic lymphadenopathy are not candidates for pelvic exenteration [156]. Although CT imaging is frequently performed in the evaluation of patients with suspected recurrent disease, differentiating tumor recurrence from radiation fibrosis may be difficult [190,191]. Several studies have evaluated the accuracy of MRI in diagnosing residual or recurrent cervical carcinoma in patients treated with radiation therapy [191–195]. On conventional spin-echo T2-weighted images, areas of recurrent tumor demonstrate increased signal intensity relative to adjacent muscle and fat, whereas radiation fibrosis remains hypointense when imaged more than 12 months after radiation therapy [191–193]. During the initial 6 to 12 months after treatment, areas of radiation fibrosis may demonstrate increased signal intensity on T2-weighted sequences due to associated inflammation, edema and increased capillary vascularity [191,192]. Although both tumor recurrence and radiation fibrosis demonstrate low signal intensity on T1-weighted sequences, the presence of an identifiable mass lesion favors recurrence [193]. Reconstitution of the normal cervical zonal anatomy or a cervix that is homogeneously hypointense is reported to have a negative predictive value of 97 percent in excluding tumor recurrence (Fig. 14.82) [192]. Conversely, the presence of a measurable cervical mass has a PPV of 86 percent in predicting tumor recurrence [192]. Fluid distention of the endometrial cavity is frequently seen in association with a homogeneously hypointense cervix following radiation therapy (see Fig. 14.82) [192]. En-

hancement of the cervix after gadolinium administration is nonspecific and can be observed in postirradiation fibrosis, inflammation, radiation necrosis, and tumor [191]. However, gadolinium-enhanced imaging has been shown to be helpful in demonstrating parametrial and pelvic side-wall recurrence (Fig. 14.83) [192]. In addition, postirradiation complications such as vesicovaginal fistulas are better depicted on gadolinium-enhanced images [181,192]. The role of dynamic gadolinium-enhanced im-

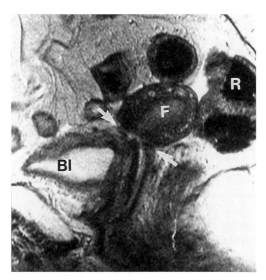

F I G . 14.82 Cervical carcinoma, postradiation changes. Sagittal T2-weighted echo-train spin-echo sequence. After radiation therapy, the cervix has shrunk and become fibrotic (*arrows*). No residual tumor is present. Note mild distension of the endometrial cavity by complex fluid (*F*) due to an associated cervical stenosis. *Bl*, bladder; *R*, rectum

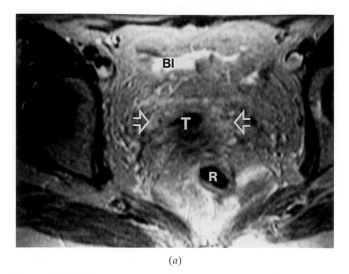
(a)

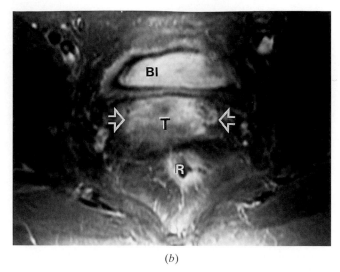
(b)

FIG. 14.83 Recurrent cervical carcinoma 12 months after radiation therapy. (a) T2-weighted spin-echo sequence, (b) postgadolinium T1-weighted fat-suppressed spin-echo sequence. There is tumor (T) recurrence at level of cervix with parametrial extension (open arrows, a,b). The tumor (T) is of intermediate signal intensity and isointense to fat on the T2-weighted image (a). After gadolinium administration, the extent of tumor (T) invasion is better delineated (open arrows, b). Bl, bladder; R, rectum

aging in diagnosing tumor recurrence has not yet been fully investigated [195]. The overall accuracy of diagnosing tumor recurrence with MRI is reported to range from 78 to 92 percent [191–193]. Because coexistence of radiation-induced fibrosis and tumor recurrence frequently occurs, MRI can be used to guide fine-needle biopsies in order to minimize sampling errors.

MRI AND PREGNANCY

Introduction

The choice of imaging techniques in pregnant patients is limited by the potential risks to the fetus. Because low-dose irradiation of a fetus may increase the likelihood of childhood cancer, the use of ionizing radiation during pregnancy should be avoided whenever possible. Ultrasound is routinely used in the evaluation of the fetus and pregnant woman because it is safe, inexpensive, and widely available. In experienced hands, ultrasound is highly accurate in the diagnosis of most complications associated with pregnancy. In recent years, several studies have reported the results of MRI in the evaluation of fetal and maternal disorders.

Safety Issues

MRI

MRI is considered safe for the pregnant patient and developing fetus. However, the potential adverse biological effects have not been thoroughly evaluated. Although a few studies have demonstrated that prolonged or high-

level exposure to electromagnetic radiation may result in disorders of embryogenesis [196] and teratogenicity [197], there is currently no evidence that undergoing an MRI examination will result in adverse effects on a fetus. In a study of 20 children who had undergone an MRI examination in utero, no hearing deficit or other disease entities that could be related to the MRI examination were found at 3-year follow-up [198]. In 1988, a report issued by the Food and Drug Administration indicated that "the safety of MRI, when used to image fetuses and the infant, has not been established" [199]. Similarly, a statement from the National Institute of Health Consensus Development Conferences on MRI indicated that "MRI should be used during the first trimester of pregnancy only when there are clear medical indications and when it offers a definite advantage over other tests." [200]. Therefore, prudence currently dictates that MRI be avoided during pregnancy, especially during the first trimester when rapid organogenesis is taking place. However, most centers do not restrict women of childbearing age from undergoing MRI after the first 10 days of the menstrual cycle.

Currently, the generally accepted medical practice requires that MRI of the pregnant patient be limited to the following indications: (1) Ultrasound has failed to establish the diagnosis or is not indicated (e.g., for neurologic or thoracolumbar disorders); (2) the results of MRI will likely affect the patient's management; and (3) the treatment of the patient's condition cannot be delayed until after delivery. The most common clinical indications for MRI are as follows: (1) assessment of placenta-related disorders, (2) evaluation of the maternal cervix or other maternal disorders (pregnancy-related or otherwise), and

(3) evaluation of fetal anomalies with equivocal ultrasound results.

Contrast Medium

Extracellular MRI contrast agents, such as gadopentetate dimeglumine, have been demonstrated to cross the placental barrier when injected into primates. These agents are then excreted by the fetal urinary tract into the amniotic cavity, and subsequently swallowed by the fetus [201]. A study performed in pregnant mice, with gadopentetate dimeglumine injected into the peritoneal cavity, failed to demonstrate any adverse effects [202]. A single case of inadvertent injection of 0.2 mmol/kg of gadopentetate dimeglumine, reported in a patient undergoing a cerebral MRI examination during early pregnancy, did not result in any apparent harmful effects to the fetus [203].

MRI versus Ultrasound

The field of view obtained with MRI is larger than that obtained with ultrasound. This facilitates anatomic orientation and allows for a global evaluation of the fetus and maternal pelvis. In contradistinction to ultrasound, image quality with MRI is not affected by the presence of air or bony structures or by maternal obesity. More importantly, MRI is less operator dependent than ultrasound, and a review of the images can be performed after the examination has been completed. Ultrasound is a real-time imaging technique, with a scan rate of up to 30 frames per second and therefore is not limited by fetal movements. Motion artifacts, however, are a significant cause of image degradation with MRI.

MRI Technique

A phased-array multicoil can be used in the early stages of pregnancy when technically feasible. In later pregnancy, MRI is usually performed in the body coil because of larger maternal body size. The examinations are usually performed with the patient lying supine on the MRI couch with the knees flexed. In late pregnancy, on occassion it may be advantageous to have the patient placed in a left posterior oblique position to avoid having maternal aortic pulsations transmitted to the fetus. When MRI is performed to evaluate maternal disorders, a combination of T2-weighted echo-train spin-echo sequences and either T1-weighted spin-echo or SGE sequences are usually obtained in the transverse and sagittal planes. When MRI is performed for fetal assessment, the effects of fetal motion on image quality must be minimized. Fetal motion begins as early as the 10th week of gestation and increases in amplitude and frequency with advancing gestational age. Several methods have been proposed to decrease fetal motion during MRI: (1) The patient may

be positioned in left lateral decubitus; (2) the examination can be performed after the mother has been recumbent for several minutes; or (3) the mother may be examined in a fasting state [204]. The use of pharmacologic agents to decrease fetal motion has also been shown to improve image quality [205,206]. More recently, the availability of fast pulse sequences with short acquisition times has significantly reduced the effects of fetal motion on image quality. Short repetition- and echo-time sequences, such as SGE sequences, can significantly diminish image degradation from motion artifacts [207,208]. The T1-weighted images obtained with SGE sequences provide excellent contrast between amniotic fluid and the placenta. Fetal contours are clearly outlined as a result of the natural contrast between the hypointense amniotic fluid and the high signal intensity of the fetal subcutaneous fat. In addition, subacute blood from a subchorionic hemorrhage, for example, can easily be detected (Fig. 14.84). T2-weighted sequences are used also in the evaluation of fetal and maternal pathology. Fast imaging techniques, such as single shot echo-train spin-echo (e.g.: HASTE) with image acquisition times of 1 second, have recently been used (Fig. 14.85). Image quality of fetuses using HASTE is excellent, and HASTE imaging may hold future clinical utility in fetal assessment. Echoplanar imaging also has been used in the evaluation of fetal anatomy [209]. Sagittal sections through the maternal pelvis frequently parallel the long axis of the fetus. However, depending on the fetal structures to be evaluated, oblique sections are often performed. In practice, a transverse section through the maternal pelvis usually is performed and oblique scans are prescribed as needed.

The Fetus

Although ultrasound is the primary modality in the assessment of fetal disorders, recent studies indicate that MRI can demonstrate the maturation of the normal brain more accurately [210]. In addition, MRI can visualize fetal anomalies not routinely detected with ultrasound [211,212].

Skull and Central Nervous System (CNS)

The fetal brain, for the most part, is unmyelinated and has a high water content, and thus is relatively hypointense on T1-weighted sequences and demonstrates increased signal intensity on T2-weighted sequences (Fig. 14.86). Similar to that of adults, the cerebrospinal fluid is hypointense on T1-weighted sequences and hyperintense on T2-weighted sequences. An area of increased signal intensity within the dorsal aspect of the fetal brain stem may be visible as early as 23 weeks with MRI. This area of increased signal intensity most probably corresponds to the initial process of myelination [213]. MRI is superior to ultrasound in assessing fetal brain maturity

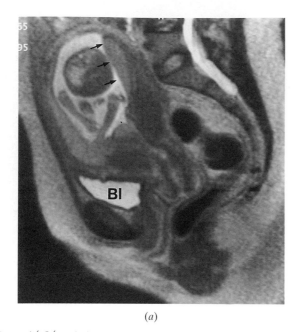

(a)

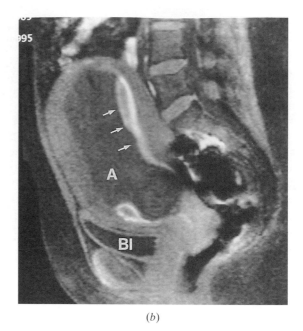

(b)

FIG. 14.84 Subchorionic hematoma. Sagittal HASTE (*a*) and fat-suppressed SGE (*b*) sequences through the maternal pelvis. A lenticular area of decreased signal intensity on the T2-weighted image (*arrows, a*) and moderately high signal on the SGE image (*arrows, b*) is consistent with a subchorionic hematoma. Note the peripheral rim of higher signal intensity on the SGE sequence indicating subacute hemorrhage. *A*, amniotic fluid; *Bl*, maternal bladder

[210]. Fetal cerebral anomalies that can be detected with MRI include anencephaly, hydrocephaly, cystic hygroma, Dandy-Walker cysts, lissencephaly, and hydranencephaly [214]. Recently, hyperintense subependymal and cortical nodules have been reported on T1-weighted se-

quences in the brains of fetuses with tuberous sclerosis, whereas antenatal cerebral ultrasound detected no abnormalities [211,212]. In another series of 22 fetuses with an abnormal cerebral ultrasound, MRI provided additional information in 6 of 22 fetuses, and in 3 cases this resulted in altered patient management [215].

Heart and Vessels

The fetal heart is routinely visible after 25 weeks of gestation. The blood in the cardiac cavities appears dark on spin-echo sequences as a result of the flow-void phenomenon. Fast imaging reduces the blurring associated with cardiac pulsations and allows visualization of the cardiac chambers and myocardium (Fig. 14.87). Using echoplanar imaging, snapshots of the cardiac cavities can be obtained at different phases in the cardiac cycle. However, electrocardiographic (ECG) gating remains technically difficult because of high fetal cardiac rates and artifacts caused by the maternal ECG [209]. The fetal aorta and inferior vena cava are readily visible anterior to the fetal spine (see Fig. 14.87). Furthermore, the umbilical cord (Fig. 14.88) carrying the umbilical vessels also can be seen.

Lungs

Fetal lungs display the signal intensity of fluid-filled structures, (hypointense on T1-weighted sequences and hyperintense on T2-weighted sequences) (see Figs. 14.86 and 14.87). Measurements of lung volume have been

FIG. 14.85 Normal fetus. Coronal HASTE sequence through the maternal pelvis. Because of short acquisition times, the gestational sac (*open arrows*) and fetal contours are clearly depicted, without motion-related artifacts. *A*, amniotic fluid; *P*, placenta; *Bl*, maternal bladder

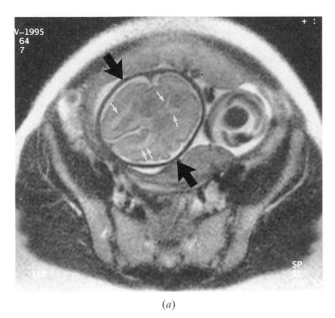

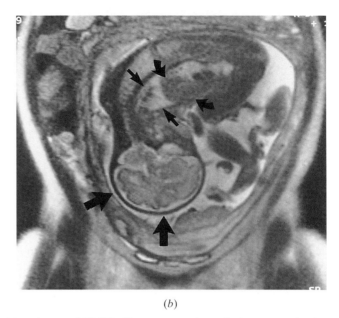

(a)   (b)

F I G . 14.86 Normal fetus. Central nervous system (CNS). Transverse (*a*) and coronal HASTE (*b*) sequences through the maternal pelvis. The contour of the fetal head (*large arrows a,b*) and the cerebral hemispheres are well-delineated. Cerebral ventricles (*small arrows, a*) are hyperintense relative to brain tissue. Fetal lungs (*arrows, b*) are of high signal intensity because of their water content. The liver (*curved arrows, b*) is of intermediate signal intensity and occupies most of the abdominal cavity. The lung-liver interface outlines the diaphragm.

performed with MRI and an exponential relationship between lung volume and gestational age has been demonstrated [216]. However, the role of MRI in diagnosing fetal lung hypoplasia remains controversial [217]. Production of surfactant begins at approximately 25 weeks of gestation. Because surfactant contains phospholipids, increasing concentrations in the third trimester may alter

the relaxation characteristics of the fetal lungs and potentially prove useful in the evaluation of lung maturity.

Abdomen

The liver, which occupies most of the upper abdomen, is readily visible on both T1- and T2-weighted sequences [205]. Liver T1 values have been shown to decrease with progressive fetal maturation [218]. On T2-weighted images, the contours of the diaphragm can be outlined by the high signal intensity of the fetal lung above and the

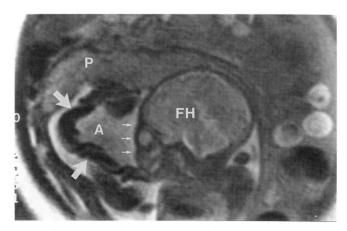

F I G . 14.87 Normal fetus. Heart and vessels. Transverse HASTE sequence through the maternal pelvis. Fetal lungs (*arrows*) are depicted on either side of the thorax. The heart is visible, and the contrast between the signal-void area generated by the circulating blood and the intermediate signal intensity of the myocardium (*small arrows*) allows assessment of ventricular wall thickness. The thoracic aorta (*long thin arrow*) is depicted as a signal-void area in front of the thoracic spine.

F I G . 14.88 Normal fetal face. Coronal HASTE sequence through the maternal pelvis shows the fetal face (*small arrows*) and a segment of the umbilical cord (*arrows*) in the amniotic fluid (*A*). *FH*, fetal head; *P*, placenta

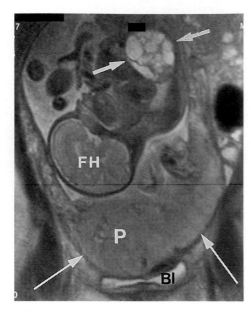

FIG. 14.89 Multicystic dysplastic kidney. Coronal HASTE sequence through the maternal pelvis. Fetal kidney (*arrows*) shows multiple high-signal-intensity cysts, which is consistent with multicystic dysplastic renal disease. In addition, a complete placenta previa is demonstrated (*long thin arrows*). *FH*, fetal head; *P*, placenta; *Bl*, maternal bladder

relatively low signal intensity of the liver below (see Fig. 14.86). The fluid-filled stomach and intestinal loops also may be seen with MRI. Meconium demonstrates a relatively high signal intensity on T1-weighted images [208].

Genitourinary Tract
With conventional spin-echo acquisitions, the normal fetal kidneys and adrenal glands are not routinely depicted [205]. The use of fast pulse sequences with diminished motion artifacts should result in improved visualization of the fetal kidneys. Renal cysts (Fig. 14.89), hydronephrosis, and the fetal bladder are easily depicted as high-signal-intensity structures on T2-weighted sequences.

Extremities
Parts of the fetal extremities are routinely depicted during the third trimester. Bony structures are of low signal intensity on T1-weighted sequences, in contrast with the intermediate signal intensity of the muscle and the high signal intensity of the subcutaneous fat. On T2-weighted images, the extremities are easily recognized as low-signal-intensity structures within the high-signal-intensity amniotic fluid (Fig. 14.90). In addition to a qualitative assessment of the fetal extremities, MRI can provide accurate measurements of their dimensions. In a recent report, MRI measurements of the fetal shoulder width during MRI pelvimetry showed significant correlation with postnatal orthopedic measurements and with birth weight [219].

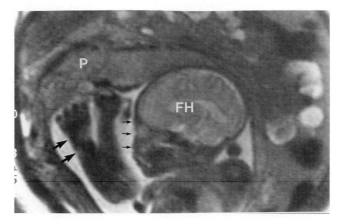

FIG. 14.90 Normal fetus. Extremities. Coronal HASTE sequence through the maternal pelvis shows the fetal face (*small arrows*) and upper extremity (*arrows*). *FH*, fetal head; *P*, placenta

Amniotic Fluid

Similar to other simple biologic fluids, normal amniotic fluid is hypointense on T1-weighted sequences and hyperintense on T2-weighted sequences (see Figs. 14.85 and 14.90). On T1-weighted sequences the dark amniotic fluid acts as a natural contrast agent outlining the fetus and placenta (Fig. 14.91). Volume measurements of the amniotic fluid can be performed with MRI, which allows detection of oligohydramnios and polyhydramnios. However, ultrasound is accurate in quantifying the amount of amniotic fluid in the majority of cases. Ex vivo studies performed on amniotic fluid have shown promising results in quantifying the concentration of me-

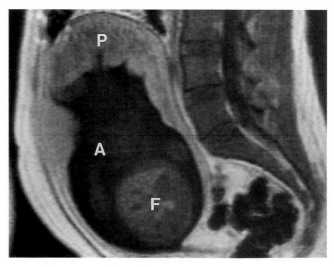

FIG. 14.91 Normal fetus. Sagittal SGE sequence through the maternal pelvis shows a gravid uterus with amniotic fluid (*A*), fetal parts (*F*), and a placenta (*P*). The low signal intensity of the amniotic fluid serves as a native contrast to outline the inner contour of the placenta.

conium in the amniotic fluid during the third trimester, but this technique is not yet used in the routine investigation of fetal distress [220].

Intrauterine Growth Retardation

Several studies have shown that quantifying the amount of fetal subcutaneous fat may be a means of diagnosing intrauterine growth retardation (IUGR) [218,221,222]. More recently, Baker et al. [223] demonstrated that a single measurement of fetal liver volume with echoplanar imaging could accurately identify fetuses with a birthweight below the 10th percentile. Furthermore, measurements of total fetal volume obtained with MRI correlated better with actual birthweight than those obtained with ultrasound [224]. Long-term, prospective studies are needed to correlate the preceding measurements with neonatal outcome before MRI can be recommended in the routine clinical assessment of fetal growth disturbances.

Pelvimetry

The use of x-ray pelvimetry has decreased steadily in the last two decades. With the advent of CT imaging, x-ray pelvimetry has largely been replaced by CT pelvimetry, which provides similar information with less ionizing radiation. Because of its safety and ability to scan in multiple planes, MRI is an ideal alternative to analog or

digital radiography [225,226]. MRI can accurately measure maternal pelvic dimensions without exposure to ionizing radiation. Furthermore, in addition to providing traditional pelvimetric measurements, MRI can clearly delineate the soft tissues of the maternal pelvis [227]. Recent reports on MR pelvimetry advocate the use of gradient-echo sequences. Advantages of gradient-echo sequences include short acquisition times and a relatively low specific absorption rate [228,229].

Placenta

Normal Appearance

The placenta can be visualized with MRI as a focal thickening along the periphery of the gestational sac as early as the 10th week of gestation. Placental tissue demonstrates intermediate signal intensity on T1-weighted sequences (slightly greater than that of myometrium), and moderately high signal intensity on T2-weighted sequences (see Figs. 14.85, 14.86, and 14.89). The placenta usually has a homogeneous appearance, and the internal architecture, including placental calcification demonstrated with ultrasound, is not visualized with MRI. Gadolinium chelates injected into the mother during an MRI examination cross the placental barrier, resulting in rapid and intense enhancement of the placenta (see earlier subsection, Contrast Medium) (Fig. 14.92). Currently, MRI is less accurate than ultrasound in the investigation of placental maturation. Indications for MRI in placental disorders are mostly limited to the diagnosis of placenta previa and placental

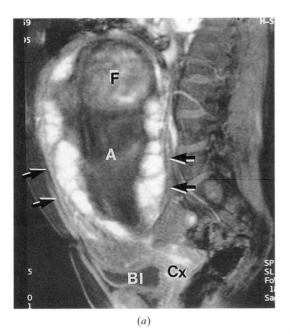

(a)

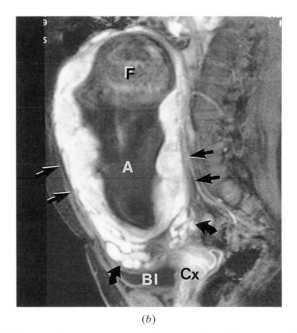

(b)

FIG. 14.92 Placental enhancement. Sagittal fat-suppressed SGE sequence (*a,b*) through the maternal pelvis obtained serially after gadolinium administration. The placenta (*arrows, a,b*) shows rapid and intense enhancement. Note enlarged uterine vessels (*curved arrows, b*) around the lower uterine segment. *A*, amniotic fluid; *F*, fetal parts; *Bl*, maternal bladder; *Cx*, cervix

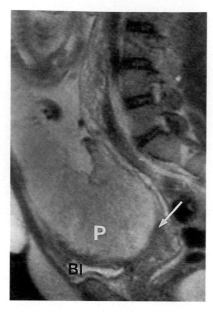

FIG. 14.93 Complete placenta previa. Sagittal HASTE image through the maternal pelvis shows that the placenta (*P*) completely covers the internal cervical os (*arrow*). *Bl*, maternal bladder

polyps, in addition to the evaluation of patients with gestational trophoblastic disease.

Placenta Previa

Placenta previa is diagnosed when the placenta covers a portion or all of the internal cervical os. Placenta previa usually presents as painless vaginal bleeding during the course of the third trimester. Ultrasound is the primary imaging modality used to diagnose placenta previa. One limitation of ultrasound is the rate of false positive diagnoses resulting from inaccurate visualization of the internal cervical os. Because of its ability to image the long axis of the entire cervical canal, MRI has been shown to be highly accurate in the diagnosis of placenta previa (Figs. 14.89 and 14.93) [230,231].

Gestational Trophoblastic Disease

Gestational trophoblastic disease (GTD) encompasses a variety of disease entities, including complete or partial hydatidiform mole, invasive mole, and choriocarcinoma. Clinically, a molar pregnancy is suspected in a patient with hyperemesis gravidarum, severe preeclampsia before 24 weeks of gestation, a large-for-date uterus, or first-trimester bleeding. Laboratory findings are diagnostic because the levels of human chorionic gonadotropin (β-hCG) are usually markedly elevated. Complete hydatidiform mole is the most common form of GTD and is characterized by trophoblastic proliferation without the development of an embryo. A partial hydatidiform mole is a distinct entity, and both mole and fetus exhibit a

triploid karyotype. Patients with partial hydatidiform mole rarely develop an invasive mole or a choriocarcinoma. However, invasive moles are seen in approximately 10 percent of patients treated for complete hydatidiform mole and are characterized by myometrial invasion. Patients present with bleeding and persistently elevated β-hCG. Approximately 50 percent of choriocarcinomas arise from a preexisting molar pregnancy. The remaining 50 percent develop after any gestational event including abortion and ectopic or term pregnancy. Choriocarcinomas metastasize most frequently to the lung.

Although some degree of myometrial invasion is present in most hydatidiform moles, evacuation of the molar pregnancy results in high cure rates. Invasive moles and choriocarcinomas are treated with chemotherapy. In addition, hysterectomy may be performed in some patients with choriocarcinomas. Because GTD is markedly sensitive to chemotherapy, high cure rates are achieved even in the presence of metastases. The serum β-hCG is a sensitive indicator of the presence of disease and has been the mainstay of patient management. A rise of plateau of the serum β-hCG level indicates persistent GTD.

The role of imaging techniques in evaluating patients with GTD is limited [232], with the diagnosis and follow-up of patients with GTD is primarily based on β-hCG testing. The main role of imaging is (1) to distinguish between a normal pregnancy and GTD, (2) to assess the degree of myometrial invasion in patients with invasive moles or choriocarcinomas, and (3) to assess regional and metastatic disease in choriocarcinomas. In addition, imaging techniques may be used to evaluate patients with recurrent GTD. On ultrasound the typical appearance of a hydatidiform mole is a soft tissue mass containing numerous cystic spaces that distends the endometrial cavity, without evidence of a fetus. This appearance, however, is nonspecific and may be seen in hydropic degeneration of the placenta or missed abortions. In addition, large theca lutein cysts of the ovaries may be present. CT imaging is most commonly used to screen for distant metastases.

There is little data on the role of MRI in the evaluation of patients with GTD. In complete hydatidiform moles, MRI demonstrates a heterogeneous mass with multiple cystic spaces distending the endometrial cavity (Fig. 14.94). A rim of hypointense myometrium may be visible at the periphery of a molar pregnancy [233]. In persistent GTD, a uterine mass displaying mixed signal intensity on T2-weighted images may be seen. Complete or partial disruption of the junctional zone was noted in all 9 cases of persistent GTD reported by Hricak et al. [234], but only in 13 of 21 cases reported by Barton et al. [235]. On T1-weighted MR images, the mass is isointense to the myometrium but often exhibits foci of high signal inten-

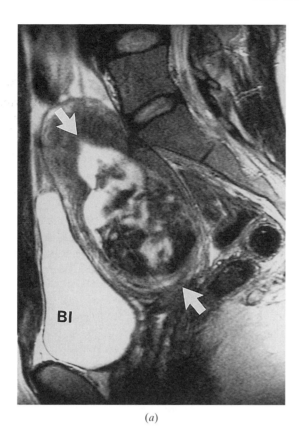

(a)

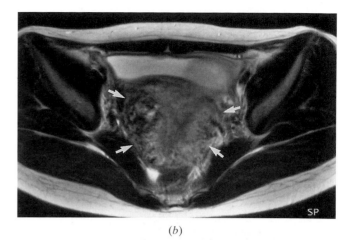

(b)

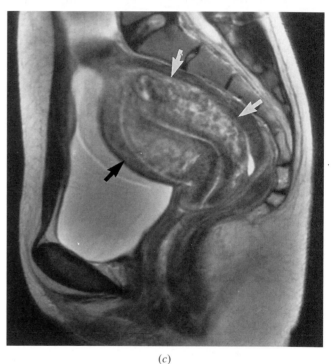

(c)

FIG. 14.94 Hydatidiform mole and invasive mole. Sagittal T2-weighted echo-train spin-echo image (a) in a patient with a partial hydatidiform male. A large heterogeneous mass is seen within the endometrial cavity (arrows) in a patient with elevated serum b-hCG levels. Note that there is no definite evidence of myometrial invasion. Transverse (b) and sagittal (c) T2-weighted echo-train spin-echo images in a second patient who has an invasive mole. Note that in distinction from the patient with the hydatid mole there is diffuse heterogeneous high signal intensity of the myometrium consistent with invasion (arrows b,c). Bl, bladder

sity corresponding to areas of hemorrhage. The mass is hypervascular and enhances intensely after gadolinium administration. Some foci of myometrial invasion may be detected only on gadolinium-enhanced images [236]. In addition, multiple, enlarged vessels are frequently visualized. On follow-up, the resolution of these findings correlates well with decreasing levels of serum β-hCG. Theca-lutein ovarian cysts often demonstrate high signal intensity on T1-weighted sequences due to associated hemorrhage. Although there is considerable overlap in the imaging characteristics between invasive moles and choriocarcinomas, Ha et al. [237] found in a small series of patients that choriocarcinomas presented as well-defined hemorrhagic masses, whereas invasive moles were seen as poorly defined infiltrative masses (Fig. 14.94).

Placental Polyps

Placental polyps represent polypoid placental tissue retained after delivery or abortion and may result in life-threatening hemorrhage. Placental polyps demonstrate high signal intensity on T2-weighted images and enhance to a greater extent than the normal myometrium following gadolinium administration [238].

The Maternal Side

The Uterus

Uterine Changes During Pregnancy. The size and appearance of the uterus alters considerably during the various stages of pregnancy. Early in pregnancy, the uterus has an appearance similar to that of the nongravid uterus but is mildly enlarged. The intrauterine gestational sac is visualized as early as the 6th week of gestation. As the uterus enlarges with fetal development, it takes on a more globular configuration. There is also progressive thinning of the myometrium with loss of the zonal differentiation between the inner and outer myometrium. At full term, the myometrium has become a thin stripe of relatively low signal intensity. An increase in the number and size of parametrial vessels is usually observed during pregnancy.

Uterine rupture is a rare but serious complication of pregnancy that is associated with a high rate of maternal and fetal mortality. The diagnosis of uterine rupture with MRI has recently been reported [239].

Postpartum Uterus. The greatest reduction in size of the uterine corpus and cervix occurs within 1 week postpartum, with the uterus gradually returning to its normal size by 6 months (Fig. 14.95). Willms et al. [240] performed serial MRI examinations on 14 healthy women who had undergone uncomplicated vaginal delivery. The presence of acute or subacute blood in the endometrial cavity was a common occurrence in the immediate postpartum period and resolved within 1 week [241]. During the early postpartum period, the myometrium was of intermediate and heterogeneous signal intensity on T2-weighted sequences. In none of the 14 subjects studied was the junctional zone visualized before 2 weeks following delivery. By 6 months there was complete reconstitution of the junctional zone. However, the junctional zone remained prominent with somewhat ill-defined borders. In addition, Willms et al. [240] found the outer cervical stroma, or smooth-muscle layer, to be hyperintense on

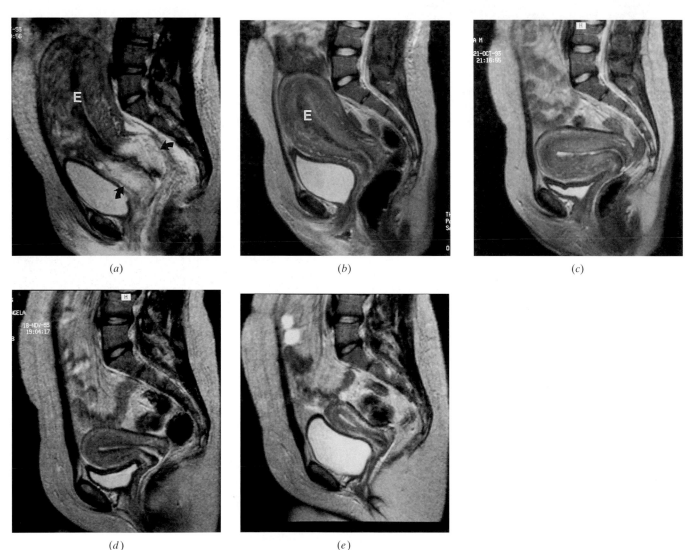

(a)   (b)   (c)

(d)   (e)

F ig . 14.95 Postpartum uterus. Sagittal T2-weighted echo-train spin-echo sequence (*a*) 24 hours, (*b*) 1 week, (*c*) 1 month, (*d*) 2 months and (*e*) 6 months after delivery. Acute and/or subacute blood is shown within the endometrial cavity (*E*) in the first week postpartum (*a*,*b*). The outer cervical stroma or smooth-muscle layer is hyperintense (*curved arrows, a*) in the first 30 hours after delivery. The inner fibrous stroma, however, remains hypointense throughout the postpartum period (*a*–*e*). The myometrium is of intermediate and heterogeneous signal intensity during the early postpartum period (*a*–*c*). By 6 months, complete reconstitution of the junctional zone (JZ) is evident (*e*). Note the gradual decreases in size of the uterus from (*a*) to (*e*).

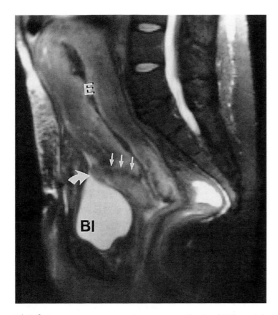

FIG. 14.96 Postcesarean section uterus. Sagittal T2-weighted fat-suppressed echo-train spin-echo sequence in a patient 5 days after cesarean section. A hypointense scar is visible in the lower uterine segment (*small arrows*), as well as a bladder flap (*curved arrow*). The low signal intensity of the endometrial cavity (*E*) due to the presence of acute and/or subacute blood and the lack of zonal differentiation of the myometrium are normal findings in the early postpartum period. *Bl*, bladder

T2-weighted images within the first 30 hours following delivery. The fibrous stroma, however, remained hypointense throughout the postpartum period. Ancillary findings included a small amount of free pelvic fluid and prominent myometrial vessels that resolved within 6 weeks.

Postcesarean Section. In women undergoing cesarean section, the incision is typically seen as an area of moderately high signal intensity on both T1- and T2-weighted sequences, although the signal intensity may be variable (Fig. 14.96) [241]. These signal characteristics suggest the presence of a subacute hematoma within the myometrium at the incision site. The presence of a myometrial defect may indicate a uterine dehiscence. A hematoma of the bladder flap, which is formed by incision of the peritoneal reflection that covers the uterus, is a normal finding postpartum and is particularly common when a low transverse incision is used [241]. Parametrial edema or masses are not usually seen after uncomplicated cesarean sections and may raise the possibility of abscess formation [241].

Leiomyoma. Uterine leiomyomas demonstrate the same imaging characteristics during pregnancy as in the nongravid uterus. However, because of continued estro-

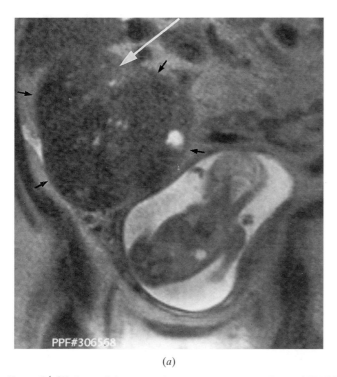

(a)

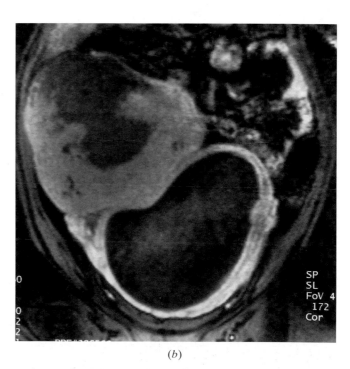

(b)

FIG. 14.97 Large leiomyoma in a pregnant uterus. Coronal HASTE (*a*) and coronal gadolinium-enhanced fat-suppressed SGE (*b*) images. An 8 cm leiomyoma arises from the right superolateral aspect of the uterus. The leiomyoma is low in signal intensity and well-defined on the HASTE image (*arrows, a*) which is the typical appearance for a leiomyoma. Ill-defined subtle high signal intensity (*long white arrow, a*) is appreciated on the T2-weighted image (*a*), which corresponds to a region of lack of gadolinium enhancement on the gadolinium-enhanced fat-suppressed SGE image (*b*). Clear definition of the uterine origin of the mass was appreciated on images obtained in multiple planes. Gadolinium was administered in this patient because of clinical concern of malignant disease. Note that even though data acquisition is 20 seconds using the breath hold SGE sequence (*b*), fetal motion blurs out definition of the fetus. In contrast the one second data acquisition of HASTE freezes fetal motion rendering the fetus clearly defined.

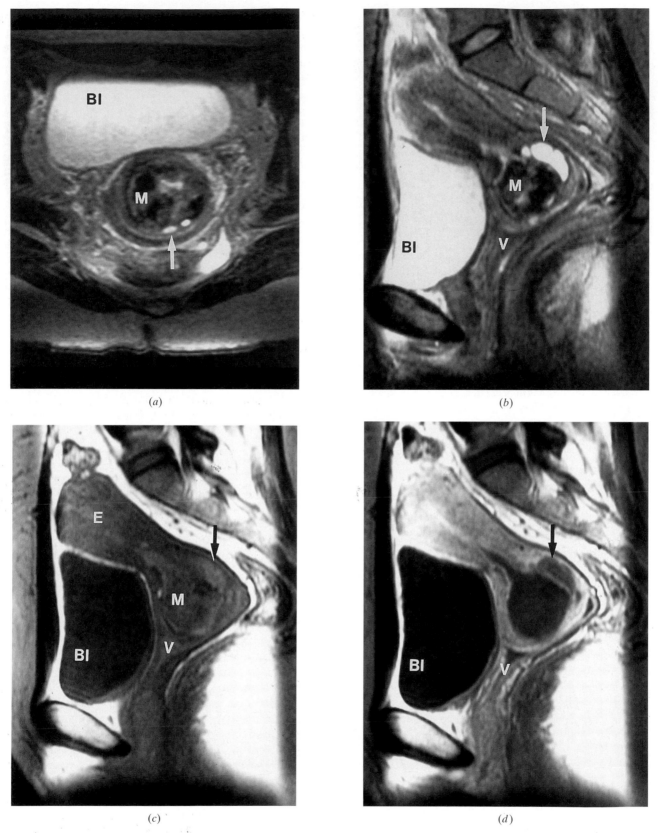

FIG. 14.98 Aborting pregnancy mimicking a cervical pregnancy. Transverse (*a*) and sagittal T2-weighted echo-train spin-echo sequences (*b*) and sagittal unenhanced (*c*) and contrast-enhanced T1-weighted spin-echo (*d*) sequences. A heterogeneous mass (*M*) is seen distending the endocervical canal (*a–c*). The mass compresses nabothian cysts (*arrow, a–d*) present in the dorsal aspect of the cervix. Lack of enhancement of the mass following gadolinium administration (*d*), and the absence of a decidual reaction of the cervix excludes a cervical pregnancy (*d*). *Bl*, bladder; *E*, endometrium; *V*, vagina

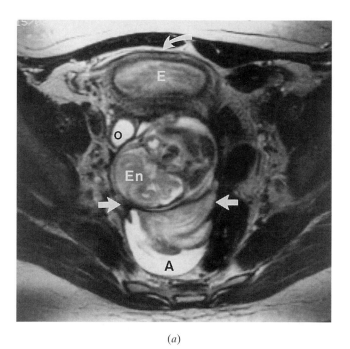

(a)

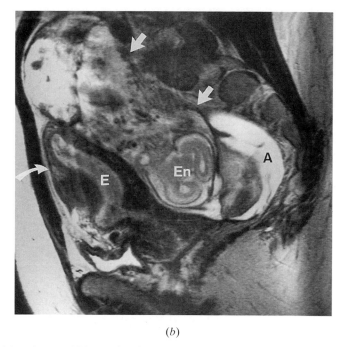

(b)

F IG. 14.99 Abdominal pregnancy with encephalocele. Transverse (*a*) and sagittal T2-weighted echo-train spin-echo (*b*) sequences. A gestational sac (*arrows, a,b*) is identified posterior to a nongravid uterus (*curved arrow, a,b*). An encephalocele (*En*) is seen at the level of the fetal head. *A*, amniotic fluid; *E*, endometrium; *O*, right ovary (Courtesy of Dr. Leslie Scoutt, Yale University, New Haven, Connecticut)

gen stimulation, uterine leiomyomas tend to enlarge during pregnancy. With rapid growth, they may outgrow their vascular supply, resulting in hemorrhagic infarction and necrosis (Fig. 14.97). Precise mapping of all leiomyomas should be performed with ultrasound early during pregnancy because evaluation will become more difficult during the second and third trimesters. When the gestational contents preclude accurate assessment with ultrasound, MRI is indicated. As in the nongravid uterus, MRI is more accurate than ultrasound in determining the size and location of leiomyomas. Multiple and large leiomyomas are accompanied by a higher incidence of malpresentation, whereas leiomyomas in the lower uterine segment may preclude vaginal delivery.

Complex Ectopic or Multiple Pregnancies. In the presence of multiple pregnancies or in pregnancies situated in the cornua or cervix (Fig. 14.98), MRI may facilitate the diagnosis by depicting the entire uterine cavity on each imaging plane. Several reports have supported the complementary role of endovaginal ultrasound and MRI in the evaluation of this group of patients [242,243]. MRI may also be useful in the diagnosis of an abdominal pregnancy (Fig. 14.99).

The Cervix

Evaluation of the cervix is an important aspect of the ultrasound examination during pregnancy. However, during the second and third trimesters, fetal parts may

obscure the cervix when the maternal bladder is empty. Conversely, an overdistended bladder may compress and elongate the cervix, masking a cervical incompetence or leading to a false positive diagnosis of placenta previa. With MRI the entire cervix, including the internal and external cervical os, can be visualized regardless of the degree of bladder distension.

Cervical Changes During Pregnancy. During pregnancy, the cervical canal often fills with high-signal-intensity mucus, whereas the stroma becomes hypertrophic and edematous. At the time of cervical effacement, immediately before term, the cervical lumen becomes wider, and the stroma cannot be distinguished from the lumen on T2-weighted sequences [244].

Cervical Incompetence. Premature delivery occurs in 10 percent of all pregnancies and significantly contributes to perinatal mortality. The role of the cervix in the pathogenesis of premature delivery remains controversial. In normal pregnancies, the cervix remains firm and closed while uterine smooth muscle is relaxed. The cervix dilates and softens when labor begins. Cervical incompetence is recognized as a contributor to premature delivery. The diagnosis of cervical incompetence may be difficult and usually is based on digital examination or ultrasound findings. A recent multicenter study performed on 2,531 low-risk patients examined with transvaginal ultrasound at 24 and 28 weeks of gestation, found

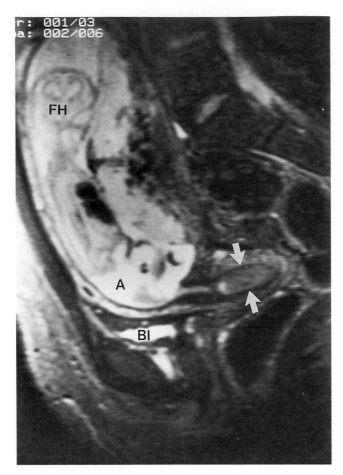

r: 001/03
a: 002/006

FH

A

Bl

FIG. 14.100 Cervical carcinoma and pregnancy. Sagittal T2-weighted fat-suppressed echo-train spin-echo sequence through the maternal pelvis. A well-defined mass (*arrows*) is shown in the lower aspect of the cervix. The mass is confined to the cervix and represents a Stage I cervical carcinoma. *A*, amniotic fluid; *Bl*, maternal bladder; *FH*, fetal head (Courtesy of Dr. Leslie Scoutt, Yale University, New Haven, Connecticut)

a close correlation between the length of the cervix and the risk of delivery before 35 weeks of gestation [245]. Although MRI allows for detailed visualization of the cervix on T2-weighted sagittal sections of the uterus, little data is available on the MRI evaluation of cervical incompetence during pregnancy. Shortening of the cervix and an increase in the signal intensity of the cervical stroma during the third trimester have been described [244].

Cervical Carcinoma. The association of cervical carcinoma with pregnancy raises difficult management issues. MRI is currently the best imaging modality for evaluating pregnant patients with cervical carcinoma (Fig. 14.100). (See the earlier subsection, Cervical Carcinoma, in the section on Malignant Disease of the Uterine Corpus and Cervix for a complete discussion on the role of MRI in the staging of cervical carcinoma.)

The Adnexa

Normal Changes During Pregnancy. Corpus luteal cysts, the most common adnexal masses encountered during pregnancy, regress by about 16 weeks of gestation. Corpus luteal cysts usually measure less than 6 cm in size and do not enlarge during pregnancy. Nonhemorrhagic corpus luteal cysts have the characteristic appearance of fluid-filled structures with MRI, demonstrating low signal intensity on T1-weighted sequences and high signal intensity on T2-weighted sequences.

Pregnancy-Related Complications. (The role of MRI in the diagnosis of ectopic pregnancy is discussed in Chapter 15 on the Adnexa.)

The incidence of ovarian vein thrombosis is approximately 1 per 600 deliveries. It is often associated with postpartum endometritis and occurs most commonly in the right ovarian vein [241,246]. The diagnosis of ovarian vein thrombosis is frequently difficult with ultrasound. MRI can be instrumental in diagnosing ovarian vein thrombosis because of its ability to image in a plane parallel to the course of the vessel.

Adnexal Masses in Pregnancy. The discovery of an adnexal mass during pregnancy poses a diagnostic challenge. Indeed, both the physical examination and ultrasound are of limited value because of the presence

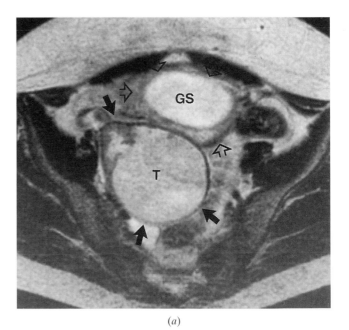

GS

T

(a)

FIG. 14.101 Ovarian cystadenocarcinoma and pregnancy. Transverse T2-weighted echo-train spin-echo (*a*), sagittal T1-weighted spin-echo (*b*), and transverse fat-suppressed T1-weighted spin-echo (*c*) sequences through the maternal pelvis. A right adnexal mass (*arrows, a–c*) is shown dorsally and caudally relative to the gravid uterus (*open arrows, a–c*).

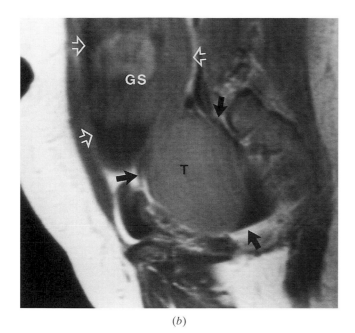

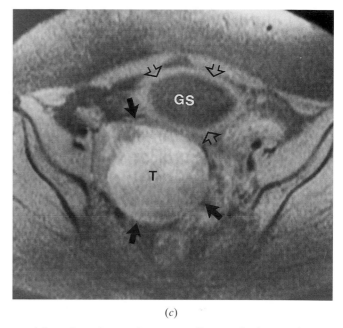

(*b*)   (*c*)

F ı g . 14.101 (*Continued*) The mass contains solid and cystic components. A Stage I ovarian carcinoma was diagnosed at histopathology. *GS*, gestational sac; *T*, maternal ovarian tumor (Courtesy of Dr. Leslie Scoutt, Yale University, New Haven, Connecticut)

of the gravid uterus. Although the most common adnexal mass in a pregnant patient is a corpus luteal cyst, more clinically significant adnexal masses must be excluded. Because of the increased pressure in the pelvic cavity, adnexal masses may become symptomatic during pregnancy as a result of extrinsic compression, hemorrhage, or torsion. Under these circumstances, MRI can be invaluable in the localization and characterization of these masses (Fig. 14.101) [247].

REFERENCES

1. Hricak H: Current trends in MR imaging of the female pelvis. Radiographics 13:913–919, 1993.

2. Chang YC, Hricak H: Current status of MR imaging of the female pelvis. Crit Rev Diagn Imaging 29(4):337–356, 1989.

3. Hricak H: MRI of the female pelvis: A review. AJR Am J Roentgenol 146(6):1115–1122, 1986.

4. Smith RC, Reinhold C, McCauley TR, et al: Multicoil high-resolution fast spin-echo MR imaging of the female pelvis. Radiology 184:671–675, 1992.

5. deSouza NM, Hawley IC, Schwieso JE, Gilderdale DJ, Soutter WP: The uterine cervix on in vitro and in vivo MR images: A study of zonal anatomy and vascularity using an enveloping cervical coil. AJR Am J Roentgenol 163:607–612, 1994.

6. Nghiem HV, Herfkens RJ, Francis IR et al: The pelvis: T2-weighted fast spin-echo MR imaging. Radiology 185:213–217, 1992.

7. Smith RC, Reinhold C, Lange RC, McCauley TR, Kier R, McCarthy S: Fast spin-echo MR imaging of the female pelvis. Part I. Use of a whole-volume coil. Radiology 184:665–669, 1992.

8. Constable RT, Gore JC: The loss of small objects in variable TE imaging: Implications for FSE, RARE, and EPI. Magn Reson Med 28:9–24, 1992.

9. Hricak H, Finck S, Honda G, Goeranson H: MR imaging in the evaluation of benign uterine masses: Value of gadopentetate dimeglumin-enhanced T1-weighted images. AJR Am J Roentgenol 158:1043–1050, 1992.

10. Constable RT, Anderson AW, Zhong J, Gore JC: Factors influencing contrast in fast spin-echo MR imaging. Magn Reson Imaging 10:497–511, 1992.

11. Jolesz FA, Jones KM: Fast spin-echo imaging of the brain. Top Magn Reson Imaging 5(1):1–13, 1993.

12. McCauley TR, McCarthy S, Lange R: Pelvic phased array coil: Image quality assessment for spin-echo MR imaging. Magn Reson Imaging 10:513–522, 1992.

13. Mark AS, Hricak H: Intrauterine contraceptive devices: MR imaging. Radiology 162:311–314, 1987.

14. Haramati N, Penrod B, Staron RB, Barax CN: Surgical sutures: MR artifacts and sequence dependence. J Magn Reson Imaging 4(2):209–211, 1994.

15. Lee JKT, Gersell DJ, Balfe DM, Worthington JL, Picus D, Gapp G: The uterus: In vitro MR anatomic correlation of normal and abnormal specimens. Radiology 157:175–179, 1985.

16. Demas BE, Hricak H, Jaffe RB: Uterine MR imaging: Effects of hormonal stimulation. Radiology 159:123–126, 1986.

17. McCarthy S, Tauber C, Gore J: Female pelvic anatomy: MR assessment of variations during the menstrual cycle and with use of oral contraceptives. Radiology 160:119–123, 1986.

18. Langlois LP: The size of the normal uterus. J Reprod Med 4(6):220–228, 1970.

19. Jones HW, Jones GS, eds. Gynecology (3rd ed.). Baltimore: Williams & Wilkins, pp. 1–8, 1982.

20. Jones HW, Jones GS, eds. Gynecology (3rd ed.). Baltimore: Williams & Wilkins, pp. 46–68, 1982.

21. Schwalm H, Dubrauszky V: The structure of the musculature of the human uterus: Muscles and connective tissue. Am J Obstet Gynecol 94:391–404, 1966.

22. Brown HK, Stoll BS, Nicosia SV, et al: Uterine junctional zone: Correlation between histologic findings and MR imaging. Radiology 179:409–413, 1991.

23. Bloom W, Fawcett DW: A Textbook of Histology. Philadelphia: WB Saunders, pp. 894, 1975.

24. Lange RC, Duberg AC, McCarthy SM: An evaluation of MRI contrast in the uterus using synthetic imaging. Magn Reson Med. 17(1):279–284, 1991.

25. McCarthy S, Scott G, Majumdar S, et al: Uterine junctional zone: MR study of water content and relaxation properties. Radiology 171:241–243, 1989.

26. Haynor DR, Mack LA, Soules MR, Shuman WP, Montana MA, Moss AA: Changing appearance of the normal uterus during the menstrual cycle: MR studies. Radiology 161:459–462, 1986.

27. Wiczyk HP, Janus CL, Richards CJ, et al: Comparison of magnetic resonance imaging and ultrasound in evaluating follicular and endometrial development throughout the normal cycle. Fertil Steril 49(6):969–972, 1988.

28. Kasai M: Clinical application of magnetic resonance imaging (MRI) in uterine disease. Acta Obstet Gynaecol Japn 42(7):711–718, 1990.

29. Mitchell DG, Schonholz L, Hilpert PL, Pennell RG, Blum L, Rifkin MD: Zones of the uterus: Discrepancy between US and MR images. Radiology 174:827–831, 1990.

30. Scoutt LM, Flynn SD, Luthringer DJ, McCauley TR, McCarthy SM: Junctional zone of the uterus: Correlation of MR imaging and histologic examination of hysterectomy specimens. Radiology 179:403–407, 1991.

31. Reinhold C, McCarthy S, Bret PM et al: Diffuse adenomyosis: Comparison of endovaginal US and MR imaging with histopathologic correlation. Radiology 199:151–158, 1996.

32. Hricak H, Alpers C, Crooks LE, Sheldon PE: Magnetic resonance imaging of the female pelvis: Initial experience. AJR Am J Roentgenol 141:1119–1128, 1983.

33. Hirano Y, Kubo K, Hirai Y, et al: Preliminary experience with gadolinium-enhanced dynamic MR imaging for uterine neoplasms. Radiographics 12:243–256, 1992.

34. Yamashita Y, Harada M, Sawada T, Takahashi M, Miyazaki K, Okamura H: Normal uterus and FIGO Stage I endometrial carcinoma: Dynamic gadolinium-enhanced MR imaging. Radiology 186:495–501, 1993.

35. Ito K, Fujita T, Uchisako H, et al: MR imaging of the uterus: Findings from high-resolution multisection dynamic imaging with a surface coil. AJR Am J Roentgenol 163:873–879, 1994.

36. Hricak H, Kim B: Contrast-enhanced MR imaging of the female pelvis. J Magn Reson Imaging 3:297–306, 1993.

37. Scoutt LM, McCauley TR, Flynn SD, Luthringer DJ, McCarthy SM: Zonal anatomy of the cervix: Correlation of MR imaging and histologic examination of hysterectomy specimens. Radiology 186:159–162, 1993.

38. Togashi K, Nishimura K, Itoh K, et al: Uterine cervical cancer: Assessment with high-field MR imaging. Radiology 160:431–435, 1986.

39. Weinreb JC: Explanation for the MR imaging appearance of the periprosatic and uterovaginal venous plexus (abstract). Radiology 169(P):138, 1988.

40. Hricak H, Stern JL, Fischer MR, Shapeero LG, Winkler ML, Conley GL: Endometrial carcinoma staging by MR imaging. Radiology 162:297–305, 1987.

41. Sheth S, Hamper UM, Kurman RJ: Thickened endometrium in the postmenopausal woman: Sonographic-pathologic correlation. Radiology 187:135–139, 1993.

42. Varner RE, Sparks JM, Cameron CD, Roberts LL, Soong S: Transvaginal sonography of the endometrium in postmenopausal women. Obstet Gynecol 78:195–199, 1991.

43. Lin MC, Gosink BB, Wolf SI, et al: Endometrial thickness after menopause: Effect of hormone replacement. Radiology 180:427–432, 1991.

44. Lyons EA, Levi CS: Ultrasound in the first trimester of pregnancy. Radiol Clin North Am 20:259–270, 1982.

45. Fleischer AC, Shah DM, Entman SS: Sonographic evaluation of maternal disorders during pregnancy. Radiol Clin North Am 28:51–58, 1990.

46. Togashi K, Kawakami S, Kimura I, et al: Uterine contractions: Possible diagnostic pitfall at MR imaging. J Magn Reson Imaging 3:889–893, 1993.

47. Togashi K, Kawakami S, Kimura I, et al: Sustained uterine contractions: A cause of hypointense myometrial bulging. Radiology 187:707–710, 1993.

48. Moghissi K: Effects of steroidal contraceptives on the reproductive system. In Hafez E (ed.). Human Reproduction. Hagerstown: Harper & Row, pp. 529–537, 1980.

49. Zawin M, McCarthy S, Scoutt L, et al: Monitoring therapy with a gonadotropin-releasing hormone analog: Utility of MR imaging. Radiology 175:503–506, 1990.

50. Togashi, ed: MRI of the Female Pelvis. Tokyo: Igaku-Shoin, p. 33, 1993.

51. Arrivé L, Chang YC, Hricak H, Brescia RJ, Aufferman W, Quivey JM: Radiation-induced uterine changes: MR imaging. Radiology 170:55–58, 1989.

52. De Muylder X, Neven P, De Somer M, Van Belle Y, Vanderick G, De Muylder E: Endometrial lesions in patients undergoing tamoxifen therapy. Int J Gynecol Obstet 36:127–130, 1991.

53. Neven P, De Muylder X, Van Belle Y, Vanderick G, De Muylder E: Hysteroscopic follow-up during tamoxifen treatment. Eur J Obstet Gynecol Reprod Biol 35:235–238, 1990.

54. Fornander T, Rutqvist LE, Cedermark B, et al: Adjuvant tamoxifen in early breast cancer: Occurrence of new primary cancers. Lancet 1:117–120, 1989.

55. Cohen I, Rosen DJ, Tepper R, et al: Ultrasonographic evaluation of the endometrium and correlation with endometrial sampling in postmenopausal patients treated with tamoxifen. J Ultrasound Med 12(5):275–280, 1993.

56. Ascher SM, Johnson JC, Barnes WA, Bae CJ, Patt RH, Zeman RK: MR imaging appearance of the uterus in postmenopausal women receiving tamoxifen therapy for breast cancer: Histopathologic correlation. Radiology 200:105–110, 1996.

57. Kaufman RH, Binder GL, Gray PM Jr., Adam E: Upper genital tract changes associated with exposure in utero to DES. Am J Obstet Gynecol 128:51–59, 1977.

58. Ascher SM, Scoutt LM, McCarthy SM, Lange RC, DeCherney AH: Uterine changes after dilatation and curettage: MR imaging findings. Radiology 180:433–435, 1991.

59. Golan A, Langer R, Bukovsky I, Caspi E: Congenital anomalies of the müllerian system. Fertil Steril 51:747–755, 1989.

60. Buttram VC: Müllerian anomalies and their management. Fertil Steril 40(2):159–163, 1983.

61. Sorensen SS: Hysteroscopic evaluation and endocrinological aspects of women with müllerian anomalies and oligomenorrhea. Int J Fertil 32:445–452, 1987.

62. Moore KL, ed. The Developing Human. Clinically Oriented Embryology. (2nd ed.). Philadelphia: WB Saunders, pp. 220–258, 1977.

63. Buttram VC Jr., Gibbons WE: Müllerian anomalies: A proposed classification. (an analysis of 144 cases). Fertil Steril 32(1):40–46, 1979.

64. Pellerito JS, McCarthy SM, Doyle MB, Glickman MG, DeCherney AH: Diagnosis of uterine anomalies: Relative accuracy of MR imaging, endovaginal sonography, and hysterosalpingography. Radiology 183:795–800, 1992.

65. Valdes C, Malini S, Malinak LR: Ultrasound evaluation of female genital tract anomalies. Am J Obstet Gynecol 149:285–292, 1984.

66. Valdes C, Malini S, Malinak LR: Sonography in the surgical management of vaginal and cervical atresia. Fertil Steril 40(2):263–265, 1983.

67. Ellart D, Houze de L'Aulnoit D, Corette L, Delcroix M, Brabant G: Apport de l'échographie pelvienne au diagnostic des malforma-

tions du tractus utéro-vaginal. J Gynecol Obstet Biol Reprod 19:967–978, 1990.

68. Carrington BM, Hricak H, Nuruddin RN, Secaf E, Laros RK, Hill EC: Müllerian duct anomalies: MR imaging evaluation. Radiology 176:715–720, 1990.

69. Wagner BJ, Woodward PJ: Magnetic resonance evaluation of congenital uterine anomalies. Semin Ultrasound CT MR 15(1):4–17, 1994.

70. Woodward PJ, Wagner BJ, Farley TE: MR imaging in the evaluation of female infertility. Radiographics 13:293–310, 1993.

71. Doyle MB: Magnetic resonance imaging in müllerian fusion defects. J Reprod Med 37(1):33–38, 1992.

72. Strübbe EH, Willemsen WN, Lemmens JA, Thijn CJ, Rolland R: Mayer-Rokitansky-Küster-Hauser Syndrome: Distinction between two forms based on excretory urographic, sonographic, and laparoscopic findings. AJR Am J Roentgenol 160:331–334, 1993.

73. Griffin JE, Edwards C, Madden JD, Harrod MJ, Wilson JD: Congenital absence of the vagina. Ann Intern Med 85:224–236, 1976.

74. Winter JS, Kohn G, Mellman WJ, Wagner S: A familial syndrome of renal, genital, and middle ear anomalies. J Pediatr 72(1):88–93, 1968.

75. Chawla S, Bery K, Indra KJ: Abnormalities of urinary tract and skeleton associated with congenital absence of vagina. Br Med J 1:1398–1400, 1966.

76. Wentz AC: Congenital anomalies and intersexuality. In Jones HW III, et al. (eds.). Novak's Textbook Of Gynecology (11th ed.). Baltimore: Williams & Wilkins, pp. 140–181, 1988.

77. Togashi K, Nishimura K, Itoh K, et al: Vaginal agenesis: Classification by MR imaging. Radiology 162:675–677, 1987.

78. Reinhold C, Hricak H, Forstner R, et al: Primary amenorrhea: Evaluation with MR imaging. Radiology. (In press.)

79. Fedele L, Dorta M, Brioschi D, Giudici MN, Villa L: Magnetic resonance imaging of unicornuate uterus. Acta Obstet Gynecol Scand 69:511–513, 1990.

80. Rennell CL: T-shaped uterus in diethylstilbestrol (DES) exposure. AJR Am J Roentgenol 132:979–980, 1979.

81. van Gils APG, Tham RTOTA, Falke THM, Peters AAW: Abnormalities of the uterus and cervix after diethylstilbestrol exposure: Correlation of findings on MR and hysterosalpingography. AJR Am J Roentgenol 153:1235–1238, 1989.

82. Hricak H, Chang YC, Cann CE, Parer JT: Cervical incompetence: Preliminary evaluation with MR imaging. Radiology 174:821–826, 1990.

83. Lawrence R, Shapiro MD: Disorders of female sex differentiation. In Blaustein A (ed.). Pathology of the Female Genital Tract (2d ed.). New York: Springer, pp. 420–450, 1982.

84. Saenger P: Abnormal sex differentiation. J Pediatr 104(1):1–17, 1984.

85. Gambino J, Caldwell B, Dietrich R, Walot I, Kangarloo H: Congenital disorders of sexual differentiation: MR findings. AJR Am J Roentgenol 158:363–367, 1992.

86. Atri M, Nazarnia S, Aldis AE, Reinhold C, Bret PM, Kintzen G: Transvaginal US appearance of endometrial abnormalities. Radiographics 14:483–492, 1994.

87. Hulka CA, Hall DA, McCarthy K, Simeone JF: Endometrial polyps, hyperplasia and carcinoma in post-menopausal women: Differentiation with endovaginal sonography. Radiology 191:755–758, 1994.

88. Jones HW, Jones GS, eds: Gynecology (3rd ed.). Baltimore: Williams & Wilkins, pp. 222–229, 1982.

89. Parsons AK, Lense JJ: Sonohysterography for endometrial abnormalities. J Clin Ultrasound 21:87–95, 1993.

90. Jones HW, Jones GS, eds: Gynecology (3rd ed.). Baltimore: Williams & Wilkins, pp. 245–253, 1982.

91. Kliewer MA, Hertzberg BS, George PY, McDonald JW, Bowie JD, Carroll BA: Acoustic shadowing from uterine leiomyomas: Sonographic-pathologic correlation. Radiology 196:99–102, 1995.

92. Rader JS, Binette SP, Brandt TD, Sreekanth S, Chhablani A: Ileal hemorrhage caused by a parasitic uterine leiomyoma. Obstet Gynecol 76:531–534, 1990.

93. Gross BH, Silver TM, Jaffe MH: Sonographic features of uterine leiomyomas: Analysis of 41 proven cases. J Ultrasound Med 2:401–406, 1983.

94. Karasick S, Lev-Toaff AS, Toaff ME: Imaging of uterine leiomyomas. AJR Am J Roentgenol 158:799–805, 1992.

95. Dudiak CM, Turner DA, Patel SK, Archie JT, Silver B, Norusis M: Uterine leiomyomas in the infertile patient: Preoperative localization with MR imaging versus US and hysterosalpingography. Radiology 167:627–630, 1988.

96. Zawin M, McCarthy S, Scoutt LM, Comite F: High-field MRI and US evaluation of the pelvis in women with leiomyomas. Magn Reson Imaging 8(4):371–376, 1990.

97. Weinreb JC, Barkoff ND, Megibow A, Demopoulos R: The value of MR imaging in distinguishing leiomyomas from other solid pelvic masses when sonography is indeterminate. AJR Am J Roentgenol 154:295–299, 1990.

98. Panageas E, Kier R, McCauley TR, McCarthy S: Submucosal uterine leiomyomas: Diagnosis of prolapse into the cervix and vagina based on MR imaging. AJR Am J Roentgenol 159:555–558, 1992.

99. Hricak H, Tscholakoff D, Heinrichs L, et al: Uterine leiomyomas: Correlation of MR histopathologic findings, and symptoms. Radiology 158:385–391, 1986.

100. Mark AS, Hricak H, Heinrichs LW, et al: Adenomyosis and leiomyoma: Differential diagnosis with MR imaging. Radiology 163:527–529, 1987.

101. Mittl RL, Yeh I, Kressel HY: High-signal-intensity rim surrounding uterine leiomyomas on MR images: Pathologic correlation. Radiology 180:81–83, 1991.

102. Yamashita Y, Torashima M, Takahashi M: Hyperintense uterine leiomyoma at T2-weighted MR imaging: Differentiation with dynamic enhanced MR imaging and clinical implications. Radiology 189:721–725, 1993.

103. Horie Y, Ikawa S, Kadowaki K, Minagawa Y, Kigawa J, Terekawa N: Lipoadenofibroma of the uterine corpus: Report of a new variant of adenofibroma (benign müllerian mixed tumor). Arch Pathol Lab Med 119(3):274–276, 1995.

104. Jones HW, Jones GS, eds. Gynecology (3rd ed.). Baltimore: Williams & Wilkins, pp. 334–345, 1982.

105. Hamlin DJ, Fitzsimmons JR, Pettersson H, et al: Magnetic resonance imaging of the pelvis: Evaluation of ovarian masses at 0.15 T. AJR Am J Roentgenol 145:585–590, 1985.

106. Azziz R: Adenomyosis: Current perspectives. Obstet Gynecol Clin North Am 16:221–235, 1989.

107. Owolabi TO, Strickler RC: Adenomyosis: A neglected diagnosis. Obstet Gynecol 50:424–427, 1977.

108. Benson RC, Sneeden VD: Adenomyosis: A reappraisal of symptomatology. Am J Obstet Gynecol 76:1044–1061, 1958.

109. Molitor JJ: Adenomyosis: A clinical and pathological appraisal. Am J Obstet Gynecol 110:275–284, 1971.

110. Bird CC, McElin TW, Manalo-Estrella P: The elusive adenomyosis of the uterus—revisited. Am J Obstet Gynecol 112:583–593, 1972.

111. Reinhold C, Atri M, Mehio A, Zakarian R, Aldis AE, Bret PM: Diffuse uterine adenomyosis: Morphologic criteria and diagnostic accuracy of endovaginal sonography. Radiology 197:609–614, 1995.

112. Muse KN: Cyclic pelvic pain. Obstet Gynecol Clin North Am 17:427–440, 1990.

113. Israel SL, Woutersz TB: Adenomyosis: A neglected diagnosis. Obstet Gynecol 14:168–173, 1959.

114. Bohlman ME, Ensor RE, Sanders RC: Sonographic findings in adenomyosis of the uterus. AJR Am J Roentgenol 148:765–766, 1987.

115. Bulic M, Kasnar V, Dukovic I: Use of ultrasound in the diagnosis of genital endometriosis. Jugosl Ginekol i Perinatol 26:33–34, 1986.

116. Fedele L, Bianchi S, Dorta M, Arcaini L, Zanotti F, Carinelli S: Transvaginal ultrasonography in the diagnosis of diffuse adenomyosis. Fertil Steril 58:94–97, 1992.

117. Fedele L, Bianchi S, Dorta M, Zanotti F, Brioschi D, Carinelli S: Transvaginal ultrasonography in the differential diagnosis of adenomyoma versus leiomyoma. Am J Obstet Gynecol 167:603–606, 1992.

118. Ascher SM, Arnold LL, Patt RH, et al: Adenomyosis: Prospective comparison of MR imaging and transvaginal sonography. Radiology 190:803–806, 1994.

119. Brosens JJ, DeSouza NM, Barker FG, Paraschos T, Winston RML: Endovaginal ultrasonography in the diagnosis of adenomyosis uteri: Identifying the predictive characteristics. Br J Obstet Gynaecol 102:471–474, 1995.

120. Togashi K, Nishimura K, Itoh K, et al: Adenomyosis: Diagnosis with MR imaging. Radiology 166:111–114, 1988.

121. Togashi K, Ozasa H, Konishi I, et al: Enlarged uterus: Differentiation between adenomyosis and leiomyoma with MR imaging. Radiology 171:531–534, 1989.

122. Hill EC, Pernoll ML: Benign disorders of the uterine cervix. In DeCherney AH, Pernoll ML (eds.). Current Obstetric & Gynecologic Diagnosis & Treatment (8th ed.). Norwalk, CT: Appleton & Lange, pp. 713–730, 1994.

123. Yamashita Y, Takahashi M, Katabuchi H, Fukumatsu Y, Miyazaki K, Okamura H: Adenoma malignum: MR appearances mimicking nabothian cysts. AJR Am J Roentgenol 162:649–650, 1994.

124. Stromme WB, Haywa EW: Intrauterine fetal death in the second trimester. Am J Obstet Gynecol 85:223–233, 1963.

125. Ansari AH, Reynolds RA: Cervical incompetence: A review. J Reprod Med 32:161–171, 1987.

126. Goodman A: Premalignant & malignant disorders of the uterine corpus. In DeCherney AH, Pernoll ML (eds.). Current Obstetric & Gynecologic Diagnosis & Treatment (8th ed.). Norwalk, CT: Appleton & Lange, pp. 937–953, 1994.

127. Requard CK, Wicks JD, Mettler FA Jr. Ultrasonography in the staging of endometrial adenocarcinoma. Radiology 140:781–785, 1981.

128. Choyke PL, Thickman D, Kressel HY, et al: Controversies in the radiologic diagnosis of pelvic malignancies. Radiol Clin North Am 23:531–549, 1985.

129. Cowles T, Magrina JF, Masterson BJ, Capen CV: Comparison of clinical and surgical staging in patients with endometrial carcinoma. Obstet Gynecol 66:413–416, 1985.

130. Shepherd JH: Revised FIGO staging for gynecological cancer. Br J Obstet Gynaecol 96:889–892, 1989.

131. Boronow RC, Morrow CP, Creasman WT, et al: Surgical staging in endometrial carcinoma: Clinical-pathologic findings of a prospective study. Obstet Gynecol 63:825–832, 1984.

132. Nolan JF, Huen A: Prognosis in endometrial cancer. Gynecol Oncol 4:384–390, 1976.

133. Chen SS, Lee L: Retroperitoneal lymph node metastases in Stage I carcinoma of the endometrium: Correlation with risk factors. Gynecol Oncol 16:319–325, 1983.

134. Figge DC, Otto PM, Tamini HK, Greer BE: Treatment variables in the management of endometrial cancer. Am J Obstet Gynecol 146:495–500, 1983.

135. DiSaia PJ, Creasman WT, Boronow RC, Blessing JA: Risk factors and recurrent patterns in Stage I endometrial cancer. Am J Obstet Gynecol 151:1009–1015, 1985.

136. Piver MS, Lele SB, Barlow JJ, Blumenson L: Para-aortic lymph node evaluation in Stage I endometrial carcinoma. Obstet Gynecol 59:97–100, 1982.

137. Chen SS, Rumancik WM, Spiegel G: Magnetic resonance imaging in Stage I endometrial carcinoma. Obstet Gynecol 75:274–277, 1990.

138. Mayr NA, Wen BC, Benda JA, et al: Postoperative radiation therapy in clinical Stage I endometrial cancer: Corpus, cervical and lower uterine segment involvement—patterns of failure. Radiology 196:323–328, 1995.

139. Worthington JL, Balfe DM, Lee JK, et al: Uterine neoplasms: MR imaging. Radiology 159:725–730, 1986.

140. Walsh JW, Goplerud DR: Computed tomography of primary, persistent, and recurrent endometrial malignancy. AJR Am J Roentgenol 139:1149–1154, 1982.

141. Balfe DM, Van Dyke J, Lee JK, Weyman PJ, McClennan BL: Computed tomography in malignant endometrial neoplasms. J Comput Assist Tomogr 7:677–681, 1983.

142. Posniak HV, Olson MC, Dudiak CM, et al: MR imaging of uterine carcinoma: Correlation with clinical and pathologic findings. Radiographics 10:15–27, 1990.

143. Gordon AN, Fleischer AC, Dudley BS, et al: Preoperative assessment of myometrial invasion of endometrial adenocarcinoma by sonography (US) and magnetic resonance imaging (MRI). Gynecol Oncol 34:175–179, 1989.

144. DelMaschio A, Vanzulli A, Sironi S, et al: Estimating the depth of myometrial involvement by endometrial carcinoma: Efficacy of transvaginal sonography vs. MR imaging. AJR Am J Roentgenol 160:533–538, 1993.

145. Yamashita Y, Mizutani H, Torashima M, et al: Assessment of myometrial invasion by endometrial carcinoma: Transvaginal sonography vs. contrast-enhanced MR imaging. AJR Am J Roentgenol 161:595–599, 1993.

146. Artner A, Bosze P, Gonda G: The value of ultrasound in preoperative assessment of the myometrial and cervical invasion in endometrial carcinoma. Gynecol Oncol 54:147–151, 1994.

147. Teefey SA, Stahl JA, Middleton WD, et al: Local staging of endometrial carcinoma: Comparison of transvaginal and intraoperative sonography and gross visual inspection. AJR Am J Roentgenol 166:547–552, 1996.

148. Carrington B, Hricak H: MRI staging of endometrial and cervical carcinoma. Curr Imaging 3:8–15, 1991.

149. McCarthy S: Gynecologic applications of MRI. Crit Rev Diagn Imaging 31(2):263–281, 1990.

150. Hricak H, Hamm B, Semelka RC, et al: Carcinoma of the uterus: Use of gadopentetate dimeglumine in MR imaging. Radiology 181:95–106, 1991.

151. Sironi S, Colombo E, Villa G, et al: Myometrial invasion by endometrial carcinoma: Assessment with plain and gadolinium-enhanced MR imaging Radiology 185:207–212, 1992.

152. Olson MC, Posniak HV, Tempany CM, Dudiak CM: MR imaging of the female pelvic region. Radiographics 12:445–465, 1992.

153. Hricak H, Rubinstein LV, Gherman GM, Karstaedt N: MR imaging evaluation of endometrial carcinoma: Results of an NCI cooperative study. Radiology 179:829–832, 1991.

154. Lien HH, Blomlie V, Tropé C, Kærn J, Abeler VM: Cancer of the endometrium: Value of MR imaging in determining depth of invasion into the myometrium. AJR Am J Roentgenol 157:1221–1223, 1991.

155. Scoutt LM, McCarthy SM, Flynn SD, et al: Clinical Stage I endometrial carcinoma: Pitfalls in preoperative assessment with MR imaging. Radiology 194:567–572, 1995.

156. Popovich MJ, Hricak H, Sugimura K, Stern JL: The role of MR imaging in determining surgical eligibility for pelvic exenteration. AJR Am J Roentgenol 160:525–531, 1993.

157. Kahanpää KV, Whalström T, Gröhn P, Heinonen E, Nieminen U, Widholm O: Sarcomas of the uterus: A clinicopathologic study of 119 patients. Obstet Gynecol 67:417–424, 1986.

158. Shapeero LG, Hricak H: Mixed müllerian sarcoma of the uterus: MR imaging findings. AJR Am J Roentgenol 153:317–319, 1989.

159. Pattani SJ, Kier R, Deal R, Luchansky E: MRI of uterine leiomyosarcoma. Magn Reson Imaging 13(2):331–333, 1995.

160. Goodman A, Hill EC: Premalignant & malignant disorders of the uterine cervix. In DeCherney AH, Pernoll ML (eds.). Current Obstetric & Gynecologic Diagnosis & Treatment (8th ed.). Norwalk, CT: Appleton & Lange, pp. 921–936, 1994.

161. Jones HW, Jones GS (eds.). Gynecology (3rd ed.). Baltimore: Williams & Wilkins, pp. 185–207, 1982.

162. Hricak H, Quivey JM, Campos Z, et al: Carcinoma of the cervix: Predictive value of clinical and magnetic resonance (MR) imaging assessment of prognostic factors. Int J Radiat Oncol Biol Phys 27:791–801, 1993.

163. Hricak H, Powell CB, Yu KK, et al: Invasive cervical carcinoma: Role of MR imaging in pretreatment work-up—cost minimization and diagnostic efficacy analysis. Radiology 198:403–409, 1996.

164. American Joint Committee on Cancer. Manual for Staging of Cancer (3rd ed.). Philadelphia: Lippincott, pp. 151–153, 1988.

165. van Negell JR Jr., Roddick JW Jr., Lowin DM: The staging of cervical cancer: Inevitable discrepancies between clinical staging and pathologic findings. Am J Obstet Gynecol 110:973–977, 1971.

166. Averette HE, Dudan RC, Ford JH Jr. Exploratory celiotomy for surgical staging of cervical cancer. Am J Obstet Gynecol 113:1090–1096, 1972.

167. Lagasse LD, Creasman WT, Shingleton HM, Ford JH, Blessing JA: Results and complications of operative staging in cervical cancer: Experience of the Gynecologic Oncology Group. Gynecol Oncol 9:90–98, 1980.

168. Mayr NA, Tali ET, Yuh WTC, et al: Cervical cancer: Application of MR imaging in radiation therapy. Radiology 189:601–608, 1993.

169. Yuhara A, Akamatsu N, Sekiba K: Use of transrectal radial scan ultrasonography in evaluating the extent of cervical cancer. J Clin Ultrasound 15:507–517, 1987.

170. Magee BJ, Logue JP, Swindell R, McHugh D: Tumor size as a prognostic factor in carcinoma of the cervix: Assessment by transrectal ultrasound. Br J Radiol 64:812–815, 1991.

171. Vick CW, Walsh JW, Wheelock JB, Brewer WH: CT of the normal and abnormal parametria in cervical cancer. AJR Am J Roentgenol 143:597–603, 1984.

172. Walsh JW, Goplerud DR: Prospective comparison between clinical and CT staging in primary cervical carcinoma. AJR Am J Roentgenol 137:997–1003, 1981.

173. Togashi K, Nishimura K, Sagoh T, et al: Carcinoma of the cervix: Staging with MR imaging. Radiology 171:245–251, 1989.

174. Sironi S, Belloni C, Taccagni GL, DelMaschio A: Carcinoma of the cervix: Value of MR imaging in detecting parametrial involvement. AJR Am J Roentgenol 156:753–756, 1991.

175. Hricak H, Lacey CG, Sandles LG, Chang YC, Winkler ML, Stern JL: Invasive cervical carcinoma: Comparison of MR imaging and surgical findings. Radiology 166:623–631, 1988.

176. Rubens D, Thornbury JR, Angel C, et al: Stage IB cervical carcinoma: Comparison of clinical, MR, and pathologic staging. AJR Am J Roentgenol 150:135–138, 1988.

177. Kim SH, Choi BI, Lee HP, et al: Uterine cervical carcinoma: Comparison of CT and MR findings. Radiology 175:45–51, 1990.

178. Sironi S, De Coblli F, Scarfone G, et al: Carcinoma of the cervix: Value of plain and gadolinium-enhanced MR imaging in assessing degree of invasiveness. Radiology 188:797–801, 1993.

179. Subak LL, Hricak H, Powell CB, Azizi L, Stern JL: Cervical carcinoma: Computed tomography and magnetic resonance imaging for preoperative staging. Obstet Gynecol 86(1):43–50, 1995.

180. Kim SH, Kim SC, Choi BI, Han MC: Uterine cervical carcinoma: Evaluation of pelvic lymph node metastasis with MR imaging. Radiology 190:807–811, 1994.

181. Semelka R, Hricak H, Bohyun K, Forstner R, Bis K, Ascher S, Reinhold C: Pelvic fistulas: Appearance on MR images. Abdom Imaging. 22:91–95, 1997.

182. Baudouin CJ, Soutter WP, Gilderdale DJ, Coutts GA: Magnetic resonance imaging of the uterine cervix using an intravaginal coil. Magn Reson Med 24:196–203, 1992.

183. deSouza NM, Scoones D, Krausz T, Gilderdale DJ, Soutter WP: High-resolution MR imaging of Stage I cervical neoplasia with a dedicated transvaginal coil: MR features and correlation of imaging and pathological findings. AJR Am J Roentgenol 166:553–559, 1996.

184. Milestone BN, Schnall MD, Lenkinski RE, Kressel HY: Cervical carcinoma: MR imaging with an endorectal surface coil. Radiology 180:91–95, 1991.

185. Kaji Y, Sugimura K, Kitao M, Ishida T: Histopathology of uterine cervical carcinoma: Diagnostic comparison of endorectal surface coil and standard body coil MRI. J Comput Assist Tomogr 18(5):785–792, 1994.

186. Yamashita Y, Takahashi M, Sawada T, Miyazadi K, Okamura H: Carcinoma of the cervix: Dynamic MR imaging. Radiology 182:643–648, 1992.

187. Lien HH, Blomlie V, Kjorstad K, Abeler V, Kaalhus O: Clinical Stage I carcinoma of the cervix: Value of MR imaging in determining degree of invasiveness. AJR Am J Roentgenol 156:1191–1194, 1991.

188. Vanzulli A, Sironi S, Pellegrino A, et al: MRI in Stage I carcinoma of the uterine cervix: Evaluation of residual uninvolved myometrium and pericervical tissues. Eur Radiol 4:190–196, 1994.

189. Greco A, Mason P, Leung AW, Dische S, McIndoe GA, Anderson MC: Staging of carcinoma of the uterine cervix: MRI-surgical correlation. Clin Radiol 40(4):401–405, 1989.

190. Heron CW, Husband JE, Williams MP, Dobbs HJ, Cosgrove DO: The value of CT in the diagnosis of recurrent carcinoma of the cervix. Clin Radiol 39(5):496–501, 1988.

191. Ebner F, Kressel HY, Mintz MC, et al: Tumor recurrence versus fibrosis in the female pelvis: Differentiation with MR imaging at 1.5 T. Radiology 166:333–340, 1988.

192. Hricak H, Swift PS, Campos Z, Quivey JM, Gildengorin V, Goranson H: Irradiation of the cervix uteri: Value of unenhanced and contrast-enhanced MR imaging. Radiology 189:381–388, 1993.

193. Weber TM, Sostman HD, Spritzer CE, et al: Cervical carcinoma: Determination of recurrent tumor extent versus radiation changes with MR imaging. Radiology 194:135–139, 1995.

194. Flueckiger F, Ebner F, Poschauko H, Tamussino K, Einspieler R, Ranner G: Cervical cancer: Serial MR imaging before and after primary radiation therapy—a 2-year follow-up study. Radiology 184:89–93, 1992.

195. Yamashita Y, Harade M, Torashima M, et al: Dynamic MR imaging of recurrent postoperative cervical cancer. J Magn Reson Imaging 1:167–171, 1996.

196. Beers GJ: Biological effects of weak electromagnetic fields from 0 Hz to 200 MHz: A survey of the literature with special emphasis on possible magnetic resonance effects. Magn Reson Imaging 7:309–331, 1989.

197. Tyndall DA, Sulik KK: Effects of magnetic resonance imaging on eye development in the C57BL/6J mouse. Teratology 43(3):263–275, 1991.

198. Baker PN, Johnson IR, Harvey PR, Gowland PA, Mansfield P: A three-year follow-up of children imaged in utero with echo-planar magnetic resonance. Am J Obstet Gynecol 170:32–33, 1994.

199. US Food and Drug Administration: Magnetic resonance diagnostic device: Panel recommendations and report of petitions for MR reclassification. Fed Reg 53:7575–7579, 1988.

200. Magnetic Resonance Imaging Consensus Conference. JAMA 259(14):2132–2138, 1988.

201. Panigel M, Wolf G, Zeleznick A: Magnetic resonance imaging of the placenta in rhesus monkeys, Macaca Mulatta. J Med Primatol 17:3–18, 1988.

202. Rofsky NM, Pizzarello DJ, Weinreb JC, Ambrosino MM, Rosenberg C: Effect on fetal mouse development of exposure to MR imaging and gadopentetate dimeglumine. J Magn Reson Imaging 4(6):805–807, 1994.

203. Barkhof F, Heijboer RJ, Algra PR: Inadvertent i.v. administration of gadopentetate dimeglumine during early pregnancy [letter]. AJR Am J Roentgenol 158(5):1171, 1992.

204. Weinreb JC, Yuh WTC: Obstetrics. In Stark DD, Bradley WG, Jr. (eds.). Magnetic Resonance Imaging (2nd ed.). St. Louis: Mosby, pp. 1987–2021, 1992.

205. Weinreb JC, Lowe T, Cohen JM, Kutler M: Human fetal anatomy: MR imaging. Radiology 157:715–720, 1985.

206. Tomá P, Lucigrai G, Dodero P, Lituania M: Prenatal detection of an abdominal mass by MR imaging performed while the fetus is immobilized with pancuronium bromide. AJR Am J Roentgenol 154:1049–1050, 1990.

207. Powell MC, Worthington BS, Buckley JM, Symonds EM: Magnetic resonance imaging (MRI) in obstetrics. II. Fetal anatomy. Br J Obstet Gynaecol 95(1):38–46, 1988.

208. Benson RC, Colletti PM, Platt LD, Ralls PW: MR imaging of fetal anomalies. AJR Am J Roentgenol 156:1205–1207, 1991.

209. Stehling MK, Mansfield P, Ordidge RJ, et al: Echo-planar imaging of the human fetus in utero. Magn Reson Med 13:314–318, 1990.

210. Naidich TP, Grant JL, Altman N, et al: The developing cerebral surface: Preliminary report on the patterns of sulcal and gyral maturation—anatomy, ultrasound, and magnetic resonance imaging. [Review]. Neuroimaging Clin N Am 4(2):201–240, 1994.

211. Sonigo P, Elmaleh A, Fermont L, Delezoide AL, Mirlesse V, Brunelle F: Prenatal MRI diagnosis of fetal cerebral tuberous sclerosis. Pediatr Radiol 26(1):1–4, 1996.

212. Werner H Jr., Mirlesse V, Jacquemard F, et al: Prenatal diagnosis of tuberous sclerosis: Use of magnetic resonance imaging and its implications for prognosis. Prenat Diagn 14(12):1151–1154, 1994.

213. Girard N, Raybaud C, Poncet M: In vivo MR study of brain maturation in normal fetuses. Am J Neuroradiol 16(2):407–413, 1995.

214. Okamura K, Murotsuki J, Sakai T, Matsumoto K, Shirane R, Yajima A: Prenatal diagnosis of lissencephaly by magnetic resonance image. Fetal Diagn Ther 8(1):56–59, 1993.

215. Yuh WT, Nguyen HD, Fisher DJ, et al: MR of fetal central nervous system abnormalities. Am J Neuroradiol 15(3):459–464, 1994.

216. Baker PN, Johnson IR, Gowland PA, Freeman A, Adams V, Mansfield P: Estimation of fetal lung volume using echo-planar magnetic resonance imaging. Obstet Gynecol 83(6):951–954, 1994.

217. Harstad TW, Twickler DM, Leveno KJ, Brown CE: Antepartum prediction of pulmonary hypoplasia: An elusive goal? Am J Perinatol 10(1):8–11, 1993.

218. Smith FW, Kent C, Abramovich DR, Sutherland HW: Nuclear magnetic resonance imaging: A new look at the fetus. Br J Obstet Gynaecol 92:1024–1033, 1985.

219. Kastler B, Gangi A, Mathelin C, et al: Fetal shoulder measurements with MRI. J Comput Assist Tomogr 17(5):777–780, 1993.

220. Borcard B, Hiltbrand E, Magnin P, et al: Estimating meconium (fetal feces) concentration in human amniotic fluid by nuclear magnetic resonance. Physiol Chem Phys 14:181–191, 1982.

221. Stark DD, McCarthy SM, Filly RA, Callen PW, Hricak H, Parer JT: Intrauterine growth retardation: Evaluation by magnetic resonance. Work in progress. Radiology 155:425–427, 1985.

222. Smith FW: The potential use of nuclear magnetic resonance imaging in pregnancy. J Perinat Med 13:265–276, 1985.

223. Baker PN, Johnson IR, Gowland PA, et al: Measurement of fetal liver, brain and placental volumes with echo-planar magnetic resonance imaging. Br J Obstet Gynaecol 102(1):35–39, 1995.

224. Baker PN, Johnson IR, Gowland PA, et al: Fetal weight estimation by echo-planar magnetic resonance imaging. Lancet 343(8898):644–645, 1994.

225. Stark DD, McCarthy SM, Filly RA, Parer JT, Hricak H, Callen PW: Pelvimetry by magnetic resonance imaging. AJR Am J Roentgenol 144:947–950, 1985.

226. Weinreb JC, Lowe TW, Santos-Ramos R, Cunningham FG, Parkey R: Magnetic resonance imaging in obstetric diagnosis. Radiology 154:157–161, 1985.

227. Sigmund G, Bauer M, Henne K, DeGregorio G, Wenz W: A technic of magnetic resonance tomographic pelvimetry in obstetrics. [German]. *Technik der kernspintomographischen Beckenmessung in der Geburtshilfe*. Rofo. Fortschritte auf dem Gebiete der Rontgen-

strahlen und der Neuen Bildgebenden Verfahren 154(4):370–374, 1991.

228. Wright AR, English PT, Cameron HM, Wilsdon JB: MR pelvimetry—a practical alternative. Acta Radiol 33(6):582–587, 1992.

229. Urhahn R, Lehnen H, Drobnitzky M, Klose KC, Gunther RW: Ultrafast pelvimetry using Snapshot-FLASH-MRT—a comparison with the Spinecho and FLASH techniques. [German]. *Ultraschnelle Pelvimetrie mittels Snapshot-FLASH-MRT—Vergleich mit der Spinecho- und FLASH-Technik*. Rofo. Fortschritte auf dem Gebiete der Rontgenstrahlen und der Neuen Bildgebenden Verfahren 155(5):432–435, 1991.

230. Powell MC, Buckley J, Price H, Worthington BS, Symonds EM: Magnetic resonance imaging and placenta previa. Am J Obstet Gynecol 154(3):565–569, 1986.

231. Kay HH, Spritzer CE: Preliminary experience with magnetic resonance imaging in patients with third-trimester bleeding. Obstet Gynecol 78:424–429, 1991.

232. Wagner BJ, Woodward PJ, Dickey GE: [From the Archives of the AFIP]. Gestational trophoblastic disease: Radiologic-pathologic correlation. Radiographics 16:131–148, 1996.

233. Powell M, Buckley J, Worthington B, Symonds E: Magnetic resonance imaging and hydatidiform mole. Br J Radiol 59:561–564, 1986.

234. Hricak H, Demas BE, Braga CA, Fisher MR, Winkler ML: Gestational trophoblastic neoplasm of the uterus: MR assessment. Radiology 161:11–16, 1986.

235. Barton JW, McCarthy SM, Kohorn EI, Scoutt LM, Lange RC: Pelvic MR imaging findings in gestational trophoblastic disease, incomplete abortion, and ectopic pregnancy: Are they specific? Radiology 186:163–168, 1993.

236. Yamashita Y, Torashima M, Takahashi M, et al: Contrast-enhanced dynamic MR imaging of postmolar gestational trophoblastic disease. Acta Radiol 36(2):188–192, 1995.

237. Ha HK, Jung JK, Jee MK, et al: Gestational trophoblastic tumors of the uterus: MR imaging—pathologic correlation. Gynecol Oncol 57(3):340–350, 1995.

238. Kurachi H, Maeda T, Murakami T, et al: MRI of placental polyps. J Comput Assist Tomogr 19(3):444–448, 1995.

239. Hamrick-Turner JE, Cranston PE, Lantrip BS: Gravid uterine dehiscence: MR findings. Abdom Imaging 20:486–488, 1995.

240. Willms AB, Brown ED, Kettritz UI, Kuller JA, Semelka RC: Anatomic changes in the pelvis after uncomplicated vaginal delivery: Evaluation with serial MR imaging. Radiology 195:91–94, 1995.

241. Woo GM, Twickler DM, Stettler RW, Erdman WA, Brown CE: The pelvis after cesarean section and vaginal delivery: Normal MR findings. AJR Am J Roentgenol 161:1249–1252, 1993.

242. Ginsburg ES, Frates MC, Rein MS, Fox JH, Hornstein MD, Friedman AJ: Early diagnosis and treatment of cervical pregnancy in an in vitro fertilization program. Fertil Steril 61(5):966–969, 1994.

243. Bassil S, Gordts S, Nisolle M, Van Beers B, Donnez J: A magnetic resonance imaging approach for the diagnosis of a triplet cornual pregnancy. Fertil Steril 64(5):1029–1031, 1995.

244. McCarthy SM, Stark DD, Filly RA, Callen PW, Hricak H, Higgins CB: Obstetrical magnetic resonance imaging: Maternal anatomy. Radiology 154:421–425, 1985.

245. Iams JD, Goldenberg RL, Meis PJ, et al: The length of the cervix and the risk of spontaneous premature delivery. National Institute of Child Health and Human Development Maternal Fetal Medicine Unit Network. N Engl J Med 334(9):567–572, 1996.

246. Simons GR, Piwnica-Worms DR, Goldhaber SZ: Ovarian vein thrombosis. [Review]. Am Heart J 126:641–647, 1993.

247. Curtis M, Hopkins MP, Zarlingo T, Martino C, Graciansky-Lengyl M, Jenison EL: Magnetic resonance imaging to avoid laparotomy in pregnancy. Obstet Gynecol 82(5):833–836, 1993.

CHAPTER 15

ADNEXA

S. M. ASCHER, M.D., E. K. OUTWATER, M.D., AND C. REINHOLD, M.D.

THE ADNEXA

The implementation of recent MRI innovations such as high resolution T2-weighted echo-train spin-echo, breath-hold gadolinium-enhanced fat-suppressed spoiled gradient-echo (SGE), and breathing-independent T2-weighted half Fourier single-shot turbo spin-echo (HASTE) have significantly increased the diagnostic utility of MRI for imaging adnexal disease. MRI is capable of diagnosing adnexal masses as cystic or solid, characterizing the components as hemorrhagic, fatty, or soft tissue, and detecting small peritoneal-based disease. In many clinical situations, MRI is more accurate than computed tomography (CT) imaging or ultrasound in these determinations. This chapter addresses the current MRI techniques for imaging the adnexa and discusses how these techniques can be utilized for evaluating common gynecologic conditions.

■ THE OVARY

NORMAL ANATOMY

Ovarian position, appearance, and physiology are functions of age. In the neonate the ovaries develop from gonadal primordia and lie in the false pelvis. They migrate during the first year of life to reside in the ovarian fossa, a region demarcated by the bifurcation of the common iliac vessels superiorly, the obliterated umbilical artery anteriorly, and the internal iliac vessels and ureter posteriorly. The ovarian position, however, may vary, influenced by parity and/or the degree of distention of adjacent bladder and bowel. The ovaries may also be surgically transferred to the abdomen or upper pelvis in patients with cervical cancer who are to undergo radiation therapy. This procedure, termed ovarian transposition, avoids radiation ablation of the ovaries and hence early menopause in reproductive age women affected with cervical cancer.

The ovary has several fixed attachments and/or relationships to adjacent structures. The superior aspect of the ovary is the attachment site of the ovarian suspensory ligament. This ligament anchors the ovary to the lateral pelvic side wall and contains the ovarian vessels. The superior aspect of the ovary is associated intimately with the fimbriae of the fallopian tube. The inferior aspect of the ovary is supported by a thickening of the broad ligament, the proper ovarian ligament, which connects the ovary with the fallopian tube and lateral uterus. The anterior aspect of the ovary is contiguous with the mesovarium, a fold of peritoneum that traverses the fallopian tube and ovary, whereas the posterior aspect of the ovary faces the ureter and is called the free border. The medial and lateral ovarian surfaces are related to the fallopian tube and parietal peritoneum, respectively.

At birth the ovaries are small, but during the period

of gonadal activity they enlarge and may weigh in excess of 8 grams. Diminution in ovarian size begins after the age of 30 years. Following menopause, the ovaries atrophy and weigh less than 2 grams [1].

The ovary is divided histologically into a cortex and medulla. The cortex contains follicles in different stages of maturation, whereas the medulla of the ovary is composed of stromal cells, lymphatics, blood vessels, and nerves. Most of the 400,000 follicles present at birth degenerate, though a few will develop into graafian follicles each month [1]. Subsequently, one of the graafian follicles matures and releases an ovum, and in doing so it becomes a corpus luteum. If pregnancy does not occur, the corpus luteum involutes and degenerates into a corpus albicans.

MRI TECHNIQUE

To optimize image quality and limit bowel motion, patients should be required to fast at least 4 to 6 hours prior to imaging. Alternatively, an antiperistaltic drug (1 mg of glucagon, intramuscularly) may be given. Although respiratory artifact is less problematic in the pelvis than in the abdomen, techniques that reduce respiratory motion such as breath-hold imaging, compression belts, imaging in the prone position, and respiratory compensation should be employed as needed. Flow-related artifacts are amenable to saturation pulses. These usually are placed superior and inferior to the imaging volume. Finally, patients should void prior to imaging. This improves patient comfort and decreases motion artifact.

The torso phased-array surface coil has significantly improved evaluation of the pelvis [2]. The coil's configuration boosts the signal-to-noise ratio two to three times in the central region of the imaging volume compared to conventional body coil imaging [3]. This in turn leads to improved spatial resolution when smaller fields of view and/or increased matrix size are employed. However, as with many MRI advances there are trade-offs. Most significant is the artifact caused by the fat beneath the coil. Because of the coil's near field sensitivity profile, the fat is high in signal intensity and motion-related phase ghosting may obscure thorough evaluation of the adnexa [4]. Techniques to moderate this effect include (1) placing nonselective saturation pulses over the anterior and posterior subcutaneous fat, (2) employing chemically selective excitation-spoiling fat-suppression sequences, (3) using breath-hold imaging, (4) shifting the phase-encoding gradient into the right-left direction for axial imaging or superior-inferior direction for sagittal imaging, and/or (5) postprocessing the data with a filter to homogenize the signal intensities [5,6].

T2-weighted echo-train spin-echo, T1-weighted spoiled gradient-echo, excitation-spoiling fat-suppres-

sion, and fat-water opposed-phase techniques, combined with intravenous gadolinium as needed, are the mainstays of MRI of the adnexa. The advent of echo-train spin-echo, including breath-hold techniques, allows high-resolution (512-matrix) T2-weighted images to be acquired in multiple planes without unduly prolonging examination time. T1-weighted fat-suppressed imaging helps to characterize adnexal lesions. These techniques are especially useful for distinguishing between hemorrhagic masses and lipid-containing lesions that may mimic each other on T1- and T2-weighted sequences [7–11]. Finally, intravenous gadolinium may be useful in selected patients. Specifically gadolinium-enhanced fat-suppressed SGE imaging helps to distinguish viable tissue from debris, hemorrhage, or clot, all of which may appear similar on unenhanced T1- and T2-weighted images [12–14]. Currently, fat-suppressed SGE images can be acquired in a 20-second breath-hold. This sequence is the most sensitive technique for the detection of small-volume peritoneal-based disease from ovarian cancer and can contribute to shorter exam times. Gadolinium-enhanced T2-weighted images of the pelvis may be acquired in the setting of an abdominopelvic survey in an effort to limit total exam time. This protocol allows the entire abdomen to be scanned first and includes dynamic evaluation of the liver followed by a pelvic exam. On the T2-weighted images concentrated gadolinium in the dependent portion of the bladder is low in signal intensity because of T2* effects.

MR urography can be incorporated into a comprehensive MRI exam. This is accomplished with a heavily T2-weighted sequence such as breathing-independent T2-weighted HASTE images. Alternatively, gadolinium-enhanced fat-suppressed SGE imaging demonstrates the urinary tract well.

The routine use of oral and/or rectal contrast agents for evaluating the adnexa is controversial. Although most clinical work is performed without exogenous intraluminal agents, one group of investigators found that use of a negative oral agent increased diagnostic confidence in the evaluation of gynecologic disease [15].

However, at the present time cost/benefit and outcome studies regarding the routine use of oral agents are not available.

NORMAL OVARY

MRI can demonstrate both ovaries in the majority of patients [16]. Reported variations in ovary detection reflects differences in imaging systems. At low field strength with the use of a body coil and conventional spin-echo technique, both ovaries were identified in almost 90 percent of patients [16]. Ovaries may be detected in almost 100

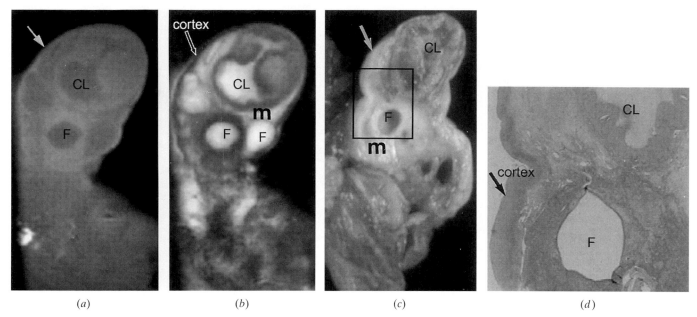

(a) (b) (c) (d)

F IG . 15.1 High resolution specimen images of the normal ovary. T1-weighted (a) and T2-weighted echo-train spin-echo (b) images, gross specimen photograph (c) and specimen photomicrograph (d) of a normal ovary in a woman of reproductive age. T2-weighted images highlight ovarian zonal anatomy: an outer rim of low signal intensity circumscribing an inner region of high signal intensity. These areas correspond to the cortex (*arrows, a–d*) and medulla (*m,b,c*), respectively, on the gross specimen photograph and photomicrograph. Follicles (*F,a–d*) are also seen. On the T2-weighted image they possess a uniform and thin low-signal-intensity rim versus the high signal intensity of their contents. In contrast, an involuting corpus luteum possesses ("*CL*",*a–d*) an uneven and focally thickened intermediate-signal-intensity periphery. This is typical of the luteinized cell lining of involuting corpus lutea. (Parts *a, b,* and *c* are reprinted with permission from Outwater EK, Schiebler ML: Magnetic resonance imaging of the ovary. Radiol Clin North Am 2:245–274, 1994)

percent of patients using a phased-array multicoil and higher-spatial-resolution echo-train spin-echo on high field MR systems.

The appearance of the normal ovary is a function of the hormonal milieu. In women of reproductive age, the ovaries are larger and the majority (85%) demonstrate zonal anatomy on T2-weighted images; which are lower signal intensity of the cortex and relatively higher signal intensity of the medulla (Fig. 15.1). After intravenous gadolinium, the ovarian stroma typically enhances less than the myometrium. In contrast, postmenopausal ovaries are smaller and zonal anatomy is less common, observed in approximately 28 percent of patient. Postmenopausal ovaries usually demonstrate enhancement equal to that of myometrium [17]. On T1-weighted images the ovarian stroma in both pre- and postmenopausal ovaries is homogeneously isointense with the uterus. Follicles within the ovary are low to intermediate in signal intensity on T1-weighted images, high in signal intensity on T2-weighted images, and demonstrate rim enhancement after intravenous administration of gadolinium (Fig. 15.2). Ovaries that have been surgically transposed have similar imaging characteristics to normal ovaries (Fig.

15.2). Transposed ovaries should not be mistaken for metastatic disease. Surgical history can clarify the imaging findings.

Ovarian cysts are common, regardless of hormonal status. In one study, 17 percent of asymptomatic postmenopausal ovaries contained at least one cyst [18]. Simple functional ovarian cysts (follicular, corpus luteal, or corpus albicans cysts) are low to intermediate in signal intensity on T1-weighted images and are high in signal intensity on T2-weighted images. The cyst walls are commonly low in signal intensity on T2-weighted images. Mural enhancement is variable, and may be slightly irregular (Fig. 15.3). Specifically, thickened and intensely enhancing walls are typical of corpus lutea [19]. Although wall irregularity may be seen with involuting luteal cysts, this feature is worrisome for neoplasm. Occasionally, follow-up studies may be necessary to distinguish between the two. Corpus luteal cysts are prone to hemorrhage. When hemorrhagic they are intermediate to high in signal intensity on T1- and T2-weighted images and occasionally may be confused with endometriomas, though the latter usually display profound T2-shortening (Fig. 15.4) [20].

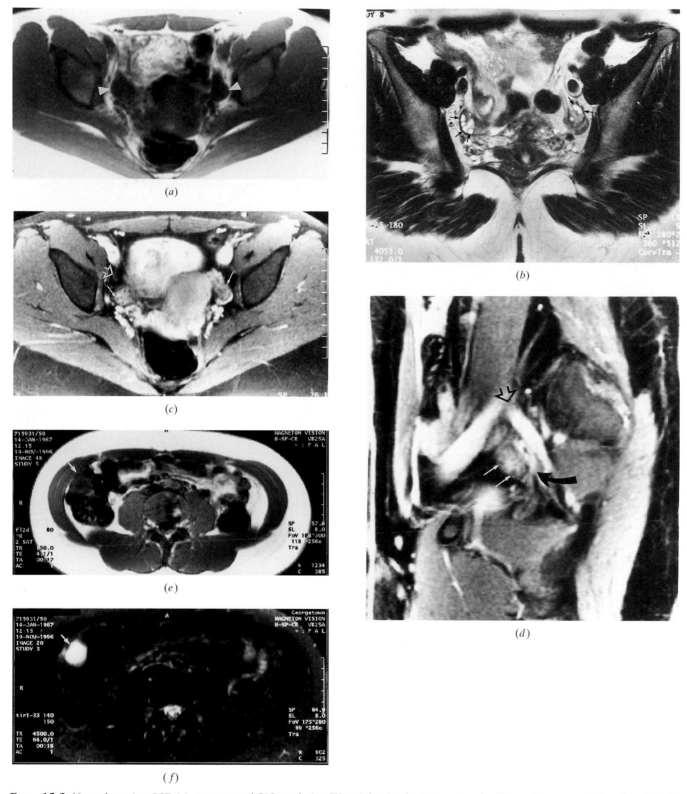

F IG. 15.2 Normal ovaries. SGE (*a*), paracoronal 512-resolution T2-weighted echo-train spin-echo (*b*), and transverse (*c*) and sagittal (*d*) gadolinium-enhanced fat-suppressed SGE images of a woman with normal ovaries. The ovaries reside in the ovarian fossa and are intermediate in signal intensity on the unenhanced T1-weighted image (*arrowheads, a*). On the T2-weighted image (*b*), follicles are identified as high-signal-intensity structures (*arrows, b*). After contrast the ovarian parenchyma enhances, whereas the follicles (*arrows, c,d*) are signal-void areas. The enhanced images show some of the anatomic boundaries of the ovarian fossa: the bifurcation of the common iliac vessels superiorly (*open arrow, d*), obliterated umbilical artery anteriorly (*open arrow, c*), and the internal iliac vessels posteriorly (*curved arrow, d*). SGE (*e*) and T2-weighted echo-train spin-echo (*f*) of a transposed normal right ovary (*arrow, e,f*) in a woman with cervical cancer treated with radiation therapy.

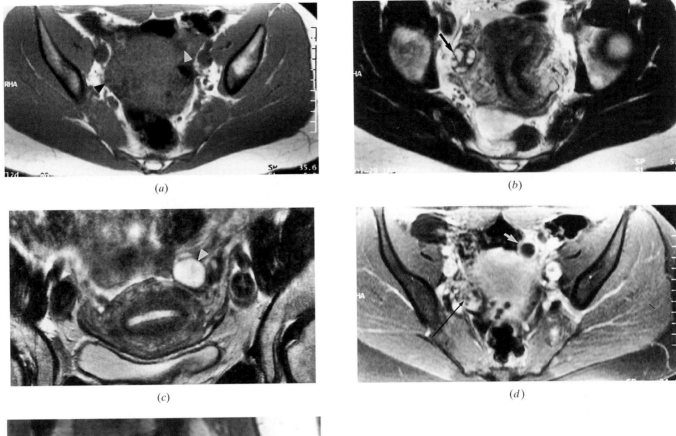

(a)

(b)

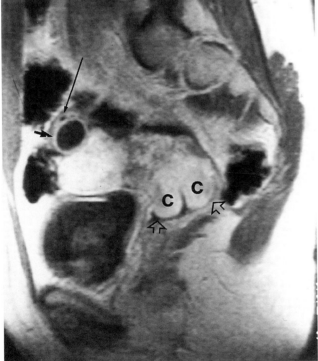

(c)

(d)

(e)

Fig. 15.3 Normal ovary with a functional cyst. SGE (*a*), transverse (*b*) and coronal (*c*) 512-resolution T2-weighted echo-train spin-echo, transverse (*d*) and sagittal (*e*) gadolinium-enhanced fat-suppressed SGE images in a woman with normal ovaries. On the unenhanced T1-weighted image (*a*), the ovary is largely isointense to the uterus save for several follicles and the functional cyst, which are lower in signal intensity (*arrowheads, a*). The high-resolution T2-weighted images (*b,c*) show the follicle-laden right ovary (*arrow, b*) and a cyst-containing left ovary (*arrowhead, c*). The cortex containing the follicles is lower in signal intensity than the medulla. Following contrast, the ovarian parenchyma enhances, including the rims of the follicles (*long arrow, d,e*) and cyst (*short arrow, d,e*). The remainder of the left ovary is draped around the functional cyst. Simple functional cysts are low to intermediate in signal intensity on T1-weighted images, high in signal intensity on T2-weighted images, and have variable mural enhancement following contrast administration. Note that the cervical lips (*"c",e*) protruding into the vaginal fornices (*open arrows, e*) are well seen with the contrast-enhanced fat-suppressed SGE technique.

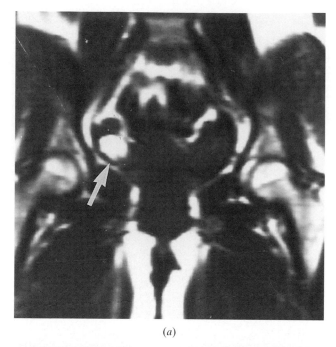

(a)

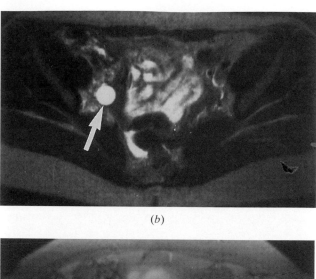

(b)

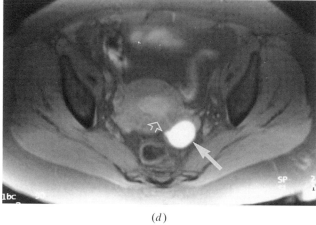

(d)

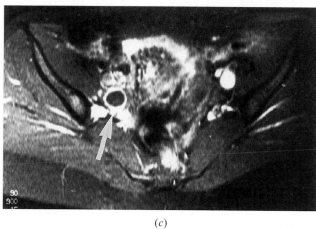

(c)

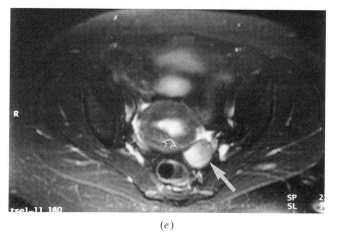

(e)

FIG. 15.4 Hemorrhagic cyst. Coronal T1-weighted spin-echo (*a*), transverse T2-weighted echo-train spin-echo (*b*), and gadolinium-enhanced fat-suppressed SGE (*c*) images in a patient with pelvic pain. A high-signal-intensity right adnexal mass is observed on the unenhanced images, which is suggestive of a hemorrhagic cyst or an endometrioma (*arrow, a,b*). There is some irregularity of the cyst rim inferiorly on the T1-weighted image. Following contrast, there is marked mural enhancement (*arrow, c*). Irregularity and marked enhancement reflect the vascularized lining of corpus lutea, but is not pathognomonic; endometriomas may behave similarly. The nonuniformity of the rim should not be mistaken for papillary projections, a finding suggestive of neoplasm. At laparoscopy, a hemorrhagic cyst was found. Transverse fat-suppressed SGE (*d*) and T2-weighted fat-suppressed echo-train spin-echo (*e*) images in a patient with endometrial carcinoma and a left adnexal hemorrhagic cyst. Hemorrhagic cysts can mimic endometriomas with high signal intensity on T1-weighted images (*arrow, d*) and heterogeneous high signal intensity on T2-weighted images (*arrow, e*). Note the focus of endometrial carcinoma that thins the junctional zone (*open arrow, d,e*).

CONGENITAL ABNORMALITIES

Disorders of sexual differentiation affect the ovaries and include complete and mixed gonadal dysgenesis as well as true and pseudohermaphroditism. (These entities are discussed more fully in Chapters 14 on the Uterus and Cervix and Chapter 13 on the Female Urethra and Vagina, respectively.) As the appearance of the external genitalia may be ambiguous, cytogenetic, biochemical, and radiologic studies are important for gender assignment and appropriate surgical or hormonal treatment. MRI is used to demonstrate the internal reproductive organs [21]. It can identify the presence or absence of normal ovaries, streak gonads, and/or ovotestes. MRI may also be used to detect gonadoblastoma, which occurs in up to one-third of patients with mixed gonadal dysgenesis [21,22].

MASS LESIONS

Benign Masses

Functional Cysts

Functional cysts are most common in women of reproductive age and include follicular cysts, corpus luteum cysts, or corpus albicans cysts. Their presence reflects normal ovarian physiology. The imaging features of simple functional cysts were discussed earlier. When complicated, functional cysts must be distinguished from ovarian neoplasms. The most useful feature for differentiating between the two is the presence of papillary projections. These are seen with ovarian tumors, but not with functional cysts. If papillary projections are suspected on unenhanced scans, administering gadolinium will confirm their presence and establish the diagnosis of an ovarian neoplasm (Fig. 15.5) [23]. The presence of papillary projections alone is not diagnostic of malignancy, though they are more common in borderline and malignant lesions [1,24]. Other criteria associated with an increased likelihood of malignancy in a cystic adnexal mass include advanced patient age, elevated CA-125 level, presence of solid components, and increased size.

Mature Cystic Teratoma

Mature cystic teratoma, or dermoid cyst, is the most common ovarian neoplasm. Depending on the series, this particular neoplasm comprises between 26 and 44 percent of all ovarian tumors [1]. Although cystic teratomas can occur in patients of all ages, the peak incidence is between the ages of 20 and 29 years. About 10 percent are bilateral [1]. These benign neoplasms are composed of varying amounts of endodermal, mesodermal, and ectodermal tissue. Typically, they are unilocular, lined with ectoderm, and filled with desquamated keratin and sebum, a lipid-laden material secreted by sebaceous glands. Occasionally, they may contain septae. Other elements that may be found within dermoid cysts include hair, teeth, skin, cartilage, bone, muscles, fat, bronchus, salivary gland, neural tissue, thyroid, pancreas, and retina [25]. In rare instances, lipid elements are confined to the cyst wall [26].

The tumors tend to grow slowly, and patients are frequently asymptomatic. However, when the tumors are large, patients may complain of symptoms related to mass effect such as pelvic pressure or pain. Complications of mature cystic teratoma include torsion, infection, rupture, and in less than 3 percent of cases, malignant transformation [1]. Malignancy is more common in postmenopausal women. In contrast to the embryonal tissues of immature teratoma (a malignant germ-cell tumor of the ovary), malignant tumors that arise in mature cystic teratomas resemble typical adult neoplasms. Squamous cell carcinoma is the most common malignant cell type and accounts for approximately 90 percent of cases. The remainder of cases are adenocarcinoma, sarcoma, melanoma, or other rare histologies. The prognosis for patients with malignant transformation of a benign dermoid cyst is poor, with most patients dying within one year of diagnosis [1].

Benign cystic teratomas can be managed conservatively. Treatment options include cystectomy, oophorectomy, or salpingo-oophorectomy. For girls and women of reproductive age who wish to preserve their fertility, cystectomy is adequate. This is especially true in cases with bilateral involvement.

The MRI features of cystic teratomas are well-described and include fat or sebum within the cyst that parallels the signal intensity of fat on all pulse sequences; fat-water chemical shift artifact (present in up to 62 percent of cases [8]); fat-fluid and/or fluid-fluid levels; layering debris; low-signal-intensity calcification (teeth); and soft tissue protuberances called Rokitansky nodules or dermoid plugs attached to the cyst wall [16,27,28]. Standard T1- and T2-weighted sequences may suggest the diagnosis of cystic teratoma, but exploiting the precessional frequency differences between fat protons and water protons with chemically selective fat saturation techniques improves diagnostic confidence (Fig. 15.6) [7,8,11]. In one study, the characterization sensitivity for teratomas with fat suppression imaging (92%) was superior to the statistically derived sensitivity of nonfat-suppressed T1- and T2-weighted imaging (77%) using multivariate image analysis [8]. These investigators also found fat saturation techniques were 100 percent specific and 96 percent accurate for the diagnosis of teratoma [8]. Alternatively, in- and out-of-phase imaging techniques may be used to assess fat-water interface cancellation [29]. A theoretical advantage of this approach is that it is more sensitive than frequency-selective fat saturation

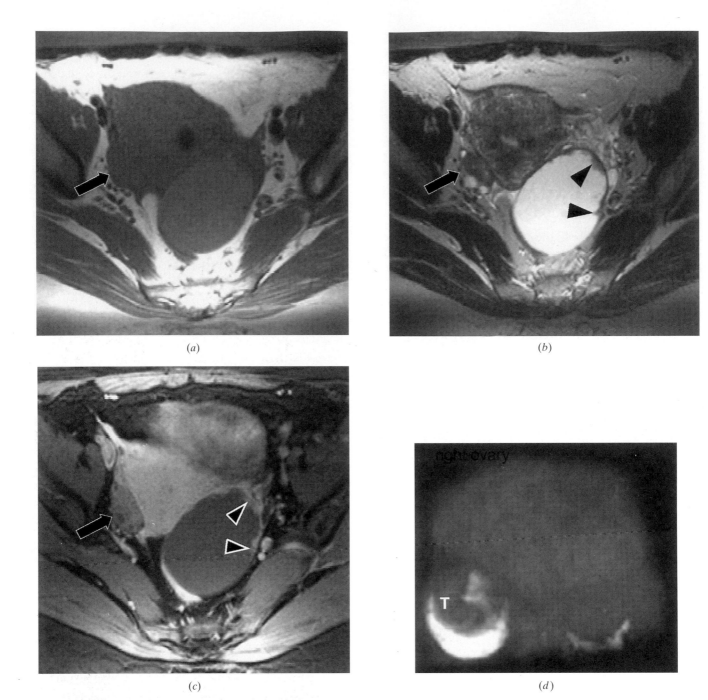

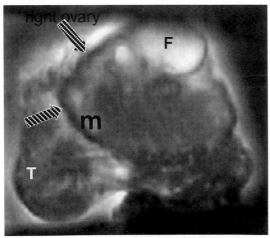

Fig. 15.5 Normal right ovary and left ovarian serous cystadenocarcinoma. T1-weighted spin-echo (*a*), T2-weighted echo-train spin-echo (*b*), gadolinium-enhanced fat-suppressed SGE (*c*), specimen T1-weighted spin-echo (*d*) and T2-weighted spin-echo (*e*) images in a 40-year-old woman with a left adnexal mass. The normal right ovary (*arrow, a–c*) contains several follicles that have enhancing rims following contrast. Note that the ovarian stroma enhances less than adjacent myometrium. The specimen right ovary image accentuates the difference in signal intensity between the ovarian cortex (*hatched arrow, e*) low signal intensity, and the ovarian medulla (*"m", e*) high signal intensity. Note the adjacent normal coiled fallopian tube (*"T", d,e*). In contrast, the left ovary has been replaced by a primarily cystic mass. Apparent thickening of the wall of the cyst (*arrowheads, b*) is confirmed on the postgadolinium image, which demonstrates enhancing papillary projections (*arrowheads, c*). *F*, follicle (Parts *b, c, d,* and *e* are reprinted with permission from Outwater EK, Mitchell DG: Normal ovaries and functional cysts: MR appearance. Radiology 198:397–402, 1996)

techniques to the presence of small amounts of fat within voxels [11].

MRI may be especially helpful in the evaluation of a pregnant woman with an adnexal mass; the increased accuracy of lesion characterization can limit surgical intervention to only those cases in which surgery is mandatory (Fig. 15.7) [30,31]. If the mass is a dermoid cyst, it is at increased risk for rupture with subsequent chemical peritonitis. MRI can establish the correct diagnosis, and appropriate management can be instituted. To date, the overwhelming majority of studies have shown no untoward effects of diagnostic MRI on the human fetus [32].

Cystadenomas

Serous cystadenomas are common, accounting for 20 percent of benign tumors of the ovary [1]. They occur in

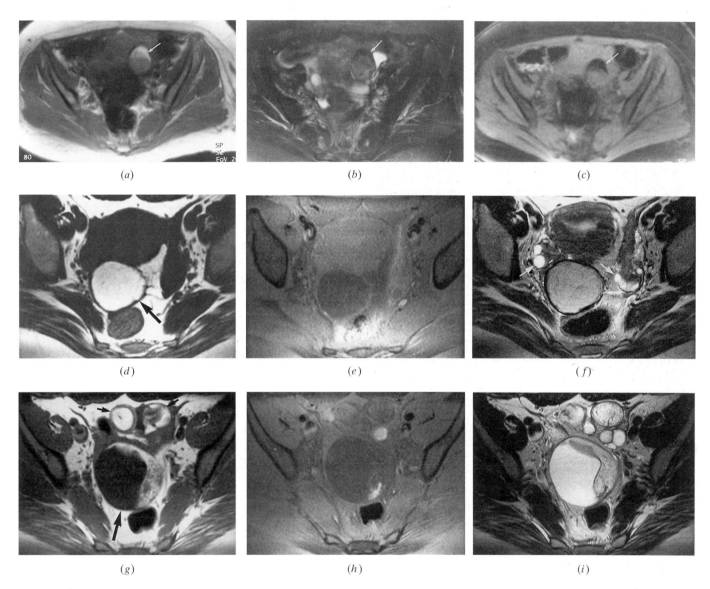

F IG. 15.6 Dermoid. SGE (*a*), 512-resolution T2-weighted fat-suppressed echo-train spin-echo (*b*), and fat-suppressed SGE (*c*) images in a woman with a left adnexal mass. On the nonsuppressed image, a high-signal-intensity component similar to the pelvic and subcutaneous fat is noted in the nondependent portion of the mass (*arrow a*). Although this is suggestive of a lipid-containing mass, methemoglobin may appear similarly. On the fat-suppressed sequences (*b,c*) this area diminishes in signal intensity (*arrow, b,c*) comparable to the pelvic, marrow, and subcutaneous fat, confirming the diagnosis of a dermoid cyst. T1-weighted spin-echo (*d*), T1-weighted fat-suppressed spin-echo (*e*) and 512-resolution echo-train spin-echo (*f*) images in a second patient. An exophytic right ovarian dermoid is present that is uniformly high in signal intensity on the T1-weighted image (*arrow, d*) and suppresses uniformly on the fat-suppressed image (*e*). Follicles are well-shown in both ovaries (*arrows, f*) on the high-resolution image, and the exophytic nature of the dermoid is clearly demonstrated. T1-weighted spin-echo (*g*), T1-weighted fat-suppressed spin-echo (*h*) and 512-resolution echo-train spin-echo (*i*) images in a third patient with bilateral dermoids. A large right (*large arrow, g*) and two smaller left (*small arrows, g*) ovarian dermoids are present. The signal intensities of the dermoids are complex on T1- (*g*) and T2-weighted (*i*) images due to a mixture of substances they contain.

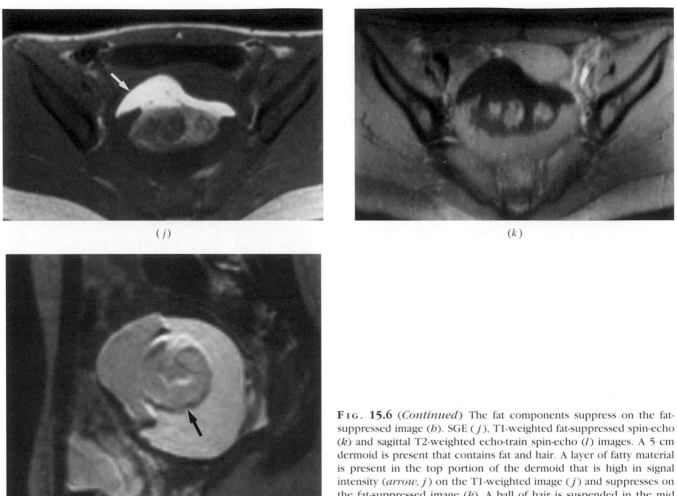

(j)

(k)

(l)

FIG. 15.6 (*Continued*) The fat components suppress on the fat-suppressed image (*h*). SGE (*j*), T1-weighted fat-suppressed spin-echo (*k*) and sagittal T2-weighted echo-train spin-echo (*l*) images. A 5 cm dermoid is present that contains fat and hair. A layer of fatty material is present in the top portion of the dermoid that is high in signal intensity (*arrow, j*) on the T1-weighted image (*j*) and suppresses on the fat-suppressed image (*k*). A ball of hair is suspended in the mid portion of the dermoid (*arrow, l*). (*j-l* courtesy of Ann B. Willms).

women aged 20 to 50 years and are bilateral in 20 percent of the cases. In contrast, their malignant counterparts develop in older women and are more frequently bilateral [33]. They are usually unilocular thin-walled cysts, but multiple locules and papillary projections have also been described [34]. Psammoma bodies, small whorled calcified structures, strongly suggest a serous neoplasm, but do not differentiate between benign and malignant tumors. Serous cystadenomas are treated by cystectomy or unilateral salpingo-oophorectomy. They do not recur or metastasize.

On MRI, the cyst fluid is similar to water or urine: very low in signal intensity on T1-weighted images and very high in signal intensity on T2-weighted images. If complicated by hemorrhage, the signal characteristics are altered due to shortening of both T1- and T2-relaxation times. When thin-walled, serous cystadenomas may be indistinguishable from simple functional ovarian cysts. Alternatively, multiloculated serous cystadenomas may

mimic malignant ovarian tumors or fallopian tube pathology (Fig. 15.8). If papillary projections are suspected on unenhanced images, administration of gadolinium is useful to confirm their presence.

Mucinous cystadenoma is a common ovarian neoplasm which, like serous cystadenoma, accounts for 20 percent of benign ovarian tumors. They are more common after age 40 and are bilateral in 5 percent of the cases [1]. The cysts tend to be multiloculated and lined by columnar mucinous cells of the endocervical or intestinal type [1]. Most mucinous cystadenomas are smaller than 10 cm, but lesions up to 50 lb have been reported [1]. Treatment is similar to that for serous cystadenoma.

The MRI appearance of mucinous cystadenoma reflects its protein content: multiple locules of varying signal intensity on both T1- and T2-weighted sequences. Hemorrhage within a locule is not uncommon (Fig. 15.9) [34]. If papillary projections are identified, a malignant mucinous neoplasm must be considered.

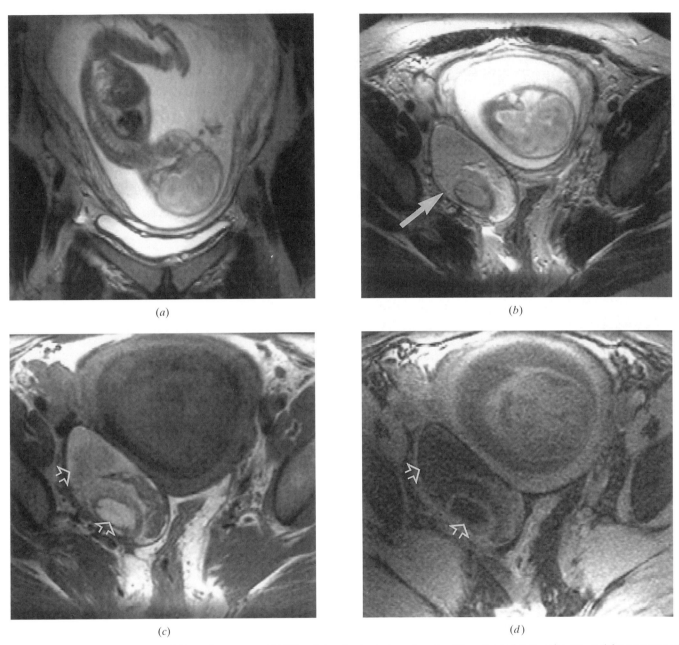

(a)

(b)

(c)

(d)

Fig. 15.7 Dermoid cyst. Coronal (*a*) and transverse (*b*) T2-weighted echo-train spin-echo, T1-weighted spin-echo (*c*), and fat-suppressed SGE (*d*) images in a young woman with a 22-week gestation. The T2-weighted images show the gravid uterus (*a,b*) and a complex right adnexal mass (*arrow, b*). Note that the mass does not have signal features of simple fluid. The T1-weighted images with and without fat suppression show a loss of signal intensity of the lipid component (*open arrows, c,d*), which establishes the diagnosis of a dermoid cyst.

Endometriosis

Endometriosis is a common entity affecting women of reproductive age. It is estimated to occur in 15 percent of the general female population and in 31 percent of women undergoing laparoscopy [1,35]. Histologically, endometriosis is composed of ectopic endometrial glands, cellular stroma and, in some cases, smooth muscle fibers. The endometrial glands respond to ovarian hormones and show secretory changes in the second half of the menstrual cycle and decidual transformation during pregnancy [36]. The diagnosis may be difficult to establish if, after repeated hemorrhages, the tissues are modified leaving only glands lined by flattened epithelium or cysts completely devoid of epithelium: endometriotic cysts and endometriomas, respectively. Endometriomas are the most common manifestation of the disease process and are well-shown on MRI. The term usually is reserved for lesions associated with the ovaries. The cysts are thick-walled with extensive fibrosis and adhesions to adjacent structures. Malignant transformation of endome-

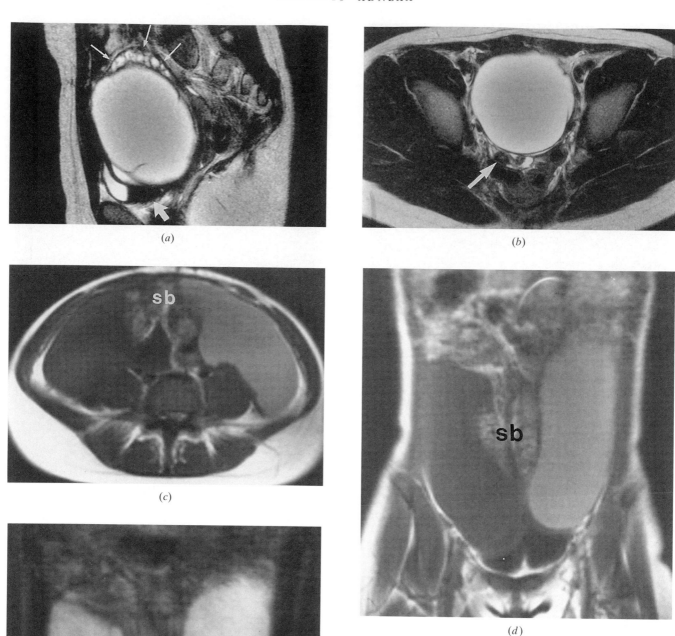

(a)

(b)

(c)

(d)

(e)

FIG. 15.8 Serous cystadenoma. Sagittal (*a*) and transverse (*b*) 512-resolution T2-weighted echo-train spin-echo images in a 10-year-old girl with precocious puberty. A large septate mass occupies the pelvis. Note the pubertal-sized, follicle-containing ovary draped over the mass (*long arrows, a*). The signal-void area in the dependent portion of bladder reflects the T2* effects of concentrated gadolinium (*short arrow, a*). The ovarian mass displaces the uterine corpus and cervix (*arrow, b*) posteriorly. At surgery a benign serous cystadenoma was resected. Transverse (*c*) and coronal (*d*) T1-weighted spin-echo, and coronal (*e*) T2-weighted spin-echo images in a second young girl who presented with an enlarging abdomen. Bilateral cystic masses originate in the pelvis and extend into the abdomen. The right-sided mass has signal characteristics suggesting a transudate, whereas the left-sided mass has signal characteristics of an exudate. Septations are more conspicuous on the T2-weighted image (*arrows, e*). At surgery, bilateral serous cystadenomas were found; the left-sided one was complicated by hemorrhage, accounting for its imaging features. Note the small bowel (*"sb",c,d,e*) compressed between the two masses.

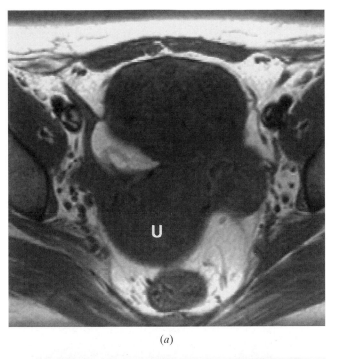

(a)

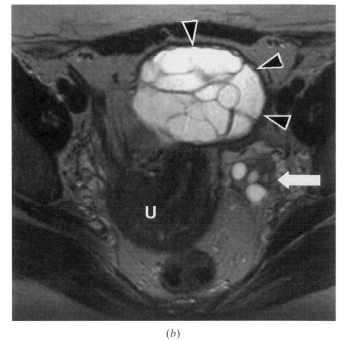

(b)

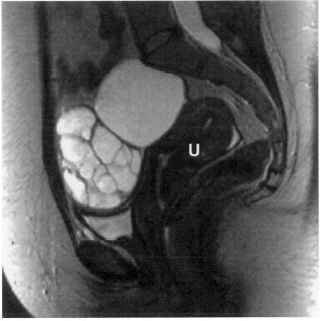

(c)

FIG. 15.9 Mucinous cystadenoma. T1-weighted spin-echo (a), T2-weighted echo-train spin-echo (b), and sagittal T2-weighted echo-train spin-echo (c) images. Multiple internal cysts and septations are typical findings in mucinous cystadenoma. The low signal intensity fibrotic wall of the mass (*arrowheads, b*) and the adjacent normal left ovary (*arrow, b*) are noted. The sagittal image (c) demonstrates displacement of the uterus (*uterus = u,a–c*) posteriorly by the mass.

triosis has been reported but is rare, occurring in less than 1 percent of patients with endometriosis [36]. The tumors most likely to arise in endometriosis are endometrioid carcinoma, clear-cell carcinoma, and carcinosarcoma [1].

The clinical manifestations of endometriosis are protean. Some women experience debilitating pelvic pain (dysmenorrhea, dyspareunia, lumbar, or rectal) and/or infertility, whereas others have minor discomfort; still others are asymptomatic [37]. Although almost any organ

of the body may be involved, intraperitoneal sites of endometriosis are far more common, and in decreasing order of frequency include the ovaries, uterine ligaments, cul-de-sac, uterine serosal surface, fallopian tubes, rectosigmoid, and urinary bladder [35–40]. The disease is diagnosed, staged, and often treated surgically, especially laparoscopically. Staging is based on a point scale that takes into account the site and depth of implants, and degree of adhesions. At surgery, endometriosis implants have a variable appearance: the classic appearance of black and blue-black or the atypical appearance of white, yellow, red, and brown. These differences reflect varying amounts of hemosiderin and other blood breakdown products [36]. Adhesions typically involve the peritoneum and omentum and, if dense enough, may preclude laparoscopic evaluation of the pelvis ("frozen pelvis"). In addition to surgical management, many patients receive medications such as oral contraceptives, GnRH agonists, danazol, or progestins to help inhibit the growth of endometrial tissue.

The noninvasive diagnosis of endometriosis has been elusive. Ultrasonography is limited [41–43]. Transvaginal sonography has a reported accuracy of 42 percent for characterizing endometriomas [44]. In another study the sensitivity of ultrasound for detecting focal implants was poor (11%) [42]. Conventional CT imaging has not fared well either. Limited contrast resolution coupled with ionizing radiation precludes routine use of this modality in reproductive age patients suspected of having endometriosis [45].

MRI also has been used for the evaluation of endometriosis [27,46–50]. Initial reports described cysts that were high in signal intensity on T1-weighted images and demonstrated a gradient of low signal intensity (shading) on T2-weighted images (Figs. 15.10 and 15.11). These cysts were surrounded by a low-signal-intensity thick fibrous capsule composed of hemosiderin-laden macrophages and were adherent to surrounding organs [46]. Using a body coil and conventional spin-echo sequences, early studies demonstrated limited success for evaluating endometriosis: 64 to 71 percent sensitivity and 60 to 82 percent specificity. MRI had difficulty identifying intraperitoneal endometrial implants and extraovarian endometrial adhesions [48,49]. Furthermore, MRI findings did not correlate with the surgically determined severity of disease [48]. These studies addressed the ability of MRI to detect both endometriomas and endometrial implants. More recent work limited their investigation to identifying and characterizing adnexal masses. Using criteria of multiple masses of very high signal intensity on T1-weighted

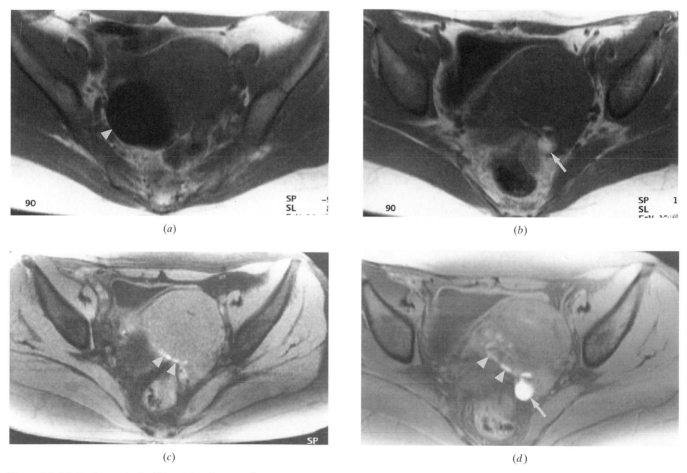

(a)

(b)

(c)

(d)

FIG. 15.10 Endometriosis. T1-weighted spin-echo (*a,b*), fat-suppressed SGE (*c,d*), T2-weighted echo-train spin-echo (*e*), and contrast-enhanced T1-weighted fat-suppressed spin-echo (*f*) images in a patient with bilateral adnexal masses on transvaginal ultrasound. The right adnexal mass is low in signal intensity on the unenhanced image (*arrowhead, a*) and does not enhance following contrast (*arrowhead, f*). Its wall is barely perceptible and without appreciable enhancement. This constellation of findings is consistent with a functional ovarian cyst. Note the enhancing right ovarian parenchyma draped anteriorly to the cyst (*open arrow, f*).

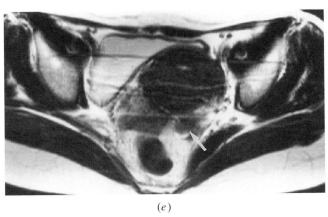

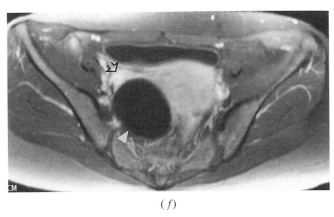

(e)   (f)

F IG . 15.10 (*Continued*) There is also a high-signal-intensity mass applied to the left ovary on the T1-weighted image (*arrow, b*), which is more conspicuous on the fat-suppressed image (*arrow, d*). The mass shows shading on the T2-weighted image (*arrow, e*), which is consistent with an endometrioma. Note that the small endometrial implants applied to the uterine serosa are well-seen with fat-suppression technique (*arrowheads, c,d*).

images or any mass with very high signal intensity on T1-weighted images and low signal intensity (shading) on T2-weighted sequences, yielded an overall sensitivity, specificity, and accuracy of 90, 98, and 96 percent, respectively [50]. Others have reported only moderate success in distinguishing endometriomas from other hemorrhagic lesions [20]. Blood products, irrespective of etiology, have similar imaging appearance. Extracellular methemoglo-

bin causes T1-shortening, while deoxyhemoglobin, intracellular methemoglobin and proteinaceous material cause T2-shortening. Endometriomas have variable mural enhancement with gadolinium and as such can be confused with other ovarian processes such as hemorrhagic cysts and tubo-ovarian abscesses [12,51].

Water and lipid suppression have been shown to improve the specificity for ovarian masses [7]. Hemor-

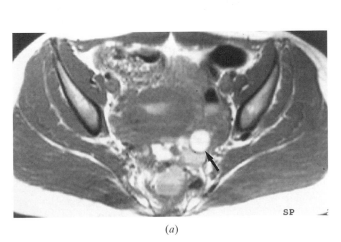

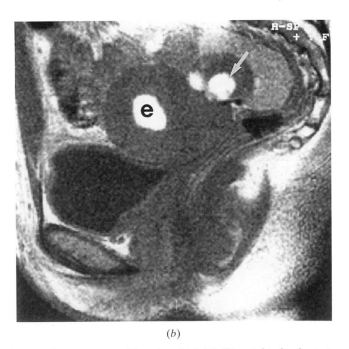

(a)   (b)

F IG . 15.11 Endometriosis. Transverse (*a*) and sagittal (*b*) T1-weighted spin-echo, transverse (*c*) and sagittal (*d*) T2-weighted echo-train spin-echo, transverse T1-weighted fat-suppressed spin-echo (*e*) and transverse (*f*) and sagittal (*g*) gadolinium-enhanced T1-weighted fat-suppressed spin-echo images in an adolescent girl with amenorrhea and pelvic pain. High-signal-intensity endometriomas on the conventional T1-weighted images demonstrate characteristic shading on the T2-weighted images (*arrow, a–d*). With the addition of fat suppression, small endometriosis implants that were indistinguishable from pelvic fat on non-suppressed images become more conspicuous (*arrows, e*).

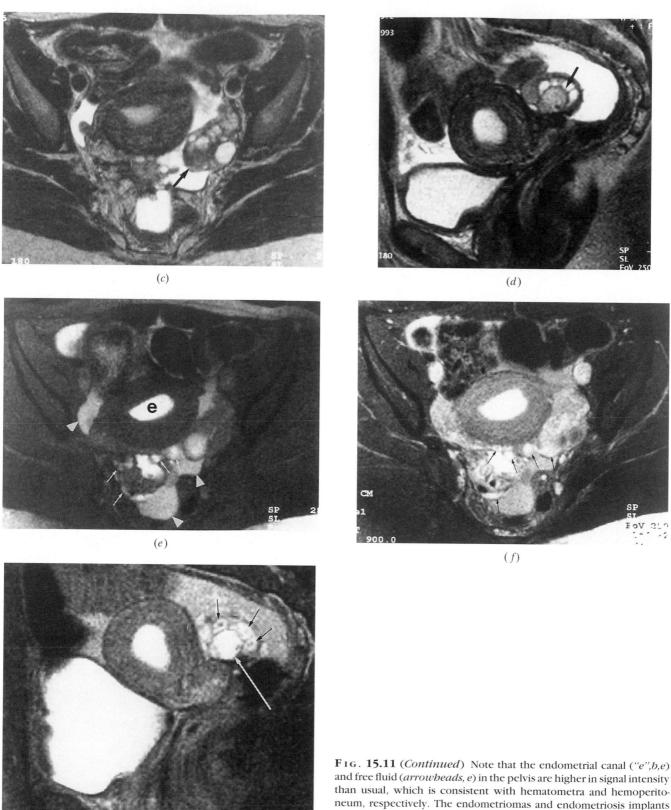

(c)

(d)

(e)

(f)

(g)

FIG. 15.11 (*Continued*) Note that the endometrial canal (*"e",b,e*) and free fluid (*arrowheads, e*) in the pelvis are higher in signal intensity than usual, which is consistent with hematometra and hemoperitoneum, respectively. The endometriomas and endometriosis implants have variable enhancement after contrast administration (*arrows, f*). Note the enhancing follicle rims (*short arrows, g*) surrounding the endometrioma (*long arrow, g*). This patient had cervical atresia and retrograde menses, which presumably account for this patient's endometriosis. Surgery confirmed endometriosis and hemorrhagic free pelvic fluid; the hysterectomy specimen revealed cervical agenesis.

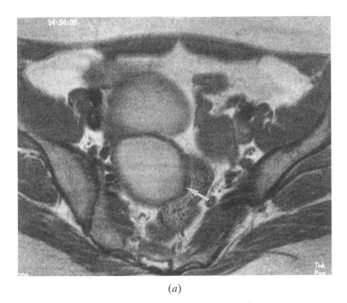

(a)

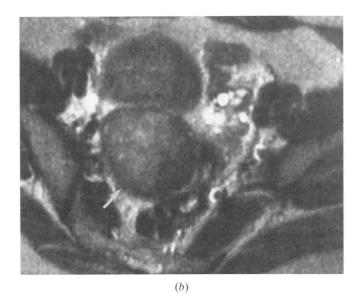

(b)

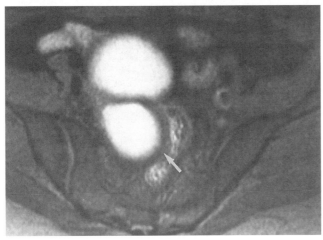

(c)

FIG. 15.12 Endometriosis. T1-weighted (*a*), T2-weighted (*b*), and T1-weighted fat-suppressed (*c*) spin-echo images in a 30-year-old woman with complex pelvic masses on transvaginal sonography. On the nonsuppressed T1- and T2-weighted images, the signal characteristics of the pelvic masses are suggestive of endometriomas. The addition of chemically selective fat suppression causes rescaling and narrowing of the dynamic signal intensity range and renders the masses higher in signal intensity than surrounding tissue. The diagnosis of endometriosis is now more easily established. Note the thick low-signal-intensity hemosiderin-laden and/or fibrotic rim that surround the endometriomas (*arrow, a–c*). (Reprinted with permission from Ascher SM, Agrawal R, Bis KG, et al: Endometriosis: Appearance and detection with conventional and contrast-enhanced fat-suppressed spin-echo techniques. J Magn Reson Imaging 5:251–257, 1995)

rhagic lesions become more conspicuous on T1-weighted fat-suppressed images by removing competing high signal intensity from adjacent fat. Additionally, fat suppression narrows the dynamic signal intensity range, thereby highlighting subtle differences between tissues (Fig. 15.12) [9]. Using frequency-selective fat suppression, one group of investigators reported an overall sensitivity of 77 percent and a specificity of 78 percent for the detection of endometriosis. In evaluating the subset of endometriomas larger than 1 cm, these values rose to 91 and 94 percent, respectively. Significant gains also were noted for detection of small endometriomas (Fig. 15.13) [9]. These findings have been corroborated by others [51,53]. Implant detection remains problematic, and variable MRI appearances have been described [46,48,50–52]. One study reported that some implants exhibit ill-defined enhancement following gadolinium, but this was neither sensitive nor specific (Fig. 15.14) [51]. The MRI

appearance of solid fibrotic endometriosis also has been described: intermediate-signal-intensity masses studded with high-signal-intensity foci on T1-weighted images; low-signal-intensity masses on T2-weighted images; and enhancement following intravenous contrast (Fig. 15.15). Identification of the high-signal-intensity foci helps to distinguish this form of endometriosis from peritoneal metastases [54]. Ancillary findings in patients with endometriosis include adhesions (spiculated low-signal-intensity stranding and/or obscuration of organ interfaces) and/or dilated fallopian tubes (Fig. 15.16) [23].

Polycystic Ovary Disease

Polycystic ovary disease is a hormonally mediated disease that may be seen in association with Stein-Leventhal syndrome: hirsutism, amenorrhea, and infertility. There is failure of the normal cyclical changes of both follicle-stimulating hormone (FSH) and luteinizing hormone

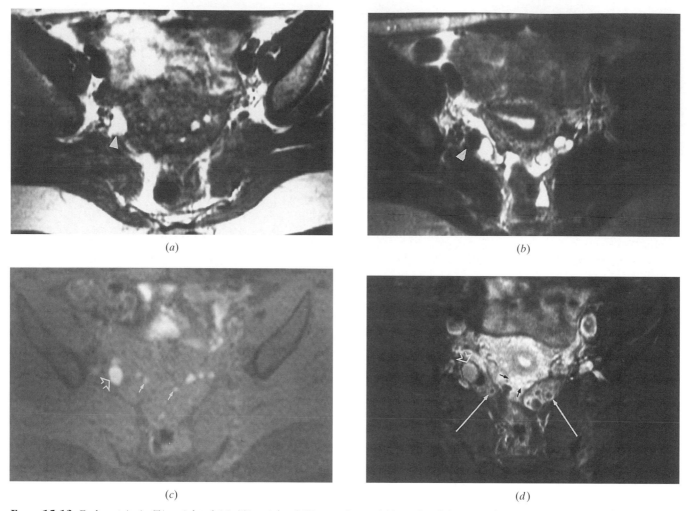

(a)   (b)

(c)   (d)

FIG. 15.13 Endometriosis. T1-weighted (a), T2-weighted (b), unenhanced (c), and gadolinium-enhanced (d) T1-weighted fat-suppressed spin-echo images in a 39-year-old woman with pelvic pain. Endometriosis was not prospectively suggested on the nonsuppressed conventional spin-echo images. Fat suppression highlights the endometriomas (*open arrow, c*) and endometrial implants (*solid arrows, c*) applied to the serosa of the posterior uterus. Following contrast, the ovarian parenchyma and right endometrioma rim (*open arrow, d*) and follicle rims (*long solid arrows, d*) enhance. The endometrial implants remain high in signal intensity following gadolinium (*short solid arrows, d*). Retrospectively, the right endometrioma (*arrowhead, a,b*) and serosal implants can be identified. (Parts *a, b,* and *c* are reprinted with permission from Ascher SM, Agrawal R, Bis KG, et al: Endometriosis: Appearance and detection with conventional and contrast-enhanced fat-suppressed spin-echo techniques. J Magn Reson Imaging 5:251–257, 1995)

(LH). Hormone imbalance leads to chronically stimulated, but unruptured follicles in the subcapsular region of the ovaries. There is also hypertrophy of the ovarian stroma and capsule [1,55]. The MRI findings in polycystic ovary syndrome include multiple peripheral ovarian cysts within a thickened fibrotic superficial cortex (Fig. 15.17). Ovarian enlargement is not universal, but the disease is always bilateral. Care must be taken to distinguish polycystic ovary disease from normal ovaries with multiple functional cysts. The cysts in polycystic ovarian disease are similar in size with homogeneous high signal intensity on T2-weighted images, whereas func-

tional cysts tend to vary in size and on occasion may have signal characteristics consistent with prior hemorrhage [23].

Theca-Lutein Cysts

Massive bilateral ovarian enlargement secondary to multiple theca-lutein cysts is associated with increased levels of human chorionic gonadotropin (β-hCG). This usually occurs in the setting of gestational trophoblastic disease (GTD). Of women with GTD, 25 to 33 percent develop theca-lutein cysts [56]. The ovaries are edematous and congested, harboring numerous multilocular cysts that

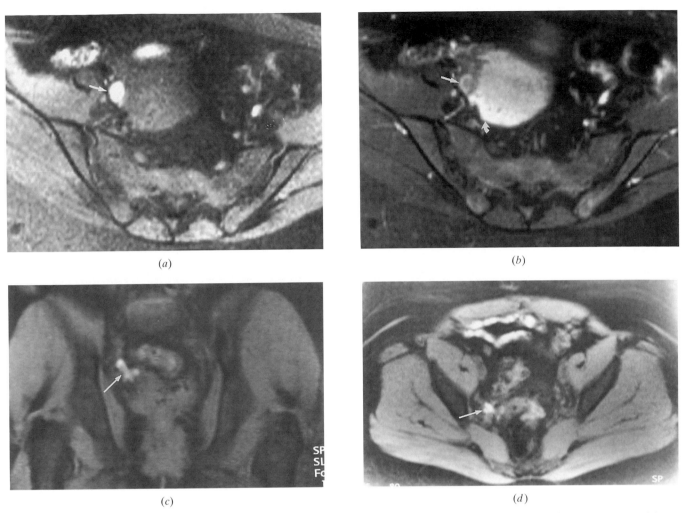

F IG . 15.14 Endometriosis. T1-weighted fat-suppressed spin-echo images before (*a*) and after (*b*) gadolinium administration in a 35-year-old woman with increasing pelvic pain. A right adnexal mass has high signal intensity on the unenhanced image, which is consistent with blood (*arrow, a*). Following contrast the rim enhances (*arrow, b*). This finding has been observed in both endometriomas and hemorrhagic cysts. Note the intense enhancement along the posterior uterine serosa (*curved arrow, b*). At surgery this region was studded with endometriosis implants. Ill-defined enhancement may be useful as an ancillary sign of endometriosis, although it may not be a sensitive or specific finding. Coronal (*c*) and transverse (*d*) fat-suppressed SGE images in a second patient with right sciatic pain. An irregular, 1.5-cm high-signal-intensity focus (*arrow, c,d*) of endometrial implant is in the right pelvis immediately adjacent to the sciatic nerve. Note the linear radiation of fibrotic tissue that extends from the mass and presumably tethers the sciatic nerve.

may measure up to 4 cm in diameter. Ovarian enlargement is usually asymptomatic, but patients may present with acute abdominal pain if there is hemorrhage into the cyst or if the cyst ruptures or torses. The presence of theca-lutein cysts up to 4 months after molar evacuation can be normal and should not be used as evidence of persistent or recurrent disease. Similar ovarian pathology can be seen in the ovarian hyperstimulation syndrome, a condition that occurs in women undergoing ovulation induction for infertility.

Theca-lutein cysts have a variable appearance on MRI. They are low to high in signal intensity on T1-weighted sequences and high in signal intensity on T2-weighted sequences [57,58]. The diagnosis of GTD is suggested if there is an accompanying hypervascular endometrial mass distorting the uterus (Fig. 15.18). When theca-lutein cysts are seen in association with the ovarian hyperstimulation syndrome, simple or hemorrhagic ascites is evident (Fig. 15.19). An intrauterine or extrauterine gestation(s) can occasionally be demonstrated.

Parovarian Cysts and Peritoneal Cysts

Virtually all types of ovarian tumor or cyst can arise in the broad ligament or parovarium. When cystic, they

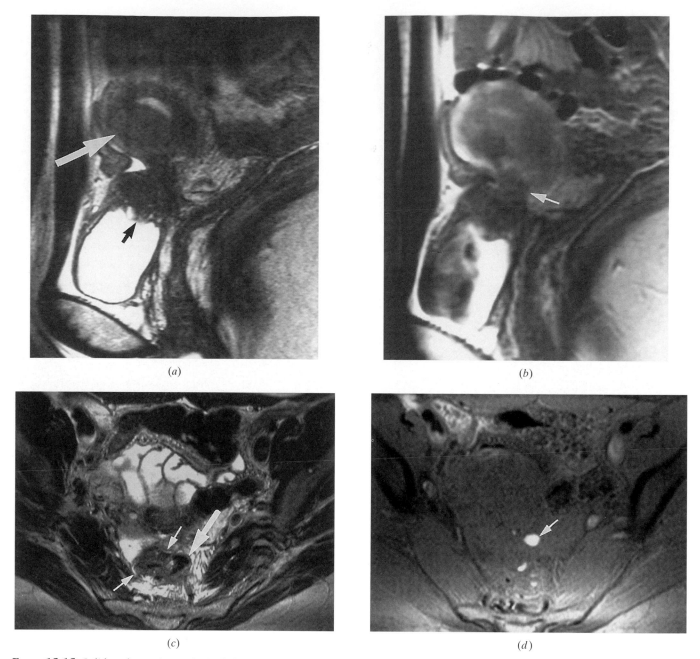

(a)

(b)

(c)

(d)

FIG. 15.15 Solid endometrioma. Sagittal 512-resolution T2-weighted echo-train spin-echo (*a*) and sagittal gadolinium-enhanced T1-weighted spin-echo (*b*) images. A 4-cm ill-defined mass is present that invades the dome of the bladder (*arrow, a*) and the anterior myometrium (*arrow, b*). The mass is low in signal intensity on T1-weighted (not shown), T2-weighted (*a*), and gadolinium-enhanced T1-weighted (*b*) images. Diffuse adenomyosis of the uterus is noted (*large arrow, a*). Cystoscopic biopsy had suspected the diagnosis of sarcoma. The correct diagnosis was made on the MRI study and confirmed at surgery. Solid endometrioma in a second patient on a 512-resolution T2-weighted echo-train spin-echo image (*c*). A low-signal-intensity mass is demonstrated (*arrows, c*) that invades the outer wall of the upper rectum (*large arrow, c*). A T1-weighted fat-suppressed spin-echo image (*d*) at the same tomographic level demonstrates a 1-cm endometrioma as a high-signal-intensity focus (*arrow, d*).

are commonly lumped together under the heading of parovarian cysts [1]. Data from surgical series suggests that parovarian cysts may account for 10 to 20 percent of adnexal masses [59]. Hydatid cysts of Morgagni are a common subset and arise from müllerian vestiges. They occur at the fimbriated ends of the fallopian tubes where they may be multiple and/or bilateral. Most are asymp-

tomatic unless complicated by torsion. The cysts are round or ovoid structures that are low in signal intensity on T1-weighted images and high in signal intensity on T2-weighted images. They may be indistinguishable from ovarian cysts [59].

Peritoneal pseudocysts are ascitic collections contained by mesothelial-lined adhesions. They are seen

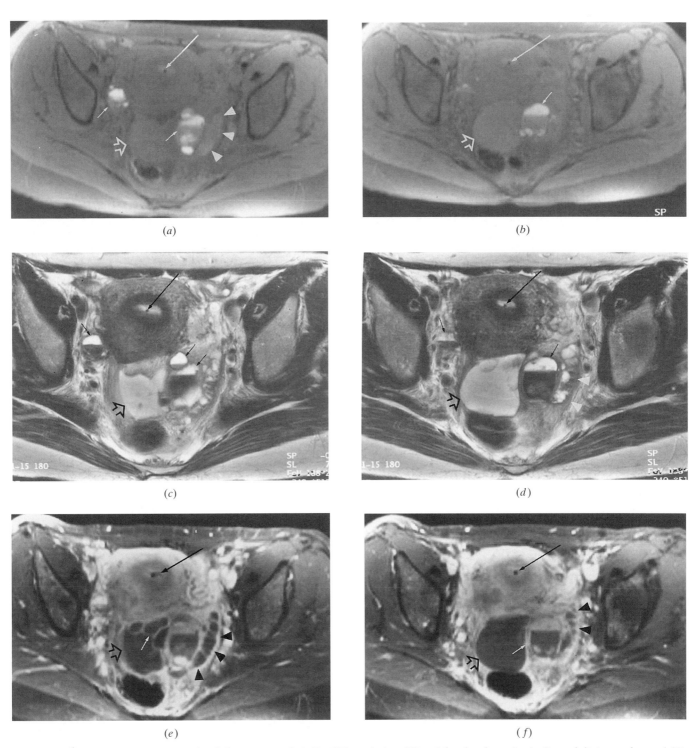

FIG. 15.16 Endometriosis. T1-weighted fat-suppressed (*a,b*), 512-resolution T2-weighted echo-train (*c,d*), gadolinium-enhanced T1-weighted fat suppressed (*e,f*), sagittal T2-weighted echo-train (*g*), and coronal gadolinium-enhanced T1-weighted fat-suppressed (*h*) spin-echo images in a 42-year-old woman with a 2-month history of pelvic pain, an elevated CA-125, and complex adnexal masses on transvaginal sonography. Bilateral adnexal masses have high-signal-intensity components on T1-weighted images, which demonstrate shading with fluid-fluid levels on T2-weighted images consistent with endometriomas (*short solid arrows, a–d*). Note the serpentine left hydro/hematosalpinx (*arrowheads, a,d–f,h*). Posterior to the uterus is a polygonal fluid collection (*open arrow, a–f,h*). Following contrast, both the rims and septations of the masses (*short solid arrows, e–h*) enhance as do the walls of the dilated left fallopian tube (*arrowheads, e,f,h*).

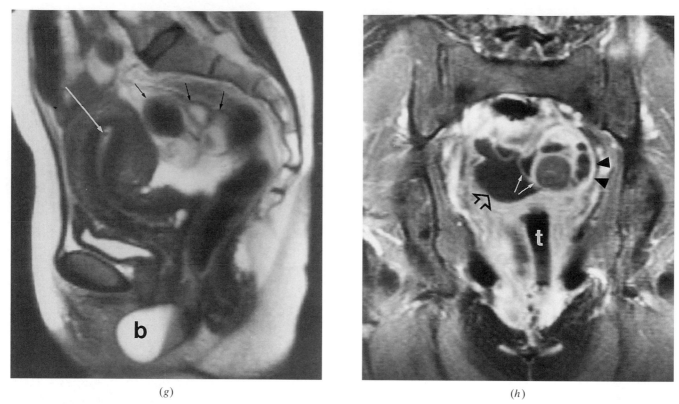

(g)   (h)

F I G . 15.16 (*Continued*) The polygonal fluid collection has similar enhancement characteristics. Orthogonal views confirm the findings. Note the IUD within the endometrium (*long solid arrow a–g*), Bartholin-duct cyst ("*b*",g) and tampon ("*t*",h). At laparoscopy, bilateral endometriomas, endometriosis implants, left hydro/hematosalpinx, adhesions, and a peritoneal pseudocyst behind the uterus were found. MRI can add specificity to the finding of an elevated CA-125.

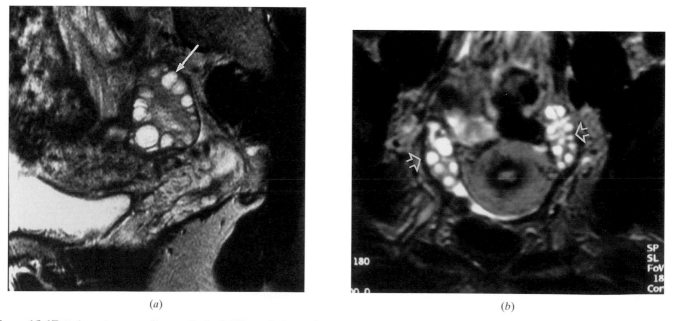

(a)   (b)

F I G . 15.17 Polycystic ovary disease. Sagittal 512-resolution echo-train spin-echo image (*a*) demonstrates a mildly enlarged ovary that contains multiple, similar-sized cysts (*arrow, a*). Paracoronal T2-weighted echo-train spin-echo image (*b*) in a second patient shows enlargement of the ovaries bilaterally (*open arrows, b*) with multiple similar-sized peripheral cysts. Central ovarian tissue is low in signal intensity, reflecting increased medullary cellular stroma.

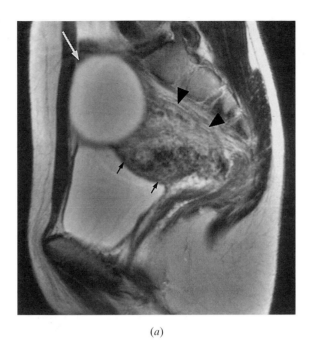

(a)

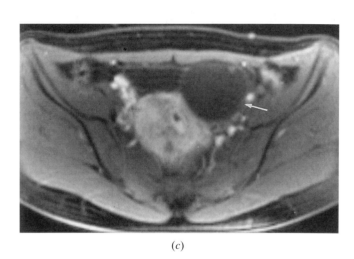

(b)

FIG. 15.18 Theca-lutein cysts. Sagittal (*a*) and transverse (*b*) 512-resolution T2-weighted echo-train spin-echo, and gadolinium-enhanced fat-suppressed SGE (*c*) in a woman with an invasive mole. The combination of an infiltrating endometrial mass and enlarged and cystic ovaries (*long arrow, a–c*) should suggest the diagnosis of gestational trophoblastic disease. Note the high signal of myometrium in the area of marked molar invasion (*arrowheads, a*) versus the area where it is relatively spared (*short arrows, a*). Whereas theca-lutein cysts are present in up to one-third of woman with gestational trophoblastic disease, they also occur in other conditions associated with elevated human chorionic gonadotropin (β-hCG) levels.

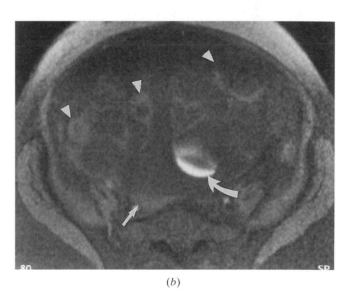

(c)

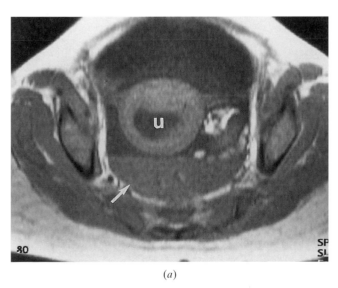

(a)

(b)

FIG. 15.19 Theca-lutein cysts. SGE (*a*), fat-suppressed SGE (*b*), transverse (*c–f*) and sagittal (*g*) T2-weighted echo-train spin-echo images in a patient on ovulation induction medicine who presented with acute pain and hypotension. Bilateral multilocular ovarian cysts (*arrowheads, b–g*) are identified in association with a gravid uterus ("*u*",*a,e,f,g*) and marked free abdominopelvic fluid. Some of the cysts are complicated by hemorrhage, which is best seen on the fat-suppressed images (*curved arrow, b*).

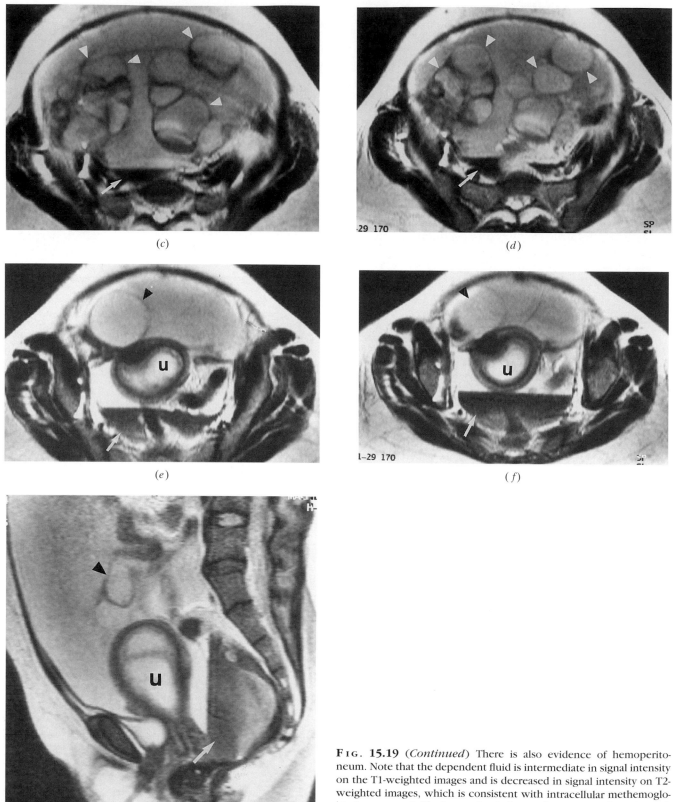

(c)

(d)

(e)

(f)

(g)

FIG. 15.19 (*Continued*) There is also evidence of hemoperitoneum. Note that the dependent fluid is intermediate in signal intensity on the T1-weighted images and is decreased in signal intensity on T2-weighted images, which is consistent with intracellular methemoglobin (*arrow, a–g*). The hyperstimulation syndrome is a well-recognized, life-threatening complication of ovulation induction therapy for infertility.

most commonly in patients with prior abdominopelvic surgery and/or women with endometriosis. Their signal intensity is variable and may mimic other conditions. A distinguishing feature of pseudocysts is their walls: They are formed by adjacent structures rather than a true discrete wall and, as such, have an irregular shape. This is especially well-seen on postcontrast images (see Fig. 15.16). Septations may be present. In one study MRI was found to be more useful than either CT imaging or ultrasound for diagnosing peritoneal pseudocysts [60].

Benign Solid Tumors

The most common solid benign tumors to affect the ovary are derived from stromal cells: fibromas and thecomas. They may be purely fibroblastic, purely lipid-laden thecal tumors, or a combination of the two. Because the histologic appearance of fibromas and thecomas overlap, the term "fibrothecoma" is often applied to this spectrum of tumors. Pure thecomas are most common in peri- and postmenopausal women. In 15 percent of patients there is coexisting endometrial hyperplasia, and up to 29 percent of patients have endometrial carcinoma [1]. Although symptoms may be nonspecific, such as abdominal pain or discomfort, postmenopausal women with pure thecomas can present with postmenopausal bleeding. In contrast, pure fibromas are most common in women under the age 50 years, most of whom are asymptomatic. Ascites has been reported in some patients with ovarian fibroma. Meigs syndrome, which is ascites and right pleural effusion in the setting of ovarian fibroma, is very rare [1]. Fibrothecomas are treated by surgical excision.

The MRI appearance of fibromas and thecomas is similar: intermediate in signal intensity on T1-weighted images and very low in signal intensity on T2-weighted images (Fig. 15.20). Because their signal approximates nondegenerative leiomyomata, fibrothecomas may be difficult to distinguish from pedunculated fibroids. Use of multiple imaging planes combined with noting small follicular cysts surrounding the mass should establish the diagnosis of a solid ovarian neoplasm. Fibrothecomas show negligible enhancement following intravenous gadolinium [61].

Ovarian Torsion

Ovarian torsion has its highest incidence before puberty and during pregnancy [62]. An underlying adnexal mass, especially a dermoid, predisposes to ovarian torsion. Patients usually present with acute onset of abdominal pain but often have a history of episodic pain, which presumably reflects twisting and untwisting of the ovary. The degree of torsion is variable (i.e., it may involve only the vein, or it may involve both the artery and vein). Typically, venous flow is first compromised; the involved ovary becomes enlarged and congested. Arterial compromise results from edema and/or progressive twisting. If torsion is complete, gangrenous, hemorrhagic necrosis of the ovary and any underlying mass, if present, ensues. Complete torsion requires immediate surgical attention.

The largest MRI series to describe complete ovarian torsion in patients with an associated adnexal tumor reported three findings that were considered diagnostic: (1) an adnexal protrusion that was continuous with the uterus or to which engorged blood vessels converged, (2) thick straight blood vessels that draped around the lesion, and (3) complete absence of enhancement. The protrusion on the involved side is believed to be the

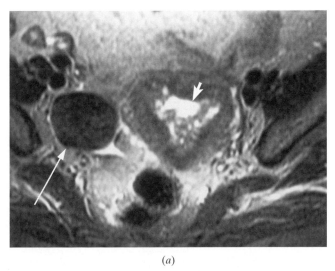

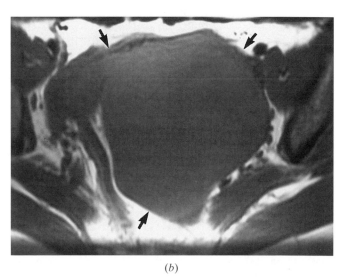

(a)   (b)

F i g . 15.20 Fibroma/thecoma. T2-weighted spin-echo image (*a*) demonstrates a 3-cm right ovarian fibroma (*long arrow, a*) that is well-defined and very low in signal intensity. Changes in the uterus (*arrow, a*) are due to adenomyosis and recent dilation and curettage for endometrial hyperplasia. T1-weighted spin-echo (*b*), sagittal 512-resolution T2-weighted echo-train spin-echo (*c*), and gadolinium-enhanced T1-weighted spin-echo (*d*) images in a second patient with ovarian fibroma.

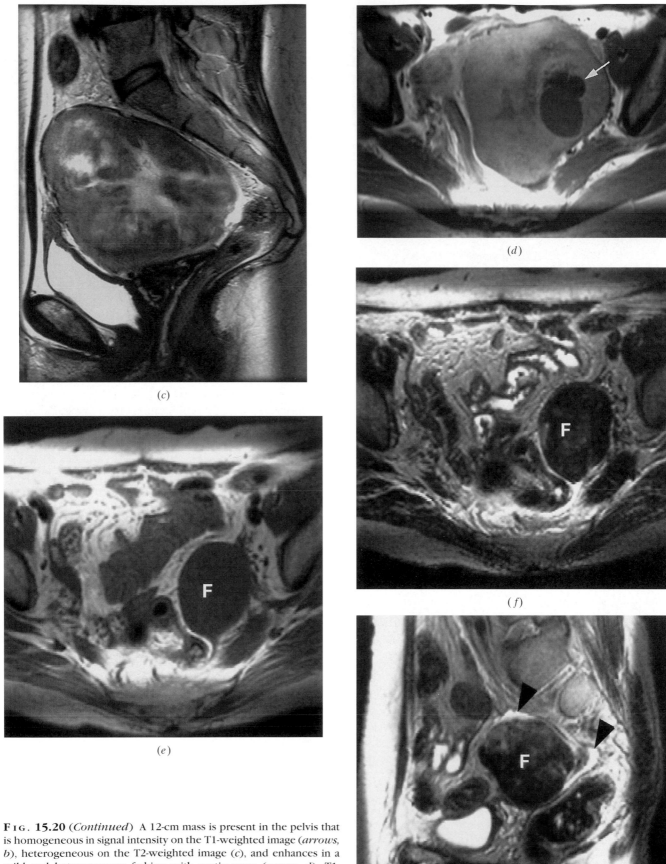

(c)

(d)

(e)

(f)

(g)

F I G . 15.20 (*Continued*) A 12-cm mass is present in the pelvis that is homogeneous in signal intensity on the T1-weighted image (*arrows, b*), heterogeneous on the T2-weighted image (*c*), and enhances in a mild and heterogeneous fashion with cystic areas (*arrow, d*). T1-weighted spin-echo (*e*) and transverse (*f*) and sagittal (*g*) T2-weighted echo-train spin-echo images in a third patient with a left ovarian fibroma ("*F*",*e–g*). The tumor is well-defined and low in signal intensity on T1-weighted (*e*) and T2-weighted (*f,g*) images. A small volume of pelvic fluid (*arrowheads, g*) is noted posterior and adjacent to the mass.

twisted edematous pedicle that connects the lesion with the uterus or engorged blood vessels. The second criteria reflects veins on the surface of the tumor distal to the torsion, whereas lack of enhancement indicates complete interruption to blood flow. An incomplete or partial torsion will still show some enhancement. The torsion knot is primarily low in signal intensity on T1- and T2-weighted images (Fig. 15.21), but may have scattered areas of high signal intensity representing hemorrhage and/or vascular congestion [23,63]. Others have observed a high-signal-intensity ring surrounding the adnexal mass on T1-weighted images, but this is nonspecific and can be seen with subacute hematoma from any cause [64]. Finally, the MRI appearance of massive ovarian edema, a forme fruste of ovarian torsion secondary to intermittent twisting, has been described. The ovary is markedly enlarged with high signal intensity on T2-weighted images [65]. In another report, massive ovarian edema mimicked

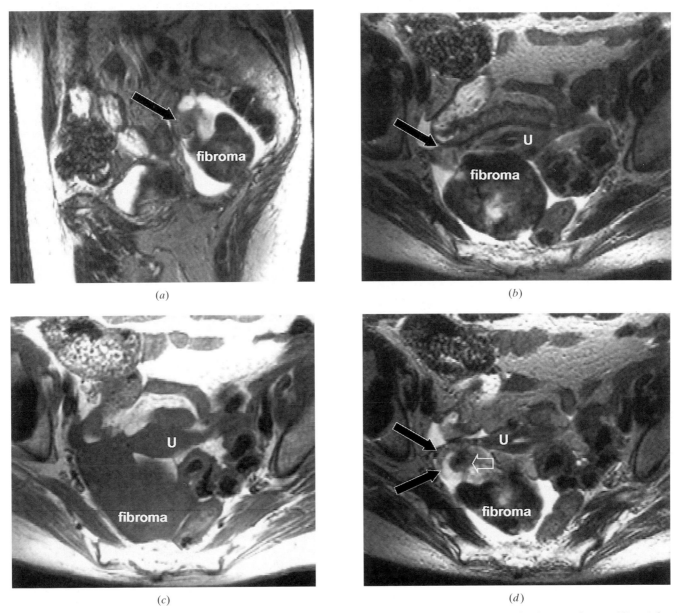

(a)   (b)

(c)   (d)

FIG. 15.21 Ovarian torsion. Sagittal (*a*) and transverse (*b*) T2-weighted echo-train spin-echo, T1-weighted spin-echo (*c*), T2-weighted echo-train spin-echo (*d*) and gadolinium-enhanced fat-suppressed SGE (*e*) images in a patient with pelvic pain. Unenhanced T1- and T2-weighted images show a primarily low-signal-intensity mass, that represents a fibroma in the cul de sac. The right fallopian tube is enlarged, edematous, and applied to the uterus; this appearance has been termed *protrusion* and is suggestive of torsion (*arrows, a,b,d,e*). Within the convoluted tube is the low-signal-intensity torsion knot (*open arrow, d*). Following contrast, the tube wall (*anterior arrow, e*), torsion knot (*posterior arrow, e*), and fibroma enhance, excluding complete arterial compromise. *u,* uterus. T1-weighted fat-suppressed spin-echo (*f*) and sagittal 512-resolution T2-weighted echo-train spin-echo (*g*) images in a second patient with ovarian torsion.

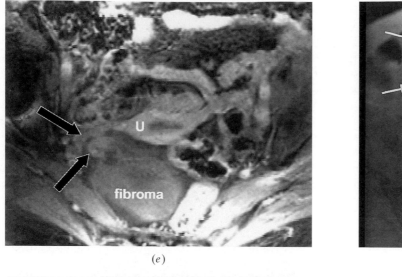

(e)

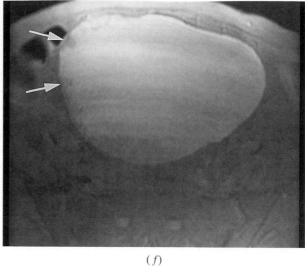

(f)

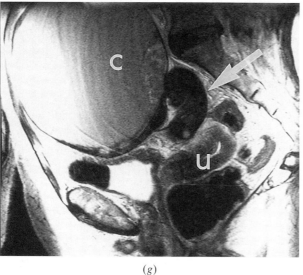

(g)

FIG. **15.21** (*Continued*) A large hemorrhagic cyst is shown on the T1-weighted fat-suppressed image that contains small peripheral excrescences (*arrows, f*). The sagittal plane image demonstrates a dilated blood-filled fallopian tube (*large arrow, g*). The low signal intensity of the blood is consistent with deoxyhemoglobin or intracellular methemoglobin reflecting acute blood. A gradation of signal intensity in the large hemorrhagic ovarian cyst is seen, representing layering of blood products. *u*, uterus, *c* cyst

a simple ovarian cyst on unenhanced spin-echo images [66].

Extrauterine Pregnancy

The incidence of ectopic pregnancy is increasing. The ovaries and fallopian tubes are the most common sites for an extrauterine gestation. Most ectopic pregnancies are diagnosed by transvaginal ultrasound with only a few anecdotal reports of the MRI features [67,68]. Theoretical advantages of MRI over transvaginal ultrasound include a larger field of view and superior spatial resolution. In one MRI report of patients with rare forms of ectopic pregnancy, an enhancing tree-like region within a hemorrhagic mass was identified. This area corresponded to villous-containing fibrin strands in a remnant of fetoplacental tissues and appeared to be a unique MRI finding in cases of ectopic pregnancy [69].

Malignant Masses

Primary Ovarian Carcinoma

Ovarian carcinoma is the leading cause of death from gynecologic cancer in the United States [70]. There are 24,000 new cases per year, and 13,600 women die annually from their disease [71]. The rate of ovarian cancer increases with age; 61 years is the median age at diagnosis. Although cancer of the ovary is more common in Caucasian women, recent trends indicate a slight decrease in their age-adjusted incidence rate compared with an increase in rate in African-American women. Epidemiologic studies have identified endocrine and genetic factors in the carcinogenesis of ovarian cancer. Recognized risk factors include lower parity, delayed onset of childbearing, infertility, and a positive family history. Birth control pills appear to be protective. Some environmental factors (industrial exposure to carcinogens) have been implicated in the development of ovarian cancer, but no unambiguous associations have been established [70]. The overall 5-year survival rate (37%) for ovarian cancer is poor. Survival depends on stage at diagnosis: 81 percent for localized disease versus 21 percent for spread outside the pelvis [70]. Unfortunately, most women present with advanced disease.

Most primary ovarian neoplasms are derived from either coelomic surface epithelium, ovarian stroma and/ or sex cords, or germ cells (Table 15.1 [72]). Tumors with ovarian histology may also arise from the peritoneal lining in patients status post bilateral oophorectomy. Surface epithelial tumors account for up to 75 percent of all ovarian neoplasms and up to 95 percent of malignant ovarian neoplasms [72]. The most common surface epithelial neoplasms include serous, mucinous, endometrioid, clear-cell and undifferentiated histologies. These epithelial tumors, except for the undifferentiated cell type, are further subdivided into benign lesions, borderline or low malignant potential (LMP) lesions, and overtly malignant lesions (carcinoma). Benign lesions have been discussed previously. Borderline neoplasms are a group of tumors that have an excellent prognosis despite some shared histologic features of cancer [70]. The absence of destructive growth (invasion) differentiates borderline tumors from their frankly cancerous counterparts. Of the sex cord-stromal tumors, granulosa-cell neoplasms have malignant potential. Tumors consisting of predominantly theca cells are invariably benign. Dysgerminomas, yolk-sac (endodermal sinus) tumors and immature teratomas are the malignant ovarian germ-cell tumors. A brief discussion of the different histological types of ovarian tumors follows.

Approximately 40 percent of serous tumors are either borderline lesions or frankly malignant, and as a group account for almost half of all ovarian malignancies [72]. Whereas bilaterality is seen in only 20 percent of patients with benign serous tumors, it is seen in 50 percent of malignant lesions. Microscopic and macroscopic papillary projections are characteristic, and psammoma bodies are seen in up to 30 percent of them [71]. The tumors are predominantly unilocular cysts, but solid elements, hemorrhage, and necrosis occur with increasing frequency in tumors with increasing atypia.

Mucinous ovarian cancer is an aggressive process, and spread beyond the ovary at initial presentation is not uncommon. Not surprisingly, these tumors tend to be the largest of the ovarian malignancies. Bilaterality is associated with higher stage disease. The tumors are multilocular with mucin-filled cysts of variable size. The septae separating the locules may be thick or thin. Solid elements, hemorrhage, and necrosis may all exist within a single specimen.

Endometrioid tumors invariably are invasive carcinomas. Unlike serous and mucinous cystadenocarcinomas, malignant tumors are bilateral in only 25 percent of cases [71]. They may arise de novo, but can also originate in foci of endometriosis. Although associated with endometrial hyperplasia or carcinoma in up to one third of cases, the prevailing assumption is that the ovarian tumor is an independent primary lesion and not a metastatic focus.

Table 15.1 Prevalence of Ovarian Tumors

Tumors of Surface Epithelium	Germ-Cell Tumors	Sex Cord-Stromal Tumors	Metastatic Tumors
General: 70–75% of all ovarian tumors, 95% of malignant ovarian tumors	General: 15–20% of all ovarian tumors, 1% of all malignant ovarian tumors	General: 10% of all ovarian tumors, 2% of all malignant ovarian tumors	General: 5% of all ovarian tumors (common primaries: gastrointestinal, breast, lymphatic, and pelvic)
Serous tumors (60% are benign): 30% of all ovarian tumors, 40% of all malignant tumors	Benign teratoma: 95% of all germ-cell tumors	Granulosa and thecal-cell tumors: 5% of all ovarian tumors	
Mucinous tumors (80% are benign): 20–25% of all ovarian tumors, 10% of all malignant tumors	Dysgerminoma: 2% of all malignant ovarian tumors, 50% of malignant germ-cell tumors		
Endometrioid carcinoma: 20% of all malignant tumors	Endodermal sinus tumor: second most common malignant germ cell tumor		
	Immature teratoma: very rare		

The tumors are typically a mixture of cystic and solid elements, although occasionally a purely solid lesion is found. Papillary projections are relatively infrequent.

Clear-cell neoplasms are similar to endometrioid tumors in that they are nearly all invasive. That fact notwithstanding, their prognosis is better than that for patients with other ovarian cancers, and most women present with local disease. Unlike clear-cell carcinoma of the cervix or vagina, they are not associated with in utero exposure to diethylstilbestrol (DES) [71]. The tumors are frequently unilocular with mural nodules and grossly may mimic a serous neoplasm. Clear-cell carcinoma has the lowest frequency of bilaterality, 13 percent [70].

Undifferentiated carcinomas cannot be categorized into one of the aforementioned groups, but they most closely resemble serous or endometrioid carcinoma. Patients with undifferentiated ovarian cancer have the poorest outcome of any of the epithelial neoplasms and present with widespread disease.

Granulosa-cell tumors arise from sex cord-stromal cells and are divided into two subtypes: the adult form that occurs in post menopausal women and the much rarer juvenile form that occurs in prepubertal girls and young women. These neoplasms elaborate estrogen causing sexual precocity in girls, menorrhagia or irregular bleeding in reproductive-aged women, and resumption of menses in postmenopausal women. Endometrial hyperplasia and/or polyps may result from increased estrogen levels. Moreover, up to 15 percent of postmenopausal women with this tumor have a simultaneous endometrial carcinoma [61]. In rare instances, a granulosa-cell tumor will produce androgens and cause virilization. Malignant tumors tend to recur locally, as late as 10 years after initial removal.

Of the germ-cell malignancies, dysgerminoma is the most common and occurs in adolescents and young adults. They are usually solid, and 80 percent are unilateral. Similar to their seminoma counterpart, these tumors are radiosensitive. Endodermal sinus tumors have an age distribution similar to that of dysgerminomas and are also solid. The tumor is aggressive with rapid growth and a poor prognosis. Immature teratomas are rare. Unlike the mature forms with recognizable adult elements, the tumor is composed of embryonic elements. It favors early transgression of the ovary, and most patients have invasion into adjacent organs and distant metastases at the time of clinical presentation.

Lack of a discrete ovarian capsule facilitates tumor spread. Up to 85 percent of patients with epithelial ovarian carcinoma have peritoneal disease at the time of initial presentation [70]. Exfoliated cancer cells follow the normal circulation of peritoneal fluid. Although the cells favor the right subdiaphragmatic region for implantation, all intraperitoneal surfaces including the omentum (e.g., "omental cake") and serosa are at risk. In addition to exfoliation and implantation, disease spreads via the retroperitoneal lymphatics that drain the ovary. Lymphatics follow the ovarian blood supply, and malignant cells lodge in the para-aortic lymph nodes up to the level of the renal hilum. Lymph channels also promote spread laterally through the broad ligament and parametrium to terminate in the lymph nodes of the external iliac, obturator, and hypogastric chains. Lymph node involvement correlates with stage of disease. Spread of sex cord-stromal and germ-cell tumors is similar.

Most patients present with abdominal pain and distension due to malignant ascites and/or a large intra-abdominal mass. Nonspecific gastrointestinal and genitourinary symptoms may also be reported. Patients are surgically staged according to the Federation International of Gynecology and Obstetrics (FIGO) system (Table 15.2 [23]). Complete surgical staging includes total abdominal hysterectomy with bilateral salpingo-oophorectomy, retroperitoneal and para-aortic lymph node

Table 15.2 FIGO Staging of Primary Ovarian Carcinoma

Stage	Description
I	Tumor limited to the ovaries
IA	Tumor limited to one ovary No tumor on the external surface; capsule intact Tumor present on the external surface, and/or capsule ruptured
IB	Tumor limited to both ovaries; no ascites No tumor on the external surface; capsules intact Tumor present on the external surface, and/or capsule ruptured
IC	Tumor at either stage IA or IB, but with obvious ascites present or positive peritoneal washings
II	Tumor involving one or both ovaries with pelvic extension
IIA	Extension and/or metastases to the uterus and/or fallopian tubes
IIB	Extension to other pelvic tissues
IIC	Tumor at either stage IIA or stage IIB, but with obvious ascites present or positive peritoneal washings
III	Tumor involving ovaries with intraperitoneal metastases outside the pelvis, and/or positive retroperitoneal nodes
IV	Growth involving ovaries, with distant metastases or Pleural effusion is present, with positive cytology or Metastasis to liver parenchyma

sampling, omental excision, peritoneal and diaphragmatic biopsies, and cytologic evaluation of peritoneal washings. Although 5-year survival correlates with tumor stage, differences have been reported in survival rates for patients with the same FIGO stage. This likely reflects inadequacies in surgical staging with many cases being understaged [73,74]. This limitation notwithstanding, laparotomy remains the preferred staging modality. Additionally, it allows for simultaneous tumor debulking, which has both therapeutic and prognostic significance.

Treatment options for patients with ovarian cancer include cytoreductive surgery, chemotherapy, radiotherapy, or a combination thereof. Unfortunately, most patients with advanced disease are incurable regardless of treatment approach. Residual disease after initial surgery and tumor grade are the most important prognostic factors, though FIGO stage, age, and histologic tumor subtype also affect outcome. Routine second-look surgery is controversial. In the strictest sense, second-look laparotomy refers to systematic reexploration of the peritoneal cavity and retroperitoneum in asymptomatic patients who have completed a planned course of chemotherapy. Advocates cite that the majority of patients with no clinical or radiographic evidence of disease still have cancer at reexploration [70]. Yet, there is no evidence that second-look surgery is a therapeutic procedure. Furthermore, there is no evidence that any form of subsequent therapy prolongs survival [75]. Recently, the National Institutes of Health consensus conference took a firm stand, stating that *routine* second-look surgery is no longer recommended [76]. The only group that benefits from reexploration are those with microscopic or minimal disease; patients with recurrent disease greater than 2 cm are not surgical candidates [77]. These findings underscore the need for a noninvasive test that reliably identifies patients known not to benefit from reoperation [77].

MRI has been found to be at least equivalent and in some cases superior to CT imaging for the evaluation of ovarian malignancy [78]. Ovarian cancer has a variable appearance on MRI: It may be entirely cystic or entirely solid, but it is usually a combination of the two. Most tumors are low to intermediate in signal intensity on T1-weighted sequences and high in signal intensity on T2-weighted sequences. Gadolinium administration facilitates detection of solid and necrotic elements and omental and peritoneal implants, especially when used in combination with fat-suppressed SGE (Fig. 15.22). Malignant ascites is present in cases of advanced disease and may enhance on late postcontrast images [79].

MRI findings are not specific for any particular cell type, but some imaging features are more typical of one histology than another. For example, the presence of papillary projections suggests a serous cystadenocarcinoma. Papillae appear as intermediate-signal-intensity excrescences within a cystic lesion and enhance follow-

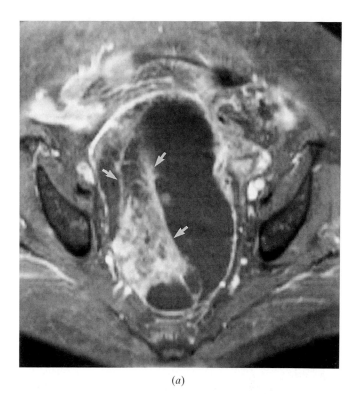

(a)

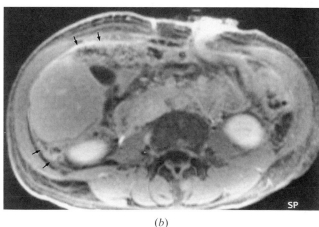

(b)

FIG. 15.22 Metastatic ovarian carcinoma. Gadolinium-enhanced T1-weighted fat-suppressed spin-echo (*a*) and gadolinium-enhanced fat-suppressed SGE (*b*) images in two women with pelvic masses. The combination of fat suppression and intravenous gadolinium highlights the internal architecture of cystic masses. A predominance of enhancing solid elements (*arrows, a*) favors malignancy. This technique is also useful for demonstrating small peritoneal-based metastases (*arrows, b*). (Part *a* is reprinted with permission from Semelka RC, Lawrence PH, Shoenut JP, et al: Primary ovarian cancer: Prospective comparison of contrast-enhanced CT and pre- and postcontrast, fat-suppressed MR imaging with histologic correlation. J Magn Reson Imaging 3:99–106, 1993)

ing contrast (Fig. 15.23). Mucinous tumors of the ovary may mimic multiple simple cysts, but frequently they have imaging features similar to those of mucin-laden tumors elsewhere: intermediate to high in signal intensity on T1- and T2-weighted images. Hemorrhage within portions of the tumor is not infrequent. The septae between cysts enhance after contrast (Fig. 15.24). Pseudomyxoma peritonei is a complication of mucin-producing tumors, generally of low malignant potential. Locules of variable-signal-intensity mucin coat the peritoneal and serosal surfaces and may indent adjacent structures. The MRI findings of pseudomyxoma peritonei from a mucinous ovarian neoplasm are indistinguishable from those of

pseudomyxoma peritonei secondary to a ruptured mucin-producing appendiceal tumor (see Chapter 7 on the Peritonal Cavity). Clear cell carcinomas tend to be large unilocular masses with solid mural elements (Fig. 15.25).

In contradistinction to epithelial ovarian tumors, granulosa-cell tumors are predominantly solid lobulated adnexal lesions. On T1-weighted images they are intermediate in signal intensity and become heterogeneously

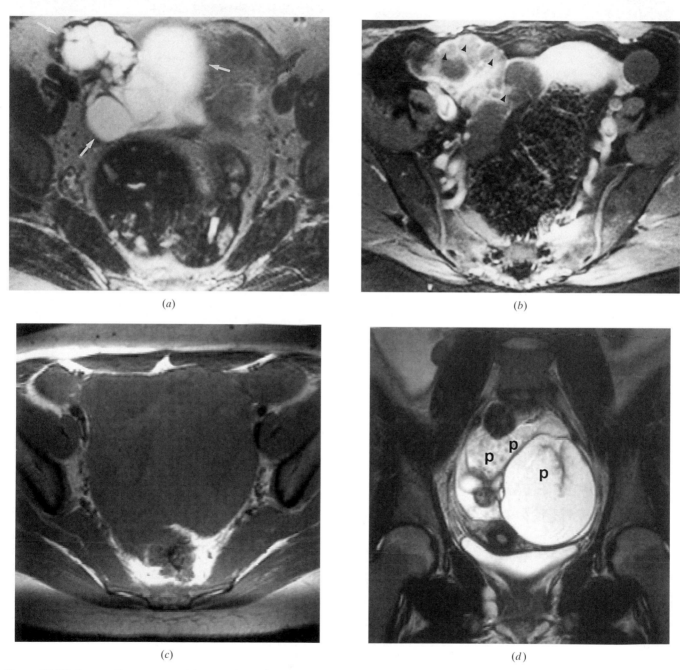

(a)

(b)

(c)

(d)

FIG. 15.23 Low malignant potential serous cystadenocarcinoma. T2-weighted echo-train spin-echo (*a*) and gadolinium-enhanced fat-suppressed SGE (*b*) images in women with a right adnexal mass. A lobulated mass replaces the right ovary (*arrows, a*). Following contrast, small internal papillary projections (*arrowheads, b*) enhance, which is a characteristic of low malignant potential (borderline) neoplasms. Transverse T1-weighted (*c*), coronal (*d*) and transverse (*e*) T2-weighted echo-train, and gadolinium-enhanced T1-weighted (*f*) spin-echo images in a second patient, a 19-year-old woman with a low malignant potential serous tumor.

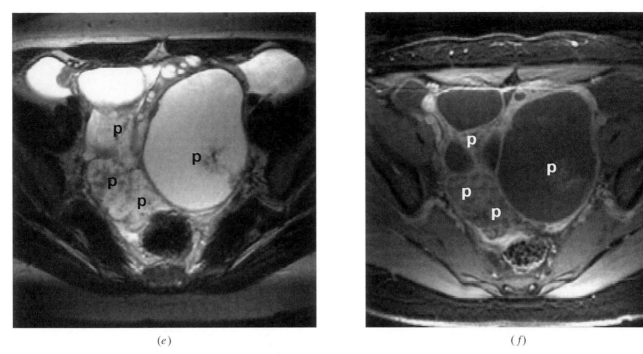

(e)   (f)

F IG. 15.23 (*Continued*) Complex bilateral adnexal masses are noted. The T2-weighted images suggest the presence of papillary (*"p",d-f*) projections. After gadolinium administration, the papillary projections show marked enhancement (*"p",f*). Contrast administration helps to differentiate between vascularized solid elements and debris within cystic masses.

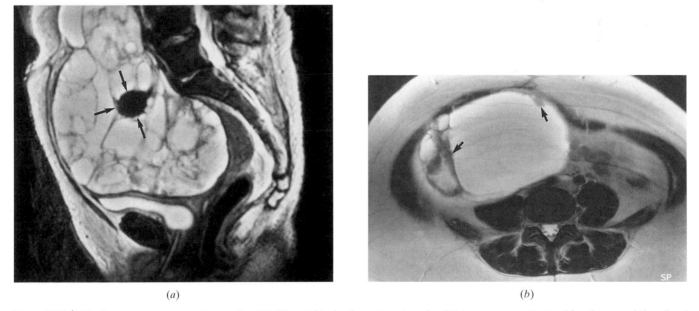

(a)   (b)

F IG. 15.24 Mucinous cystadenocarcinoma. Sagittal T2-weighted echo-train spin-echo (*a*) image in a patient with a large multiloculated mucinous cystadenocarcinoma. One of the locules is complicated by hemorrhage; intracellular methemoglobin is low in signal intensity on T2-weighted images (*arrows, a*). Hemorrhage into a tumor locule is common with mucinous neoplasms. Transverse 512-resolution T2-weighted echo-train spin-echo (*b*), coronal HASTE (*c*) and transverse gadolinium-enhanced fat-suppressed SGE (*d*) images in a patient with advanced mucinous ovarian cancer. A large cystic mass with septations and nodules (*arrows, b*) is applied to the uterus (*arrow, c*).

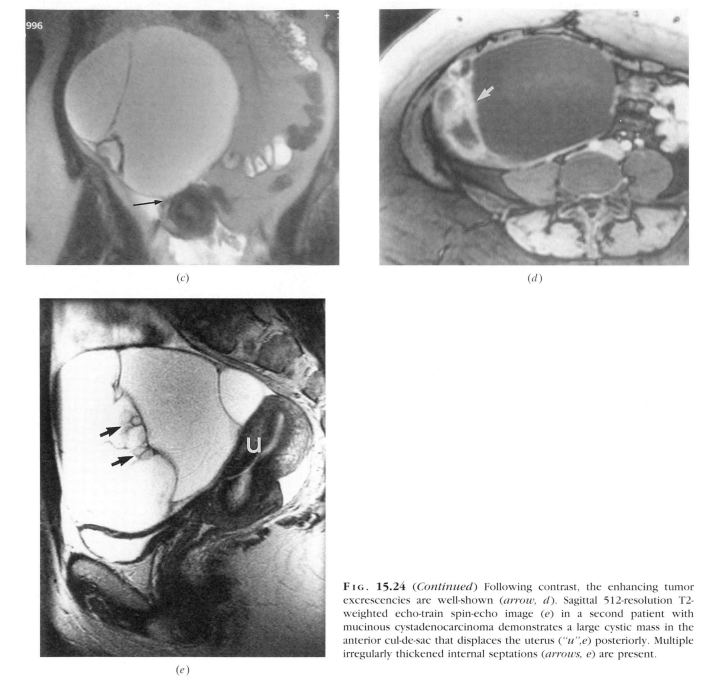

(c)

(d)

(e)

FIG. 15.24 (*Continued*) Following contrast, the enhancing tumor excrescencies are well-shown (*arrow, d*). Sagittal 512-resolution T2-weighted echo-train spin-echo image (*e*) in a second patient with mucinous cystadenocarcinoma demonstrates a large cystic mass in the anterior cul-de-sac that displaces the uterus (*"u",e*) posteriorly. Multiple irregularly thickened internal septations (*arrows, e*) are present.

high in signal intensity on T2-weighted images. After contrast, the solid elements enhance and small necrotic foci stand out as signal-void areas (Fig. 15.26). Granulosa-cell tumors have a propensity for local invasion. Sacral involvement is not uncommon and is well-shown on sagittal and paracoronal images. Germ-cell tumors have a variable appearance, but are often quite large due to their aggressive nature (Fig. 15.27). Small amounts of fat should suggest the diagnosis of an immature teratoma.

The strengths of MRI lie in its ability to determine the origin of a pelvic mass [12,80], and, if it is ovarian, to further classify it into neoplastic versus nonneoplastic and malignant versus benign (Fig. 15.28). Studies report accuracy rates of 60 to 99 percent for such determinations [8,34,81–83]. For characterizing an adnexal mass as malignant, primary and ancillary criteria have been established. In one study statistical analysis yielded the following five significant criteria of malignancy: (1) size larger than 4

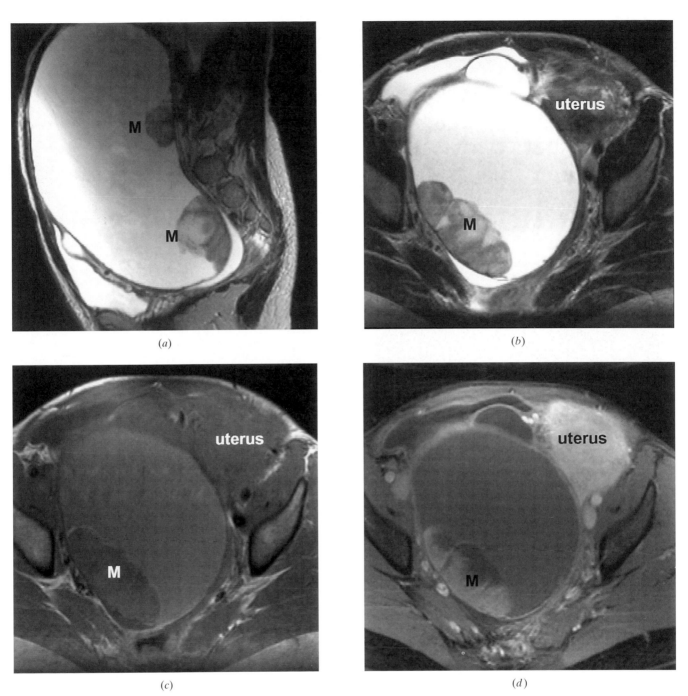

F I G. **15.25** Clear cell carcinoma. Sagittal (*a*) and transverse (*b*) T2-weighted echo-train spin-echo, T1-weighted spin-echo (*c*) and gadolinium-enhanced fat-suppressed SGE (*d*) images in a 51-year-old woman with an ovarian mass. A large primarily unilocular cystic lesion with peripheral masses ("*M*",*a*–*c*) arises from the pelvis. The masses enhance following contrast ("*M*",*d*). This appearance is typical of clear-cell carcinoma.

cm, (2) solid mass or large solid component, (3) wall thickness greater than 3 mm, (4) septa thicker than 3 mm and/or presence of vegetations or nodularity, and (5) necrosis. Four ancillary criteria of malignancy were also statistically formulated in this study: (1) involvement of pelvic organs or side wall; (2) peritoneal, mesenteric, or omental disease; (3) ascites; or (4) adenopathy. When gadolinium-enhanced T1-weighted and unenhanced T1- and T2-weighted images were collectively analyzed, the presence of at least one of the primary criteria coupled with a single criterion from the ancillary group correctly characterized 95 percent of malignant lesions (Fig. 15.29)

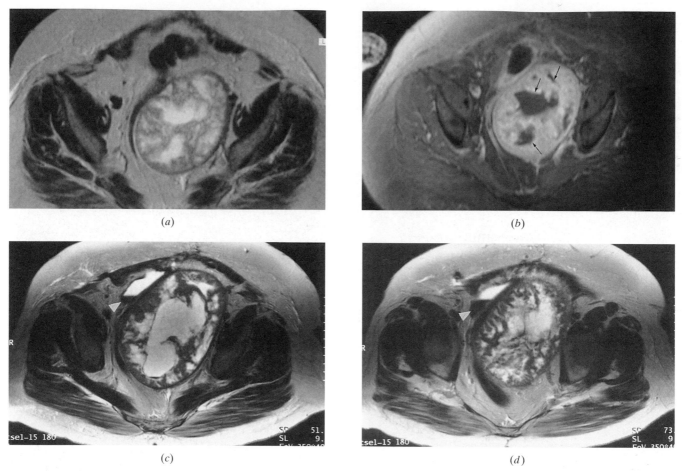

FIG. 15.26 Granulosa cell tumor. T2-weighted echo-train spin-echo (*a*), gadolinium-enhanced fat-suppressed SGE (*b*) images in a woman with a granulosa-cell ovarian tumor. The tumor is heterogeneous on the T2-weighted image, and following contrast the solid elements enhance. Necrotic foci interspersed in an otherwise solid mass is a common feature of granulosa-cell tumors (*arrows, b*). Transverse 512-resolution T2-weighted echo-train spin-echo (*c,d*) images 9 months later show interval growth of tumor and increasing necrosis. Note that the bladder is displaced anterolaterally by the mass. Low signal intensity in the dependent portion of the bladder reflects excreted concentrated gadolinium (*arrowhead, c,d*).

[84]. These rates reflect improvements in lesion characterization associated with intravenous contrast, and have been reproduced by others [78,85]

The role of MRI in evaluating an adnexal mass is emerging. Currently, patients with a pelvic mass on physical exam and/or transvaginal sonography usually undergo additional noninvasive testing to assess for malignancy including serum tumor markers (CA-125), duplex Doppler ultrasound, and immunoscintigraphy or CT imaging or MRI. CA-125 is the most useful commercially available marker for epithelial ovarian cancer. Its strength is in monitoring patient response to therapy. It performs less well in the workup of a new mass [86]. In postmenopausal women with an asymptomatic pelvic mass, an elevated serum CA-125 (>65 U/mL) is only 78 percent specific for ovarian cancer. Specificity is lower for premenopausal women because pregnancy, uterine fibroids,

endometriosis, and pelvic inflammatory disease can all cause CA-125 elevation [87]. Duplex ultrasound also suffers from high false positive rates [88–90]. A prospective study comparing duplex transvaginal ultrasound, MRI, and serum CA-125 levels reported that the highest accuracy was achieved with MRI [23]. Two other studies comparing transvaginal ultrasound to contrast-enhanced MRI for characterizing adnexal masses found that the accuracy of MRI was significantly better than for transvaginal ultrasound: 95 versus 88 percent and 99 versus 68 percent, respectively [81,82]. Another prospective study reported that MRI was more accurate than ultrasound or CT imaging in differentiating benign from malignant tumors [83]. In comparison to immunoscintigraphy, MRI had a higher sensitivity for detecting individual sites of tumor: 81 versus 50 percent, respectively [91].

For staging purposes, including lymph node assess-

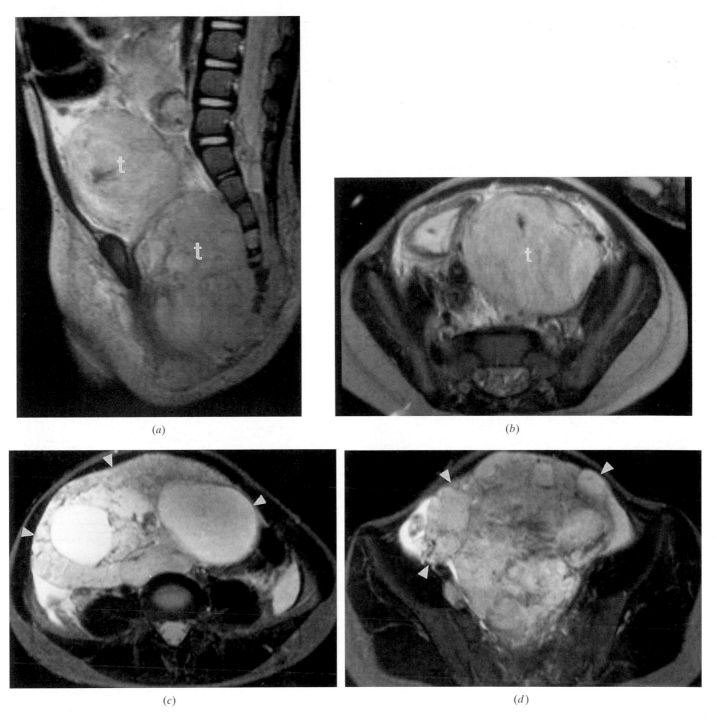

(a)

(b)

(c)

(d)

F IG. 15.27 Germ cell carcinomas. Sagittal (*a*) and transverse (*b*) T2-weighted echo-train spin-echo images in a young girl with an endodermal sinus tumor. A large tumor originated in the ovary but has spread contiguously into the abdomen and spine (*t,a,b*). These tumors tend to be solid and are very aggressive, with rapid growth and a poor prognosis. T2-weighted fat suppressed echo-train spin-echo (*c,d*) and contrast-enhanced fat-suppressed SGE (*e,f*) images in a second patient who has an abdominopelvic immature teratoma. A complex cystic and solid mass occupies the abdomen and pelvis (*arrowheads, c–f*). Immature teratomas are composed of amorphous embryonic elements. This accounts for their markedly disorganized appearance and contrasts with the more regular and recognizable elements associated with mature teratomas. T1-weighted spin-echo (*g*), T2-weighted echo-train spin-echo (*h*), T1-weighted fat-suppressed SGE (*i*), and gadolinium-enhanced T1-weighted fat-suppressed SGE (*j*) images in third patient who has complex right adnexal masses. The two masses have variable amounts of fatty elements, which are high in signal intensity on the conventional T1-weighted spin-echo image and suppress on the fat-suppressed images (*short arrows, g,i*). Note that some of the high-signal-intensity foci in the larger mass retain their high signal intensity on the fat-suppressed images, which is consistent with coexisting hemorrhage (*long arrow, g,i*). The smaller posterior mass shows nearly complete suppression on the fat-suppressed image (*arrowheads, i*). Following contrast, there is a profusion of solid tissue enhancing in the larger mass (*open arrows, j*). The smaller mass does not enhance appreciably, which is consistent with a cystic structure (*arrowheads, j*).

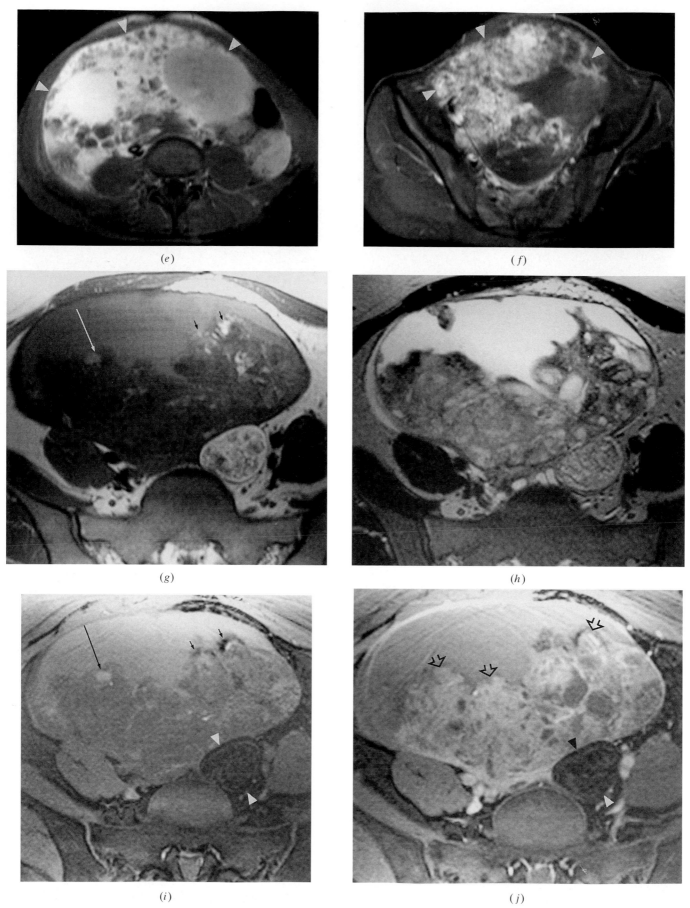

(e)

(f)

(g)

(h)

(i)

(j)

F IG . 15.27 (*Continued*) Extensive solid elements in a fat-containing mass are atypical of a dermoid cyst and should raise the suspicion of an immature teratoma. This was proven at surgery, whereas the posterolateral mass turned out to be a mature teratoma (dermoid cyst). (*g–j* were reprinted with permission from Outwater EK, Dunton CJ: Imaging of the ovary and adnexa: Clinical issues and applications of MR imaging. Radiology 194:1–18, 1992)

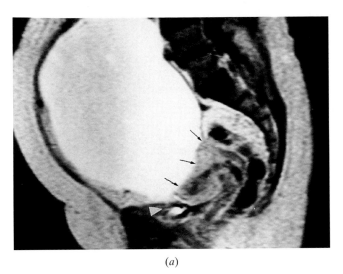
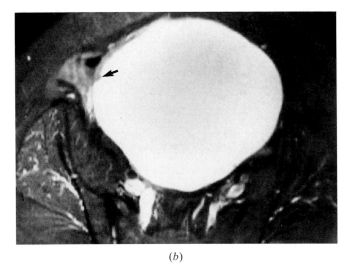

(a) (b)

FIG. 15.28 Ovarian carcinoma. Sagittal 90-second postgadolinium SGE (*a*) and gadolinium-enhanced T1-weighted fat-suppressed spin-echo (*b*) images. A high-signal-intensity lesion on both nonsuppressed (*a*) and fat suppressed (*b*) images accurately characterizes its hemorrhagic contents. The sagittal plane delineates the relationship of the mass to the uterus (*arrows, a*) and bladder (*arrowhead, a*). Multiplanar MR images are superior to other cross-sectional studies in defining the origin of a pelvic mass and its relationship to adjacent structures. Note the mural nodule along the sidewall (*arrow, b*). (Reprinted with permission from Semelka RC, Lawrence PH, Shoenut JP, et al: Primary ovarian cancer: Prospective comparison of contrast-enhanced CT and pre- and postcontrast, fat-suppressed MR imaging with histologic correlation. J Magn Reson Imaging 3:99–106, 1993)

ment, MRI using T1-weighted, T2-weighted, and gadolinium-enhanced T1-wieghted spin-echo sequences perform moderately well with an overall accuracy of 77 percent and is comparable to CT imaging (Figs. 15.30 and 15.31) [92]. Contrast-enhanced breath-hold T1-weighted fat-suppressed SGE technique outperforms unenhanced spin-echo techniques [93]. Specifically, MRI reliably demonstrates the primary tumor as well as macroscopic (>1 cm) metastases to the peritoneum, omentum, and bowel (Fig. 15.32) [78,93]. Enhancement of ascites on delayed images (15 minutes after contrast) suggests peritoneal

carcinomatosis [79]. MRI has proven to be an excellent predictor of nonresectability, with positive and negative predictive values of 91 and 97 percent, respectively [92]. Detection of small mesenteric and bowel implants remains problematic. Currently MRI cannot replace staging laparotomy, but it can identify patients with significant recurrent disease in whom reexploration may not be beneficial (Fig. 15.33). Accuracies of up to 83.3 percent for detecting recurrence have been reported [94]. In another study using recurrent tumor longer than 2 cm as indicative of inoperability, MRI was 82 percent accurate in

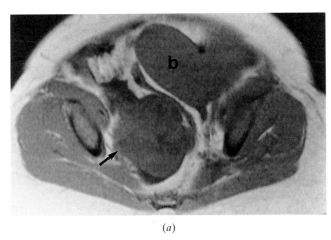
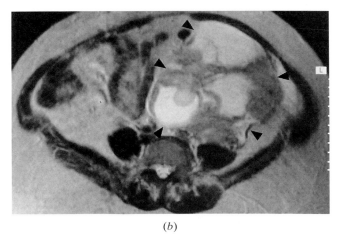

(a) (b)

FIG. 15.29 Ovarian carcinoma. SGE (*a*), 512-resolution T2-weighted echo-train spin-echo (*b,c*), transverse (*d*), and coronal (*e*) gadolinium-enhanced SGE images and MIP MR urogram (*f*) in a patient with ovarian cancer. A primarily solid mass is seen in the pelvis (*arrow, a,c*), whereas a more cystic mass (*arrowheads, b*) is noted in the left lower abdomen. Gadolinium enhancement improves identification of the solid components (*arrow, d,e*).

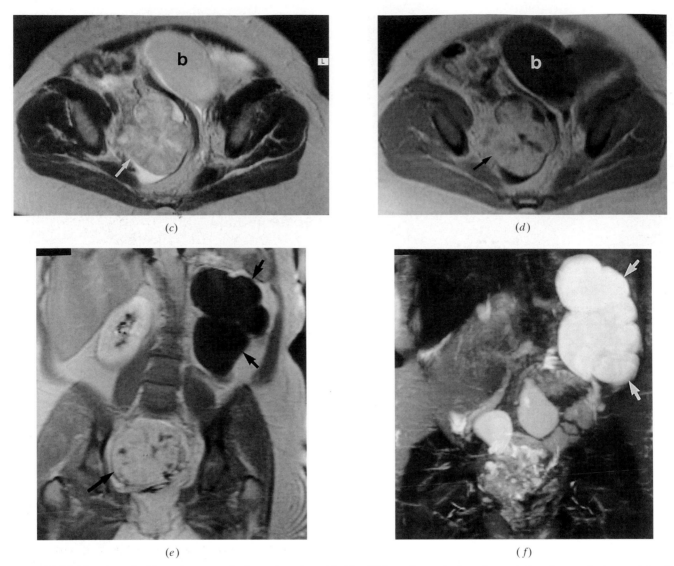

FIG. 15.29 (*Continued*) The pelvic mass displaces the urinary bladder (*"b",a,c,d*) anteriorly and superiorly, whereas the lower abdominal mass compresses the ureter. Dilation of the intrarenal collection system is well-shown on the postcontrast coronal SGE image and the MIP reconstruction (*short arrows, e,f*).

stratifying which patients would not benefit from second-look surgery [95].

Other Primary Tumors

Virtually any type of soft tissue tumor can arise in the ovary. Leiomyoma is the most common mesenchymal neoplasm, but leiomyosarcoma is sometimes observed. Other primary ovarian sarcomas are rare.

Primary extranodal ovarian lymphoma is a controversial entity. Normally, the ovary lacks lymphocytes, but rare cases of primary ovarian lymphoma have been reported [1]. Extrapolating from descriptions of extranodal lymphoma elsewhere in the body, primary ovarian lymphoma would be expected to be a primarily solid homogeneous intermediate-signal-intensity mass on T1-weighted images that is mildly hyperintense on T2-weighted images.

Metastases

Metastases to the ovaries account for 10 percent of all ovarian malignancies. In decreasing order of frequency, the most common primary tumors to involve the ovaries are gastrointestinal, pancreas, breast, and uterine carcinomas [96]. Functioning ovaries are at increased risk for metastatic disease. Several modes of spread exist: lymphatic or hematogenous route, serosal implantation of exfoliated malignant cells, or contiguous extension from adjacent organs. The term Krukenberg's tumor is reserved for metastases to the ovaries in which malignant signet-ring cells invade an abundant and hypercellular stroma

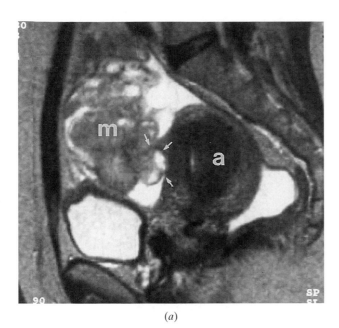
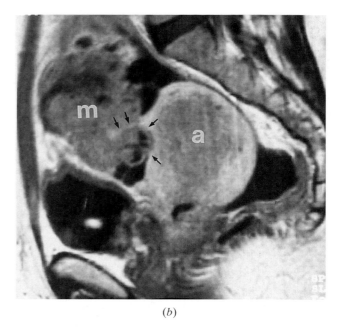

(a)   (b)

F IG. 15.30 Stage II serous cystadenocarcinoma. Sagittal T2-weighted (*a*) and gadolinium-enhanced T1-weighted (*b*) spin-echo images. A complex mass ("*m*",*a,b*) is anterior to, but also indents the uterus (*arrows, a*). Following contrast the solid elements, including the masses scalloping the uterus (*arrows, b*), enhance. There is a moderate amount of ascites. Serous adenocarcinoma is usually unilocular, but solid elements, hemorrhage, and necrosis occur with increasing frequency with higher grade tumors. Incidental note is made of adenomyosis ("*a*",*a,b*) affecting the posterior uterine corpus.

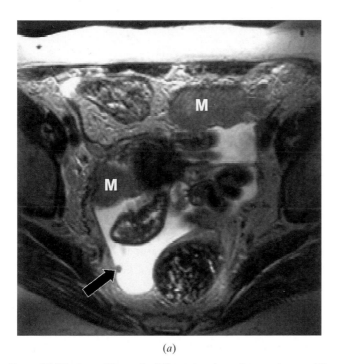
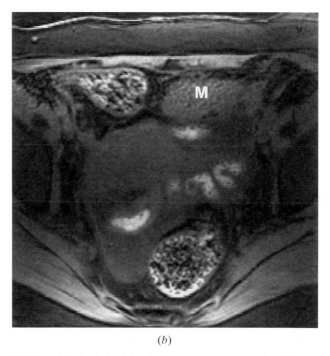

(a)   (b)

F IG. 15.31 Stage III poorly differentiated ovarian carcinoma. T2-weighted echo-train (*a*), T1-weighted fat-suppressed (*b*), and gadolinium-enhanced T1-weighted fat suppressed (*c*) spin-echo images in a 69-year-old woman with advanced ovarian carcinoma. The peritoneum is diffusely thickened and has superimposed nodules (*arrow, a*). Peritoneal metastases are most conspicuous in the setting of ascites on T2-weighted images (*arrow, a*) and following contrast administration on T1-weighted fat-suppressed images (*arrows, c*).

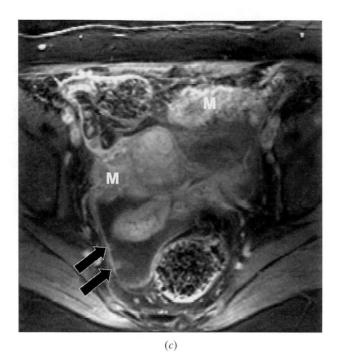

(c)

FIG. 15.31 (*Continued*) Note the larger metastatic masses distributed in the pelvis ("*M*",*a*-*c*). Contrast-enhanced T1-weighted fat-suppressed technique increases staging accuracy of ovarian carcinomas.

[1]. The offending neoplasm is usually gastric in origin, but breast, colon, pancreas, and gallbladder carcinomas can all give rise to this type of ovarian metastasis. Krukenberg's tumor has a poor prognosis, with a 90 percent mortality rate 1 year after discovery of ovarian masses [92]. Grossly, the ovaries are enlarged but retain an ovoid or reniform shape. The tumors are usually solid, but cystic areas are not uncommon. Involvement is typically bilateral.

Ovarian lymphoma is usually part of a disseminated disease process. Tumors vary in size but on the average are large (15 cm). In the majority of patients there is bilateral involvement (Fig. 15.34). Microscopically, lymphoma that involves the ovary is of the non-Hodgkin type: small noncleaved cell, which is most common in children and young adults; or large cell, which is most common in adults. Because ovarian disease usually signals widespread involvement, patients undergo combination therapy: tumor excision and chemotherapy and/or radiotherapy.

In most instances, the MRI findings of metastases to the ovary are nonspecific, underscoring the need for clinical history in evaluating adnexal masses (Fig. 15.35). The largest series to the present describing the MRI appearance of Krukenberg's tumors found that most were bilateral, oval-shaped, solid masses with sharp margins (Fig. 15.36). An unusual feature on T2-weighted images was peripheral or randomly distributed low signal inten-

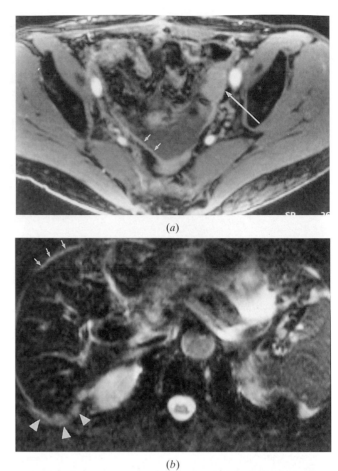

(a)

(b)

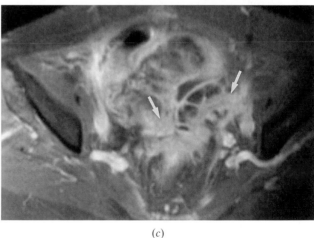

(c)

FIG. 15.32 Peritoneal-based metastases. Gadolinium-enhanced fat-suppressed SGE (*a*) image in a woman with ovarian cancer metastatic to the peritoneum. The involved peritoneum enhances and is thickened (short arrows, a). A larger discrete peritoneal-based mass is also identified (*long arrow, a*). T2-weighted fat-suppressed echo-train spin-echo (*b*) and gadolinium-enhanced fat-suppressed SGE (*c*) images in a second patient with diffuse disease. Note the metastatic thickening of the peritoneum surrounding the liver (*short arrows, b*). Tumor nodules indent and scallop the posterior aspect of the right lobe of the liver (*arrowheads, b*). Following contrast, peritoneal disease in the pelvis enhances (*arrows, c*). The combination of fat suppression and gadolinium is the most sensitive technique for assessing peritoneal based metastases.

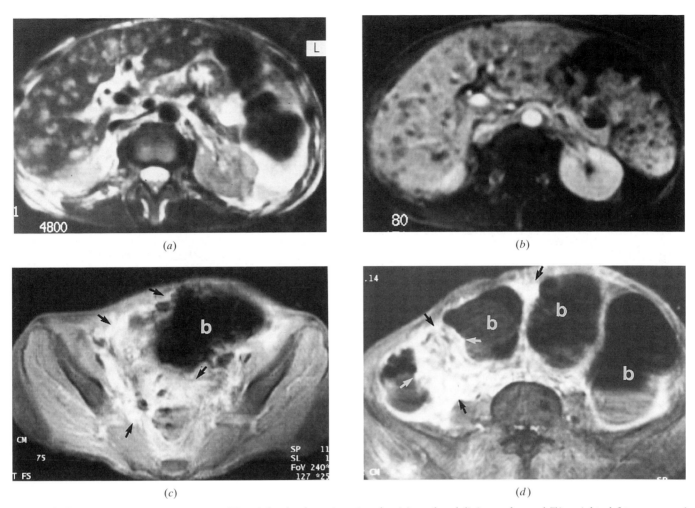

(a)

(b)

(c)

(d)

F IG. 15.33 Recurrent ovarian carcinoma. T2-weighted echo-train spin-echo (*a*), and gadolinium-enhanced T1-weighted fat-suppressed spin-echo (*b*) and fat-suppressed SGE (*c,d*) images in a patient with a history of ovarian carcinoma status posttransabdominal hysterectomy, bilateral oophorectomy, omentectomy, lymphadenectomy, peritoneal sampling, and adjuvant chemotherapy. The patient presented with complaints of bowel obstruction. Diffuse liver metastases and dilated loops of bowel (*"b",c,d*) are identified. Enhancing recurrent ovarian cancer of the peritoneum and serosa encases the colon (*arrows, c,d*) and causes distal large bowel obstruction. MRI is useful for identifying which patients may benefit from second-look surgery. No therapeutic benefit for patients with recurrent disease greater than 2 cm have been demonstrated, although debulking surgery may provide symptomatic relief.

sity that corresponded histopathologically to dense collagenous stroma. This imaging finding is rare in primary ovarian neoplasm, and when present should suggest the diagnosis of Krukenberg's tumor [97]. After gadolinium administration, the solid elements in Krukenberg's tumors enhance.

INFLAMMATION

Pelvic Inflammatory Disease/Tubo-Ovarian Abscess (PID/TOA)

Pelvic inflammatory disease (PID) is the generic term applied to many pelvic infections. It is relatively common: an estimated 1 million American women have PID each year [98]. Although antibiotics have modified the clinical and pathological aspects of this condition, it remains responsible for a significant percentage of cases of secondary sterility by occlusion or stenosis. The frequency of PID is inversely proportional to improved hygiene and socioeconomic status. The use of an intrauterine device (IUD) increases the risk of PID: up to 50 percent of PID patients have been IUD wearers [99]. Ascending infection is the mechanism of spread, and organisms that have been implicated include chlamydia trachomatis, *Neisseria gonorrhoeae*, bacteroides, and both gram-positive and gram-negative aerobic and anaerobic bacteria. One group of investigators has reported Actinomyces as the offending organism in up to 87 percent of patients with IUDs who have PID [100]. Tubo-ovarian abscess (TOA) is a well-recognized complication of PID. It occurs in the

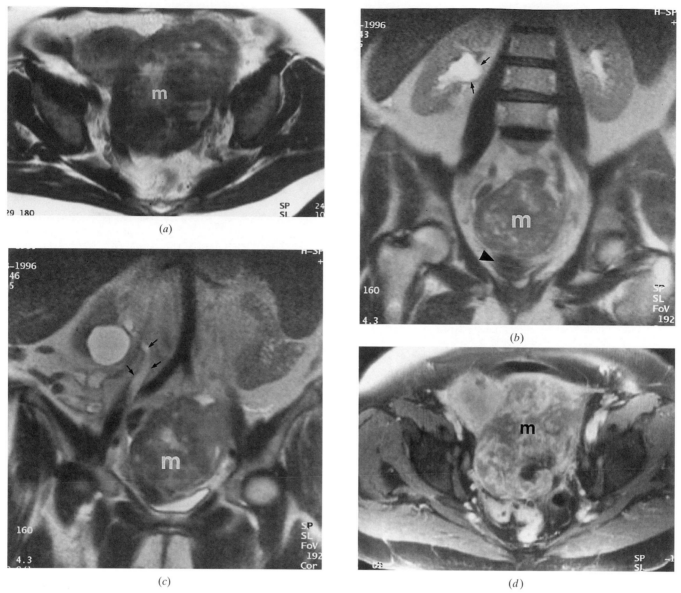

F IG. 15.34 Disseminated lymphoma. Transverse 512-resolution T2-weighted echo-train spin-echo (*a*), coronal HASTE (*b,c*), and transverse gadolinium-enhanced fat-suppressed SGE in a woman with disseminated lymphoma. Primary lymphoma of the ovary is rare, and ovarian involvement usually is seen in the setting of diffuse disease. A large mass (*"m",a–d*) occupies the pelvis and obstructs the right distal ureter. Contiguous coronal HASTE images highlight the pelvocaliectasis and proximal ureterectasis (*arrows, b,c*). Following contrast, the lymphomatous mass enhances. The uterus is displaced inferiorly (*arrowhead, b*). Discrete ovaries were not identified on any of the imaging sequences. At surgery, disseminated non-Hodgkin lymphoma with invasion of the adnexa was found.

setting of marked tubal necrosis with abscess formation that overflows the tubal wall to invade the ovary.

Patients with PID present with fever and abdominal pain. Tenderness on pelvic examination exacerbated by cervical motion is a classic sign. A palpable adnexal mass suggests a coexisting TOA. Uncomplicated cases of PID usually respond to conservative therapy, whereas patients with TOA also may require surgical drainage. Patients with chronic TOA may have a more indolent clinical course, and diagnosis may not be established until surgical resection of an apparent cystic adnexal mass.

Most cases of PID/TOA are diagnosed clinically or with the aid of transvaginal ultrasound. MRI, however, can demonstrate tubal involvement, and if present, an adnexal abscess. Multiple imaging planes show a tortuous enlarged fluid-filled tube, a hydro- or pyosalpinx, especially on T2-weighted images. An apparent aggregate of cysts on a transverse image may be shown to be a

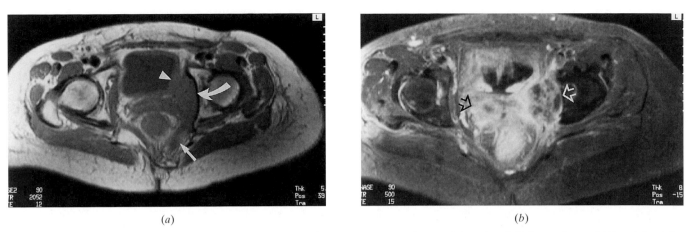

FIG. **15.35** Recurrent müllerian duct cancer metastatic to the ovaries. Proton density (*a*) and gadolinium-enhanced T1-weighted fat-suppressed spin-echo (*b*) images in a woman with recurrent müllerian-duct cancer. Note the left pelvic mass, which invades the obturator externus muscle (*curved arrow, a*). Associated thickening of the left bladder wall (*arrowhead, a*) and levator ani muscle (*straight arrow, a*) suggests that the imaging findings may be related to previous radiotherapy. However, at a slightly higher level following contrast, bilateral adnexal masses demonstrate heterogeneous enhancement consistent with metastases to the ovaries (*open arrows, b*). The bladder and obturator internus muscles do not enhance similarly and are not involved by tumor. Uterine carcinoma is one of the more common primary tumors to metastasize to the ovaries.

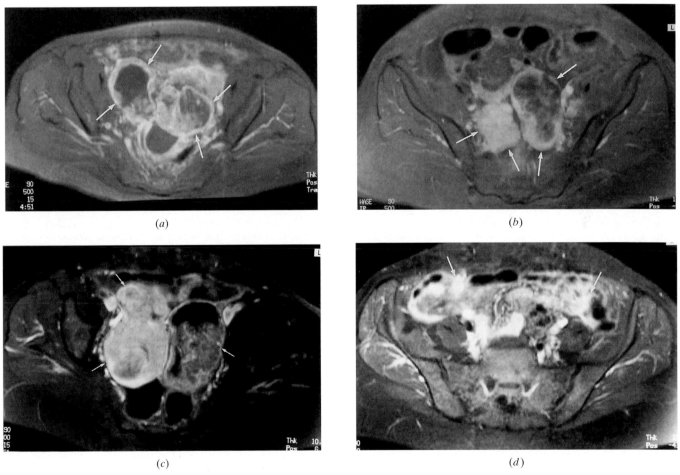

FIG. **15.36** Krukenberg's tumor. Gadolinium-enhanced T1-weighted fat-suppressed spin-echo (*a–d*) images in patients with malignant signet-cell metastases to the ovaries, Krukenberg's tumor. The most common malignancies to cause Krukenberg's tumor are gastric, pancreas (*a*), breast, colon (*b–d*) and gallbladder carcinomas. Involvement is often bilateral; the ovaries are enlarged but retain an ovoid or reniform morphology (*arrows, a–c*). The metastases are primarily solid though cystic regions are common. Gadolinium-enhanced T1-weighted fat-suppressed technique demonstrates the ovarian involvement, as well as any coexisting peritoneal disease (*arrows, d*).

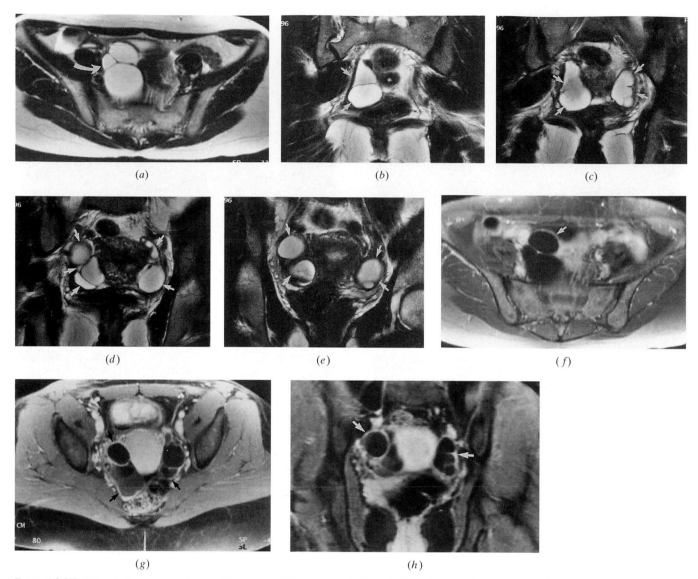

FIG. 15.37 Pelvic inflammatory disease. Transverse (*a*) and coronal (*b–e*) 512-resolution echo-train spin-echo and gadolinium-enhanced transverse (*f,g*) and coronal (*h*) fat-suppressed SGE images in a patient with acute pelvic pain and fever. A complex cystic right adnexal mass is seen (*curved arrow, a*). On a lower section (not shown) a similar mass was seen on the left. Coronal images demonstrate that the masses are not ovarian cysts but the inflamed dilated fallopian tubes folded upon themselves (*arrows, b–e*), which flank the uterus. Following contrast the tube walls enhance and further demonstrate that the masses are not adjacent discrete cysts, but rather continuous structures (*arrows, f–h*).

dilated, folded cylindrical structure on sagittal or coronal images. The signal intensity of the tubal contents varies depending on the presence and degree of hemorrhage [27]. A continuous thin ridge of solid tissue along the periphery of the involved tube represents normal mucosal projections. However, an ectopic pregnancy or fallopian tube carcinoma should be considered in the presence of discrete solid elements [101]. After gadolinium administration, the wall of the tube enhances (Fig. 15.37).

PID complicated by TOA appears as an adnexal fluid collection that is adherent to or replaces the ovary. The signal intensity of the fluid collection is variable. In the absence of hemorrhage or significant protein, the fluid will be low in signal intensity on T1-weighted images and high in signal intensity on T2-weighted images. Contents that are more complicated result in an increased signal intensity on T1-weighted images and the collection may closely resemble an endometrioma [61]. Greater perilesional enhancement is appreciated of a TOA on gadolinium-enhanced fat-suppressed images. Recently, a 1- to 3-mm hyperintense rim in the innermost portion of the abscess on T1-weighted images has been described. This rim, which showed marked enhancement following intravenous contrast, corresponds to a layer of granulation tissue admixed with focal fresh hemorrhage [102]. A similar rim has been seen in patients with ovarian torsion. Peritubal and periovarian inflammation can be identified as low-signal-intensity curvilinear strands within the high-signal-intensity fat on T1-weighted images. Both the inflammatory strands and the walls of the abscess enhance after contrast. Fat-suppressed SGE imaging highlights this enhancement (Fig. 15.38). Lesser inflammatory changes are observed with chronic TOA (Fig. 15.38).

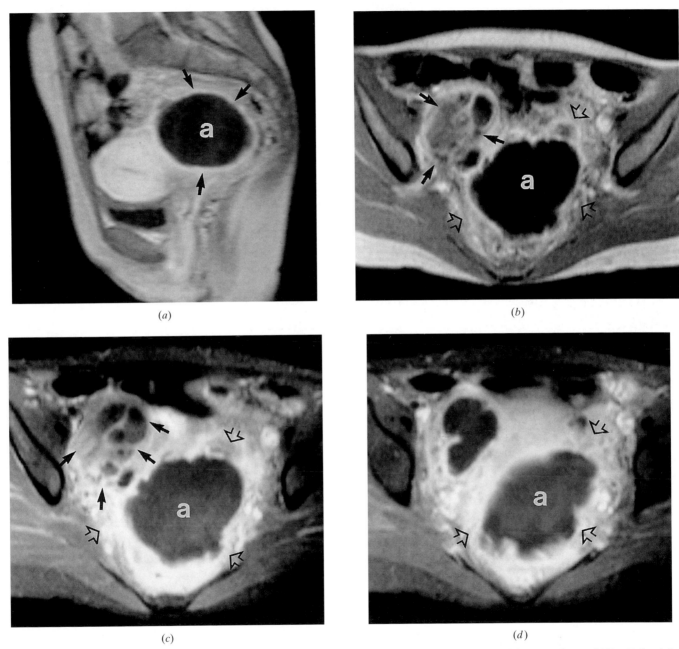

(a) (b)

(c) (d)

FIG. 15.38 Tubo-ovarian abscess. Sagittal (*a*) and transverse (*b*) gadolinium-enhanced SGE and gadolinium-enhanced T1-weighted fat-suppressed spin-echo (*c,d*) images in a woman with fever and a fluctuant adnexal mass on bimanual exam. A large loculated abscess occupies the posterior pelvis ("*a*",*a–d*). The right ovary is enlarged and is also invested with an abscess (*solid arrows, b,c*). The well-formed abscess capsules (*arrows, a*) and septations enhance markedly, as does the inflammation in the surrounding fat (*open arrows, b–d*). The associated inflammatory changes are more conspicuous on the fat-suppressed images. Tubo-ovarian abscess is a well-recognized complication of PID and whereas most cases of PID can be managed conservatively, the presence of an abscess usually necessitates surgical intervention. SGE (*e*), sagittal fat-suppressed SGE (*f*), and transverse (*g,h*) and sagittal (*i*) 512-resolution T2-weighted echo-train spin-echo images in a young woman with chronic low grade fever and pain and a pelvic mass. A complex cystic adnexal mass displaces the uterus to the right.

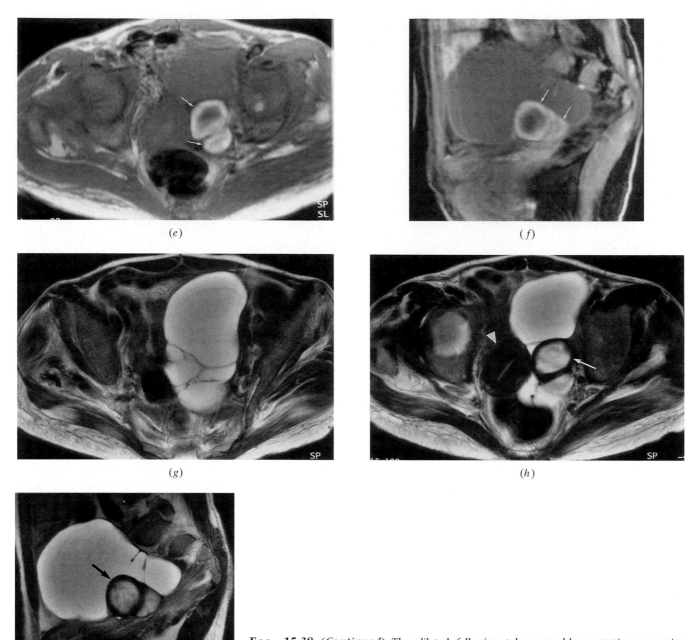

FIG. 15.38 (*Continued*) The dilated fallopian tube resembles septations coursing through the posterior aspect of the mass. The hydrosalpinx contains hemorrhage that has high-signal-intensity rims on T1-weighted images (*arrows, e,f*) that become low in signal intensity on T2-weighted images (*arrow, h,i*). This is consistent with intracellular methemoglobin. (*uterus = arrowhead, h*).

Pelvic Varices

Pelvic venous congestion is a common, albeit frequently overlooked, cause of chronic pelvic pain. In one laparoscopic study, 91 percent of women complaining of chronic pelvic pain had dilated veins of the broad ligament and ovarian plexi as their sole pelvic abnormality [103]. Pelvic varices usually affect multiparous women of reproductive age, but may affect young multiparous women. Women complain of a dull ache that is exacerbated by activity. Venography and duplex ultasound are the most common methods to suggest this diagnosis. However, MRI can detect pelvic varices as part of a comprehensive exam. On unenhanced images, large serpiginous structures surround the uterus and adnexa. The varices enhance after gadolinium administration and are well-shown on gadolinium-enhanced fat-suppressed

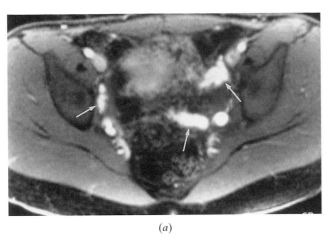 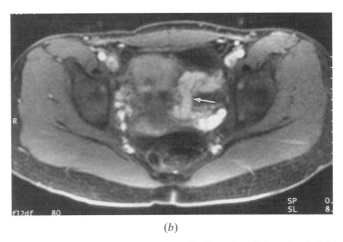

(a)   (b)

F I G . 15.39 Pelvic varices. Transverse 45-second postgadolinium fat-suppressed SGE image in a patient with chronic pelvic pain. Pelvic varices, left greater than right, show marked enhancement after intravenous gadolinium administration (*arrows, a,b*). The concurrent use of fat suppression increases the conspicuity of the dilated vessels by removing the competing high signal intensity of fat. Pelvic varices are a common, though rarely recognized, cause of chronic pelvic pain. In imaging a patient with pelvic pain of unknown etiology, the presence or absence of varices should be noted.

SGE images obtained within 2 minutes of contrast injection (Fig. 15.39).

■ FALLOPIAN TUBES

The fallopian tubes arise from the müllerian ducts. Initially the tubes are vertical, but they assume their normal nearly horizontal position as they accompany the ovaries during migration. The fallopian tubes occupy the superior aspect of the broad ligament and measure approximately 10 to 12 cm in length and 0.4 to 0.9 mm in diameter. They are divided into four segments (from medial to lateral): (1) the interstitial portion, (2) the isthmus, (3) the ampulla, and (4) the infundibulum including the fimbria. The tubal wall possesses longitudinal folds, mucosal rugae, whose size and number increase from the interstitial portion to the infundibulum. Histologically, the wall of the fallopian tube consists of serosa, muscularis, submucosa, and mucosa. The mucosa contains ciliated cells that aid the ovum in its journey to the endometrial cavity.

MRI TECHNIQUE

The techniques outlined for imaging the ovaries also apply to imaging the fallopian tubes. Multiplanar high-resolution (512-matrix) T2-weighted echo-train spin-echo and post gadolinium T1-weighted fat-suppressed spoiled gradient-echo images are effective. No MRI specific techniques to assess tubal patency in women are currently available, although research in an animal model is ongoing [104].

NORMAL MRI APPEARANCE OF THE FALLOPIAN TUBES

The normal fallopian tubes are not routinely imaged, although their location can be inferred by knowing their relationship to the ovaries, uterus, and pelvic ligaments (Fig. 15.40).

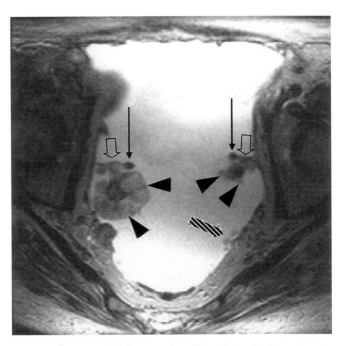

F I G . 15.40 Normal fallopian tubes. T2-weighted echo-train spin-echo in a patient with metastatic ovarian papillary serous cystadenocarcinoma (*arrowheads*). The normal fallopian tubes (*solid arrows*), attached to the broad ligaments (*open arrows*) are well-seen in the setting of marked ascites. Peritoneal-based metastases are similarly highlighted (*hatched arrow*).

CONGENITAL ABNORMALITIES

Aplasia of the tube is associated with unicornuate uterus. Tubal hypoplasia and atresia are uncommon. (See Chapter 14 on the Uterus and Cervix for a full discussion of congenital anomalies.)

MASS LESIONS

Benign Masses

Benign diseases that affect the ovaries and/or uterus often affect the fallopian tubes as well. These include endometriosis, leiomyomata, and teratoma. Regardless of location, the pathologies are similar and as such, the MRI findings of tubal involvement would be expected to parallel those described in other locations in the genital tract.

Hydrosalpinx

Occlusion of the fimbriated end of the fallopian tube produces distension and results in a hydrosalpinx. The tube may be distended by simple fluid, or it can be filled by bloody or infected fluid, hematosalpinx, and pyosalpinx, respectively. The most common etiology of hydrosalpinx is salpingitis (see PID described earlier), though any process that obstructs the tube (adhesions from surgery, endometriosis, pelvic tumor) can cause tubal occlusion. The findings on MRI are discussed earlier and include a serpentine adnexal mass with contents that vary depending on the complexity of the fluid distending the tube. Gadolinium-enhanced fat-suppressed SGE im-

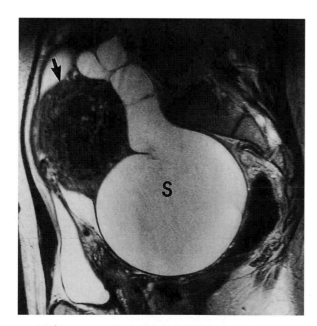

FIG. 15.41 Hydrosalpinx. Sagittal 512-resolution T2-weighted echo-train spin-echo image demonstrates a large hydrosalpinx (*S*). Adenomyosis of the uterus (*arrow*) is also present.

ages highlight associated inflammatory changes as well as the tube wall (see Fig. 15.37). The dilated fluid-filled tubes are high in signal on T2-weighted images. On transverse images hydrosalpinges often resemble multiple cystic lesions, and multiplanar imaging is useful for demonstrating the tubular morphology of hydrosalpinges (Fig. 15.41).

Malignant Masses

Primary Fallopian Tube Carcinoma

Primary fallopian tube malignancies are rare. They account for about 0.5 percent of all malignant tumors of the genital tract with an incidence in the United States of 3.6 million women per year [99]. Adenocarcinoma is the most common histology. Fallopian tube carcinoma affects older women with an average age of 65 years at presentation. Symptoms are nonspecific: abdominal pain, abnormal vaginal bleeding, and discharge. Prognosis is poor with less than 50 percent of patients surviving more than 5 years. This likely reflects early spread of disease through the fimbriated end of the tube or by penetration through the wall, with simultaneous lymphatic spread to regional nodes and near and distant organs. Survival correlates with tumor burden at the time of diagnosis. Tumor may be staged according to the FIGO system. Alternatively, some clinicians advocate a Duke's staging system similar to that used for bowel malignancy (Table 15.3 [99]). Treatment is primarily surgical with adjuvant chemotherapy.

The MRI features of primary fallopian tube carcinoma have been described. The most common finding is a small solid mass that is low in signal intensity on T1-weighted images and high in signal intensity on T2-weighted images. Following contrast, the tumor enhances (Fig. 15.42). Peritumoral ascites and hydrometra are associated findings. Hydrosalpinx is not always present [101]. The combination of T2-weighted images and

Table 15.3 Staging of Fallopian Tube Carcinoma

Stage	Description
0	Carcinoma in situ
I	Tumor extending into the submucosa and muscularis but not penetrating to the serosal surface of the fallopian tube
II	Tumor extending to the serosa of the fallopian tube
III	Direct extension of the tumor to the ovary and/or endometrium
IV	Extension of tumor beyond the reproductive organs

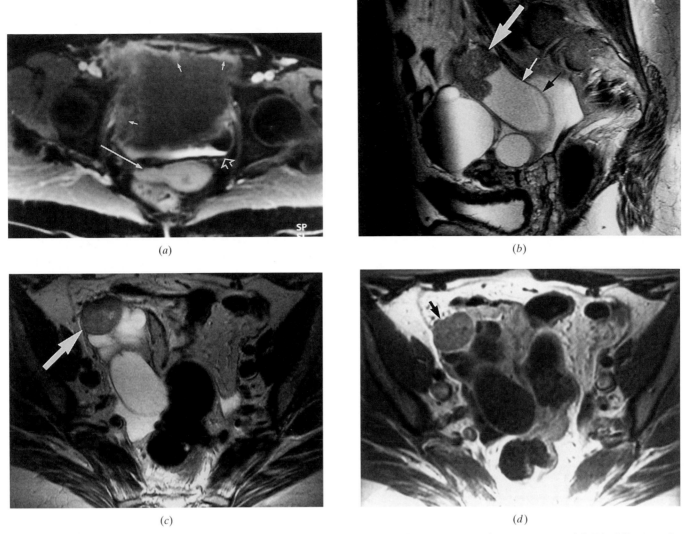

(a)

(b)

(c)

(d)

F IG . 15.42 Fallopian tube adenocarcinoma. Gadolinium-enhanced fat-suppressed SGE image (*a*) demonstrates a solid right fallopian tube cancer (*long arrow, a*) and multiple peritoneal metastases (*short arrows, a*). The bladder (*open arrow, a*) contains high-signal-intensity gadolinium. Sagittal (*b*) and transverse (*c*) 512-resolution T2-weighted echo-train spin-echo, and gadolinium-enhanced T1-weighted spin-echo (*d*) images in a second patient. The fallopian tube is shown as a dilated tubular structure (*arrows, b*) that contains solid tumor components (*large arrow, b,c*). Heterogeneous enhancement of the tumor nodules is present (*arrow, d*) after gadolinium administration.

gadolinium-enhanced T1-weighted fat-suppressed im-ages allow good delineation of the primary tumor and metastases.

Metastases

Metastatic disease to the fallopian tube is more common than primary tumors and usually represents direct exten-sion from ovarian, endometrial, or cervical carcinomas. Involvement of the fallopian tube from extragenital tu-mors are rare, but can occur in the setting of breast or gastrointestinal cancers. No series addressing the appear-ance of fallopian tube metastases have been published, but anecdotal reports suggest that they can mimic metas-tases to the ovaries. Solid nodules within the involved tube help to establish the diagnosis (Fig. 15.43).

INFLAMMATION

Salpingitis
(The epidemiologic, clinical, and MRI findings of salpin-gitis are discussed in the ovary section under the heading Pelvic Inflammatory Disease/Tubo-Ovarian Abscess.)

FUTURE DIRECTIONS

Continued research to develop an MRI equivalent of hys-terosalpingography is underway and may propel MRI to the imaging forefront in the workup of infertility.

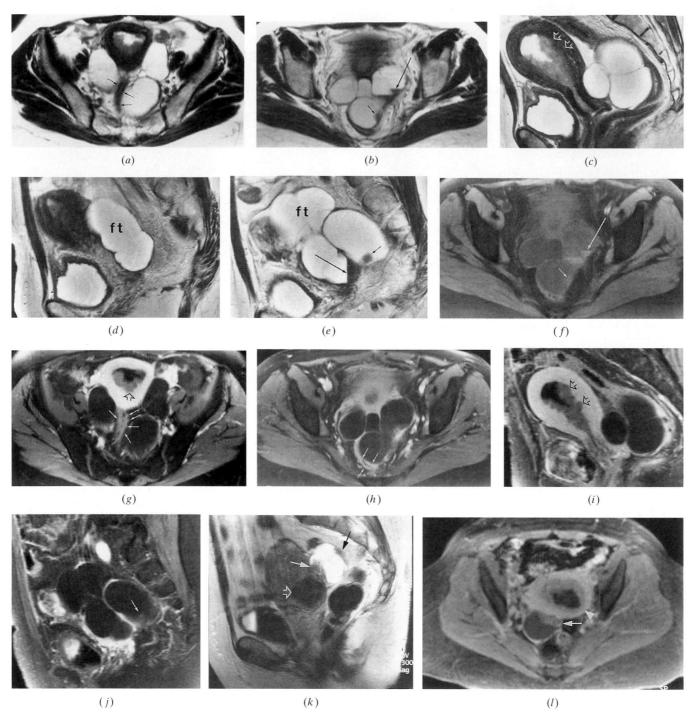

(a) (b) (c)

(d) (e) (f)

(g) (h) (i)

(j) (k) (l)

F IG. 15.43 Endometrial carcinoma metastatic to the fallopian tubes. High-resolution transverse (a,b), midline sagittal (c), right sagittal (d), left sagittal (e) T2-weighted echo-train spin-echo, transverse fat-suppressed SGE (f), and transverse (g,h) and sagittal (i,j) gadolinium-enhanced fat-suppressed SGE images in a woman with metastatic mixed papillary serous and clear-cell endometrial carcinoma complaining of a change in bowel habits. The endometrium is expanded and contains intermediate- and high-signal-intensity elements on the T2-weighted image. The junctional zone is effaced posteriorly (*open arrow, c*). Bilateral adnexal cystic masses compress and surround the sigmoid colon (*arrows, a*). On the right parasagittal image the adnexal cysts appear in continuity with a dilated fallopian tube ("*ft*",*d*), a hydrosalpinx. Similar findings are noted on the left. *ft,e*, fallopian tube. In addition, the contents of the left tube appear complex; there is blood dependently (hematosalpinx) (*long arrow, b,e,f*) and nodularity of the tube wall (*short arrow, b,e,f*). The ovaries (not shown) were displaced anteriorly and superiorly by the diseased tubes. Following contrast, the viable endometrial tumor enhances and scallops the posterior myometrium (*open arrows, g,i*). The compressed wall of the sigmoid colon is tethered to, and adherent to the dilated fallopian tubes (*solid arrows, g,h*). Note an enhancing metastatic nodule in the fallopian tube (*arrow, j*). Sagittal gadolinium enhanced 512-resolution T2-weighted echo-train spin-echo (k) and transverse gadolinium-enhanced fat-suppressed SGE (l) images in second patient who has invasive endometrial carcinoma metastatic to the right fallopian tube. There is a complex fallopian tube metastasis. The solid components are intermediate in signal intensity on the T2-weighted image (*solid arrows, k*). After contrast, the endometrial carcinoma enhances less than adjacent normal myometrium (*arrowhead, l*). Intravenous gadolinium administration is mandatory to accurately assess myometrial invasion. The solid portions of the fallopian tube metastasis also enhance (*solid arrow, l*). Incidental note is made of an intramural fibroid (*open arrow, k*).

CONCLUSION

MRI of the ovaries and adnexa is a robust technique. Multiplanar imaging allows the origin of a pelvic mass to be determined, especially in cases where ultrasound is ambiguous or confusing. It can also characterize lesions with the use of chemically selective excitation-spoiling fat-suppression sequences alone and in combination with intravenous gadolinium. Currently, MRI can delineate the origin of an adnexal mass and diagnose dermoids, endometriomas, fibromas, and hydrosalpinx with confidence. In pregnant women, MRI can contribute important diagnostic information about adnexal masses and may spare expectant mothers unnecessary surgery. Similarly, MRI has been shown to be cost-effective in managing women with a variety of gynecologic conditions. In one study, a savings of $63 per patient as a group and $1,736 per patient in the group already scheduled to undergo surgery was calculated when the MRI findings were incorporated into treatment plans [105]. At present MRI cannot supplant surgical staging for ovarian cancer in most cases. However, in patients for whom surgery is contraindicated, MRI can estimate tumor burden. Furthermore, as routine second-look laparotomy becomes obsolete, MRI can accurately stratify patients into those who may benefit from reexploration, from those who may not.

REFERENCES

1. Zaloudek C: The ovary. In Gompel C, Silverberg SG (eds.). Pathology in Gynecology and Obstetrics, Philadelphia: Lippincott, pp. 313–413, 1994.

2. Smith RC, Reinhold C, McCauley TR, et al: Multicoil high resolution fast spin-echo MR imaging of the female pelvis. Radiology 184:671–675, 1992.

3. Hayes CE, Dietz MJ, King BF, et al: Pelvic imaging with phased-array coils: Quantitative assessment of signal-to-noise ratio improvement. J Magn Reson Imaging 2:321–326, 1992.

4. McCauley TR, McCarthy S, Lange R: Pelvic phased array coil: Image quality assessment for spin-echo MR imaging. Magn Reson Imaging 10:513–522, 1992.

5. Outwater EK, Mitchell DG: Magnetic resonance imaging techniques in the pelvis. Magn Reson Imaging Clin N Am 2:161–188, 1994.

6. Tempany MC, Fielding JR: Female Pelvis. In Edelman RR, Hesselink JR, Zlatkin MB (eds.). Clinical Magnetic Resonance Imaging. Philadelphia: WB Saunders, pp. 1432–1465, 1996.

7. Kier R, Smith RC, McCarthy SM: Value of lipid- and water-suppression MR images in distinguishing between blood and lipid with ovarian masses. AJR Am J Roentgenol 1992:158:321–325.

8. Stevens SK, Hricak H, Campos Z: Teratomas versus cystic hemorrhagic adnexal lesions: Differentiation with proton-selective fat-saturation MR imaging. Radiology 186:481–488, 1993.

9. Sugimura K, Okizuka H, Imaoka I, et al: Pelvic endometriosis: Detection and diagnosis with chemical shift MR imaging. Radiology 188:435–438, 1993.

10. Chan TW, Listerud J, Kressel HY: Combined chemical-shift and phase-selective imaging for fat suppression: Theory and initial clinical experience. Radiology 181:41–47, 1991.

11. Mitchell DG: Chemical shift magnetic resonance imaging: Applications in the abdomen and pelvis. Top Magn Reson Imaging 4:46–63, 1992.

12. Thurnher S, Hudler J, Baer S, Maricek B, vonSchulthess GK: Gadolinium-DOTA enhanced MR imaging of adnexal tumors. J Comput Assist Tomogr 14:939–949, 1990.

13. Hricak H, Kim B: Contrast-enhanced MR imaging of the female pelvis. J Magn Reson Imaging 3:297–306, 1993.

14. Hamm B, Laniado M, Saini S: Contrast-enhanced magnetic resonance imaging of the abdomen and pelvis. Magn Reson Q 6:108–135, 1990.

15. Haldermann-Heusler RC, Wight E, Marincek BM: Oral superparamagnetic contrast agent (ferumoxsil): Tolerance and efficacy in MR imaging of gynecologic diseases. J Magn Reson Imaging 4:385–391, 1995.

16. Dooms BC, Hricak H, Tscholakoff D: Adnexal structures: MR imaging. Radiology 158:639–646, 1986.

17. Outwater EK, Mitchell DG: Normal ovaries and functional cysts: MR appearance. Radiology 198:397–402, 1996.

18. Levine D, Gosink B, Wolf SI, et al: Simple adnexal cysts: The natural history in postmenopausal women. Radiology 184:653–659, 1992.

19. Outwater EK, Dunton CJ: Imaging of the ovary and adnexa: Clinical issues and applications of MR imaging. Radiology 194:1–18, 1995.

20. Outwater EK, Schiebler ML, Owens RS, et al: MRI characterization of hemorrhagic adnexal masses: A blinded reader study. Radiology 186:489–494, 1993.

21. Gambino J, Caldwell B, Dietrich R, et al: Congenital disorders of sexual differentiation: MR findings; AJR Am J Roentgenol 158:363–367, 1992.

22. Secaf E, Hricak H, Gooding CA, et al: Role of MRI in the evaluation of ambiguous genitalia. Pediatr Radiol 24:231–235, 1994.

23. Outwater EK, Schiebler ML: Magnetic resonance imaging of the ovary. Radiol Clin North Am 2:245–274, 1994.

24. Granberg S: Relationship of macroscopic appearance to the histologic diagnosis of ovarian tumors. Clin Obstet Gynecol 36:363–374, 1993.

25. Thickman D, Gussman D: Magnetic resonance imaging of benign adnexal conditions. Magn Reson Imaging Clin N Am 2:275–289, 1994.

26. Yamashita Y, Hatanaka Y, Torashima, et al: Mature cystic teratomas of the ovary without fat in the cystic cavity. AJR Am J Roentgenol 164:613–616, 1994.

27. Mitchell DG, Mintz MC, Spritzer CE, et al: Adnexal masses: MR imaging observations at 1.5 T with US and CT correlation. Radiology 162:319–324, 1987.

28. Togashi K, Nishimura K, Itoh K, et al: Ovarian cystic teratomas: MR imaging. Radiology 162:669–673, 1987.

29. Yamashita Y, Toraxhima M, Hatanaka Y, et al: Value of phase-shift gradient-echo MR imaging in the differentiation of pelvic lesions with high signal intensity at T1-weighted imaging. Radiology 191:759–764, 1994.

30. Curtis M, Hopkins MP, Zarlingo T, et al: Magnetic resonance imaging to avoid laparotomy in pregnancy. Obstet Gynecol 82:833–836, 1993.

31. Kier R, McCarthy SM, Scoutt LM, et al: Pelvic masses in pregnancy: MR imaging. Radiology 176:709–713, 1990.

32. Colleti P, Sylvestre PB: Magnetic resonance imaging in pregnancy. Magn Reson Imaging Clin N Am 2:291–307, 1994.

33. Morrow CP, Townsend DE: Tumors of the ovary: General considerations, classification of the adnexal mass. In Morrow CP, Townsend DE (eds.). Synopsis of Gynecological Oncology. New York, Wiley, pp. 231–255, 1987.

34. Ghossain MA, Buy JN, Ligneres C, et al: Epithelial tumors of the ovary: Comparison of MR and CT findings. Radiology 181:863–870, 1991.

35. Olive DL: Schwartz LB: Endometriosis: N Engl J Med 328:1759–1769, 1993.

36. Gompel C, Silverberg SG. Endometriosis. In Gompel C, Silverberg SG (eds.). Pathology in Gynecology and Obstetrics (4th ed.). Philadelphia: Lippincott, pp. 425–431, 1994.

37. Fukaya T, Hoshiai H, Yajima A: Is pelvic endometriosis always associated with chronic pain: A retrospective study of 618 cases diagnosed by laparoscopy. Am J Obstet Gynecol 169:719–722, 1993.

38. Clement PB: Endometriosis, lesions of the secondary mullerian system, and pelvic mesothelial proliferations. In Kurman RJ (ed.). Blaustein's Pathology of the Female Genital Tract (3rd ed.). New York: Springer-Verlag, pp. 516–559, 1987.

39. Williams TJ: Endometriosis. In Mattingly RF, Thompson JD, (eds.). Te Linde's Operative Gynecology (6th ed.). Philadelphia: Lippincott, pp. 257–286, 1985.

40. Rock JA: Endometriosis. In Rasenwaks Z, Benjamin R, Stone ML (eds.). Gynecology: Principles and Practice. New York: Macmillan, pp. 559–576, 1987.

41. Coleman BG, Arger PH, Hulhern CB Jr: Endometriosis: Clinical and ultrasonic correlation. AJR Am J Roentgenol 132:747–749, 1979.

42. Friedman H, Vogelzang RL, Mendelson EB, et al: Endometriosis detection by US with laparoscopic correlation. Radiology 157:217–220, 1985.

43. Berland LL, Lawson TL, Albarelli JN, Foley WD: Ultrasonic diagnosis of ovarian and adnexal disease. Semin Ultrasound 1:17–29, 1980.

44. Yamashita Y, Torashima M, Hatanaka Y, et al: Adnexal masses: Accuracy of characterization with transvaginal US and preocontrast and postcontrast MR imaging. Radiology 194:557–565, 1995.

45. Sawyer RW, Walsh JW: CT in gynecologic pelvis disease. Semin Ultrasound, CT MR 9:122–142, 1988.

46. Nishimura K, Togashi K, Itoh K, et al: Endometrial cyst of the ovary: MR imaging. Radiology 162:315–318, 1987.

47. Nyberg DA, Portal BA, Olds MO, et al: MR imaging of hemorrhagic masses. J Comput Assist Tomogr 11:664–669, 1987.

48. Arrive L, Hricak H, Martin MC: Pelvic endometriosis: MR imaging. Radiology 171:687–692, 1989.

49. Zawain M, McCarthy SM, Scoutt L, Comite F: Endometriosis: Appearance and detection at MR imaging. Radiology 171:693–696, 1989.

50. Togashi K, Nishimura K, Kimura I, et al: Endometrial cyst: Diagnosis with MR imaging. Radiology 180:73–78, 1991.

51. Ascher SM, Agrawal R, Bis KG, et al: Endometriosis: Appearance and detection with conventional and contrast-enhanced fat-suppressed spin-echo techniques. J Magn Reson Imaging 5:251–257, 1995.

52. Togashi K: MRI of the female pelvis. Tokyo: Igaku-Shoin, pp. 207, 1993.

53. Ha HK, Lim YT, Kim HS, et al: Diagnosis of pelvic endometriosis: Fat-suppressed T1-weighted vs. conventional MR images. AJR Am J Roentgenol 163:127–131, 1994.

54. Siegelman ES, Outwater EK, Wang T, Mitchell DG: Solid pelvic masses caused by endometriosis: MR imaging features. AJR Am J Roentgenol 163:357–361, 1994.

55. Franks S: Polycystic ovary syndrome. N Engl J Med 333:853–861, 1995.

56. Soper JR, Hammond CB, Lewis JL Jr: Gestational trophoblastic disease. In Hoskins WJ, Perez CA, Young RC (eds.). Principles and Practice of Gynecologic Oncology. Philadelphia: Lippincott, pp. 795–825, 1992.

57. Hricak H, Demas BE, Braga CA, et al: Gestational trophoblastic neoplasm of the uterus: MR assessment. Radiology 161:11–16, 1986.

58. Barton JW, McCarthy SM, Kohorn EI, et al: Pelvic MR imaging findings in gestational trophoblastic disease, incomplete abortion, and ectopic pregnancy: Are they specific? Radiology 186:163–168, 1993.

59. Kier R: Nonovarian gynecologic cysts: MR imaging findings. AJR Am J Roentgenol 158:1265–1269, 1992.

60. Kurachi H, Murakami T, Nakamura H, et al: Imaging of peritoneal pseudocysts: Value of MR imaging compared with sonography and CT. AJR Am J Roentgenol 160:589–591, 1993.

61. Carrington B: The adnexae. In Hricak H, Carrington BM (eds.). MRI of the Pelvis. London: Appleton & Lange, pp. 185–228, 1991.

62. Jain KA: Magnetic resonance imaging findings in ovarian torsion. Magn Reson Imaging 13:111–113, 1995.

63. Kimura I, Togashi K, Kawakami S, et al: Ovarian torsion: CT and MR imaging appearances. Radiology 190:337–341, 1994.

64. Kawakami K, Murata K, Kawaguchi N, et al: Hemorrhagic infarction of the diseased ovary: A common MR finding in two cases. Magn Reson Imaging 11:595–597, 1993.

65. Lee AR, Kim KH, Lee BH, et al: Massive edema of the ovary: Imaging findings. AJR Am J Roentgenol 161:343–344, 1993.

66. Hall B, Printz D, Roth J: Massive ovarian edema: Ultrasound and MR characteristics. J Comput Assist Tomgr 17:477–479, 1993.

67. Bader-Armstrong B, Shah Y, Rubens D, et al: Use of ultrasound and magnetic resonance imaging in the diagnosis of cervical pregnancy. J Clin Ultrasound 17:283–286, 1989.

68. Rafal RB, Kosovsky PA, Markisz JA: MR appearance of cervical pregnancy. J Comput Assist Tomogr 14:482–484, 1990.

69. Ha HK, Jung JK, Kang SK, et al: MR imaging in the diagnosis of rare forms of ectopic pregnancy. AJR Am J Roentgenol 160:1229–1232, 1993.

70. Ozols RF, Rubin SC, Dembo AJ, Robboy S: Epithelial ovarian cancer. In Hoskins WJ, Perez CA, Young RC (eds.). Principles and Practice of Gynecologic Oncology. Philadelphia: Lippincott, pp. 731–794, 1992.

71. Wagner BJ, Buck JL, Seidman JD, McCabe KM: Ovarian epithelial neoplasms: Radiologic-pathologic correlation. Radiographics 14:1351–1374, 1994.

72. Sutton CL, McKinney CD, Jones JE, Gay SB: Ovarian masses revisited: Radiologic and pathologic correlation. Radiographics 12:853–877, 1992.

73. Young RC, Decker DG, Wharton JT, et al: Staging laparotomy in early ovarian cancer. JAMA 250:3072–3076, 1983.

74. McGowan L, Lesher LP, Norris HJ, Barnett M: Mistaging of ovarian cancer. Obstet Gynecol 65:568–572, 1985.

75. Friedman JB, Weiss NS: Sounding board: Second thoughts about second-look laparotomy in advanced ovarian cancer. N Engl J Med 322:1079, 1990.

76. NIH Consensus Development Panel on Ovarian Cancer. Ovarian cancer: Screening, treatment and follow-up. JAMA 273:491–496, 1995.

77. Miller DS, Spiritos NM, Ballon SC, et al: Critical assessment of second-look exploratory laparotomy for epithelial ovarian carcinoma. Cancer 69:502–510, 1992.

78. Semelka RC, Lawrence PH, Shoenut JP, et al: Primary ovarian cancer: Prospective comparison of contrast-enhanced CT and pre- and postcontrast, fat-suppressed MR imaging with histologic correlation. J Magn Reson Imaging 3:99–106, 1993.

79. Arai K, Makino H, Yagi H, et al: Enhancement of ascites on MRI following intravenous administration of Gd-DTPA. J Comput Assist Tomogr 17:617–622, 1993.

80. Weinreb JC, Barkoff ND, Megibow A, Demopoulos RD: The value of MR imaging in distinguishing leiomyomas from other solid pelvic masses when sonography is indeterminate. AJR Am J Roentgenol 154:295–299, 1990.

81. Yamashita Y, Torashima M, Hatanaka Y, et al: Adnexal masses: Accuracy of characterization with transvaginal US and precontrast and postcontrast MR imaging. Radiology 194:557–565, 1995.

82. Komatsu T, Konishi I, Mandai M, et al: Adnexal Masses: Transvagi-

nal US and gadolinium-enhanced MR imaging assessment of intra-tumoral structure. Radiology 198:109–115, 1996.

83. Smith FW, Cherryman GR, Bayliss AP, et al: A comparison of the accuracy of ultrasound imaging, X-ray computerized tomography, and low field MRI diagnosis of ovarian malignancy. Magn Reson Imaging 6:225–227, 1988.

84. Stevens SK, Hricak H, Stern JL: Ovarian lesions: Detection and characterization with gadolinium-enhanced MR imaging at 1.5 T. Radiology 181:481–488, 1991.

85. Thurnher SA: MR imaging of pelvic masses in women: Contrast-enhanced vs. unenhanced images. AJR Am J Roentgenol 159:1243–1250, 1992.

86. Olt GJ, Berchuck A, Bast RC: Gynecologic tumor markers. Semin Surg Oncol 6:305–313, 1990.

87. Malkasian GD Jr, Knapp RC, Lavin DJ, et al: Preoperative evaluation of serum CA-125 levels in premenopausal and postmenopausal patients with pelvic masses: Discrimination of benign from malignant disease. Am J Obstet Gynecol 159:341–346, 1988.

88. Hamper UM, Sheth S, Abbas FM, et al: Transvaginal color Doppler sonography of adnexal masses: Differences in blood flow impedance in benign and malignant lesions. AJR Am J Roentgenol 160:1225–1228, 1993.

89. Karlan BY, Raffel LJ, Crvenkovic G, et al: A multidisciplinary approach to the early detection of ovarian carcinoma: Rationale, protocol design, and early results. Am J Obstet Gynecol 169:494–501, 1993.

90. Schneider VL, Schneider A, Reed KL, et al: Comparison of doppler with two-dimensional sonography and CA 125 for prediction of malignancy of pelvic masses. Obstet Gynecol 81:983–988, 1993.

91. Low RN, Carter WD, Saleh F, Sigeti JS: Ovarian cancer: Comparison of findings with perfluourocarbon-enhanced MR imaging, In-111-CYT-103 immunoscintigraphy, and CT. Radiology 195:391–400, 1995.

92. Forstner R, Hricak H, Occhipinti KA, et al: Ovarian cancer: Staging with CT and MR imaging. Radiology 197:619–626, 1995.

93. Low RN, Sigeti JS: MR imaging of peritoneal disease: Comparison of contrast-enhanced fast multiplanar spoiled gradient-recalled and spin-echo imaging. AJR Am J Roentgenol 163:1131–1140, 1994.

94. Prayer ALM, Kainz C, Kramer J, et al: CT and MR accuracy in the detection of tumor recurrence in patients treated for ovarian cancer. J Comput Assist Tomogr 17:626–632, 1993.

95. Forstner R, Hricak H, Powell CB, et al: Ovarian cancer recurrence: Value of MR imaging. Radiology 196:715–720, 1995.

96. Blaustein A: Metastatic carcinoma in the ovary. In Blaustein A (ed.). Pathology of the Female Genital Tract. New York: Springer-Verlag, pp. 705–715, 1982.

97. Ha HK, Baek SY, Kim SH, et al: Krukenberg's tumor of the ovary: MR imaging features. AJR Am J Roentgenol 164:1435–1439, 1995.

98. McCormack WM: Pelvic inflammatory disease. N Engl J Med 330:115–118, 1994.

99. Gompel C, Silverberg SG. The fallopian tube. Gompel C, Silverberg SG (eds.). Pathology in Gynecology and Obstetrics. Philadelphia: Lippincott, pp. 284–311, 1994.

100. Burkman R, Schlesselman S, McCaffrey L, et al: The relationship of genital tract actimomycetes and the development of pelvic inflammatory disease. Am J Obstet Gynecol 143:585–589, 1982.

101. Kawakami S, Togashi K, Kimura I, et al: Primary malignant tumor of the fallopian tube: Appearance at CT and MR imaging. Radiology 186:503–508, 1993.

102. Ha HK, Lim GY, Cha ES, et al: MR imaging of tubo-ovarian abscess. Acta Radiol 36:510–514, 1995.

103. Gupta A, McCarthy S: Pelvic varices as a cause for pelvic pain: MRI appearance. Magn Reson Imaging 12:679–681, 1994.

104. Lee F, Grist T, Nelson KG, et al: MR hysterosalpingography in a rabbit model. J Magn Reson Imaging 6:300–304, 1996.

105. Schwartz LB, Panageas E, Lange R, et al: Female pelvis: Impact of MR imaging on treatment decisions and net cost analysis. Radiology 192:55–60, 1994.

INDEX